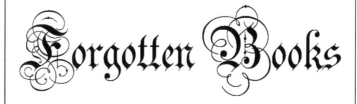

ISBN 978-0-243-32560-3
PIBN 10793642

Forgotten Books is a registered trademark of FB &c Ltd.
Copyright © 2018 FB &c Ltd.
FB &c Ltd, Dalton House, 60 Windsor Avenue, London, SW19 2RR.
Company number 08720141. Registered in England and Wales.

For support please visit www.forgottenbooks.com

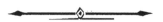

# CLINICAL GYNÆCOLOGY

## MEDICAL AND SURGICAL

### FOR STUDENTS AND PRACTITIONERS

BY

EMINENT AMERICAN TEACHERS

EDITED BY

JOHN M. KEATING, M.D., LL.D.,

AND BY

HENRY C. COE, M.D., M.R.C.S.,

PROFESSOR OF GYNÆCOLOGY, NEW YORK POLYCLINIC

ILLUSTRATED

PHILADELPHIA

J. B. LIPPINCOTT COMPANY

1895

PRINTED BY J. B. LIPPINCOTT COMPANY, PHILADELPHIA, PA., U. S. A.

# PREFACE.

THE impulse which has been given to the clinical teaching of medicine and surgery during the past ten years by the establishment of numerous post-graduate schools throughout the country has been communicated to recent text-books, in which the practical has largely superseded the theoretical. The practitioner at the present day is not only keenly alive to the fact that immense advances have been made in medicine since his student-days, but is filled with the laudable ambition to keep abreast of them. To enable him to do this, information must be imparted to him in a clear, concise, and more or less dogmatic form. This is the object aimed at in the present volume, which represents the combined experience of a number of clinical teachers selected by the former editor as men who, while disposed to be conservative, were none the less progressive and free from hobbies. The success which has attended the publication of the volumes of the *International Clinics* led the publishers to believe that a work on gynæcology treated from a clinical stand-point would find a place in the voluminous literature of diseases of women.

Owing to the untimely death of Dr. Keating, the completion of the work devolved upon the present editor, who has as far as possible carried out the plans and wishes of his lamented predecessor. While seeking to preserve that coherence which is desirable in a text-book, he has in the main allowed each contributor to consult his own judgment with regard to the arrangement and phraseology of his article, believing that in this way the individuality of each would be best preserved. In view of the needs of the student and busy practitioner, especial attention is given to diagnosis and treatment, the sections on pathology being less extended than in most text-books on gynæcology.

Especial care has been taken in the preparation of the illustrations, a large proportion of which have been drawn or photographed for this work under the immediate supervision of the contributors. Occasionally illustrations from other sources have been used, when particularly useful and appropriate. Numerous cuts of various gynæcological instruments have been kindly lent by surgical instrument makers, to whom a grateful acknowledgment is due.

The editor takes this occasion to fulfil a promise made to the late Dr. Keating. It was the latter's expressed wish, when he recognized the fact that he would be unable to complete this work, that he should not be held responsible for any views contained in it regarding the destruction of the living fœtus which might appear to be contrary to the tenets of the Catholic Church.

The introductory pages will be read with mournful interest as the last words of a gifted teacher whose voice and pen exercised a potent influence upon the medical world for over a quarter of a century. To those who have felt their spell in the past his latest utterances will appeal with peculiar force.

# CONTENTS.

## CHAPTER III.

## CHAPTER IV.

## CHAPTER V.

# CHAPTER VI.

# CHAPTER VII.

# CHAPTER VIII.

# CHAPTER IX.

# LIST OF ILLUSTRATIONS.

## PLATES.

# FIGURES.

# INTRODUCTORY.

BY WILLIAM GOODELL, M D.

ONE advantage accruing to the writer of an introductory lies in the circumstance that he is not limited to any given text or narrowed down to a special topic. Untethered to thesis or to theme, he can range at large over the whole field of the subject-matter, and treat it pretty much as he pleases. Now as a mentor he can preach his homily, now as a pupil he can con his hornbook.

In this survey of gynæcology I shall not hesitate to borrow from my previous writings on the subject, without credit and without stint. I shall also use the pronoun of the first person, not from egotism, but in order to invest my own views with that personality which the editor has urged all his collaborators to assume. Nor, on occasions, shall I hesitate to show myself a "proselyte of the gate,"—one who does not wholly yield up his own creed to all the articles of orthodox medical belief, or subscribe to all the obligations of its ritual.

With the ancients the Golden Age was in the past. With us it looms as the promise of the future; and, indeed, a great future lies before us. At the brink of the twentieth century let us look back upon the one that is fading away; and a wonderful one it truly has been. In every department of art and of science it has been a century of marvellous progress. When one considers the amazing discoveries made and making in it, when one takes into account its crowning intellectual achievements, one cannot but feel that this dying century—dying from age, but immortal in other attributes —is not one hundred years merely, but centuries, in advance of the last one. As one of the results of this age of unrestful progress, at every turn of the hour-glass some cherished scientific creed is found wanting, some accepted philosophic dogma is proved a heresy, and not a tradition stands unchallenged. Hence the seeker after truth often has to unlearn as well as to learn.

Nor, in these stirring times and runnings to and fro upon the face of the earth after knowledge, has the science of medicine lagged behind. Every branch of it has been leavened with the yeast of progress, but perhaps in this general ferment no single branch has gained more than that of gynæcology. The present work is in itself a striking voucher for this fact. Twenty years ago there did not exist, to my knowledge, any

systematic work like this.   There were, it is true, encyclopædias of general
medicine, but there was no collection of monographs on special medical
branches.   Gynæcology then lagged as a mere appendage to obstetrics, and
the teaching of it was limited to a few perfunctory lectures delivered at the
close of the curriculum.   Later, these chairs were divided, and, if I am not
in error, I was the first teacher in this country who bore the specific title
of professor of gynæcology.   Since its recognition as a special branch of
medicine, gynæcology has grown commensurately with the age.   So marked
is its advance that all literature treating of this branch of medicine ages
rapidly, shortly becoming as obsolete as last year's almanac, which shows
what was, but not what is.

To illustrate the law that the knowledge of the past vanishes before the
progress of the day and is "east as rubbish to the void," Drummond, in
one of his charming essays, writes as follows: "But yesterday, in the University of Edinburgh, the greatest figure in the faculty was Sir James Y.
Simpson, the discoverer of chloroform.   The other day his successor and
nephew, Professor Simpson, was asked by the librarian of the University
to go to the library and pick out the books on his subject that were no
longer needed.   His reply to the librarian was this: 'Take every text-book
that is more than ten years old, and put it down in the cellar.'"   To replace those books which have outlived their usefulness is the object of this
new work of which I stand as introducer.

Let us for a moment consider the phenomenal gains which gynæcology
has made within the past few years,—that is to say, since it was weaned from
obstetrics and east upon its own resources.   Ovarian cysts are now removed
with a percentage of mortality far below that of any other capital operation.
By the ingenious posture devised by Trendelenburg, which appeals to the
sight as well as to the touch, difficult operations are readily and safely
performed which formerly either were not undertaken or were abandoned
after being begun.   Thanks to this posture and to an improved technique,
the removal of fibroid tumors of the womb, which had long been the bug-
bear of the profession, is now the leading operation of the day.   The old
theories of extra-uterine conception have been overthrown by the simpler
one of tubal origin from tubal disease.   We do not yet know whether the
ciliary movement propels the ovum along the tube into the womb, or merely
repels the intrusion of spermatozoa.   But we do know that when this
movement is arrested by disease the ovum is liable to be detained in the
tube and to be inseminated there.   This knowledge has led to marvellous
results, both in anticipating mischief and in snatching women from the
very jaws of death.   The belief that cellulitis lies at the bottom of most
female ailments, and that local applications and the hot-water douche are
its cure-all, has been consigned to the limbo of false creeds.   The crucial
test of surgical research—an appeal to touch and to sight which cannot be
gainsaid—has shown that cellulitis is almost a myth, and that what have
long been deemed exudation tumors and inflammatory deposits in the

areolar tissue are tubal and ovarian lesions. Yet error dies hard, for "truth new-born looks a misshapen and untimely growth," and there are a few medical Uzzahs who still perilously uphold their tottering theory of cellulitis.

This discovery marks an era in gynæcology, for since then the true conception of salpingitis in all its forms, the significance of adherent tubes and ovaries, and the meaning of a fixed womb have all been grasped fully and intelligently. The sufferers from these diseases are no longer the victims of that hap-hazard and unsuccessful course of treatment which aimed at everything and at anything but the true cause. Owing to vast improvements, Porro's operation and the Cæsarean section are no longer relegated to experts, but are in emergency cases successfully performed by the general practitioner. Uterine cancer, the presence of which until very lately signed the death-warrant of the sufferer, is now treated with such immediate and remote results as far to surpass the most sanguine expectations. To the gynæcologist no operation, it seems to me, can give more unalloyed pleasure than a hysterectomy which holds out the promise of rescuing his patient from the clutches of so horrible a disease. Chronic endometritis, formerly so intractable as to be the opprobrium of the profession, now yields to the nimble use of the curette followed by gauze packing.

The employment of catgut has been a decided gain in gynæcology. As a buried suture it hinders the occurrence of hernia in the scar of an abdominal section, and in plastic operations it gives great help in the coaptation of deep raw surfaces. As a short-lived ligature thrown around ovarian and tubal pedicles, in operations which cannot be made wholly aseptic, it saves the patient from those sinuses and fistulæ which often follow the use of the lasting silk ligature. Through the genius of Emmet tears of the cervix are no longer mistaken for ulcerations, and the operation of trachelorrhaphy not only has restored health to many invalids, but also has lessened greatly the cases of uterine cancer. The term "ulceration of the cervix," in fact, has been banished virtually from gynæcological literature, and its use is now the shibboleth which marks the mildewed drone of the busy medical hive. Complete lacerations of the perineum and uro-genital fistulæ of every kind now rarely fail to yield to measures adopted for their repair.

Gynæcology also has gained within the last two years a useful generic term—cœliotomy—which accurately defines operations hitherto incorrectly termed laparotomies. For this much-needed word we are indebted to our scholarly and industrious statistician, Dr. R. P. Harris. Another term greatly needed in the English language is an acceptable one to denote the act of removing the ovaries. The word *spaying* is offensive, because it has hitherto been applied to this operation in the lower animals —especially in the sow. In the male the analogue to this operation is called *castration*. In default of a better word, this term *castration* is employed by European medical writers to indicate indifferently the removal both of the testicles and of the ovaries, and I see no good reason why we should not follow their example.

One of the grandest discoveries in the treatment of the nervous phase of woman's diseases is the rest-cure, for which we owe a large debt of gratitude to Weir Mitchell. Formerly there were in every city, town, and hamlet sofa-ridden and bed-ridden women who were doomed to hopeless invalidism under the label of "weak spine," of "spinal irritation," of "irritable womb," or of "chronic ovaritis." So countless were these cases, in the young and in the old, in the married and in the single, in the fruitful and in the barren, so much misery was entailed both on the sufferer and on her kin, so many homes were blighted, so powerless was the medical profession to give help, that the pathetic lament of the Hebrew prophet could not have been better applied than to this great and wide-spread scourge : "Is there no balm in Gilead? is there no physician there? why then is not the health of the daughter of my people recovered?" Yet now I think myself safe in the assertion that very few of these cases are incurable, and that no other discovery in medicine has raised so many women from their beds and restored them to lives of active usefulness. It is the miracle of modern therapeutics.

Gynæcology has gained also by its losses, by casting off its exuviæ, by unlearning much of its traditional teaching. It has learned to unlearn the grandmotherly belief that the climacteric is an entity, and that, as such, it is responsible for most of the ills of matronhood, and especially for menorrhagia. True, it must be conceded that as an entity—as a mere suppressant of menstruation—it does seem to disturb the vaso-motor system, and through it to cause many perturbations, such as numbness and tingling and sweating of the skin, flashes of heat and shivers of cold, emotional explosions, and a large group of nervous symptoms. It can also lay claim to being an important factor in the causation of insanity. But, contrary to the prevalent lay belief, rarely can true uterine hemorrhages or other uterine discharges be traced to the climacteric as a cause in itself. They come, we know now, not from the climacteric, but from the cancers, the polypi, the fibroids, the sarcomatous tumors, the papillary growths, and the fungoid vegetations of the climacteric period. Yet many a poor woman has lost her health, her life indeed, through her own and her physician's traditional belief that her hemorrhages or her other vaginal discharges were "critical" and due to the "change of life," as it is popularly called,—a misnomer which has too often led to indolent diagnosis and to slovenly therapeutics.

Until very recently the orthodox teaching has been that woman must not be subjected to a surgical operation during her monthly flux. Our forefathers, and especially our foremothers, from time immemorial, have thought and taught that a menstruating woman is unclean, and that her presence pollutes religious rites, turns milk sour, spoils the fermentation in the wine-vats, and does much other mischief in various ways. Influenced by hoary tradition, physicians very generally postponed all operative treatment until the flow had ceased, even when there was danger in the delay. Now, while physicians do not select this period for surgical relief, they have found, through careful and painstaking research, that all operations, save possibly some of those upon the womb itself, can with impunity be performed during the continuance of the flow.

The great gains in gynæcology have produced corresponding ones in cognate surgery. Hence come the various operations devised for the cure of ventral hernia. From this source has sprung the scientific treatment of appendicitis, of perityphlitis, and of all intestinal and visceral lesions. To gynæcology is due the revival of symphyseotomy, which has now secured a foothold and promises to stay as a most beneficial obstetric operation. Other triumphs might be recounted, both intrinsic and extrinsic, but I forbear repeating oft-told tales.

Nor should we overlook the progress which gynæcology has made in the profession at large. A few years ago all operations upon the female reproductive organs were referred to specialists. At the present day most of these operations, and especially the plastic ones, are performed either by the family physician or by the local surgeon. Time was when I was overburdened with cases of uro-genital fistula, while for clinical illustration I had always on hand more than enough typical cases of the minor female lesions. Of late it was a rare circumstance for a case of vesico-vaginal fistula to present itself to my clinic, and the cases of badly-torn cervix or of complete laceration of the perineum were getting few and far between. In consequence of the early repair of the torn cervix, cancer of the womb is, in my experience, not so frequent a disease as formerly. Of course these changes are due not only to a more widely diffused skill in repairing female lesions, but also to greater skill in preventing them. On the other hand, an ever-increasing number of cœliotomies at every clinic and private hospital shows how alert the family physician is to have his patient seek for such aid as he himself cannot give.

But, granting all these magnificent triumphs, in which every gynæcologist takes pride, there remain problems not fully solved, and much is yet to be learned. One question not yet satisfactorily answered is, what effect upon a woman has the removal of her ovaries? Unquestionably there usually follow the annoyances of the change of life. These, in my experience, are long spun out, because when menstruation has been abruptly and artificially stopped the change of life, especially in young women, takes a longer time to become fully established than when the menopause has been naturally established. Consequently, months may elapse—nay, even years —before the victim of the operation escapes from the perspirations, the flashes of heat, the skin-tinglings, the numbness of the extremities, the nerve-stress, the nerve-storms, and all other vaso-motor disturbances which are so hard to bear. My experience also coincides with that of Hegar, who says that "the artificial menopause induced by the operation is often attended with more serious complications than those which are not rarely observed in the natural change of life." [1]

Then, again, the unwelcome fact cannot be ignored that mental disturbance may be traced directly to the ablation of the ovaries. This is manifested by morbid brooding, by low spirits, by melancholy, by suicidal impulses, and even by insanity. Every ovariotomist has met with such painful episodes in his practice, and has greatly regretted that it had fallen to his lot to operate upon the unfortunate woman. Glaevecke, who has made extensive researches on this point, goes so far as to say that " in almost all cases the mind becomes more or less affected, and not infrequently melancholia results." [2] Keith has stated [3] that ten per cent. of his patients who recover from hysterectomy subsequently suffer from melancholia or from other forms of mental disease. Yet this result must have come in his cases not so much from the removal of the womb, which is merely a muscular bag, as from the associated ablation of the ovaries, of which the womb physiologically is only the appendage.

Whether this deplorable event is due directly to the nerve-shock of the operation itself, together with its emotional environment, whether to the abrupt cessation of an habitual flow, or whether to the absolute need of the ovaries for mental equilibration, is yet an open question. We know, however, that sexuality is a potent factor in woman, as well as in man, and that even certain sexual functions, such as coition, menstruation, gestation, parturition, and lactation, of themselves tend not infrequently to disturb the mental poise. I am disposed, however, in a measure to attribute the attacks of insanity in those women who have lost their ovaries to their brooding over the thought that they are unsexed; and if brooding may be deemed in itself a mental aberration, Glaevecke's sweeping statement is not an extravagant one.

But, above all, the burning question is, Does the removal of the uterine appendages affect the sexual sense of the woman or in any way unsex her? Here we have an embarrassing diversity of opinion. Some operators contend that in these respects castration does not change her at all; others that it does so, and often very decidedly. The truth in such cases usually lies in the mean, as I shall try to show.

In my " Lessons in Gynæcology" and in my early teachings I maintained that after puberty the removal of the ovaries and of the tubes does not unsex a woman,—at least not to a greater extent than castration after puberty unsexes the man. In the one the ability to inseminate is lost; in the other, the capability of being inseminated; but in both the sexual feelings remain pretty much the same. Males who have lost their testes after the age of puberty are said to retain indefinitely the power of erection and even of ejaculation, the fluid being, of course, merely a lubricating one. The

---

[1] British Medical Journal, December, 1886, p. 1280.
[2] New York Medical Journal, July 20, 1889, p. 73.
[3] Ibid., p. 73.

amorous proclivities of the steer are the scandal of our highways. Alive to these facts, Oriental as well as Chinese jealousy demands in a eunuch the complete ablation of the genital organs. Not only are the testes, therefore, removed, but also the scrotum and the penis flush with the pubes. Hence, to avoid the soiling of his clothes, every eunuch carries a short silver tube, which he inserts merely in the pubic meatus whenever he passes his water.[1] I contended further that, apart from cessation of menstruation and from inevitable sterility, the woman after castration remains unchanged, having the same natural instincts and affections, that the sexual organs continue excitable, and that she is just as womanly and as womanish as ever. I held that the seat of sexuality in woman had long been sought for, but in vain. The clitoris had been amputated, the nymphæ had been excised, the tubes and ovaries had been extirpated, yet the sexual desire had survived these mutilations. The seat had not been found, because sexuality is not a member or an organ, but a sense,—a sense dependent on the sexual apparatus not for its being, but merely for its fruition. My inference was that the physical and psychical influence of the ovaries upon women had been greatly overrated. In the popular mind a woman without ovaries is not a woman. Even Virchow contends that "on these two organs [the ovaries] depend all the specific properties of her body and her mind, all her nutrition and her nervous sensibility, the delicacy and roundness of her figure, and, in fact, all other womanly characteristics." This statement I held to be true in so far as the ovaries are needful for the primary or rudimental development of woman; but not true when once she is developed, for then they are not essential to her perpetuation as woman.

In time, however, I slowly found out that the removal of the ovaries does blunt and often does extinguish ultimately the sexual feeling in woman, although the removal of the testes after puberty is said not to impair the virile sense of the male. The truth of this random opinion, however, I very much doubt, despite the ribald satires of Juvenal, the gross pleasantries of the "Lettres Persanes," and the maudlin sentiment indulged in by De Amicis, and by other travellers, even about the eunuchs of Oriental palaces, who are castrated in infancy. Unquestionably, the secretion and the retention of the seminal fluid are in themselves the great aphrodisiacs. Otherwise we cannot explain the changed behavior of Abelard towards Héloïse after his forcible castration. Overlooking the effect of such a mutilation, sentimentalists have judged too harshly of Abelard and have lavished too one-sided a sympathy upon Héloïse.

Giving up, perhaps erroneously, the analogy of a castrated woman to a castrated man, in my more recent teachings I adopted that of the menopause, as suggested by Koeberlé. I accepted his analogy, although I could

---

[1] North American Medico-Chirurgical Review, May, 1861, p. 500; New York Medical Record, June, 1870, p. 190; Medical and Surgical Reporter, April 24, 1875, p. 329; "Dictionnaire en Trente," article "Eunuque;" Universal Medical Journal, November, 1893, p. 329.

not accept wholly his inference, that woman is not affected sexually by the natural cessation of her menses. Koeberlé sums up his opinion in the following words : " In my own experience the extirpation of both ovaries causes no marked change in the general condition of those who have been operated on. They are women who may be considered as having abruptly reached the climacteric. Their instincts and affections remain the same, their sexual organs continue excitable, and their breasts do not wither up."[1]

A riper experience, of which time was the main element, has led me still further to modify my views on this subject. Undoubtedly the natural change of life when fully established, but not until it is fully established, does very sensibly dull and deaden the sexual sense of woman, which ultimately disappears in her long before virility is extinguished in man. Reveillé-Parise, in his excellent treatise on old age, enlarges on this fact, and makes the period of gradually lessening sexual feeling in woman to last from the age of forty-five to that of fifty, when this sense is usually lost.[2] Nor is the survival of the sexual feeling after the menopause so essential to the woman, because when menstruation ceases she loses the power of procreation, which is retained to an advanced age by the man. This is a wise provision of nature, for did the sexual sense of the wife outlast that of the husband it could not be gratified. Sensible in herself of these changes in her sex, a gifted French authoress makes one of her heroines say, with italicized emphasis, " *Men* may forget the course of years; they may love and become parents at a more advanced period than we can, for nature prescribes a term after which there seems to be something monstrous and impious in the idea of [our] seeking to awaken love. . . . Yes ! age closes our mission *as women* and deprives us of our sex." Now, what happens in the natural change of life holds good in that artificially produced, with this important difference, that in the latter the sexual feeling is sooner lost. I am willing to concede that in some women, by no means in all, whose health has been so crippled as to quench all sexual feeling, there is after castration a partial recovery of the lost sense whenever health has been regained. Yet even in these cases, so far as I can ascertain,—for women are loath to talk about these matters,—the flame merely flares up, flickers, and soon goes out.

My own large experience would lead me to the conclusion that in the majority of women who have been castrated the sexual impulse soon abates in intensity, much sooner than after a natural menopause, and that in many cases it wholly disappears. This tallies with Glavaecke's verdict, that " in most of the cases the sexual desire is notably lessened and in many cases is extinguished." In corroboration of this statement I could cite many cases in point, but, as I have done so elsewhere,[3] I shall not repeat them here. In other sexual characteristics I have not found in these women any marked

---

[1] Nouveau Dictionnaire de Médecine et de Chirurgie, tome xxv. p. 487.

[2] Traité de la Vieillesse, chap. ix.

[3] The Medical News, December 9, 1893, p. 653.

changes, either physical or psychical. Their affections seem to remain the same, their breasts do not flatten or wither up, they do not become obese, abnormal growths of hair do not appear on the face or on the body, and the tone of their voice and its quality are not changed. In one word, there has not been in a single one of my cases a tendency towards any characteristic of the male type. If any change has taken place, it has been in the direction of old-maidhood.

In close relation with this subject four questions press to the front, and grave ones they are:

(*a*) Do chronic diseases of the appendages often lead to a fatal issue?

(*b*) To restore health to the woman suffering from such diseases of the appendages, is it needful invariably to invoke the aid of surgery?

(*c*) After an abdominal section has been made, and after adhesions have been separated, must the now free appendages always be removed?

(*d*) Is castration of the female a warrantable operation for the cure of insanity or of epilepsy?

To the first question I answer that the death-rate from chronic diseases of the appendages is greatly overrated, so much so that, in my opinion, more deaths result from the operation of removing the tubes and the ovaries, in the hands of even the most successful gynæcologist, than from the disease itself. In my experience, after the patient has safely passed through the acute stage of the inflammatory attack, her life is in very little danger. Chronic diseases of the appendages usually affect the well-being of the woman, but they ordinarily do not threaten her life in any other way than by the wear and tear of prolonged discomfort. This may shorten her days, but fatal attacks of peritonitis, even in leaky pus-tubes, are the exception. Paradoxical as it may seem, the life of a woman with but one ailing appendage is in greater danger than the life of a woman with both her appendages diseased. The explanation is a simple one: parturition very generally relights a chronic inflammation of the pelvic structures; but, when both appendages are diseased, pregnancy rarely takes place.

To restore the health of a woman whose appendages are diseased, or to relieve her from her sufferings, a surgical operation is by no means always necessary. Many women with adherent tubes and ovaries, and, for the matter of that, some even with pus in these organs, suffer either no inconvenience whatever or very little indeed from that condition *per se*. There are, again, others who have pains and aches at their monthly periods only. Let, however, their health break down, say from influenza, from malaria, from overwork, or from nerve-strain; then symptoms may arise from their hitherto latent pelvic lesions. Yet in most of these cases, if the woman can be restored to her former condition of health—that is to say, to that which she enjoyed just before the final break-down—she will lose her local symptoms and become symptomatically well. On this matter I can speak positively, for many a patient has been sent to my private hospital to have her distinctly damaged tubes and ovaries removed, who has

been restored to health without the use of the knife. Now, by the term
"restored to health" I do not mean that the treatment has always released
the adherent appendages, but that it has freed the woman from every pain
and restored her fully to all her social and domestic duties and pleasures.
She has been cured so well as to be able to row, to swim, to dance, to take
long walks, to ride on horseback, and to exercise in the gymnasium; and
what better vouchers of good health than these can be given?

I shall go yet further, and assert that even women with all the subjective and objective symptoms of ovarian or of tubal abscess have been
cured by me without any operation whatever, the pus having disappeared
either through absorption or through inspissation.   What is still more
strange, in a few cases of abscess of both uterine appendages—very few, I
acknowledge—the treatment by massage, electricity, local applications, and
by a general building up of the system was followed by conception, pregnancy, and parturition.   These were cases in which I did not advocate castration until other means had been tried, but all had been sent to me by
their physicians for the purpose of having their appendages removed. Nor
do I stand alone in this opinion.   At a meeting of the American Gynæcological Society,[1] Dr. Robert A. Murray gave a clinical report of six cases
of double pyosalpinx.   He had treated them by Polk's method of uterine
drainage, and the women all afterwards conceived and bore healthy children.
In the discussion following the reading of this paper, Dr. George M. Edebohls stated that he had known a number of cases of true pyosalpinx to get
well, the women afterwards becoming pregnant.

I come now to two cases in which I unwisely urged castration. Probably I have had more, but I cannot recall them.   Each one had the fixed
sausage-like tubal tumor on either side.   Yet each patient, to my great
surprise, conceived and bore children.   The one, a patient of my friend Dr.
D. Murray Cheston, first consulted me and afterwards a gynæcologist of
world-wide renown, who corroborated my diagnosis of double pus-tubes and
doomed her, as I had doomed her, to hopeless sterility.   The puerperal convalescence was stormy and at one time threatening; but she ultimately got
well, and is now pregnant for the second time.   The other case is a standing joke of my friend Professor Parvin, who knew the circumstances.   The
patient presented characteristics analogous to those of the preceding case,
and I urged an operation.   This she luckily refused to undergo, and more
than a year afterward she gave birth to twins.   Of course, the rejoinder
will be made that my diagnosis, although shared by other specialists besides
myself, was a faulty one.   But I can unhesitatingly reply that had the
objector made the examination he inevitably would have followed it by an
abdominal section, and as inevitably would have removed both adnexa,
as I certainly should have done had I opened the abdomen.

Now, in these cases either the pus was confined to the ovaries or, as I

---

[1] Transactions of the American Gynæcological Society, 1893, pp. 345, 346.

inferred from the sausage-like form of the tumors, it lay sealed up in the tubes, and the closed lumen of one of them was, by returning health, fully reopened. The possibility of a closed-up tube regaining its bore is, I know, strongly disputed, even ridiculed, and *a priori* reasoning would certainly justify the doubt. Yet it is well known that solid uterine fibroids of stony hardness and of several pounds' weight will occasionally, through retrograde metamorphosis, greatly lessen in size and even wholly disappear. At the meeting of the Obstetrical Society of London held June 7, 1893, Doran and others referred to forty such cases, and I myself have in my practice met with three analogous ones. In one of them, after a merely exploratory incision, a large uterine fibroid wholly disappeared. Why, then, may not the thin tubal barriers and septa also break down and melt away? I have read somewhere, but the reference has escaped me, that, in order to prevent conception in a case of narrow pelvis, both tubes were ligated, yet without establishing sterility. On the other hand, great disorganization of the ovaries is not incompatible with conception and pregnancy, for it appears that a very small amount of ovarian stroma goes a great way. Menstruation often continues, however diseased or damaged the ovaries may be, and Atlee reports two cases in which, one ovary having been removed, the other became so cystic as to need *repeated tappings*, yet each woman not only menstruated, but conceived and gave birth to a child.[1] In one of these cases a cyst of the sole ovary, the other having been removed many years previously, was tapped twice before conception, twice before delivery, seven times afterwards, and then was extirpated. Robertson[2] mentions a remarkable case in point, which occurred in his practice. He extirpated both the ovaries, which were diseased, from one of his patients, yet she afterwards conceived and gave birth to a child. His explanation is that he must have left unwittingly a scrap of healthy ovarian tissue in one of the stumps. But, on the other hand, the ovum could not have descended into the womb unless the lumen of one of the tubes had reopened at the point where it had been sealed up by the adhesive inflammation set up by the ligature. A number of years ago I had a case of intraligamentary cyst of the right ovary. After its removal, which was attended with much difficulty, the left tube and ovary were found firmly embedded by adhesions to the pelvic wall and to the surrounding viscera. In view of the shock under which my patient was laboring, and of the desperate character of the adhesions, I did not dare to detach and remove this appendage. Yet, not many months later, this lady, who hitherto had been sterile, conceived and bore a healthy child. Dr. B. F. Baer has had an analogous but still more remarkable case.[3] In this case, the womb and both appendages being firmly bound down by adhesions, he " by great effort"

---

[1] Atlee, Ovarian Tumors, pp. 38, 39.

[2] British Medical Journal, September 27, 1890, p. 722.

[3] Annals of Gynæcology and Pædiatry, January, 1894, p. 232.

released the womb, tore the left ovary and tube " piecemeal from their position," and ligated their " shreddy pedicle." " The right appendages were
found in an almost similarly diseased condition, and when they were dissected loose they also were in shreds, the tube having been torn off about
two inches from the uterus." Dr. Baer wished to remove them, but he was
not permitted to do so by a physician present, who was the brother of the
patient. Fifteen months later the woman gave birth to a child at full
term.

With regard to the third problem : supposing ordinary therapeutic measures fail, and the physician is driven to surgical interference, must he, after
breaking up the adhesions, always extirpate the now free uterine appendages? Most surgeons contend not only that the diseased appendage
should be removed, but also that both appendages should be extirpated,
even if one alone is damaged. This advice is given on the ground that
the healthy one is liable in its turn to become affected. My own course
under such circumstances would be, never to remove the healthy appendage unless the menopause had been already established, or unless there
existed a good reason for hastening it on. On the other hand, should
both ovaries be intrinsically diseased and their tubes contain pus, I should
always remove both uterine appendages in their totality, no matter what
the age of the patient might be. Generally, however, the pus is limited to
the tubes, and in that case sometimes one ovary, barring its adhesions,
which, of course, must be broken, is healthy enough to be left behind. In
such a case, the tube alone, if possible, should be removed, and not the
healthy ovary or the healthy ovaries—if both happen to be sound. Further,
rather than wholly remove all ovarian stroma, I should try in such cases
to leave behind at least a small fragment. For in several of my cases in
which a piece of ovary not larger than a bean was left behind, no menstrual
or sexual changes whatever took place in the women. Should the uterine
appendages be merely adherent, and not intrinsically diseased to any extent,
I should, as a rule, during active menstrual life, release them, and perhaps
extirpate the worse of the two, but not both of them.

My reasons for this conservative treatment are that the complete extirpation of these organs, as I have shown before, tends to destroy the sexual
feeling, to disturb the mental equilibrium, and to produce prolonged nervous perturbations, all of which come from the abrupt and untimely suspension of menstruation. There is yet another very excellent reason for
this advice. The majority of physicians and all laymen look upon women
deprived of their ovaries as unsexed. Just as with castration in the male,
so the analogous operation in the female is deemed a sexual mutilation to
which common consent attaches a stigma. No woman would marry a
eunuch, and few men would wed a woman deprived of her ovaries. In
my own practice I have known of several very sad cases of marriage en-
gagements broken off, of marital infidelities, and of bitter estrangement
between husband and wife, all of which would have been avoided had one

ovary been spared, or, indeed, had a mere fragment of one been left behind. A third good reason for conservative surgery lies in the fact that fertility may continue. Polk, Schroeder, and Martin, its champions *par excellence*, and others,[1] have published cases in which after a mere fragment of an ovary had been spared, and indeed after resection of the oviducts, conception and parturition took place.

Upon the question of the removal of the uterine appendages for the cure of insanity and of epilepsy I have very few words to say, but they are all based upon cases occurring in my own practice. If the insanity is limited to periodic outbreaks, strictly ovarian in their character and with the menstrual flux as a storm-centre; if the epileptic fits are preceded by an ovarian aura,—that is to say, if they pivot around the monthly period and appear at no other time,—the removal of the appendages, by suppressing a pernicious menstruation, usually will bring about a cure. But when the organs are extirpated merely as a panacea *per se* for these mental and neural disorders, irrespective of an ovarian origin, the operation affords no relief. At the same time I frankly confess that, in order to stamp out insanity, I am strongly inclined to advocate the legal castration of every man and of every woman who is the unfortunate victim of this hereditary curse.

The causes of ill health in women from functional injuries are so well known that it would be a thankless task to enumerate them. Neither shall I enlarge upon the subject of tight lacing or of woman's dress, for the medical profession is powerless against the Moloch of fashion. Its disinterested warnings in this direction are, like those of Cassandra, truthful but unheeded. But other causes not so patent exist, to which a brief reference may be made.

One cause is, unquestionably, a faulty mode of education. The chief strain of reproducing the species falls on woman, and her share in this cardinal matter is complex, while man's share is single and simple. To this end he merely secretes and ejaculates the semen, but she ovulates, she menstruates, and she conceives. To this end she bears the burdens of gestation, of parturition, of lactation, and of maternity. For this great end she needs the utmost perfection of physical development. Therefore the growth and the well-being of her body should be at least as carefully looked after as the growth and the well-being of her mind. It should be a co-education of body and mind, the one helpful to the other. But this essential concordat in female education is not sufficiently well maintained. From the age of eight to that of fourteen our daughters spend too much of their time in the unwholesome air of the recitation-room or in poring over their books when they should be at play. Then, just as the menstrual period is beginning, just as puberty is struggling to assert itself, comes the series of examinations which selects the most ambitious girls and promotes them to the com-

---

[1] Transactions of the American Gynæcological Society, 1893, pp. 175, 457; American Journal of Obstetrics, December, 1893, p. 807.

plex curriculum of the high schools. Four years of hard study and intellectual rivalry now follow,—four precious years, very needful for the perfect development of the reproductive organs and for the full establishment of their functions, but spent in an endless antagonism between brain-growth and body-growth. Hence especially our public schools and also our boarding-schools and female colleges are liable to become the hot-beds of forced and sickly girls. As a result, the chief skill of the dressmaker seems to be directed towards concealing the lack of organs needful alike to beauty and to maternity, and the highly cultured girl of to-day becomes the barren wife or the invalid mother of to-morrow, or she has all the natural human instincts partly, or indeed wholly, educated out of her. So commonly do I find ill health associated with brilliant scholarship, so often is it the case that she who wins an honor is a "victor who hath lost in gain," that one of the first questions I put to a young lady seeking my advice for shattered health is, "Did you stand high at school?" This break-down in school-girls comes from a combination of causes. It is due to the mode and quality of their education, to long confinement in impure air, to the close-fitting female dress, and to an unwholesome diet of cakes and candies. It is, perhaps, especially due to an utter disregard in most educational institutions of the catamenial week, when by their own sensations and feelings women are, as they call themselves, "*unwell.*" They are then by their own showing literally *unwell*, and are therefore as unfit for exhausting brain-work as for fatiguing body-work.

Thus far I have sketched the school-girl of the day, from early childhood up to sickly maidenhood. Released now from her school-desk, this weary, worn-out, rest-needing girl launches into the dissipations of society. Within a few years, it may be, she becomes engaged to some unwary youth, who, bewitched by her face and charmed by her intelligence, sees not the frail body and the butterfly down. He weds her to find that, "fair by defect and delicately weak," she has brought him a dower of ill health, and that she has dared to assume the duties and responsibilities of a married life with undeveloped reproductive organs, and with a large outfit of back-aches and spine-aches and headaches. Unequal to the obligations of marriage, she at first tolerates them, then loathes them. Soon repugnance merges into aversion and hate. The husband is driven to unfaithfulness, and finally the domestic drama too often ends in separation or in divorce. Should pregnancy ensue, a big-headed child and a narrow pelvis endanger her life and that of her offspring. Should the child survive, it is suckled by aliens. Cursed with a puny frame and with a too highly organized brain, it is, like the cherubs of the old masters, all head and no body. But this is not all. "There is but little difficulty," says the leech in "The Fair Maid of Perth," "in blighting a flower exhausted from having been made to bloom too soon." The young girl—this hot-house plant—wilting under the double strain of wifehood and motherhood, remains ever after an invalid.

In one word, it is to the present cramming and high-pressure system of education, together with its environment, that I attribute much of the menstrual derangements, the sterility, and the infecundity of our women, the absence of sexual feeling, the aversion to maternity, the too often lingering convalescence from a first labor, which is frequently the only one, and the very common inability to suckle their offspring. From this cause come most of my unmarried patients with nerve-prostration, with their protean mimicry of uterine symptoms,—unmarried often because they are not well enough to wed. If woman is to be thus stunted and deformed to meet the ambitious intellectual demands of the day, if her health must be sacrificed upon the altar of her education, the time may come when, to renew the worn-out stock of this Republic, it will be needful for our young men to make matrimonial " incursions into lands where educational theories are unknown."[1]

Another grave fault of the times, one which makes many invalids, is the lack of that "foster-nurse of nature," repose. Fashion compels its votaries to be on the go day and night without cessation. To keep up her social and domestic duties every ambitious mother must live more or less at high pressure. Younger women exhaust their vitality on fads and cults and literary clubs and on a mania to be omniscient. So ingrained in our women has the lack of repose become—this hustle and bustle of American life—that one notes it in their voice, in their manners, and in their carriage.

One word here with regard to the sewing-machine. While I do not believe all that is laid to its charge, yet its treadle motion does undoubtedly lead to pelvic and to portal congestion. In spite of myself, I have become convinced that a woman who herself works this machine as a trade cannot escape from some uterine derangement. Even its domestic use is not unattended with risk, because, although intermittent, it is liable to be too prolonged. Many a woman is laid up by her spring and autumn bout with it. By its noise and by the tension of mind and of body that it demands, the sewing-machine wears also on the nerves. The strain is great, for the brain, the eyes, the fingers, and the feet have all to be on the alert to act in unison. With the old-fashioned needle, the woman could at times gain repose. She could sit at ease, and think and dream and build castles in the air. The sewing-machine has great virtues, and we cannot well dispense with it; but it certainly does not conduce to repose.

Undoubtedly some of the worst forms of women's diseases come from the three following causes : the specific infection of wives by their husbands, criminal abortion, and the prevention of conception.

So long as society condones in man such lapses from virtue as it peremptorily and pitilessly condemns in woman, so long as a chaste woman is willing to take to herself an unchaste husband, so long will young men indulge in illicit sexual pleasures. As a too common result, they, soon

---

[1] Puberty and Adolescence, by T. S. Clouston, Edinburgh Medical Journal, July, 1880, p. 9.

after their marriage, often on the honey-moon journey, unwittingly infect their wives with the venereal disease which years before they may have caught, and of which they honestly deemed themselves cured. Specific blood-poisoning in all its harrowing forms will occasionally be met with ; but gonorrhœal infection is far more common,—so common in some classes of society as to be a veritable matrimonial scourge. From this cause come very many cases of sterility, miscarriage, oöphoritis, and salpingitis of every kind and degree, pelvic and intestinal adhesions, chronic ill health, and even death.

Criminal abortion is, alas! another too frequent cause of impaired health. Being performed without antiseptic precautions, generally by illiterate persons of either sex, sometimes by the woman upon herself or by the unskilled hand of a sympathizing neighbor, it slays its thousands. Of those who fortunately escape with their lives, many do so after an attack of peritonitis, which is liable to entail on them the lasting lesions of this disease. Even should peritonitis not occur, endometritis usually will, or involution is arrested and the enlarged and heavy womb is liable to displacement.

But the most common of these three causes of ill health in women is the prevention of conception,—a deplorable practice which, like the plague of the frogs, creeps into our " houses and bedchambers and beds." It comes from the dainty dilettanteism of our women, which shrinks from having its patrician pleasures and æsthetic tastes disturbed by the cares of maternity. It comes from fashion, from cowardice, from indolent wealth and shiftless poverty. It comes from too high a standard of living, which creates many artificial wants and demands many expensive luxuries. I am amazed at the very low standard of morality with regard to the sexual relations obtaining in the community. So low, indeed, has it fallen that I have known clergymen either themselves practising preventive measures or else abetting their wives in them, and physicians of repute teaching their patients how to avoid having offspring. To these detestable practices do I attribute in a great measure much of the ill health of our married women. Why is it, asks a layman, J. Parton, that " in the regions of the United States otherwise most highly favored, nearly every woman under forty is sick or sickly?" Why is it, I ask, that the waiting-rooms of our gynæcologists are crowded with so many querulous and complaining women,—women with groin-aches, backaches, headaches, and spine-aches, women either without sexual feeling or else too weak to indulge in it? Why do so many women break down either shortly after marriage or very soon after the birth of their first child? It is, I answer, because the majority of them, false to their moral and physical obligations, are trying either not to have children or to limit their number. It is because, by an immutable law of nature, there appears to be no harmless way by which " the seed of another life" can be made unfruitful. It is because the wife, sinning the most and most sinned against, suffers the most. Be the mode of prevention what it may, so much engorgement and hyperplasia and disorganization of the uterine structures and appendages are apt to take place in those women who keep themselves sterile, that their health breaks down and they are liable to lose all sexual desire. Then, when they advance in age and there comes that inevitable yearning and need for offspring, they find to their dismay that they cannot conceive, and they repeat the despairing cry of Rachel. What physician is there of ripe years who has not been importuned by women, hitherto wilfully barren but now longing for children, to undo the mischief caused by such practices?

There is another phase to this many-sided evil, an ethical one, any allusion to which in a strictly medical work may seem, at first blush, out of place. But health and happiness are so correlated that what harms the one hurts the other. Statistics show that divorces are multiplying in this land in far greater ratio than the gain in population. In the New England States the increase is so alarming as to arouse the attention of patriots and philanthropists. Every year the divorces granted in these States break up over two thousand families. But these figures do not tell the whole tale of disrupted households, for they do not include the many cases of voluntary separation between husband and wife, or of applications for divorce which were denied by the courts. While it is true that so high a divorce rate does not prevail in the other States, yet, to our shame, it is steadily increasing all over the Union. For instance, a few years ago Congress appropriated ten thousand dollars to bear the expense of an inquiry into the working of marriage and divorce laws in the United States. The official report was made to Congress on February 20, 1889. It shows that 328,716 divorces were granted in the twenty years between and including 1867 and 1886. A single State, Illinois, granted 36,072 divorces in that time. Ohio followed closely with 26,367, and Indiana with 25,193. The total in all the States for the year 1886 was 25,535. In the year 1867 the number of divorces granted was 9837. The increase, therefore, in twenty years was about 157 per cent. But in the same years the population increased about 65 per cent., which shows that the evil of divorce is increasing more than twice as fast as our population. From statistics lately published by the clerk of Cuyahoga County, in which Cleveland is situated, it appears that during the past year 1080 cases of divorce were put upon record in the courts,—viz., one divorce in seven marriages.[1]

Now, why are there so many ill-mated marriages? Why these unhappy homes and broken households? What mean these separations between man and wife? I answer, they mean the violation of one of nature's immutable laws. Sex is a profound fact which underlies all the relations of life and the fabrics of society, and it cannot be ignored. The love interchanged between man and woman is no mere operation of the mind, no sheer intellectual process. However pure this passion may be, it is neces-

---

[1] National Reform Documents of 1890 and 1894; New York Observer, October 26, 1893; The Congregationalist, July 27, 1893.

2

sarily an alloy, made up, like ourselves, of body and mind, the grosser mould so interfluxed with the more ethereal that the one finds its most passionate expression in the fruition of the other. The sexual instinct is given to man for two reasons, to perpetuate the species and to rivet the tie between husband and wife, not only by offspring but by mutual endearment. The conjugal relation is therefore twofold in its nature: it has a moral as well as a physical expression, the two so interwoven that it is impossible to dissociate the one from the other without doing moral as well as physical harm.

The causes of domestic infelicity and ill-mated marriages are, then, to my mind, clear enough. The grossness of the carnal union is redeemed by its purpose, the moral union in which is involved the desire for offspring. Deprive the marriage tie of these qualities, strip it of the family idea, and it loses its cohesiveness in intense personality and self-asserting individualism. Now, when a wife is too sickly to admit the approaches of her husband or to respond to them; when she receives them on sufferance, or absolutely refuses to entertain them, as I have known many a wife to do; when she soils the marriage-bed with the artifices and equipments of the brothel, and quenches all passion by cold-blooded safeguards; when she consults her almanac and puts off an ardent husband to stated times and seasons,—when a wife, I say, behaves in so unwifelike a way, can it be otherwise than that estrangement or jealousy should take place? Can a home with such an environment be a happy one? Would not most husbands be tempted to seek elsewhere those pleasures which are denied them at home? These are nature's reprisals; these, indeed, her never-failing retributions.

The ill health and childlessness of our women are sources of national weakness at which every patriot may well take alarm. Searching statistical inquiries show that the birth-rate of our native population is steadily and alarmingly lessening. By the ill health of our women, and by their resorting to criminal abortion and to the use of preventive measures, the American family is growing smaller and smaller, and the good old original Anglo-Saxon stock of our country—its brains, its bone, and its sinew—is rapidly dwindling towards extinction. For instance, from the records of six generations of families in some New England towns the following facts were gleaned: "It is found that the families composing the first generation had on an average between eight and ten children; the next three generations averaged about seven to each family; the fifth generation less than three for each family. The generation now coming on the stage is not doing so well as that." In Massachusetts the average family has numbered as low as less than three persons. Other States have not yet made such searching statistical inquiries, but there is no doubt that an alarming diminution in the Anglo-Saxon stock is taking place all over our country. In view of these facts let us read two lessons from ancient history and take warning from them.

Time was when every prolific Roman matron received a civic reward.

Then she would exhibit her children, as Cornelia did her twelve, and proudly say, "These be my jewels." Five hundred and twelve years elapsed from the foundation of Rome before the first formal divorce was granted, and the divorcer till his death was pursued by the obloquy of his fellow-citizens. In those days nothing could withstand the onset of the Roman legion. Then Rome ruled the known world. But, as Mommsen tells us, "In the time of Julius Cæsar celibacy and childlessness became more and more common; the family institution fell. The Latin stock in Italy underwent an alarming diminution." Divorces were now obtained on the flimsiest grounds. Criminal abortion was practised on the slightest pretext; nay, indeed, it was lauded as a praiseworthy domestic economy. Marcus Aurelius foresaw the danger and tried to stem the evil, but, being a pagan and a doctrinaire, he failed. So prevalent had this crime become in Juvenal's day that he levelled one of his most biting satires against it. In it he says that it was most commonly resorted to by the Roman ladies lest pregnancy should mar their beauty or spoil their figure. They termed the unborn child the shameful burden (*indecens onus*), and got rid of it lest its growth should disfigure their belly with scars (*ne rugis ventrem Lucina notaret*). But national sins beget national woes, and the Roman empire overrun by Northern hordes perished for want of men.

Once the family institution was deemed the palladium of Hellas. The contemporary of Plato, of Socrates, and of those heroes who fell at Thermopylæ "prided himself on the number of his sons who could fight for his country, and boasted of the number of his daughters who could hold the distaff." Then Greece, for her superb heroism and magnificent pluck, won the admiration of the world. Her navies swept the Mediterranean, and her colonies studded its coasts. But (alas! these buts) one century and a half before the Christian era the serried ranks of the Macedonian phalanx quailed before the Roman legion, and the Greek became a vassal. Why this dire disaster? Because Greece, spoiled by prosperity and warped by vain philosophy, could not brook to have its classic tastes and æsthetic cults interrupted by family cares and family ties. Polybius, her own countryman and historian, writes that "the downfall of Greece was not owing to war or to the plague, but mainly to a repugnance to marriage and to a reluctance to rear large families, caused by an extravagantly high standard of living."

Now, what happened to Rome, what happened to Greece, may yet befall our own beloved country. It may die for lack of Anglo-Saxon men. The hour of need may come when, after great national calamities, after portentous reverses, the genius of this Republic, disordered by an imperial grief like that of the Roman emperor, may catch the burden of his cry, "Give me back, O Varus, give me back my legions."

In the treatment of the diseases of women at the present time there seems to me to be a tendency to lay too much stress upon lesions of the reproductive organs. Too little heed is therefore given to the nerve-element, and, as a natural sequence, the surgical antennæ of the medical profession, always too keenly sensitive, vibrate most vehemently at the approach of an ailing woman. This trend of the profession to appeal to the knife as the great panacea for woman's diseases is seen everywhere. It prevails alike in city, town, village, and hamlet. It asserts itself in every medical discussion, and stands out in bold relief upon the pages of every medical journal. This, in my opinion, is the *great medical error of the nineteenth century*. It has been eloquently scored by Professor Parvin in his presidential address before the American Gynæcological Society. "There is a glamour," he says, "about successful surgery—a flashing of swift fame, a glitter of gold and a promise of financial felicity, as well as the conscious pride of success and of instant relief—that may mislead, operations being done that might have been averted by judicious hygiene, and patient, wise medical treatment. It is useless to deny that unnecessary operations, sometimes sexual mutilations, are done, and that many women are saved from them by changing their professional adviser."

While in the main agreeing with Professor Parvin, I cannot believe that mercenary motives induce the profession to perform needless "sexual mutilations" and "unnecessary operations." It is not the greed for gold, but errors of judgment and mistaken diagnosis, which are due to the fact that woman, through her sensitive organization, is a bundle of perplexing contradictions. More pitiful than man and more long-suffering, her anger is more cruel and her jealousy more relentless. Feebler than man, an appeal to her affections will make her surpass him in sheer muscular endurance. Who can nurse her kin so untiringly and with so little rest as even a frail woman can? What father can equal a mother in fondling and soothing a sick and fretful child through the weary night watches? What man can undergo the sheer fatigue, the strain and stress, that a woman will for those she loves? Even in her pleasures, her physical amusements, she will through keen enjoyment often out-tire the strongest man. As Dumas the elder writes in one of his historical novels, "It is perfectly true that with regard to dancing, concerts, promenades, and such matters a woman is far stronger than the most robust porter." In one word, she is a creature of impulse and of emotion. But all nerve-strains, whether arising from the emotions, from the affections, or from the passions, have their reactions, and very strange and very misleading reflexes come from the loss of brain-control over insubordinate lower nerve-centres. For what is hysteria but nerve-misrule and the panic of the brain at incompetent control? The secret and sanctity of woman's inner life lie in her affections, and what disturbs them disturbs the nerves, and through them their environment of flesh and blood. These unruly nerve-lights flashing and fading at their own will and without control in the different organs of the body the most careless observer may sometimes plainly see, for the clue is then as secure as the steps of a geometrical problem. But then, again, the symptoms are more frequently obscure. Often they are as misleading as the lapwing's flight. To construe such symptoms, to unfold their sense, and to paraphrase them so as to gain a true conception of their character, will often demand a deep acquaintance with human life and a keen insight into the most secret springs of its action.

Again, what is very perplexing, uterine symptoms are by no means always present in cases of uterine disease; and, what is still more bewildering, when so-called uterine symptoms are then present, they need not come from the uterine disease. The nerves are mighty mimes, the greatest of mimics, and they cheat us by their realistic personations of organic disease, and especially by their life-like imitations of uterine disease. Hence it is that even seemingly urgent uterine symptoms may be merely nerve-counterfeits of uterine disease. In fact, the time has come when we must give up the belief, which with many amounts to a creed, that the womb is at the bottom of nearly every female ailment.

Nerve-strain, or nerve-exhaustion, comes largely from the frets, the griefs, the jealousies, the worries, the bustles, the carks and cares, of life. Yet, strangely enough, the most common symptoms of this form of nerve-disorder in women are the very ones which lay tradition and dogmatic empiricism attribute to ailments of the womb. They are, in the usual order of their frequency, *great weariness*, and more or less *nervousness* and *wakefulness;* inability to walk any distance, and a bearing-down feeling; then headache, nape-ache, and backache. Next come scanty, or painful, or delayed, or suppressed menstruation; cold feet and an irritable bladder; general spinal and pelvic soreness, and *pain in one ovary*, usually the left, or in both ovaries. The sense of exhaustion is a remarkable one: the woman is always tired; she spends the day tired, she goes to bed tired, and she wakes up tired,—often, indeed, more tired than when she fell asleep. She sighs a great deal, she has low spirits, and she often fancies that she will lose her mind. Her arms and legs become numb so frequently that she fears palsy or paralysis. Nor does the skin escape the general sympathy. It becomes dry, harsh, and scurfy, and pigmentary deposits appear under the eyes, around the nipples, and on the chin and forehead. Blondes are likely to get a mottled complexion, and brunettes to be disfigured by brown patches or by general bronzing. Sometimes the whole complexion changes to a darker hue, and an abnormal and disfiguring growth of hair appears on the face. There are many other symptoms of nerve-strain, but, since they are not so distinctly uterine in expression, and therefore not so misleading, I shall not enumerate them.

Now, let a nervous woman with some of the foregoing symptoms recount them to a female friend, and she will be told that she has "womb disease." Let her consult a physician, and, especially if she has backache, bearing-down feelings, an irritable bladder, and pain in the ovaries, he will assert the same thing, and diligently hunt for some uterine lesion. If one be found, no matter how trifling, he will attach to it undue importance, and treat the womb heroically as the erring organ. If no visible or tangible disease of the sexual organs be discoverable, he will lay the blame on the invisible endometrium or on the unseeable ovaries, and continue the local treatment. In any event, whatever the inlook or the outlook, a local treatment more or less severe is bound to be the issue.

Yet these very exacting symptoms may be due wholly to nerve-strain, or (what is synonymous) to loss of brain-control over the lower nerve-centres, and not to direct or to reflex action from some supposed uterine disorder. Neither, for that matter, may they come from some real, tangible, and visible uterine lesion which positively exists. Thus it happens that a harmless anteflexion, a trifling leucorrhœa, a slight displacement of the womb, a small tear of the cervix, an insignificant rent of the perineum, or, what is almost always present, an ovarian ache, each plays the part of the will-o'-the-wisp to allure the physician from the bottom factor. To these paltry lesions—because they are visible, palpable, and ponderable, and because he has by education and by tradition a uterine bias—he attributes all his patient's troubles ; whereas a greater and a subtler force, the invisible, impalpable, and imponderable nervous system, may be the sole delinquent. The sufferer may be a jilted maiden, a bereaved mother, a grieving widow, or a neglected wife, and all her uterine symptoms—yes, every one of them —may be the outcome of her sorrows, and not of her local lesions. She is suffering from a sore brain, and not from a sore womb.

Fortunately for my own reputation and for that of my medical brothers who have thus erred, this grave error of diagnosis is not without excuse. For, as has been shown, the symptoms of nerve-strain—the reflexes of grief, of love, of neglect, of remorse, of jealousy, and of unrest—so closely simulate those of even coarse uterine lesions that the nerve mimicries very readily may be mistaken for the symptoms of actual organic disease. Nor, indeed, are they always distinguishable the one from the other ; for the marvellous kinship between mind and matter is a tangled skein unravelled yet in the dead-house or in the laboratory.

I have seen intolerable itching of the genitalia produced by jealousy, excessive vaginismus forbidding sexual intercourse following exacting literary work, an almost fatal vomiting starting from the shock of bad news, and extremely irritable bladders without number caused by every passion the female breast is capable of harboring. Several cases I have personally known of women who for months had been treated for supposed uterine or ovarian disease, when their whole trouble was remorse at having had illicit intercourse or at having resorted to criminal abortion. I could spin out to an interminable length this list of cases illustrating the close and often very perplexing kinship between the brain and the reproductive organs, but time and space forbid.

In the interpretation and the treatment of such cases as the foregoing we may well take a lesson from the ancients, who were often wiser in their generation than we are in ours. They recognized the influence of the mind upon the body, and did not omit moral therapeutics. In the Charmides of

Plato, Socrates makes the Thracian Zamolxis say, " That, as it is not proper to attempt to cure the eyes without the head, nor the head without the body, so neither is it proper to cure the body without the soul, and that this is the reason why many diseases escape the Greek physicians. . . . For all things, both the good and the bad, proceed from the soul to the body and to the whole man and flow from thence, . . . and that it is therefore requisite to attend to that point first, and especially if the parts of the head and the rest of the body are to be in a good state." Zamolxis, wisely with his light, used incantations for treating the disorders of the mind, concurrently with medicines for the ensuing ailments of the body. Such sterling good sense evidently made him a very successful practitioner, for after death he was enrolled among the gods.

Savages observe this duality of treatment by their herb-teas and sweat-baths, made mysterious by the pow-wows of the wizard and by the thaumaturgic pranks of the medicine-man. The incantations used by civilized nations at the present day—and I name them with all reverence—are alms, vows, spells, charms, shrines, pilgrimages, exorcisms, Christian science, the faith-cure, the laying on of hands, and other like forms of moral therapeutics, which unquestionably have cured and will cure so long as they produce dominant impressions. The legitimate incantations of medical therapeutics are now pretty much limited to distractions, diversions, travel in foreign lands, isolation, hypnotism, massage, electricity, and, above all, the personal magnetism of the physician, however exerted, for this is the kernel of the treatment and the greatest of incantations.

Sometimes in these cases an operation acts the part of an incantation. The dread of the knife and the shock of the operation distract the mental attitude of morbid concentration; while the enforced rest in bed gives a chance to the worn-out brain to regain strength and to assert its supremacy over the mutinous lower nerve-centres. This leads me to think that in a large majority of operations upon trifling tears of the cervix and on incomplete lacerations of the perineum, the good which may accrue comes less from the repair of those organs than from the mental distraction and the enforced rest. But this kind of incantation—the surgical variety—does not always work well; indeed, it often, very often, makes matters worse. One striking example was that of a lady who saw her only child run over and beheaded by a locomotive. Her health began at once to fail, and she took to her back, with the hackneyed symptoms of weariness, wakefulness, a bearing down, an irritable bladder, and many other canonical uterine reflexes. These were attributed, by an excellent and a conscientious physician, to a torn cervix and to a torn perineum, which were accordingly repaired. But the added shock of the two operations made her very much worse. For these reasons I must confess to becoming far less inclined than formerly to operate on trifling lesions of the reproductive organs, and especially on small tears of the perineum, the repair of which is painful, unnerving, and generally of doubtful expediency. I have grown very sceptical as to the influence of such lesions upon the general health, and have come to the belief that even in bad cases it is greatly overrated. In my experience the mistake usually made in these cases is that of attributing to the lacerations the mock uterine symptoms of nerve-prostration. About this there can be no error, for I have over and over again, without any surgical treatment whatever, cured of all their ailments patients who had been sent to me for the very purpose of undergoing some operation on the womb, on the perineum, or even on the ovaries themselves.

Another reason why operations are often needlessly performed comes from another harlequin trick of the nerves. In many cases when riotous they billet themselves, like an insolent soldiery, on some maimed organ, and hold high revel there. For instance, a woman, hitherto in perfect health, may have an adherent or a dislocated or a sensitive ovary, or she may have a torn cervix, or a lacerated perineum, or a narrow cervical canal, or a slight displacement of the womb,—lesions which may not have given her any appreciable trouble whatever. But let her nervous system become unstrung, and at once, through disturbances in the circulation both of the nerve-fluid and of the blood, there set in vesical, uterine, or ovarian symptoms so exacting as to demand relief. Nor are the sexual organs the only ones thus affected. Every weakened organ in the body is liable to such functional storms. The stomach rejects its food, the bowels either refuse to act or else become very loose, the heart loses its rhythm and beats irregularly or tumultuously, the vocal cords relax and the voice cannot be raised above a whisper, and almost every sphincter muscle in the body behaves as if it were insane. I have known a lady in her nervous attacks to become as jaundiced as if she had the liver of a Strasburg goose. Even the eyes, which before may not have exhibited to their owner any visual defect, now blink painfully at the light or cause violent headaches which glasses alone can allay.

Just as headache does not necessarily mean brain disease, ovary-ache, groin-ache, and backache do not necessarily mean ovarian disease. Nerve-strain and these aches are, it is true, correlatives; but the middle term which connects them is merely a disturbance in the circulation. Yet time and again—and I say this deliberately—have ladies been sent to me to have their ovaries taken out, when the whole mischief had started from some mental worry. Their ovaries were sound, but their nerves were not, and no operation was needed for their cure. As angels, according to the Schoolmen of the Middle Ages, fly from point to point without traversing the intervening distance, so with like swiftness the physician of the present day jumps from any distinctly female ache to an ovarian conclusion without the delay of any intermediate misgivings. The ache is in the back; then, he argues, it is probably ovarian It is in the groin; then of course it is ovarian. It is in the head; but extremes meet, and surely it also comes from the ovaries. I indeed have seen a painful nose, as well as a red one, attributed to the ovaries, and treated canonically by the hot vaginal douche and by uterine applications.  From this wide-spread bias and pernicious haste, the removal of the ovaries has degenerated into a busy industry, by which, in city and in country, very many women have been and are being mutilated both needlessly and on the slightest provocation.

So misleading, indeed, are the symptoms of a jaded brain or of other nerve-strain under the uterine guise in which they often masquerade, that when a jilted girl, a bereaved mother, or a grieving wife consults her physician, he, unless on his guard, will be more likely to minister to a womb diseased than to a mind diseased.  Such cases, even when associated with actual uterine disease, are not bettered by a merely local treatment.  Nor are medicines by themselves of much avail.  What these invalids need are the incantations of the rest-cure, massage, electricity, and strict seclusion.  Hope should be infused into every case, and, above all, there must be imported into its treatment the personality of the physician.  It was not the staff of Elisha that awakened the dead child, but death was quickened into life when the prophet threw himself upon its body and breathed into it of his own intense vitality.

In conclusion, the riper my experience the more firmly am I convinced that in the treatment of woman's diseases the possibility of a nerve-origin or of a nerve-complication should be the *fore*-thought and not the *hind*-thought of the physician.  I therefore have arrived at a very short gynæcological creed : I believe that the physician who recognizes the complexity of woman's nervous organization and appreciates its tyranny will touch her well-being at more points, and with a keener perception of its wants, than the one who holds the opinion that woman is woman because she has a womb.

# CHAPTER I.

## METHODS OF GYNÆCOLOGICAL EXAMINATION AND GENERAL OUTLINES OF DIFFERENTIAL DIAGNOSIS.

BY WILLIAM H. BAKER, M.D., AND FRANCIS H. DAVENPORT, M.D.

### VERBAL HISTORY.

WHEN a patient presents herself for advice and treatment, the first essential to a full understanding of her case is a complete history. This embraces more than a mere detail of her pelvic symptoms. It should, in the first place, include a brief reference to her general family history, the presence of any hereditary taint or constitutional tendency, and possibly the cause of death of her immediate female relatives. Then the patient's general condition of health during childhood up to puberty is a legitimate object of inquiry, the occurrence of any severe illnesses during that time being noted.

We now inquire into the phenomena connected with the menstrual life,— the time of the first appearance of the catamenia, its regularity or irregularity, and in what the irregularity, if such is present, consists; the length of time the flow lasts on an average, the number of napkins used, the occurrence of pain and its duration, and the presence of intermenstrual pain. It is of decided advantage to make these inquiries precise and minute, and many points of importance in the case will be elucidated by them.

The amount of the flow can be approximately estimated by knowing the number of napkins used, in how many thicknesses they are folded, how many are soaked through so that the stain appears on the outside, and whether, in addition to what is on the napkin, there are clots which pass during defecation or micturition; some inferences of value may be drawn from the color and odor of the discharge.

So, too, with regard to pain. The mere fact of its occurrence is not sufficient. Its real significance can be judged only by knowing the exact time of its appearance with reference to the flow, the duration and period of greatest intensity, its seat, and especially its character, its relation to the amount of the flow, and the occurrence of accompanying reflex symptoms, such as headache, nausea and vomiting, chills, diarrhœa, or frequency of micturition.

The same careful questioning should be employed in regard to leucor-

26

rhœa, its amount, character, odor, and irritating properties, whether it necessitates wearing a napkin or not, and at what part of the menstrual month it is most profuse.

Pain, as one of the most common and significant symptoms, should be very minutely inquired into. The time of its occurrence, its aggravation by exercise or at certain times of the day or the month, the seat of greatest intensity, its character, whether sharp or lancinating or a dull, heavy ache, whether steady or paroxysmal,—all these and many other facts are of importance. Even with the most minute inquiry, the variety of pains, combined with the inability of the average woman to describe them accurately, renders the whole subject very confusing. Much can be gained by a more systematic and thorough investigation of this important symptom.

The functions of the bladder and rectum should not be overlooked. Frequency of micturition, inability to hold the urine, or, on the other hand, to pass it, and pain before or during the act, or smarting and burning following it, are the most common bladder symptoms. Constipation is so exceedingly common with women that it is practically the rule. But, as it may arise from various causes, the practitioner who contents himself with noting its occurrence, without going further and asking as to its cause, makes a blunder. It may arise from a sluggish condition of the bowels, being a symptom accompanying indigestion. It may be caused by pressure of the retroverted uterus, or of exudates, or of enlarged tubes or ovaries, on the upper part of the rectum; or it may be the result of a ruptured or sundered perineum, being due to an inability to expel the contents of the full rectum.

If the patient has had children, the character of the labors, whether instrumental or not, should be noted, also any accidents during pregnancy or the puerperium.

Of equal, and in some cases of more, importance are the symptoms affecting other organs, and the nervous system generally. Too often these are neglected in favor of the more obvious local symptoms. But when it is remembered that it is a common experience to find serious local lesions and at the same time almost no symptoms primarily affecting the organ involved, but profound disturbances of the general nervous system, it is evident that we cannot with impunity neglect this important inquiry. Certain organs are very often functionally disturbed in a reflex way from pelvic disease, notably the alimentary canal, the heart, and the special nerve-centres. Flatulence, constipation, indigestion, nausea and vomiting, palpitation, and irregularities of the circulation, as shown by congestion of the head, coldness or numbness of the extremities, and neuralgiæ of various nerves, are all expressions of these functional disturbances which may be the result of some pelvic disorder.

An important line of inquiry relates to the amount of physical exercise which the patient can take, what special forms of mental exertion tire her, and whether her disposition is affected.

It will be readily understood that it is not necessary in every case to go so fully into the patient's general history as the foregoing implies; but it may be necessary, and in a large proportion of cases it is wise to question thus closely.

The first interview between the patient and the physician is an important one, and it is a very good rule of practice to allow the patient time and opportunity to state her case fully. Not only *what* she says, but also the manner in which she says it, will give the physician an insight into her disposition and character which will enable him to treat her more intelligently and successfully. Then, too, it will be a great satisfaction to the patient to have had the opportunity to say all that she wished to the doctor.

A printed form for case-taking, while not essential, is yet an aid. It both saves time and suggests objects of inquiry which might be overlooked, and is of great advantage for the subsequent study of one's cases. It may be simple or complex. Possibly it is a good thing to have two sets, one for routine cases and one for cases of greater interest.

FORM I.

| Examined. | Name, Residence, and Nativity. | Age. | Social Condition. | Children. | Abortions. | Duration of Illness. |
|---|---|---|---|---|---|---|
|  |  |  |  |  |  |  |
| History and Symptoms. |  |  |  |  |  |  |
| Diagnosis. |  |  |  |  |  |  |
| Treatment. |  |  |  |  |  |  |

FORM II.

*NAME* . . . . . . . . . . . . . . . . . . . . . . . . *Reg. No.* . . . . . . . . .

**MENSTRUATION** *began at* . . . . . . . . *Always regular after* . . . . *until* . . .

| CATAMENIA FORM NOW | CHARACTER | COLOR | FETOR | DUR. OF FLUX | INTERVAL | PAIN |  |
|---|---|---|---|---|---|---|---|
| Prof. Nor. Scanty. | Clots. Nor. | ——— | ——— | . . Days | . . Days | | Bef. dur. after. |
| Prof. Nor. Scanty. | Clots. Nor. | ——— | ——— | . . Days | . . Days | | Bef. dur. after. |

*REMARKS:* . . . . . . . . . . . . . . . . . . . . . . . . . . . . . . . . . . . .
*Last menstruation* . . . . . . . . . *days* . . . . . . . . . . *mos.* . . . . . . . *years ago.*
**LEUCORRHŒA** *began* . . . . . . . *days, months, years ago. Whitish, yellowish, greenish, watery, fetid, odorless, acrid. No.* . . . . . . . . . . . *Napkins used daily. Most severe before, after menstruation.*

**PAIN** *began . . . . . . days, months, years ago, in supra-pubic, right, left, groin, lumbar, sacral region. CHARACTER: Feeling of weight, weakness, forward pressure, dragging, aching, bearing down, expulsion, and is constant, paroxysmal, with exacerbations, radiating to back, front, down right, left thigh. Has not increased steadily up to present time. Is not increased, diminished, during menstruation, defecation, micturition, coition, motion, sitting.*

**MARRIED** *. . . . . months, years. Number of children . . . . . First, . . . . . months, years ago. Last, . . . . months, years ago. Number now living . . . . . Number of miscarriages . . . . First, . . . months, years ago. Last, . . . months, years ago. Last one . . . . . months, years ago. Period of utero-gestation: 1st, . . . . ; 2d, . . . . ; 3d, . . . . Last labor natural, tedious, rapid, instrumental. In labor . . . . . hours.*

**URINE.** *Amount increased, normal, diminished. Color: light, dark, clear, turbid sediment. Micturition not frequent and with no pain. Bearing down, constant, paroxysmal, scalding, lancinating.*
    *EXAMINATION: Color, . . . . . ; Reaction, . . . . . ; Sp. Gr., . . . . . ; No Albumin . . . Microscope . . . . . . . . . . . . . . . . . . . . . . . . . . . . . .*

*DIGESTIVE SYSTEM:* . . . . . . . . . . . . . . . . . . . . . . . . . .
*CIRCULATORY* " . . . . . . . . . . . . . . . . . . . . . . . .
*RESPIRATORY* " . . . . . . . . . . . . . . . . . . . . . . . .
*NERVOUS* " . . . . . . . . . . . . . . . . . . . . . . . .
*URINARY* " . . . . . . . . . . . . . . . . . . . . . . . .

**FAMILY HISTORY:**

**PREVIOUS HISTORY:**

**PRESENT ILLNESS:**

**PHYSICAL EXAMINATION:**
    *GENERAL APPEARANCE: . . . . . . . . . . . . . . . . . . . . . . . .*
    *HEART: . . . . . . . . . . . . . . LUNGS: . . . . . . . . . . . . .*
    *ABDOMEN: . . . . . . . . . . . . . . . . . . . . . . . . . . . . . .*
    *VULVA: . . . . . . . . . . . . . . . . . . . . . . . . . . . . . . .*
    *PERINEUM: . . . . . . . . . . . . . . . . . . . . . . . . . . . . . .*
    *VAGINA: . . . . . . . . . . . . . . . . . . . . . . . . . . . . . .*
    *VAGINAL VAULT: . . . . . . . . . . . . . . . . . . . . . . . . . .*
    *DOUGLAS'S POUCH: . . . . . . . . . . . . . . . . . . . . . . . . .*

**UTERUS.** *SIZE: . . . . . . . . . . . . . SHAPE: . . . . . . . . . . . . . .*
    *CONSISTENCY: . . . . . . . . very, slight, not, sensitive . . . . . . . . . . . .*
    *POSITION: . . . . . Mobility, normal, slight, absent . . . . . . . . . . . .*
    *CERVIX . . . . . . . . . . . . . . . . . . . . . . . . . . . . . . .*

**PELVIC PERITONEUM AND CELLULAR TISSUE:**
    *FALLOPIAN TUBES: . . . . . . . . . . . . . . . . . . . . . . . . . .*
    *OVARIES: . . . . . . . . . . . . . . . . . . . . . . . . . . . . . .*
    *BROAD LIGAMENTS: . . . . . . . . . . . . . . . . . . . . . . . . .*
    *BLADDER: . . . . . . . . . . . . . . . . . . . . . . . . . . . . . .*
    *ANUS: . . . . . . . . . . . . . . . . . . . . . . . . . . . . . . .*
    *RECTUM: . . . . . . . . . . . . . . . . . . . . . . . . . . . . . .*
    *DIAGNOSIS: . . . . . . . . . . . . . . . . . . . . . . . . . . . . .*

FORM III.

DATE.                                                    No.

| | Age. | Nativity. | Single—Married—Widow. | Occupation. |
|---|---|---|---|---|
| | | | | |

PRESENT COMPLAINTS AND THEIR DURATION.

1. *History:*
   Family History
   Previous Diseases

MENSTRUATION.
{ First appearance
  Regularity
  Duration
  Amount and character
  Pain, before, during,
     or after
  Confined to bed
  Last appearance

PAIN.
{ In head
  In back
  In abdomen
  In legs
  During coitus
  In sitting
  In standing
  In walking

Date.      Pregnancy      Labor.      Puerperium.

VAGINAL LABORS.
{ At full term

  Premature

DISCHARGE.
{ Amount
  Character
  Persistence
  Duration

  Urination

  Defecation

Appetite                     Digestion
Cause of illness (supposed by patient)

2. *Status Præsens:*
   General Condition
   Condition of the Nervous System
   Constitution
   Breasts

   Abdomen

   Vulva
   Perineum
   Vagina
   Broad Ligaments
   Tubes
   Ovaries
   Douglas's Pouch
   Bladder
   Urethra
   Rectum
   Complications

UTERUS.
{ Position
  Size
  Mobility
  Shape
  Depth of Cavity
  Secretion

CERVIX.
{ Position
  Shape
  Length
  Density
  Secretion
  Internal Os
  External Os
  Lacerated

3. *Diagnosis:*

4. *Treatment and Progress:*

Form I. represents one which has been found of practical use, especially for out-patient work or routine cases in office practice.

FIG. 1.

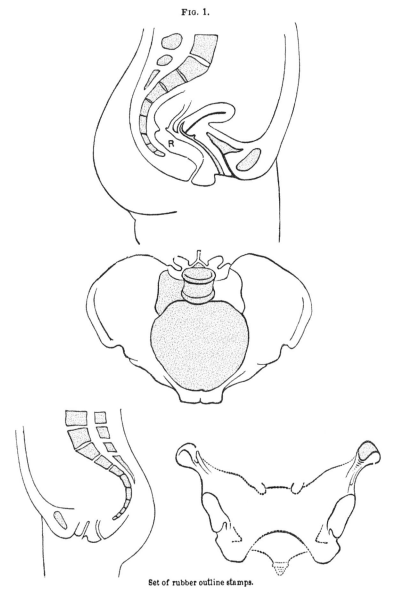

Set of rubber outline stamps.

Forms II. and III. are more elaborate, and enable the busy practitioner with a minimum expenditure of time to get a large number of important facts in a convenient form for reference. A useful adjunct to the case-book is a set of rubber outline stamps of the pelvis in various sections (Fig. 1), in which a sketch of a tumor or a displacement can be drawn, thus serving as an aid to the memory and a standard of comparison if changes in the condition occur.

In the majority of cases no correct inferences as to the nature of the trouble can be deduced from the verbal statements of the patient. The disorders of menstruation, leucorrhœa, pains of various kinds and degree, and general nervous disturbances are common to so many pelvic disorders that any differential diagnosis based on them alone is impossible.

## PHYSICAL EXAMINATION.

A physical examination is, therefore, essential in a large proportion of cases. The only general exception to this rule is in the case of young girls. It is most often for irregularities of menstruation or for leucorrhœa that young unmarried women consult the gynæcologist, and it is in such affections, which are very frequently dependent upon the general health, that hygienic measures and drugs will accomplish a great deal and local treatment may be entirely omitted. In fact, only when such measures have been faithfully tried and found ineffectual, or when there is clear evidence that there is such pelvic trouble that other treatment will not reach it, is an examination justifiable, and even then it may be best to examine by the rectum or under ether, as will be described later.

In all other cases which come to the physician with any suspicion of local disease the bimanual examination, so called, should be made; and a word of warning is in place here as to the neglect of it. If the specialist sometimes lays himself open to the charge of making unnecessary examinations, the general practitioner is certainly often wilfully culpable in the other direction. When it is remembered that by far the larger proportion of distinctly gynæcological cases come first to the family physician, it will be seen what a grave responsibility rests upon him. Two causes operate to the prejudice of the patient: first, the too frequent tendency either to delay or to dispense altogether with the vaginal examination; and, second, the lack of knowledge as to the proper methods of making such an examination. The sad results of the neglect to examine are nowhere more forcibly shown than in cases of beginning cancer in women at the menopause, where the favorable time for operation is lost through the unwillingness of the practitioner to see in the irregular hemorrhages anything more than a symptom of the "change of life." Better make ten unnecessary examinations than neglect one and lose a patient.

## VARIOUS POSITIONS FOR EXAMINATION.

There are five positions in which a woman may be placed for purposes of examination or treatment. They are: 1, the dorsal; 2, Sims's, or the semi-prone; 3, the erect; 4, the knee-chest; and 5, Trendelenburg's.

The dorsal position, as its name implies, is the one in which the woman lies upon her back with the knees drawn up and separated, and the heels placed upon the edge of the table, or on stirrups. It is the position in which the abdomen is palpated, the visual inspection of the vulva is made, and the bimanual examination of the pelvic organs is practised.

## BIMANUAL EXAMINATION.

This method of examination is the key-stone of all gynæcological work, and its correct performance is so essential that it will be described in considerable detail. First, as to the preparation of the patient. She should be instructed to have all the clothing loose. If seen at home, she should be clothed in a loose wrapper without corsets; if at the office, all tight and constricting bands should be loosened. It is not enough for her merely to loosen the buttons of the dress-waist; the lower fastenings of the corsets, and the skirt and other bands, should be so far undone that the clothing would slip off if not held up. Anything short of this will often materially interfere with a satisfactory examination, especially when we examine in the semi-prone or Sims's position. The effect of a single constricting band is, as will be readily seen, first, to crowd the contents of the lower half of the abdomen downward, thus displacing the uterus somewhat and preventing the hand that is making pressure over the abdomen from sinking down into the pelvis; and, second, to nullify wholly or in part the effect of Sims's position. The essential feature of the latter is the admission of air into the vagina, and, unless the abdominal walls are absolutely free to fall forward, this can occur to only a limited extent. Any one who has attempted to obtain a view of the cervix or to pack the vagina when the clothing is not loose, and has then observed the change when the tight bands were all removed, will appreciate the importance of this detail, and realize why it is so strongly insisted upon.

If possible, the bowels and the bladder should be emptied shortly before the examination; in fact, a full rectum may so encroach upon the vagina as to render the bimanual examination exceedingly unsatisfactory.

It is best, if possible, to use a table for this examination. It has the advantage of being of a convenient height, so that the surgeon may examine without stooping, and affords a firm, hard surface, into which the patient does not sink as into a bed or lounge. The special form of table is of no particular consequence. It may be simple or elaborate to suit the physician's taste. If the practitioner is in general practice, or does general surgery, one of the numerous adjustable chairs which admit of the patient's being arranged in several different positions will be found useful. Various adjuncts to the table, such as a movable top for raising the patient's buttocks so as to exaggerate Sims's position, or stirrups for the feet, while possibly convenient, are not essential. (Fig. 2.)

The table should be about four feet long, two feet wide, and two and one-half feet high, an inch or two lower at the end where the patient's head

3

will lie than at the other, and fitted with easy-rolling casters, so that its position with reference to the light may be readily changed. It should be covered with a thin mattress or folded quilt, so as to be comfortable for the patient, and over all a sheet should be thrown. Patients rarely object to being placed upon a table so arranged.

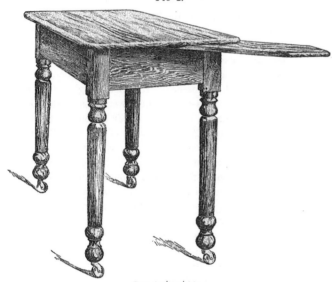

Examination-table.

When the patient is ready, she should be instructed to stand upon a chair or stool placed in front of the table, and, raising the clothing behind, to sit upon its edge. She should then lie down with the head on the pillow and the heels separated perhaps a foot and a half and resting on the edge of the table or supported by stirrups. The lower part of the body is then covered over with a sheet, and the clothing is pushed up above the knees. This enables the patient to spread the knees easily apart, which facilitates the examination. The hips should be brought down as near the edge of the table as is possible and at the same time leave room for the heels without slipping.

The hands of the physician require some attention. They should be scrupulously clean, especial care being bestowed upon the finger-nails. These should be cut short and rounded, both for the sake of cleanliness and to avoid hurting the patient. The hands should also be warm. Some lubricant is necessary, but the particular form may be left to the taste and judgment of the doctor. The most cleanly is soap, as it and any secretions which may cling to the finger may be most easily washed off after the examination, and the hands left in a perfectly clean condition for a second patient. The only objection to soap is that it is occasionally irritating to a very sensitive mucous membrane. Vaseline, carbolated or plain, or any smooth ointment, may be used. Simple ointment perfumed with oil of bergamot has been found very satisfactory.

The patient and the physician are now prepared for the bimanual examination. The patient lies in the dorsal position, with the knees drawn up and abducted, and the physician stands directly in front of her. The bimanual examination, as its name implies, is the method of exploring the contents of the pelvis with one or more fingers of one hand in the vagina and the other hand making counter-pressure over the abdomen. The object is to find out what lies between, and to note the size, shape, and condition of the various organs and structures. How this examination can be made with the patient lying on the side, as has been recommended in English text-books, it is difficult to see. Certainly no such thorough exploration can be made as with the patient on the back.

*Digital Examination of the Vagina.*—As the most important factor in the bimanual examination is the education of the touch, the same hand should always be used, except for special reasons. The left forefinger has been the one usually preferred, and for this choice there are one or two good reasons. If one is engaged in obstetrical work, the importance of keeping the right forefinger, which is the one usually used for vaginal examinations, surgically clean will be recognized at once, hence the left should be reserved for gynæcological work. This reason is less potent in these days of elaborate antiseptics in midwifery, but it still has weight. The strongest reason in favor of the left index finger is that it leaves the right hand free for the use of instruments. It not infrequently happens that it is necessary to perform some minor manipulation or even a serious operative procedure by the aid of touch alone. If the sense of touch of the left forefinger is acute, it will be of the greatest assistance in accurately determining the various structures, while the right hand remains free for the use of the necessary instruments. A score of applications of this principle will occur to every operator.

The left index finger, then, should be the one chosen for the vaginal examination. Having been well lubricated, it should be passed in under the sheet until it enters the vulva. It is rarely necessary at this stage of the examination to raise the sheet in order to introduce the finger, for, if the patient is lying as she should, the entrance to the vagina will be in the median line a short distance above the level of the table. The patient will feel grateful for any consideration of her feelings which the physician may show her. It is well to remember that the entrance to the vulva in most women (very stout women are an exception) is very near the table as they lie on the back. It is a good rule, therefore, to point the finger downward, so as to strike the cleft between the buttocks below the level of the introitus, thus avoiding the sensitive clitoris and meatus urinarius. The vagina, too, is more easily entered over the perineum, and there is not the danger of pushing the hair which sometimes grows luxuriantly around the vulva before the finger into the vagina. All these points, though seemingly insignificant, will be found to be of practical value, especially in the examination of nervous women.

Every little detail which will lessen the nervous strain which is inseparably connected with this trying ordeal will be very gratefully appreciated by the patient, and will repay the physician amply for the pains taken. Quietness of manner and movement, the avoidance of rough manipulation, thoroughness of examination combined with quickness in diagnosis of existing conditions, and a regard for the patient's feelings of modesty, are all points which well merit attention and study.

The finger is passed over the perineum slowly and carefully into the vagina. A little rotary motion will aid in its passage if the vagina is narrow or dry; and if there is a spasmodic contraction of the constrictor vaginæ muscle, which may sometimes cause considerable difficulty to the entrance of the finger, turning the palmar surface of the finger downward and making firm pressure on the perineal body will so inhibit the action of the constricting muscle that the finger will easily pass in.

The position in which the other fingers of the hand are held is important. Most text-books on gynæcology describe and figure the remaining fingers as folded upon the palm, but a very little consideration will show that this arrangement is not the best. The broad surface of the folded fingers is opposed to the perineum and the projecting folds of the buttocks, and it is impossible that the forefinger should reach as high in the vagina as it ought. If, however, the fingers are extended downward along the cleft of the nates, over the anus, then only the web between the index and middle fingers is opposed to the perineum, and the finger can be pushed up to its fullest extent. (Fig. 3.)

In this way considerable is gained in the length of the examining finger. At first thought it might seem as if with this arrangement the side of the forefinger would be opposed to the cervix, and the part of the pelvis reached by its sensitive tip be limited to the left side. But, using the buttock as a point of resistance, the finger can be so rotated that its palmar surface

FIG. 3.

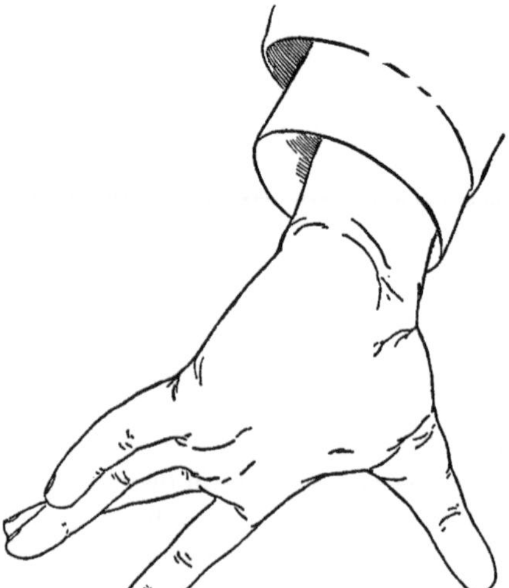

Position of examining hand.

will be directed upward and the whole vaginal vault can be reached and palpated, even the right side, though naturally less perfectly than the left. By reversing the hands, as will be spoken of later, the examination can be made thorough.   Practice will so increase the flexibility of the index finger at the metacarpo-phalangeal joint that this method will become more and more easy.

Certain facts can be ascertained by the examining finger alone.   The condition of the perineum can be told in a general way, though its exact status can be determined only by visual inspection.   The shape and length of the vagina and the condition of its walls can be approximately made out and valuable inferences drawn.   Unusual dryness or heat of the vagina, excessive development or absence of the rugæ, and the presence of swellings or cicatrices, may be quickly noted.

Fig. 4.

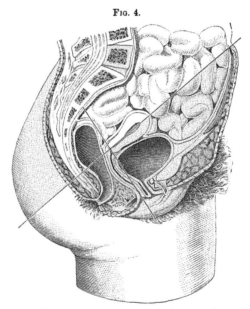

Relation of axis of normal uterus to that of the vagina.

*Palpation of the Cervix.*—At the upper end of the vagina, projecting to a greater or less extent into its lumen, is felt the cervix uteri.   Its normal shape is conical, with an opening at its extremity.   It is easily distinguished from the surrounding vaginal walls by its greater hardness.   It may vary within normal limits in length and shape and in the size of the os uteri. It may also be very markedly changed by parturition and by disease, so as to present a variety of forms.   It softens as a result of pregnancy, so that in the later stages it can hardly be distinguished from the walls of the vagina; to a less degree as the result of profuse hemorrhages.   It grows hard from cicatricial contraction following lacerations at labor and as a result of chronic inflammatory processes.

*Normal Position of the Cervix.*—The normal position of the cervix is with its long axis about at right angles to the long axis of the vagina. (Fig. 4.) This is shown to be the case by the fact that when the finger is introduced into the vagina and is pushed well up into the posterior cul-de-sac, the os uteri comes opposite the ball of the finger. (Fig. 5.) If the cervix has a faulty position, either because the whole organ is tipped over backward or the cervix is bent forward, the neck will come to lie in the axis of the vagina, and the os will impinge upon the tip of the index finger. (Fig. 6.)

FIG. 5.

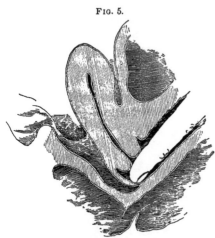

Examining finger with cervix in normal position.

*Condition of the Os Uteri.*—Certain facts with regard to the os can also be found out by the examining finger. Its size varies greatly, the os being rendered patulous as a result of parturition, by endocervicitis, or endometritis, or the presence of polypi. It may have been torn during labor,

FIG. 6.

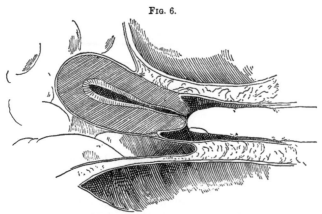

Examining finger with cervix in abnormal position.

so that the anterior and posterior lips are separated by a deep sulcus, and still further deformed by hypertrophy and eversion, or it may be divided into several irregular nodules by a stellate laceration. The mucous membrane immediately around the os, which is normally smooth, may be eroded, and may present a roughened surface to the examining finger, or it may be studded with little shot-like bodies, the so-called ovula Nabothi.

*Palpation of the Cul-de-Sac.*—The depressions around the cervix, where the vagina is reflected over on to the cervix, are called respectively the anterior, posterior, and lateral cul-de-sacs. The finger can be passed much farther behind the uterus than in front or at either side. Posteriorly the finger meets with no resistance, unless the body of the uterus or one of the appendages is displaced backward, or there is a tumor or other swelling present. Usually there is only the soft, yielding rectum, the loose connective tissue, and the peritoneal folds in Douglas's cul-de-sac. On deep pressure, especially if they are in a state of tension, the utero-sacral ligaments may be made out. Anteriorly the vaginal cul-de-sac is much shallower and the attachment of the bladder to the uterus more intimate, so that the finger cannot make much impression. So, too, at the sides; the broad ligaments come down so far on the body of the uterus that they present an effectual hinderance to any very deep pressure.

The most that the unaided finger can do in palpating the surroundings of the uterus is sometimes to recognize the resistance caused by the body of the uterus, either in front or behind, to note an increased area of its lower segment when enlarged, to feel the lower contours of swellings at either side or behind the uterus, to determine their points of greatest sensitiveness, the smoothness or roughness of their outline, their density or elasticity, to get a little idea as to their size, and to note the presence of pulsating vessels.

These are the more obvious things which the finger can find out alone, and, as will be readily seen, it practically amounts to a palpation of merely the vagina and the lowest border of the pelvic organs. For any satisfactory or proper knowledge of the condition of the pelvic viscera in their completeness, the assistance of the other hand is essential.

*Bimanual Examination—Use of the Hand on the Abdomen.*—As soon as the forefinger of the left hand is inserted into the vagina, the right hand should be carried under the sheet and clothing and placed upon the abdomen over the pubes. The object to be sought is to ascertain the condition of the organs which occupy the pelvis and in certain pathological states encroach upon the lower abdomen. To this end the right hand depresses the abdominal walls downward towards the inlet of the pelvis, and the examiner by making counter-pressure with the finger in the vagina seeks to determine the presence and size of any solid bodies which may be between them.

*Bimanual Palpation of the Uterus.*—The first point to be ascertained is the position of the uterus. The direction in which the cervix points, as determined by the finger in the vagina, will give us a clue, but, as will be seen in the chapter on displacements, it may be a misleading one, unless controlled by the information furnished by the external hand. Thus, if the cervix is found pointing in the axis of the vagina, it may mean anteflexion of the cervix or retroversion of the whole organ, two entirely different conditions. Which is present can often be determined only by the bimanual examination.

To ascertain the position of the uterus, the left forefinger is placed underneath the cervix, its tip being in the posterior cul-de-sac. The cervix is then gently tilted upward and at the same time the abdomen is depressed. If the conditions are favorable and the uterus is in its normal position, the examiner will be conscious of a solid body between the two. The fundus is usually not to be appreciated as a distinct rounded mass, but merely as an indefinite resistant body whose outlines are far from clearly made out.

FIG. 7.

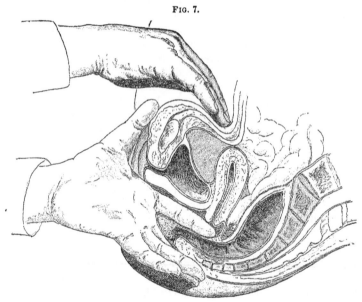

Bimanual examination.

Often even this feeling is wanting, and the presence of the uterine body in its normal place is shown by the fact that on pressure the cervix impinges on the finger, and every impulse given to the body above is directly transmitted to the cervix.

If the body of the uterus is not found in its normal position, it should be sought for either in front of or behind the cervix. If found in front, with the finger in the anterior cul-de-sac, as if it were palpating the bladder, it is anteverted, and can be felt by the hand outside if pressure is made lower down over the pubes.

If retroversion is present, the body cannot usually be felt bimanually, but is recognized by the examining finger as a resistant mass in the posterior cul-de-sac.

The relation of the body to the cervix, or the existence of a flexion, is made evident by the presence of a bend at the junction of the cervix and the body.

The second point to be determined is the size of the uterus. A slight increase in the size of the body, as is found, for example, in areolar hyperplasia, is not usually very definitely made out. When the uterus is enlarged from pregnancy or the presence of tumors, the resistant area of the lower segment of the uterus is larger, and the finger may notice this more or less clearly all around the cervix. To feel the enlarged fundus, the right hand should palpate a larger segment of the surface of the abdomen. This suggests a difficulty which often meets the beginner, where on the abdomen to make counter-pressure. That depends, of course, upon the size of the uterus. When of normal size, a point between the umbilicus and the pubes just above the margin of the growth of the pubic hair would in a large proportion of cases be the best; but if the finger in the vagina detects signs of enlargement, the hand should be carried higher and swept around to the sides, and instead of the tips of the fingers the whole palmar surface should be used. In this way the large rounded outline of the uterus may be readily detected.

*Bimanual Examination of the Appendages.*—It is often a difficult matter to palpate the normal tubes and ovaries. Success presupposes lax abdominal walls and a distensible vagina, and a delicate touch. Unless they are enlarged by disease, the finger in the vagina alone cannot appreciate these organs. They are so small and movable that, unless steadied by the hand on the outside, they recede before the finger and offer no resistance. When felt, the tubes are two cord-like bodies which run towards either side of the pelvis from the upper angles of the uterus. As they lie in the upper part of the broad ligaments, they are often difficult to reach. They can be felt to slip under the finger and to dip somewhat downward and backward as they are palpated farther from the uterus.

The ovaries are small oval bodies which lie below the tubes, behind the broad ligaments, and back of the plane of the uterus. To palpate them the finger must be carried towards the side of the pelvis and the lateral cul-de-sac pushed as far before the finger as possible. The outside hand makes counter-pressure so as to meet as nearly as possible the tip of the finger in the vagina, and then both finger and hand are together drawn downward and towards the median line and the structures are carefully palpated as they pass between them.

The ovary is recognized as a small, elastic, movable body, about the size of a pecan-nut, which slips from between the fingers. When enlarged or prolapsed, it is lower and nearer the uterus, and is more easily felt. A method of examining the ovary through the rectum will be spoken of later.

*Use of the Right Forefinger.*—While the left forefinger is the one which it is wise to make use of in the majority of cases for the vaginal examination, yet in certain cases the right should be used. It will readily be seen that the left side of the pelvis can be thoroughly explored only with the left forefinger.  The same is true of the right side.  When, therefore, our first examination shows some obscure trouble with the right side, the right forefinger should be used in the vagina and the left hand on the abdomen.  The better trained both hands are, the better equipped will the physician be for the diagnosis of obscure pelvic disease.

*Use of Two Fingers in the Vagina.*—Where there is any doubt about the diagnosis, especially where there is a question of the relation of growths and swellings to the uterus or its appendages, it is often of advantage to use two fingers.  There is no objection to this in most married women, especially if they have borne children.  But where the entrance to the vagina is small, the introduction of two fingers is usually too painful to be attempted without ether.  Two fingers will be found particularly useful in the bimanual reposition of a retroverted or flexed uterus.

*Bimanual Examination of Virgins.*—It is a question of great importance to the practitioner, under what circumstances he should make a physical examination in the case of young girls.  There is no doubt that there has been, and is at the present time, altogether too little regard paid to the feelings of young unmarried women.  On very slight pretext, perhaps merely some menstrual irregularity, a vaginal exploration has been made and local treatment carried out, where general treatment and attention to hygiene would have accomplished the same result.

A good rule is, if there is any doubt as to the wisdom of examining, to give the patient the benefit of the doubt.  Examine only when either the present symptoms are of such a character that some serious trouble not amenable to general measures is almost a certainty, or after a fair trial of other means of treatment has shown their futility.

In certain cases of amenorrhœa, where girls have passed well beyond the age when this function is usually established, and especially if there have been menstrual molimina, it is important to satisfy one's self as to the existence of atresia hymenalis.  In such cases it is not necessary to introduce the finger through the opening in the hymen, as the tip of the sound will demonstrate the presence or absence of atresia without causing the patient any pain or rupturing the hymen.

In other cases where an examination is imperative, it is often possible to avoid rupturing the hymen by examining by the rectum.  This will be spoken of more in detail later.  Not infrequently in the case of virgins it is best to give ether.  This gives perfect relaxation and permits of a thorough examination without pain.

*Difficulties of the Bimanual Examination.*—It may be well to speak here of certain difficulties which attend the bimanual examination in some cases, and how, if possible, to overcome them.

One is rigidity of the abdominal muscles.  This may be from extreme sensitiveness, the result of disease of the pelvic organs,—a sensitiveness which is not confined to the lower abdomen, immediately over the affected parts, but may extend over the whole abdomen. The fear of pressure starting pain, which it is certain to do in these cases, causes the patient to render her abdominal muscles perfectly rigid. In such cases the only remedy is to obtain perfect relaxation by means of ether.

In other cases this rigidity is not from pain, but from a nervous dread of it. This is most often found in unmarried women of a nervous temperament. They involuntarily contract their abdominal muscles, and are apparently unable by the exercise of their will-power to relax them. In such cases there are one or two simple expedients which may be tried. It is well to divert the patient's attention as far as possible from what you are doing by asking her questions about herself and her symptoms. This, combined with a quiet manner, will do much to relieve the tension of mind and body from which such patients suffer. Tell them to breathe with the mouth open and quietly and deeply. Where a single fact is to be ascertained, as, for example, the position of the uterus, one opportunity of depressing the abdominal walls is all that may be necessary. This may sometimes be obtained by asking the patient to take a deep inspiration and then to let the breath out completely. At the moment when the abdominal walls sink as the diaphragm rises, the hand may follow and depress them sufficiently to gain the desired information.

In fat women the bimanual examination is often very unsatisfactory. In addition to the thickness of the abdominal walls, which prevents satisfactory palpation with the external hand, the examining finger finds difficulty in reaching the pelvic organs, owing to the fat about the thighs and nates. In such cases, for information about the uterus we must resort to the sound, and for the more obscure pelvic disorders anæsthesia is essential.

### VISUAL INSPECTION OF THE EXTERNAL GENITALS.

In hospital and dispensary practice, the class of women who come for examination are liable to have some disease of the external genitals, either venereal in character or the result of want of cleanliness. A visual inspection of the external genitals is therefore a wise precaution, and it is well to make this the first step in the examination. With private patients to whom the whole procedure is a shock, it is well to make the bimanual examination first; then, before the patient changes to the semi-prone position, to look at the vulva. There are a great many facts which can be ascertained by this inspection. In the first place, any abnormalities of structure, such as atresia of the hymen or variation from its normal form, hypertrophy of the clitoris or labia, swelling of the vulvo-vaginal gland of one or both sides, the presence of papillary growths, of venereal ulcers or eruptions, may be immediately noted. The cause of obstinate pruritus may be recognized from the discovery of pediculi pubis. Painful micturition may call attention to the meatus urinarius and a caruncle may be found.

The most important, because the most necessary, information which can be gained by the visual examination is that regarding the condition of

the perineal body and the vaginal outlet generally. A fairly correct idea
as to whether it is intact or not may be gained by the examining finger, but
the extent and character of the tear, if such is present, can be told only by
the sight. If the external perineum is torn down to or involving the sphincter ani, that becomes apparent at once on exposing the vulva. The vaginal
outlet gapes, and there is usually a prolapse of the anterior vaginal wall.
This is, however, by no means the most frequent tear ; more often the lateral
attachments are torn away on one or both sides, while the external perineum
is practically intact. Such a lesion is liable to be overlooked. It is recognized by passing the finger within the vulva and pressing the lower part
of the vagina downward and outward. If the attachments of the levator
ani muscle on one or both sides have been torn away, the finger lies in a
sulcus, and the vulva can be stretched widely open so as to expose at least
a third or a half of the vagina. In many cases where with the parts at
rest there may be no evidence of prolapse of the vaginal walls, if the
patient is asked to strain there will be a very evident protrusion, especially
of the bladder-wall.

In this visual inspection of the parts the condition of the anus should
not be neglected, as various diseases of the rectum and anus are frequent
causes of complaint referred to the pelvic organs, or are associated with
other symptoms of pelvic disease.

### EXAMINATION IN THE SEMI-PRONE POSITION.

The semi-prone or Sims position, as it is called, is the position which
the patient assumes in order that Sims's speculum may be used. This
speculum, which is also called the duck-bill speculum, is merely a perineal
retractor. Its principle is to draw back the perineal body so that air shall
enter the vagina, and in order that this may occur the patient must be in a
suitable position.

She must be on her left side, with the left arm thrown out behind her,
the chest nearly flat upon the table, and the right hand and arm hanging
over its edge. The hips should be near the lower left-hand corner of the
table, the body diagonally across it, so that the right shoulder is near its
right-hand edge, the thighs flexed upon the body, and the right knee drawn
up more than the left, but lying close to it. For comfort, there should be
a foot-rest extending out from the table at an angle of forty-five degrees
with the lower edge. (Fig. 8.)

In this position even more than in the dorsal it is imperative that the
clothing should be loose. In order that air should enter the vagina, the
abdominal viscera should have a chance to recede towards the diaphragm,
and a single tight band will prevent this.

In this position, with Sims's speculum the walls of the vagina may be
examined, the condition of the cervix noted, and any instrumentation of
the uterus may be proceeded with. All forms of treatment can also be
carried out in this position.

FIG 8.

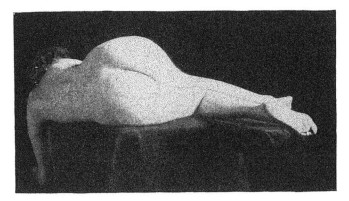

Sims position.  (Potter.)

FIG. 9.

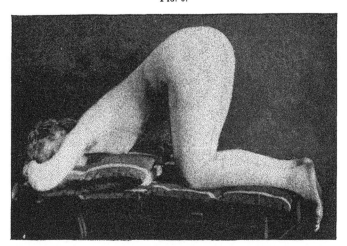

Knee-chest position.  (Potter.)

### EXAMINATION IN THE ERECT POSTURE.

This is occasionally necessary; fortunately, not often, as it is naturally an unpleasant position for the woman. It is of value in determining the degree of prolapse in its slighter forms. These slight variations from the normal are not appreciable when the patient is examined in the dorsal position, even if she is told to bear down; but if she stands, the degree to which the cervix approaches the vulva can be easily measured with the finger. The patient should be directed to stand erect, either with the feet slightly apart or with one foot placed upon a low stool or the round of a chair. A sheet is placed around her, reaching to the floor. The physician, kneeling on one knee, passes one hand beneath the clothing and inserts the forefinger into the vagina. If the patient is then requested to strain down, the degree of prolapse, if any be present, can be readily noted.

### THE KNEE-CHEST POSITION.

This position is of more value in treatment than in diagnosis, but even for treatment it is of very limited application. Almost its sole use is in bringing the aid of gravity to the reposition of a backward displaced uterus. In this position the abdominal viscera fall forward towards the diaphragm, and if the perineum is retracted upward the vagina fills with air and the uterus is carried upward in the pelvis. It does not, however, tend to become anteverted spontaneously, as many have supposed, and as the figures in many text-books would lead us to imagine, but puts the parts in the most favorable condition to effect reposition by manual or instrumental means. To insure the desired result, the knee-chest position must be correctly assumed, as shown in Fig. 9.

The patient kneels upon the table, the thighs are kept perpendicular, and the back slopes down evenly. The arms are spread out so as to allow the upper part of the chest to lie flat upon the table, and the head rests upon one cheek. The errors which most frequently occur in assuming this position are that the thighs are not held perpendicularly, and the back is hunched up. The back should rather sway downward, so as to be somewhat concave, a position which relaxes the abdominal muscles.

### THE TRENDELENBURG POSITION.

There is one other position which in recent years has grown in favor as a position for operating,—viz., the Trendelenburg. In this position the knees are raised high above the head, so that the body slants upward from the shoulders. (Fig. 10.)

This allows the abdominal viscera to gravitate towards the diaphragm, and in operations on the pelvic viscera through an abdominal incision enables the surgeon to see the field of operation and thus to control his work.

It is rapidly becoming popular in all abdominal operations, and tables specially constructed are now considered essential in all well-appointed operating-rooms.

Where it can be secured, there should be a slight bending of the thighs

FIG. 10.

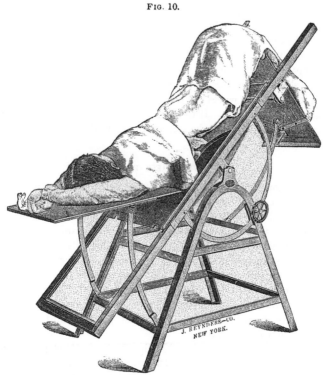

Patient in Trendelenburg position, on Cleveland's table.

upon the abdomen, thus slightly relaxing the abdominal muscles. (*Vide* also Figs. 19, 20, and 21, Chapter XI.)

### EXAMINATION WITH THE SPECULUM.

A speculum is an instrument by the aid of which we are enabled to look into the vagina and to treat various pathological conditions which we find. There is an infinite variety of specula, which act on different principles and have various degrees of merit.

As the first use to which a speculum would be put would naturally be to enable the physician to see the upper end of the vagina, and especially the cervix uteri which projects into it, a simple tube would suggest itself as the best means. Hence one of the oldest forms of the speculum is the cylindrical. (Fig. 11.) Cylindrical specula were made of various substances,—hard rubber, glass, or metal,—and served their original purpose well enough.

When, however, the various conditions, not only of the vagina and vaginal surface of the cervix, but of the canal of the uterus itself, began to be treated, this form of speculum was found wanting. Its introduction was painful, it gave a very limited view, and it was too narrow at the lower end to admit of any satisfactory manipulation of instruments. It has, therefore, fallen almost entirely into disuse.

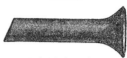

FIG. 11.

Cylindrical speculum.

The cylindrical speculum is used with the patient on the back. The clothing should be loose and the knees spread well apart. As, owing to the close attachment of the vagina to the pubic arch, there can be very little distention upward, all enlargement of the entrance to the vagina must be by stretching the vagina laterally and depressing the perineal body. It is important to remember this, as otherwise great pain may be caused by drawing upon the meatus urinarius or pinching the soft parts against the rami of the pubic arch. It is also important to remember that at first the direction of the vagina is downward towards the hollow of the sacrum, and that the speculum must be inserted accordingly.

The labia majora are separated with the fingers of one hand, and the bevelled point of the well-oiled speculum is gently inserted into the vaginal entrance, depressing steadily the perineal body, and is gradually passed in with a rotating motion. It is then pushed up to the end of the vagina, and the lower end is depressed so as to bring the cervix into its lumen, care being taken so to turn it that the longer side shall fit into the deeper posterior cul-de-sac. It is evident that the cervix alone can be seen well, the walls of the vagina being in view only when the speculum is being introduced or withdrawn. It is a very imperfect method of examination, and is described here merely because in case of the necessity arising for using a cylindrical speculum it is well to know how to use it correctly.

*Valvular Specula.*—The next important variety of speculum was constructed with the idea of having blades which would lie close together when introduced through the narrow entrance of the vagina, and then be capable of expansion after it was in place, so as to expose the upper part of the vagina and the cervix to view; hence the large number of bivalve, trivalve, and even quadrivalve specula. These are a distinct improvement on the cylindrical form, because they permit a much more thorough and natural view of the vault of the vagina and give more room at the opening for the use of instruments.

As the best example of this class of instruments may be mentioned Goodell's (Fig. 12), Nott's (Fig. 13), and Brewer's (Fig. 14).

These are used with the patient in the dorsal position. The labia majora are parted and the entrance to the vagina is exposed; the speculum is then well oiled, and is introduced with the blades closed and the long axis of the blades perpendicular. Pressure is made downward so as to depress the

FIG. 12.

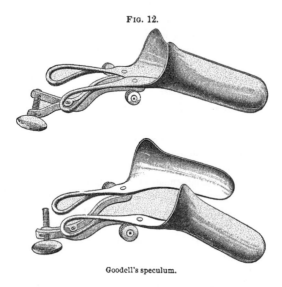

Goodell's speculum.

perineum, and the point is gradually inserted, the blades are turned so as to raise the anterior wall and depress the posterior, and are separated by the

FIG. 13.

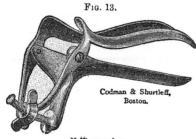

Codman & Shurtleff,
Boston.

Nott's speculum.

screw or spring at the handle. In this way a very good view of the cervix may be obtained, and the various methods of treatment may be carried out. This is a satisfactory form of speculum to use where one has not an assistant and needs to use two hands. Its disadvantages are that its introduction is painful when the entrance of the vagina is small, that it is liable to pinch and hurt the patient, that if the vagina is lax its folds fall in between the blades of the speculum so as to prevent a good view of the cervix, and that, even with the best constructed variety, the amount of room at the entrance is encroached upon by the speculum itself.

*Sims's Speculum.*—The necessity of contriving an instrument which would open the vagina and at the same time not interfere with the view of the anterior wall of the vagina led Sims to construct the speculum which is called by his name. He believed that cases of vesico-vaginal fistula which had been formerly considered incurable could be cured by operation, and the problem of getting at the field of operation was solved by his recognizing that in certain positions of the body, if the perineum was retracted, air would enter and balloon out the vagina, and the whole canal could be easily reached. This is, of course, most evident with the patient in the knee-chest position, but this is a position which is trying for her, and which she cannot maintain for any length of time. Sims saw, however, that in the semi-prone position the same

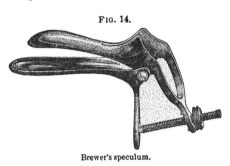

FIG. 14.

Brewer's speculum.

result is attained in a less marked but still perfectly satisfactory degree. This is the position that has been described, and is one which is comfortable to the patient.

All that is needed to expose the vagina and cervix, when once this position has been assumed, is a perineal retractor, and that is virtually what Sims's speculum is. It has two blades connected by a slender shank (Fig. 15); these blades are of different widths, and one is slightly longer than the other. The narrow blade is about as wide as the average forefinger, and can be introduced unless the opening in the hymen is very small or the hymen itself very tense. The broader one is useful in lax and large vaginæ, or for operating where a great deal of room is needed.

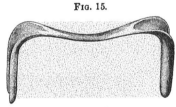

FIG. 15.

Sims's speculum.

There are small Sims's specula made for small vaginæ, and broad ones for operating.

It is at once evident what are the advantages of this form of speculum. As it hugs the posterior vaginal wall, it takes up the minimum quantity of room in the canal and permits an unobstructed view of the vault of the vagina and cervix. It stretches the entrance of the vagina as wide open as possible in the only direction in which it can yield, and this allows a large, free space for the manipulation of instruments. It is the only speculum through which it is possible to do most of the operations on the cervix and body of the uterus. It is the easiest of all specula to introduce, and the semi-prone position is the least trying one of any to the patient.

The only disadvantage which can be with any show of reason urged against it is that it necessitates the presence of an assistant. While this is true in certain cases, yet experience will show that a large proportion of the ordinary every-day treatment of gynæcological cases can be successfully carried out with this speculum without an assistant. We are convinced that this objection has been allowed to have too much weight. If the essential features of the semi-prone position are borne in mind, there will be much less difficulty than is generally supposed. Having the clothing absolutely loose about the waist is necessary in order that the vagina may fill with air. The Sims position should be studied and the patient made to assume it accurately. The patient can assist by holding up the right buttock with her right hand. If all these conditions are rendered favorable, the cervix will in the majority of cases be easily brought into view, and most of the simpler forms of treatment, such as applications to the cervix and vagina, tamponing the vagina, and the adjustment and care of pessaries, can be carried out. Where both hands are needed, some one of the forms of self-retaining specula which will be spoken of later may be used.

FIG. 16.

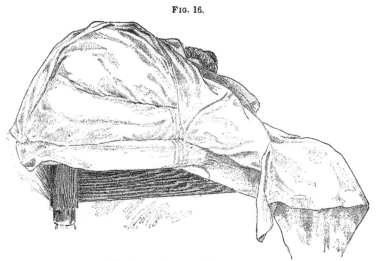

Patient prepared for use of Sims's speculum.

We come now to a description of the method of using Sims's speculum. The semi-prone position has been described, and it is only necessary to insist again upon the fact that the secret of the intelligent use of this form of speculum depends largely upon the correctness of the position. The patient should be covered with a sheet, which should come well down over the feet, but is gathered up upon the right hip, so as to expose the buttocks. These are best covered with two towels, so arranged that one shall be placed over each buttock, their approximate edges meeting in the middle line and the free edges tucked away under and over the thighs. They should be pinned to some article of clothing above, or tucked securely in. In this way the patient is thoroughly covered, and only the entrance to the vagina need be exposed when the speculum is used. (Fig. 16.)

A good light is most essential. A north exposure is best, for the sun-light is so dazzling as to obscure the view, and the window should be high enough to allow the light to fall over the operator's shoulders. A bay-window is bad, as it gives cross-lights.

Where good daylight cannot be secured, artificial light serves admirably; any apparatus for illuminating, whether by oil, or gas, or electricity, can be used, provided only that it is so arranged as to be adjustable. It should be capable of being raised or lowered, or of being moved to the right or left, to suit different patients.

When the patient has been placed in a good position, with the towels arranged, the nurse should take her place at the patient's back, facing the physician, her left arm resting on the patient's thigh and the hand raising the right buttock. To do this helpfully, she should carry the hand well over, so as to hold up the labium majus and the hair and expose the hymen.

FIG. 17.

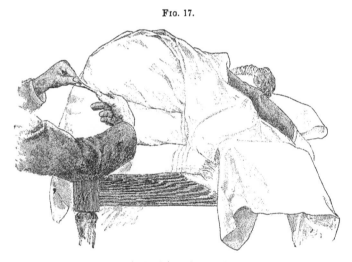

Method of introducing speculum.

Having warmed and well anointed the speculum so that it will easily slip in, the physician should hold it with the left hand by one blade, and gently insert the forefinger of the right hand into the vagina just far enough for the first joint to be within the hymen. This will protect the sensitive parts of the vulva from being pressed upon, and at the same time serve as an entering wedge for the speculum. The beak of the blade of the speculum should then be carried in on the finger, gentle pressure being made on the heel of the blade by the thumb. (Fig. 17.) Slight traction is to be made backward, so as to depress the perineum, it being remembered that only in this way can room be gained. The speculum should hug the posterior vaginal wall, and it should be borne in mind that the direction of the vagina at first is backward towards the promontory, or even the hollow, of the sacrum. If the speculum is merely pushed in in the supposed direction of the uterus, it will impinge on the anterior wall and will be arrested by its folds.

It is carried well up into the posterior cul-de-sac, gentle traction on the perineum being made all the time, and is then given to the nurse to hold, who should grasp it by the shank, the back of the blade resting in the hollow between the thumb and the hand. (Fig. 18.) This is the most

FIG. 18.

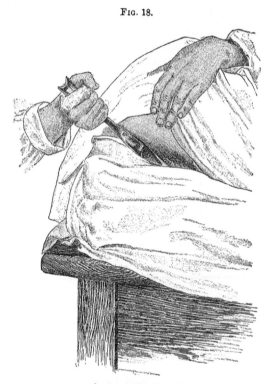

Method of holding speculum.

convenient way to hold the speculum, as the physician can easily grasp the free blade and change the position if necessary, while it is much less tiring to the nurse.

If the cervix does not easily come into view, the difficulty is usually because the anterior wall obscures it. This must be depressed, for which purpose a so-called depressor is used (Fig. 19), or, what is quite as convenient and serves the additional purpose of cleansing the vagina, a cotton-stick armed with a wad of cotton. (Fig. 20.)

If the anterior wall is pushed forward in the direction of the bladder, and the beak of the speculum is tilted somewhat forward as well, the cervix is usually well exposed. Its peculiarities may then be noted and conclusions drawn as to the existence of disease.

First as to its shape. It is normally conical in shape, the os being a small oval opening at its end. There are variations within normal limits, some cervices being long and narrow, others short and thick. The most common variation from the normal is the small conical cervix with

FIG. 19.

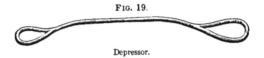

Depressor.

a small os, which is commonly met with in cases of anteflexion of the cervix, or of the body and cervix. This seems to be due to an arrest of development. If the patient has borne children, the changes in the shape of the cervix are various and well marked. As a rule, the os is enlarged, and in a not inconsiderable proportion of cases such a laceration has occurred as materially to alter the appearance of the cervix. If the tear is of moderate extent, not extending beyond the crown of the cervix, there is apt to be some eversion of the cervical mucous membrane, which presents a deep-red granular appearance. If of greater extent, there is a fissure extending over the crown of the cervix towards the junction of the vagina

FIG. 20.

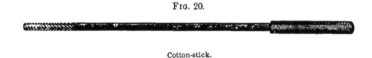

Cotton-stick.

and cervix, sometimes on one side, sometimes on both. This makes a sharp division line between the anterior and the posterior lip. The angles of the tear are usually partially filled with cicatricial tissue. Under certain conditions marked eversion occurs, so that the anterior or the posterior lip, or both, are rolled out and become hypertrophied. When this takes place, the everted torn surfaces and the cervical canal are red and granular and secrete mucus. This used to be called ulceration, but is now known as erosion. When the mouths of the glands become occluded and the secretions are retained, what are called retention cysts or "ovula Nabothi" are formed.

The normal color of the cervix is pink. When the pavement epithelium which covers the vaginal portion is lost, there is present the red inflamed-looking surface described above. This same red appearance is characteristic of the everted and eroded membrane which is due to a laceration. Under certain conditions this raw-looking surface is covered with a

thin covering of membrane which has a cloudy-red color and is very apt
to have semi-transparent spots showing through it. This is nature's attempt to reproduce on this eroded surface a normal covering. It is in
reality a thin cicatricial tissue, and the transparent spots are the retention
cysts showing through.

This thin covering may be formed also as a result of treatment applied
to the lacerated cervix, but when thus produced it is not apt to be permanent, but breaks down when treatment is suspended. If there is passive
congestion of the uterus, which may arise from a number of causes, the
pink color changes to red or even purple.

The normal secretion of the uterus is of a clear, viscid character, like
the white of an egg. In amount it is enough to fill the cervical canal and
to lubricate the vagina. When examined with the speculum there should
not be enough, if the uterus is healthy, to be seen projecting from the
mouth of the womb. When excessive in amount it is occasionally clear,
but more often becomes cloudy and even yellow. Such a change usually
denotes a catarrhal condition of the endometrium, so-called cervical or corporeal endometritis, and, if severe, the mucus is seen hanging in a clump or
mass from the cervix, and may be exceedingly difficult to dislodge. It is
very tenacious, and often cannot be wiped off with the cotton-stick, but

FIG. 21.

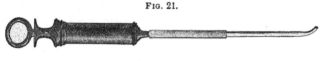

Uterine syringe.

must be drawn out with a syringe. A syringe especially adapted for this
purpose is figured here. (Fig. 21.)

*Self-retaining Specula.*—As has been already stated, the chief objection to Sims's speculum for purposes of diagnosis and treatment, as distinguished from its use for operations, is the necessity of having an assistant.
It has been pointed out that the importance of this objection has been
overestimated, since with the patient's assistance a large proportion of the
simpler forms of manipulation can be perfectly carried out with this instrument. To adapt it still more widely, the use of self-retaining specula
has been advocated, and numerous instruments planned with this object in
view have been devised.

It is self-evident that to be of value the point of attachment of the
speculum must be the patient's body, since if the instrument is fastened to
the table any movement of the patient will instantly disturb the relations
and throw the cervix out of view. This renders a large number of self-
retaining specula practically useless.

Of those constructed on the right principle, probably the best is Cleveland's self-retaining speculum. It is simple, easy of application, not painful

to the patient, and fulfils all the indications. The essential features are a strap buckled around the waist, to which a second strap is attached, which comes down over the coccyx and is attached to the speculum. This is composed of two blades, connected by a short shank, so that when one blade is in the vagina the other lies flat against the coccyx. The strap passes through one slot in the end of the free blade and a second at the connecting middle piece, so that if traction is made on

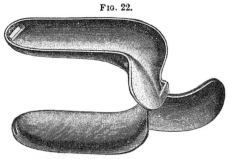

Cleveland's self-retaining speculum.

it the perineum will be retracted. Each blade has a flange for holding up the right buttock. (Fig. 22.)

Fig. 23.

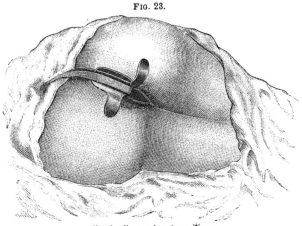

Cleveland's speculum in position.

This speculum has proved in practice to be a thoroughly satisfactory one. Fig. 23 shows it in position.

### USE OF THE PROBE OR SOUND.

The uterine sound is a long, slender, more or less flexible instrument which is inserted into the uterine canal to determine its direction, depth, and calibre, and exceptionally may be used for replacing the organ. The probe is a more delicate instrument, and is a safer one to use where the position and depth of the uterus are to be ascertained. The sound may be made of copper which is silver-plated. The probe is best made of pure silver, at least the end, so as to admit of being bent easily. (Fig. 24.) The sound is notched at the extremity, and marked with inches and fractions of an inch for convenience in measuring the depth. The probe is smooth.

FIG. 24.

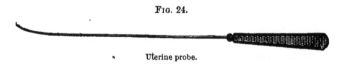

Uterine probe.

To determine the calibre of the canal it is well to have sounds of two or three different sizes. A Simpson's sound (Fig. 25) and a Peaslee's sound (Fig. 26) are sufficient, as any canal which will admit the last is sufficiently patulous.

The question as to when and how often to use the probe or sound is

FIG. 25.

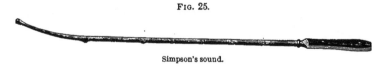

Simpson's sound.

an important one. Many writers on gynæcology would restrict its use to the rarest occasions, and almost condemn it altogether. They hold that injury is done to the lining membrane of the uterus, and that infection is likely to be carried and inflammation of the endometrium set up by its use. That this is a possible danger is true, but, as the simplest rules of cleanliness and disinfection will guard against this, it ought not to have much effect. The fact is that with increasing skill in diagnosis the necessity for the employment of the probe or sound grows less, until the more ex-

FIG. 26.

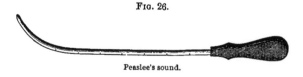

Peaslee's sound.

perienced gynæcologist will restrict its use almost entirely to determining the calibre of the canal, and, in obscure cases, its depth.

Not so, however, with the beginner. With him it is a valuable aid to diagnosis, and, provided it is used antiseptically, there is very little danger from its use. I am of the opinion that more serious results would follow from neglecting its use, in the way of mistakes in diagnosis, than from its use, in the form of endometritis or sepsis. Impress upon the mind of the young practitioner the necessity of absolute cleanliness and the avoidance of violence, and that he should not forget the possibility of pregnancy, and he should be encouraged to use the probe and the sound.

After a thorough visual inspection of the vault of the vagina and the vaginal portion of the cervix with the speculum, if the symptoms call for a further examination to determine the size of the uterus, the probe should be passed. Where the abdominal muscles are thin and relaxed and the uterus freely movable, any marked enlargement of the organ can be fairly well estimated by the bimanual examination. Minor degrees of enlargement, especially in women who are stout, cannot be appreciated, nor will the bimanual examination always give us a correct idea of the position of the body of the uterus. The various conditions which may render this difficult have been spoken of before. So, too, in irregular enlargements of the uterus, such as are due to fibroids, the depth and direction of the canal may be very obscure. To clear up these points the probe is necessary.

It should be first bent to correspond to the supposed curve of the canal as found by bimanual examination. If there is a probability that the

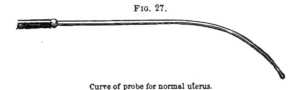

Fig. 27.

Curve of probe for normal uterus.

uterus is in its normal position, it should be given a moderate curve, somewhat as is represented in Fig. 27. Should the uterus be anteverted or flexed, a sharper curve should be given. (Fig. 28.) If retroverted,

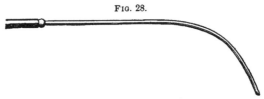

Fig. 28.

Curve of probe for anteflexed uterus.

the curve should be lessened somewhat. (Fig. 29.) If retroflexion exists it should have more nearly the normal curve.

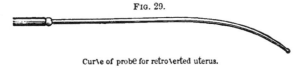

Fig. 29.

Curve of probe for retroverted uterus.

After it has been bent as desired, it should be dipped in a solution of corrosive sublimate or quickly passed through a flame. The vagina should be swabbed out with a corrosive sublimate solution, and any mucus in the canal should be drawn out with the uterine syringe. The probe should then be gently passed into the canal, and carried through the internal os to the fundus, where it will meet with an elastic resistance.

To measure the depth, the finger may be carried into the vagina and placed against the probe; then both probe and finger are withdrawn, and the number of inches is read off by comparison with the sound. A better way is to grasp the probe just at the os externum with the locking forceps and to withdraw both.

The passage of the probe, if carefully done, is usually painless. If there is any pain, it is when the point is passing the internal os. This is particularly apt to be the case if the patient suffers from dysmenorrhœa. Sometimes the pain is very severe. If skilfully done, and there is no unusual hyperæmia of the uterine mucosa, no blood should follow the passage of the probe. If the canal is narrow, or the most suitable curve has not been secured, a drop or two may follow without exciting any suspicion of disease of the endometrium. If considerable blood follows, such a complication is probable.

There are certain difficulties which may be met with in this procedure. In the first place, the curve may not be the right one. If the probe does not enter readily, it is well to withdraw it and either straighten it or give it a sharper curve. Which to do will depend upon the greater probability of one or another form of displacement being present. If there is a forward displacement, the curve will probably need to be made greater; if a backward, less. After considerable skill has been acquired in the use of the instrument, if the difficulty is with the curve, the delicately trained sense of touch will suggest the right change to make.

In one displacement there is a peculiar difficulty,—viz., in anteflexion of the neck. Here there is a more or less acute angle at the internal os, around which it is difficult to get the point of the probe. This may be often overcome by passing the probe as far as the internal os with the concavity backward (Fig. 30), and then giving it a half turn, which allows the point to enter the canal and pass up to the fundus. (Fig. 31.) In acute anteflexion, after the point has passed the internal os, it will facilitate its farther introduction to carry the handle backward towards the speculum. Only the very gentlest pressure must be used.

A second difficulty in passing the probe is that its point may catch on the folds of the mucous membrane of the cervix and be arrested. This is likely to occur near the internal os. In such cases counter-traction with the tenaculum will sometimes straighten out the canal so that the probe will pass. The tenaculum (Fig. 32) should be embedded firmly in the tissues of the anterior lip of the cervix on its vaginal aspect, not in the canal, which is more sensitive and more likely to tear out. It should be carried into the muscular substance so as to insure a firm hold. If the probe still catches, the blunter sound should be used, which will be less likely to be caught in such folds.

A third difficulty may be a narrowness of the canal, especially at the internal os. This is rarely so marked as to prevent the introduction of

FIG. 31.

FIG. 30.

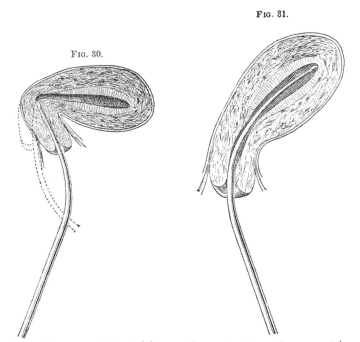

Passage of probe in anteflexion: first step.     Passage of probe in anteflexion: second step.

the fine probe, but it is sometimes contracted to that extent, and in any case it may make the opening hard to find. Occasionally it is only after the patient has been etherized that the probe can be passed.

Still a fourth difficulty is tortuousness of the canal. This is found in uteri which are the seat of fibroids, and an accurate measurement of the

FIG. 32.

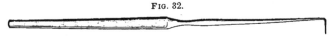

Tenaculum.

direction and depth of the canal is well-nigh impossible. No stiff instrument can be relied upon to reach the fundus. This difficulty may generally be overcome by using a small flexible bougie or gum-elastic catheter which will accommodate itself to the curves. This will enable us to measure the depth, but will not show the direction of the canal. An ingenious instrument for this purpose is Jennison's flexible sound. It is a coil of wire covered with rubber, with a handle of hard rubber near one end. When the longer end is carried into a curved canal the shorter end will describe the same curve, but in the opposite direction. (Fig. 33.) The knowledge

FIG. 33.

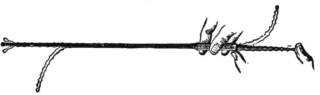

Jennison's sound.

thus gained is often of advantage in determining the position of a tumor which impinges more or less upon the uterine cavity.

There is one other use of the sound which must be alluded to here, but more in the way of warning than of commendation. This instrument is recommended in many text-books as a means of replacing a retroverted or retroflexed uterus. The advice has even been given to replace the uterus forcibly every day with the sound until it will stay of itself. Such a procedure, or even the occasional use of the sound for this purpose, cannot be too strongly deprecated. It is dangerous to use a stiff, unyielding instrument to pry forward a misplaced uterus. If the uterus is free, other simpler measures will answer the purpose; if it is adherent, the attempt to straighten it can result only in injury and the possible setting up of dangerous inflammatory trouble. Repositors—instruments made with special reference to this manœuvre—are bad enough, but the sound is distinctly worse.

### INSPECTION OF THE ABDOMEN.

In a certain proportion of cases with which the gynæcologist has to deal the inspection of the abdomen is of importance. This applies especially to abdominal tumors,—primarily those which have their origin in the pelvic organs, and secondarily those of abdominal origin. It is hardly ever called for where the disease is confined to the pelvis.

Where the patient gives a distinct history of a swelling in the abdomen, such as would warrant us in believing that there may be a tumor present, inspection had better be the first step in our examination. It is less of a shock to a sensitive woman than the vaginal examination, and paves the way for it, if it should prove necessary.

A woman is often unconscious of the existence of a considerable swelling in the abdomen, especially if it be unaccompanied by pain. The method of dressing which obtains in civilized countries permits of some enlargement of the lower abdomen without its being apparent, and the abdominal viscera will sometimes admit of considerable encroachment upon their normal space without resenting it by disturbance of function.

There are symptoms, however, which, in the absence of any direct evi-

dence of swelling, would suggest the possibility of a tumor. Sometimes
there is the suggestion of increased pressure in the pelvis, on account of
bladder and bowel symptoms, frequent or difficult micturition, and constipation. Sometimes nausea is associated with enlargement of the uterus,
usually caused by pregnancy, sometimes by other conditions. Shortness of

Fig. 34.

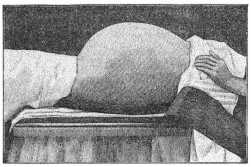

Outline of abdomen in ascites. (Kelly.)

breath on exertion, palpitation of the heart, sense of fulness after taking
food in small quantities, flatulence, swelling of the feet and ankles, and
pains in the legs are other hints of abdominal pressure.

Occasionally the patient is conscious of a weight shifting from one side
to the other on turning, or of an inability to lie on one side or the other
on account of discomfort in the lower abdomen.

Fig. 35.

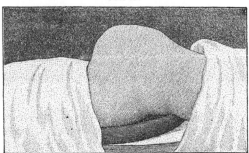

Outline of abdomen in ovarian cyst: side view. (Kelly.)

For the inspection of the abdomen the patient should lie on the table,
on her back, with her feet in a chair, or raised a little if the legs are short
and the abdominal walls are made too tense. The skirts and drawers should
be loosened and pushed down, and the undervest pushed up to a level with
the lower ribs, so as completely to expose the whole surface. On looking
at the abdomen, its contour will suggest certain things. If the enlargement

is due to ascites (Fig. 34), it will be flattened at the top, symmetrical, bulging at the sides; if to pregnancy or an ovarian tumor (Figs. 35 and 36), it will

FIG. 36.

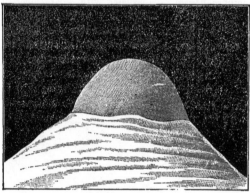

Ovarian cyst from below. (Kelly.)

be prominent in the middle, falling rapidly off at the sides; if to a fibroid (Fig. 37), there will usually be irregularities of the outline.

FIG. 37.

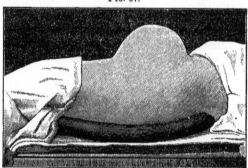

Outline of abdomen in case of myoma uteri. (Kelly.)

*Palpation of the Abdomen.*—Having previously warmed his hands, the physician should thoroughly palpate the abdomen, in order to discover any solid mass, if such be present. A little gentle manipulation is often of value to overcome muscular rigidity and to permit the outline of any swelling to be accurately made out. This rigidity of the muscles may be so pronounced as to simulate a tumor, and this mistake should be guarded against. The size, consistency, and relations of the tumor can be ascertained by palpation. If there is a growth, the practised touch will show whether it has a smooth or an irregular surface, whether it arises in the pelvis, and sometimes whether it is in the median line and continuous with the uterus or has its origin on one side.

The hand on the surface will recognize movements within the mass if pregnancy of over five months' standing is the cause of the tumor. Pressure will reveal painful spots or areas, and will also give the varying degrees of resistance due to variations in density. The mobility of the growth can be tested by deep pressure and attempts to dislodge it from one side to the other or upward.

Certain special manipulations are of great use in this examination. Pressing both hands deep into the pelvis from the sides will enable the operator to detect the head of the fœtus in the pregnant uterus, if that is the presenting part, and will also help to solve the question of the connection of certain tumors with the uterus or its appendages. With one hand under each flank, the contents of the abdomen may be pressed forward and upward and unusual resistance be detected. A movable kidney may be palpated by compressing the sides of the abdomen below the ribs, with one hand at the back and the other at the front. Some little light on the question of the presence or absence of adhesions may be gained by sliding the abdominal wall over the surface of a swelling. If it moves freely and causes no pain, the chances are that there are no adhesions.

If there is present a distinct enlargement of the abdomen, and on careful palpation no tumor is found, ascites is the most probable cause. A considerable degree of ascites may, however, mask the existence of a small tumor.

*Percussion of the Abdomen.*—A good deal of aid in the determination of the character of the swelling is given by percussion. The area of dulness is of the greatest importance in distinguishing between a tumor and ascites. The broad rule is that in the former the dulness extends over the front of the abdomen, the percussion at the sides being resonant, while the reverse holds true of ascites. Here the fluid gravitates to the lowest part of the abdominal cavity, and the intestines are floated upward. There are, of course, exceptions, such as cases where the ascitic fluid is walled off from the general peritoneal cavity by adhesions, and the fluid remains on top and gives a dull note; but the rule holds good. Percussion enables us to define with greater accuracy the height to which a tumor rises in the abdomen, its size, and its outline.

A modification of percussion gives us a method of discriminating between solid tumors and cysts or free fluid in the abdomen. Free fluid or thin-walled cysts will give the characteristic wave of fluctuation. Usually this may be easily appreciated by placing one hand flat on one side of the abdomen and gently tapping the other side, when a distinct impulse will be felt on the palm of the opposing hand. Sometimes, especially in fat subjects, a wave will be transmitted over the surface of the abdomen from one hand to the other, and will simulate true fluctuation. This may be cut off by having an assistant make light pressure with the edge of the hand on the median line of the abdomen.

The absence of such a wave is not necessarily proof of the solid nature of a tumor, as in very tense-walled cysts no fluctuation can be felt.

*Auscultation of the abdomen* is of value only in the differential diagnosis of pregnancy from other varieties of abdominal tumor. The detection of the fœtal heart will settle the diagnosis so far as that condition is concerned. The placental souffle is a more indefinite sign and of less diagnostic value.

*Measurements of the Abdomen.*—It is sometimes important to take accurate measurements of the abdomen as a matter of record and for convenience of judging of the rate of growth of tumors. To be of value, certain fixed points should be chosen. The most convenient are the umbilicus, the anterior superior spines of the ilium, and the symphysis pubis. The following measurements, taken at regular intervals, will give a satisfactory and sufficiently reliable record of the growth of a tumor: the circumference of the abdomen at a point midway between the umbilicus and the lower edge of the sternum, the same at the umbilicus, the same halfway from the umbilicus to the upper border of the symphysis, the distance from the umbilicus to the right anterior superior spine of the ilium, that from the umbilicus to the left spine, and that from the umbilicus to the symphysis.

### BIMANUAL EXAMINATION THROUGH THE RECTUM.

This method of examination has been referred to in speaking of the examination of virgins, where the hymen is so rigid as to make the vaginal method impossible or inadvisable. It is the sole method that we can employ when we have to deal with a case of atresia or absence of the vagina. In atresia of the hymen, the condition found on examination usually makes the rectal examination unnecessary, as the bulging hymen and the presence of a tumor rising above the brim of the pelvis tell the story. In atresia of the vagina, if partial, palpation through the rectum will give valuable information as to its extent and the changes in the structures beyond which it has involved. In absence of the vagina, the question of the condition of the uterus, tubes, and ovaries becomes of prime importance. The first point to be ascertained is whether the uterus is present; if so, in what degree of development. It should be remembered that it may exist in any degree, from the slightest swelling in the median line to normal size. The question of the formation of an artificial vagina depends in a large measure upon the size of the uterus. If of normal size, or nearly so, it may be considered advisable to attempt the often very difficult task of opening up the septum between the bladder and the rectum, thus rendering coitus and even impregnation possible.

The presence or absence of ovaries has an important bearing upon the future welfare of the patient. If present, they are probably functionally active, and the periodical changes which occur in them may be accompanied by such pain that an operation for their removal is justifiable. Their absence gives an additional reason for not attempting the formation of a vagina.

The rectal examination is also of the greatest value in the diagnosis of obscure pelvic affections, especially the relations of swellings of the various organs to each other. It would probably be the testimony of all gynæcologists that with enlarged experience they practise this method more and more, and learn to depend upon the information which it gives.

The student and young practitioner should become familiar with it, and should employ it when possible. Like the vaginal examination, it requires a good deal of practice to gain the necessary skill. The conditions are different, and it is not always easy to distinguish the several organs.

It is essential, of course, that the rectum should be empty. If this has not previously been attended to, an enema should be given at the time. The left forefinger may be used as in the vaginal examination, and, having been well lubricated, should be pressed firmly against the anus. If the patient is requested to strain down as though at stool, it will facilitate the entrance of the finger. It should first be passed upward and forward towards the vagina, then with a slight rotary motion carried farther in. When about two-thirds of the finger has entered, the cervix uteri is usually felt as a round hard body impinging upon the rectum. This is often mistaken for the fundus by those unfamiliar with this mode of examination, and many an error in diagnosis has been made in this way. Just beyond this the finger encounters a fold of the rectum which seems to bar the way, and there may be a little difficulty in finding the lumen. This fold is on the anterior wall, and if the finger is hooked around it and carried forward, it will enter another segment of the rectum and reach the level of the body of the uterus. It will surprise the beginner to find how with gradual upward pressure the finger will reach higher and higher as the perineum is pushed up, and how the contents of the upper pelvis can be palpated.

The procedure is now the same as in bimanual examination per vaginam. The right hand placed on the abdomen and exerting counter-pressure will both steady and depress the pelvic viscera so that the information desired can be gained.

The advantages which the rectal examination affords are that the finger can reach higher than in the vagina and has a much more extensive lateral sweep, the result of which is that the whole of the posterior surface of the uterus can be satisfactorily mapped out and the tubes and ovaries more thoroughly reached.

To complete this method of examination, and to enlarge its scope, the tenaculum may be used to draw the uterus down. This not only enables the finger to reach higher on the uterus, but displaces the ovaries sufficiently to make their palpation easy and thorough. The tenaculum, or, better, the double-hook forceps, is caught firmly in the anterior lip of the uterus, and traction is made on it until the cervix approaches the vulva, a procedure which may be carried out without affecting the integrity of the pelvic structures. This is then given to an assistant to hold, and the bimanual examination is carried out as before. To render this method of examination possible without an assistant, Kelly, of Baltimore, has devised a tenaculum

5

which has a grooved handle, which can be held by the free fingers of the
left hand without slipping.

## THE RECTO-VESICAL EXAMINATION.

This method of examination, which, as its name implies, makes use of
both rectum and bladder, is of use only where the vagina is absent, and has
for its object the determination of the condition of the uterus and its appendages in cases of absence or atresia of the vagina. With the finger of one
hand in the rectum, and of the other hand in the bladder (after previous
dilatation), the structures lying between can be examined in a perfect
manner. It is not always necessary to introduce the finger into the bladder; sometimes a sound will serve the purpose equally well.

## EXAMINATION OF THE URETHRA AND BLADDER.

The fact of the intimate vascular and nervous connection of all the
pelvic viscera is forcibly brought home to the physician by the very frequent association with uterine troubles of symptoms referable to the urinary organs. Complaints of pain either before, during, or after the act
of micturition, inability to hold the urine or a frequent desire to pass it,
leaking on cough or exertion, a feeling of weight and discomfort over the
pubes,—these and other symptoms are very commonly part of the patient's
history, and if not volunteered should be carefully inquired for.

Since they are so common, the best methods of examining the condition
of the urethra and bladder should be familiar to the practitioner.

It would seem hardly necessary to refer in this connection to the importance of an examination of the urine, yet this is often overlooked by the
specialist, and important information is thereby neglected. It will often
clear up a doubtful diagnosis or suggest some effective mode of treatment.
It should be thorough, both chemical and microscopical, and its method
should be perfectly familiar to the practitioner.

Some knowledge of the condition of the lower part of the urethra may
be gained by visual inspection. The most common conditions that we find
that give rise to trouble are polypi, prolapse of the urethral mucous membrane, and urethral caruncle. Loss of tissue, due to ulcerative processes
which are the result of venereal disease, or lupus, or epithelioma, are also
occasionally found. Stricture of the lower part of the canal is sometimes
met with.

The presence of these conditions is easily determined by the sense of
sight. Visual inspection will also show the condition known as urethrocele, if such exists. This, as its name implies, is a stretching of a portion
of the urethra so as to form a pouch which is seen to bulge into the vagina.
Cystocele, or prolapse of the anterior vaginal wall, as has been said before,
becomes apparent on separating the vulva and asking the patient to strain
down.

Some bladder and urethral affections may be recognized by the examination with the finger. Unusual sensitiveness of any portion of the urethra can be demonstrated by pressure with the finger. This is most often found at the neck of the bladder. A stone, if of any considerable size, may be detected by palpating the bladder through the vagina, and the position of the uterus with reference to the bladder can be made out bimanually.

For the examination of the condition of the urethra more elaborate methods are necessary. One of the most common conditions found is acute urethritis, the result of gonorrhœal infection. The symptoms are frequent and painful micturition, with a discharge of pus from the urethra, in severe cases of blood. In mild cases, or in the later stages of more severe ones, the presence of pus may not be readily demonstrable. To detect a small quantity it is best to wipe gently the meatus with cotton to remove any pus or mucus which may have come from the vagina, and then inserting the finger in the vagina, to withdraw it slowly, making firm pressure on the urethra from the neck of the bladder towards the meatus. If pus is present it will be squeezed out and appear between the folds of the meatus.

The existence of sensitive areas in the urethra, especially at the vesical neck, where they are most commonly found, may be determined by the passage of a sound. While the urethra is normally sensitive to the passage of any instrument, yet the pain on reaching any inflamed spot, or touching a fissure at the neck, is so much more acute that this sign is fairly reliable. The passage of a sound or catheter will also determine the presence of a stricture, a condition which, though rare in comparison to its occurrence in the male, is yet occasionally met with.

For the determination of the exact condition of the lining membrane of the urethra the endoscope is necessary. This, as its name implies, is an instrument which enables us to see the mucous membrane either directly or reflected in a mirror. As the urethra can be stretched without undue violence so as to admit the average-sized forefinger, a simple tube may serve as an endoscope. The urethra can be gradually dilated with Simon's plugs (Fig. 38), for instance, the inner plug withdrawn, and the tube left *in situ*.

FIG. 38.

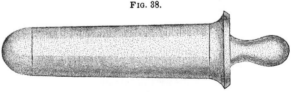

Simon's urethral plugs.

Through this the whole urethra may be inspected, the field being illuminated by light thrown from a head-mirror. The neck of the bladder being placed in the field first, the tube may be slowly withdrawn, and each successive part examined as it rolls into view. Such a thorough examination, of course, presupposes that the patient is under ether.

This method will give us information as to the presence of a fissure at the neck of the bladder or an ulcerated surface anywhere in the course of the canal. But if the trouble, as is more often the case, is due to hyper-

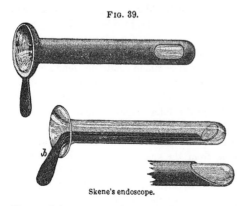

FIG. 39.

Skene's endoscope.

æmia of the mucous membrane, or dilatation of the blood-vessels, the pressure of the large tubes will drive out the blood and prevent the recognition of the true condition. Therefore a smaller tube is essential, and the most satisfactory endoscope is that known as Skene's. (Fig. 39.) It consists of three parts: first, a small glass tube, closed, looking like a miniature test-tube; second, a section of a tube, with a small mirror set at an angle at one end and a handle at the other; third, two hard-rubber specula large enough to hold the glass tube, one with an opening on the side, the other with a bevelled opening at the end.

The method of using it is as follows. The glass tube is inserted into the urethra until it passes within the vesical neck. The small mirror is then passed into the tube, and by means of a head-mirror the light is thrown in. As the handle of the speculum mirror is turned, all parts of the neck of the bladder and the urethra may be successively examined and any abuor- malities detected. Although the tube is small, the pressure may still affect to some extent the blood-supply. To avoid this difficulty the hard-rubber tube with the open end may be used instead, and as it is slowly withdrawn and different parts of the canal come into view, the condition of the blood-vessels may be noted. A frequent occurrence is a varicose condition of the veins, especially at the vesical neck, which can be seen radiating from the centre in the field of vision.

With this tube applications by means of cotton or spray through an atomizer may be made to the whole canal. Where there is some localized condition, such as ulceration, and it is desirable to confine the application to the immediate spot, the affected area may be brought into view by means of the hard-rubber tube with the side opening, and the appropriate treat- ment applied directly to the diseased membrane.

### DIGITAL EXAMINATION OF THE BLADDER.

This procedure is sometimes necessary under the following circum- stances. The examination of the urine suggests the presence of some foreign growth, the character, size, and location of which can be determined only by the sense of touch. Fortunately, the urethra in women during the child-bearing period is sufficiently dilatable to admit an average forefinger without doing undue damage either in the way of lacerations or resulting incontinence. Dilatation should be begun with Simon's instruments, and carried slowly forward by using successive sizes, until the largest has been passed. The forefinger can then usually be inserted. The narrowest part of the urethra is at the meatus. This may be stretched so tightly that to avoid a bad tear into the surrounding tissues it is well to make two or three small nicks at the sides.

With the finger in the bladder, counter-pressure may be made over the pubes and the whole interior of the viscus explored, irregularities or morbid growths detected, their seat made out, and their size estimated. Small calculi or other foreign bodies which may have eluded detection with the sound can in this way be felt.

The visual inspection of the interior of the bladder by means of the cystoscope is hardly one of those methods of examination which come within the scope of the ordinary practitioner: it presupposes special skill and opportunities. It is considered at length in the chapter on Diseases of the Bladder.

### PALPATION OF THE URETERS.

Simon, of Heidelberg, Pawlik, and Kelly have all contributed to our knowledge of diseases of the ureters and the methods by which they may be recognized. The normal ureters can be made out in the favorable subject for nearly two-thirds of their length, about half of this being situated in the pelvis and half within the abdomen. The pelvic portion before it reaches the broad ligament can be palpated through the anterior vaginal wall, and is recognized as a flattened cord, embedded in the loose cellular tissue, running from the bladder laterally and upward and backward towards the base of the broad ligament. Counter-pressure must be made through the abdominal walls. The rest of the pelvic portion can be made out by introducing a ureteral catheter through the urethra and bladder into the ureter, carrying it up to or over the brim of the pelvis, and then examining by the rectum.

At the brim and for a short distance above towards the kidney it can be felt through the abdominal wall while the catheter remains in place.

The method of catheterizing the ureters, as described by Dr. Kelly, is essentially as follows. After emptying the bladder with a catheter, it is distended with from five to seven ounces of a blue aniline solution. The posterior wall of the vagina is retracted with a speculum and the ureteral catheter (Fig. 40) is introduced. Its point is made to impinge on the anterior vaginal wall, and, with the tip of the finger making counter-pressure, the ureteral eminence is sought for. When this is felt, the catheter is withdrawn a little, and its point swept downward, outward, and backward in the direction of the prominence. This is repeated till the tip catches, when it is turned towards the posterior lateral wall of the pelvis and carefully introduced until its point reaches the pelvic wall.

To carry the catheter up over the brim of the pelvis and even to the pelvis of the kidney, the bladder is emptied, and, with the index finger in the rectum, the catheter is lifted up over the pelvic brim and on through the abdominal portion.

FIG. 40.

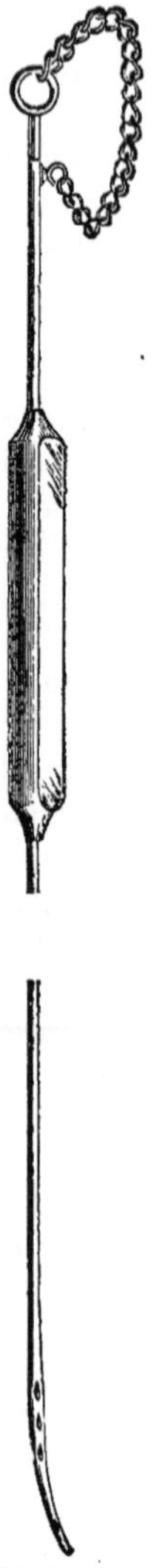

### EXAMINATION OF THE RECTUM AND ANUS.

What has been said about the importance of affections of the urinary apparatus in connection with diseases of women applies with equal force to diseases of the rectum. The troubles to which the anus and rectum are liable should be understood, as they are very often caused by pre-existing pelvic disease or are complications, and women, for obvious reasons, are much more apt to consult the gynæcologist than the rectal specialist for such affections. The examination *per rectum* of the pelvic organs has been spoken of; it now remains to describe the methods of examining the rectum and anus for disease of those structures.

*Methods of Examination.*—Visual inspection of the anus will reveal the presence of external hemorrhoids. By stretching open the anus and asking the patient to strain, considerable more of the rectal mucous membrane may be brought into view. A fissure may in this way be detected. So, too, the lower opening of a fistula, if such exist, may be seen.

Digital eversion of the rectum, as recommended by Mundé, can be used for examining the lower part of the rectum. It is applicable only in women with relaxed vaginal walls, or with torn or sundered perinea, or when the patient is under ether. The patient is placed in Sims's position. The forefinger of the right hand is then inserted into the vagina and pressure is made on the posterior vaginal wall backward and outward towards the anus. It is as though one were trying to push the finger through the posterior vaginal wall out of the anal orifice. (Fig. 41.) The effect is to expose the lower segment of the rectum, especially anteriorly.

For any but the lowest part of the rectum a speculum is necessary. The best rectal speculum for the lower rectum is Ives's (Fig. 42), of which there are three sizes, the largest being the best for general use.

Kelly's ureteral catheter.

For the inspection of the higher rectum ether is usually necessary, as most instruments require forcible stretching of the sphincter ani. Sims's speculum may be used, and in many cases is a very satisfactory instrument. It is better to give ether, but it may be used without. The patient should be placed in an exaggerated Sims's position,—that is, the hips should be raised higher than usual. Some examining-tables

FIG. 41.

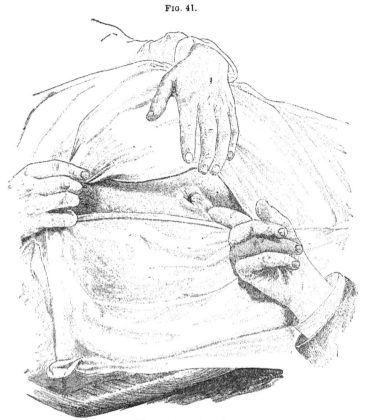

Digital eversion of the rectum.

provide for this. Where they do not, a pillow may be placed under the hips and the same result attained.

The speculum, well lubricated, is then slowly passed in and the posterior wall retracted just as in the vaginal examination. The air enters and balloons the rectum, and two-thirds of the circumference of the bowels can be well seen. Traction on the anterior wall will expose the posterior wall, but not so well.

FIG. 42.

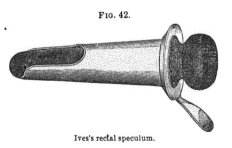

Ives's rectal speculum.

Illumination can be obtained by reflected

light from a head-mirror, or a small incandescent electric light can be introduced into the rectum.

### EXAMINATION OF THE INTERIOR OF THE UTERUS.

Where the symptoms of which the patient complains and the results of our bimanual and speculum examination make it evident that the trouble is seated within the uterus, an exploration of its interior is essential to a thorough understanding of the case, and to neglect it is criminal. Our modern methods of investigation and the employment of aseptic precautions make this an easy and safe procedure, and the practitioner who contents himself with conjectures as to what the trouble is, and treats the symptoms without seeking to investigate the cause, fails completely in his duty to his patient.

The most common symptom which would lead us to suspect trouble inside the womb is hemorrhage. The paramount importance to the patient of knowing whether this proceeds from a simple hyperplastic endometritis, from a benign tumor like a fibroid, or from malignant disease, is too apparent to need mention; yet men of good standing in the profession, who have had the recent thorough training of our best schools, will allow hemorrhage from the uterus to go on, and will be satisfied to attempt to check it by tampon and ergot, without once suggesting that it is better to find out the cause.

Some degree of dilatation must precede any attempt to learn anything about the condition of the endometrium. Sometimes nature has accomplished this sufficiently for our purpose. After an abortion the canal is usually sufficiently patulous to admit a curette, sometimes even a finger; so, too, prolonged hemorrhage from any cause may so soften and dilate the tissues that an instrument may be passed in. But usually the internal os presents an effectual barrier to any satisfactory exploration, either by the finger or instrument. Some method of dilatation must, therefore, be used.

The method to be employed will vary with the object which we wish to accomplish. If we merely wish to enlarge the canal enough to pass in a curette and scrape, and provide adequately for subsequent drainage, one method will be sufficient. If, on the other hand, we wish to explore the cavity of the uterus with the finger, a more elaborate method is necessary.

The first object is much the more frequent. We are constantly meeting with cases in which we either know from the history that there is some foreign body in the uterus, such as the retained products of conception, or suspect some degenerative change in the lining membrane. To make a diagnosis it is only necessary to pass in a curette and scrape away a bit of the membrane.

Such dilatation can be best accomplished rapidly by instruments. Ether had better be employed, as it is a painful process, and the details can be more thoroughly carried out if the surgeon knows that he is not inflicting pain.

The patient may be placed either in Sims's position or on the back, and the vagina thoroughly washed out with a corrosive sublimate solution of 1 to 2000. The anterior lip is then seized with the double-hooked forceps (American bullet-forceps, Fig. 43) and held firmly. The direction of the canal is now tested by the probe or small sound. This having been ascertained,

FIG. 43.

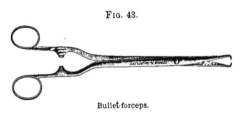

Bullet-forceps.

the canal is dilated by a series of graduated dilators. There are several different sets of such dilators, some steel, some hard rubber, with varying curves and of different shapes. A thoroughly satisfactory form is Hanks's hard-rubber dilators, which come in a set of six, embracing twelve numbers, from nine to twenty. (Fig. 44.) The smallest will usually readily pass the internal os, and the largest secures sufficient dilatation to admit of thorough curettage and drainage.

They should be rendered aseptic and should be carefully passed in, one number after another, each number being allowed to remain in position long enough to overcome the muscular spasm to some extent. The length of time required for the full dilatation

FIG. 44.

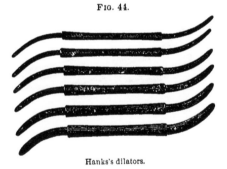

Hanks's dilators.

varies with the amount of muscular rigidity or the character of the tissue, especially at the internal os. If the cervix is softened by disease or long-continued hemorrhage, the dilators may be passed in as rapidly as they can be manipulated. If the internal os is fibrous and rigid, it may be a long process. Sometimes it is impossible to pass the larger numbers until some dilating instrument has been used.

If the tissues have yielded readily, the curette may be used immediately.

FIG. 45.

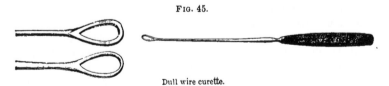

Dull wire curette.

The best for diagnostic purposes is the dull wire curette. (Fig. 45.) This may be bent to suit the direction of the canal, and then passed in until it has reached the fundus of the uterus. It should then be withdrawn and the whole interior of the uterus scraped, especial attention being given to the angles where the Fallopian tubes open, as disease is sometimes either limited to, or is most marked at, those points. Any scrapings which may be brought away by the curette should be carefully inspected. A good method is to float them in water, which will help to solve their true character, whether they are blood-clot, hyperplastic endometrium, or bits of new growth. If there is doubt as to their true nature they should be submitted to the microscope.

Where it is impossible to effect sufficient dilatation with Hanks's or similar dilators, some one of the steel, branched dilators may be used. It may be necessary to use this in order to pass the highest numbers of the series, or the os internum may show so marked a tendency to contract on the withdrawal of the last number that some more efficient means of paralyzing the muscular contractions may be advisable.

A very satisfactory instrument—perhaps the best—is Goodell's modification of Ellinger's. (Fig. 46.) This should be rendered thoroughly aseptic

FIG. 46.

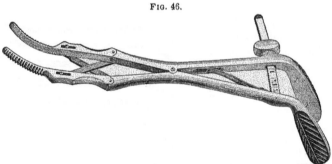

Goodell's modification of Ellinger's dilator.

and then passed in and the blades separated slowly but firmly. Too much force should not be used, as rupture of the cervical tissues has been known to occur. As the parts yield to slow, firm pressure, what is gained may be held by the screw on the ratchet. It is unwise to use this screw to effect the dilatation, inasmuch as it is impossible to appreciate the degree of force that we are employing in this way. Compressing the handles with the hands is a much safer way and completely under the control of the operator. From five to twenty minutes may be consumed in overcoming an obstinate stricture of the internal os.

When the blades are separated, the resulting opening is oval in shape and the giving way of the tissues is mainly in one direction. It is, therefore, well to turn the blades in different directions in the canal, so as to dilate thoroughly all parts. With this instrument sufficient room may be always gained to admit of thorough curetting and provide for subsequent free drainage.

Sometimes the introduction of the finger is called for. Fortunately, this is not often required, for, except after an abortion or when the tissues are very much softened, it is a very difficult matter and not always satisfactory. Even if the finger is forced by the internal os, the contraction of the muscular ring is so firm that it benumbs the sense of touch and renders the recognition of the condition of the endometrium exceedingly difficult. In the unimpregnated uterus, or where the cavity of the womb has not been dilated by disease, there is not room for the end of the finger, and the method of dilatation by instruments, while it may be effectual at the internal os, leaves the cavity of the uterus practically untouched.

For these reasons it is a fortunate occurrence that the exploration of the interior of the uterus with the finger is seldom called for. The most common condition which demands it is the recognition of the presence of a small fibroid in the uterine wall, too small to be appreciated bimanually, or so situated that it does not materially alter the shape of the uterus as a whole. Such a tumor may give rise to hemorrhage, and the curette fail to give any evidence of its presence. With the finger, however, inside the uterus, it is possible to thoroughly palpate the uterine wall and fundus and appreciate any unusual thickness.

The best method of securing adequate dilatation, where it can be carried out, is forcible stretching under ether in the manner described, first with graduated dilators, then with Ellinger's powerful instrument, taking enough time to overcome the rigidity of the strong uterine muscles. This may be done on the side or on the back. Whichever position is used, there should be constant antiseptic irrigation, and, as this can be more satisfactorily carried out on the back with the patient on a Kelly's pad, that position is more generally used. When the dilatation seems sufficient, the forefinger of the left hand, having been rendered absolutely aseptic, should be carried into the uterine canal. Traction is made by an assistant on the anterior lip by means of a vulsellum forceps, while the fundus is grasped through the abdominal wall over the pubes with the operator's right hand and firmly pressed down upon the finger.

If the finger enters readily, the condition of the lining membrane should be quickly investigated, any roughness noted, polypi sought for, and the thickness of the various parts of the uterine wall be appreciated by the bimanual examination. This should be done immediately and with as much speed as is consistent with thoroughness, for the uterus contracts very quickly and the finger is either benumbed or forced out.

If the finger does not readily pass in, it is of little use to spend much time in forcing an entrance, as the tissues are too rigid to yield to the finger. It should be withdrawn and fresh dilatation with the instrument be tried.

In case repeated attempts at this fail, there is one procedure which may be tried,—namely, dilatation with tents. Tents have so deservedly fallen into disrepute that one hesitates to recommend them under any circumstances, but under the conditions above indicated their use is justified.

Given a case where the digital exploration of the interior of the uterus seems demanded, and dilatation with instruments has failed because of the rigidity of the tissues,—under those conditions, with the observance of proper precautions, tents may be used. The tents commonly employed are of three kinds,—sponge, laminaria, and tupelo. The first (sponge) should never under any circumstances be placed in the uterus, as there is too much danger of sepsis, and the difficulties can be overcome with those that are less dangerous.

Of the two kinds remaining, the laminaria (Fig. 47) are the smallest and smoothest and dilate the most in proportion to their size. Therefore, their use is indicated when there is a small canal, with great rigidity of the

FIG. 47.

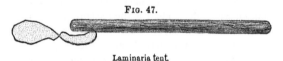

Laminaria tent.

os internum. A size as large as may be expected to go in without the use of too much force should be selected. The vagina should be thoroughly swabbed out with a 1 to 2000 solution of corrosive sublimate, and a pledget of cotton soaked in the same solution passed into the uterine canal and its walls disinfected. The tent should be thoroughly scrubbed with a brush dipped in the bichloride solution before introduction.

The anterior lip of the uterus is seized with a double hook and held firmly, while the tent is grasped with a pair of uterine forceps and carried well in through the internal os. Should it be forced out immediately, as is sometimes the case, a second smaller one may be carried in by its side, and the vagina then plugged with iodoform gauze. These tents may be left in from twelve to twenty-four hours, by which time they will have dilated to their full size, and under the same precautions as have been before described the exploration of the uterus may be carried out.

When the canal is patulous enough to admit a good-sized tupelo tent (Fig. 48) it has certain advantages. The surface is rougher, and it therefore holds better after it is introduced, and its expansive action is more

FIG. 48.

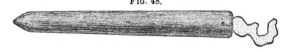

Tupelo tent.

gentle than that of the laminaria. A single large-sized one will give full dilatation. It has, too, the great advantage over the laminaria that it can be put through the dry sterilizer without injury, and thus be rendered more aseptic; hence where it can be employed it should be, being dipped into a bichloride solution just previous to introduction.

The pain, which is apt to be quite severe for a few hours at least, may be controlled by morphine, and it is, of course, absolutely necessary that the patient should remain in bed during the whole time that the tents are in position.

### GENERAL OUTLINES OF DIFFERENTIAL DIAGNOSIS.

In diseases of women more than in most branches of medicine the diagnosis is dependent upon the physical examination. The principal symptoms of which women complain are common to too many different affections to enable us to draw correct inferences from them as to the particular trouble which causes them; therefore our history must in the majority of cases be supplemented by an examination.

While the importance of the physical examination is thus emphasized, it is not for a moment intended to minimize the value of the information to be gained by a careful questioning of the patient and an attentive hearing of her own statement. The subjective symptoms can only be ascertained in this way, and the digital and instrumental examination serves the double purpose of interpreting and correcting the facts thus given and adding such information as the employment of the different senses furnishes.

The successful diagnostician in this department of medicine will be the man who recognizes the value of the patient's account of herself, both its exaggerations and its limitations, and who has so trained his senses that he is able to employ them to the best advantage in the physical examination. He must possess a good knowledge of human nature, especially important in dealing with women, keen judgment as regards the value of evidence, an accurate sense of touch, and skill in the use of instruments.

Having in this general way indicated the two methods of examination and shown their mutual interdependence, it is now our purpose to go a little more into detail, and indicate the value of the various symptoms of which the patient complains and of the conditions which our physical examination reveals. There are two classes of symptoms, subjective and objective: subjective, those of which the patient is conscious; objective, those which the physician can appreciate by his senses. The subjective symptoms may be direct, affecting the organ or organs which are the seat of the disease, or reflex, affecting other organs of the body at a distance.

These distinctions cannot, of course, always be closely maintained. Thus, the symptom leucorrhœa is both subjective—the patient being conscious of a feeling of moisture—and objective when the discharge escapes from the vagina and is seen. Still, it may in a general way serve as a basis for their consideration.

*Pain.*—Of the purely subjective symptoms the most common is pain. It is usually the first to attract the woman's attention and lead her to consult a physician, and is often the most obstinate to treat and the last to disappear; at the same time it is of comparatively little value as an aid to a differential diagnosis. There are comparatively few kinds of pain, either as regards character, intensity, or time of occurrence, which can be of use in distinguishing various forms of disease. Physicians are too vague in their inquiries, and women are too unobserving or ignorant to help much. We will briefly mention the more common kinds of pain complained of, and note their significance as far as they have any.

First as regards character. Most women, when questioned as to the character of the pain of which they are conscious, will describe it as a dull heavy ache. This is especially true of backache, which is probably the most common form we meet with. So, too, of pain low down over the pubes and across the lower abdomen. This is also the kind of pain felt in the groins and the thighs and hips. Such pain, whether constant or only supervening on exercise or after fatigue, suggests some chronic trouble,—congestion, displacement, laceration, or remote results of acute inflammation. Even the chronic ache may vary in character, and in consequence afford us some suggestion of value. Thus, pain in the back, confined to a small area at about the junction of the lumbar and sacral vertebræ, and of a more burning character, is suggestive of some trouble with the cervix uteri, such as endocervicitis, more often laceration, rarely cancer. A bearing-down pain, or feeling of weight and pressure as it is described, when less pronounced, is caused by a lack of harmony between the uterus and its supports, —an increase in the weight of one, or a loss of integrity in the other.

Sharp pain is usually symptomatic of some acute condition, either inflammatory or of neuralgic origin, or due to spasmodic contraction of muscular fibres. If in the abdomen and associated with fever, it suggests localized or general peritonitis; if without fever, either neuralgia or a peculiar hyperæsthetic affection of the abdominal walls that simulates peritonitis. If coincident with the menstrual flow, it has a special name, dysmenorrhœa, which, however, throws no light upon its causation.

When we come to consider pain as regards its intensity, we are met at the outset with the difficulty that, owing to the personal equation, it is impossible to form any estimate in a given case of how severe the pain really is. This is notably true of women. There are no fixed rules for judging whether a pain of which a patient complains is sufficiently intense to warrant the expression of suffering or to effect the disability which she is laboring under, or whether the nervous system is so reduced in strength below the normal standard that it reacts to a really slight stimulus. Two factors will help us to form a correct judgment in this matter: first, the relation of pain to other symptoms of which the woman complains; and, second, her manifestation of pain when she is not being noticed, or when her attention is distracted from herself. Severe pain is rarely present as the sole symptom; there are usually accompanying symptoms which should be more or less consistent with the complaint of pain that is made. The desire for sympathy or a tendency towards hysteria, which is so common with women, will lead them either to manufacture a pain out of whole cloth or to exaggerate a mild one.

The seat of pain is a symptom of more value. Something has been said on this point when speaking of the character of the pain. When situated in the lower abdomen,—a very common complaint,—if in the median line, just above the pubes, it usually indicates some uterine trouble; if at the sides, just above Poupart's ligament, in what is recognized even by the laity as the ovarian region, it suggests trouble with the appendages. Formerly all such pain was called ovarian. With our more intimate knowledge of the pathology of the appendages and the diseases which affect them, we know that pain in that region *may* be from ovarian disease, but is more likely to be tubal in its origin, and is quite likely to have its seat in the peritoneum which invests the pelvic organs. Pain in the back has been spoken of. Pain in the hips and thighs extending as far as the knee is usually a symptom of pressure in the pelvis.

From what has been said of pain, it will be seen that though it is the most common symptom of which women complain, yet, taking it all in all, by itself it throws very little light on the diagnosis.

*Disorders of Menstruation.*—The next most common group of symptoms relates to abnormalities of the menstrual function. These are amenorrhœa, oligomenorrhœa, menorrhagia, and dysmenorrhœa. Here we find rather more definite hints of value as to the causative trouble than was the case with pain. Let us examine them with a little more detail. Amenorrhœa is a very common complaint. In the primitive form it has to do with young women in whom this function has not appeared, and who are either suffering in some way to suggest that its non-appearance may be the cause, or, while free from suffering, have so far passed the age at which it usually appears as to excite suspicion that there may be some trouble. Here the differential diagnosis is of importance, as upon it depends the question whether a physical examination is necessary or not. If there are absolutely no symptoms, especially if there have been no abdominal pains occurring monthly, the case may for the time being be treated by general tonic and hygienic measures. If there is suffering, especially of a periodical character, a simple examination to determine the presence or absence of any abnormality, such as absence of the uterus or atresia of the vagina, should be made.

Acquired amenorrhœa has a variety of obvious causes which should be carefully considered, and which the patient's history may throw light upon. The most frequent of these is pregnancy; and as it is often for the patient's supposed interest to conceal this condition, it should not be overlooked. Atrophy of the uterus following child-birth, change of climate, especially when accompanied by a sea-voyage, and obesity are other frequent causes of amenorrhœa.

Oligomenorrhœa is necessarily a relative term, and its true significance is not so readily appreciated. It seems to depend upon general conditions much more than upon local. It is, therefore, of little value in differential diagnosis. It is, of course, often the preliminary stage of acquired amenorrhœa, and as such is significant of the same conditions.

Menorrhagia varies in importance as a symptom with the time of life at which it occurs. It is not at all uncommon in young girls, and is then usually an expression of some general condition incident to adolescence. It may be caused by anæmia, which is in turn the result of overstimulation of the brain, lack of exercise, and neglect of proper hygienic conditions, or it may occur in apparently healthy girls, presumably a symptom of local congestion. It is rarely the result of gross local pathological changes: hence a physical examination is rarely càlled for. Usually general tonic and hygienic measures suffice for its relief.

In middle life, especially after marriage and child-bearing, other causes of menorrhagia develop. Prominent among these are endometritis, fibro-myomata and polypi of the uterus, and general debility. Which of these is the cause must be decided by a physical examination. In general it may be affirmed that the menorrhagia due to endometritis is more apt to show itself by prolonged menstruation, and that due to fibroids or polypi by a profuse flow more hemorrhagic in its character.

Menorrhagia occurring at or about the time of the menopause, while possibly dependent upon that change and a symptom of it, is yet so sus-picious of either fibroid or malignant disease, that a vaginal examination should never be neglected.

Closely connected with menorrhagia, and dependent upon very much the same conditions and open to the same interpretations, is metrorrhagia, or hemorrhage from the uterus occurring between the menstrual periods. This, however, is so abnormal that the thorough investigation of the cause should never be neglected. Endometritis and fibroids may give rise to this symptom in their later stages. To them must be added as causes pregnancy and its complications, and malignant growths. These latter are apt to be accompanied by metrorrhagia from the beginning, while the former usually begin with menorrhagia. Other symptoms must be taken into considera-tion in distinguishing between these various causes, the presence of a tumor, the usual signs of pregnancy, and the occurrence of pain and foul discharge being significant of one or the other; but the physical examination must settle the question.

The last of the abnormalities of menstruation is dysmenorrhœa. This has been referred to when speaking of pain, but may be considered a little more fully here. The time at which the pain occurs is of some diagnostic importance. If it comes on a day or two before the appearance of the flow, it is more likely to be due to some general disturbance of the circula-tion or nervous supply of the pelvic organs, especially the ovaries or uterus, and may be usually characterized as neuralgic or congestive dysmenorrhœa. If it comes on with the flow, lasts for a day or two, and then ceases, it is usually due to some condition of the canal of the uterus, and is perhaps fairly well named obstructive dysmenorrhœa. A subdivision of this variety is where the flow is painless at its onset, but as it becomes more profuse shows a tendency to clot, and the efforts of the uterus to expel the clots are accompanied by severe cramp-like pains. This may be called the spasmodic form. The character of the pain is not so suggestive. Almost all kinds are accompanied by pain in the back and lower abdomen and bearing down, the congestive being almost wholly of this character, and, as a rule, milder. In the obstructive form the pain is usually very much more severe, more concentrated in the uterus, and accompanied by reflex symptoms, as nausea and vomiting. The agony is sometimes intense, the patient being almost thrown into convulsions. The most common physical condition found on examination in these cases is anteflexion of the body or the neck or of both. The next most common cause is an extremely sensitive condition of the internal os, sometimes accompanied by endocervicitis, sometimes not.

*Leucorrhœa.*—The next symptom which we have to consider is leucorrhœa, under which head we include all discharges from the vagina except blood. Very little of value can be drawn from the statements of patients, as women differ widely in their estimate of what constitutes a discharge. Some women are rendered miserable by the slightest suspicion of moisture about the vulva, while others have well-marked leucorrhœa without noticing it at all. Vaginal leucorrhœa is thin, creamy, non-viscid, and, as a rule, not very profuse. If due to acute vaginitis, it is accompanied by heat and swelling of the vulva and vagina, and, when gonorrhœal in origin, not infrequently by urethritis. When chronic, the heat and redness disappear, and the thin creamy discharge sometimes changes to a thick smegma-like secretion which clings to the walls of the vagina.

Cervical leucorrhœa, if merely an abnormal amount of the natural secretion of the glands, is clear like the white of an egg, viscid, and non-irritating. A thick, opaque, or yellowish discharge which makes its appearance in clumps at intervals, often only when some straining occurs, as during micturition or defecation, or on cough or other exertion, is characteristic of endocervical catarrh. When the endometrium is affected the discharge is usually thinner than where it is purely cervical, is very apt to be of a brownish color, due to some admixture with blood, and may have a slight odor. When the secretion from the uterus is markedly purulent it suggests tubal disease.

A watery discharge is usually associated with one of three conditions,—pregnancy with escape of liquor amnii, or hydatiform mole, fibroid of the uterus, or hydro-salpinx with periodical escape of the contents of the tube. The differential diagnosis between these conditions must be made from the history of the case and the physical examination.

A foul-smelling discharge may arise from the retention of the normal secretions. This may occur as a result of atresia following operations; more frequently it denotes either the decomposition of material, as the retained products of conception, or the breaking down of abnormal growths, such as fibroids, or malignant disease.

*Enlargements.*—A patient very quickly becomes conscious of any enlargement of the external genitals. If acute and accompanied by pain, it is most often a swelling of the vulvo-vaginal gland, either a cyst or an abscess, and occupies the lower part of the labium majus of the affected side. Other swellings of the external genitals may be hæmatoma of the vulva, to which the history will clearly point, hernia, chronic hypertrophy of one or both labia majora due to syphilis, and primary epithelioma of the clitoris or vulva. Swellings of the vagina are due to a prolapsed uterus presenting at the vulva, or prolapse of the anterior or posterior vaginal walls, or a foreign growth, such as a fibroid polypus, which has become extruded into the vagina, or rarely an extensive epithelioma of the cervix which has filled up the vagina and can be seen at the vulva. Moderate enlargements of the uterus are not recognized by the patient as such. The symptoms to which they give rise are an increased feeling of weight in the pelvis, backache, pain in the thighs with interference with locomotion, increased amount of leucorrhœa, and frequency of micturition. These are the local symptoms. Quite as common and as important are the reflex symptoms to which uterine enlargements give rise—nausea and vomiting, headache, sensitiveness and swelling of the breasts, flatulence, constipation, and general nervous disturbances. These are often the only symptoms, the local manifestations being absent. The most common causes of enlargement of the uterus are pregnancy, subinvolution and chronic metritis, fibroids and malignant disease. The history and physical examination will enable one to decide between these. Abdominal enlargements have been spoken of in treating of the methods of examination. The rules for deciding between the more common causes—ascites, fibroid and ovarian tumors—were there given in detail.

*Disturbances of Function.*—Those of menstruation have already been discussed. There remain to be mentioned coitus, defecation, and micturition.

Painful coitus is called dyspareunia. The most common cause of this is such extreme sensitiveness of the introitus vaginæ that intercourse is impossible. In such cases the slightest touch is followed by severe cramps and intense pain, and the examination with the finger is often impossible This is characterized as vaginismus, and has various causes. Attempts at intercourse may also be painful where there is no vaginismus present. A very thick and rigid hymen may present an insuperable obstacle to intercourse. So, too, an abnormally small vulva and vagina of the infantile type may be a cause. Congenital malformations, such as atresia of the hymen or vagina, must also be taken into consideration. In the absence of all these conditions, coitus may be possible, but is accompanied by pain, which is then usually due to abnormal sensitiveness of the uterus, its appendages, or surrounding tissues. What special condition is present in the individual case can only be determined by a vaginal exploration. To complete the subject, it is only necessary to allude to those cases where coitus is followed, not by local pain, but by general nervous phenomena,—cramps, fainting, headache, palpitation of the heart, and nausea.

Disturbances of the function of defecation are very common. Constipation may be said to be almost the rule with women, and a more precise knowledge of its various forms will be of material aid in judging its cause and applying appropriate measures for its relief.

The term itself is of varying significance among women. Some understand by it a difficult movement, even though it occurs every day and at a regular time. Another woman would not call herself constipated, even though she did not have an evacuation for two or three days, provided that it occurred then without the use of medicine. Still another considers that her bowels act naturally, even though she is obliged to use some artificial means every day, provided such means are effectual.

This lack of precision among the laity is supplemented by a failure on the part of the profession to discriminate between the different kinds of constipation. There is one form which depends upon a sluggish condition of the bowels, due perhaps to a loss of muscular power in the walls of the intestines or to inefficient innervation. In this form the bowels fail to propel their contents along, and the rectum remains empty. There is, therefore, no desire to have a movement. There is another form where the trouble seems to lie in the upper part of the rectum. Fæces accumulate in the descending colon and the sigmoid flexure, but fail to enter the rectum. The cause is usually some pressure within the pelvis or the rectum, due to a displacement of the uterus or to some enlargement either of the uterus or its appendages, or to adhesions and consequent immobility of any of the pelvic organs. Still a third form is that where the bowels do their work properly and the fæces are satisfactorily carried along to the rectum, but the expulsive power seems to be at fault. The patient cannot use force enough to expel the contents of the rectum, unless the bowels are very loose. The most common cause of this is a weakening of the muscular structures which constitute the floor of the pelvis by lacerations during parturition. It is not necessary that the perineum, as such, should be torn if the muscular attachments are sundered or even only stretched, this loss of power may result. A relaxed condition of the vaginal walls and pelvic outlet may occasionally occur in women who have never borne children, in connection with general debility, with the same result.

The last special form of constipation is that associated with affections of the anus, such as hemorrhoids, fissure, or fistula, where the pain that is sure to be occasioned by the act of defecation prevents the proper relaxation of the sphincter.

This last form of constipation suggests the second functional disturbance of which we should take cognizance,—viz., pain. Painful defecation is most often due to troubles of the anus, as spoken of above. Not infrequently it causes pain higher up, first generally in the lower abdomen, and second in certain organs, such as the womb, or one of the ovaries, most often the left. The cause of this pain is sometimes obscure, in other cases it seems to be occasioned by the pressure of the fæces upon a displaced and sensitive ovary, or a swollen tube, or even upon the body of the retro-displaced womb.

In a few cases it seems as though the pressure against the sensitive cervix where it impinges upon the rectum has been sufficient to evoke pain. Sometimes the mere act of straining is followed by discomfort throughout the pelvis which may in some cases persist for hours.

To determine which of these various forms of constipation is present, a thorough examination of the pelvic organs by the vagina or rectum, often by both, is necessary.

The disturbances of the function of micturition which are suggestive are frequency of the act and pain accompanying it. Sometimes frequent micturition is merely a habit, and expressive of the nervous temperament of the woman. Perhaps the most common cause is pressure on the bladder from a displaced or enlarged uterus, or some growth or swelling which prevents the proper vesical distention. Irritation or inflammation of the urethra, especially if it has extended to the neck of the bladder, is an exceedingly common cause, and cystitis is, of course, always accompanied by this disturbance of function. Alteration in the character of the urine by which it becomes irritating even to a healthy mucous membrane may cause frequency of the act.

Pain accompanying micturition may for purposes of diagnosis be considered as occurring before, during, or after the act. If before, it is usually symptomatic of some affection of the bladder itself which may extend from the bladder side so as to involve the neck, in which case the very beginning, as marked by the relaxation of the sphincter, is painful. If a little later in time of occurrence, giving the sensation of an intense burning at the vesical neck and running down the urethra, it suggests fissure or ulceration of the neck of the bladder, with or without urethritis. If the pain is felt only as the urine passes from the urethra, some cause at its mouth should be looked for, as a caruncle, ulcerative process, polypi, or prolapse of the mucous membrane. Irritation about the vulva may cause pain during or after micturition from the urine trickling over the sensitive surface. The closure of the sphincter vesicæ at the end of the act may give rise to severe cramp-like pain, just as its relaxation at the beginning. Examination of the urine will often throw light on obscure cases.

*Reflex Symptoms.*—The last set of symptoms which we have to consider in this connection opens a very wide field of investigation. They are the reflex symptoms, those which affect other organs than those primarily the seat of the trouble. It may be truly said that there is scarcely an organ of the body which may not be and is not sometimes functionally disordered as a result of disease of the pelvic organs. Even the eye and the ear are not exempt from this law. Sometimes these symptoms are wholly a result of the pre-existing pelvic conditions; sometimes they have been present before and are only aggravated by it. In either case it becomes the difficult task of the physician to solve the problem of the mutual relationship of the

local and the general symptoms, or of the pelvic lesion to the remote manifestation. Sometimes this is not so difficult. One most obvious example
of a reflex symptom directly dependent upon the pelvic condition is the
nausea of pregnancy, but the greater part of such phenomena are much
more obscure. All that will be attempted here is in a very general way to
point out a few of the more common reflex symptoms we meet with in the
course of our every-day experience.

The digestive system is perhaps the most easily affected; certainly
patients complain most often of the various aberrations of function to which
the stomach and bowels are subject. The nausea of pregnancy has been
alluded to, but this symptom may be associated with other pelvic troubles.
This is especially true of those conditions which are characterized by an increased size of the uterus, such as myomata or chronic metritis. Diseases of
the ovary may be accompanied by nausea, and the nausea of dysmenorrhœa
illustrates again the close connection between the uterus and the stomach.

Other disturbances of function are very common. The various forms
of dyspepsia, flatulency, and constipation or diarrhœa need only to be
mentioned to be recognized as the most frequent accompaniments of uterine
disease.

The circulatory system has its share of reflex symptoms, which express
themselves in palpitation, dizziness, fainting, tingling or numbness, especially in the extremities, flushing incident to the menopause, and other
irregularities of the circulation.

The manifestations on the part of the nervous system are manifold.
Neuralgia in various parts of the body, headaches of various forms, cramps
and pareses, and sleeplessness indicate but in a general way some of the
forms in which pelvic disease may show itself in remote portions of the
body.

Not less striking are the mental disturbances which accompany the diseases we are treating of. Irritability, loss of self-control, from its incipient
stages up to well-marked hysteria, inability to concentrate the attention,
forgetfulness and confusion of thought, are a few of the most evident manifestations.

The foregoing brief sketch of the general forms of reflex symptoms
merely enumerates what may occur. The important point for the physician
to decide in the given case is how far such symptoms are the cause of
or dependent upon the so-called diseases of women. This is often very
difficult, especially when the local symptoms are either absent or so overshadowed by the general and remote symptoms as to be overlooked. The
innate skill of the practitioner and a wide experience show their real value
here.

Certain almost axiomatic truths may be here set down for our guidance.
Where pelvic symptoms have preceded the reflex manifestations, even
though the former may have nearly or wholly disappeared, it is safe to
suspect the local trouble as the cause. This is more apt to be the case if

the first trouble followed some acute affection of the pelvic organs, as
gonorrhœa, a miscarriage, an attack of pelvic peritonitis, or a difficult or
abnormal labor.    Again, if the reflex symptoms are aggravated at the times
of menstruation out of proportion to the normal effect upon the nervous
system, it is sufficient to warrant the supposition that the uterus or its
appendages may be at fault.

If the ordinary treatment for the various functional disturbances of
which we have been speaking fails, it is the part of prudence to look to
some other organ or set of organs for the source of the difficulty; and there
is none which is so likely to be the cause as the sexual organs.

If we find evidences of trouble, such as chronic inflammations, enlargements, lacerations, disturbances of function, it is our duty, even though we
may not be able to trace the connection between such affections and the
symptoms present, to treat and, if possible, to cure such difficulties, feeling
sure that, if we cannot relieve all the symptoms, we have contributed to the
patient's well-being by rectifying what we have actually found out of order,
and have so far improved her condition that she is more likely to recover
permanently.

# CHAPTER II.

## GYNÆCOLOGICAL TECHNIQUE.

BY HUNTER ROBB, M.D.

### I.

IMPORTANCE TO THE SURGEON OF A BACTERIOLOGICAL TRAINING—SEPSIS AND WOUND-INFECTION—MICRO-ORGANISMS CONCERNED—ASEPSIS—ANTISEPSIS.

THE number of those who do not believe it necessary to observe stringent precautions in operative surgery or who are content to confine themselves to methods which have been proved to be faulty is now, fortunately, very small, and is diminishing every day, so that we may safely say that every prominent surgeon is now working on practically the same lines, being anxious to discover and to carry out any measure which promises to aid the speedy healing of the wounds which he makes and to obviate the danger of infection.

Among the brilliant results to be obtained from the study of bacteriology, none seems at the present time more important than the establishment on a scientific basis of a thorough technique for surgical operations.

It will obviously be impossible for a surgeon to have any fixed rules by which he may be guided unless he has first obtained a true conception of the meaning of the terms sepsis, asepsis, and antisepsis, and is determined at all costs to apply his knowledge practically to his every-day work. While the majority of our operators of to-day may theoretically appreciate the dangers of wound-infection, and have read or heard of the various means that are to be taken to prevent it, there are comparatively few who are consistent in the technique which they employ.

It is by no means unusual to hear a surgeon remark that he has performed an "aseptic" operation, or that he always operates "under strictly aseptic precautions," when his technique, as actually observed by one trained in bacteriology, is found to be wofully defective.

The practical scientific application of an aseptic and antiseptic technique can be thoroughly carried out only by observing every even the most minute detail the utility of which has been proved by bacteriological experiment. In order to become familiar with these details, and to be able to appreciate them fully, the surgeon should have at least an elementary training in bacteriology. If he has not had this training,—and, unfortunately, it has not as yet been possible to secure it at the majority of medical schools, —he must accept and carry out in his work principles which have been laid down by those who have had the opportunity of submitting their methods to the test of bacteriological criticism. Any one who has been trained in a bacteriological laboratory will have exalted ideas of *surgical cleanliness*, and cannot fail to see the many inconsistencies that occur during the majority of operations. While these inconsistencies may to many appear trifling, in reality they are only too often responsible for the introduction of infectious material into the wound. One would think that an operator, after taking every precaution to render his own hands surgically clean, would avoid bringing them in contact subsequently with objects which have not been previously sterilized, and yet it is by no means uncommon to see those who are regarded as " careful men" touching with their hands the face or hair, or permitting them to come in contact with some non-sterile article—such, for example, as a blanket which protects the patient— just prior to or during an operation, and proceeding with their work without thoroughly cleansing the hands again. If such errors in technique be committed by the operator himself, he can scarcely expect his assistants and nurses to exercise proper precautions.

I remember seeing a surgeon leave the operating-table, while performing an abdominal section, to pick up an unsterilized instrument which he wished to bend at a certain angle and employ in order better to expose the parts. In doing this he used as a support a table and a chair that happened to be near at hand, but which were unsterilized. After having bent the instrument to the desired shape, the surgeon proceeded to employ it immediately without making any attempt to sterilize either it or his hands. I have also seen a nurse, who was assisting with the handling of the sponges at an abdominal section, take her handkerchief from her pocket, wipe her nose with it, and at once continue with her duty of passing the sponges to the assistant surgeon. On another occasion I saw a surgeon open an abdomen, and, after himself examining the structures of the pelvic cavity, invite two professional brethren who were looking on to do the same, and they were actually permitted to introduce their hands into the wound after having simply washed them for a minute or two with soap and water in a soiled basin. At another time an assistant, after drawing a ligature between his teeth, proceeded to thread the needle with it for the surgeon to use in the abdominal wound. Some surgeons have even been guilty of holding the scalpel between the teeth in the course of an operation.

It would hardly be necessary to mention such glaring instances of faulty technique were it not for the fact that errors as bad as these have been observed in men who are considered leaders, and to whose lot it falls to instruct others in surgery. While the surgical judgment and skill of such men may be undoubted, the technique they employ is dangerous and pernicious. Even after we have become thoroughly imbued with the importance of

aseptic work, and have made the most careful preparations before our operations, the technique will never be perfect unless we have schooled ourselves
to provide against the unforeseen dangers which are constantly turning up
in the operating-room. Every operator of experience, no matter how conscientious and careful, has met with fatal cases in his practice due to faulty
methods, and has had inflammation with pus-formation at or near the site
of the wound which he has made.

He who is thoroughly conversant with the conditions which underlie
suppuration in wounds and septic processes generally, knows only too well
how many are the loop-holes for infection, and to him it seems really
remarkable that such cases do not occur more frequently. It is not improbable, especially in conditions of lowered resistance where the cells and
tissue-fluids of the body do not exercise their normal germicidal power, or
do so only in a feeble way, that infection may occur, even though all possible precautions have been taken by the surgeon and his assistants. Experiments have shown that no method has yet been discovered by which
the skin can be rendered absolutely sterile, and that the cutaneous glands
contain, even after the most careful disinfection of the surface, micro-
organisms which in a proper "soil" are capable of giving rise to inflammation and suppuration. Though it may be true, as has been contended
by good men, that every wound made by the surgeon contains micro-
organisms, we may assume that under ordinary circumstances the resisting
powers of the patient will be sufficient to prevent their growth and development. Experience, however, has taught us that there are several kinds
of bacteria which under certain conditions possess such virulence, that
when introduced into the tissues even of a perfectly healthy individual they
are capable of setting up violent local or general infections. And it is
only right that every surgeon shall do everything in his power to prevent the ingress of such bacteria. While admitting then that infection
following an operation must, with our present knowledge, be sometimes
attributed to a lowered systemic resistance and to no fault on the part of
the operator or his assistants, it must be understood that this is a very
rare occurrence, and that in nearly every septic case a rigid analysis of the
technique employed will bring to light some sin of omission or of com-
mission to account for it. I believe that a perfect technique can ultimately be attained by submitting every step to the test of bacteriological
examination, and the surgeon who works on these lines will, *cæteris paribus*, undoubtedly obtain the best results in his own operations, and, what is
perhaps hardly less important, will be able by his teaching and example
to inculcate in others principles by the adoption of which much loss of life
may be prevented.

That some surgeons do not seem to pay much attention to a careful
technique and yet obtain good results is no argument against the carrying
out of thoroughly scientific procedures. As a matter of fact, a careful
investigation of their results and those of their followers compared with

those of aseptic surgeons and their students will, if a sufficient number of parallel cases be taken, certainly show the inferiority of the older methods. Statistics showing uniformly good results from operations in which no precautions were taken will usually be found to be based on too limited a number of cases to be of much value.

The term *sepsis*, or *septic infection*, includes nearly all the surgical infections, general or local, resulting from bacterial invasion. The symptoms are due, as a rule, not so much to the direct effect of the bacteria themselves as to the action of their chemical products. When the bacteria have gained entrance into the general circulation and have multiplied there (and several varieties are capable of doing this), we have a general blood-infection which often proves fatal. With or without extensive multiplication of the micro-organisms in the blood, the system may be overwhelmed with the bacterial poisons. This condition is called *acute septicæmia*. Localization of pyogenic bacteria in the organs, especially when they have been transported there by infectious emboli, gives rise to multiple abscess-formation. This condition is called *pyæmia*. These terms are, of course, only relative, and it is customary to speak of infections in which the two conditions are combined as cases of *septico-pyæmia*.

Under the head of *local infections* we at the present day group together all those so-called "accidents" which befall wounds : suppuration, traumatic fever, hospital gangrene, wound-diphtheria, and erysipelas. All of these, though met with much less often than of old, are still occasionally seen. The rarity of their occurrence is to be attributed to the improvement in operative technique and the less frequent infection of wounds. The phenomena resulting from the absorption into the general circulation of the products appearing after the local growth of micro-organisms, especially putrefactive forms, have been included under the term *sapræmia* or *toxæmia*, but it is not possible to make any sharp distinction between sapræmia and septicæmia. The importance of recognizing clearly the distinction between a purely local infection and a general infection of the blood and organs with bacteria will be easily understood. In the former case the symptoms produced are in direct proportion to the amount of poison absorbed, and, if this absorption has not been too great, they will all disappear with the subsidence of the local infection. In a general infection, on the other hand, fresh poison is being constantly produced by the bacteria distributed everywhere through the body, so that local therapeutic measures can then be of no avail.

General septicæmia, or pyæmia, may be set up by almost any of the micro-organisms which have pyogenic properties,—*i.e.*, which are capable of giving rise to local suppuration. The organisms most frequently met with in surgical experience are the *staphylococcus pyogenes aureus*, the *streptococcus pyogenes*, and the *bacterium coli commune*. Less frequently we have to deal with the *staphylococcus epidermidis albus*, the *staphylococcus pyogenes albus*, the *staphylococcus pyogenes citreus*, the *gonococcus of Neisser*, the

FIG. 1.

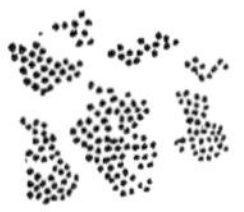

Staphylococcus pyogenes aureus

FIG. 2

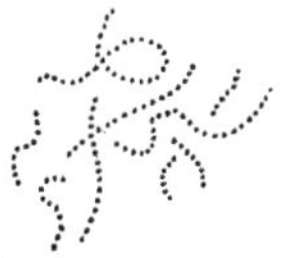

Streptococcus pyogenes.

FIG. 3.

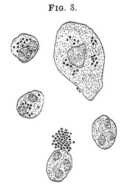

Gonococcus.

FIG. 4

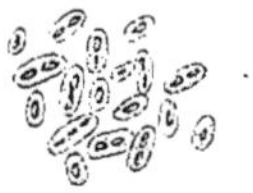

Micrococcus lanceolatus

FIG. 5.

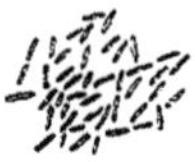

Bacillus coli communis.

FIG. 6.

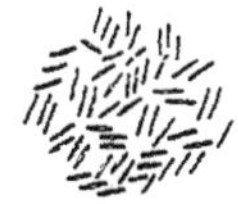

Bacillus pyocyaneus.

· FIG. 7.

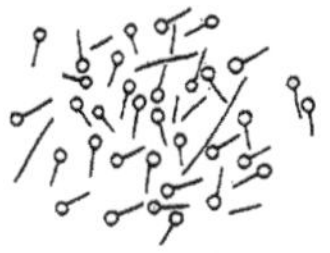

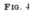

Bacillus tetani.

FIG 8.

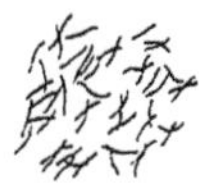

Bacillus tuberculosis.

*bacillus of green pus* (bacillus pyocyaneus), and the *micrococcus lanceolatus* (diplococcus pneumoniæ).

It will be as well, perhaps, to describe briefly the principal micro-organisms which concern us in our work, and especially the *pyogenic* bacteria. The forms chiefly concerned in suppurative processes are cocci. Of these the staphylococcus, of which several varieties have been isolated, distinguished by differences both in their chromogenic properties and in their pathogenic power, has been found more frequently than any other associated with acute phlegmons.

The *staphylococcus pyogenes aureus* (Ogston, Rosenbach, *et al.*), or *golden staphylococcus*, is the most important form for the surgeon, and is more common than any other. It is widely distributed in nature, its presence having been repeatedly demonstrated upon the skin of healthy persons, in the secretions of the mouth, beneath the finger-nails, in the air, especially in that of hospital wards, in the water, and elsewhere.

It can thus be easily understood how readily it can come in contact with the field of operation. The cocci grow in grape-like bunches, but in the tissues are also seen in pairs or in groups of four. (Fig. 1.) They stain well in the ordinary aniline dyes, and also by Gram's method.

The staphylococcus aureus grows well on all the culture media of the laboratory, and forms, especially when allowed to grow slowly with free access of air, large golden-yellow masses.

Its pathogenic power is variable, some varieties being much more virulent than others. Its pyogenic properties for human beings have been clearly proved by the experiments of Garré, who rubbed into the uninjured skin of his left forearm a pure culture of this organism. Four days afterwards a large carbuncle, which was surrounded by isolated furuncles, appeared at the site of the inoculation. The inflammation thus established ran the usual course, and it was only after several weeks that the skin healed over completely. Seventeen scars remained as a lasting proof of the success of the experiment.

When cultures of this coccus are injected into the vein of a rabbit's ear, the animal dies after a certain period of time (which varies according to the virulence of the particular culture used), with symptoms of acute septicæmia, and at the autopsy necroses or small abscesses are found in the various organs.

In human beings this organism has been isolated from suppurating foci of all kinds and in all situations. It is the most frequent cause of superficial and deep abscesses as well as of acute osteomyelitis, and has often been recognized as the infectious agent in acute ulcerative endocarditis and general septicæmia following operations or childbirth.

The *staphylococcus pyogenes albus*, while resembling the aureus in form, can be distinguished from it in that it grows as a white coating on the culture media, and moreover is possessed of less virulence. It has in some instances been found as the only micro-organism present in acute abscesses, but, as a rule, it is associated with other pyogenic cocci, most frequently with the staphylococcus pyogenes aureus.

The *staphylococcus epidermidis albus* is so called because it is always present, even under normal conditions, in the human skin. According to Welch, it is often found in parts of the epidermis deeper than can be reached by any known method of cutaneous disinfection save the application of heat, and he therefore regards it as a nearly constant inhabitant of the epidermis. This coccus resembles very closely the staphylococcus pyogenes albus, and is distinguished from it only by minor cultural differences and by its lower virulence. It has frequently been found in wounds the healing of which did not appear to be at all delayed; but experiments have proved that it sometimes causes suppuration along the line of the stitches and in the track of a drainage-tube. In a series of forty-five laparotomy wounds examined by Dr. Ghriskey and myself, where every aseptic precaution had been observed, bacteria were found in thirty-one, or sixty-nine per cent. of the whole; in only fourteen were the results of the cultures negative. In nineteen cases we found the staphylococcus epidermidis albus, in five the staphylococcus pyogenes aureus, in six the bacterium coli commune, and in three only the streptococcus pyogenes.

Cultures made also in a large number of cases from the hands and from the surface of the abdomen showed that, even after the application of the different methods recommended for surface disinfection, the staphylococcus epidermidis albus still remained, and that, too, in such a condition as to be capable of developing on the ordinary media.

The *staphylococcus pyogenes citreus* (Passet) is characterized by its lemon-yellow growth on agar-agar. It has been found alone in abscesses, and must be looked upon as a pyogenic micro-organism, although it occurs much more rarely than any of the other forms.

The *streptococcus pyogenes* grows in chains consisting of from four to ten or more cocci, each individual coccus being somewhat larger than those seen in cultures of the staphylococcus. (Fig. 2.) This organism stains well by all the ordinary methods. In culture media it grows very differently from the staphylococcus, forming, as a rule, minute pin-point colonies. The streptococcus is one of the most important micro-organisms with which the surgeon has to deal. It has long been known that erysipelatous inflammations are due to the so-called *streptococcus erysipelatosus;* it is doubtful, however, whether this coccus can be distinguished from the ordinary streptococcus pyogenes. In fact, the differentiation of streptococci into distinct species or varieties has thus far met with little success. The streptococcus is found sometimes in acute abscesses, but not so frequently as the staphylococcus pyogenes aureus, with which it is often associated in acute suppurative processes.

External inflammations due to the streptococcus are characterized especially by their spreading character and erysipelatous redness. The streptococcus pyogenes is one of the most frequent causes of post-operative peritonitis. It has been proved to be the etiological factor in many cases of ulcerative endocarditis as well as of acute septicæmia in human beings, and it is a well-known fact that the pseudo-membranous anginas complicating scarlet fever and measles are, as a rule, due to this organism. It has been found in some forms of acute broncho-pneumonia, sometimes in acute pleurisy and empyema, and occasionally in acute osteomyelitis. Comparatively recent researches have shown an interesting relation to exist between the streptococcus pyogenes and the different forms of puerperal infection. Döderlein has shown that in the pathological secretions from the vagina immense numbers of organisms, and generally streptococci, are present. His work was based upon the study of the vaginal secretions from nearly two hundred women, about one-half of which were found to be abnormal; in ten per cent. of the pathological secretions he was able to demonstrate the presence of the streptococcus pyogenes; inoculation experiments proved that in at least fifty per cent. of these the organism was pathogenic for animals.

It is not difficult, then, to understand how after labor, when the parts are wounded, organisms can enter the circulation and give rise to a general infection, the infectious agent being not infrequently the streptococcus pyogenes. Clivio and Monti have demonstrated the presence of streptococci in five cases of puerperal inflammation of the peritoneum. Czerniewski found the same organism in the lochia of thirty-three out of eighty-one women suffering from puerperal fever, while in those of fifty-seven healthy women he was able to find it only once. In ten fatal cases he demonstrated its presence in the organs of the body after death. Such observations as these, and many more might be cited, are sufficient to impress upon us the importance of preventing the access of the streptococcus to open wounds. The organism is of very wide distribution, and it is only strange that more patients in surgical and obstetrical practice do not become infected by it. It may be that in many cases, having led a saprophytic existence, it has lost some of its virulence, and is not capable of setting up pathological processes unless it happens to enter a soil particularly suited for its development. Any one who has examined a drop of the fluid exudate from the abdominal cavity in a case of streptococcus peritonitis, and has seen the myriads of cocci present in a single microscopic field, will appreciate somewhat the developmental power of this organism.

From what has been said, the danger of going from a case of erysipelas or of streptococcus phlegmon to a surgical operation or an obstetrical case will be sufficiently evident. Even with every antiseptic precaution more or less danger will be incurred, and one should never take the risk unless it is absolutely unavoidable. To go to such a case without thorough disinfection would be criminal.

The *micrococcus gonorrhœæ*, or *gonococcus*, was discovered by Neisser in 1879. It is found in the gonorrhœal discharge and in the secretions from the eyes in cases of gonorrhœal ophthalmia. According to some, it is always present in the joints in gonorrhœal rheumatism, and Councilman has demonstrated its presence in the muscular structures of the heart in a case of myocarditis following gonorrhœa. It is usually to be seen lying within the pus cells or attached to the surface of the epithelial cells. (Fig. 3.) Its specific character has been proved by inoculation into man. It is extremely difficult to grow outside of the body, and will not develop at all on the ordinary culture media. A mixture of human blood-serum and agar-agar has been found to give the best results.

Very considerable pathogenic importance has been attributed to this organism, and many gynæcologists are ready to assert that nearly all inflammations of the tubes and ovaries in women are due to its agency. That it does play an important part in the etiology of these affections there can be but little doubt, but whether so extreme an opinion is justifiable remains still uncertain. The clinical history of the patient is occasionally of some assistance, but in the vast majority of cases it is difficult to determine positively whether a pelvic abscess has or has not been preceded by an attack of gonorrhœa.

The *micrococcus lanceolatus* is also known as the *diplococcus pneumoniæ* and as the *pneumococcus*. It was discovered by Sternberg, and also independently by Pasteur. It has been studied thoroughly by Fraenkel, Weichselbaum, Weleh, and others.

It is an oval or lancet-shaped encapsulated diplococcus which often grows out into short chains, and has on that account been called by Gamaléia the streptococcus lanceolatus. (Fig. 4.) It is present normally, either with or without virulence, in the saliva of nearly all human beings, and is the cause of the acute septicæmia (sputum septicæmia) which frequently results in rabbits from the inoculation into them of small quantities of human sputum. It is the causative factor in acute lobar pneumonia and also in many cases of acute broncho-pneumonia, and has been recognized as having given rise to many of the acute inflammations of the serous membranes of the body,—pleuritis, pericarditis, peritonitis, endocarditis, and meningitis. It is now known to be a definite pus-producer, and has been found more than once in acute abscesses, in empyema, in suppurative otitis media, in quinsy, and in suppurative polyarthritis. It is a rapidly growing micro-organism, but is rather difficult to cultivate outside the body; it easily succumbs under adverse circumstances, and is extremely variable in its virulence.

The *bacillus coli communis*, or *bacterium coli commune*, is constantly present in the fæces of man and of the higher animals. It is a bacillus about one and four-tenths micro-millimetres in thickness and two or three micro-millimetres in length. (Fig. 5.) It is pathogenic for mice, rabbits, and guinea-pigs, and recently has been proved to be of great importance as an etiological factor in many of the inflammatory processes which occur in human beings. It appears to be the cause more often than any other organism of acute suppurative peritonitis, especially where there has been any communication between the lumen of the gastro-intestinal canal and the peritoneal cavity. It has also been found in localized abscesses, in suppurative infections of the liver and gall-bladder, in acute hemorrhagic pancreatitis, in cystitis, in pyelitis, and in other conditions. It is interesting to note that in the infections due to this organism and to the micrococcus lanceolatus we have to deal with pathological lesions resulting from the action of bacteria which we normally carry about with us in the exposed cavities of our bodies.

The *bacillus pyocyaneus* was first isolated in pure cultures by Gessard, in 1882, from pus having a green or blue color. (Fig. 6.) The organism is widely distributed, and " epidemics of blue pus" are not infrequently seen in hospitals. For some time it was thought not to possess any pathogenic power, but was believed to be simply a concomitant of the pyogenic bacteria. It is generally conceded now, however, that this micro-organism is pyogenic as well as chromogenic in its action, and it has been found to be capable of setting up a general infection in rabbits. Comparatively recently it has been demonstrated that general infection with the bacillus pyocyaneus sometimes occurs in human beings.

The *bacillus tetani* is an anaërobic bacillus discovered by Nicolaier, and first isolated in pure culture by Kitasato. (Fig. 7.) Its natural habitat is the soil. It is commonly present in the fæces of herbivorous animals. The organism is not a pus-producer, and does not become distributed over the body, but develops *in loco*, and it is to the absorption of its toxines into the general system that the symptoms of the disease are due. Fortunately, tetanus is a rare complication in gynæcological surgery.

The *bacillus tuberculosis* does not belong to the group of pyogenic organisms, and only rarely has to be considered in the infection of wounds. (Fig. 8.) As it is concerned, however, in a certain proportion of cases of peritonitis and in some diseases of the genitalia, the author has thought it advisable to mention it here.

The properties of this bacillus are so well known that it is unnecessary to describe here its history or its general characteristics. It may reach the peritoneum through the blood-current, from the intestines, or through the lymphatic channels from above. In the genitalia the organisms are deposited in the tissues, as a rule, from the blood-current, but it is believed that they may sometimes enter from below,—*e.g.*, by direct contagion during coition.

When, after an abdominal section, the patient has died without having exhibited the characteristic symptoms of septicæmia, the death has not usually been attributed to septic infection, but rather has been supposed to be due to "heart-failure," shock, pneumonia, suppression of the urine, or some other more or less satisfactory cause. But when a patient dies even less than twelve hours after an operation we cannot positively exclude sepsis as the cause of death until the fact has been proved by an autopsy made by a competent pathologist and bacteriologist.

Autopsies are on record at which none of the local lesions which attend septic inflammation were demonstrable to the naked eye, yet where the examination of cover-slips made from a small amount of fluid in the pelvic cavity showed that organisms were present in large numbers, and tubes of nutrient agar-agar inoculated with the same fluid gave the characteristic growths.

Experiments have shown that the poisoning resulting from a peritoneal infection is sometimes so intense as to cause death before the appearance of any marked local reaction in the peritoneum. In the fatal cases in which it has been impossible to secure a complete autopsy, even where during life the ordinary symptoms of such a condition were absent, we have not the right to state positively that death was not due to septic infection.

It is undoubtedly more comforting to the operator to attribute the result to any cause other than this, since he is naturally unwilling to think that his technique has been faulty. Those surgeons who are best able to judge are perhaps most ready to admit the possibility of infection of the wound through some slip during the operation, since it is they who realize the manifold ways in which such an accident might occur.

In practising *asepsis* we aim at bringing about that condition in which there is complete absence of septic material,—a condition which, of course, can be insured only by excluding all pathogenic micro-organisms from the site of operation.

By this we do not mean to say that in the most complete asepsis to which we attain there is always a sterile wound; on the contrary, as we have already stated, it is probable that most fresh wounds contain a certain number of organisms, but these either are non-virulent or are present in too small numbers to give rise to the phenomena of sepsis.

The maintenance of an aseptic condition is certainly one of the most important points to be aimed at in formulating a technique of operative surgery. It is true that an ideal technique which will be aseptic from a bacteriological stand-point, and which will protect our wounds so as to prevent the ingress of even a single bacterium, is scarcely ever possible, at least at the present day; but those who control their technique by bacteriological experiments, and strive in every way to approach as nearly as possible to such an ideal, constantly aiming at perfect cleanliness in their work, will undoubtedly obtain better results than those who have no such standard.

In practising *antisepsis* we employ the various means which have been devised for destroying bacteria or for so inhibiting them in their action as to render them incapable of giving rise to infection. The agents which are employed to bring about this condition are known as antiseptics and disinfectants.

Strictly speaking, antiseptics must be classed separately from disinfectants, the latter term applying only to those agents which kill pathogenic or putrefactive organisms, and which may consequently be termed true germicides, the former to the agents which arrest putrefaction or fermentation, but which do not necessarily destroy the micro-organisms. A deodorant does away with bad smells, but does not necessarily have either disinfectant or antiseptic powers.

While bacteriologists have shown us that infection from the air is comparatively rare, they have also demonstrated that it is most frequently brought about by contact. We can thus readily understand the comparative uselessness of the carbolic spray, and the importance of preventing the introduction of bacteria which are much more likely to be carried into the wound from the instruments or the hands of the operator and his assistants.

The association of laboratory with operative clinical experience must continue; we have learned much, but there is a promise of still greater progress to be reached in this way. While deprecating the adoption of methods based solely upon laboratory experiments, experience having too often shown the inexpediency of such a procedure, the author would insist most strongly upon the necessity of the harmonious working together of the surgeon and clinician with the bacteriologist, believing that each and all will in this way gain new facts and new points of view.

But in our enthusiasm for asepsis and aseptic methods we must not by any means lose sight of the importance of a perfected mechanical technique.

Besides depending upon the presence or absence of the seed,—the bacteria, —the question of infection or immunity is influenced to a great extent by the condition of the soil,—the tissues and fluids of the individual. Our more modern knowledge of wounds and wound-infection should by no means tend to make us belittle the skill of the surgeon, and at the same time it should stimulate him to increase his operative precision.

Linear incisions, the avoidance of any rough handling of the tissues and of the use of irritating fluids in the wounds, the filling of dead spaces with substances having their origin in the body (serum, moist blood-clot, known to have definite germicidal power), the abbreviation of the time required for operations, the maintenance of hygienic surroundings, and the adoption of every means for strengthening the vital resistance of the patient,—all contribute largely to a surgeon's success.

## II.

### PRINCIPLES OF STERILIZATION—DRY AND MOIST HEAT—FRACTIONAL STERILIZATION—CHEMICAL DISINFECTION.

By the term *sterilization*, as employed in connection with surgical technique, we properly mean a process which brings about the absolute and complete destruction of bacteria.

The most reliable way of destroying infectious material is by the use of the actual flame; but this, of course, can be applied in only a few instances, and, fortunately, we have other agents from which to make our choice: 1. Heat, (a) dry and (b) moist. 2. Chemical disinfectants.

Any or all of these methods may be supplemented by mechanical means, —washing, rubbing, brushing, scraping, and the like.

One may well allow one's self to be guided by the modes of procedure adopted in bacteriological laboratories, for there the best methods of sterilization have been elaborated, inasmuch as the technique employed in the sterilization of culture media, to be of any use at all, must obviously be devoid of flaws. As we shall see, however, the laboratory methods are to be used only as a guide, for many ingenious modifications of them have to be introduced in order to render possible their practical application to operative surgery. As a rule, those micro-organisms which do not form spores (vegetative bacteria) are killed at a comparatively low temperature (58° to 65° C., or 136°–150° F.), while the destruction of spore-containing bacilli requires higher temperatures and stronger chemical solutions. Fortunately, the ordinary pyogenic cocci do not, so far as we know, form spores, and so are easily destroyed, in this way differing from the tetanus-bacillus and the tubercle-bacillus, which belong to the second category.

It goes without saying that, before any further attempt is made to proceed to the sterilization of an article, all extraneous material is as far as possible to be removed by the ordinary mechanical methods. In my remarks upon the different methods of sterilization to be employed I shall disregard those which may still be considered to be *sub judice*, and only those procedures will be described which have proved themselves by their effectiveness and the reasonableness of their cost to be suitable for recommendation to the practical surgeon.

*Sterilization by fire*—i.e., by means of the actual flame—is used by the surgeon only on very rare occasions, except for doing away with worthless and dangerous objects, such as soiled dressings, and need not be discussed at length here.

For the carrying out of *sterilization by means of dry heat* a "hot-air sterilizer" is required. This consists of an oven made of sheet-iron with double walls, and fitted with shelves, on which the articles to be sterilized are placed. (Fig. 9.) The heat is supplied by a rose or tulip gas-burner beneath, and the temperature is registered by a thermometer which passes through the roof of the oven. To kill the ordinary vegetative (non-spore-forming) bacteria, exposure to dry heat at a temperature of 100° C. (212° F.) for one hour and a half is sufficient, but where spores exist a temperature of 140° C. (284° F.) for three hours is necessary. Unfortunately, the process of sterilization by means of dry heat destroys many substances of vegetable or animal origin, so that, even in the disinfection of metal instruments, it has been supplanted by more convenient and speedy methods. Dry heat does not permeate the substance to be sterilized nearly so thoroughly as steam heat, and is in consequence much more difficult to control. It still, however, finds an important application in the sterilization of glassware.

In *sterilization by means of moist heat*, one of the quickest agents which we possess is *boiling water*. The ordinary pyogenic cocci and other vegetative bacteria are killed by it in from one to five seconds, while anthrax spores succumb in about two minutes; and while it is true that there are spores which are much more resistant, these are not pathogenic for human beings, so that we may safely say that exposure to the action of briskly boiling water for from fifteen to thirty minutes will almost certainly insure complete disinfection.

*Sterilization by steam* is another simple and practical method. To insure success an apparatus must be used in which all the air is expelled from the chamber by the steam and an even temperature of 100° C. (212° F.) can be maintained throughout.

Several kinds of steam-sterilizers have been recommended. One of the cheapest and most convenient is the copper sterilizer of Arnold, made by Wilmot Castle & Co., Rochester, New York. (Fig. 10.) This is especially

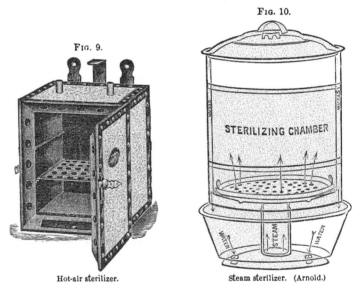

Fig. 9.

Fig. 10.

Hot-air sterilizer.

Steam sterilizer. (Arnold.)

useful for sterilizing bandages and gauze dressings, and is so generally known that it need not be described here.

Another form which may be mentioned is the tall, cylindrical Koch sterilizer constantly seen in bacteriological laboratories. (Fig. 11.) In hospitals or other places where large quantities of clothing and other material have to be sterilized at one time, large steam disinfectors must be set up.

One of the most ingenious methods of insuring complete disinfection is that known as *fractional* or *discontinuous sterilization*. If a fluid is kept at a temperature of 100° C. in a steam sterilizer for twenty minutes, all vegetative forms of bacteria will be destroyed. If this fluid is then kept for twenty-four hours at the ordinary room or body temperature, any spores which have escaped destruction (certain spores are known to resist a two hours' exposure to streaming steam) at the first heating will have developed into vegetative forms, and can then be killed by a similar exposure on the second day. If the process be repeated for a third time, one can be reasonably sure of having secured a completely sterile fluid. Tyndall, Pasteur, and others have shown that complete sterilization is practicable with the use of much lower temperatures (60° C., or 140° F.) if the process is repeated on three or four successive days.

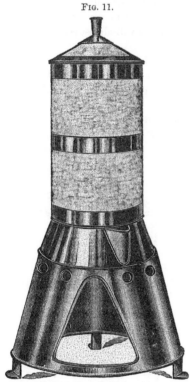

Fig. 11.

Cylindrical steam sterilizer. (Koch.)

While, as we have said, steam sterilization, where applicable, is a most reliable and satisfactory method, we can see at once that its universal employment is out of the question. For example, to use steam heat for the disinfection of the hands of the operator and of his assistants is impossible, neither can it be employed for the body of the patient to be operated upon. Again, it must not be used in the sterilization of objects made of leather or rubber, as these substances are destroyed by it.

On no subject in surgery have the opinions of men changed so much, perhaps, as on the value and sphere of usefulness of the "individual antiseptic," and the zeal of imperfect knowledge is responsible for much of the opprobrium which has been thrown by some upon the "antiseptic" treatment of wounds. The ideal chemical disinfectant will be one that can be readily employed for a variety of purposes, so as to be generally useful in practice; it should be easily soluble in water, and inexpensive; it should possess active germicidal powers, and not simply lead to the arrest of the development of bacteria; it should exert a sufficient action within a reasonably short space of time; it should not injure the substances to be disinfected, and should be of such chemical composition that it cannot be easily decomposed or rendered inert by chemical combination with the substances to be disinfected; and, finally, it should not endanger those who handle it, or possess any very unpleasant odor. A careful study of the properties of the ordinary chemical disinfectants in use will soon convince any impartial observer of the many deficiencies of the best of them when judged by this standard.

*Carbolic acid* is a powerful antiseptic, but a dangerous one. In fact, there are no antiseptics of much power which can with impunity be poured into a wound. The day has come when we must relegate the use of antiseptics to the period before an operation, and rely during the operation on the maintenance of an aseptic condition. *Antisepsie avant l'opération, asepsie pendant* (Terrillon).

Carbolic acid is a fairly stable body, and has the advantage of being readily soluble in water (up to the strength of five per cent.) with the aid of heat. If the solutions are made with cold water, it is advisable to add an amount of alcohol or glycerin equal to that of the acid employed. Carbolic acid, besides being a disinfectant, is also a deodorizer and a local anæsthetic. It is well to keep a two-and-a-half-per-cent. and a five-per-cent. solution always on hand. The dressing recommended by Keith for cœliotomy wounds consisted of one part of pure carbolic acid mixed with fifteen parts of glycerin, but it is now no longer employed.

*Corrosive sublimate* (mercuric chloride, $HgCl_2$) for a long time has occupied a prominent place in the list of disinfecting agents, but the deductions drawn from the experiments at first made with it have been proved to be incorrect. Koch asserted that a single application of it for but a few minutes, without any previous preparation of the objects to be disinfected, guaranteed an absolute disinfection even in the presence of the most resistant organisms. Gärtner and Flügge, Behring, Tarnier, and Vignal thought they had shown that the yellow staphylococci were killed in from a few seconds to as many minutes by exposure to the action of a 1 to 1000 solution of corrosive sublimate; but after Geppert had drawn attention to the fallacies of these early experiments, our views on the value of bichloride of mercury as a disinfectant underwent a material change. Geppert showed that the principal source of error lay in the failure to guard against carrying over, together with the bacteria which had been exposed to its action, enough of the sublimate to prevent the growth and development of the organisms in the nutrient media to which they were transferred for the purpose of determining whether or not they had been killed. He found, by precipitating the mercury with a solution of ammonium sulphide and thus converting it into the insoluble and inert sulphide, that the pyogenic bacteria had not only not been killed, but that they often still possessed the power of setting up disease in animals.

In order to see how far these objections were applicable to surgical disinfection, Abbott has repeated the experiments with sublimate in Professor Welch's laboratory, with particular reference to the pyogenic organisms, observing most carefully the precautions indicated by Geppert. He found that even under the most favorable conditions a given amount of sublimate had the property of rendering inert only a given number of individual organisms, the process being a definite chemical one, consisting in a combination of the sublimate with the protoplasm of the bacterial cell. He also found that the disinfecting power of the sublimate is profoundly influenced by the proportion of albuminous material in the medium containing the bacteria, and that while certain organisms (yellow staphylococci) after exposure to sublimate may undergo a temporary alteration, these effects may be made to disappear by successive cultivations in normal media.

The extreme toxicity of sublimate is so well known and generally appreciated that it would scarcely be necessary to mention it were it not for the fact that many undoubted and probably some unsuspected cases of death from sublimate-poisoning have occurred following the irrigation of wounds with too strong solutions of this substance. Besides showing the general toxic effects, the experiments relating to the local injury done to the tissues by chemical disinfectants are full of interest, inasmuch as it has been definitely proved that the local necroses caused by these chemical irritants favor the multiplication of the micro-organisms of suppuration. Dr. Halsted has shown that irrigation of fresh wounds with a solution of bichloride of mercury as weak as 1 to 10,000 is followed by a distinct line of superficial necrosis which can easily be demonstrated under the microscope, and it is readily conceivable that solutions even much more dilute may render inert those delicate processes by means of which the cells and tissue-fluids exert a germicidal power. The ill effects, then, whether general or local, which may follow from its toxicity, to say nothing of its inefficiency, would seem absolutely to preclude the use of corrosive sublimate for irrigation in the case of fresh wounds. Moreover, it must now, even as an agent for the external disinfection of inanimate objects, rank much lower than formerly. As, however, it is required for certain purposes, it is well to keep a supply on hand. The most convenient strength for a stock solution is five per cent., which can be made by dissolving with the aid of heat fifty grammes (seven hundred and seventy grains) of sublimate and an equal amount of common salt in one litre (thirty-three and one-half ounces) of distilled water. From this the solutions required for use can be made in a moment by dilution with a proper amount of water: thus, twenty cubic centimetres (five and one-half drachms) of the stock solution with the addition of enough distilled water to make one litre (thirty-three and one-half ounces) give approximately a 1 to 1000 solution. The use of distilled water and the addition of salt are necessary in their preparation, since otherwise, if sublimate solutions are allowed to stand, the mercuric salt is gradually transformed into an inert oxychloride.

*Potassium permanganate*, in solutions varying in strength from 1 to 100 to 1 to 10, possesses some germicidal power. This is materially enhanced by an after-treatment with *sulphurous* or *oxalic acid*. It has been suggested that its effects are due to processes of oxidation. Reference will be made to the mode of its application when we deal with the disinfection of the skin.

*Other chemical disinfectants*, such as solutions of boric acid, naphthol, chloral, and salicylic acid, are of questionable usefulness, and, as will be seen when we treat of the methods advised for practical disinfection, are of extremely little value; they may therefore be dispensed with by the surgeon in his operations. Preparations of cresol, lysol, and other coal-tar derivatives may sometimes be convenient as deodorizers, but are not to be relied upon as disinfectants.

## III.

### PRACTICAL APPLICATION OF THE PRINCIPLES OF STERILIZATION—OPERATING SUITS—PREPARATION OF THE SURGEON AND HIS ASSISTANTS.

The principles to be followed by the surgeon in formulating for himself a scientific technique have been already indicated. The necessity of paying attention to the most minute details has been insisted upon, and enough has been said to show that the smallest slip may invalidate the whole procedure. But, however well trained and skilful he himself may be, it is easy to understand how dependent an operator is upon those about him for the prevention of technical errors. It is only by choosing assistants who are thoroughly imbued with the strictest ideas of asepsis, who are willing to learn, and who are enthusiastic in their work, that he can hope for much aid from them. And after a surgeon has surrounded himself with desirable and faithful assistants, he will find it advantageous repeatedly to review and drill them in the minor points. Above all, he should by setting a good example endeavor to keep everything up to the mark and thus to establish a system of intelligent routine. Any good work necessarily involves a great deal of drudgery, and in the technique of the newer surgery the lazy man has no place.

A daily bath and especial attention to personal hygienic measures are essential to all who work in the operating-room. The tax on the physical powers of those who operate several times a week is by no means light, and it is only with the best care of his personal health that a surgeon, even when naturally strong, will be able to maintain his full physical vigor.

It will be necessary to provide for the operating-room a sufficient number of suits especially adapted for the purpose, and made of some material which can be easily sterilized. For, now that we know the dangers of infection by contact, it would seem essential that not only the surgeon but all his assistants should wear at every operation thoroughly clean sterilized suits. During an operation the sleeve or some other portion of the dress may come in contact with the field of operation, or one of the surgeons may accidentally touch the clothing of one of his fellows, and thus, if the suits are not sterile, pathogenic micro-organisms may readily be introduced into a wound. It is safer and better that all should put on a complete change of costume rather than simply draw on a sterilized coat and pair of trousers over the ordinary clothes, as has been recommended by the German school. The former plan also offers many advantages, for not only are the warm out-door clothes exchanged for thin, cool garments, which are far better suited for the temperature of the operating-room, but the ordinary clothes run no risk of being soiled or of carrying away on them the disagreeable odor of the fumes of the anæsthetic. Besides this, such suits afford much better protection against infection and are not nearly so cumbersome and awkward to work in as a sheet or a rubber apron. They are best made of some white material that can be easily and thoroughly washed. Twilled muslin, costing about thirteen cents per yard, is perhaps the most serviceable for this purpose. The suits should be made to fit comfortably, and should be fairly loose, so as not to impede the movements in any way. They can be made in one piece like a bathing-suit, with buttons down the front, and with a belt attached to the waist. The sleeves of the jacket should extend to just above the elbow-joint. It is more usual, however, to have them made in two separate parts, consisting of a shirt (or jacket) and a pair of trousers. The jacket can be made to button either down the front or down the back, the former arrangement being probably the more convenient. The trousers should not be long enough to allow the bottoms to drag on the floor. To sterilize these suits it is not sufficient to trust to the washing that has been given them in the general laundry, as even after this they could easily contain infectious material from coming in contact with the hands of those employed in ironing and folding them. In order to do away with this source of danger, it is necessary that they should be thoroughly sterilized before they are worn. This can be done by wrapping them in a towel or by placing them in bags made of butcher's linen and then exposing them to the streaming steam of the sterilizer for half an hour. They can then be taken out of the sterilizer and allowed to dry on a clothes-line which either has been sterilized or is covered with sterilized cloths or towels. Or they may be hung over the backs of chairs or spread out on tables which have been protected in a similar manner. After they have been thoroughly dried they may be put away in dry sterilized towels or bags until they are required for use. The nurse or assistant who attends to the sterilization of these suits should, of course, after the process is completed be careful not to nullify the results in putting them away. Danger can be easily avoided by protecting the hands with rubber gloves which have been soaked in a 1 to 500 aqueous solution of bichloride of mercury before being used. The sterilization should be done some time before the suits are required for use, so that they may have time to become thoroughly dry, a process which will generally be found to take three or four hours.

The operator, his assistants, and the nurses should wear white canvas shoes with low tops and rubber soles. They are clean and noiseless, and by their employment the soiling of the street shoes during an operation is avoided. They can be easily cleaned by washing them off with hot water, and a coating of pipe-clay will give them a very neat appearance.

When putting on the operating suits, care must be taken to allow the hands to come in contact with the clothing as little as possible. All the ordinary clothing should be first removed, then the white shirt and trousers are carefully put on, the shoes being adjusted last of all.

In hospitals there should be a dressing-room adjoining the operating-room. Too much attention cannot be paid to the minor points of personal cleanliness. It is important to keep the head and face scrupulously clean. The hair of the head should not be allowed to grow long, and should be kept as free as possible from dandruff. It has been suggested that the surgeon will do well to moisten the hair before an operation, since particles of dust might easily fall down from his head into the open wound, and thus, particularly if some inflammatory condition of the scalp were present, might produce a dangerous infection. If he is willing, the surgeon had best be clean shaven. A moustache is perhaps allowable, but a heavy beard should never be permitted in close proximity to an open wound. The finger-nails should be kept well trimmed, for a long nail at times does a great deal of injury by scratching and otherwise injuring the tissues. They should not be cleaned with the blade of a knife, as this will wound the matrix. A bit of wood or ivory shaped like a toothpick, or even a match shaved down, will answer very well.

Since Eberth in 1875 demonstrated the presence of large numbers of bacteria in normal sweat, many experiments have been made in this direction, and as a result our ideas with regard to surgical disinfection of the skin have been more or less completely overturned. Several different kinds of bacteria have been found upon the surface of the human body, and a whole bacterial flora for this region has been described. Attempts have been made to determine whether or not any particular kind or kinds of bacteria are constantly present there. The results of the European investigators on this point are more or less at variance. Bordoni has even advanced the view that groups of men in every country have a peculiar bacterial flora of their own upon the body surface, and that the flora varies with the occupation. The experiments made in the Pathological Laboratory of the Johns Hopkins University have been rewarded with the isolation of a form of bacterium which has been found to be almost constant in the skin. This variety is a white staphylococcus, and has been named by Professor Welch the staphylococcus epidermidis albus, about which I have already spoken. The significance of these investigations, as bearing upon the disinfection of the hands and forearms of the surgeon and his assistants, can hardly be overestimated, and I cannot but feel that the question of this disinfection has not even now received the consideration which it deserves. The gist of the matter is contained in the following sentences which I have taken from Dr. Welch's article: "Since the institution of bacteriological control as a test of the sufficiency of surgical technique, many methods before believed to be reliable have been proven to be faulty. We are past the days when an ordinary washing of the hands with soap and water followed by a dash of sublimate solution sufficed to put them in a condition to enter a clean wound. Numerous experiments that have been made with a view of ascertaining the best methods of accomplishing the sterilization of the hands show that it is indeed a difficult matter to effect it, and especially to insure the destruction of micro-organisms which lie beneath the finger-nails."

Fürbringer, in an extended series of experiments in 1888, found that a preliminary cleansing with soap and water together with a vigorous use of the brush was even more important than the subsequent employment of a disinfectant solution. His method of disinfecting the hands is as follows. (1) The nails are kept short and clean. (2) The hands are washed and scrubbed thoroughly for one minute with soap and hot water. (3) They are next washed for one minute in alcohol at 80° C. (176° F.), in order to remove all fatty and oily substances. (4) They are then scrubbed for one minute in a warm solution of carbolic acid (two per cent.) or of sub-limate (1 to 500).

I fully concur with Fürbringer's suggestion that the effects of cleansing with soap and brush, the water used being as hot as it can be borne, are of more value than those obtained from the employment of the disinfectant solution. In this mechanical removal of organisms we have therefore an agent of the first importance. The author has demonstrated this many times in the following way. Cultures were taken from the hands before the scrubbing was begun, and then several times again at different periods of the process, the results showing that the longer we scrub with soap and water the smaller the number of bacteria which are left. Cultures taken after scrubbing for ten minutes always showed a less number of bacteria than those taken after five minutes' work had been done on the hands.

The inefficiency of chemical disinfectants to which we have referred in the preceding section has shown the necessity of bringing about as thorough a removal of the bacteria as is possible by the mechanical action of the scrubbing, and of not trusting too much to these uncertain chemical agents, which henceforth must play a subordinate *rôle* in disinfection.

Not only, then, the operator and his assistants, but all those who in any way aid in the handling of the materials that are employed during an operation, must be very thorough with the cleansing of their hands. A French surgeon has gone so far as to state that in ninety-nine cases out of a hundred, when infection takes place, it occurs during the operation, from the instruments, the hands of the surgeon, the sutures, the sponges, the dressings, or from the patient herself.

Fürbringer's method, when conscientiously carried out, yields fairly good results, but it has been shown that if the mercury is precipitated with ammonium sulphide, and scrapings taken from the skin which has been thus prepared are placed in nutrient media, the presence of numerous living bacteria can nevertheless often be demonstrated.

After applying bacteriological tests to the methods usually employed, I have found the following to be the most reliable. The operating-room suit with the short sleeves having been put on, the hands and forearms are scrubbed vigorously for ten minutes by the watch with a stiff brush pre-viously sterilized by steam and with green soap, the water used being as hot as can be borne and being changed at least ten times. In order to avoid any possible contamination from the necessity of turning the spigots off and on with the hands, I have recently had constructed an arrangement by means of which this can be done equally well with the feet. The excess of soap is washed off in hot water, and the hands and forearms are then immersed for two minutes in a warm saturated solution of permanganate of potassium, which should be well rubbed into the skin with the aid of a sterilized swab. They are next washed in a warm saturated solution of oxalic acid until the stain of the permanganate has completely disappeared. Experiments made by Dr. Mary Sherwood in the Pathological Laboratory of the Johns Hopkins University have shown that in this process the oxalic acid and not the permanganate of potassium is the essential disinfecting agent. The hands and forearms are then rinsed off in sterilized lime water, next in sterilized water or sterilized salt solution, and finally are immersed in a solution of bichloride of mercury (1 to 500) for two minutes.

At the risk of repetition, it must be insisted again that after the hands and forearms have been once prepared they must on no account be allowed to come in contact with objects which are not sterile, or the whole work will be undone, since " a chain is no stronger than its weakest link."

Just before beginning the operation the hands and forearms should be well rinsed in sterilized salt solution, to remove any excess of the bichloride. After these procedures have been employed, cultures made from the scrapings underneath and around the nails, even after precipitation of the mercury, almost always yield negative results. It is to be remembered that little or nothing certain can be attained unless each step is conscientiously carried out. In fact, if practised in a slipshod manner, an elaborate technique does more harm than good, by deceiving us with a sense of security which is unwarranted.

The use of sterile rubber gloves to protect the hands after they have been sterilized will often prove of the greatest convenience, for with their aid we can without much fear of contamination often perform the needful manipulations about the patient before the operation begins. After the patient is well arranged and all is ready, we remove the gloves, and after washing the hands once more in the bichloride solution (1 to 500) and again in the salt solution, we can proceed with our work.

The strict observance of all these details may seem to be a tedious and an almost endless task, but when we consider how important it is to obtain and preserve a condition of surgical cleanliness, we shall not grudge any time or trouble spent upon them, and in a short while it will become a matter of routine work.

There are many other points connected with this subject to which we might refer. Thus, should the operator perspire, the moisture should be removed from his face by a nurse with a towel before any drops have been allowed to fall into the wound. Talking should be avoided over the field of operation, as saliva and its accompanying micro-organisms may by some

accident gain access to the wound.   If he can avoid it, the surgeon should
never operate when he is suffering from coryza, or from a catarrh which is
accompanied by mucous secretions.   The handling of a pocket-handkerchief
makes a break in the technique,—a point always to be remembered.   It
would be impossible to enumerate here all the contingencies which the
aseptic surgeon has to meet, and he must trust to his common sense to teach
him to apply consistently the principles upon which his whole technique is
based.

IV.

THE PREPARATION OF PATIENTS FOR OPERATIONS, MAJOR AND MINOR
  —MEANS EMPLOYED TO OBTAIN AN ASEPTIC FIELD.

It is advisable to have a patient who is to undergo an abdominal section,
or, in fact, any operation, under careful observation for some few days, in
order that we may form some idea as to the condition of her viscera or
of any particular idiosyncrasy which she may have, and may be able to
follow out any indications by which her general condition may as far as
possible be improved, and her powers of resistance proportionately increased.
In some cases rest in bed for a few days prior to an operation will be of
decided advantage.

In ordinary cases the patient should take a daily bath for one or two
days prior to the operation.   She should also receive a daily vaginal douche
of a warm one- to three-per-cent. aqueous solution of carbolic acid.   The
former will usually be strong enough for abdominal cases, and it is perhaps
better not to use the three-per-cent. solution even in all plastic cases, as it
not infrequently gives rise to pain.   The bowels should be opened daily.
This can be accomplished by gentle laxatives,—e.g., the citrate of magnesium, a seidlitz powder, or the compound liquorice powder.   Twelve to
twenty-four hours before the operation a good purge is given, and two or
three hours before the patient is placed on the table the rectum should be
thoroughly emptied by a large enema of soap and warm water.   If the enema
is omitted or is not given in such a way as to prove effectual, the bowels are
liable to be moved while the patient is on the table, and thus, especially in
plastic cases, the progress of the operation may be very much delayed.   The
doctor should give explicit directions to the nurse in regard to this matter.

Light, nourishing food should be taken, and nothing that is liable to
upset the stomach should be allowed.   The patient is generally permitted to
have any kind of soft food which seems to agree with her during the two
or three days preceding the operation, except that during the last twenty-four
hours she is restricted to such things as broths made from chicken or mutton,
although at times stewed fruits are allowed.   As a rule, unless she is very
weak and requires stimulants or nourishing broths, nothing should be
taken by the mouth after midnight.   Shortly before the patient is anæsthetized the bladder should be emptied, and if the urine cannot be voided
naturally, she should be catheterized.

In urgent cases, such as those of suppurative peritonitis or of extra-uterine pregnancy where rupture has taken place, there is, as a rule, little or no time for any preparation before the anæsthetic is administered. In any case, however, an enema should be given.

The further preparation of the patient for an abdominal section is about as follows. On the night preceding the operation the abdomen and pubes, after being thoroughly shaved, are scrubbed with soap and water, next with equal parts of alcohol and ether, in order to remove all oily and fatty substances, and finally with a solution of bichloride of mercury (1 to 500).

The field of operation is now covered with a thin poultice of green soap, which is allowed to remain on for from one to three hours, according to the degree of sensitiveness of the skin. The soap is removed by scrubbing the parts with a brush and hot water, so as to get rid of as much epithelium as possible. A large compress wrung out of a warm bichloride solution (1 to 1000) is then applied to the abdomen and is held in place with a bandage.

To summarize, the abdomen may be rendered practically sterile in all cases if the following procedures are adopted:

1. A bath of soap and water and a vaginal douche of a one-per-cent. solution of carbolic acid are given daily for three days before the operation.

Fig. 12.

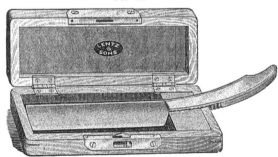

Robb's aseptic razor, with case.

2. Shaving the hair of the abdomen and pubes on the night preceding the day of the operation. (Fig. 12.)

3. Thorough scrubbing of the parts with (a) soap and water, (b) alcohol and ether, (c) bichloride of mercury (1 to 1000).

4. The application of a poultice of green soap for from one to three hours.

5. Removal of the soap by scrubbing with brush and hot water.

6. The application of a compress of bichloride (1 to 1000), kept on until the patient is brought to the operating-table.

The nurse in charge of the case must see that the patient is properly attired before leaving the ward and that every precaution is taken to avoid all danger of her becoming chilled. Over the fresh night-gown a warm wrapper should be drawn. Long stockings which reach well above the knees are desirable for warmth as well as for the avoidance of unnecessary exposure.

After the patient has been anæsthetized and placed upon the operating-table, the compress is removed and the following additional details are carried out:

1. The field of operation is scrubbed with soap and warm sterile water.

2. It is sponged again with alcohol and ether.

3. In some cases it is washed with solutions of permanganate of potassium and oxalic acid, as in the disinfection of the hands, with subsequent irrigation with warm sterile water or salt solution.

4. Irrigation with one litre of a solution of bichloride of mercury (1 to 1000).

5. Irrigation with sterilized salt solution, to remove any excess of sublimate.

Of the rules for diet and preliminary preparations for both major and minor operations we have spoken above. We should aim at as thorough an aseptic technique in plastic work as in abdominal surgery. While, in the majority of instances, errors in technique are not so often associated in these so-called minor cases with disastrous consequences as when the same errors have been committed in abdominal sections, yet there are many instances on record of death from sepsis following a simple plastic operation; and could we properly analyze the list of cases in which the cause of death has been attributed to pneumonia, to lesions of the kidney or other organs, their number would undoubtedly be much augmented. In not a few obscure cases in which death has followed a plastic gynæcological operation, a thorough autopsy, with a careful bacteriological examination, has clearly demonstrated that death was due to an infection with pyogenic bacteria. Many of the cases which we have been inclined to regard as cases of acute nephritis are now known to be cases of infection with associated acute lesions of the kidney. I may cite a case here which recently came under my notice, where it was possible to show beyond doubt that pyogenic micro-organisms had found an entrance at the site of a perineal operation. A woman, fifty-eight years of age, six weeks after a perineorrhaphy gradually developed symptoms suggestive of a nephritis. Examination of the urine showed the presence of albumen and of hyaline and granular casts. She gradually grew worse, and died a week later in coma. At the autopsy minute abscesses were found in the heart muscle, in the liver, spleen, kidneys, and intestines, and agar-agar Esmarch tubes made from these organs gave in every case a pure culture of the staphylococcus pyogenes aureus. The portal of entrance was found to have been the deep perineal tissues, where, just beneath the line of the wound, small collections of pus were found. Death has more than once followed as a result of apparently trivial operations upon the uterus, cervix, and vagina, and this fact should teach us that no operation, however insignificant it may seem, should be lightly undertaken or be carried out without due regard for the dangers of infection. As a rule, it is difficult to have the field of operation thoroughly clean and to keep it so during these minor operations. Still, although this is even more difficult to accomplish than in abdominal cases, the attempt must be made.

On the previous evening the parts are carefully shaved and scrubbed with soap and water, and are washed off with water, and afterwards with a solution of bichloride of mercury (1 to 1000).

After the patient has been placed upon the operating-table, the vagina, perineum, and external genitalia are to be thoroughly scrubbed with oleine soap and sterilized distilled water. This should take at least from three to five minutes. A liberal supply of soap should be used, and it should be well rubbed into the skin. In order to cleanse the vagina, a small oblong piece of soap is introduced well into the cavity and the suds are rubbed thoroughly into the walls, or a large piece of absorbent cotton, held with a sponge-holder or bullet forceps, can be used as a swab. The excess of soap having been washed off with warm sterile water, the external parts are rinsed with a litre of warm aqueous solution of bichloride of mercury (1 to 1000), and finally with sterilized water or salt solution. If there are large, protruding hemorrhoids and a considerable surface of the rectal mucous membrane is exposed, great caution is necessary in using the bichloride of mercury, as it is easily absorbed and may give rise to toxic effects. Under these circumstances it is well to wash out the rectum with a solution of permanganate of potassium (1 to 1000) morning and evening for two days before the operation, while on the morning of the operation soap and water only are employed, and the parts are finally rinsed off with sterilized water. The maintenance of asepsis throughout the operation will be discussed more fully later on.

V.

GYNÆCOLOGICAL INSTRUMENTS—METHODS OF STERILIZATION—INSTRU-
MENT TRAYS—CARE OF THE INSTRUMENTS AFTER OPERATIONS.

The more modern principles of treating wounds have led to certain marked modifications in the surgeon's armamentarium, and in no part, perhaps, has the change been so pronounced as in the kind of instruments used in operative work. The day of instruments with elaborately carved wooden and ivory handles is past, and complicated trocars and tubular needles no longer have a place in our instrument cases. The present tendency is to simplify their construction as much as possible and to use no greater variety than is absolutely necessary. It is wonderful how much can be done by the trained hands and fingers of a surgeon with a very few instruments, even with a scalpel and a few pairs of forceps. The choice of instruments must necessarily vary with the predilections and training of the individual operator. Certain main principles, however, should always be kept in mind. The surgeon need not encumber himself with such instruments as are seldom needed, or with a multitude of so-called "surgical conveniences" and "automatic appliances." He should, however, always provide himself with a liberal supply of the instruments in daily use, in order to be prepared for emergencies. None should be retained which do not permit of easy sterilization. Knives should have smooth metal handles, and handle and blade should be in one piece. Instruments with grooves, depressions, and notches are to be avoided. Good hæmostatic forceps with smooth blades can now be obtained, and are just as effectual as the old ones with grooved faces. All scissors, forceps, needle-holders, and the like should have simple articulations, so that the different parts are readily separable. An instrument with permanent joints cannot be kept surgically clean, and should therefore not be tolerated. A surgeon will find it to his advantage to have his instruments well nickel-plated, as they have a much better appearance and do not rust easily, and, besides, stand better the wear and tear of repeated sterilizations. Since the nickel-plating, however, even when double, has been proved to be not so valuable as was at first hoped, and instruments which are in constant use have soon to be replated, those which are used every day need not be nickel-plated, for by the methods of sterilization now recommended there is comparatively little danger of rust. But for those which are not so often used, nickel-plating is advantageous, since it protects them from the action of the air.

Instruments made of aluminium have been recommended, but they are undesirable for the following reasons : (1) they are too expensive ; (2) they are too soft ; (3) they will not stand repeated sterilization.

In a hospital one nurse or assistant should be given the full charge of the instruments and must be held responsible for their proper sterilization and preservation. In private practice the surgeon must give the instruments his personal attention ; and even in hospitals he will do well to watch closely the assistant to whom they are intrusted, in order to be sure that the constant careful attention which is absolutely necessary is being paid to them. It is important to write out lists of the instruments that are required for the different operations and to keep them where they can be easily consulted on each day of operation, so that none of the necessary ones will be forgotten. These lists should be divided into two parts, the first containing the instruments which are sure to be required, the second those which may possibly be needed under certain circumstances, and which should therefore be prepared, although they may be set aside until they are called for.

The problem of discovering a simple and effectual way of sterilizing metal instruments has been a difficult one. Many methods have been employed, but none is more satisfactory than that introduced by Schimmel-busch, to be described presently. The exposure of the instruments to the flame of a Bunsen burner or a spirit-lamp is an effectual way of sterilizing them, but the method has many disadvantages. The time required and the danger of overheating as well as blackening the instruments, besides at the same time of dulling them, make it useless except on rare occasions or when, perhaps, a single scalpel or needle is required for immediate use. The hot-air sterilizers, which have been introduced especially for the sterilization of metal instruments, have been found to be unsatisfactory for this purpose. To make sure that the instruments are completely sterile, it is necessary to keep them in the hot-air sterilizer at a temperature of from 150° to 180° C. (300° to 350° F.) for at least two hours. When one remembers that at least twenty minutes or half an hour is necessary to bring the sterilizer to this temperature, and that another half-hour will be required to allow the instruments to cool down, it will be seen that fully three hours are required for the whole process. Of course this objection may be obviated by following the recommendation of Poupinel, who suggests that the instruments should be placed in tight metal boxes and sterilized on the day before the operation, being then allowed to remain in the boxes until just before they are needed. But in any case the inconvenience is great, and still another serious objection is found in the fact that, in spite of the greatest care, instruments thus treated will almost surely rust, even when the new "ventilated" disinfecting ovens are employed. Attempts to shorten the time required for sterilizing by hot air have given unfavorable results, and it has also been proved that exposure to a temperature above 180° C. is deleterious to the temper of the steel and affects the hardness and sharpness of the cutting instruments.

Some surgeons prefer to sterilize the instruments by means of steam, and employ the Arnold or some other steam sterilizer. The instruments are put in bags made of "bird's-eye" or "towel" linen, which are then placed in the sterilizer and exposed to a temperature of 100° C. for an hour. The mouths of the bags are provided with draw-strings, by means of which they can be lifted from the sterilizer, and the instruments are turned out into the trays, which have been sterilized and which contain enough sterile water to cover them completely. If the instruments are allowed to dry in the sterilizer, they are almost sure to rust or to become discolored. · The time of sterilization may be somewhat reduced if an autoclave is used; but all these methods of sterilization by steam are also open to the objection that they not only require too long a time but are also apt to injure the instruments.

From what we have already said with regard to disinfection by chemical agents in Section II. it will be readily understood why, if only on the grounds of the injury done to the tissues, the method so much in vogue formerly, of simply placing the instruments in a solution of carbolic acid for a short time before the operation, must be discarded. But, besides this serious objection, solutions of carbolic acid which are concentrated enough to have any decided germicidal power may be injurious to those who handle the instruments. In addition to the grave local lesions set up in the hands of susceptible individuals, instances of carboluria and of the occurrence of severe general symptoms of carbolic-acid poisoning have more than once

8

been noted simply from the effects of handling instruments kept soaking in the solutions during prolonged operations.

Instead, therefore, of employing dry heat or steam, or trusting to chemical solutions, surgeons during the past few years have had recourse to the boiling of the instruments in water and other fluids. The French writers have recommended boiling glycerin and oil of various kinds, but the use of these need not be discussed here, since in simple boiling water we have an efficient and speedy disinfectant for instruments. Five minutes suffice for complete sterilization. The most serious objection to the use of plain water, which has been very warmly recommended by Dandrohn, Redard, and others, lies in the serious damage done to the instruments. If they are placed in ordinary cold water and boiled, they will often be found to be studded with spots or even covered thickly with rust. The danger can to a great extent be avoided if the water be boiled for some time before the instruments are placed in it, and the addition of some alkali to the boiling water is a sure preventive, the one best suited for the purpose, as shown by Schimmelbusch, being ordinary washing-soda (sodium carbonate).

Fig. 13.

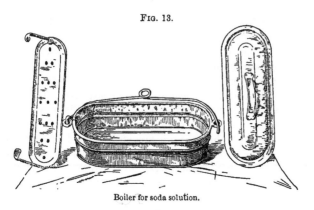

Boiler for soda solution.

The method employed by Schimmelbusch for sterilizing instruments is by far the most convenient and effective for general employment, and has been used for some time in many operating-rooms with universally satisfactory results. It was first introduced into von Bergmann's clinic in Berlin, and, while free from objection from a bacteriological stand-point, has the additional advantages of requiring very little time, of being inexpensive, and of entirely doing away with the danger of rust. Soda also adds to the disinfectant power of the boiling water. Repeated experiments made to test the efficacy of the method have shown that a boiling one-per-cent. soda solution kills all known pyogenic organisms in from two to three seconds, while anthrax spores are all destroyed after an exposure of two minutes. The procedure is as follows. The instruments (which have been thoroughly cleansed after the preceding operation) are boiled for five minutes in a one-per-cent. solution of carbonate of sodium. Any vessel can be made to serve for this purpose if one is operating in a private house, but in hospitals and operating-rooms it is convenient to have a specially constructed apparatus made of copper, agate-ware, or nickel. This consists of an oblong boiler fitted with a cover. The heat beneath can be supplied by Bunsen burners ("wreaths") or by a spirit-lamp; or, where these cannot be obtained, the boiler can be set directly upon a stove. The size of the boiler required will depend, of course, upon the amount of work to be done. In hospitals one of large size will be necessary, but in private practice or in small operating-rooms a boiler twenty to forty centimetres (eight to sixteen inches) long, fifteen to twenty centimetres (five and a half to eight inches) wide, and ten to twelve centimetres (four to four and a half inches) deep will answer every purpose. (Fig. 13.) In making the soda solution, one soon learns how much, approximately, of the dry soda to add to a given amount of water without actually weighing it; but, to save time and insure accuracy, a concentrated solution of known strength may be kept ready, so that by simply diluting it a one-per-cent. solution may be made whenever it is

FIG. 14.

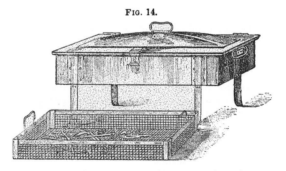

Improved boiler, with wire basket containing instruments.

required. In order to facilitate the introduction and removal of the instruments, a flat wire basket which fits into the boiler will be found very convenient. (Fig. 14.) After they have been boiled for five minutes the wire basket containing the instruments is removed, and the latter are turned out into sterilized trays which contain sufficient warm sterilized water to cover them. Instead of simple water, a cold (previously boiled) one-per-cent. soda solution may be used in the trays, or a solution which contains one per cent. of soda and one per cent. of carbolic acid. The addition of the latter would seem, however, to be entirely unnecessary. Between operations which follow one another in rapid succession, or if some of the instruments by chance have come in contact with non-sterile material during an operation, they may, after being carefully washed in cold water, be quickly re-sterilized in the boiling soda solution. The procedure should be actually timed by a watch kept hanging up in the operating-room.

The most satisfactory vessels to keep the instruments in at the time of the operation are trays made of thick glass. At present, however, good ones are not made in this country, but must be imported from abroad, and are quite expensive. They offer the advantage of being readily rendered sterile, and at the same time of presenting a cleanly appearance. On account of the cost, great care must be exercised while sterilizing them, and also when washing them in hot water, else they are liable to be broken. Glass dishes are best sterilized by means of dry heat, but, besides the length of time required and the risk of breakage, the bulkiness of the glass-ware which is used renders the procedure very inconvenient in practice. The smooth surface of glass dishes, which can easily be kept perfectly clean, makes it possible to render them sterile by mechanical means supplemented by sufficiently strong solutions of bichloride of mercury. They are first washed thoroughly with water and then filled to the brim with an aqueous solution of bichloride of mercury (1 to 500), which is allowed to remain in them for an hour before they are needed for use. Just before the operation they are finally rinsed out well with sterile water, and after being placed upon the table are filled with enough sterilized water or salt solution to cover the instruments. If they are required for a second operation following closely upon the first, they may be cleansed by rinsing them out with cold water to which hot water is cautiously added, then with a 1 to 500 bichloride solution, and lastly with sterilized salt solution. To clean them before putting them away after the operations are over for the day, they are washed out thoroughly with soap and warm water and are then turned upside down and allowed to drain until they are perfectly dry.

If glass dishes cannot be obtained, trays made of hard rubber, agate-ware, or porcelain may be substituted for them. They can be sterilized in the same way as the glass dishes.

The instruments which have been used should first be washed in cold water, in order to remove all pus, blood, or tissue-particles. They are next immersed in hot soda solution and thoroughly scrubbed with soap and brush. After being rinsed off they are wiped dry with a soft towel and polished with a piece of chamois skin. Finally, they are boiled for five minutes in a one-per-cent. soda solution and carefully wiped dry, after which they may be put away in their proper places in the instrument case. Instruments thus carefully and regularly treated will never rust and will always be clean and bright.

In all these manipulations instruments with cutting edges should be handled with particular care, in order that they may not be dulled. The edges should not be allowed to come in contact with hard surfaces, as they would do if they were roughly handled and carelessly dumped into the trays. Great care is also necessary when wiping off the blades. In those instruments the parts of which are connected by means of the French lock it is especially important that no moisture should be allowed to remain in the joints, and the numbers on the several parts should be carefully noted, so that those which correspond may be joined together. Neglect of this simple rule will soon ruin the instruments. Force should never be exercised in adjusting them, as the pivots are delicate and the slightest roughness will prevent their accurate apposition, so that after a short time the joints will become so loose as to be quite useless.

The instrument cases are described in Section XI.

When a surgeon wishes to carry sterilized instruments with him to avoid the necessity of sterilizing them at a private house, they should be boiled in the one-per-cent. soda solution and placed in sterilized bags, which are then placed in closely fitting metal boxes made for the purpose, the latter having been previously sterilized by dry heat; the boxes are to be left unopened until the time of the operation. It is probably safe, however, to carry the sterilized instruments in the sterilized bags with the other things in the telescope valise, omitting the use of the metal box. The ordinary case or loose bag formerly employed for carrying instruments should, of course, no longer be used. It will, as a rule, be found more convenient, even for operations in private houses, to carry a small apparatus for sterilizing instruments; but, as a matter of fact, we can find in almost any house a vessel in which they can be boiled.

## VI.

### ASEPTIC SUTURES, LIGATURES, AND CARRIERS—SUTURE MATERIALS— STERILIZATION AND PRESERVATION OF THE VARIOUS KINDS.

We have a variety of materials from which to select our sutures and ligatures. The substances commonly employed are the cable twist silk, silkworm-gut, catgut, silver wire, kangaroo tendon, and horse-hair, and of these silk, silkworm-gut, and catgut are most frequently used. No one suture material will suffice for all purposes, although silk can be made available for the majority of cases. Whatever we use, the main point is that it shall be sterile, and, as we shall see later, we may have a material which at first sight appears in every way adapted for our purpose, and yet presents such apparently insuperable difficulties in the way of rendering it sterile that, unless some newer and more effective method is devised, surgeons will have to consider the advisability of giving up its use entirely. The material must also be smooth and pliable but not brittle, and it is but natural that, *cæteris paribus*, we should choose something not too costly and which is easily obtainable. If I were asked to state my preference in regard to the materials in ordinary use, I would, on the ground of the bacteriological experiments made by Dr. Ghriskey and myself, place them in the following order: (1) silkworm-gut, fine and coarse; (2) surgeon's cable twist silk, Nos. 1, 2, 3, 4, and 5; (3) silver wire, fine and coarse; (4) catgut, sizes a, b, c, d, and e. Since, however, silk is the material most commonly used, we will take it up first.

When using the surgeon's cable twist, five sizes are to be kept in stock. No. 1 (fine) is very necessary when carriers are to be employed. The carrier is of the greatest convenience, as it does away with the necessity of having a large number of needles and also facilitates quickness in the performance of an operation. It consists of a piece of silk fifty centimetres (nineteen inches) in length, and is prepared in the following way. The surgeon passes the two ends through the eye of the needle from opposite directions. A nurse then holds the needle, or it may be allowed to hang down over the side of the hand while the two ends are tied snugly in a knot, and slight traction being made on the loop thus made, the knot is securely fixed in place immediately behind the eye of the needle. As the operator passes the needle through the tissues, each suture, as it is to be introduced, is threaded by an assistant through the loop of the carrier, and is thus drawn into its place. One has not to employ this method long for the introduction of interrupted or continuous sutures in order to appreciate its advantages.

The next size of silk sutures (No. 2) is used for superficial sutures which are to bring the skin and subcutaneous tissues in apposition. Sizes Nos. 3 and 4 are employed for deep sutures which are to approximate muscular tissues. Size No. 5 (heavy) is used in the ligation of pedicles or whenever a heavy ligature is necessary for any other purpose. Instead of Nos. 3, 4, and 5 of the surgeon's cable twist, we have found that the best quality of gum silk will answer every purpose. The ligatures are wound on glass reels, and it will be found that by the adoption of a routine method of arranging them much confusion will be avoided. The glass reels are placed in "ignition test-tubes," a piece of non-absorbent cotton being placed in the bottom of the tube, upon which the reels rest. Each tube for an abdominal operation should contain four reels, one of the heavy silk, one of silk of intermediate weight, one of No. 2, and one of the fine silk for the carrier. The first reel holds four heavy ligatures, each one metre (thirty-nine inches) in length. These ligatures may be wound separately, but it is generally better to wind them together, as they can then be more conveniently removed from the reel, and four is the usual number required for one operation. On the second reel should be wound ten "intermediate" or deep ligatures, each forty centimetres (sixteen inches) in length. The third reel is for ten superficial ligatures, each forty centimetres in length ; the fourth holds eight fine ligatures (for carriers), each fifty centimetres (nineteen inches) in length. This number of carriers will be necessary, as it is important to have one for each of the several·needles of different sizes which are likely to be required in the course of the operation. After the silk has been cut into the required lengths, the strands are bunched into fours and wound together (not separately) on the glass reels. The full reels are placed in the heavy glass tubes, the mouth of each tube being plugged with ordinary cotton batting. The empty tubes, plugged with cotton, should have been previously sterilized in the hot-air oven. Absorbent cotton should not be used for this plug, as it will take up moisture from the air, and fungi will be much more likely to grow through it. The tubes with the ligatures in them are to be sterilized in the Arnold steam sterilizer for one hour the first day and for half an hour on each of the two succeeding days. It is perhaps not absolutely necessary to sterilize them more than twice, but it is safer to adopt the routine method of sterilizing on three successive days. When the ligatures have thus been rendered aseptic, they will remain so indefinitely if the tubes are kept well plugged and in a dry place. Instead of the arrangement mentioned above, the different sizes of ligatures may be kept in separate tubes, and each tube will then have to be opened only when the particular size of suture which it contains is required. If the plug of cotton is carefully held by its outside surface and is immediately replaced when one reel is taken out, the others will not be contaminated, provided that we are careful either to allow the reels which we require to roll out of the tube into the solution prepared for them, or else (and this is perhaps the safer way) to remove them from the tube by means of a pair of sterilized forceps. If, however, there should be the least suspicion that the ligatures on the remaining reels have become contaminated during this manipulation, the tube with its contents must again be steamed in the sterilizer for an hour. The tubes can be kept in glass jars like those employed by confectioners, each jar as well as each tube being provided with a label bearing the date of sterilization. Some surgeons prefer to re-sterilize their silk ligatures immediately before every operation. This can easily be done by placing the tubes in the Arnold sterilizer. Silk ligatures will not, however, bear steaming many times, as the procedure if repeated too often will render them brittle. The glass cases which have been recommended by so many, in which the ligatures are kept wound on reels, the ends being allowed to come out through small openings, are very objectionable. (Fig. 15.) The ligatures, more particularly the protruding ends, are almost certain to become contaminated, and none of the devices which have been suggested for overcoming this difficulty have proved satisfactory. Their use is therefore to be condemned. The still older custom of keeping ligatures in antiseptic oils and fluids is even more reprehensible.

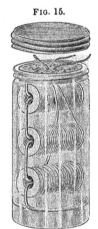

FIG. 15.

Glass jar for ligatures (not recommended).

*Silkworm-gut* is a substance which is excellently adapted for being employed as a suture material, and it is a pity that it does not admit of more universal application. It has a smooth surface, is compact and free from interstices, and in consequence sutures of silkworm-gut may be allowed to remain in position longer than silk sutures without injury to the tissues. This is, of course, of great advantage in such a wound as we have, for example, after a perineorrhaphy, and in fact in all cases in which it is desirable that the sutures shall remain in position for more than a few days. Silkworm-gut is easily introduced and moulds itself readily to any desired position in a wound. When properly applied, it does not produce the same constriction of the tissues as either silk or silver wire, but acts more like a supporting splint. The sutures can be very easily removed when desired, and experiments have shown that silkworm-gut resists the invasion of bacteria much better than silk or catgut which has been left in for the same length of time. It is best employed in two sizes, the coarse and the fine, and may be bought in bundles of one hundred strands, at a cost of seventy-five cents a bundle. It is sometimes stained red, but this procedure is not necessary, although by it the ligature is rendered more easily visible. In preparing them for use, the twisted ends of the strands having been cut off, a dozen ligatures, folded once, are placed lengthwise in each of the glass tubes in which they are to be kept. The methods which we described for the sterilization and preservation of silk sutures will apply equally well to sutures of silkworm-gut. They should be placed in a sterilized tray containing sterile water or salt solution half an hour before the operation. This renders them more pliable, and they are not so likely to break as when they are used perfectly dry. Any silkworm-gut remaining after an operation can be rinsed off and re-sterilized for another time by repeating the process described above. As a rule, it is better not to make a complete knot when employing silkworm-gut, but to use instead only the first stroke of the surgeon's knot, which will hold quite well. The advantage of this is that the threads lie flat, and the sutures can afterwards be tightened or loosened at will, and thus the parts be kept in perfect apposition without any constriction of the tissues.

Silver wire has no advantages over silkworm-gut as a suture material. It is less desirable inasmuch as it is more expensive and is more apt to injure the tissues. It can be bought in different sizes, and generally comes wound on spools. It can be sterilized by steam heat, by dry heat, or by boiling in the one-per-cent. solution of soda.

Catgut would be an almost ideal material for sutures, but, unfortunately, we have as yet no thoroughly reliable method of rendering it absolutely sterile without at the same time making it so weak as to unfit it for our purpose. When properly handled, it supports the tissues for a sufficient length of time to allow of a thorough approximation of the parts, and when it has served its purpose the suture is absorbed. Just as soon, then, as we have a reliable method for sterilizing catgut which will not at the same time destroy its other necessary properties, we shall indeed have a ligature material of great value. Different specimens of catgut vary greatly, and, although some of the methods of sterilization which are advocated are perhaps effective in the majority of instances, it will often happen that a few of the strands are not rendered sterile; and many cases of suppuration or death following operations have been directly traceable to the use of catgut ligatures.

I shall now describe three of the most reliable methods of preparing catgut, although it must be understood that none of them is free from fault, and that for the present I must advise against its use.

(1) The catgut is soaked in an aqueous solution of bichloride of mercury (1 to 1000) for one hour, and afterwards in oil of juniper for forty-eight hours. It is then transferred to absolute alcohol, which is changed every month. The glass bottles in which it is kept should be provided with tops which are screwed on; they should have been previously sterilized by steam, and should contain enough alcohol to more than cover the strands of catgut.

(2) Von Bergmann was accustomed to place the catgut, wound on reels, in ether for twenty-four hours, in order to remove any fatty substances from it. He then transferred it to a one-per-cent. solution of corrosive sublimate in eighty-per-cent. alcohol, which was changed daily for two or three days. The sublimated alcohol was then poured off and the reels covered with ordinary alcohol.

(3) The third and perhaps the best method is as follows. Six strands of catgut, each forty centimetres (sixteen inches) long, are wound on a glass reel. A number of these reels are placed in a bottle of ninety-five-per-cent. alcohol, care being taken that the catgut is completely covered, some slight allowance also being made for evaporation. The mouth having been plugged with cotton, the bottle is placed in a water-bath, which is heated until the alcohol boils. The heating is repeated on three successive days. The stopper is then put on, being protected with paraffin or rubber protective, unless the ligatures are required for immediate use. When required, some of the reels may be taken from the bottle by means of a pair of sterilized forceps. If it is thought preferable, the strands on each reel may be all of the same calibre, in which case it will be advisable to have a complete series of reels in the same bottle.

When applying ligatures it is of the greatest importance, as has been previously pointed out, to avoid any undue constriction of the tissues which might lead to obstruction of the circulation and diminish the normal resistance of the parts. The manipulation of the sutures and ligatures is too often a weak point in the technique of surgeons. The ligatures are often cut into lengths just before the operation, and the ends are not infrequently allowed to hang down over the edge of the dish in which they are arranged. Sometimes they are brought in contact with an unsterilized object in being passed from the instrument-table to the operator, and even after they have reached his hands the ligatures are still often in great danger of becoming infected, so that it may be truthfully said that where a large number of ligatures are employed during an operation it is indeed a wonder that they can be all kept aseptic.

## VII.

The early surgeons, and particularly those in hospital practice, laid great stress upon the dexterous application of many complicated bandages and dressings, and looked with some pardonable pride upon their parallels and angles, their reverses from straight lines, and the even, smooth dressings which were then considered an essential part of a good surgical technique. As a matter of fact, the application of the non-sterile dressing of those days often did more harm than good, and we can hardly be surprised that many surgeons were led to believe that they could obtain better results from treating wounds by exposure to the air than by covering them with gauze and bandages,—results which we are less likely to question since it has been proved how much greater are the dangers of infection by contact than those of infection from the air. The various efforts to obtain a more satisfactory method of dressing wounds need not be discussed here. Many of us still remember the treatment by the *earth dressing*, so lauded by Addinell Hewson. In studying the statistics of wounds which have been treated in this way, one is struck by the number of cases in which the patients subsequently died of lockjaw, and to-day a surgeon would be thought very rash if he applied to the wound, without sterilization, a substance known to be the natural habitat of the tetanus-bacillus.

The occlusive dressing has been much employed, and not without reason, inasmuch as it imitates more or less closely nature's own method. It has, indeed, its peculiar dangers, but, as will be shown later, it is very valuable both in abdominal and in perineal surgery.

When a wound is not to be closed hermetically, it is important to apply a dressing which, while being itself free from pathogenic bacteria, will prevent the access of micro-organisms from the outside, and at the same time will thoroughly absorb the secretions from the wound and prevent their subsequent decomposition. A great variety of substances have been recommended for their absorptive power, among them straw, bran, sand, ashes, tan-bark, tow, moss, wood, and sawdust, but no one of these is so useful or so generally applicable as cotton or gauze, which has been made capable of absorption by the removal of all fatty substances from it. Good absorbent cotton can be bought for from forty to sixty dollars per hundred pounds. It is generally sold in rolls, each weighing one pound. Common cheese-cloth one yard wide costs about five dollars per hundred yards. For dressings it can be cut into lengths of two metres or of two yards and boiled for half an hour in a one-per-cent. solution of carbolic acid and soda, and then thoroughly rinsed in sterile water. The manufacturers have reaped bounteous harvests from the preparation of the host of so-called "antiseptic gauzes," made by saturating absorbent gauze with solutions of bichloride of mercury, carbolic acid, boric acid, salicylic acid, and cyanide of mercury and zinc. But now we know that all these methods of disinfection are inefficient, and even if the materials are in a sterile condition when packed by the manufacturers, the numerous subsequent handlings which they undergo before they come in contact with a wound would almost certainly lead to contamination. And if contamination can occur so easily in this way, surely nothing need be said of the many instances where "antiseptic gauze" has been thrown beneath the buggy seat, or at the bottom of not over-clean boxes or bags, to be placed a short time afterwards as a dressing upon a wound which it is meant to protect.

The surgeon of to-day does not need to acquaint himself with these fancy preparations, except to learn to avoid them. Only in rare instances do we require a gauze impregnated with antiseptic substances (vide permanganate and iodoform gauze). It will generally be sufficient if we render our gauze and cotton free from pathogenic micro-organisms before applying them to wounds. The methods are not complicated, and surgeons are to be congratulated upon the immense simplification of dressings and of the ways of applying them which have been given to us through the recent advances in our knowledge of the different modes of infection and of the way in which it is to be avoided.

Absorbent cotton, absorbent gauze, and bandages should be sterilized by means of steam in the Arnold sterilizer. Exposure for three-quarters of an hour to steam at 100° C. serves to render all these substances, if not packed or rolled together too tightly, absolutely sterile. It is best to sterilize the dressings shortly before each operation, and in large operating-rooms where several cases are operated upon daily it is necessary to have several steam sterilizers. They are made in such numbers now that they are comparatively inexpensive.

But the question will be asked, How will the application of simple sterile gauze to wounds, in the absence of chemical substances, prevent the decomposition of the secretions from the wound which are taken up by the dressing? The answer is so simple that it seems strange that we should only recently have appreciated it. One of the first requisites for the growth of micro-organisms is moisture. Bacteria do not multiply in dry substances. Good gauze and cotton permit of the constant evaporation of moisture from them, and so prevent bacterial growth. They do not remain damp long after being removed from the sterilizer, so that the dressings may be applied almost immediately after the sterilization has been completed. It is rather better, however, to place the dressings, which have been exposed to the steam, in a drying chamber for a short time before they are used. The uselessness of employing dressings which have been impregnated with antiseptics becomes easily apparent when we consider that, in the first place, the presence of powerful antiseptics in sufficient concentration to have any germicidal effect would irritate the skin and the wound, and, secondly, that antiseptics are quite inactive in dry gauzes when there is but little exudation, and therefore, in order to obtain any benefit

from them, the dressing would have to be applied wet, whereas, as we have
said, the dryness of the gauze constitutes in itself a great safeguard.

In order to have a stock of thoroughly dry and sterile cotton always on
hand, the absorbent cotton may be cut into pieces of convenient size and
securely wrapped in a towel or in a piece of gauze several layers thick.
The bundle, securely but not too tightly fastened, is then sterilized by
steam for forty-five or sixty minutes, and, after being allowed to dry in
the air in a room where there is no dust, is kept until required for use in
a closed glass jar or in a tin box. Sterilized gauze may be preserved in
the same way. Before opening these sterilized packs, the hands should
either be disinfected or covered with rubber gloves taken from a jar of five-
per-cent. carbolic acid solution, or the pack may be removed with sterilized
forceps. If any cotton or gauze is left over after the package has been
opened, it may be again wrapped up and re-sterilized.

In order to prevent contamination of the field of operation, it is necessary to surround it with sterilized gauze or towels. The latter are made of
the ordinary towelling, with perfectly plain hemmed edges. They are to be
sterilized by steam, and, if desired, a good supply of them may be kept in
covered glass jars filled with a 1 to 500 sublimate solution or a three-per-cent.
carbolic acid solution, so that they are ready at all times. (Fig. 16.) When
they are to be used where they will come in con-
tact directly or indirectly with the field of operation, they must first be rinsed in sterile water.

FIG. 16.

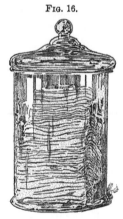

Towels in a three-per-cent carbolic acid solution.

*Iodoform gauze* is occasionally required for
various purposes, and may be prepared in the following manner. Plain gauze is cut into lengths
of three hundred centimetres (about three yards)
each and folded lengthwise. For the iodoform
mixture enough castile soap is mixed with two
hundred cubic centimetres (about six ounces) of
a one-per-cent. aqueous solution of carbolic acid
to make good suds; forty-five cubic centimetres
(about twelve drachms) of powdered iodoform are
then added, and the whole is thoroughly mixed.
The quantities given above will be sufficient for
the preparation of three metres of gauze. The
gauze is immersed in the mixture, which must
be well rubbed into the meshes. It is then
rolled up and placed in a covered glass dish and sterilized in the Arnold
steam sterilizer. In cutting pieces of gauze off for use, the hands must be
sterilized, or sterilized rubber gloves must be worn, and a pair of sterilized
scissors used. Such precautions as these are very important if we wish to
prevent any possibility of contamination. When the iodoform gauze is
to be used for dressing plastic cases, it is convenient to have it cut into
strips ninety-four centimetres (thirty-six inches) long and eight centimetres

(three inches) wide. Each strip is rolled up separately, and several of these rolls are preserved in a sterilized glass jar. When required for use, they can be taken out with sterilized forceps.

*Permanganate gauze* is not infrequently used for dressings, and does a great deal to diminish the odor that is so objectionable in cases of cancer of the cervix and uterus, and elsewhere where there is any bad-smelling discharge. The ordinary gauze is cut into lengths of one hundred centimetres (thirty-nine inches) each, folded lengthwise, sterilized for one hour, and then saturated with a one-per-cent. aqueous solution of permanganate of potassium (ten grammes (one hundred and sixty grains) of the crystals of permanganate of potassium to one thousand cubic centimetres (thirty-three and a half ounces) of hot water). The gauze is cut and rolled in the same way as the iodoform gauze, and should be preserved in a colored glass jar.

*Subiodide of bismuth* may also be rubbed into gauze which is to be used for plastic cases. For three hundred centimetres (three yards nine inches) of gauze a mixture of 45,0 (about twelve drachms) of pure subiodide of bismuth with one hundred and fifty cubic centimetres (about five ounces) of water and thirty cubic centimetres (about one ounce) of glycerin will be sufficient.

*Tampons of lamb's wool* are especially useful when a non-absorbent material is desired. Such a tampon is very elastic and serves excellently as a support. A piece of wool thirty centimetres long and three centimetres wide (ten inches by one inch) is twisted over three fingers so as to form a loop. Round it at this point a piece of stout linen thread is tied, the ends being left free. The tampons are then steamed in the Arnold steam sterilizer and kept in aseptic glass jars.

*Tampons of absorbent cotton* are made in very much the same way. The cotton, as it is taken from the roll, is cut into pieces measuring twenty by ten by two centimetres (eight by four inches by half an inch), and, each piece being folded once, a thread is attached to the loop, and the ends are rounded off with scissors. The tampons are then sterilized and kept in aseptic glass jars.

*Bandages* are always being required, and a good supply made from gauze and flannel should be kept on hand. They should be of different widths, and in order

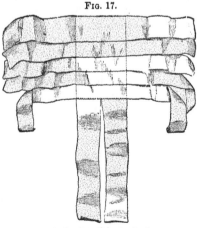

Fig. 17.

Modified Scultetus bandage.

to insure straight margins should be cut by " drawn thread." Besides these, the ordinary *T bandage* and the modified *Scultetus bandage* (Fig. 17) should be always kept in stock. All bandages are to be sterilized in the steam sterilizer in the way described above for dressings of the same material.

*Sponges* either may be made from sterilized gauze, or the ordinary marine sponges may be used. The gauze used for this purpose is the same as that used for dressings. Sponges may also be made by wrapping cotton somewhat loosely in squares of gauze, the corners being brought together and tied at the top with thread. (Fig. 18.) When gauze is employed for sponges, the edges should not be cut, but should be folded over and hemmed, as otherwise loose threads are liable to be left in the field of operation. Such sponges can be made of various sizes, and can be easily sterilized by means of steam heat immediately before the operation. Or a supply may be sterilized and then kept in a jar of a solution of corrosive sublimate (1 to 500) till just before the operation, when they are to be removed from the solution and thoroughly rinsed in sterile water or in sterile salt

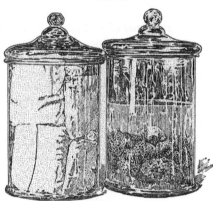

FIG. 19.

FIG. 18.

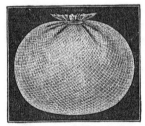

Sponge made of cotton and gauze.

Sponges and towels in glass jars.

solution. In buying marine sponges, the cheap reef sponges and those that are in the rough will serve every purpose. They generally arrive packed so tightly together as to form almost a solid mass. They should first be carefully separated, placed in a muslin bag, and well pounded, to remove all particles of sand and other foreign materials. They are then rinsed out in water several times. A very good way is to place them in a basin or pail and allow the water to run in upon them from a tap for several hours. They are next soaked in a saturated solution of permanganate of potassium, are afterwards decolorized in a solution of oxalic or of sulphuric acid, and are then left for twenty-four hours in an aqueous solution of hydrochloric acid, made strong enough to taste slightly sour. After this they are again soaked in water until the washings are clear. They are next placed in a bichloride solution (1 to 500) for twelve hours, and finally are rinsed in warm water and preserved in covered glass jars containing a three-per-cent. aqueous solution of carbolic acid, the solution being changed every week. (Fig. 19.) When required for use, the sponges may be taken out, after the hands have been thoroughly sterilized, and dropped into a sterilized pitcher which contains sterilized water. The excess of carbolic acid is then squeezed out, the water being changed two or three times. The sponges are then placed in basins containing sufficient sterile salt solution to cover them completely.

The gauze sponges are easily sterilized, and are so inexpensive that they need never be employed more than once, and consequently are far preferable to marine sponges. The latter, however, have the advantage of being more elastic and pliable, and are therefore more desirable for abdominal cases, and indeed in abdominal surgery we cannot entirely dispense with them. Unfortunately, we cannot sterilize them by steam without ruining them. Although they are rather expensive, they should be thrown away after they have been used once, since the possibility of rendering them sterile after they have been covered with purulent and bloody substances is, to say the least, problematical. Schimmelbusch, in dealing with the sterilization of marine sponges, does not recommend boiling them in water or soda solution, for under such a procedure the sponges contract and become hard, but he says that if, after being thoroughly cleansed, they be placed in a bag and immersed for half an hour in a one-per-cent. solution of soda (which has been boiled, and afterwards removed from the fire and allowed to cool to 85° or 90° C. (185°–194° F.) ), they will be quite sterile. The sponges, with care, will stand this treatment several times. As we have said, it is far better never to use them a second time; and, at any rate, sponges which have once been employed should never be admitted to an operation without being sterilized in this way.

## VIII.

ASEPTIC DRAINAGE—GLASS AND RUBBER DRAINAGE-TUBES—GAUZE DRAINS—CARE OF RUBBER MATERIALS—RUBBER DAM—RUBBER TUBING—RUBBER GLOVES.

Our ideas regarding the necessity for and the efficacy of drainage in abdominal surgery have undergone during the past few years the most radical changes. The time was when we did not close the wound of an abdominal section without inserting a large tube which reached well down among the tissues. It was then thought that infected cases—such, for instance, as pelvic abscesses—could never recover without drainage, and that even in the cleanest cases it was always well to insert the tube for at least a few hours, until the so-called serous oozing had ceased, in order not to tax too severely the absorptive power of the peritoneum. Now that our attention has been called to the importance of taking more pains with the minute operative details, since we have recognized the necessity of checking all hemorrhage, even from the smaller bleeding points, of avoiding any infection of the field from the contents of abscesses or of the intestines, and of making a careful peritoneal toilette, above all, since we have understood the effects of any rough handling of the tissues, we have come to look upon the necessity for drainage as being the exception rather than the rule. Whereas a few years ago nearly ninety per cent. of all cases were drained, now we drain only from ten to fifteen per cent.; and indeed, from bacteriological examinations made in a large number of cases, it has been proved that, even under the most favorable conditions and with the personal attention of trained assistants, it is extremely difficult to prevent the access of pyogenic micro-organisms into the tube. We have pointed out that the presence of the white staphylococcus in the skin is a constant menace where the way to the wound is kept open by a tube, and it was found that the dressing of the drainage cases led almost invariably, after two or three times, to bacterial contamination. Whereas we used to be afraid to close the abdominal wound completely, on account of the danger of sepsis, we now close it in every case possible, and rather hesitate, from fear of infection, to drain the abdomen. The objections to the insertion of drainage-tubes have been formulated recently by Dr. Welch[1] as follows:

"(1) They tend to remove bacteria which may have gotten into a wound from the bactericidal influence of the tissues and animal juices. (2) Bacteria may travel by continuous growth or in other ways down the sides of a drainage-tube, and so penetrate into a wound which they otherwise would not enter. We have repeatedly been able to demonstrate this mode of entrance into a wound of the white staphylococcus found so commonly in the epidermis. The danger of leaving any part of the drainage-tube exposed to the air is too evident to require mention. (3) The changing of dressings necessitated by the presence of drainage-tubes increases in proportion to its frequency the chances of accidental infection. (4) The drainage-tube keeps asunder tissues which might otherwise immediately unite. (5) Its presence as a foreign body is an irritant and increases exudation. (6) The withdrawal of tubes left for any considerable time in wounds breaks up forming granulations,—a circumstance which both prolongs the process of repair and opens the way for infection. Granulation tissue is an obstacle to the invasion of pathogenic bacteria from the surface, as has been proved by experiment. (7) After removal of the tube there is left a track prone to suppurate and often slow in healing." To these Professor Halsted has added an eighth,—viz., "Tissues which have been exposed to the drainage-tube are suffering from an insult which more or less impairs their vitality and hence their ability to destroy or inhibit micro-organisms."

When an abdominal wound became infected subsequently to an operation, it was formerly thought that this result was due to micro-organisms already present, it may be, in a pelvic abscess or in the secretions about the uterine adnexa. Undoubtedly this mode of wound-infection may occur, but it should be remembered that in a very large proportion of cases of pyosalpinx the pus is sterile, any organisms which had before been present being dead. This has been proved many times by examination of smear cover-

---

[1] Maryland Medical Journal, 1891.

glass preparations and the study of cultures made at the time of the operation. Unless bacteriological examinations have been made of such secretions or accumulations of pus, it is impossible to feel sure that an infection which has followed the operation has come from within.

There are cases, however, in which drainage is still indispensable, and the surgeon has to decide on the safest and best means of employing it.

Where tubes are employed, those made of glass, introduced by Koeberlé, of Strasburg, with slight modifications, are the best, as they can be easily rendered sterile by being allowed to remain for an hour in a 1 to 500 bichloride solution. These tubes are straight, of a length varying from twelve to fifteen centimetres (five to six inches), and with a diameter of eight, ten, or twelve millimetres (three-tenths to one-half inch). Tubes curved at the end are also valuable where it is necessary to drain Douglas's pouch over the convex surface of a tumor.

Every tube should be perforated with from nine to twelve holes, one millimetre (one-twenty-fifth of an inch) in diameter, beginning from the inner end and extending for one-third the length of the tube. When the diameter of such holes is larger than one millimetre, portions of the omentum and the small intestines are very apt to work through them into the lumen of the tube, and thus an artificial strangulated hernia may be formed, giving rise to severe pain and vomiting, with hemorrhage and sloughing.

The tube should be placed in such a position that it will carry off the fluid which accumulates in the most dependent portion of the pelvis. This is best accomplished by inserting it in the cul-de-sac of Douglas, so that the inner part lies just behind the uterus, gently resting on the floor of the pelvis, while the more external portion rests in the abdominal incision from four to eight centimetres above the symphysis pubis.

*Capillary drainage* can be obtained through the glass tube by means of a piece of wick, gauze, or cotton. If one of these substances be thoroughly sterilized and carefully placed in the tube, so that drainage can take place from the bottom, it will insure a steady capillary flow of fluid from the pelvis to the outside.

A drain made of ordinary lamp-wick thoroughly sterilized is the most efficient; next to this narrow strips of gauze, twisted into rolls just large enough to enter the tube easily, are to be preferred.

Other means of draining the pelvis from above are employed. In some cases of wide-spread injury to the cellular tissue of the pelvis it is impossible to check the bleeding and drain satisfactorily by means of the glass tube alone. Under these circumstances it is often possible to effect both objects by packing long strips of a five-per-cent. iodoform gauze, three centimetres (one inch) in width, behind and on each side of the uterus, the ends being brought out at the lower angle of the wound. Firmer pressure can be made and drainage secured by folding or coiling the gauze, as it is placed in the pelvis, in the form of a spiral, one end being brought out through a drainage-tube. The pressure on the tube, and through this on

9

the gauze packed in the pelvis, can be regulated by tightening or loosening the abdominal binder.

A pack introduced in this way can be removed with very little disturbance by slightly raising the tube and pulling the gauze out through it layer by layer. There is thus no danger of drawing out intestines or omentum with the dressing.

If the tube be placed in a proper position, so that capillary drainage be provided for in some such way as we have described, there will not only be a continuous flow from the peritoneal cavity to the outside, but the tube will not need cleansing as frequently as has been generally thought necessary.

It is useless to remove the dressings every hour or two and expose the patient to the risk of a septic infection by repeatedly cleaning out the tube. A tube which has been put in properly can safely be left to care for itself for a period of from twelve to twenty-four hours, after which time it will be necessary to uncover it in order to remove the overlying dressings which have become saturated by the discharges.

In fifty cases thus drained, this point has been tested by allowing the tubes to remain undisturbed for from twenty-four to forty-eight hours, and in no case was a single unfavorable symptom observed.

The importance of perfect cleanliness in dressing the tube is not usually sufficiently appreciated. Hands, instruments, and dressings employed must be as thoroughly aseptic as at the time of the operation, if we wish to avoid the danger of introducing infection from without.

For the purpose of cleaning out the tube, the tube-forceps devised by Dr. Kelly has proved very valuable in facilitating rapid and cleanly work. The instrument is provided with two very slender tapering handles, crossing like scissors, the blades below being furnished with rat-teeth to hold the little ball of cotton which is to be carried down to the bottom of the tube. The blades are fastened by a new style of lock devised for the purpose.

A piece of sterilized cotton, sponge, or gauze small enough to pass easily down to the bottom of the tube is grasped in the forceps, gently guided down into the pelvis, and again withdrawn, bringing up with it the secretions, the process being repeated with a fresh pledget until the tube is dry.

This is a better method than the use of a suction apparatus, which is not efficient, is soon contaminated, and is difficult to sterilize so as to render it fit for further use.

It is necessary at each dressing, after cleaning the tube, to rotate it at least two or three times. It will sometimes be found, as we have said above, especially where the perforations are of somewhat large calibre, that pieces of omentum as large as a split pea have become firmly fixed in the holes in the tube, forming veritable omental herniæ. Sometimes all the holes on one side will thus be choked. If gentle rotation and traction fail to effect a release of the omentum, the tube must be carefully lifted up far enough to permit of a ligature being passed on the outside of it around each little hernial mass in turn ; after the ligature has been tied the tube should be cut loose with a pair of delicate long-bladed scissors or with a slender knife. If the intestine should be caught in this way, it must be released by traction and careful pressure from the outside of the tube, made by means of a small piece of cotton or gauze in the grasp of the tube-forceps.

To decide how long the tube shall be left in the abdomen is in some cases a difficult matter. It must be borne in mind that the tube is inserted for the purpose of drainage, and that, its function being over, it should be removed as soon as the flow of fluid is not more than enough to wet the plug in it. This point may be reached in from twelve to twenty-four hours, or in some instances not until the fourth or fifth day. The early removal of the tube relieves the patient of discomfort and consequent mental anxiety; it also allows the fresh tissues in the track of the tube to come together, so that immediate union is promoted and the liability to ventral hernia at a later date is diminished.

If there is but a scanty flow of serum on the dressing about it, and the general condition of the patient is good, the tube may be removed without fear, and any slight secretion left to the care of the peritoneum. If, on the other hand, the pulse and temperature are of such a character as to occasion anxiety, the pulse being 120 or more and the temperature over 100° F., although the discharge may be but slight, it is better not to remove the tube and close the wound until the flow has entirely ceased.

When the tube has been removed and a slight discharge still remains, we may keep the track open by inserting a piece of twisted gauze, which is changed once in twelve or twenty-four hours, a few grains of the iodoform and boric-acid powder (1 to 7) being dusted into the wound at each dressing. This procedure, while allowing the sinus to close up gradually, at the same time provides for the carrying off of any noxious fluids which would otherwise tend to accumulate. Where there exists a free purulent discharge from the first, the tube should not be removed until one or two weeks have passed, otherwise we are liable to have a formation of pockets of pus in the pelvis.

Another more gradual method of removing the tube may be employed when the discharge is rapidly diminishing and does not amount to more than a few teaspoonfuls in twenty-four hours. At each dressing the tube may be rotated and raised from one to two centimetres. Before its final removal the tube should be cleansed as thoroughly as possible and rotated to make sure that the intestines are free. The thumb is then placed over the end, and the tube, being grasped between the first and middle fingers, is slowly and gently removed. As soon as it is out, the wound is dried and the provisional sutures drawn up, thus closing the track of the tube in the abdominal wall. The provisional sutures consist of one or two passed through both sides of the abdominal incision round the tube, and left loose until they are required for this purpose.

*Drainage by means of the gauze bag* also gives very good results. A gauze pack made up of several strips of sterilized gauze is inserted into a long, narrow gauze bag and used as the tube: this causes a rapid removal of the fluid by capillary attraction.

Two useful canons in gynæcology are: (1) drain rarely, and only when absolutely necessary, and (2) when employing drainage let it be thorough.

*The rubber dam* is also a useful adjunct to our stock of dressing materials. Where a glass tube is employed for the purpose of drainage after an abdominal section, it is convenient to have a strip of sterilized rubber dam twenty-four centimetres (ten inches) wide (of the same kind as that used by dentists, or a little thicker) and long enough to extend from the symphysis pubis to the umbilicus. A slit is made down the middle of this, through which the top of the drainage-tube projects. After the gauze has been packed into the drainage-tube and the cotton placed immediately over it, the ends of the rubber dam are folded in over the cotton. Over this comes an additional layer of absorbent cotton, and a bandage is applied to cover the whole. The rubber dam thus holds the dressing immediately over the tube in place and tends to prevent the penetration of any fluids beyond this limit. Since the rubber comes in such close contact with the wound and the abdominal cavity, it is, of course, very necessary that it should be thoroughly sterilized. To effect this it may be boiled for five minutes in a one-per-cent. soda solution and afterwards preserved in a glass jar containing a 1 to 20 aqueous solution of carbolic acid. When required for use it is removed from the jar with the necessary precautions, and then rinsed off in sterile warm water before being placed in position.

*Rubber tubing*, besides being used sometimes for drainage, is convenient for constricting the uterus while a myoma is being removed from it. It comes in several sizes, and costs about twenty-five cents per metre. It can be sterilized in soda solution and kept till it is needed in the same way as the rubber dam, in a stoppered glass bottle containing a five-per-cent. aqueous solution of carbolic acid. In order to make quite sure that it is perfectly sterile, it will perhaps be best to boil the piece about to be used in a one-per-cent. soda solution just before the operation. Rubber dam and rubber tubing should not be kept in solutions of sublimate, owing to the chemical action exerted upon them by this substance.

*Rubber gloves*[1] are not employed so widely as they should be. It is probable that the chances of infection would be very much diminished if the assistants were required to wear them at operations, since they can be rendered absolutely sterile, which is not necessarily true of the skin of the hands. Their use by the operator himself would also facilitate the performance of a great deal of minor work without any inconvenience resulting therefrom. If the gloves are worn after being sterilized by being boiled in a one-per-cent. soda solution, it will be necessary to scrub the hands and forearms only once or twice, and, as we have pointed out above, their use will often prevent contamination. The gloves may be kept after steriliza-

---

[1] These gloves may be bought of the Goodyear Rubber Company, New York.

tion in an aqueous solution of bichloride (1 to 1000) until required for use. The excess of sublimate may then be washed off in sterile water. They will stand sterilization in soda solution many times without injury. They come in different sizes, and it is best to wear a pair which fit the hands very loosely, in order to facilitate putting them on and off. Those with the long wristlets are the most serviceable, as they protect a considerable portion of the forearms. When putting the gloves on or taking them off, care should be exercised, on account of their delicate structure, not to handle them roughly. If one experiences any difficulty in getting them on, they can be filled with the solution contained in the vessel until the fingers of the glove become distended, after which they can be slipped on quite easily. The hand is then held up and the solution is allowed to run out. If they stick at all when one attempts to remove them, they should be gently turned inside out. After the operations are over for the day, the gloves may be washed off thoroughly, hung up to dry, and afterwards put away, to be sterilized in soda solution immediately before the next operation.

## IX.

FLUIDS FOR IRRIGATION—PLAIN STERILE WATER—ANTISEPTIC FLUIDS FOR IRRIGATION—STERILE PHYSIOLOGICAL SALT SOLUTION—ANTISEPTIC POWDERS—IODOFORMIZED OIL—BICHLORIDE CELLOIDIN—IODOFORMIZED CELLOIDIN.

It is the custom of many surgeons to irrigate the abdominal cavity after almost every operation, while others use this method only in those cases where fluid has escaped into it during the removal of a tumor, or where the bleeding from the separated adhesions has been marked. The substances which have been used for this purpose are plain hot water, sterile salt solution, and a variety of so-called antiseptic solutions. The routine treatment of irrigating every case cannot now be considered a necessary practice. Where the structures are non-adherent and there have been no complications, there would seem to be no indication for its employment, but after the removal of a mass which contains bloody or purulent fluid, or where a great deal of oozing has occurred as a consequence of the separation of dense adhesions, irrigation may sometimes be useful. If the fluid that has escaped be of a septic nature, the advantage of irrigating the pelvic cavity under these circumstances will be doubtful, and it is not unreasonable to suppose that when such material has escaped into the abdominal cavity, attempts to remove it by irrigation are quite as likely to spread it farther about between the coils of the intestines and into parts of the abdominal cavity whence it would be impossible to remove it by any subsequent sponging. If solutions containing germicidal drugs are used for irrigating the abdominal cavity, there is not only the uncertainty that the drug may not prove of sufficient strength to destroy the septic material which remains, but there is also the danger of causing local lesions, as well as of subsequent results from the absorption of toxic chemical substances. Fortunately, in the majority of cases the fluid which is contained in old abscess-cavities in the pelvis does not contain living organisms. This fact has been proved by cultural experiments, and explains why in these cases infection has not occurred, though pus has escaped at the time of the operation. When it happens that, during the removal of an ovary for malignant disease, it ruptures and the contents of the tumor escape into the pelvic cavity, it is above all things necessary to remove the escaped particles of tumor material, so that the formation of metastases upon the peritoneal surface may be prevented. For the reasons given above, all material which has escaped should as far as possible be removed by sponging; but when this is impossible we have to fall back upon irrigation with some bland and non-irritating fluid.

In selecting a fluid for abdominal irrigation we naturally look for one that promises the best possible results with the minimum possible amount of harm, and up to the present time none has proved more satisfactory than the warm sterile normal salt solution. Of its advantages and of the way of preparing it we shall speak in a few moments. The fluid which has perhaps been most generally used is plain water. It can easily be rendered sterile by boiling it in a clean vessel just before the operation. It is well to have two vessels, one of sterilized water which has been allowed to cool, and the other containing water still hot. When required for irrigation, the water from the two vessels is mixed until the proper temperature is obtained (43°–48° C. (110°–118° F.) ). The water should be in a perfectly clean pitcher or graduate, and from this it is poured into the abdominal cavity.

With plain sterile warm water we are able not only to cleanse the abdominal cavity but also to stimulate the circulation and thus in a measure overcome the tendency to shock. The principal objection to the use of plain water for irrigation is that it has a definite deleterious effect upon the tissues. It is a fact well known to microscopists that when fresh animal tissues are examined in plain water the cells are seriously altered, and, as has been shown by repeated experiments, the red and white blood-corpuscles are injured or completely broken up by its action.

The use of solutions of sublimate and carbolic acid for irrigation of the peritoneal cavity must now be unhesitatingly condemned, both on account of the local necrotic effects which are produced and because of the danger of general intoxication. The experiments which have been made with dilute solutions of sublimate upon the abdominal cavity of dogs are too well known to need description here; yet there are abdominal surgeons who will persist in pouring this poison into the abdominal cavity, notwithstanding the fact that autopsies have proved that the patients sometimes died afterwards with intestinal ulceration and peritonitis, or with lesions of the heart and kidneys, of which there was no evidence before the operation.

Of the milder antiseptic solutions, such as one-half- to two-per-cent. solutions of boric acid, Thiersch's solution of salicylic acid, and the like, it may be said that they possess no advantages over the simple solution of common salt. This is made to correspond in specific gravity very closely with the normal serum of the blood, whence the term " normal" or " physiological" salt solution. It is prepared by dissolving six grammes (ninety grains) of sodium chloride in each litre (thirty-three and a half ounces) of distilled water. This solution is filtered into a clean flask which may hold about three litres. The flask is plugged with non-absorbent cotton, the top of the plug being securely wrapped in a gauze bandage in order to prevent the deposition of dust on the rim of the flask. After being heated over a Bunsen flame until the fluid boils, it is immediately transferred to an Arnold steam sterilizer, already heated to 100° C., and allowed to remain there for half an hour. The process is repeated on the two following days. The fluid is to be used at a temperature of 43° C. (110° F.) or as high as 48° C. (118° F.). It can be made up in quantities of one dozen flasks or more, and kept all ready for use.

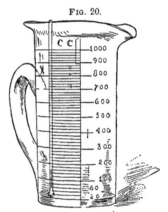

FIG. 20.

Glass jar with thermometer attached. (Robb.)

When required, two flasks are taken, one containing cold and the other hot solution, and their contents are mixed in a sterile glass graduate to which a thermometer is attached, and which holds from five hundred to one thousand cubic centimetres. (Fig. 20.) This jar must, of course, have been rendered perfectly sterile in the same way as the glass trays for the instruments. The gauze and plug having been removed with due precautions, the cold salt solution is first poured into the thermometer jar and then enough of the hot solution is added to raise it to the proper temperature. The thermometer affords the best means of testing the temperature of the water, and the hand of the assistant or nurse should not be relied upon. Such loose determinations are inaccurate, and, what is more important still, the hands may contaminate the fluid. This is a detail of importance, and the careful observance of it should be insisted upon.

The solution is poured into the abdominal cavity directly from the glass

FIG. 21.

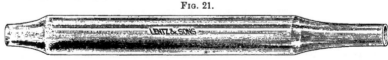

Glass douche nozzle. (Robb.)

graduate, or it can be siphoned through a glass or hard-rubber nozzle attached to a piece of rubber tubing, or, if preferred, a new Davidson syringe, previously sterilized in boiling soda solution, with a glass nozzle attached, may be employed. The Davidson syringe suitable for this purpose can be bought without the usual attachments for the irrigating end, and so be less expensive. The glass nozzle can be readily attached to the end of the tube, and the lumen being so much larger than that of the ordinary nozzles which come with these syringes will permit a much larger flow through it; besides this, the nozzle being of glass can be much more easily sterilized. (Fig. 21.)

In performing plastic operations, not only is irrigation very necessary, but its use dispenses with the necessity of sponging. A constant stream can be employed and be so regulated as to keep the field of operation free from the blood that would otherwise obscure it and hamper the operator. The fluids used for this purpose are either warm sterile water or, better still, sterilized normal salt solution. The solution is placed in a sterile glass jar (Fig. 22) fitted with a piece of rubber tubing which is provided with a hard-rubber syringe stopcock by which the current is controlled. If a glass stop-

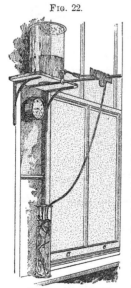

Fig. 22.

Aseptic apparatus for irrigation.

cock can be used it will be still more satisfactory, as it is rather easier to clean and sterilize. Instead of a glass jar, a rubber bag large enough to contain two litres may be used. Such rubber bags are sold under the name of fountain syringes, and are to be rendered sterile in the manner described for other rubber materials.

The *powders* most frequently employed in gynæcological surgery consist of iodoform and boric acid, either alone or in combination. The iodoform, when used alone, should be well rubbed up, as it is very apt to become lumpy, and it should be lightly dusted over the surface of the wound. Iodoform, perhaps, is the best germicidal powder that we have. The boric acid is frequently employed in the same manner as the iodoform. The chief objection to using powders at all is, that, while the substances may perhaps preserve their germicidal power when in solution, it is difficult to have them perfectly sterile when in the form of the dry powder. Iodoform and boric acid in combination in the proportion of one part of powdered iodoform to seven parts of powdered boric acid is a valuable mixture and one often employed, since it possesses the advantage of being non-irritating. After an operation it is well to dust this powder just along the line of the incision or on the gauze which protects it. After an abdominal section, when we wish to close the wound immediately, we protect it first with the occlusive dressing shortly to be described, and then incorporate the iodoform and boric powder with the celloidin after it has been poured over the gauze. In plastic cases we dust the powder well over the field of operation, and also use a small quantity of it each time after catheterizing the patient, the powder being dusted over the field of operation and the external genitalia.

Some patients are extremely susceptible to the toxic effects of iodoform, even when very small quantities are employed. Under these circumstances we can use either the boric powder alone or a powder composed of one part of subiodide of bismuth to seven parts of boric acid. The powders should be kept in sterilized glass vessels, and when they are to be applied to a wound are shaken from a special flask that has first been sterilized. Such a powder-box can be cheaply and easily made by covering the mouth of a bottle, made of glass or metal, with a piece of wire screen. The meshes should not be too coarse, or the powder will escape too freely. (Fig. 23.)

On account of the danger of poisoning by iodoform, salol has been recommended as a substitute for it.

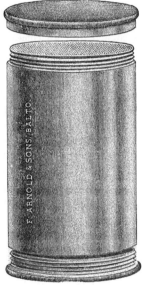

FIG. 23.

*Iodoformized oil,* which is a combination of oil and iodoform powder, often employed locally, can be mixed according to the following recipe. The oil (olive oil or oil of sweet almonds) is sterilized in a flask, plugged with cotton, for an hour on three successive days, and iodoform powder in the proportion of one part to four parts of oil is added just before the preparation is to be used. In making this combination it will be necessary to use a sterilized glass rod and dish, and in order to insure asepsis Böhm has suggested that the iodoform powder should be first carefully washed in an aqueous solution of sublimate and afterwards dried.

Aseptic powder-flask. (Robb.)

*Occlusive dressings* are frequently used to protect wounds. The solution which is perhaps most often used for this purpose in abdominal cases is that known as *bichloride celloidin.* The advantage of such a dressing, as has already been stated, lies in the fact that it not only protects the wound from infection from without, but will remain in place for a considerable length of time, and in a measure acts as a splint, allowing of a certain amount of movement on the part of the patient without any disturbance of the wound.

Bichloride celloidin (1 to 16,000) may be made according to the following formula :

℞ Ether (Squibb's),
    Absolute alcohol āā, 200 cubic centimetres (6½ ounces);
        Of a solution made of 1 gramme (15 grains) of bichloride crystals dissolved in 40 cubic
        centimetres (11 drachms) of absolute alcohol, 1 cubic centimetre (16 minims).
    Mix, and add of Anthony's "Snowy Cotton" enough to give the solution the consistence of simple syrup.

To the skin of some patients the bichloride in this strength will act as an irritant, and in such cases it is better to use a similar preparation of the strength of 1 to 32,000.

The occlusive dressing is simple and gives satisfactory results. The method of procedure is somewhat as follows. After the wound has been closed and the skin in the line of the incision and the sutures have been dried, they are covered with a piece of sterile cheese-cloth. This is fixed in its place by being saturated with the celloidin mixture, which can be evenly distributed over the surface of the gauze with a sterilized glass spatula. Over it is dusted some of the mixture of iodoform and boric acid powder (1 to 7). A second piece of gauze, considerably larger than the first, is next applied, over which more celloidin is poured and more of the powder of iodoform and boric acid is dusted on. The dressing soon becomes dry and fixed, and over all comes a mass of sterilized absorbent cotton, which is held in place by a binder. A wound which has been covered with this dressing may be left for a week or more, if everything goes well. When the dressing is to be removed, it should be well softened either with warm sterile water or with a 1 to 40 aqueous solution of carbolic acid applied on lint or cotton. This should be allowed to remain over the dressing for an hour or so before any attempt at removal is made, but, if necessary, the dressing may be loosened in a few minutes by pouring ether over it.

*Iodoformized celloidin* may be used in the same manner as the bichloride celloidin. It is made as follows:

> ℞  Absolute alcohol, 200 cubic centimetres (6½ ounces);
> Iodoform powder, 50 grammes (12½ drachms);
> Mix, and add ether, 200 cubic centimetres (6½ ounces).

Mix, and add of Anthony's "Snowy Cotton" enough to give the solution the consistence of simple syrup.

When making any of these celloidin mixtures, absolutely dry graduates and bottles must be used. These may be obtained by rinsing them out first with absolute alcohol, then with pure ether, the latter being then allowed to evaporate. In the preparation there must be as little exposure to the air as possible. The "snowy cotton" is to be added in small pieces, and the bottle well shaken after each addition. Wide-mouthed flasks are the most convenient for the purpose.

## X.

CERTAIN PROCEDURES SOMETIMES NECESSARY BEFORE AND AFTER OPERATIONS, WHICH MUST BE CONDUCTED ASEPTICALLY—HYPO-DERMIC INJECTIONS — EXPLORATORY PUNCTURES — CATHETERIZA-TION—BLADDER-WASHING—URETERAL CATHETERIZATION.

Of the ordinary precautions to be taken in choosing a site for a hypodermic injection, and of the anatomical structures to be avoided, it is not necessary to speak here. These points have been fully treated of in other works, and, as a rule, the suggestions made therein are carefully noted and acted upon. Unfortunately, hitherto sufficient attention has not been paid to the need of aseptic methods in making the ordinary hypodermic puncture, and it is a very common occurrence for even a good physician to take a hypodermic syringe from its case, dissolve a tablet in water, immediately fill the syringe, and at once plunge the needle into the subcutaneous tissues. It is more than probable that the risk of puncturing a vein, of injecting the periosteum, and the like, is no greater than is the danger of setting up an infectious process, so that one of the most important points to be attended to is that the puncture be made aseptically. That the danger of sepsis is by no means merely hypothetical is evidenced by the large number of cases of hypodermic puncture which have been followed by abscess formation or localized phlegmons, and we have only to refer to the recent monograph of Fraenkel, of Hamburg, on gas phlegmons, in which he reports two cases of fatal spreading gangrene following hypodermic puncture, to illustrate further the danger which lurks beneath this ordinarily simple operation. The importance of sterilizing the hypodermic syringe after using it upon one patient before employing it again is shown by the cases on record in which erysipelas, anthrax, and tuberculosis have actually been transmitted through the medium of the hypodermic syringe. The sources of infection to be particularly remembered in giving hypodermic injections are the following: (1) the syringe and its needles, (2) the fluids to be injected, (3) the skin of the patient, (4) the hands of the operator. Although the dangers of an infection from the two last-named sources are not very great, yet the careful surgeon will disinfect both his own hands and the skin of his patient before introducing the hypodermic needle. Fortunately, solutions of drugs, such as quinine, antipyrin, and apomorphine, sometimes used for hypodermic injections, possess a certain amount of antiseptic power which tends to prevent the development and multiplication of pyogenic bacteria in them. On the other hand, solutions of the drugs in most common use, such as atropine, morphine, cocaine, and ergotine, favor the development of bacteria, and when kept too long, or if made without proper precautions, are frequently found to be swarming with micro-organisms, with the result that not only are their medical properties sometimes impaired, but thousands of micro-organisms may be placed in the subcutaneous tissues; and even though the greater number of them may be harmless, at other times there may be pyogenic bacteria present which will give rise to the formation of local abscesses which are likely to prove very troublesome and even dangerous to life.

Fluids used for hypodermic injections should be sterile. When hypodermic injections of a drug are given only rarely, it is best to make up a fresh solution each time. In private practice, where the tablets are so much used, a very simple expedient enables us to make a practically sterile solution at a few minutes' notice. A dessertspoonful of water is held over a lamp until the water boils. A tablet is then allowed to roll from its phial into the spoon. This immediately dissolves, and we have a practically sterile solution. Of course, where the drug is one which is injured by a temperature of 100° C. (212° F.), the best we can do is to have the water boiled and allowed to cool somewhat before the tablet is placed in it.

Even in hospitals, where stock hypodermic solutions must be kept in the operating-room, it is best not to make too large a quantity at once. In the case of the majority of solutions which have been prepared aseptically the addition of from two to three drops of pure carbolic acid to thirty cubic centimetres (one ounce) of the solution will prevent the development of bacteria and at the same time will not be sufficient to do any injury. Cocaine may be dissolved in various menstrua, but keeps best in a 1 to 10,000 solution of corrosive sublimate.

The sterilization of hypodermic syringes has been and is still a difficult problem : the complexity of the instrument, and especially the inaccessibility of the piston, render it by no means easy to free from germs. The ingenious syringe of Koch has no piston and is easily sterilized, but it is too inconvenient for practical use, and the many improvements suggested have as yet failed to give us a satisfactory instrument. The syringes made entirely of glass with asbestos pistons, if they are well made, are very satisfactory for a time, but the asbestos piston soon gets out of order. In the case of the ordinary glass syringe the piston should be withdrawn from the barrel and both placed in a 1 to 20 solution of carbolic acid, which will render them sterile. Hot water should afterwards be drawn through the syringe just before it is used. Metal syringes, as well as the needles, can be boiled in a one-per-cent. soda solution. Hypodermic needles made of platinum can be rendered perfectly sterile by heating them in the flame of a Bunsen burner or of an alcohol lamp, but exposure of the ordinary needles to the flame soon ruins them.

*Exploratory puncture and paracentesis* are not so frequently resorted to as in former days, chiefly because major operations with our present methods are not accompanied with much greater risks. It is still occasionally necessary, however, to draw off the fluid from the abdomen in cases of pleurisy, ascites, or in other conditions, either for purposes of diagnosis or for the relief of the patient. The needle, trocar, or rubber tubes used should be sterilized in a one-per-cent. soda solution, and the skin of the patient as well as the hands of the operator prepared according to the principles already laid down.

*Catheterization* of the female bladder is so simple a procedure that it seems almost superfluous to do more than mention it in a text-book on gynæcological technique. But, although simple enough, there is probably no operation which is so often done improperly, and the nurse or physician has been responsible over and over again, through oversight or carelessness, for the setting up of a serious infection of the bladder, or even of fatal suppuration in the kidneys or their pelves. The normal urine is probably always sterile, bacteria being discharged through the kidney only when there are lesions in the renal parenchyma. In the majority of cases of infection of the urinary passages the pathogenic bacteria have gained entrance from below. It is interesting to note, too, that one of the most frequent organisms found in connection with cystitis, pyelitis, and pyelonephritis is the bacillus coli communis. The staphylococcus, streptococcus, and proteus vulgaris are also sometimes present in cases of cystitis. These facts should teach us the importance of thoroughly cleansing the external parts before we undertake the catheterization of the bladder. The physician should not only always take care himself, but also instruct the nurse to make sure, that no possible precaution for the prevention of infection is neglected.

For catheterization the patient lies in the dorsal position, with the knees somewhat separated. A sheet or blanket is thrown over the hips and extends to the knees, leaving the vulva exposed. "Catheterization in the dark" is no longer justifiable. The labia are held apart with a gauze sponge, and the meatus urinarius and the parts around it are thoroughly cleansed with a cotton sponge and warm boric acid solution before the catheter is inserted. One great difficulty in the way of an aseptic catheterization of the male has lain in the impossibility of sterilizing the gum-elastic catheters, which are still often used, without at the same time injuring them. Fortunately, in the female this difficulty has been obviated by the introduction of the simple glass catheter (Fig. 24), which is easily rendered sterile by being

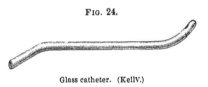

FIG. 24.

Glass catheter. (Kelly.)

well scrubbed with soap and water and afterwards being placed in a five-per-cent. solution of carbolic acid for a few minutes. A number of them may be cleaned at the same time, if desired, and kept in a 1 to 20 solution of carbolic acid (Fig. 25.) Whenever one is needed, it is removed from the jar and placed in a basin containing a warm boric acid solution. If by chance a glass catheter is not available, rubber or silver catheters may be employed after having been boiled in the one-per-cent. soda solution. For a lubricant, sterilized oil or glycerin may be used. If the glass catheter be used, no lubricant is necessary. It has been suggested that the urethra should be washed out carefully with some sterile fluid before catheterization, inasmuch as this takes away a certain number of bacteria. In the female it has been shown that the chances of contamination from the urethra, in the absence of a definite urethritis, are very slight.

FIG. 25.

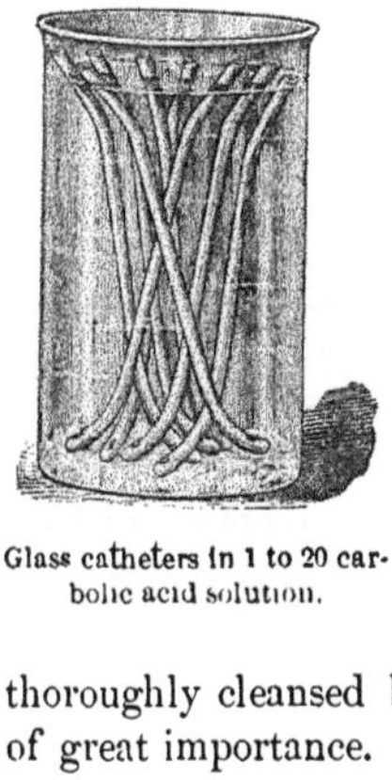

Glass catheters in 1 to 20 carbolic acid solution.

After a catheter has once been used it should be thoroughly cleansed before it is put away ; and here mechanical means are of great importance. The outside should be scrubbed with brush and soap, and hot water or soda solution should be syringed through it until the lumen is thoroughly clean.   The catheter is then placed in a jar containing a 1 to 20 solution of carbolic acid until again required for use.

*Irrigation of the bladder* is often indicated, and for this purpose a sterilized solution of boric acid or normal salt solution is generally used.   The warm solution is filtered into a sterilized rubber bag or fountain syringe, the end of the conduit tube from the bag being attached to the end of the sterilized glass catheter, and, after the urine has been drawn off, is allowed to run slowly into the bladder, the stream being controlled by a pinch-cock placed on the tube.   The tube is disconnected from the end of the catheter after about a pint has run in, or sooner if the patient complains of pain, and the bladder allowed to empty itself.   The process may be repeated two or three times until the washings are clear.   If desired, a two-way catheter may be employed, especially if the distention of the bladder is at all painful.

*Catheterization of the ureters* will not be described in detail here.   It is necessary here simply to mention that the instrument, the hands of the operator, and the external genitalia are disinfected thoroughly according to the methods already described.

## XI.

### THE GYNÆCOLOGICAL OPERATING-ROOM —OPERATING-TABLE—INSTRUMENT-CASES AND OTHER FURNISHINGS.

Only in a hospital can we expect to have an ideal operating-room; at times we must content ourselves with a room fitted up at the patient's house, but this is at the best but a poor substitute.

*The operating-room* in a hospital should, while being within a convenient distance of the wards, be so located that the patients in them will not be disturbed by any of the unavoidable noises belonging to it, nor be annoyed by the smell of the fumes of the anæsthetic.   There should be good-sized windows at the sides and in the roof, so arranged that most of the light comes from the north.   It will be of advantage to have several smaller rooms adjoining the operating-room,—a dressing-room for the operator and his assistants, a store-room for supplies, a room in which the anæsthetic is administered, and another in which the patients may remain, if necessary, until they have had time to recover somewhat from its effects. A water-closet with bath-room attached should be near at hand, and a photographic dark room with water-supply is a great convenience, as it is often desirable to make photographs of unusual conditions upon the spot while the operation is in progress.   These smaller rooms may be arranged on either side of the corridor at the end of which the operating-room is situated, the room where the patient is anæsthetized being provided with a second door which communicates directly with the operating-room.   The corridor can, if it be absolutely necessary, be also used as a waiting-room.   If only two rooms are available, the one most favorably located as regards the distribution of the light and the water-supply should be employed as the operating-room, while the second room is used for a supply-room, in which the anæsthetic can also be given.

The operating-room of a general hospital should be sufficiently large to satisfy all requirements, more especially those which will facilitate the efforts for the maintenance of an aseptic technique. One measuring 26' 9" by 25' 8", or 18' 0" by 26' 6", will answer every purpose where the number of operations does not exceed three or four daily. Everything about the room should be as simple and plain as possible and of such material and shape as will admit of a thorough mechanical cleansing and bear repeated washings with hot soda solution. The floor should be tiled or made of hard wood which has been paraffined. The walls and ceiling are best plastered with King's cement, which should be coated with white enamel paint. The corners of the room should be rounded, in order to do away with crevices and nooks from which dust will be hard to remove. The walls and floor can thus be scrubbed whenever necessary without injury. There should be arrangements for a good supply of light for operations by night or on dark days. The electric light will be found most convenient. A movable incandescent lamp with reflector is very useful for throwing a light directly into the abdomen during an abdominal section, especially where it is desired to find small bleeding points. A gas supply and fittings for the Bunsen burners are necessary. The room should be heated by the general heating apparatus of the hospital, but, where it can be obtained, an open fireplace in addition will be of value. The temperature, which should be about 70° F. (21° C.), should be carefully regulated, a thermometer being always kept suspended in the room.

*The operating-table* may either be of wood, or have a glass top supported by legs made of metal. It can be made of quartered oak finished in paraffin, and both the top and the legs should be perfectly plain, in order that they can be easily and thoroughly cleansed. A table forty-four inches (one hundred and twelve centimetres) long, twenty-one inches (fifty-four centimetres) wide, and thirty-one inches (eighty centimetres) high will be of a convenient size. It is well to have the two legs at one end provided with rubber casters, so that while standing firm with the two ends level at other times, the table can be easily wheeled in any direction desired. The top is made of one-inch oak with rounded edges. There should be no grooves in which dust or foreign material may lodge. For an abdominal section a chair should be placed at the lower end of the table at such an angle that the top of the back will be caught beneath the lower edge of the table, so that the patient's feet rest upon the chair during the operation. When performing a plastic operation, the operator sits astride of this chair (Fig. 27). The table devised by Dr. Kelly is very complete and can be used for any kind of operation. It is thirty-two inches high, twenty-one inches wide, and forty-four inches long.[1] The objection to such a table is that

---

[1] A full description of this table will be found in the catalogue of Charles Lentz & Sons.

it is expensive and requires a considerable amount of time to keep it clean. The surgical table devised by Dr. Halsted can be employed for abdominal and plastic work, as well as for ordinary surgical operations. This table is in reality a shallow wooden sink supported by four legs, the sink being twenty-four centimetres (ten inches) wider and forty centimetres (sixteen inches) shorter than the board of the stretcher, shortly to be described, which is placed upon it. By shifting the board the spaces at the side which serve as gutters can at any moment be made as wide as desired. The floor of the sink drains to a hole in the centre, beneath which is placed a large galvanized iron can for the reception of fluids and waste materials. This should be emptied and disinfected at the end of each operating-day.

Fɪɢ 27.

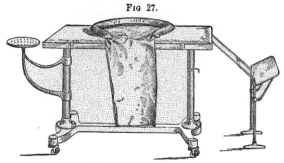

Dr. Kelly's operating-table.

*Tables for holding the basins or glass vessels* may be made of the same kind of wood as the operating-table, or they may be made of metal supports with glass tops. They should be on casters, which will allow of their position being changed as often as desired. The semicircular table devised by Dr. Halsted is convenient, as it will hold the vessels containing the instruments and dressings, while at the same time it hedges off the operator and his assistants from the by-standers. One or two receptacles (made of iron or wire, which can be easily sterilized) for soiled dressings and sponges should be placed in the operating-room.

An instrument-case, constructed somewhat like a book-case, for holding the instruments when not in use, is a very necessary piece of furniture. It should be simply constructed, so as to permit of being easily and thoroughly cleaned. Those made of plain quartered oak are the most satisfactory. The wood should not be thick, and the shelves should be perfectly plain, without trimmings. The shelves are best made of light wood covered on the upper surface with a thin piece of glass, or they may consist entirely of wood or glass. They should be so arranged that any one of them can be pulled out separately, and the instruments be thus exposed without the necessity of touching them with the hands. (Fig. 28.) The instrument-case should be large enough to hold all the necessary instruments, and no cupboard should be placed beneath it, as it will render the case more diffi-

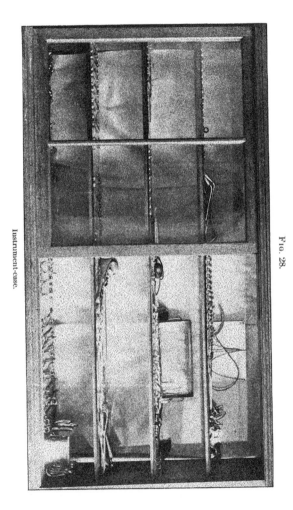

Fig. 28.

Instrument-case.

cult to clean and also increase the risk of contamination. It should have casters attached to it, so that its position can be changed as often as it is necessary to clean the floor beneath it.

*A good water-supply and conveniences for the disinfection of the hands* are necessities in every operating-room, and an abundance of hot and cold water must be always at hand. Arranged on one side of the room there should be several marble basins, in order that the water may be changed rapidly and as frequently as is necessary. One or two large sinks will be necessary for cleansing the instruments and vessels between operations, and these should contain the solutions in which the glass dishes are immersed before a second operation. It will be better to have the basins with the attachments freely exposed, so that they can be easily kept clean. The glass vessels in which the hands are rinsed off during the operation should be placed on a small table close to the operator, and should contain either warm sterile water or salt solution. If glass basins are not obtainable, those lined with porcelain will serve every purpose.

A table for holding the glass jars, glass dishes, and glass basins when not in use should occupy one of the corners of the room. It may be made of the same kind of wood as the instrument-case, and should be of the simplest possible construction.

The *sterilizers* can be arranged on tripods on a shelf at one end of the room with the Bunsen burner under them, so that they are ready for use at short notice.

*Stretchers* upon which patients are moved from place to place in the hospital are of many kinds. The one which I have found to be most satisfactory is two hundred and eleven and one-half centimetres (one hundred and five inches) long, forty and one-half centimetres (sixteen inches) wide, and sixty-five centimetres (twenty-six inches) high. The tires of the wheels are covered with rubber. The board on the top is detachable, with two holes at either end which fit the hands; it measures one hundred and eighty-six centimetres (seventy-two inches) in length and fifty-five centimetres (twenty-one inches) in width, and with the patient on it can be easily lifted on or off the operating-table by two persons.

*The operating-room of a private hospital* can be arranged in very much the same manner as that belonging to a general hospital, but, of course, everything will be on a much smaller scale. So large a room will not be needed, as it will not be necessary to allow more space than that which is actually required for the fittings of the room and for those engaged in the work. The question of space for spectators will not have to be taken into consideration. The room should be situated in one of the upper stories, as far distant as possible from the other rooms of the house. One at the back of the house with a northern exposure, containing as many windows as possible, will be preferable on account of the light, and it will be a decided advantage if it have a skylight, which will not only give us light from above, but can also be opened after an operation and thus

10

afford speedy and thorough ventilation.   Two smaller rooms are better than a single large room, as a great many things which should not be in the operating-room itself may be kept in the second room, which can communicate with it by a door-way which need have no door.   The walls of the room should be painted with white enamel paint, as this can be washed without injury.   The floor may be covered with linoleum, and this should extend up the walls of the room for one or two feet.   The floor can then be thoroughly scrubbed without injuring either it or the ceiling of the room below.   The fittings of the room should approximate as nearly as possible to those described for a large operating-room.   The basins in which the hands are washed and sterilized should be conveniently situated.

In order to have as much space as possible in the operating-room, the doors should be made to open towards the outside.   The same care is to be exercised in the cleansing of the room as with the operating-room in a general hospital, and once a week, as a matter of routine, it will be advisable to scour thoroughly the walls and the entire furniture.

It is possible to arrange a small private operating-room at comparatively little cost.   Time was when both operator and patient avoided hospital operating-rooms, as they seemed to be hot-beds of infection.   Now a surgeon will never operate, if he can avoid it, outside of his own well-regulated operating-room.   However, even with the utmost care infection will sometimes occur, and too often a series of cases in which suppuration follows the operation are still met with.   In such instances the whole paraphernalia of the operating-room, including instruments, furniture, ligatures, sutures, and dressings, are to be thoroughly overhauled and re-sterilized.   There has been some fault in the technique, and as all the good boys in the school suffer for one bad one, so everything in the operating-room must be re-sterilized in order that the one source of danger may not be passed over.

## XII.

### THE ORGANIZATION OF OPERATIONS—THE MAINTENANCE OF AN ASEPTIC TECHNIQUE DURING OPERATIONS.

Now that we have completed the description of the preparation of the different materials which come into play in our operative technique, it may be well to describe briefly the method of properly organizing operations, whether major or minor, and to show how, after starting into surgical work with an aseptic field, sterilized instruments, hands, and dressings, the aseptic condition is to be maintained.

In order to do the best work, the surgeon should surround himself with a sufficient number of well trained assistants and nurses, and keep them with him for some time, until they have become used to his particular methods of working.   No matter how well-trained the individual members of the corps may be, the whole cannot move satisfactorily unless all have worked together long enough for each to have learned his own particular duties and the precise relation of his own actions to those of others about him, so that his attention may not be distracted. To borrow an expression from the foot-ball field, it is essential that the operator and his assistants shall do "good team work." It is necessary, therefore, in starting in to do regular operative work in hospitals, large or small, that the surgeon shall clearly define the exact duties of those about him. It is important that this shall be done at the start, and then, as experience in the course of time teaches, as it always does, that improvements in methods and in the distribution of duties can be made with advantage, the necessary changes may gradually be introduced. When a systematic routine has been once established, surgical work becomes a pleasure, and any operation can be done with but very few hitches and with a minimum of trouble. A surgeon who has accustomed himself to this orderly method of procedure will naturally avoid operations outside of his own operating-room, but will nevertheless, in case the necessity arises, be the better prepared for conducting operations in private houses, or in other places where the dangers of breaking the technique become great.

We shall proceed to describe, therefore, as a type, the order of events in an ordinary abdominal section—undertaken, let us say, for the removal of an ovarian cyst, of adherent adnexa, or for a hysterectomy—in a well-conducted operating-room. We shall suppose that the patient is a young and strong woman, of good constitution, in fair condition for operation, who has been under observation for some days, parts of which have been spent in bed, in order to accustom her to the recumbent position which will have to be maintained for a few days following the operation. She has had a general bath besides two antiseptic vaginal douches each day. A specimen of urine taken by catheter has been carefully examined and has been found to show no striking abnormalities. During this preliminary surveillance the diet has been limited to soft, easily-digested food, and the bowels have been kept freely opened. If abdominal hysterectomy is to be performed, especial attention must be paid during these days to the cleanliness of the vagina and cervix, inasmuch as after removal of the uterus the dangers of infection of the peritoneal cavity from below are very great. The vagina in such cases must be repeatedly cleansed with soap and water and the douches be more frequent and thorough. Attempts to disinfect the cervical canal and cavity of the uterus are perhaps in some cases justifiable.[1]

The operation is to be done sharply at 9 A.M., an excellent operating hour in a hospital. The day before the operation the patient's abdomen

---

[1] One thorough method of doing this is to curette the internal surface of the uterus and cervix several days before the operation, and after curettement go gently over the surface of the uterine mucosa with the small point of the Paquelin cautery, packing the uterine cavity immediately afterwards with a strip of ten-per-cent. iodoformized gauze. The vagina is thoroughly douched twice daily and loosely packed with strips of iodoform gauze. Such radical measures are, however, only rarely to be adopted even in cases where the uterus is to be removed at the operation.

has been prepared in the way directed in Section IV., special attention having been given to the cleansing of the folds round the umbilicus. On the evening preceding the operation a purgative has been administered, followed by an enema in the morning. The bladder has just been emptied by catheter, and the vagina, rectum, and external genitalia have received a final thorough washing. Nothing has been given by mouth since midnight. The patient, attired in a fresh night-gown, flannel undervest, stockings, and warm wrapper, is now taken from the ward to the operating-room on a stretcher, where she should arrive at least half an hour before the time set for the operation. She is put to bed in a small room adjoining the operating-room, where the anæsthetic will be given by one of the assistant surgeons.

In the mean time the nurse has been doing her work. She is in operating-room garb, and her hands and arms have been thoroughly disinfected. She has consulted her instrument-list and has seen that everything is prepared and in good condition. The knives all have keen edges, and these and other things made of metal or rubber are boiling in a one-per-cent. soda solution. The gauze, sponges, and dressings have been sterilized by steam and are in the drying chamber, and an abundant supply of sterilized towels is at hand. The temperature of the room has been properly regulated.

The operating-table is prepared in the following way. A folded blanket, or, better still, a felt pad, large enough to cover it, is placed upon the table. Over this is spread a rubber sheet, which in turn is covered with a fresh white sheet. The head of the patient is to rest upon a small hair-pillow or upon an air-pillow, and the rubber ovariotomy pad is placed in position.

Some surgeons prefer to employ the Horn-Martin or the Trendelenburg position for their operations. The operating-table used by Martin is somewhat shorter than usual, and as the patient lies upon it the buttocks are placed near the edge and the legs are allowed to hang down. The surgeon sits on a chair between the patient's thighs, and is thus able to hold them steady without being obliged to support them. Besides the fact that the position is somewhat awkward, there is the objection that a larger incision is required in order to expose the pelvic structures than would otherwise be necessary. The advantages claimed for the table are (1) the facility given for making the first incision by the tension of the abdominal wall, (2) the inclination given to the pelvis of the patient, by which the examination and manipulation of the organs are rendered easier, and (3) the saving of fatigue to the surgeon, who is able to sit down during the entire operation.

To Frau Horn, Dr. Martin's head operating-room nurse, belongs the credit of suggesting a further improvement in the construction of the table. A section of the middle portion of the top is so arranged that it can be let down, thus permitting the abdominal dressing to be applied with greater facility.

The Trendelenburg position, in which the pelvis is elevated, has been considered to be of especial value in exposing the pelvic contents to view. While the patient is in this position the intestines are not so likely to obstruct the necessary manipulations, because by the action of gravity they are naturally displaced upward towards the thorax. We have found this position to be inconvenient and in the majority of cases unnecessary. Another somewhat serious objection to its adoption lies in the fact that it favors the spreading about among the intestines of any fluids that may be present in the pelvis, thus increasing the danger of the carriage of septic material into the abdominal cavity.

Besides these preparations, the various basins which will be required are conveniently arranged on the side tables. The sterilized salt solution and a plentiful supply of distilled water in large granite-ware vessels are being heated over Bunsen burners. When these matters have been attended to, the nurse gives her hands a second disinfection, after which she must not touch anything which might contaminate them, but must leave it to the assistant nurse or attendant to do anything which necessitates the handling of unsterilized articles.

The surgeon and his assistants have arrived in good time; in their dressing-room they have removed their ordinary clothes and have put on their operating-suits; they have then entered the operating-room long enough before the operation to give themselves ample time to complete the disinfection of their hands and forearms. None of them must have been in contact with septic material for the forty-eight hours preceding. Any visitors who are admitted are to put on over their ordinary clothing the long, loosely-fitting, freshly-washed linen dusters with which they have been supplied. The partially anæsthetized patient is now put upon the table, the hips being placed over the rubber pad which is to conduct the waste fluids over the side of the table into a large vessel. (Fig. 29.) The night-gown and undervest are rolled up over the elbows to hold the arms still. The final disinfection of the abdomen now takes place. The assistant nurse hands to one of the surgeons a basin of warm water, scrubbing-brush, and green soap, and the parts are once more thoroughly cleansed. The soapsuds are rinsed off with sterile water, and the surface of the abdomen is

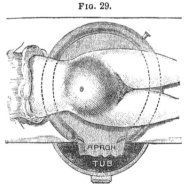

FIG. 29.

Rubber ovariotomy pad in position.

next sponged (sterilized gauze sponges being used) with ether or strong alcohol. After a further washing with a 1 to 1000 sublimate solution, the excess of sublimate is washed off with sterilized water or salt solution.

The sides of the abdomen are well covered with a piece of sterilized gauze, over which towels are laid, the upper part of the abdomen and the lower part of the thorax being also protected by sterilized towels. The field of operation itself is to be covered with a piece of sterilized gauze which has had an opening made in it down the middle, so that when the edges are pulled apart the line of the abdominal incision will be easily exposed. Finally, the adjacent parts of the patient's body and of the operating-table are completely covered with sterilized towels, and the operation will be done through the artificial opening in the gauze over the abdomen. The assistant at the head of the table completes the anæsthesia, and the patient is ready for the first incision.

The arrangement of the different instruments and other accessories is deserving of mention. The operating-table is placed so that a good light shall, when the surgeon is in position, fall upon the field of operation. The surgeon stands, of course, upon the right of the patient, and his first assistant stands opposite him upon the left side. The latter holds hæmostatic forceps in his hand all ready to check the hemorrhage, and also attends to the sponging.

In order to do the most satisfactory work, the surgeon will require a liberal number of helpers. He should have, as a rule, three, four, or even five, assistant surgeons, besides two nurses. Directly opposite him should stand the first assistant, and on either side of the table there should be an assistant. One of these should have entire charge of the instruments and ligatures, while the other should look after the sponges and dressings which may be required during the operation. The first assistant should assist the operator directly, and unless his hands are occupied in holding apart the structures, or in other manipulations, the sponges and instruments should generally be passed to him.

The assistant to whom the administration of the anæsthetic is intrusted should give his undivided attention to this duty.

A fifth assistant is of especial value if cultures have to be made or any microscopical work is necessary during the operation. The head nurse in the operating-room watches for any opportunity to be of service to the surgeon and his assistants. She must, as we have said, touch nothing which is not sterile, and indeed there is no necessity for her to contaminate her hands, as to the second nurse are relegated all duties which involve the handling of any articles which have not been rendered aseptic.

About the operation itself it is necessary to make here only a few general remarks; the special points will be considered separately when the methods of the different abdominal operations are discussed. The incision should be made in the median line with a sharp scalpel, starting midway between the umbilicus and the symphysis pubis and being carried towards the latter. It should not, however, extend quite to the symphysis pubis, and care must be taken that the bladder shall not be injured. The first stroke of the knife cuts down to the superficial fascia. After the hemorrhage has been checked, this is divided exactly down to the linea alba. Next come two fibrous layers, between which is a variable amount of fat; after which there is a thin layer of fat directly above the peritoneum. The assistant should keep the parts clean by pressing a sponge firmly along the line of incision and then removing it quickly. The sponge is never to be rubbed along the line of the wound. After the tissues have been separated down to the peritoneum, this is lifted up with a pair of dissecting forceps. The assistant opposite the operator now with a second pair of forceps takes hold of another portion of the peritoneum at a short distance from the first forceps, and, while he raises it, the operator divides the peritoneum very carefully at a point between the two forceps. This precaution is necessary in order to avoid any possibility of injuring the intestines. At the moment the peritoneal cavity is opened, air will enter, and the intestines, unless they are adherent, will fall away from the parietal peritoneum, making its further section free from danger. After the peritoneum has been divided for the full length of the incision through the skin, the abdominal structures are palpated with the left hand, and after a careful examination it will be possible to decide whether or not it will be advisable to enlarge the incision further. If this is thought necessary, there should be no hesitation in doing so, as a better exposure will thus be obtained and all the manipulations will be much expedited.

If cysts have to be punctured and evacuated, great care should be taken that none of the contents gain entrance into the peritoneal cavity. This is particularly important if the cyst be papillomatous, since the fragments which escape may become implanted upon the peritoneum and give rise to malignant metastatic growths. Before the sac is punctured it is well to place a large sponge or piece of gauze round it, to absorb any fluid which we might otherwise not be able to catch. Should any fluid or particles of papillomatous growths, in spite of our efforts, have been carried into the abdominal cavity, they must be carefully sponged out. A collection of pus which has been opened into must always be well walled off from the peritoneal cavity.

After the diseased parts have been excised and the pedicle firmly ligatured, the surgeon makes the peritoneal *toilette*. If there has been no escape of fluid and no free oozing into the abdominal cavity, it is not necessary to employ any irrigation, and it will be sufficient if the peritoneal cavity be sponged dry, particularly the portion posterior to the uterus. To do this the uterus is held well forward with the left hand, so that the fingers of the right can thus be carried well down into the cul-de-sac. All ligatures should now be well inspected before the ends are cut off, and if there is little or no oozing and the pedicle does not retract from the ligature, the latter may be cut off about one centimetre from the knot.

When adherent structures are to be removed the technique to be carried out is more difficult than when they are free. It is in these cases that the longer abdominal incisions are required. Fortunately, adhesions are more rare now than of old, since patients submit to an operation earlier and the previous puncture of the abdomen for diagnostic purposes or for drawing off fluid is less common.   If the intestines obstruct the field of operation, they can be kept out of the way by pushing them back and covering them with a large sponge or with a large piece of sterilized gauze wrung out of hot water or hot salt solution.   The adherent structures are to be separated by gently working the adhesions loose with the fingers, every precaution being exercised in doing this to avoid any laceration of the abdominal organs, particularly of the intestines and bladder.   If we find it impossible to separate the structures at any one place in this way, we proceed to make attempts to do this at various points until we find a place where the adhesions are less firm.   This will frequently require a good deal of time, but it pays to "make haste slowly," since in the great majority of cases grave injuries can be thus avoided.   If there should be much hemorrhage following such removal, it can frequently be checked by washing the peritoneal cavity with hot sterilized salt solution, or often, if the adhesions are fresh, simple pressure made with a sterilized sponge will arrest the bleeding.   Where the adhesions are old and firm and the hemorrhage is persistent, the bleeding points must be ligated.   In desperate cases of bleeding from the uterus, where all the ordinary means have failed, the hemorrhage can generally be checked at once by tying the ovarian or uterine arteries, or by packing the pelvic cavity with ten-per-cent. iodoform gauze which has been wrung out of very hot salt solution.   If there be troublesome oozing over a large area, it is often possible to control it by applying the tip of the Paquelin cautery lightly over the bleeding surface.   After the bleeding has been checked, the peritoneal cavity is to be washed out with warm sterile salt solution and all clots removed.

The abdominal cavity is closed by first uniting the peritoneum by means of a continuous ligature.   (The question of drainage has already been discussed in Section VIII.)   The skin and muscular surfaces are then brought together with deep sutures of silkworm-gut and silk.   If Halsted's subcutaneous suture is employed, the stitching of the muscular and skin surfaces can be done separately.   After the wound has been properly closed, we have to decide upon the most suitable method of dressing it.   The following procedure has yielded very satisfactory results.   After the sutures have been tied, the field of operation is well washed off with sterilized salt solution and then sponged dry, care being taken to disturb the line of incision as little as possible.   A strip of sterilized gauze (single thickness) twenty-one by ten centimetres (eight by four inches) is placed over the incision.   Enough bichloride celloidin (1 to 16,000 or 1 to 32,000) is poured over the gauze to saturate it thoroughly, and is then smoothed out with a sterile glass spatula.   This is better than employing the fingers for this purpose, since the celloidin adheres to them and is troublesome to remove.   As soon as the piece of gauze has been covered with this adhesive dressing, a powder consisting of iodoform and boric acid (1 to 7) is freely dusted over it. Over this is placed a second piece of gauze, twenty-one by eighteen centimetres (eight by seven and a half inches). This is fixed in the same manner as the first with the celloidin, and over it more of the powder of iodoform and boric acid is applied. This dressing dries in a few minutes. Finally, several pieces of absorbent cotton are to be applied and held in position by the many-tailed bandage. The wound is now well protected from any infection from the surrounding skin, which would be more likely to take place if any but a fixed dressing were employed. The advantage of the second strip of gauze is that it protects a wide area of the skin around the wound, while the first strip covers the incision itself. In ordinary cases the wound need not be disturbed for a week or more. When the dressing is to be removed, it will generally be necessary to moisten it thoroughly by applying to it for an hour a pad of absorbent cotton which has been soaked in sterile water or in a 1 to 40 carbolic acid solution. If this is not done, and we wish to remove it quickly and without causing pain, ether may be poured directly upon the dressing, which, as a rule, can then be readily removed. If the dressing still adheres to the stitches, we can cut them free from the gauze and remove them later. In removing the cutaneous sutures the loop is to be cut below the point where the celloidin and powders are encrusted, and at a point where the suture is moist and pliable. In this way we avoid dragging the ragged and rough part through its whole track (Fig. 30).[1] The subcu-

Fɪɢ. 30.

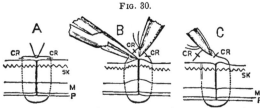

Removal of the abdominal suture. *A* shows the suture *in situ*, passing through skin, muscle, and peritoneum. *CR*, *CR* are the little masses of incrustation of hardened lymph discharged from the suture-track. *B* shows the removal of the suture, elevated and cut below the crust. *C* shows the direction in which it is to be pulled out.

taneous suture probably has the advantage of lessening the chances of stitch-hole infection. After the stitches have been removed, the dry dressing of iodoform and boric acid powder (1 to 7) or subiodide of bismuth powder is applied to the wound. Over this it is better to place a piece of plain sterilized gauze, and if there is any tendency to separation of the edges of the wound it will be well to apply an additional strip about six centimetres (two and a half inches) in width over the surface, the whole dressing being kept in place with cotton and the many-tailed bandage. Dr. Halsted prefers to dress the wound of an abdominal section with strips of sterile gutta-percha tissue (or protective, as it is called), which are applied

---

[1] American Journal of the Medical Sciences, vol. ci. page 53.

immediately along the line of incision, thus protecting the granulations which form : he believes that the removal of ordinary dressings into which the granulations have grown is very injurious to the wound. In his dressings no powders or celloidin are applied, but pieces of dry sterilized gauze and cotton are placed over the protective, the whole being held in place by an abdominal bandage.

Where the operation is to be upon the perineum, upon the vagina, or upon the uterus through the vagina, the external genitalia and adjoining parts will require more careful preparation. All the hair should be shaved off and the parts should be thoroughly scrubbed twice daily with soap and hot water for two or three days, and on the

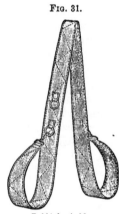

Fig. 31.

Robb's leg-holder.

morning of the operation they should be thoroughly cleansed with alcohol and ether and afterwards with sublimate solution. The bladder and rectum are, of course, to be thoroughly emptied before this cleansing. The patient is anæsthetized, brought to the operating-table, and placed in the dorsal position. The legs are flexed on the abdomen, and may be conveniently held in place with the simple leg-holder shown in the figure (Fig. 31). The external genitalia and the vagina are again scrubbed with soap and warm water, and the skin about the parts and over the thighs is irrigated thoroughly with a 1 to 1000 solution of sublimate and afterwards with sterile water. The parts are then protected with a large piece of gauze, in which a hole is cut large enough to expose thoroughly the perineum and vaginal outlet. The operation is then proceeded with. If a continuous stream of sterile water or salt solution be kept playing over the field of operation, sponging will be unnecessary, and the operation will thus progress more speedily.

## XIII.

POST-OPERATIVE CARE—POSITION IN BED—DIET—VOMITING—RECTAL FEEDING—SHOCK—PAIN AND RESTLESSNESS—CONSTIPATION—CATHETERIZATION — CONVALESCENCE — REMOVAL OF STITCHES — DRESSINGS SUBSEQUENT TO OPERATIONS — HEMORRHAGE — INTESTINAL OBSTRUCTION AND INFECTION.

Immediately after the operation has been finished and the dressings have been applied, the patient, not yet entirely recovered from the anæsthetic, is removed to the bed where she is to remain until convalescence. The after-care of operative cases is naturally of very great importance, and mistakes in treatment are often attended by the most serious results. The nurse in charge should be one who has had special experience in abdominal work, and none should be chosen who are not specially fitted for the post. At first the patient is to be kept quietly in bed in the recumbent position, and she must be closely watched until she has fully regained consciousness. Of the dangers from vomiting during the semi-unconscious stage it is scarcely necessary to speak. When it occurs, the head should be turned on one side and the nurse should have a basin ready to place beneath the patient's chin for the reception of vomited or mucous material, so that any soiling of the night-dress and of the bedclothes may be avoided. Every precaution must be taken to sustain the strength of the patient and to keep her warm and comfortable. Exposure to draughts or allowing her to become chilled in this condition of lowered resistance may easily prove to be the exciting cause of a serious bronchitis or pneumonia. Hot cans are to be placed round her in the bed, care being taken that the skin shall not be burned. This may easily be avoided by placing a blanket between the cans and the surface of the body. Neglect of this simple measure has before now led to serious superficial burns, which have delayed convalescence and have proved a source of much annoyance to both physician and patient.

It is extremely difficult to lay down definite rules regarding the food and drink to be ordered after abdominal operations. Where a plastic operation has been performed upon the perineum and cervix, the problem is comparatively simple, and after the early nausea has disappeared a light soft diet may very soon be allowed ; but where the patient has undergone an abdominal section the greatest care has to be exercised. With ordinary simple cases a light soft diet may be given after the first twenty-four hours, but where the operation has been a serious one, or where the viscera have been much disturbed, the woman must be kept as quiet as possible, and frequent feeding by the way of the stomach cannot be permitted for some days. In all such cases a great deal of tact and patience will be required. Milk is not a good substance to give by the mouth after abdominal sections in the majority of cases. In the first place, it is not easily digested in the stomach, and the curd remaining may pass along the intestines and act as an irritant. In the second place, milk very often causes flatulence and produces much discomfort. Peptonized milk would be free from this objection ; but patients, as a rule, complain of its bitter taste, and it is difficult to get them to take it more than once or twice. During the first six or twelve hours it will be found preferable, if there be any vomiting, to give the patient by mouth nothing except small quantities of toast-water or of warm water, from one to two teaspoonfuls every fifteen or twenty minutes. This frequency of administration is generally not only tolerated, but is very comforting to the patient, from the fact that it tends to relieve the thirst which is complained of, and sometimes will diminish the vomiting as well. It will occasionally be desirable to give nutritive enemata at intervals of three or four hours. They should not be given more frequently than this, for fear of rendering the rectum intolerant of them. The enema should consist of milk with whiskey or brandy, together with the white of egg and a little common table salt. The following proportions make a good combination, and the enema may be given by means of a hard-rubber syringe or through a rectal tube :

> ℞ Peptonized milk, 80 cc. (℥i) ;
> Whiskey, 30 cc. (℥i) ;
> The whites of two eggs ;
> Common table salt, 1,50 (grs. xxiv.).

The rectum should be thoroughly irrigated once or twice daily with warm physiological salt solution, which will keep it clean, so that the nutritive enemata will be better absorbed.

Often, besides the warm water and toast-water, fifteen to twenty drops of sherry with one or two teaspoonfuls of soda-water, given at frequent intervals, will be retained by the stomach. This method of treatment can be kept up for the first day or so. After this, if the patient is still willing to take a fluid diet and there is no vomiting, the quantity of the liquids may be gradually increased. At the end of the third day we may begin with small quantities of milk and lime-water by the mouth, if the patient cannot take the peptonized milk. It is better to give this in the proportion of two parts of milk to one part of lime-water, slowly increasing the quantity of the former each day and diminishing the amount of the latter until the patient is taking three parts of milk to one part of lime-water. It is unwise to give cold water to drink to quench the thirst, and the custom of allowing the patient to suck ice is not a good one, as neither is nearly so efficacious as warm water, and the patient is never satisfied, but is always asking for more. Besides this, the ingestion into the stomach of much cold water or ice soon causes nausea, and may thoroughly upset the stomach and thus add considerably to the discomfort of the patient. If she still complains of distressing thirst, an enema consisting of five hundred cubic centimetres (one pint) of tepid water may be slowly administered. This may be repeated if necessary, and is generally most satisfactory in its results. If the patient does not vomit at all, or only at infrequent intervals, after some six or twelve hours, home-made beef-tea or beef-jelly, in teaspoonful doses, either concentrated or diluted, may be given.

The above treatment applies to those cases which proceed easily and rapidly towards recovery. When, however, the vomiting is persistent and aggravated, it becomes a most troublesome symptom, and one which taxes severely the ingenuity of the surgeon and of the nurse. The vomiting which follows anæsthesia may sometimes be relieved by allowing the patient to rinse out the mouth with warm water, a procedure which will often help to relieve the thirst, which is at times almost unbearable. While the nausea and vomiting continue, the head should rest on a level with the body or be only slightly elevated on a small pillow. As a rule, the vomiting due to the anæsthetic is over by the end of eighteen or twenty-four hours, and when this symptom continues after the third day, and particularly where the fluid is expelled without much apparent effort, in too many cases peritonitis is to be feared. After the second or third day, if there still be a great deal of nausea, it may sometimes be relieved by giving two or three tablespoonfuls of very hot water containing 0,24–0,30 (four or five grains) of bicarbonate of sodium to 30 cc. (one ounce) of water. This may be repeated every hour or so, and where it does not succeed, a mustard leaf may be applied over the epigastrium. In a certain number of cases the washing out of the stomach may be of service.

The vomiting which accompanies a marked septic condition, such as a general or a localized peritonitis, is, however, most resistant to treatment. In the majority of cases this symptom is aggravated instead of being relieved by the administration of drugs especially directed against it, and the treatment of the accompanying constipation or tympany is more likely to stop the vomiting. Occasionally (but only as a last resort) it may be necessary to give a hypodermic injection of morphine over the epigastrium for the relief of the severe retching, if there is reason to fear that it will otherwise soon exhaust the patient.

In those cases where the operation has been a long one, or where the viscera have been much disturbed, it becomes necessary to employ unusual methods of stimulation to tide the patient over the stage of shock until she reacts. Into the question of the true nature of "shock" and the phenomena of "reaction" we shall not go now. What little is known about them can be obtained from the text-books on general surgery. The treatment may be briefly outlined as follows. The patient should be kept warm ; she should be enveloped in blankets, and hot-water cans or hot sand-bags should be applied round the trunk and thighs and to the soles of the feet. Stimulating applications may be cautiously made over the epigastric region, and if necessary the legs and forearms may be enveloped in cloths wrung out of hot water; while in alarming cases hypodermic injections of ether, brandy, whiskey, or camphor are given every few minutes or every half-hour, according to the urgency of the symptoms.

Nearly every patient is restless and suffers more or less pain during the first twenty-four hours after an operation. Not every complaint must be met with drugs, and a skilful nurse can do much to relieve many of the little discomforts of which the patient complains. A slight change in position, made by putting a soft pad or pillow under the head and shoulders or under the bend of the knees, so that the legs are supported in a flexed position, will often do much to effect this. The arms, legs, and chest may be sponged with warm alcohol or with soap and warm water. After the first day, if the patient is still restless and there is no contra-indication, it will do no harm to transfer her once in the twenty-four hours from one bed to another which has been already prepared and dressed with warm clean linen. This, if done in the evening, very often succeeds in giving the patient a good night's sleep. Convalescence is promoted also by frequent spongings and by rubbing the body with alcohol. If, in spite of our efforts, the patient continues to be very restless, especially at night, the administration of an enema consisting of 3,0–4,0 (48–64 grains) of bromide of potassium with from 15,0 to 30,0 (℥ss–℥i) of milk of asafetida may be tried, and if necessary repeated in an hour or two. If the restlessness still persists, or if the patient suffers severe pain, it may be necessary to give morphine in doses of 0,010–0,016 ($\frac{1}{6}$–$\frac{1}{4}$ grain), which may be repeated according to the effect produced. Morphine, however, should never be used unless all other measures fail. It is much better to encourage the patients to control themselves and to bear the pain, telling them that it will not last long, and that they will be in every way much better if they can endure it for a short time without taking medicine for its relief. The routine employment of morphine is to be condemned. The healing always proceeds better without it, and there is little doubt but that the surgeon is often directly responsible for the formation of the morphine habit. Unfortunately, the practice of giving this drug as a matter of course after operations is apparently becoming more and more wide-spread. It is popular, perhaps, because it affords immediate comfort to the patient and to the surgeon. It is not an infrequent practice of surgeons to keep their patients under the influence of morphine for the two or three days subsequent to the operation. Its use is occasionally a necessity, but in the vast majority of cases I feel sure that a patient does not require any sedative at all after an operation, especially if we enlist on our side her own moral support. The danger of using morphine after operations lies in the fact that after a short time the patient not only feels the necessity of its repeated use, but is also much more difficult to manage; she becomes restless and fretful, complaining loudly of the most trivial suffering, and her *morale* suffers so much that at times her mind becomes unbalanced. In the after-care of over one thousand cœliotomies, only in rare instances have I found it necessary to give a dose of morphine, and even then in some of the cases in which it was given there was more than once occasion to regret its employment.

In the majority of cases it is well that the bowels should be opened on the second or third day after an abdominal operation. The giving of medicines by the mouth for this purpose is often contra-indicated, especially in the cases in which there is much nausea. The most satisfactory method consists in the administration on the second day of an enema consisting of five hundred cubic centimetres (one pint) of soapsuds and warm water, given as high up as possible. To do this, the rectal tube having been introduced well up into the rectum, to the external end a small glass funnel is attached, into which the mixture of soap and water is poured and allowed to run slowly into the bowel. Sometimes a litre can be introduced in this way. If the enema has not been effectual, it may be repeated after three or four hours, or an enema may be given consisting of warm water, oil, and turpentine in the following proportions:

Plain warm water, 500 cc. (Oj) ;
Oil, 60 cc. (℥ii) ;
Turpentine, from two teaspoonfuls to a tablespoonful.

This may be repeated once or twice at intervals of two or three hours, but generally the first enema is followed by a satisfactory evacuation of the bowels. If preferred, the first enema may consist of from 120 to 180 cc. (℥iv–℥vi) of warm olive oil or glycerin, to soften any fecal matter that is in the rectum, and then an hour or so later it may be followed by a second made of soapsuds and warm water. Sometimes an enema consisting of a pint of warm soapsuds and water mixed with 30,0 (℥i) of Epsom salt will act where others have failed. If, however, there are no contra-indications to the giving of medicine by the mouth, in addition to using the enema we may give by mouth about one-third of a bottle of the effervescent citrate of magnesium, to be repeated every two hours until the bowels have been opened. Some, again, prefer a Seidlitz powder to be taken on the second morning after the operation, and in other cases it may be advisable to give calomel in doses of from 0,10 to 0,30 ($\frac{1}{6}$–$\frac{1}{2}$ grain) every two to three hours at night, to be followed by a Seidlitz powder on the next morning. The compound liquorice powder is a favorite laxative with some surgeons.

If the employment of these measures fails to produce an evacuation of the intestinal contents, the existence of an obstruction of the bowels is to be suspected, and the question of resorting to operative measures has to be considered.

After the bowels have been thoroughly opened, the patient may complain of a feeling of weakness, and sometimes, indeed, there is a considerable degree of prostration. In order to counteract this condition it may be necessary to give a warm enema containing a stimulant, one consisting entirely of peptonized milk with the addition of brandy or whiskey being often very useful. After plastic operations upon the perineum it is, of course, absolutely necessary that there should be no straining at stool, and after each movement the parts must be carefully cleansed, on account of the dangers of infection. Fuller particulars regarding the after-care of these operations will be found in the section which treats *in extenso* of the operations themselves.

*Catheterization* of the patient at stated intervals after an operation is advised in most of the text-books. This procedure is, however, by no means always necessary. As a rule, the urine need not be drawn off for at least six or eight hours, if this is done immediately after the operation, before the patient leaves the table. It is a good plan to wait until the patient has expressed a desire to micturate and has been allowed to attempt to void her water voluntarily without success before employing the catheter. If she is encouraged to try to pass her urine, in some instances catheterization will not be necessary at all. During the first twenty-four hours the secretion of urine is scanty, and it would therefore seem unnecessary to draw it off more frequently than every six or eight hours. The trouble-some cystitis which sometimes follows catheterization may generally be avoided by the exercise of the proper precautions, as I have already shown in an earlier section. In plastic cases it is particularly important, of course, that catheterization be done aseptically and that the field of oper-ation be not irritated by urine.

In every case for a certain time after an abdominal section the patient should remain in the recumbent position as much as possible. The main-tenance of such a position, of course, is particularly desirable if the drainage-tube has been employed, lest the structures be injured or the tube displaced. After the first ten or twelve hours immediately follow-ing an ordinary abdominal section, if there is no contra-indication, the patient may with safety be placed on her side for a few minutes at a time, while the back is supported by pillows. This, indeed, may often be permitted even earlier, if the drainage-tube has not been used and if the patient has vomited but little. The change of position from the back to the side, if it adds to the comfort of the patient, may be made every two or three hours during the day and night. While the patient is lying on her side the back and legs may be well rubbed with alcohol, after which the bed will not feel so uncomfortable when the dorsal position is resumed. As a rule, the patient should not be allowed to sit up in bed until the six-teenth or eighteenth day after an abdominal operation, and even then the first attempts should be limited in duration to a few minutes, and should not be made without the use of the bed-rest to support the back and head. Gradually the time may be prolonged, until at the end of the third week the patient may be allowed to get out of bed; but on the first day she should simply be wrapped in a blanket and placed in a rolling- or rocking-chair for ten or fifteen minutes, and at the expiration of this time should be put to bed again. On the next day, if the first getting up has not tired her too much, she may be allowed to sit up a little longer; and on the third day the time may be extended to an hour or perhaps more, and increased every day until she can sit up all the morning and finally during the entire day. About the end of the fourth week she may be allowed to walk, but for only a few steps at a time. She should, however, avoid going up- and down-stairs and lifting anything for some days. The observance of these precautions is important, for if they are neglected many patients will sub-sequently complain a great deal of the backache and general weakness which often follow a too early getting about. Before the patient is permitted to get out of bed she should be furnished with an abdominal bandage (Fig. 33), which will not only tend to prevent any opening of the incision, which might be followed by a hernia, but will add a great deal to the patient's comfort by supporting the abdominal walls. This bandage should be used for from six months to a year. After it has been worn for about three weeks it need not be kept on during the night while the patient is lying quietly in bed.

After a trachelorrhaphy or a perineorrhaphy has been performed the patient is generally allowed to sit up in bed with the bed-rest or supported by pillows on the tenth or twelfth day, and on about the seventeenth day after the operation she may get out of bed. Any internal stitches may be removed at the end of the third week, and the patient can then begin to walk around slowly, provided that she is very careful not to do too much and is particularly cautious in going up- and down-stairs. After an operation upon the perineum the patient should keep in the recumbent position for the first ten hours. After this, if she is restless and complains of pain in the back, or if she desires to change her position, she may be carefully turned on her side. A small soft pillow should be placed between the knees. A bandage around the pillows will seldom be necessary, as the patient can generally be induced to keep the knees sufficiently close together, and if she is told to keep the internal surface of one as nearly as possible op-

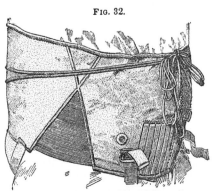

Fig. 32.

Abdominal bandage in position.

posite to that of the other, there will usually be no harm done by dispensing with the bandage. The T-bandage which is applied over the line of the wound will sufficiently protect it from any injury of the parts which might otherwise be caused by movements that the patient may make in turning over. As a rule, after the first two or three days the patient may assume the position which she finds most comfortable.

In ordinary section cases where the abdomen has been closed without drainage, the stitches may be removed on the seventh or eighth day. Some of the precautions to be observed when removing the stitches have already been referred to in Section XII. Naturally, the hands are to be disinfected whenever a wound is being cared for. After the removal of the stitches the incision should be protected by some sterile non-irritating material, such as gauze impregnated with iodoform, or sterilized cotton, or else a powder consisting of iodoform and boric acid (1 to 7) may be dusted freely over the parts. Over this, again, some sterile cotton may be applied and held in place by a many-tailed bandage. This dressing need not be changed more frequently than once every two or three days, or until the wound becomes dry, after which it is only necessary to place over the line of incision a strip of sterile cotton, which can usually be dispensed with at the end of the third week subsequent to the operation.

After a trachelorrhaphy or a perineorrhaphy has been performed a strip

11

of ten-per-cent. iodoform gauze is usually left in the vagina. This should be removed within the first twenty-four hours following the operation, and under ordinary circumstances it is not necessary to reapply it. Over the external wound iodoform and boric acid powder (1 to 7) or subiodide of bismuth powder may be applied, and gauze and cotton held in place by a T-bandage, which must be changed as often as it becomes soiled. The bandage and external dressing will generally not be required to protect the parts after the external stitches have been removed.

*Tympanites,* a by no means uncommon symptom following abdominal operations, is most frequently caused by constipation, and in that case is usually relieved when the bowels are evacuated. It may give rise to severe pain, and, by causing pressure upon the diaphragm, often embarrasses the action of the heart and lungs and leads to acceleration of the pulse and respiration. One or two drops of the tincture of capsicum in a teaspoonful of warm water every half-hour for three or four doses, or fifteen to twenty drops of the essence of peppermint, will prove an effectual remedy for the more simple cases. At the same time a mustard leaf or a warm application, such as a turpentine stupe, may be applied over the epigastrium, care being taken not to leave it on long enough to cause a blister. If the tympanites still continues after the bowels have been well opened, it will be well to pass a rectal tube, which has been previously well warmed and oiled, into the bowel for a distance of fourteen inches, and thus get rid of the accumulated gases.

*Hemorrhage,* and more especially *intra-peritoneal hemorrhage,* will rarely be met with after operations, if the technique of the surgeon has been good. When, however, it does occur, and the loss of blood is considerable, the condition may soon become serious. The symptoms which follow such an accident must always be carefully watched for after any abdominal operation. The lips grow pale, the face takes on a fixed expression, the pupils are dilated, the surface of the body soon becomes covered with a clammy sweat, the extremities are cyanosed, and the patient complains of dizziness, or even loses consciousness. Where the hemorrhage is extensive, the only hope lies in reopening the wound and ligating the bleeding vessels. Hemorrhage following stitch-hole wounds seldom assumes any serious proportions.

*Peritonitis,* by which we mean an infection of the peritoneum either local or general, is always an unfortunate complication. Not every case of tympanites with distention is due to peritonitis. It is only when one gets the array of symptoms which form so striking a clinical picture—the pain, the distention, the drawn expression of the face, the pinched look about the nostrils, and the wiry pulse—that one is justified in positively diagnosing an acute peritonitis. Of stitch-hole infection we need not speak here, except to point out that the elevation of temperature which accompanies it does not usually appear before the second week.

## XIV.

OPERATIONS IN THE COUNTRY, IN PRIVATE HOUSES, OR IN OTHER
PLACES WHERE THE TECHNIQUE MUST NECESSARILY BE MORE OR
LESS IMPERFECT—THE ARMAMENTARIUM—AN IMPROVISED OPER-
ATING-ROOM—MODIFICATIONS IN TECHNIQUE.

Every time that a surgeon is called upon to operate at a distance from
the hospital or from his regular operating-room, he has to encounter many
difficulties in the way of maintaining asepsis. It is, however, just under
these circumstances that the well-trained gynæcologist who has mastered
the principles underlying surgical technique will be able to utilize this
knowledge while adapting himself to his surroundings. Even if he is
called upon to operate on the shortest notice he need never be taken by
surprise, and even if the conditions are the most primitive, so long as he
has fire, water, and vessels he is in a position to carry out an aseptic technique. Boiling water will give him sterile instruments, ligatures, and
dressings,—though there are other and better ways of obtaining these,—and
it will be possible for him to regulate his surroundings with a fair degree
of satisfaction to himself.

A surgeon who is frequently called upon to do operations away from
home will find it convenient to have a set of instruments, dressings, and
other necessaries already packed in a transportation valise, or to have these
kept apart and always sterile, so that they can be put together in a few
moments. The instruments and all the dressings should be rendered sterile
in the same manner as when preparing them for operations in the hospital.
The materials that are required can be supplied from the regular stock in
the operating-room. If one has not the advantage of an operating-room
supply to draw upon, then it will be well to furnish a room adjoining the
office, so that the materials can be kept in good order after they have
once been sterilized. Before going to an operation the instrument-list
should be consulted, and one must be particularly careful to make sure that
nothing that will be required is left out, since away from home it will not
be possible to make a requisition upon the stock instrument-case for any
article which has been forgotten. The surgeon should give the preparation
of the outfit his personal attention, or intrust it to a trained assistant or
nurse whom experience has proved to be competent. For many reasons it
is better to sterilize the instruments and dressings at the place where the
operation is to be performed, in which case it will be necessary to take
along the small soda solution apparatus (*vide* Section V.) and an Arnold
steam sterilizer. If for some reason or other this is impossible, they may
be sterilized before the surgeon sets out, and afterwards conveyed to the
place of operation under aseptic precautions. If the instruments are to
be sterilized after arriving at the house, they can conveniently be carried
arranged in compartments in a long sheet of canton flannel, which is then

rolled up and tied round the middle with a broad tape. (Fig. 33.) If
they have been sterilized at home, they may be carried in stout sterilized
bags made of butcher's linen and closed by a draw-string. It will be found
convenient to have several sizes of these bags, so that the more bulky instru-

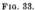

Fig. 33.

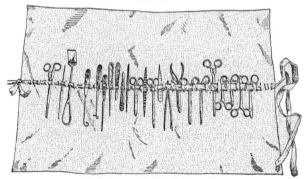

Canton flannel sheet for instruments.

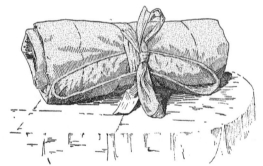

Instruments wrapped in canton flannel sheet.

ments may be kept in the larger and the knives and forceps in the smaller
ones. Three or four hard-rubber trays for the instruments should be
included in the outfit, and should be made so that they may fit into one
another ("nests") and thus not occupy too much room. Brushes for
scrubbing the hands and forearms are to be sterilized by steam and rolled
up in a sterile towel, or they may be carried in a stoppered jar containing
a 1 to 30 carbolic acid solution. Good soap in tin cases, air-tight screw-
capped bottles containing potassium permanganate and oxalic acid, and a
good supply of green or oleine soap, must not be forgotten. The sterilized gauzes, cotton, sponges, and bandages are best rolled up in sterilized
towels and enclosed in sterilized gauze or bags. It will be better to have
at the operation a few wide-mouthed sterilized glass jars which hold from
one-half to two litres and are fitted with air-tight covers. The ligatures

are carried in the large ignition tubes, which are plugged with cotton stoppers and have been sterilized in the manner before described. Several tubes may be carefully rolled up in a towel. The outfit should include a liberal supply of towels, rubber gloves, and mackintoshes.

It is well to collect everything before commencing to pack the valise, so that each item on the list may be checked off as the article is put in. The "telescope" valise will be found most serviceable and convenient. It has also the advantages of being inexpensive and of being easily cleaned, and things packed in it can be transported safely. The surgeon who has many outside calls will find it very convenient to have two or three bags always ready, one containing the necessary instruments for abdominal sections, a second those required for the ordinary plastic cases, and a third those employed in the simpler operations, such as dilatation and curettement.

In handling the articles and preparing the outfit it is essential, if they are sterilized, that the person who does this shall prepare his hands and forearms as carefully as if for an operation.

The inside of the valise, particularly the lower half, should be well protected with sterilized towels or with a piece of muslin sufficiently large to be folded entirely over the contents after they have been put in. In packing the glass-ware great care should be taken to avoid breakage upon the journey.

In order still further to preclude the possibility of any contamination during transportation, we can wrap the bags containing the instruments, cotton, towels, and trays in a piece of sterilized rubber mackintosh. After the valise has been well packed, and the top properly adjusted, it should be fastened snugly with the leather straps.

The operating-room should be chosen with special regard to two requirements,—viz., (1) that it is well lighted, and (2) that it can be easily cleaned. To select it, if possible, one of the assistants or nurses should be sent to the house a few days before the operation. The nurse, besides, should be with the patient for two or three days, in order that all the necessary preparations may be made. In case this is impossible (for example, in the country and in the practice of another physician), special instructions should be sent several days previously, in order that everything may be ready. The room chosen is to be cleared of all the ordinary furniture, carpet, and rugs; the floor and, if possible, the walls and ceiling should be thoroughly scrubbed with soap and water. All hangings are to be removed from the windows and doors, and special attention is to be given to the cleansing of the window sills, of all corners and crevices, and of the wood-work generally. For the operating-table, an ordinary plain, narrow kitchen-table that can be bought for a few dollars will answer every purpose. It should measure about three feet in length, thirty inches in height, and twenty-two inches in width. For the patient's feet to rest on, a plain wooden chair can be placed at the end of the table at such an angle that the back of the chair will be caught under the lower edge of the table. It will be necessary to have two other tables about the same size as the operating-table, on which may be placed the vessels which are to contain the instruments, ligatures, sponges, and other necessaries. When the same sort of tables as the operating-table cannot be obtained, then any two small narrow tables about the house may be used for this purpose, provided that, after being thoroughly scrubbed with soap and water and bichloride solution, they are covered with sterile towels. Six perfectly plain wooden chairs should also be ready; plush or cane-seated chairs are not suitable for this purpose. The tables and the chairs should be thoroughly scrubbed with soap and water and mopped over with a 1 to 500 aqueous solution of bichloride of mercury. After this preparation they are not to be touched until the surgeon and his assistants arrive. There should be an abundant supply of hot and cold water, which, after being boiled, should be kept ready for use in perfectly sterile vessels. Special orders must be given about the cleansing of the large tin boilers in which the water is to be kept. They should be thoroughly scrubbed out with sand-soap and water and then well rinsed out with water. The water which is to be employed for washing the hands and instruments should be thoroughly boiled some hours previous to or even on the day before the operation. If distilled water can be obtained for this purpose, it will be better. The supply-vessels in the operating-room should be provided with lids, which should be covered with sterilized towels or some other clean material, in order to avoid the slightest risk of contamination from the dust of the room. On the day of the operation one of the boilers should be placed on the stove and a sufficient quantity of water made hot again. The water should remain under the supervision of an assistant, to whom the duty of attending to the bringing of it to the operating-room should be delegated. It will not be safe to allow one of the members of the family or a servant to undertake this duty, as they might, from ignorance, be guilty of putting their hands into the pitcher, or in some other way might contaminate the water. Four to six perfectly clean china basins and pitchers, which have been thoroughly scrubbed out with soap and water and then rinsed out with 1 to 500 bichloride solution and plain hot water, will be needed to receive the hot and cold water, being afterwards covered over with sterilized towels.

*The preparation of the patient* in a private house can be as thorough as in a hospital, and the methods already advised in Section IV. should be closely followed. Where possible, the surgeon will find it best to have two nurses, one who will attend to the preparation of the patient and will have the subsequent charge of the case, and a second to attend to the details of the operating-room and to assist at the operation itself. If the operation be in the country, the surgeon should always have at least one assistant with him who has had the advantages of a practical training in modern methods, to aid him in the maintenance of an aseptic technique. This is particularly advisable for abdominal work; and if an untrained assistant is permitted to take any part in the operation, he must be thoroughly instructed as to what he is to do, and that he is to touch nothing unless especially told to do so. The nurse and the assistant should make as little noise as possible while arranging the room in which the operation is to be performed. The assistant should allow himself at least two or three hours in which to make his preparations. When he arrives at the house, the nurse should be called, and she should at once show him to the room. He first proceeds to clean his hands, and then, having dressed himself in his uniform, begins his work. The tables and chairs are put in their places, the operating-table occupying a position near a window from which the greatest amount of light will be thrown upon the field of operation. Those on which the vessels containing the instruments and sponges are to be placed are arranged at a convenient distance from it. The sterile water, which has been boiled some hours previously and allowed to cool, must be ready. The hot water which is in the boilers on the kitchen stove should be transferred to the clean pitchers by means of a perfectly clean tin ladle with a long handle, the tops of the pitchers being immediately afterwards protected with a towel or a gauze hood, and strict orders being given that under no circumstances is any one to put his hand into the water or touch the mouth of the pitcher. I have not infrequently seen both nurses and doctors test the temperature by dipping their fingers into the water in the pitcher. This, of course, is an inconsistency, and should never be permitted.

After these preparations have been made, the assistant proceeds to wash his hands and forearms before getting the instruments ready. If, however, he wears the rubber gloves and rinses them well in a 1 to 500 bichloride solution from time to time, it will not be necessary to give the hands the final scrubbing until later. The basins or trays, after being washed out with a 1 to 500 aqueous solution of bichloride of mercury and then with hot water, are now partially filled with the plain hot water and are ready to receive the instruments and ligatures. The artery forceps should all be placed in one tray and the ligatures and needles in another, while a third is devoted to the scalpels and scissors with the dissecting forceps which are first used at the beginning of an operation. Two large basins half filled with plain sterile water should be provided, the first in which the sponges can be cleaned and the other in which they are kept. On the table nearest the operator should stand two basins filled with plain hot water, so that he may rinse his hands from time to time during the operation. There should be near at hand a vessel in which the diseased structures which are to be removed can be received. The assistant now takes off the rubber gloves and then thoroughly disinfects his hands. The gloves can be placed in the bucket containing the bichloride solution and put on again if it is necessary for him to help to lift the patient on the table. The patient should not be anæsthetized until everything has been satisfactorily arranged, so that there may be no delay after she is once ready. It may be left to the assistant who has charge of making these preparations to say when the anæsthetic is to be administered, as he knows exactly how long it will take to complete them. The operator should arrive at least fifteen minutes or half an hour before the time set for the operation, and should spend this time in changing his clothes and in cleansing his hands. A nurse or one of the assistants, who may wear rubber gloves, should be ready to change the water in the basins for him. The nurse generally remains with the patient while the anæsthetic is being administered. This is best given in a room away from the operating-room, as the patient will then not be disturbed by the noise or by the sight of the preparations. The anæsthetizer will require aid in carrying the patient to the operating-room and placing her in position on the table. If the other assistant surgeons help him to do this, their hands should be protected with the rubber gloves.

The patient being on the table, the abdomen is first thoroughly cleansed in the manner previously described. This cleansing should be performed by one of the assistants who is well acquainted with the method which the operator employs for this purpose. While the abdomen is being prepared, the second assistant, who has been scrubbing his hands for the last time, should soak them thoroughly in the 1 to 500 bichloride solution for one or two minutes, and then rinse them off in the plain sterile salt solution or hot water just prior to the beginning of the operation. The abdomen having been rendered sterile and the field of operation being protected with the gauze and towels, the operator is ready to make the first incision.

If irrigation of the abdominal cavity is required, a pitcher which has been thoroughly sterilized should be ready. The most convenient vessel for this is a glass jar, the so-called thermometer-jar, which has been already referred to. If an ordinary pitcher is to be used, a sterilized thermometer is necessary in order to test the temperature of the water, as it will not be safe to trust to the impression given to the hand from the outside, and it will not be allowable to place the fingers in the water.

It requires a considerable length of time to arrange all the details that have been described, but if we hope to do an aseptic operation none of them can be neglected. Where, from the grave condition of the patient, it is necessary to operate immediately, of course it will be impossible for us to carry out every one, but in any case we should attempt to follow them as closely as possible. Naturally, even where the most careful and elaborate preparations are made, there are many more chances for the wound to become contaminated than there would be in an operating-room especially set aside for the purpose. We must, however, never fail to pay strict attention to the details, since, though we may have good luck for a while, careless habits, once formed, cannot fail sooner or later to lead to bad results.

In doing plastic operations a rubber irrigating-bag filled with warm sterile water, suspended from a nail driven into the sash of the window, may be used, by means of which a steady stream can be directed upon the parts, thus doing away with the necessity of sponging. Not so much furniture will be required for a plastic as for an abdominal operation. One table is generally sufficient for holding the vessels containing the instruments and ligatures. On a chair on the left-hand side of the operator a basin may be placed to receive the soiled instruments. These should never be allowed to touch his lap, unless it is protected by a piece of sterilized gauze or a sterilized towel. On another chair to the right of the operator may be placed a tray for holding the instruments that will be required throughout the operation. Not only does this simplify matters a good deal, but the instruments run less risk of becoming contaminated.

The after-care of cases has been outlined in Section XIII. If the operator lives too far away to make it possible for him to see the patient every day, he must of necessity intrust her to the care of a local physician, leaving with her, if possible, one of his own trained nurses. Before going away he must give full instructions regarding diet, catheterization, the administration of enemata, and the indications for changing the dressings, and provide as far as possible against any emergency which may arise.

A detailed description of all the possible chances of error and of the many precautions which must be taken to meet them would require the writing of a whole book. In this section we have attempted merely to give an outline of the general course to be pursued, leaving it to the good sense of the surgeon himself to decide upon the precise steps to be taken when other emergencies arise.

# CHAPTER III.

## OUTLINE OF GYNÆCOLOGICAL THERAPEUTICS.

BY BACHE McE. EMMET, M.D.

### GENERAL HYGIENIC CARE.

It undoubtedly falls more to the lot of the family physician than to that of the gynæcologist to have the care of the child and of the growing girl; it devolves upon the latter merely to cure the ailments which possibly might have been prevented by watchfulness and proper guidance, so that my present remarks may seem somewhat misapplied: still, we shall suppose that the gynæcologist may act as the teacher of his brother practitioner, by reason of his experience with the later life of women, in which most of the errors of childhood or adolescent life become manifest.

As regards menstruation, there is one standard which we recognize as that of perfect health, in which the functions of the genital organs are thoroughly balanced and act in perfect unison; this is the periodic flow of blood from the uterine cavity, preceded by more or less of a molimen, the whole recurring at definite intervals for each individual.

With our advancing civilization and its attendant abuses, however, the normal is but seldom adhered to, and it becomes a question how many of the deviations from our standard are harmless to the individual, and how many are pathological in character, requiring the attention of the physician.

At the present time it is rather the rule for girls who appear to be perfectly developed, when they reach the age of puberty, to have a show of menstruation and then no return for an indefinite time, or to fail to menstruate altogether. It is comparatively rare, in my experience, to find girls who, having once matured, continue regularly in the same course.

In others, again, though they develop well at the first, even after the regular flow has been established and has continued for a year or more, at some early time, before womanhood is reached, menstruation will cease without known cause, or a decided change in character will take place, either diminution of the quantity or increased frequency, or an alteration in color; or perhaps, instead of being painless, it becomes exceedingly painful.

There is still another class, sickly and delicate in aspect, with the mien of grown women, yet having the generative organs well developed, who menstruate at the time habitual to girls of their age and habits of life, and ultimately menstruate irregularly,—that is, frequently or abundantly.

170

This type of early matured girls, whom their mothers often consider in every respect strong and hardy, are so, in fact, only as regards their sexual development, owing probably to an hereditary precocious, highly developed nervous system. So far as that is concerned, there may seem but little that we can do to stay the progress of this nervous tendency, yet we may still be able to accomplish something by seeking to turn the forces of nature in a normal direction, by developing the muscular system at the expense of the nervous, so that the latter may be checked for a time.

By a systematic method of training much may be done in this respect, especially if we are watchful of the growing child and from our knowledge of the family history are enabled to foresee what is to come. There is, to my mind, no doubt that by thus developing one portion of the body and retarding the other, we would be in little danger of seeing our race of city women gradually deteriorate and, from the robust healthy type, fall to the plane of undersized, over-sensitive, nervous females. How this shall be accomplished must be determined by the individual case rather than by any strict system of rules, for many outlying questions in each family will have to be taken into account and judged for themselves.

This scheme, considered in its entirety, would embrace all points of hygiene and diet almost from infancy to puberty; nor can any rules be followed blindly without due consideration and study of the type of each girl, even though of the same family. Every girl will not, of course, partake of her mother's organization, nor yet of her father's. She may derive her type from the second generation back, and from either the father's side or the mother's; so that the physician must use good judgment and discrimination, and perhaps in this field the future medical man may find his work of prevention of disease by improving the type of man and woman from the cradle up. In all families such questions are left entirely too much to chance; the child eats what the family eat; if the food disagrees with it, the child is often thought to be at fault, and so may be put under medical care, instead of being placed on careful diet. The different degrees of development of the various portions of the alimentary tract are not fully considered; heads of families do not know that various foods suit various ages, much less do they take into account that different articles of food are disposed of in different portions of the digestive canal. We see this from infancy, from the time when the overloaded stomach rejects a surplus of milk to the period of frequent diarrhœas from untimely and ill-chosen substitutes. Nature defends herself, and the young do grow, but who knows at what cost of healthy development their various trials and tribulations are borne? This is only an indication of what prevails through childhood and adolescence. As it is with food, so also is it with exercise, rest, work, and recreation: the child is denied the benefits of pure air, is made to undertake tasks unsuited to its age, is deprived of wholesome sleep, and is begrudged the pastimes of youth. It is thought essential that she should learn to look after herself, or at a tender age she is placed in factories where the body is dwarfed, where nutrition must be imperfect, and the nervous system develops badly and is not slow to show the effects by lack of balance of the general body growth.

But here we must consider the girl when she has already developed under these unfavorable influences.  If we see her from the time of her first menstruation, we must strive to quiet any undue nervous development, which is, in fact, due to defective inhibitory force.   So far as this is indicated by over-activity of the generative organs, shown by frequent and profuse menstruation, we shall do best by adopting the derivative treatment, seeking to determine to parts of the body which are lacking in this energy the extra force of the one system, at the same time quieting the latter by the avoidance of excitants, both mental and physical.   This will include the choice of company, books, and amusements, the regulation of the portal system and bowels, and the rest of the organs themselves.

The first aim of derivative treatment is to influence the muscular system.   Calisthenics, bathing, massage, riding, boating, and tennis, if practised with judgment and in moderation, may develop the body and overcome the results of improper care before puberty.

Those girls who grow up to all appearance physically well developed, but in whom the generative organs have not developed at the same pace, should receive a good share of the physician's care as well.   The question must of necessity arise here also, Where lies the fault, and towards which system should we direct our energies in order to strike a proper balance? Is the fault in an over-development of the muscular structure of the body? is it in a poor supply of blood to any one part of the system, to the nerve-centres or to the generative organs, or are we to seek the cause in the nervous system itself?   These are questions which, properly or improperly answered, will determine the restoration to health of many an opening life or will doom the girl to an indifferent existence.   These matters, viewed too strictly from a specialist's stand-point, fail, I think, to receive their full consideration, and the tendency is constantly to attribute such conditions to a purely local cause; and though some good results may be attained by so biassed an opinion, we are far from producing the greatest improvement in health to which a more general view would lead.

In considering this class of cases it is essential to keep in mind that there are two sets of girls, similar in appearance, yet totally different in fact. In the one there is real physical development, in the other it is apparent only; that is, the former have firm muscles, stout bones, good color, and strong nerves, being well balanced ; these will menstruate normally and will continue to do so; the others are but a semblance of what they should be.

As puberty approaches, another effort is put forth, possibly without preliminary sensation, or else we find that it costs the girl severe suffering. She has the dragging, bearing-down symptoms, yet without the natural result of satisfying nature by the discharge of blood.  Or, she may go through what seems to be a natural period, but loses either a small amount of black blood, after a great effort, or has merely a white discharge indicating the willingness, but at the same time the utter powerlessness, of the system to accomplish its purpose. The pelvic organs, or the nerves, or both, are unfit for their task.

How can we come to the rescue of such a sufferer? We must recognize from the first where the strain has been, which part of the body has been doing more than its share under unfavorable conditions. We must seek to build up the nervous system through nutrition properly selected and judiciously adapted. The character of the blood must have our first care, its quality being improved by the use of chalybeates. The tone of the muscular system must also be improved through carefully applied calisthenics and massage. With its improvement a difference in the degree of warmth of the patient will be noticed, and when this effect on the circulation is shown, a general improvement in nutrition will be apparent.

There is a hygiene of the menstrual period, and of sexual life as well. Every girl should be told how to take care of herself during the performance of this important function. It is astounding to learn that many children are allowed to come to maturity and to have their first menstrual flow without ever having been instructed that they are to expect such a thing. Is it a wonder that they should continue to bathe and seek to rid themselves of so unwelcome a condition?. Without such a caution in anticipation of this change in a girl's life, it is small wonder, also, that the child should continue her play and be as heedless of her welfare as we see her older sisters who have had ample opportunity to know better. In many cases, no doubt, the mothers have never known trouble themselves, and cannot realize that harm should come to their daughters. Possibly they are, so to speak, examples of the "survival of the fittest," and are not so much to blame as we would infer. The experience of every day teaches us that the growing girl should not ride, dance, play tennis, skate, or swim at such times. Repeated illnesses, congestion of the uterus, tube, or ovary, with delayed or painful menstruation and evidences of inflammation, and even displacement and fixation of the uterus or ovaries, are constantly seen as the result of such imprudence, not to mention the exposure which results from witnessing athletic sports in the fall season.

I shall not speak at length of the proper time for marriage, of the fit condition for such a state, of the inadvisability of incurring frequently repeated pregnancies, and of the care during and after them, which every physician will readily appreciate. These points, of course, require ample consideration, but cannot be discussed as they should be in this place; it is sufficient if I indicate to general practitioners that they should hold themselves in great measure responsible towards the families under their care, if they fail to tender their advice in such matters.

Another burden of responsibility to which the gynæcologist is most competent to direct the general practitioner's attention, considering that the latter is morally the custodian of the family's welfare, in which he stands

as no other can, is that he should form some opinion, or have some knowledge, of the party to an alliance in which his patient is interested.   It is not
too much to hope that a judicious investigation on the physician's part or a
guarded prompting even to a father may, in many a case, save a young
girl from gonorrhœal infection which may impair her health, if it does not
threaten life.   It is undoubted that the importance of a positive cure is not
yet fully appreciated by young men who have thought themselves rid of
all trouble, and they rarely have the opportunity of ultimately knowing
that they have been the cause, though ignorantly, of childlessness, of long-
continued suffering on the part of their young wives, or even of death from
gonorrhœal salpingitis or peritonitis.

I shall say only a word, also, about the constantly growing practice of
evading pregnancy in which women in our large cities at present indulge.
They cannot be too strenuously enjoined to desist, in view of the multiple
ills which it may bring upon them.   The two forms in which it is carried
out, either by protecting themselves against it, while still allowing the husband's approach, or inducing an abortion the moment they find themselves
*enceinte*, are positively harmful, and, combined with the excessive wear and
tear of fashionable city life, surely produce, or contribute to, the many
ovarian neuralgiæ, the backaches, the pelvic weight, and the exhausted
nerves which we are so frequently called upon to treat nowadays.

The care of the woman after she has passed the active period of her
sexual life should also engage our attention.   It is not only the system at
large which requires care, by establishing the balance of the circulation,
which must be reached through the nervous system, by quieting apprehen-
sions and instituting a perfect harmony among the various vital functions,—
this is an essential and sometimes a most difficult task to assume and to
manage well,—but the sexual organs themselves need attention.   Every
physician having the responsibility of a family should direct the woman's
attention to the change of life and its attendant evils.   He should, in case
the menopause does not become established in regular form, take the matter
into consideration and satisfy himself that nothing is amiss.   Even if the
flow, after it has begun to diminish, does not steadily decrease, it would be
his duty to ascertain the condition of the endometrium; it will possibly be
found in a fungous condition which will require its removal by curettage.
To allow such a flow to persist, when nature has already announced her
readiness to end such activity, is to countenance a pathological state which
is not without its positive harmful effect, and may possibly inaugurate a
period of ill health for the woman.

Close attention should also be paid to the character of the flow, as well
as to that of any intercurrent discharge after the menopause has seemingly
been instituted, especially if menstruation has been absent for several
months.   One should bear in mind the possibility of the development of
malignant disease at the climacteric; above all, in the case of a parous woman
in whom there may have been a neglected laceration of the cervix which

has given rise to no symptoms in her earlier life. Uteri which have suffered such injury, and especially if they have been the subject of hyperplasia or chronic metritis, are not quite so ready to accede to the change demanded of them; their cell-life will not so quickly become quiescent, but, on the contrary, is often prone to assume a new activity and to develop into a pathological state. This leads me to emphasize what I have not had occasion to mention hitherto,—viz., that cases of laceration of the cervix with any degree of cystic degeneration or eversion, with congested mucous membrane, should receive attention and should be thoroughly healed or excised before the woman approaches the menopause, so as to avoid the possibility of this retrograde malignant change.

*Rest and Exercise.*—It becomes a difficult matter to state in a general way what shall be one's guide in ordering these two opposite essentials of daily life.

It will be readily seen that each condition with which we have to deal will suggest points applicable to its own care or cure, and that no positive rule can be laid down which will not admit of deviation. Still, there are general principles to be adhered to belonging to the sphere of gynæcology which may not find their application in any other branch of medicine; therefore I shall dwell for a moment upon, first, the necessity, and secondly, the limitations, of rest, considering subsequently the question of exercise.

Rest with one woman would be a day's work with another, and our daily experience shows the different views which the various classes take of it. We must adopt these in a great measure, and realize that it is rest for one woman to avoid washing or doing heavy sweeping, while for a finer organization nothing short of the bed and a darkened room will suffice. Physical rest is one thing and mental rest another; with one, we may have to consider the physical aspect alone; in the other, the body may already have rest to the point of indolence, but the mind needs repose. I shall not dilate upon this further, but shall turn to the question of rest as a necessity. It requires but a slight knowledge of the diseases of women to appreciate that in the majority of patients their suffering is due to the fulness of vessels within the pelvis, and that the more this can be overcome the greater will be the amount of relief which will follow. Hence it is desirable to favor the emptying of the blood-vessels of the hemorrhoidal, uterine, and ovarian systems by the avoidance of prolonged standing; in fact, by having the patient assume the recumbent posture for a certain time each day, in order to break in upon the long series of hours from the time of rising to that of retiring; it is even desirable to place the body not only in a prone position, with the clothing loosened, but also with the lower part of the body raised. Tilt, in this connection, speaks of the American attitude of repose instinctively assumed by those who suffer much from uterine disease, and says that several of his patients who had suffered greatly from complicated pelvic inflammation had their beds so made that the lower limbs should be higher than the pelvis. This is certainly good, and may be accomplished, in a modified degree, by placing a firm pillow beneath the hips when lying down. The rest enjoined upon a patient at the chosen time should be commensurate with the requirements of the case and not in any way arbitrary. I recently saw a woman who had a large pus-tube which felt as if it were on the point of bursting; yet to her it seemed nothing to finish up a washing and to pack a trunk before entering the hospital for operation. One patient may have a retroversion which is aggravated by defecation; she may require a half-hour's rest after the act, in order to relieve the temporary congestion or to allow an ovary which has been displaced to resume its former position. Another may have imperfect perineal support and cannot well tolerate a prolonged séance at the dress-maker's; a third may have a fibroid and perhaps has not made up her mind to apply to the surgeon; she needs rest, so that her uterus may be relieved of its congestion once or several times daily. Her tendency to metrorrhagia will be less, her dysuria will be diminished, and her headache. may be dissipated, while her swollen feet will cease aching.

Care should now be exercised not to advise too much rest, or to allow the patient to overestimate the necessity of it for herself: many a woman has become a bedridden invalid from the habit of seeking her couch on slight provocation, not knowing when to arise. It is here that the need of discrimination arises, and we should know when to advise exercise and the amount suitable to individual cases. Were we to ignore this, we should have turgid, flabby vessels with stagnant blood; the pelvic muscles especially would become soft and yielding, losing their tone; it may be, too, that the slightest effort on the woman's part will become painful, independently of any actual disease, so that these muscles will require training and coaxing by electricity and massage. This is as true of the pelvic muscles, internal and external, as it is of the muscles of the body in general.

Our patients should be told when and how much to walk, whether they may ride or drive, row or swim, dance, play tennis, use the sewing-machine, etc., each encouragement or injunction being guided by an intelligent appreciation of the necessities and requirements, as well as by the contra-indications, in any given case.

*Dietetics.*—Among the various complicating disorders of the economy which play a very important *rôle* in gynæcological cases is unbalanced nutrition, dependent upon the fact that the food taken is not properly chosen, that it is in too great quantity, that it is not properly digested, that it is not fully assimilated, or, lastly, that the various emunctories fail in their function of elimination. The resultant of any one of these different states, or of several combined, is an accumulation in the blood of deleterious material which acts as a poison upon the nervous centres and produces many symptoms which simulate those of uterine disease, or which so depreciates the system that it cannot be brought up to the proper level so that these ailments can be treated successfully.

This condition is made manifest by headache, by insomnia, by dyspepsia, by indigestion, by constipation, by neuralgia, by skin-affections,—all of which suggest a rheumatic or gouty tendency.

Evidence of this disorder is to be found mainly in the urine, but imperfect digestion is also represented by an habitually coated tongue. It is, therefore, always well to examine the urine thoroughly, as it furnishes hints to guide us in our treatment, through our knowledge of its quantity and specific gravity, the amount of urea, phosphates, or chlorides, or the presence of albumin, sugar, or bile, and by a judicious treatment of the various conditions indicated we shall more thoroughly master the situation and attain to better results in the care of our gynæcological cases than would be possible were we to overlook such important side-issues.

Excess of uric acid in the system, the most common abnormality, has a decidedly pernicious effect upon the blood, and may, I believe, even prove antagonistic to our efforts to enrich it. We constantly observe that tonics are of very little value, that it is exceedingly difficult to overcome an anæmic state, so long as the blood is overcharged with this material, and that our best results are obtained only after special attention is given to the hemorrhoidal and portal systems, by making the liver do its work properly, watching the diet, improving the digestion, and insisting upon suitable exercise. In addition, the skin must be roused to action and the kidneys flushed by the drinking of lithia or Londonderry water, and it may also be necessary to stimulate them with digitalis and potash. Should the patients go abroad, the waters of Vichy, Ems, or Contrexéville should be recommended to them. Piperazin and carbonate of lithia should not be overlooked as the great solvents of uric acid.

Concerning the habits of eating and the kind of food. It is, undoubtedly, injudicious to make only one principal meal in the day or to make each meal of one kind of food. The alimentary tract is so constructed that it can deal with several varieties at various stages of digestion, while if one kind alone is taken certain functions of the digestive system remain quiescent; so that it is far better that an average amount of each of the elements called proteids or albuminoids, fats and carbohydrates, be taken with each meal.

Then, again, we must take into account the absorption of food elements into the blood, which is more thorough the less time it lies in the intestine, subject to decomposition. But there are individual peculiarities which every physician must recognize and cater to, just as there are various needs of individuals, according to their physique and the nature of their daily work, many having fixed habits which apparently suit them individually, as their systems have become accustomed even to injurious diet. Some women will tell you that they cannot take this or that article of food. In one case eggs will always disagree, another will express an aversion for milk, which she never could digest, etc., and these dislikes have a certain amount of foundation in fact, just as we meet with one individual who cannot bear quinine and may be made wild by half a grain, while another is poisoned by even a fractional dose of calomel, and a third by strawberries, or still another by mushrooms. Some cannot eat at all in the morning; others, again, can digest best what they eat late at night.

It is not habit alone that has to do with these idiosyncrasies; we often find that some illness has been at the bottom of the trouble, a weakening or perversion of nerve-force dictating to the digestion, and indolence or invalidism marking the hours.

### GENERAL REMARKS ON LOCAL THERAPEUSIS.

Probably the oldest method of treatment for diseases of women has consisted in the more or less perfect inspection of the cervix uteri, of applications to its surface, of similar applications made within the cervical canal as far as the internal os, and of a general swabbing of the vagina with medicated substances. As notions of the pathology of pelvic disease changed from time to time, so to some extent would treatment; but as regards local medication, much the same methods have been in use for generations. Of late years, however, a great advance has been made by the use of the hot vaginal douche. The older practice was to use cold water, but there is no doubt that, as a rule, the hot effects the most good; indeed, I may safely say that the majority of American gynæcologists depend upon this treatment to meet all general indications in lieu of whatever applications or medicaments to the vaginal surface or to the neck of the uterus have been made in the past. It does, indeed, have a far more extensive field of usefulness in the pathology of women's diseases than any other one agent, and it should never be neglected, though for special local diseases of the mucous membrane of the vulva and vagina ointments and powders may still find their place to some extent. I have spoken elsewhere of Churchill's tincture of iodine as a counter-irritant, and it is true that it is mostly used for this purpose; but it is also an astringent, a hæmostatic, an aseptic, and a deodorizer, and as such it may be applied both to the vagina and to the uterine canal.

Boric acid with glycerin, solution of alum on cotton, iodoform, ichthyol, lysol and aristol, balsam of Peru, Canada balsam, and pyroligneous acid are agents which serve a good purpose as unguents or stimulating applications when we use packing within the vagina or uterus.

At the present day it is a rare practice, at least in this country, to apply any medication to the cavity of the womb. Formerly it was not so, and its surface was treated with the solid nitrate of silver, chloride of zinc, fuming nitric acid, chromic acid, persulphate of iron, or, more commonly, Churchill's tincture of iodine, which was always at hand. Theories and beliefs have changed so that the practice at the present day is thorough curettage, cleansing, and draining of the cavity. When that has been carefully done it is all that is necessary; it effects the cure by removing the cause of trouble from the endometrium, it acts as a derivative or revulsive in other cases of distant disease, or promotes drainage in salpingitis.

The gradual dilatation of the cervical canal is not held to be of the same utility for purposes of diagnosis as is the rapid and more forcible, simply for the reason that the latter is absolutely safe if we exercise proper aseptic precautions.  This applies to the use of tents as well as to the hard dilators, though, as I have said elsewhere, tupelo tents may still be used to advantage for digital exploration in some cases of uterine fibromata in which a sudden and forcible dilatation of the cervix would possibly cause rupture of the tissues.

Tampons and pessaries call for special mention as means of relief in simple displacements or in those complicated by adhesions; tampons are utilized as temporary means of support and to exert pressure which will serve to soften and stretch the organized lymph that forms bands and cords within the pelvis, while pessaries are more permanent supports of displaced organs which cannot rely upon their ligaments to hold them continuously in their normal position.

*Blisters.*—To speak of blisters in a general way may seem unsatisfactory, yet my purpose is fulfilled if I call attention to them more forcibly than is usually done and succeed in establishing their value firmly in the estimation of gynæcologists.

They may be of signal service, at times, in aborting an acute attack of localized peritonitis or one that threatens to become general.

It is more especially in the chronic form, however, that counter-irritation will yield us happy results, and it is so positive a good that no gynæcologist can afford to do without it.  The repeated use of blisters, two or three during the month, over the site of a chronic inflammation of the appendages or peritoneum will very materially aid the perplexed practitioner in the solution of a knotty case.  The capillaries and lymphatics, excited to renewed action, certainly do carry off much effused material, so that organs and parts of organs that have long been buried in exudate are recognizable in their own—perhaps distorted—shapes, yet still presenting an individuality which has been long denied them.  The feelings of the patient treated by this means, under appropriate conditions, are also such a satisfactory gauge of the benefits obtained that the realization of improvement detected by the touch seems almost superfluous.  The changes wrought are at times wonderfully speedy, but again they are slow, so that one may even despair now and then of seeing the favorable change established; but patience and repetition will bring it about and encourage us to follow on the same line.

Other methods of counter-irritation in use to-day are mostly confined to sinapisms and applications of tincture of iodine, repeating the one or the other according as we desire temporary benefit or a continuous effect; the iodine treatment is to be measured by the tolerance of the skin.

Painting the vault of the vagina and the cervix with Churchill's tincture, which is now such a routine practice and has sometimes, to the profession at large, seemed to represent the sum total of gynæcological practice, illustrates well the necessity experienced from the first for a counter-irritant to those parts. This necessity has been met by blistering the cervix, or the vaginal vault as well, by means of vesicating collodion. This is not so common a practice at the present day as it was some years ago; not because it failed to produce good results, but because better methods have superseded it. It was most frequently resorted to in cases of hyperplasia uteri (chronic metritis) commonly dependent upon injuries to the cervix during parturition. Electricity has proved to be beneficial in this condition. Moreover, a change in gynæcological therapeusis has been brought about through the better recognition of pelvic lesions, the more exact appreciation of peritonitis, and the discarding of what was once regarded as the ever-prevalent cellulitis. So we may say that internal vesication is a thing of the past.

*Bloodletting.*—Bleeding and cupping in gynæcology have also largely gone out of practice. This is somewhat to be deplored, since those who have witnessed the beneficial results attending such practice must believe that no method of the present day can quite supplant it. The drugs which are held to affect the circulatory system and the nervines which sustain and control the nervous system act imperfectly when compared with the abstrae-tion of blood at given periods; for instance, in the case of a much-engorged uterus, with a high nervous tension, which seriously interferes with the development of the menstrual flow. It may be said that there exists here a pathological condition which should be treated in advance before its manifestation becomes apparent: this is true, yet it is desirable to give immediate relief. This in former days could be accomplished by moderate bleeding from the arm or even by local abstraction. So, also, in the peri-odical returns of the molimen before the system has become accustomed to the onset of the change of life, the patient's head will feel as if ready to burst, with the vessels throbbing, the nerves excited, and hysteria impending. What better, at such times, than to adopt the old plan of an occasional bleeding, in order to establish the balance? This, of course, would not be essential if all proper contributive methods could be called to our aid at such a time to fit the subject to bear the strain.

### TREATMENT OF CONGESTION OF THE HEMORRHOIDAL SYSTEM.

In studying this condition, which plays so important a *rôle* in gynæ-cological practice, we must not ignore the fact that the obstruction offered by the liver and the heart must be overcome before the venous blood which has already been utilized can again enter the arterial system and receive new life and a fresh impulse. We must remember that the veins of the pelvis are already large and tortuous, and should any additional weight be added to the column of blood within them their size must increase con-siderably and the distress from pressure upon sensitive nerves within the pelvis must be correspondingly greater. In this way we may explain the resulting discomfort and aggravation of existing pelvic disease, especially in cases of loss of the perineum, subinvolution of the uterus, displacements, enlarged tubes and ovaries, tumors of all sorts which are not lifted above the brim of the pelvis, enlargement of the veins themselves,—the hemorrhoidal and those forming the pampiniform plexus,—and constipation.

The liver is the organ most constantly at fault, and it frequently reaches an advanced degree of torpidity and congestion before the alarm is sounded and measures are taken to correct it. So many causes contribute to bring about this state of affairs that an exhaustive consideration of them would carry us too far beyond our purpose; it must suffice to call attention to the fact and to indicate in a general way the course to pursue to overcome it.

As constipation is invariably an accompaniment of this torpor, the numerous remedies for its cure must be applied, and we must not allow ourselves to be deceived by the patients' estimate of their own condition. So constantly does it occur that they think themselves quite regular when they have an action of the bowels daily, or every other day, that we are prone to rest satisfied with their statement. Yet, if, in view of the persisting symptoms, we begin to purge them, we shall frequently recognize the fallacy of their premises.

A good way to empty the lower bowel thoroughly, which may be done nightly, is to have the patient take an enema of water, from a half-pint to a pint, as hot as she can comfortably bear it, and have her retain it all night. This will at first appear difficult, and she may expel it; but little by little she will be enabled to retain it, and the result will prove most beneficial. It is well to add to such an enema a half-drachm of inspissated ox-gall at first, and, when no more blackened fæces appear, to change to a saline, half a teaspoonful of sulphate of sodium, sulphate of magnesium, or Sprüdel salts being added to the water. This will often soften and liquefy the fæces, will cause the bowel to regain its tone, and will deplete the vessels about it. Glycerin and gluten suppositories are also good for the same purpose, one being inserted at bedtime.

Directing our attention to the liver, we should give small and repeated doses of calomel, one-tenth of a grain nightly, following it in the morning by a saline laxative, a teaspoonful of Carlsbad Sprüdel salts in half a glass of hot water on rising, or a wineglassful of Rubinat water or of Hunyádi Janos with an equal quantity of hot water. Congress water, Hathorn, and Natrolithic may be substituted. If the liver proves excessively torpid, we should begin our treatment with hot fomentations, or stupes dipped in very hot water, wrung out and applied over the liver, the patient lying upon her left side. Change the applications every half-minute, increasing the heat up to the extreme limit which she can bear, and continue the treatment for ten or fifteen minutes. Repeat every day for four or five days, or until the bile begins to be apparent in the stools; continue the calomel, or blue mass, or podophyllin and saline laxatives, such as sulphate of sodium (Glauber's salt) and sulphate of magnesium (Epsom salt). Forbid sweets and farinaceous food and wines; recommend, and insist upon, exercise; if that is impossible, employ massage of the abdomen; give lemon-juice (one or two lemons on awakening each morning), or a wineglassful of hard cider one or two years old and very tart. Send your patient to Carlsbad or Kissingen Springs for a course of the waters, or, if the difficulty is still confined to the hemorrhoidal system itself more than to the liver, she will find benefit at Marienbad or Homburg. The treatment at these places is intended to reduce plethora generally, to meet a rheumatic or gouty tendency which is so frequently engrafted upon this condition, and to build up the system at large. We have waters of a similar character in our own country, and such a "cure" might be carried out here, but not so perfectly, for at our spas there is no one in authority to establish hygienic rules, and, as the general tendency is to live freely and to keep late hours, such establishments with us fail of their purpose. Some of the waters may, however, be drunk with benefit, those of a sulphurous character, more especially, proving serviceable in abdominal plethora and obesity,—viz., the Blue Lick of Kentucky, the Sharon of New York, and various sulphur springs of Virginia.

The use of belladonna as a component of our laxative pills is also to be much commended; the addition of strychnine, as well, to any tonic which may be chosen on general grounds, and the use of ergot in suppositories, are not to be overlooked.

If the heart is also at fault (and it is a matter of common observation that functional diseases of this organ, at any rate, are frequently associated with the pelvic diseases of women, and it has even been observed that mitral disease is not an uncommon accompaniment), if it needs strengthening and regulating, fluid extract of digitalis or tincture of strophanthus is indicated. Digitalis has been frequently found useful in combination with ergot in general plethora, and it probably has an effect upon the uterus similar to that of ergot; it may, therefore, be used by itself or in combination with the latter in persons of full habit, especially when there is mitral regurgitation.

Nor must we overlook the excellent methods which almost seem too trite to rehearse here. The elevation of the body in the modified Trendelenburg's position to empty the blood-vessels of the pelvis, the use of very hot douches frequently repeated, applications made to the roof of the vagina with boroglyceride tampons, counter-irritation to the cervix by vesicating collodion to establish a serous oozing, the proper support given to the contents of the pelvis, the use of appropriate gymnastic exercises,—all these come in for their full share of attention in aiding to overcome this troublesome condition.

### MASSAGE.

Massage may be considered as combining two forces,—pressure and motion. When pressure is applied alone, its effect will be to empty the capillaries at the spot at which it is applied; if that pressure is relieved, the same capillaries will refill, to be emptied again if the pressure is repeated.

Were this process kept up for a definite time, we should have still another effect added, due to a moderate degree of nerve-stimulation produced by this repeated pressure. The result of this stimulus would be to make both voluntary and involuntary muscular fibres contract, the latter in consequence of a reflex action through the cerebro-spinal system. This continues for a time without change; but after a little these same muscular fibres will become exhausted through overstimulation, their contractile force is discharged, and then there is a relaxation, and an increased quantity of blood will be present at the point of repeated pressures (congestion).

This may be carried on to the point of destruction of vitality of the parts, causing a contusion or bruising of the muscular fibres; possibly the walls of the small vessels may be injured, so that there is an actual effusion of blood.

The effect of motion combined with any degree of pressure is to displace whatever fluids may be immediately beneath the hand, whether these are in the capillaries or are the fluids which are contained in all tissues. This displacement caused by motion is entirely different from that caused by pressure alone, in that the fluids have a momentum imparted to them. and if the same motion is repeated a second momentum is afforded, and so on until, as we readily understand, we have created a current in the fluid. Every one is familiar with the method of stimulating the heart to fresh action in syncope by rubbing the palms of the hands vigorously, thus using a reflex stimulant and forcing the blood directly to the heart.

Inasmuch as massage is designed to take the place of natural activity or to bring into healthy work parts which are, or have been, deprived of natural stimulus, we should in all respects observe physiological laws in its application, and therefore all motion of fluids should be in their natural direction. The fluids or juices of the tissues have no course, nor even those of the capillaries, so that we have only the arteries, veins, and lymphatics to heed. The larger lymphatic trunks follow approximately the direction of their neighboring veins, so that the restrictions are reduced to two. To influence the arteries and to propel the blood in them we must, of necessity, make deep pressure, while that made over the veins is, of course, much more superficial.

Pressure may be made to reach deep parts and to produce upon them effects almost similar to those at the surface; this is to be accomplished by utilizing the intermediate parts as if they formed a portion of the working hand and pressing through them. This is not so evident when pressure alone is used as when motion is added to it. Still, deep pressure may reach a nerve or its neighborhood and may effectually relieve severe neuralgia without any motion being employed.

Motion, also, may be superficial or deep. The former stimulates nerve terminations, which react and give color to the surface by affecting the inhibitory force of the blood-vessels. Deep motion, utilizing the intermediate parts as above described, will affect muscular tissue more particularly and will favor its development.

Motion, like pressure, may be extensive or limited, so that we can have gentle, slow manipulation, or violent and quick.

Massage includes friction, kneading, pounding, percussion, tapotement, vibrations, and passive movements.

The motions in massage should not be excessively slow, nor yet very rapid. I think that a good rule to adopt is, that in kneading and executing passive movements they should be no more rapid than the operator's normal breathing, say about twenty-four to the minute; that in friction and vibrations they should be made with the same rapidity as the operator's pulse, say seventy-two to the minute; and in pounding, percussion, or tapotement, at double that rate. I might, in indicating the speed, say that it should accord with the patient's normal pulse or respiration. In kneading the abdomen, the time of expiration is the best moment at which to have a fresh wave of fluid enter the heart, so that it may be pumped directly into the lungs, and the same holds true in kneading the muscles to improve the circulation and to promote assimilation; if it is done synchronously with the heart's action, it is more beneficial than if the rhythm is broken. The patient's respiration and heart-beat cannot, however, be as well adopted as a guide as that of the operator himself.

Though massage in its different forms enters into the treatment of various female affections, it is also valuable as a part of the general care of the body, to increase the activity of the blood-current, so as to bring it more frequently in contact with the oxygen in the lungs, and to promote nutrition by making the muscles work out what elements they have already taken up but have not utilized. Thus the body at large becomes more vigorous and robust, so as to respond the more effectually to therapeutics and to local treatment of the organs whose care we are considering.

*Pelvic Massage.*—It is not many years since the idea of applying massage as a part of the local treatment of women's diseases was developed. Fortunately, it has been brought to bear upon a class of ailments which usually prove most intractable, and for the treatment of which the means at our command have always been too few.

The idea had its origin, we are told, in the relief which a sergeant of the Swedish army, Thure Brandt, was enabled to afford a soldier who was suffering with prolapsus recti. No physician being at hand, he undertook to see what he could do, and conceived the idea of grasping the bowel at some point within the pelvis and gradually drawing it up. This was accomplished by placing the sufferer in the recumbent position and by repeatedly raising as much of the contents of the pelvis as could be seized with both hands. The success attendant upon this manœuvre served to direct the operator's attention to an affection akin to the one he had just attended,—viz., procidentia uteri,—and he questioned whether a like treatment would not serve a similar purpose in such cases. Opportunity favoring, he was enabled to put his theories to the test, and succeeded beyond his expectations. The report of one case induced many sufferers to seek his aid, until, in time, he achieved great fame.

Whether the manipulations necessary to effect a happy result in these cases wrought other benefits as well, such as the relief of pelvic pains and the absorption of plastic exudations, thus directing Thure Brandt's mind to extend his method to the cure of such affections, or whether it was owing to his familiarity with Swedish movements that he was impelled to make the trial,—whatever his motives, it was not long before he put it in practice, and good results were soon announced from this treatment of various chronic affections of the female pelvis.

Little by little his system was developed and enlarged, until now, in Germany especially, it is a recognized mode of practice, well calculated to produce some wonderful results if judiciously undertaken, in selected cases, and carried out with patience and with a clear perception of its indications.

Unfortunately, the method has not been much studied or put in practice in this country, and until more individual experience has accumulated we must work on the lines laid down by its originator, with such omissions or additions as may be suggested by one's own good judgment and constantly growing familiarity with the practice.

One can scarcely overestimate the amount of discretion which it is essential to exercise in utilizing this valuable aid to our treatment of the various pelvic diseases of women : this is especially true in respect to the precise recognition of the conditions which admit of its use. In other words, it is of paramount importance that we should possess the *tactus eruditus*, and should be able to make accurate palpation, to interpret symptoms correctly, to establish an exact differential diagnosis, and, further, that we acquire sufficient skill to manipulate the parts involved so as to effect good and produce no injury. It is only with such aids at our command that we may feel justified in undertaking this mode of treatment or be warranted in anticipating the results promised us by the originator of the method and by his close followers, who have had a pride in adhering strictly to his original precepts.

Many physicians who have made an attempt to avail themselves of the promised assistance which massage has yielded to others have, either through faulty judgment, misguided energy, or lack of patience, seen such harmful results ensue that they have been amazed at nature's resentment of harsh treatment; or else they have seen cases defy their efforts and the same ill train of symptoms persist, demanding protracted care or driving the patient to a confrère who may inaugurate a fresh season of applications and tampons, or to another ever ready to present the knife as a plausible, but uncertain, solution of the problem.

To him, however, who starts in well equipped in the knowledge of pelvic anatomy, and who has had experience in treating and in relieving stubborn cases by other methods, there will be given a rare opportunity to effect marked benefit, if he will bring his faculties to bear and will allow himself time to carry out the method, since it has already yielded results sufficiently encouraging to establish itself firmly in the estimation of the few who have practised it.

This treatment is applicable, and has been applied, to a great diversity of ailments: it will, therefore, serve my purpose best if I consider them in turn and state my belief and experience concerning each one.

It is quite in place here, I think, to quote Thure Brandt when he says, " Whether my local treatment, aided by general gymnastic movements, is preferable to the previous methods of the medical profession will be shown most certainly by unbiassed investigation and increasing experience. But we must emphasize the fact that the true value of a method can only be estimated correctly when it is carried out as fully as possible."

I quote this, as it is my purpose, as I intimated above, to present merely some simple definite rules to be observed in carrying out what is really only a modification of the system developed by Thure Brandt, for its incompleteness would, I know, make him unwilling to acknowledge it as his own. Still, it is with the conviction that I am doing it for the best, feeling that many physicians will give time and attention to a part of this process if they can see their way clearly to help their patients, but will discard the entire method if they are urged to carry it out in its entirety and are told that it must be that or nothing.

At the very outset I am confronted by the difficulties attending the study of this portion of our subject, for the reason that my purpose is to lay down such simple lines and clear-cut indications that the reader may be assisted, rather than confused, by statements which seem to be contradictory.

As in general massage of the body, so in that directed to the pelvic organs alone, according to the method and to the force applied, we may develop a constructive, or we may establish a destructive, tendency. In other words, we may by our manipulations, if they are gentle and are applied to the organs involved, produce a greater flow of vital fluids and help to build them up, or, if they are vigorous and centripetal, we may reduce them in size and carry from them much that has already served its purpose of nutrition, or material which is foreign and harmful. We see these two effects well illustrated as regards the deposition or the removal of fat. A skilled masseuse will almost coax fat upon a thin person, or will reduce an obese individual by a change in her method which will make the patient the envy of her fellow-sufferers.

In what cases shall we make use of pelvic massage? It may in a general way be stated that those chronic affections of the female pelvis such as persistent pain, constantly recurring congestion, displacements, deformities and fixation of organs attributable to lack of support, increased weight, peritoneal inflammation, and lymph deposits are the ones which we may hope to benefit by this method.

This will embrace quite a number of conditions which prove intractable enough to ordinary means; so that we may feel no little satisfaction if we are able to relieve a few of our patients and thus save some from the knife. Many other affections have been subjected to the same treatment, either alone or combined with the Swedish movements, but my experience has not been such as to warrant me in recommending it for other cases than the above description will cover.

As opposed to this class we may review those conditions which are entirely unsuited to such handling.

In the first place, do not attempt massage in any acute diseases nor in any acute exacerbation of a pre-existing disease. It has been advised and practised by some, in the belief that the acute stage might be shortened, but such treatment does not seem rational, as experience certainly teaches that nature demands quiet and rest during acute processes; we should, therefore, wait until such symptoms have abated.

Next in order I may mention pus-tubes and pus in any part of the pelvis, with some reservations to which I shall refer when discussing the application of the treatment.

We should never allow ourselves to practise massage in cases of pregnancy, normal, or, still less, abnormal, *i.e.*, ectopic. However, an exception may be made in favor of the early months. Should we have, for instance, a retroverted uterus, and especially if it is caught beneath the promontory or is adherent from old exudations, we should not hesitate to endeavor by manipulation to restore the organ to a good position. To do this may not be called massage, strictly speaking; still, I make a point of insisting that the mere fact of pregnancy, at any stage, should not interfere with the restoration of the womb to its proper axis. It must of necessity be limited to a period not later than the third month, otherwise the organ will be so imprisoned that the method will not avail and the subject will have to receive an entirely different consideration, which is more in the domain of obstetrics. Apart from this one condition, however, the pregnant uterus must not be tampered with by massage.

Tuberculosis of the peritoneum is another contra-indication, so are malignant growths of all descriptions anywhere within the pelvis,—in fact, every tumor, whether liquid or solid, unless it can be recognized as a hydrosalpinx, a chronic hæmatocele, or the result of a lymph exudation. This general class is to include ovarian cystomata, cysts of the broad ligament, and fibroids.

Such is the rule; and yet some physicians who have practised massage have felt justified in applying it to fibromata. It can scarcely be said to have injured them or to have made the patients worse,—in fact, it is possible to diminish the bleeding which often accompanies them,—but observation has not shown that any appreciable change takes place in the tumors themselves.

Before closing this list I would also include blennorrhagia as a contra-indication. Without any further explanation, it will readily be seen why no disturbance of the parts should take place when we have such a condition to deal with.

It seems superfluous to repeat here, while considering the topic of treatment alone, the ever-important injunction, Be sure of your diagnosis; never misplace your energy and begin to treat a case by this method until you have made the most careful and painstaking examination by all methods at your command. Anybody about to apply this treatment, however modified from the original, must observe certain rules which experience has shown to be beneficial: as each operator progresses, however, he may formulate methods for himself, just as he may adopt new forms of manipulation and reject others which seem less appropriate or successful under his hands.

The first laws to govern us are of a general nature. The patient should be "fit;" so should the physician. The woman must have her bowels thoroughly emptied some time in advance of the treatment, so that any fulness which may have been present owing to pressure upon the hemorrhoidal system shall have had time to disappear; the bladder should be empty, the patient should be in perfect repose of mind and body, she should not have just partaken of a full meal, there should be no tight clothing about the waist, and her position should be half reclining, dorsal or on the side, as one may choose for various purposes; for some, one may even adopt the genupectoral or prone posture.

The patient should be lying somewhat lower than the physician as he sits, so that his forearm shall be exactly on a plane with her body. He places himself at one side of the patient, either the right or the left as he may find it handy for manipulating, and rests his unused arm upon his knee, or, if he is sitting quite low, he may support it upon the lounge in front of the patient. For my own part, I prefer to be seated somewhat lower than the patient's couch, for the reason that I believe that I can get a better fixed point and am able to reach higher in the pelvis by allowing the elbow to rest upon the couch, thus directing the forearm somewhat upward and fatiguing it less. The arm is to be at perfect rest, and one or two fingers of the hand belonging to it are to pass within the vagina or, sometimes, within the rectum and to be "in touch" with the outer hand, which will be engaged in performing the massage through the abdominal wall. The fingers within the vagina or rectum should not take any part in the actual massage, but should remain perfectly quiet, merely giving support for the outer hand to work upon, though, of course, they must follow the movements of the latter.

These are much the same rules that have guided masseurs up to the present time. I have, however, found myself departing from them now and then, and, I have thought, with advantage, in so far that, acting upon the assumption that one hand was as intelligent as the other, I have made use of the finger within the vagina, in conjunction with the outer hand, to press out full veins, to soothe tender points, to raise displaced organs, and to assist in stretching and overcoming adhesions.

One of the first objects to aim at when we begin massage—which may almost, in fact, be said to be the corner-stone of the system—is to disgorge the blood-vessels.  As I have said elsewhere, this is much aided by gymnastic movements,—both active, on the part of the patient, and passive, produced by the physician,—and a few of them may be brought to bear very efficiently in accomplishing the purpose.  I have already spoken of the bowels being open : there should be no constipation ; that is a great point. Then the position of the patient aids us greatly ; the hips may even be raised slightly on a pillow, or considerably—even the whole trunk—by adopting the Trendelenburg posture.  It is immensely serviceable, not only for the one effect which we are considering, but also for the assistance which it gives us in replacing prolapsed organs.

To accomplish this emptying of the veins by massage we should begin with gentle upward strokes in the direction of the vessels, and as we advance we may make our motions stronger and stronger.  One of Thure Brandt's rules to adopt for all massage is, that every treatment should be gentle at first, becoming vigorous as we see how much each individual case will bear, and then tapering off with mild massage again, ending each séance as we have begun, by emptying the vessels of the pelvis, veins, and lymphatics as thoroughly as possible.

As we proceed with the treatment, we shall find, provided that the patient has stood it well, that our manipulations may become much more severe, even to the point of using extreme force and pressure with the one hand ; the finger of the other, it is understood, is to remain either in the vagina or in the rectum, as the case may be, during the entire séance, to control the work done by the outer hand.

It is wise never to approach directly a spot to which we desire to apply massage, but to circle about it, to approach and retire from it.  In this way we accustom the part to our touch, and what would seem harsh at first will be well tolerated in the course of the treatment.

It is difficult to say, in advance, how long a treatment may be necessary ; I mean both the individual one and the whole course.  For each sitting we must be guided by the strength and endurance of the patient and by the end to be gained, the time varying from twenty to forty minutes. Each séance must be brought to a close the moment the patient shows fatigue or excessive pain, and the course must naturally depend upon the nature of the case ; for instance, with firm chronic adhesions it must extend over a very long period, and the treatment should be continued after the patient is apparently cured, to make success the more certain ; but all such treatment should cease at once if any complications arise.

The few gymnastic exercises to which I allude, which may still be utilized without making such work a special feature of the treatment, for reasons stated in the opening of this chapter, are the elevating motions of the perineum, which the patient executes repeatedly, as if she were trying to close the vagina and bowels forcibly.  The sphincters or their remnants on either side, the levator ani, and the transversus perinei muscles accomplish this to perfection; and whereas it might appear that these muscles are disabled or destroyed from accidents of parturition, a few efforts to use them will prove in a gratifying way that they still have power.

A second movement is that of parting the knees against slight resistance, the patient being on her back with the knees drawn up, and then slowly bringing them together, also opposed to slight resistance offered by the maid, a nurse, or the physician. Four or five repetitions of this exercise suffice for each séance, but the contraction of the perineal muscles alone may be repeated fifteen or twenty times, or more, whenever the patient chances to be lying down. It may also be undertaken while standing, as a part of the general treatment, and the patient will find that she receives great benefit from it. This is, in fact, a motion or exercise which is automatically made in walking by every woman who suffers much from that feeling of weight or bearing down due to full pelvic vessels, and it is the relief which it affords which will cause every one to say that she much prefers walking to standing. In standing, these muscles relax; in walking, they become taut.

It must not be inferred, from what I have said in relation to the determination of blood *from* the pelvis for the improvement of certain diseased conditions, that seemingly opposite states may be improved by the reverse treatment. To some degree such a view may be held, in so far as a determination of blood to a *part* may improve its nutrition; but impelling blood to a *region* must, under all circumstances, be considered a fault, inasmuch as we cannot hold it fully under our control, and, once accomplished, it may result in a condition of congestion and stagnation. Such a state is at all times pathological.

Determining blood to a part is not for the purpose of utilizing the blood as such, but for the nutrition which it may supply, the stimulus which it may give. How much better, then, is it to improve the nerve-tone of the body at large so that it shall have the power to send the necessary amount of nutritive element to any given part, and then we may count upon this same power to give and take according to requirement!

This principle should ever be before us, that the constitution at large needs the first care, and that only when this is fully heeded can local improvement take place to good advantage. Therefore, were we to consider the question of the treatment of functional amenorrhœa, we should not attempt in any way to have blood settle in the pelvis as if it were obstructed; otherwise we should feel justified even in encouraging constipation and leaving the liver engorged. On the contrary, we determine fresh blood to the hemorrhoidal system by cathartics,—that is, a beneficial stimulus,—but we seek to have it pass rapidly along.

Massage of the pelvis really plays but a secondary part in the treatment of this condition. Some benefit can undoubtedly be effected by stimulating the parts from without by friction and massage, to determine blood to the pelvis, but much more can be accomplished, apart from general improvement of health, by good food and air, by tonics, and by well-adapted gymnastic exercises of the legs, hips, and abdomen, also by riding. Besides which, in the amenorrhœa of unmarried girls especially, it is scarcely desirable to begin with manipulations about the vagina; but, with the object of exciting the nerves within the pelvis and of urging the blood towards the uterus, it may be allowable in exceptional cases, and the method to employ is then to fix the cervix with the index finger of one hand and to make the stroking and vibratory circular motions with the free hand over the abdomen, the movements being light at first, gradually increasing in force, and then diminishing. If the patient is semi-recumbent, and the legs are raised at the same time, it will prove an advantage in forcing the blood from both portions of the body towards the pelvic cavity for the moment. Such exercises and motions may be executed for twenty minutes at a time, being repeated twice daily and during four or six days prior to the expected menses.

If the reader consults the sections on general therapeutics and electrotherapeutics he will see that we have various other resources at our command for effecting the same object, and many will undoubtedly have recourse to them in preference to the above, which often proves uncertain.

Aches, dragging and bearing-down pains, are familiar terms to us all, many of these sufferings being dependent on nothing very tangible; yet, if one questions the patient closely in such cases, the history will always show an arrested menstruation, an abortion, produced or accidental, a heavy fall, attempts to prevent conception, skating or dancing during the monthly period, etc.; all these tend, if not positively to an inflammatory condition, at least to passive engorgement, to increase of weight, and to neuralgia. Benevolent nature may seek to remedy all these evils, but the ever-recurring monthly congestion aggravates them and new troubles are constantly added.

Dysmenorrhœa is a symptom indicative of so many different affections that no gynæcologist is satisfied to treat it as a disease. This is so far the custom, however, doubtless due to the difficulty experienced by the general practitioner in singling out its special cause at the time, that we perhaps do best to consider it in this light.

In this connection, I shall only pass in review its association with such definite pathological states as are individually amenable to the treatment by massage, otherwise a study of the subject would far exceed our limits. To this I shall make but one exception, and that is, to mention membranous dysmenorrhœa; not to discuss it, however, but to point out that it should rank, if not as an independent pathological condition, at any rate as occupying a position on the border-line.

The substance of the paragraph relating to amenorrhœa may be taken almost word for word as applying to dysmenorrhœa. The most common example of dysmenorrhœa is that in the developing girl, due to a congenital flexure of the uterus. This is apt to right itself in time, as it does, in fact, during the process of the flow, and it should in any case not be regarded as an indication for manual interference. As the girl develops, provided that she is spared the many possibilities of pelvic and uterine disease, the uterus will also grow, and, if care has been bestowed on her physique and all abnormal abdominal pressure has been removed, a perfectly normal condition will probably be established. This same flexure may, however, become a decided pathological condition should the patient, through the various vicissitudes to which she is exposed, be afflicted with pelvic peritonitis or cellulitis. The evidences of this are, as a rule, more manifest in producing retroflexion and latero-flexion, as well as the versions, and sometimes, indeed, the same inflammation which eventually produces the backward displacement gives rise at one stage of its formation to anteversion, by holding the cervix uteri too far backward, thus throwing the fundus violently forward. This point must be duly weighed in the treatment; however, these various fixations being so much alike and due to one cause, I shall consider them all together under the heading of pelvic exudation.

Menorrhagia and metrorrhagia, excluding cases due to general conditions, are also so much dependent upon these outside causes that a like remark has its application here. Before dismissing this subject I should like once more to insist upon the great importance of thoroughly sifting the etiology before beginning treatment, as my mind reverts to occasional errors of diagnosis in overlooking the possibility of ectopic gestation and placenta prævia.

Subinvolution of the uterus, which always plays so active a part in the conditions just referred to, has a special place of its own in the nosological chart, with a formidable array of other affections to account for it. These are more especially referred to in the section on Electricity.

We shall now take up briefly the study of pelvic exudations, and their results in producing deformities and displacements of the uterus, tubes, and ovaries. There is one point upon which we need to lay special stress. Strange as it may seem, there are cases in which we can readily recognize extensive lymph exudations on the floor of the pelvis and about the broad ligaments, yet the woman may not have an ache or a pain in their neighborhood. Have we not all wondered, on opening the abdomen for the removal of an ovarian cystoma or pyosalpinx from one side of the pelvis, to find the tube, and perhaps the ovary, of the opposite side buried in lymph, thoroughly crippled, and that, too, when there was not a symptom to point to such a condition?

Again, we are all familiar with displacements of the uterus of which the patients never complain. We discover them in examining for other conditions on which they may have no bearing. Judged from one point of view, there is no reason whatever for interfering with such exudations or displacements. They are harmless in themselves, and may never give rise to complications. The uterus may, in fact, occupy almost any position so long as its circulation and that of the tissues about it are not disturbed.

This is just what the exudations and adhesions do, as a rule : they distort and constrict the vessels by pressure and traction, though we all see cases in which we must wonder at the absence of such symptoms. The temptation is, however, strong to set right anything that we find amiss, but it is just as often a mistake of judgment, and we run the risk of consigning the patient to a life of invalidism, while she has been quite content to go her way in ignorance, because in comfort. This is a serious matter to a woman who may be earning her livelihood or who has the care of a household upon her. She has been a useful wage-earner, and we make her perhaps a dependent invalid. This, of course, is not a certainty, but it is a possibility. Should this same woman, however, be desirous of bearing more children, the case assumes a different aspect, and we then set about our work, not so much to overcome the present abnormal condition as, indirectly, to endeavor to fulfil the patient's wish. As I have said elsewhere, it is not every one who is capable of practising massage, and it is just as true that it requires a special training and considerable experience safely to handle and replace the pelvic organs which have become bound down and are adherent to one another. According as one is content with making a slow, gradual progress in restoring such crippled organs, or aims at a brilliant immediate stroke, at the same time taking some risks and putting the woman's health in jeopardy, he is marked as either a careful, conscientious gynæcologist, much to be trusted, or an irresponsible self-seeker, unfitted to his task.

It is not my purpose to describe here in detail the many varieties of expression, so to speak, which pelvic exudations may assume. From a thin superficial layer occupying the peritoneum alone to lumps and cords and bands, from a slight traction upon the broad ligament to its blending with the caput coli or the omentum, there are so many gradations and shades that an enumeration would be tedious and their study unprofitable. So also in regard to the forms and phases of displacements with either versions or flexures. To make diagrams or to cite cases would be as simple as one's given skill to depict or to pen. It is needless : one finds no such precision ; the points are not so clear.

I have hitherto purposely said nothing about any more forcible method than is implied by the term massage ; still, we must not overlook the fact that more violent means of restoring fixed uteri have been in use by almost all gynæcologists when they have felt that they were safe in separating parts with some force, and such a method has been advocated by Schultze, to be practised with the patient anæsthetized. Though it is a common usage to tear up parts relentlessly when we have the abdominal cavity in view, it is certainly not a method which conservative surgeons, in this country at least, are prone to advocate as justifiable through the abdominal walls. It is blind and unintelligent ; what with the uncertainty of the surroundings in pelvic exudations and the unreliability of mechanical force applied when the patient is unconscious, it is far safer and more judicious to use

13

only so much force as the patient's sensations will permit and her endurance allow. Such stretching is not tearing, and in proceeding in this manner we may feel satisfied that we are not risking the rupture of a tube or the laceration of a loop of intestine.

The technique of massage for pelvic exudations, after having fully heeded all the points which were detailed in the fore part of this chapter, consists in grasping the parts between the two hands, or rather the finger of one hand within the vagina and the palmar face of the fingers of the other hand, so that we are conscious of the presence of one on the other or in direct relation to the other. In obese persons there is considerable difficulty in accomplishing this, and a great deal of patient and persistent endurance is required to gain our point; in no case shall we find that this can be done at once unless the abdominal walls are excessively flaccid. Gentle manipulation must be practised for a time to induce the abdominal muscles to yield, and little by little, when the patient's confidence is secured and the conviction is established that no suffering is to be inflicted, we shall have the satisfaction of knowing that the parts are within our grasp. I speak of pain; I do not say that we shall not give any as we proceed, but we should make our treatment so light at first that none will be felt, and when it does become necessary it is to be almost with the woman's consent. If the motions are of the right kind we shall almost remove pain; indeed, we do so, by working away the blood from the tissues and thus soothing irritated nerves.

Massage, when well carried out, is really one of the best means at our command for the treatment of uterine displacements caused by adhesions. In retroversions, for instance, if we pursue the method indicated, gradually approaching the part involved from the periphery and feeling our way so as to guard against producing pain, we shall be able by means of the finger of the left hand placed high up in the posterior cul-de-sac, with the right hand over the fundus of the uterus, so to work upon moderately thick and dense bands as to soften and stretch them a little, and, perhaps, at a single sitting, to replace the organ. It usually requires several treatments, but the same work must be repeated day by day, as the patient will bear it and as the case warrants it, until our end is attained. We compress and almost triturate such exudations. They are often exceedingly firm and unyielding; still, the pressure, constantly repeated, will promote their absorption, and in time they will be dispelled.

I have, erroneously, perhaps, described this movement as stretching; that effect does certainly enter into it, yet it is rather a pressure,—a pushing, and at the same time a soothing, motion, which does no violence.

When a certain amount of success has been obtained, or even from the time of the very first treatment, it is well to make sure that we retain what we have gained, and for that purpose to place within the posterior cul-de-sac a few aseptic tampons to do their part in holding the adhesions on the stretch and maintaining the uterus in the position secured. Little by little a point may be reached at which the fundus is well forward, and then it is that we may begin the use of a pessary, or else depend upon the ligaments themselves to continue the support, if we have been able to strengthen them at the same time and to relieve their overstretched condition; or, again, we may resort to the operation for shortening the round ligaments.

There are cases, perhaps not a few, in which we shall not succeed in parting or stretching the adhesions, and the uterus cannot be raised. I trust that due regard has been paid to all the elementary instructions hitherto given for the treatment of retroversion, and yet it may seem surprising, but still it does happen, that a uterus the fundus of which is caught beneath the promontory of the sacrum is constantly mistaken for a fixed uterus, and one physician will absolutely fail in replacing such an organ when the expert will succeed as if by legerdemain.

With all our points well taken and all our best efforts expended, we may not succeed in accomplishing what we set out to do. Surgery must then come to our aid, provided that the gravity of the case, the woman's suffering, or the unfitness of the organ for its natural function demands the extreme measure.

A few words about anteversion. It is common in text-books to find that the subject of anteversion occupies a conspicuous place and is spoken of as a disease requiring considerable attention and treatment. There is no doubt whatever that we frequently recognize this condition either as a congenital state or as a result of enlargement of the uterus, whether from pregnancy, subinvolution, or a fibroid, or that the organ is displaced by the traction of exudations; but every one with a little experience must have also noticed that this so-called displacement is never harmful in itself, that it is never a source of trouble; that it is the presence of its *cause* which is the fault to be remedied or overcome. It must, therefore, be held as unwise to attempt to treat this displacement as a disease *per se,* and the condition which we are here considering, parametritis, plays the most important part as a factor in producing it. Indurations from old parametric inflammation, or scars from lacerations of the cervix or vagina running into the same cellular tissue, are frequent causes; the first, however, will alone engage our attention, as it is the one which is to be met by the method of treatment which we are considering.

When lymph is thrown out over the pelvic peritoneal surface we can never know how far or to what extent it may be removed spontaneously. Without being familiar with the cause, we are accustomed to find that what we had plainly recognized during the acute attack as induration has already disappeared from one portion of the cavity and is firmly persistent in another, one of the regions in which it remains being the broad ligament. The old contention is not fully settled even yet, and the question as to the possibility of pelvic cellulitis having any origin other than septic is still a pertinent one. I believe that it does exist, though it is by no means as

common as it was once thought to be, when compared with pelvic peritonitis due to disease of the tubes, and that we must take it into consideration
and direct our treatment towards it as well as to the thickening of the
peritoneum.

The induration, then, which is so constantly appreciable in the broad
ligaments, and which is sometimes *not* the accompaniment of pyosalpinx,
serves, through the contraction which takes place in the exudation, to
shorten the broad ligaments, and this draws the fundus of the uterus in
the same direction. Were the inflammation on one side only, the deviation
would, of course, be in that direction ; in cases of more general peritonitis,
as there is traction on both sides, the uterus deviates little, if at all, from the
median line. This is the state of things which we find much more commonly
than thickening of peritoneum anterior to the uterus, between it and the
bladder. My impression is that it is quite exceptional to find lymph in
this region : the usual site being in the neighborhood of the tubes, a very
strong argument is furnished in favor of the majority of such inflammations being due to infection through them. But, if it is not the result
of peritonitis, we undoubtedly often do find induration beneath the peritoneum in that region, and that is cellulitis. This we are able to dissi-
pate by massage, promoting its absorption by gentle kneading and pressure ;
still preserving the wave-like motions, radiating from the outside towards
the point of most marked induration.

When the broad ligaments are the parts most involved, the greatest
care is necessary in handling them, for fear of tearing some important
organ which may have adhered to them. If the touch can accurately
determine the exact condition of affairs, there will be comparatively little
difficulty in manipulating to great advantage, so as even to detach one bend
of the tube from another, and thus gradually to free it entirely. Should
either ovary be at the same time prolapsed and adherent, it can possibly
be felt in the same manner, and it may then be detached and raised to
its normal position. This is to be done without any violence whatever,
rather pushing upon the organ from without while it is supported from
within. This we might designate as the compression and lifting, or rolling,
motion. When an ovary is adherent behind the broad ligament or in
the cul-de-sac of Douglas, as it may be even with an anteverted uterus,
we may often reach it and be able to treat it to better advantage by passing
one or two fingers into the rectum. It may even be found that we detach it
best by pressure exerted from this point without external aid ; still, one
hand over the abdomen is even here, I think, an advantage and a safeguard.

We meet with many cases in which the diagnosis may be obscure as
regards the presence of pus, or in which, though the anatomical condition
is perfectly clear, opinions may differ as to the wisdom of applying this
special mode of treatment. I do not allude to acute cases of any type,
but to those which, though chronic in form, yet present features which
ally them closely to those of an acute character. It will readily be seen

that I have reference to tubes and ovaries which are purulent foci ; more especially, however, to those cases in which we have evidence that pus is already escaping by a natural outlet.   Under such circumstances we may say here that there are a few cases in which this method may be brought to bear with some benefit, and there are others in which it would be positively criminal to tamper with it.   The distinction should be fully established between tubes which, though containing pus, find a free outlet for it, and others which retain it partially or allow an occasional discharge, however small, into the peritoneal cavity.   Again, we must exercise careful judgment as to the time at which we should undertake such treatment in one of the former cases, and whether singly or in conjunction with other appropriate methods.

Take for instance a case of uterine displacement with pelvic induration and fixation of the tubes and ovaries.   The most experienced may well be at a loss, until the effused material has been absorbed to some extent, to know, in the first place, whether pus is present at all ; in the second, whether that pus is imprisoned in the ovary or in the tube by adhesions ; and, thirdly, in case that pus is discharging *per vias naturales,* just where it comes from, and whether we may aid its escape, or are liable to aggravate the case by this treatment and see it collect anew.

We may draw our inferences, based upon a large experience with this class of cases ; still, I insist upon it that accurate diagnosis of such conditions is not possible at all stages.   Do not employ or recommend massage in a case complicated with pus, or, to modify the injunction, where pus is concealed and cannot find an external outlet.   On the other hand, I confidently say, given a case with the above conditions, with a discharge of pus through the uterine canal, all acute symptoms having subsided, massage is perfectly safe, not only for overcoming the displacement of organs, but also for the more rapid evacuation of such (presumable) abscess cavity, and, possibly, its final obliteration, preceding or following this course by curettage and drainage of the uterine cavity, and following this up by galvanism. In the same way we may venture to evacuate collections of bland fluid in the tube, if we have evidence that such an evacuation has occasionally taken place in the direction of the uterine canal.   We may then so improve the condition of the tube that these accumulations will cease.   The direction of the motions should, in these cases, of course, always be from without inward,—that is, towards the uterus.   This is the direction which it is well to follow in all massage about the uterus, on account of the possible danger of squeezing harmful fluids out of the tube into the peritoneal cavity.

### GYNÆCOLOGICAL ELECTRO-THERAPEUTICS.

Some six or seven years ago the attention of gynæcologists was drawn to a new method of treatment of diseases of women, and recorded successes and reputed facts accumulated so rapidly that the whole medical world felt that it could pin its faith to the new doctrine, and henceforth could count upon electricity as a faithful ally in the contest hitherto waged, with questionable success only, against some of the more formidable pelvic affections.

Apostoli, of Paris, to whom must ever be awarded the credit of having developed this departure in therapeutics, was, fortunately, in a position to demonstrate his procedure and to hold his cases before the professional eye so that the sceptics could believe and the seekers after truth could profit by his teaching and put into practice for themselves the various expedients which he had devised.   Thus it was not long before men of note, anxious to seize upon whatever help could be secured for the alleviation of woman's suffering and a more perfect restoration to health than had hitherto been possible, took the matter up, and have since persevered in its study.

The time which has elapsed since its inception and the continued interest which still attaches to it demonstrate more fully than could any words of praise in what general esteem this method of treatment is held.   And the study, from being tentative at first, has steadily become more and more positive, so that in the near future, I think, we may hope to see the practice estimated at its true value, the enthusiasts gradually moderating their extreme views, while those who are unwilling to depart from well-beaten paths will be brought to accept proved truths and demonstrable facts ; for it is inevitable that every new method should have its strong advocates and its detractors.   It is not to be expected that gynæcologists developed in the infancy of the art, say even twenty years ago, will turn their attention with much seriousness to a new idea of this kind,—certainly not to the extent to busy themselves about the details of its correct application ; nor is it even to be expected that they will relinquish their old methods, even though they require months to accomplish what a few weeks will do nowadays.

I am not one of those who believe that this treatment can be applied only by physicians who have made it their study for years.   I hold, as I have written elsewhere, " It will not be doubted that those of us who have been anxious to test this method of treatment have fully informed ourselves as to the nature of the supposed remedy, its intended mode of action, and the A B C of its application.   Notwithstanding the importance of being familiar with quantity, quality, resistance, ampèrage, and the minutiæ of this subject, we may still reduce the practical application of galvanism to a few simple rules : have a sufficiently powerful battery, be able to measure the force of the current, be familiar with the action of the two poles, be sure of the condition to be treated, have a correct understanding of the results to be obtained and a just appreciation of the effects produced.   Further than this, a judicious selection of the appropriate case to be subjected to such treatment, and the proper choice of instruments and mode of application, will, I think, render a man competent to solve for himself some of the questions involved, and to have an intelligent understanding of its merits and shortcomings."

There are, however, some inconveniences connected with the adoption of this mode of treatment : it requires considerable time to get all the appliances in readiness for work, it calls for special care to guard the patient against infection, and it demands the physician's close attention in applying it. Furthermore, he is destined to meet with some disappointments, in that he may either undertake too much or may even not do a little well; and another disagreeable element is, that patients will often discontinue treatment as soon as they feel improved, regardless of the fact that such relief may be but the first step in the process of cure. They urge the excuse, possibly, that they have applied for medical aid solely on account of the presence of pain or for excessive menstruation; that the partial undressing is somewhat of a nuisance, which is considerably added to by wet applications being placed over the abdomen; and that they frequently suffer with considerable prostration for a time after the treatment, and sometimes with headache. As a matter of fact, however, almost all patients feel considerable general improvement after treatment with electricity, which is undoubtedly in large part due to general stimulation; the nutrition of the body at large is also greatly improved. Apparently, this stimulus does not result in improvement of the nerve-tone alone, thus promoting the more rapid and regular evolution of nutritive processes, but seems to affect the blood and tissues themselves, causing a chemical change in their elements.

Some of the pelvic affections in which I shall advise the use of electricity, either as a destructive or as a constructive agent, to arrest growth, to promote absorption, to relieve pain, to arrest hemorrhage, sometimes in the hope of curing disease, many times as an adjunct to other methods of treatment, either preceding or following them, are: amenorrhœa, stenosis causing sterility, dysmenorrhœa, menorrhagia and metrorrhagia, subinvolution, passive engorgement of the uterus (flabby uterus), endometritis, membranous dysmenorrhœa, catarrhal salpingitis, oöphoritis, parametritis and perimetritis (plastic exudations), fibroids and malignant disease of the cervix or corpus uteri, and ectopic gestation.

*Amenorrhœa, Suppressed or Defective Menstruation.*—Amenorrhœa of the functional type is one of the affections in which we may hope for the greatest amount of good from the use of electricity. Both the galvanic and the faradic current may be used in this condition. I need not speak again of the general health and of the influence which it ever exercises upon this function, though their mutual dependence cannot be too often insisted upon. Assuming that such a view has been taken of the matter, and that all that can be effected in that line has been tried (including general electrization and static electricity), what may we do locally to promote the full development of the menstrual flow? It may be necessary either to stimulate the generative organs to a proper degree of growth by directly determining blood to the parts, or to stimulate the nerves which control this supply.

We cannot, in any given case, accurately determine that only one of these different effects is to be especially aimed at, since usually both the blood-supply and the nerve-tone are inadequate; we therefore make use of the two currents, devoting a special séance to each or using them alternately at the same sitting. This can be readily done, for neither should be used with such intensity that a patient could feel in the least prostrated by it. The mild currents are the best. If the patient is a virgin, or circumstances are such that it seems undesirable to give the treatment by the vagina, we may hope for good results by placing the negative pole of the galvanic current over the lower part of the abdomen and the positive over the lumbar region, or the negative low down over the perineum and the positive over the upper portion of the abdomen. Fifteen to twenty milliampères is quite sufficient at a time, and the duration of each treatment should not exceed ten minutes. Such applications may be made every two or three days for two or three weeks of each month until the menses appear, and then continued at somewhat longer intervals, say twice a week, during the following two or three months, according to the amount and the character of the flow.

While this is done, the faradic treatment may also be used, employing the medium coarse wire coil, so that it shall be stimulating and yet not painful, and applying it up and down the spine from the nape of the neck to the sacrum. It may also be used gently through and through the body, say the anus and the lumbar region, or the sacral region and lower abdominal: this certainly produces a marked tonic effect upon the lower bowel, stimulating it so that defecation is made more easy and constipation is overcome, and we may naturally hope to see a similar tonic effect exercised upon the uterine system.

If, now, we feel warranted in making vaginal and intra-uterine applications, we do so by using the negative pole within the uterine cavity, taking care to make the current act more especially upon the body of the uterus by having the metal portion of the electrode not longer than one to one and a half inches, and placing the positive pole over the lumbar region or even working it up all the way to the base of the skull. Here, again, it is wise to have the applications mild, say fifteen to twenty milliampères, and not to continue them over ten minutes. They may be repeated as often as indicated above and continued in the same manner. To use the faradic current, which is also beneficial here as well as externally, the bipolar electrode may be utilized, the vagina and the intra-uterine in turn, care being observed, though using the stimulating current, not to push it to the extent of giving pain. This current may also be used in mild form from within the uterine canal to the lumbar region.

It will sometimes happen that we must persevere for a long time in this treatment before securing the results which we look for, but, if we have evidence that the genital organs are normal and merely need developing, we may still push the electricity, confident that it will ultimately bring about the flow. If we once see evidence of its appearing, we should give nature an opportunity to assert herself, and discontinue the applications, to renew them as preparatory treatment before the next menses are due. Some electro-therapeutists, however, prefer to push the treatment still more vigorously during the show, but I believe it best to leave the nervous system at rest and to allow the act to complete itself, for I have no doubt that in young girls of a sensitive organization, to whom such an occurrence is a total novelty, the continuous attendance of a physician at such a time might prove a check to the full development of the function. In any event, no vaginal or intra-uterine treatment should be given at such a time.

*Galvanism in Stenosis of the Uterine Canal.*—I do not consider this the place to discuss the pathology of stenosis of the uterine canal. Its existence as an anatomical fact is denied by some, who will not take any steps to treat it, though symptoms which can evidently be referred to it alone exist which can seemingly not be met by any but direct treatment. Several forms of stenosis are amenable to this treatment,—viz., the congenital pin-hole os externum; spasmodic contraction of the internal os, without apparent disease; stenosis of the canal due to sharp flexure, forward or backward; contraction of the whole cervical canal or of the os externum only, following a faulty operation for repair of a lacerated cervix; or atresia consequent upon the use of escharotics.

These several conditions may be the cause of dysmenorrhœa or of sterility, and it is in view of the benefit which we may derive from the use of the galvanic current that we pause for a moment to consider their treatment. True it is that all sorts of dilators have been employed in just such conditions, and many times with marked benefit; from sponge and tupelo tents down to the modern improved steel dilators, each method has cases to its credit; it is, therefore, presumable that many gynæcologists will still adhere to the older methods, but surely the number will diminish if they once witness the results of carefully applied galvanism in such conditions. This is not to say that this treatment should be instituted blindly, without due consideration being given to pathological states which produce such contractions. For instance, no one should think of treating acquired anteflexion or retroflexion as a disease; that would be absurd in the extreme. Those conditions have their appropriate treatment, and, except by enthusiasts, will ordinarily not be brought within the scope of this method; though I believe, as I have elsewhere stated, that the causes of these same conditions can often be much modified by this treatment, and that it may prove a very valuable aid in removing attendant complications, for it is undoubted that the change in nutrition of the uterus wrought by galvanism is sufficient to overcome the effect of congenital flexion and to stimulate the uterine tissue to a more normal development, and the same thing may be observed in chronic acquired flexures: so that when, after a case is virtually cured in other respects, we find a tight contraction persisting at the point of flexure, the result of plastic exudation in that neighborhood, we have nothing that promises us a better prospect of overcoming it than does electrolysis. The negative pole of the galvanic current is applied to the constricted part during ten or fifteen minutes with a power of fifteen to twenty milliampères, the positive pole, in the form of a large clay or wire gauze electrode, being placed on the abdomen.

Also, in respect to other discoverable pathological conditions, if there is a spasm of the internal os when an exploring probe is passed, the cause of such irritation must be sought; it may be in the uterus, it may be in the lower bowel (fissure). Even when it is a symptom alone, or when we are unable to discover the cause of it, we may still treat it and overcome it by this same method. Such a spasm, or such a flexure, even though the cause of the latter has been removed, will give rise to persistent dysmenorrhœa. This spasm of the internal os (it may be owing to nothing more than a congenital anteflexion) will in time create disease on its own part; congestions, frequently repeated, will lead to engorgement and hypertrophy of the organ; it is also one of the most frequent causes of sterility. Probably the orgasm itself, with such an irritable point, will close the canal still more tightly and prove an effectual barrier to impregnation.

These rather simple cases are easily met by a few applications of low power and short duration, and one may frequently have the gratification of seeing women become pregnant when, without this treatment or after posterior section of the cervix, they might have remained sterile. Now, undoubtedly, similar results have followed gradual and rapid dilatation, the wearing of glass stems, and, as I said above, surgical work upon the canal; but there is not a shadow of a doubt of the proper choice of means to make in such cases. The patient runs not the slightest risk, no anæsthetic is necessary, little time is taken, there is no confinement to bed, and the cure is absolute, even though conception does not follow, which is far more than can consistently be said for the other methods.

When the canal is closed by cicatricial tissue from any cause, the only difference in the treatment is the time which it may require. The case will possibly bear a little stronger current or a longer sitting, and the treatment will stretch over a longer period.

In cases in which there exists a small uterine outlet on account of a badly-performed cervical operation, it is not necessary to apply this treatment, because usually the difficulty is mechanical rather than structural, and moderate divulsion will suffice to overcome it. Should the opening be cicatricial, however, the former mode of treatment is the proper one to adopt.

*Galvanism and Faradism in Dysmenorrhœa.*—This is a subject which covers an immense field, as shown by the variety of diseases which may give rise to the symptom. It is like a dial indicating that something is wrong within. It may seem unphilosophical to give it a prominent position when we can discuss fully the many conditions of which it is merely a signal; still, one thing has been noted by every physician, that he is often called upon to relieve dysmenorrhœa as such, and does it successfully by the ordinary anodynes, when he may never be told or have an opportunity of learning the cause of it. It is positive that with galvanism we may also, sooner or later, overcome almost every form of dysmenorrhœa; but in undertaking such a treatment we are at least enabled to study the pathology of the case by the various means at our command,—a decided gain to both patient and physician. Even with this opportunity for investigation, we may still, at times, be obliged to proceed somewhat blindly, and to apply electricity because we know that we can relieve by it. It is rather in this light that I intend to consider the treatment of dysmenorrhœa by galvanism. In the previous section we have supposed that every step has been taken which could in any way overcome any tangible disease.

One thing to be stated at the outset is, that the character of the treatment must depend upon the presence or absence of congestion in and about the uterus. On these conditions depends our choice of the pole to be passed within the uterus; the negative, having a stimulating effect, will draw blood to a part, while the positive, having a repressing, anti-congestive power, will dispel it. This may to a certain extent seem theoretical; still, the poles, when brought to bear on recently living tissue, show such effects, and the symptoms as affected by the application of galvanism certainly bear out this assumption. In the same way the negative pole may be said to give pain and the positive to allay it; the positive to produce an escharotic, drying effect, the negative a softening, liquefying one.

Given such facts, we have traced for us a pretty straight course, and, with the exception of the condition just described, amenorrhœa, we shall be most commonly called upon to use the positive pole within the uterine canal, in that most of the painful states are attributable to congestion in that region. Here, also, the current should be slight; there is no necessity for the escharotic effect; all that we need is to diminish the fulness of vessels, and by that means we shall diminish the pain.

I referred to the effect of morphine as an anodyne, comparing the ready use of it with that of galvanism. It has the advantage over the latter in its ready adaptability to an emergency. Galvanism, of course, might be employed under such circumstances; but it is not pleasant to patients to have local treatment during menstruation, therefore it is utilized as a curative means in the intermenstrual intervals only: still, it may even be used during the period, for one can secure excellent results, symptomatically, by placing the positive pole over the anus and the negative over the abdomen with a large electrode. A small dosage and frequent applications are desirable.

It may require few or many treatments to bring about the desired result. The sittings should, however, not be longer than ten or twelve minutes, with the milliampère-meter marking from ten to fifteen or twenty.

It will be seen in other paragraphs relating to special diseases how much this symptom forms a part of each pathological state.

*Galvanism in Membranous Dysmenorrhœa.*—Membranous dysmenorrhœa must be considered as the result of endometritis, notwithstanding the difficulty which we experience in reconciling the appearances with an inflammatory state. We have no better name for the condition, at any rate, and it may be as well to adopt it as to seek for a new one. This is not a disease of frequent occurrence, therefore the means advocated for its cure are not so numerous as for most other female ailments. The disease, consisting as it does in some unexplained hinderance to the normal exfoliation of the mucous membrane of the uterus, apparently does not allow the capillaries to break down and establish a free flow. The pathological cause appears to reside in the nerves which preside over the nutrition of the parts much more than it does in the endometrium itself, and we would treat it on that principle if there was tangible evidence to support this theory. We must, however, again be guided by the symptoms, and attack the spot where the disease finds expression.

As was said above, cases are too few upon which to found any really fixed rule of treatment; probably that which will best stand the test of time is thorough curettage of the lining membrane of the uterus, repeated several times in succession, in anticipation of the catamenia, followed by a thorough application of carbolic acid and packing the cavity with gauze. This effects a decided change in nutrition and brings about a healthy disposition of the tissues, so that the mucous membrane is readily thrown off at the proper time and menstruation becomes painless.

Galvanism has also some claim, however, to effecting a cure of this condition, and, as it is well to have two strings to one's bow, it should receive its share of consideration. It is best used by passing the negative intrauterine electrode to the fundus and turning on a current of from twenty-five to one hundred milliampères for from ten to fifteen minutes, repeating the treatment at intervals through the month, and resuming it if the desired improvement has not been shown at each subsequent menstruation.

*Electricity in the Treatment of Subinvolution of the Uterus.*—This is one of the conditions with which we are constantly brought in contact in gynæcological clinics, and it is one, also, which many times has baffled us and made us despair. The reason, I believe, why so much difficulty is experienced in successfully treating it depends on the neglect of physicians to ascertain fully either its cause or the complicating circumstances attending it.

We may view it as depending on a low grade of inflammation of the uterine tissue, a chronic metritis, in which the uterus has engorged vessels with inactive muscular structure and a certain amount of lymph thrown out in its substance. Such a condition of the uterus, caused probably by arrested lactation, cold, or mild sepsis, will give rise to sensations of dragging and pressure, yet the organ itself will be little sensitive.

What is necessary in such a case is to deplete the uterus by hot douches and to elevate it to its proper level in the pelvis, so as to allow a free venous return; but we may also obtain considerable assistance from electricity by making use of the faradic current, of an intensity to suit the patient, one pole being placed in contact with the cervix, the other over the abdominal or lumbar region. Faradism stimulates the uterus to contract, causing it to squeeze itself out, as it were; we must persist until a permanent effect is obtained, which may require weeks, the applications of moderate intensity being repeated, say, every two days. As we progress and find the uterus diminishing in size we may use galvanism, placing the positive pole within the uterine canal and the negative plate over the abdomen, using twenty or thirty milliampères for ten minutes at a time, and repeating this every second or third day until we find that the uterus maintains its improved condition as to size and the catamenia are more normal in all respects.

Another form which subinvolution assumes is in connection with injuries of parturition, notably of the cervix itself and in connection with tubal and ovarian diseases and pelvic exudations. Subinvolution of this variety we shall find always exists in chronic cases, and, the source of irritation of the uterus being constant, its tissues have become harder and firmer, as if to withstand the attack. The vessels, through constant distention, have become enlarged and have exuded lymph, giving to the uterus a firmer consistency as well as causing marked enlargement. Here also, without neglecting the many other means which we are in the habit of applying to the treatment of this condition, we may utilize the galvanic current. We endeavor to promote the absorption of pathological products of long standing; in order that such a process may be completed, we must first soften the uterus. Now, instead of using the positive pole, which was before used as a stimulant, we here apply the negative. This condition, you will remember, is dependent upon, or is complicated by, the injuries of parturition (notably laceration of the cervix) and by pelvic exudations. With many physicians (gynæcologists also) it has been the practice to do all that was possible for such a subinvolution by the old routine methods, then to operate upon a torn cervix, hoping to see the effect disappear when the cause was removed; and so it may, but the result is gradual and imperfect if the uterus is in the condition described above, though it is rapid and gratifying in the first form of subinvolution, where the organ is still somewhat soft. In the latter, removal of the cause proves sufficient, but in the more chronic form the process of involution is tedious. But precede the operative work by the softening influence of the negative galvanic pole (intra-uterine), using upward of sixty to eighty milliampères, for fifteen to twenty minutes, about twice a week for a variable time, according to the effect, averaging a month or six weeks, and you will find that it has effected what nature could not so speedily bring about.

The third form to which I wish to call attention is that of areolar hyperplasia. In this, not only has the lymph organized, but there is really an increase of cellular tissue, and, though the uterus may once have been enlarged, or may be so still, we may, on the other hand, find it small, the case being a more chronic one, in consequence of the contraction of the new cellular tissue. Such a condition is observed in cases of premature menopause in young women. We constantly speak of reflex symptoms depending upon a plug of cicatricial tissue at the site of an old cervical laceration, and we appreciate the causal relation between the two when we see the cure of one by the removal of the other. We often find a satisfactory explanation of existing reflex neuroses, as the whole cervix presents the appearance of cicatricial tissue. After the menopause the neurosis also usually abates. In these cases the wise surgeon will remove the cervix up to the vaginal junction; higher, if necessary. The thorn is removed, but it·has left its sting, and possibly we shall never see all the effects removed, if such a state has existed for many years. Such a case may be benefited by galvanism, as indicated above. Fortunately, all cases are not so severe. In some, there are patches of induration in the cervix; in others, there is a certain amount of stenosis; in others, the uterine body is much indurated, assuming the condition of areolar hyperplasia, while the cervix may still be soft and congested. So it is seen that each variation must be studied separately and the galvanic current applied accordingly. In the one case it is used for stimulation, in the other to induce resolution; in one it is a derivative, in the other it is a disperser, so to speak.

*Galvanism in Endometritis.*—It is not to be doubted that the common form of so-called endometritis which we meet with daily is but an expression of disease elsewhere. As a matter of fact, the endometrium is not often inflamed, though we frequently see it otherwise diseased. It is really inflamed when there is septic or infectious matter in contact with it, or when it has been touched by a corroding chemical. The lower portion of the cervical endometrium is frequently the site of capillary engorgement and erosion; when ectropion exists it is also the site of cystic disease and of granulations or vegetations. The corporeal endometrium may be congested and hypertrophied, but, with the exception of the septic, specific, and traumatic forms, its epithelium is not even removed, and it remains merely the site of growths or of change of nutrition. These are the conditions which are called endometritis,—simple, catarrhal, granular, hemorrhagic, fungous, etc.,—and as such we are called upon to treat them, and we may accomplish good results with galvanism.

In cases of general pelvic congestion there may be a uterine discharge which is nothing but the hypersecretion of the uterine follicles, caused by the almost œdematous state of the organ. Rest and free actions of the bowels usually effect a cure. It may persist and resist hot and astringent douches. The uterus may become chronically enlarged through a repetition of such processes; then the coarse faradic coil will cause the organ to regain its tone; its nutrition may also be improved by the galvanic current, the positive pole being intra-uterine, frequent applications of a mild current being used.

If there is old cystic degeneration, causing occlusion of the cervical canal, the negative pole with high intensity may need to be used repeatedly to change the tissues from their hard, unyielding, cartilaginous character to the elastic and normal. When the uterine cavity is occupied by fungosities or polypoid growths, they should, of course, be excised or removed with the curette; indeed, the hypertrophied tissues just referred to should also be excised; but, as I am now presenting only the electrical side of the treatment, we may use the positive pole with high intensity to destroy them, though it will be up-hill work to remove them without first scraping or cutting them off. When that is done, an escharotic effect may be produced upon them which is at the same time antiseptic; otherwise the ordinary surgical routine should be followed, i.e., the introduction of a gauze tampon.

In cases of hemorrhagic or fungous endometritis we, of course, curette, if the uterine cavity is entirely accessible; if not, we have recourse to the positive galvanic pole, seeking to bring it in contact with the entire surface. The electrode need not be large; in fact, it is better to have it small, so that the power may be more concentrated.

If the canal is tortuous, as it is sure to be in cases of multiple fibroids, it becomes a rather difficult matter to reach the entire surface. I have thought that we might use, under these circumstances, a flexible electrode on the principle of Otis's flexible catheter.

In these various applications we shall do well with low ampèrage,—twenty to thirty, as a rule,—and probably not more than six or eight applications will be necessary to effect a cure of the condition producing the hemorrhage, though the deeper-lying tissues may require further treatment, which will vary with the special indication. If the case is a chronic one, and the tissues are indurated, the negative pole must first be used, just as in areolar hyperplasia; and when the change in nutrition has been accomplished, the positive pole or the coarse wire coil (faradic) will become necessary to stimulate the uterus to regain its tone.

If we find the uterus in this state from chronic engorgement attending the low grade of inflammatory process in its deeper tissues, we might proceed at once with the positive pole, creating a somewhat deeper impression at the time of removing the superficial growths than would otherwise be called for, so as to establish a more marked change in nutrition and a more positive electrolytic effect at the same time that we stimulate the uterine tissue to a better tone.

Now, when we speak of septic and infectious endometritis, we understand that we are dealing with conditions very different from the above; and yet I have not the slightest doubt that both septic and infectious material may be in the uterine cavity, or pass through it, without affecting the endometrium any more than do the discharges of pus which may flow over it at any time from a pyosalpinx.

The endometrium is fairly well protected by the mucus upon its surface, and, furthermore, it is not always a congenial habitat for the septic or infectious material. We can all recall cases of septic poisoning having their origin undoubtedly in the endometrium, yet not offering any indication of its development there. In the same way we can recall cases of gonorrhœal salpingitis in patients in whom at no time was there evidence of a gonorrhœal endometritis or even vaginitis. So it must be that some mucous membranes at certain times (as do other mucous membranes habitually) furnish a poor resting-place for special microbes. Then, again, we must keep in mind that we often find the uterine mucous membrane bathed in pus and yet beneath this the mucosa will be as healthy as ever. If the treatment is conducted as advised, no harm can come of it, and it may chance that the application intended to affect one region may have a salutary influence on another; in intra-uterine galvanization, for instance, the tube, which we may suppose to be the real seat of the trouble, may, being between the poles, be benefited.

If there is a septic endometritis, and we can recognize it as such, it can only be due to putrid material within the cavity : under such circumstances it is folly to talk about galvanism and electrolysis. We must remove the offending material, flush the whole cavity with antiseptics, keep the outlet free and the drainage perfect.

But specific endometritis may, in addition to the general cleansing and use of astringents, be favorably influenced by galvanism. It has been so applied in acute gonorrhœa when the specific poison occupied the uterine canal only, and the results were surprisingly good; but the method did not serve so well if the disease had extended to the tubes, although even then there was improvement in the symptoms. Having determined that microbes could be destroyed by contact with the positive pole of the constant current, it seemed natural to make some effort to utilize the method in this affection. The current which has been used is about one hundred and twenty milliampères, the duration of application being ten minutes. No such power could be tolerated in the urethra,—scarcely more than twenty-five to thirty milliampères,—otherwise it might be good treatment there; to carry it out, one might anæsthetize the woman, but to effect any good quite a number of applications are necessary, and no patient is willing to take ether or chloroform repeatedly.

If we decide to try the galvanic treatment, it should be continued even after the gonococci are no longer to be seen.

*Galvanism in Plastic Exudations.*—The conditions in which we may feel confident of happy results in adopting this treatment are those of old parametric and perimetric exudates. It matters little how they may have occurred; they have really all resulted from inflammation, and, in the light of recent pathology, it is fair to assume that most of them have had for their cause some septic infection.

There is no gainsaying the evidence of many good observers, that cellulitis is still to be found in our clinics. A wonderful benefit has resulted from the doubt which has been thrown out as to its existence, and the fact is undisputed that a very large number of cases formerly treated as such were instances of pelvic peritonitis, which includes salpingitis of various forms and peritoneal adhesions : still, I stand with clinicians in this, rather than with impulsive surgeons who will allow no time for progressive resolution, but determine at once to remove the offending condition and then often fail to find anything or to relieve their patient.

The one important question to consider in setting out to treat these affections is, Have we any pus to deal with? If so, where is it, and in what quantity? If it is locked up in a tube, and it cannot find its way out by the uterine cavity, it is dangerous to handle, and by the application of an electric force to it we may burst the tube and set up an acute attack of inflammation. So, also, if a collection of any size is buried elsewhere within the pelvis, it is desirable to know it; it may be advisable to empty it. As a matter of fact, however, pus may be present and may give rise to no symptom whatever. It depends largely upon its age, but it must depend also upon its quantity. A small collection of long standing may be entirely free of all infecting power, may even have become cheesy and inert; but a large collection, even of the same date, may not be considered quite so innocuous; it may remain dormant, thoroughly shut in and harmless, but it would never do to ignore it as a possible mine, ready to explode.

Then the difficulty of diagnosis is often so great in these cases that we may see them many times and never learn by the touch, and even the history may never point to the fact, that there is pus present. Could we know in every case of the presence or absence of encysted pus, there would no longer be any question as to the proper action to take; removal is the one and only rational method. One must have met with such cases and have borne with the uncertainty and anxiety attending their care, and must have seen them clear up week by week, fully to appreciate the difficulties which we have at times to face. And it is no light responsibility to assume, to pronounce on the curability of such a case by galvanism or to affirm that surgery alone can restore the patient to health. The practical lesson to be gathered from what I have here said is that we should give to every patient the benefit of treatment by galvanism to cure her as far as it can be done by this means. Some make marvellous recoveries; none are made worse if cases are judiciously selected. A number of cases of poor working-women whose time is their sole capital come under the care of every gynæcologist. When the facts are fully laid before them, they much prefer the radical operation of cœliotomy, even though pain is the only active symptom, since they cannot submit to prolonged treatment; so, also, may a number of women placed in better circumstances. If so, their wish should have some weight, and the physician is not acting amiss, I think, who recommends the more heroic measure if the history points to a deterioration of the woman's health or to a recurrence of inflammatory attacks. It is more especially the chronic inert case which appeals to us for this treatment, and it is in it that we can obtain our most brilliant results.

It is usually pain which is the most prominent symptom, and it is desirable to inaugurate our treatment by seeking its removal. This is to be effected by placing the positive ball electrode, covered with clay and

14

chamois, within the vagina, having at the same time the negative clay or wire gauze electrode over the abdomen. Beginning at zero, we should work the current-strength up to thirty or forty or fifty milliampères, increasing the power in direct ratio to the supposed high organization of the exudates, and continue the application for twelve or fifteen minutes. This current-strength and mode of application will drive blood away from the parts and allay the suffering. This may be repeated every two or three days until the pain is quite gone. Should it not prove successful, we may have recourse to the fine wire faradic current with the bipolar vaginal electrode, or this may be employed at the outset. After pain has been relieved, applications should be begun with the negative pole in the vagina and the positive over the abdomen, using about the same strength as indicated above, but increasing if it is well borne and does not produce pain. The vaginal electrode should not be held long in one place if the stronger current is used. I have found that by exceeding fifty milliampères we are in danger of producing sloughing of the parts with which the electrode comes in contact for any length of time, and yet considerably higher powers may often be called for,—two hundred to three hundred milliampères,—when the action at either pole may be destructive.

But in cases of lacerated perineum and relaxed vagina a large electrode may be used, and, of course, the larger the surface over which the current is dispersed the greater may be the power. It is desirable to push the strength of the current to the utmost that the patient and the parts will bear; for, even though we may secure excellent results by low intensities and prolonged treatments, the electrolytic effects will surely be more rapid, provided that we do not produce a galvano-caustic effect at the same time, which would unfortunately delay our operations. Repeat such treatments every two or three days if a moderate dosage is employed, once a week if the current is strong. We shall witness a process of resolution going on, we shall be the better able to map out the various organs, their mobility will be restored, and their functions may be re-established. As a matter of fact, general practitioners are in a position to apply this remedy, and if they will confine themselves to low powers no possible harm can result from their treatment, while it is unnecessary to state that few are in a position to operate successfully, and all do not care to send their patients to specialists.

The wise gynæcologist will not content himself with this method alone, but will utilize other means at his command : therefore massage will come to his aid and hasten the progress of his case. The treatment can also be applied by the intra-uterine electrode, the negative being used if the canal is patent, the positive if there is a thickened endometrium as an accompaniment of the trouble outside of the uterus.

*Galvanism in Salpingitis and Oöphoritis.*—I do not intend to discuss these conditions exhaustively. In looking over the literature of gynæcological electro-therapeutics one often finds reports of wonderful cures of both these affections. Some writers combine the two under the term "salpingo-oöphoritis," and have used this term to include the various conditions in which the two organs designated are usually associated, notably the pelvic exudation which either involves them primarily or is set up by disease in one or the other. I shall treat them separately, and it is only the so-called "catarrhal" form of salpingitis which I shall consider, and the ovary when in a state of chronic congestion, so far as we are able to diagnose either condition accurately.

Whatever may be the cause of the enlargement, we are able to map out enlarged, thickened tubes which are painful to pressure. We know the appearance of these tubes; they are just such as we have seen removed dozens of times when, apparently, there was no need of the operation, since they bore no trace of any disease which could not be treated just as well by counter-irritation, tincture of iodine, and fly-blisters, not to mention curettage and drainage of the uterus. The tubal mucous membrane is swollen, sometimes it is quite thick, and possibly there is some serous or œdematous infiltration of the muscular coat. Probably the pain attendant upon this condition arises from the congestion, which is, of course, much more marked before removal than after, and because of the unyielding peritoneum enclosing the tube. Such a tube feels firm, yet elastic, like a distended appendix vermiformis.

I have little faith in the ability of any gynæcologist to insert intentionally the tip of an electrode into the uterine end of the Fallopian tube, though, of course, one may do it occasionally or by chance. Were it always possible, we should naturally have a most ready access to collections of fluid within the tube, and there would be but few cases that would not prove amenable to the galvanic treatment. If it were possible to carry the electrode within the tube, it would also prove the most valuable mode of treatment for "catarrhal" salpingitis (for want of a better name), and, short of that, we should strive to push the positive electrode up as far as possible into the uterine cornu and the negative electrode over the abdomen. A moderate current—twenty to thirty milliampères—for ten to fifteen minutes, and repeated half a dozen times, will, in most instances, relieve such a condition so that we can barely feel the tube at all, or only as a slightly indurated cord, more and more free from sensitiveness if we have succeeded in diminishing its volume by relieving the congestion. Sometimes after the galvanic treatment there will be an abundant aqueous discharge from the uterine canal; this, to my mind, would either indicate the marked good and justification of such treatment in determining the serous discharge, or else I should infer that we have to do with a case of hydrosalpinx in which there is partial occlusion of the proximal end of the tube.

A discharge of pus has also been noticed after such treatment, and on that score galvanism has been advised in pyosalpinx. I would positively discountenance it as a rule, feeling that if we have pus enclosed we should remove it by cœliotomy, and that any meddling with electricity is apt to cause rupture; but I should make an exception in favor of the few cases in which we see such a collection already finding its outlet by the uterine canal; in these I see no objection to favoring the curative process, just as I advocate massage under similar conditions. Galvano-puncture is open to serious objections. The risk taken is incomparably greater than in a cœliotomy; it must be blind work, and one can never tell if he is puncturing an adherent gut, dividing an artery, or entering the peritoneal cavity.

Oöphoritis will detain us but for a moment, and the reason is that I consider it a very difficult matter to say when we have and when we have not oöphoritis. It is impossible to determine accurately that we are dealing with an inflamed ovary and nothing else, to decide whether it is partially degenerated as well, whether it is covered with exudate or not. Pain may be present in any one of the above conditions, as well as tenderness on palpation. Enlargement of the ovary occurs in all, probably some prolapsus as well, and the history may give us no aid whatever.

In such a case, especially if it is associated with the form of salpingitis which we have been describing as catarrhal, we may feel justified in subjecting the patient to the galvanic treatment tentatively; if there is any degeneration, of course we shall not expect a change for the better, but we may hope for improvement under other circumstances. We do secure good results in treating by this means ovaries which are enlarged, heavy, and tender. Call them "congested" or "inflamed," as you will, they are certainly not adherent, and cannot be regarded as seriously diseased. In treating such ovaries, as well as such tubes, everything which may contribute to the improvement of the general condition must be enlisted to further the result, otherwise it will be doubtful. The method of applying electricity in these cases is as follows. Apply the positive ball electrode within the vagina or in the rectum, as near as possible to the enlarged and prolapsed ovary, and the negative over the abdomen, using a moderate current (fifteen to thirty milliampères), which is maintained for ten minutes, and is repeated every three or four days.

*Electricity in Ovarian and Pelvic Neuralgia.*—There are certain pains in the region of the ovaries and deep within the pelvis which it is often difficult to associate with any disease, which are, in fact, probably associated with no local pathological condition whatever, but are more likely examples of reflex neuralgiæ. The anæmic, the chlorotic, the jaded and worn, —these are they who suffer more in mind than in body, whose nervous system is racked, and who, not wilfully, yet just as positively, mislead the physician, because it is upon these poor tried and tired organs that the impress of suffering is most manifest.

How these patients are drugged! How rich a field they offer to a succession of doctors to treat "ovarian and womb trouble"! How many receive the *coup de grâce* and are mutilated! But all to no purpose; there is no local trouble to be removed; we must look for the cause of the disturbance in the general nervous system.  Still, electricity can be utilized to great advantage in just such cases.

General electrization, or static electricity, is indicated, and general massage will prove its most valuable aid under such circumstances; but its local use is also valuable.  We should, first of all, use bipolar faradization with the fine wire coil, increasing the strength of the current as it can be borne, then changing to the coarser wire coil until the parts become either benumbed or free from pain.  Either persist with this treatment or follow it shortly with the galvanic current, as in the case of subacute inflammation or congestion of the ovaries, introducing the positive clay-covered ball within the vagina and having the negative electrode over the abdomen.

*The Treatment of Uterine Fibroids by Galvanism.*—One of the first things to determine, if we hope to meet with any success in the treatment of fibroids by galvanism, is the exact character of any individual tumor. We should fully understand with what we have to deal, and not make a blind beginning and find, when it is too late, that our hopes have been over-sanguine or have been utterly misplaced.  Many errors of diagnosis have led to very strange deductions as to the value of this agent in the treatment of such growths.  Ovarian tumors have been mistaken for them, and so have inflammatory exudates, as shown by subsequent cœliotomies or by post-mortem examinations.  When it is settled that we have really a fibroid of the uterus, we must be positive of its location, whether subperitoneal, intramural, or submucous, and we must also have a fair appreciation of its quality, whether it is hard or soft, a real fibroma, a fibromyoma, or one of the soft œdematous variety.

Were it within our power to recognize accurately, from the first, the exact location and nature of the neoplasm, we might direct our treatment more intelligently or withhold what may prove wasted energy.  I am fully convinced that the older methods of uterine exploration are not sufficiently carried out at the present day.  Before the metal divulsors were in constant use, it was the practice to secure full dilatation of the uterine canal by means of the graduated sponge tent, and when that was carried to the full extent the finger was inserted and afforded us much valuable information.  With the steel dilators, however, it is seldom that the cavity is opened to that extent, nor, in fact, can it be so effectually done with rapid dilatation.  For the purpose of such examination, it is far better to use the aseptic tupelo tents, or to pack the uterine canal with aseptic gauze until we are able to introduce the exploring finger easily.

The value of such an examination cannot be overestimated; it enables us to have a perfect appreciation of all the features of a case.  If a man is indifferent in his premises, he may have a rude awakening on finding that he has tackled a case of pregnancy,—a blunder which has been committed frequently,—or the exploration may reveal to him that he has to deal with a malignant tumor.  A thorough examination will demonstrate to him the irregularities of surface, the character of the mucous membrane, perhaps the exact nature of the neoplasm, and it will aid him in judiciously laying out his plan of treatment. Then no longer will attempts be made to reduce by electrolysis an intra-uterine polypus or pedunculated fibroid, which can be benefited through this treatment only by being forced out of the womb; we shall no longer have dozens of valueless observations of hemorrhage arrested or volume diminished without knowing whether the uterine enlargement was due to a fibroid or not.

Equal care should be taken not to devote too much of our attention to a subperitoneal fibroid. There are also distinctions to be established between some of the uterine fibromata. They may be composed mostly of fibrous tissue, with abundant channels throughout their structure, they may be largely composed of muscular fibres and abundantly supplied with blood-vessels, or they may be quite soft and equally vascular. The latter are of rapid growth, are boggy, and appear to be full of serum contained in cavernous spaces; the uterus almost seems to pit on pressure, being, in fact, œdematous. This variety is different from the fibro-cystic tumor, which is composed of some hard and some entirely fluid portions. Of these different varieties, the myo-fibromata, strictly speaking, are the ones in which the most good can be accomplished; next in order stand the pure fibromata. The benefit resulting from the treatment of either will depend mainly on the greater or less vascular supply. The myo-fibromata, being more vascular, feel the impression the more, and the durability of the so-called cure will depend on how far a purely electrolytic effect has been produced. There cannot be any great change of that character in muscular tissue alone; there never is upon normal tissue. The consequence is that the durable effect (when once produced) will be most marked in the fibromata, in that an electrolytic change does absolutely take place in its substance, and the change of nutrition may continue for an indefinite time. The first will require small amounts of galvanism frequently repeated, the latter will call for high intensities and short sittings.

The soft œdematous tumors should be carefully studied, for in applying galvanism to them we may often find that we have stimulated them to new growth, or it may be that we promote what I am inclined to believe is a natural tendency on their part to break down into fluid spaces. I have never felt quite certain whether cases of this kind which have ultimately come to the operating-table presented this character originally or whether it had been brought about through the influence of the battery, but it appears evident that either the poorly vitalized tissue is stimulated to absorb more serum from the blood and to undergo fresh development, or else we fail utterly to make any impression upon it. As to the loculi, I incline strongly to the opinion that they will always be produced in fibroids of any variety if we make use of the galvano-puncture, and, as a fact, they do strongly resemble the softened or broken-down areas of tissue sometimes produced by high powers: therefore in cases of this kind I should strictly avoid such treatment, for I am fully convinced that I have seen mild cases of sepsis after galvano-puncture, which I felt might be attributed to it. Of course there will be a few cases which will require the use of the galvano-puncture, such as those in which the uterine canal cannot be reached; but, as far as is possible, that method is gradually being dropped by the more prudent gynæcologists, in view of the uncertainties attending its use.

The fibro-cystic tumors of the uterus form likewise a forbidden ground for the galvanic treatment, on account of their poor vitality and their liability to break down and produce systemic poisoning. This force does not seem at any time to threaten the dissolution of tissues which are not in themselves predisposed to take on such a change, but tumors of this character are notably prone to it, and they must go to the surgeon.

The cases reported in which fibroid tumors are said to have disappeared are, considering the large number treated, exceedingly rare. In the large majority so treated, however, there is a perceptible diminution in size, persisting for a longer or a shorter time, though the observations of the subsequent history of cases are not sufficiently abundant to establish anything very positive on this point; still, a number of cases are on record which have been seen at long intervals after such treatment, and these have shown quite uniformly that the curative effect upon the tumors, when once established, was progressive, and that the growths had diminished steadily during months, even though the treatment had been discontinued.

Of the many cases submitted to treatment, even when they are well chosen, in some, of course, the tumors are not appreciably affected in size. Probably these are more subperitoneal than interstitial; yet the patients may be much improved symptomatically by relief from pain and pressure.

It is an interesting question just what does take place in a fibroid tumor when a galvanic current is made to pass through it: whether there is principally a contraction of the arterioles and muscular fibre which controls hemorrhage and brings about a diminution of the mass, or whether it depends on the vital change in the character of the solids and fluids which enter into its composition. Judging from the effect of the galvanic current when applied to other tissues, we know that the first assumption is in great part correct, that this contraction does take place, and we can, in fact, feel the uterine mass harden and become firm under the hand. Further, we see that fluids are expressed from these masses to some extent, usually during the sitting, and frequently some hours later. As regards the second assumption, it has been definitely asserted, and proved by experiments on muscular tissue in animals, that something akin to a cooking process does take place; furthermore, in a fibroid mass removed after such an application the course of the galvanic current can be accurately traced, its mark being a decided white line in the direction of the current, to say nothing of the chemical decomposition which we know takes place at each pole. It is a fair inference that a similar change takes place *between* the poles and as far around them as the influence of the current is felt in waves or curves. We might, further, take into account the softened spots which can at times be seen in large fibroids that have been subjected to the treatment by galvano-puncture with a current of from two to three hundred milliampères, and which have had to be removed ultimately: so it may fairly be assumed that the two forces are here combined and contribute to bring about a retrograde metamorphosis and atrophy.

Before beginning this treatment for uterine fibroids, we should thoroughly cleanse the vulva, the vagina, and the uterine canal with antiseptic douches and swabs. Bichloride of mercury (1 to 3000) will serve admirably for the vulva and the vagina, and the uterine canal may be swabbed with a five-per-cent. carbolic acid solution, or an application of lysol may be made.

The patient lies upon her back, with the limbs flexed to relax the abdominal muscles. The clothing about the abdomen should all be protected from moisture. I say that the patient should be upon her back, and yet it is not easy to introduce the uterine electrode in that position; she may be asked to hold the abdominal plate firmly to the body, or it may be strapped, and she may then turn upon her side, so that the speculum may be introduced and the electrode inserted more easily. Of all the abdominal plates that I have seen, there are none which I like better than the clay and that made of brass-wire gauze. The latter may be of any size to suit the abdomen, and can then be placed within the folds of a towel wet in a bicarbonate of sodium solution. The whole should be pretty thoroughly soaked, and should be warm, so as not to shock the patient. Apostoli recommends the clay pad only, and others think that it is indispensable and spares the patient pain. Still, I have been entirely satisfied with the gauze plate and wet towel, and have found that patients did not complain of any burning sensation, and could tolerate as high as two hundred and fifty milliampères.

In choosing an intra-uterine electrode, it is better to have one of moderate length, say from one-half to three-fourths of an inch, and to slide it up and down in the canal as the local condition may require, or to have one with an insulated slide. By this means the power may be brought to bear more fully upon a given surface, and the time of the application need, therefore, not be so long. If one is about to use only a moderate current for deep electrolysis, with a prolonged sitting, it is better to use an electrode which will extend the entire depth of the canal. The best one of this kind for all purposes is the block-tin electrode introduced, I think, by Dr. Goelet; it will bear either the negative or the positive current, and is serviceable either to produce an eschar or to use in stenosis. If not made of this material, every positive electrode for use within the body should be made of platinum, otherwise it will corrode and prove injurious to the tissues.

Applications of galvanism, with the positive pole within the uterine canal, will always arrest hemorrhage, though in a very hyperæmic endometrium it would sometimes appear to have the opposite effect at first;

that is, to cause bleeding. This is, undoubtedly, at the beginning of a séance, caused either by an abrasion of a congested mucous membrane or by the uterine contraction causing blood to ooze out.

Sometimes, after removing the positive electrode, we may also observe a slight show of blood. This I have regarded as due either to the escharotic effect of the anode upon some superficial arteriole or to the resistance offered on withdrawal, especially if one has used the block-tin electrode. In the first case this ceases of itself, as a rule, or may be arrested by re-inserting the same electrode and turning on the current to a less degree than before; it will then act as a hæmostatic rather than as an escharotic. In the second instance this little mishap may be obviated, if we appreciate the resistance, by turning on for a few moments the negative current, when we shall feel that the hold has been loosened, owing to the relaxing influence of the cathode, which we see so beautifully illustrated in the treatment of cervical stenosis.

As I have said above, such applications will always arrest hemorrhage; still, we must not overlook the point that in cases of fibroids, especially the submucous, one portion of the endometrium, where they project, may be excessively hyperæmic, while another portion, far beyond, may be more nearly normal. There are cases in which it may prove a difficult matter to cauterize directly the diseased portions of mucous membrane, as we shall readily see if we consider for a moment the tortuous course of a uterine canal under such circumstances; therefore no one is in a position to argue the futility of attempting to overcome hemorrhage in such cases unless he is sure that he has been able to reach the entire lining membrane.

It is undoubtedly in the capsule of a fibroid that the greater portion of its vitality resides, as the fibrous mass itself is only slightly vascular, and the thicker the capsule or portion of myomatous tissue enveloping the neoplasm, the greater the vitality. Therefore the larger the portion of mucous membrane which we can attack in such cases the more benefit we produce, and we must, in consequence, seek to carry the positive electrode over all the sinuosities and pockets of the lining membrane of the uterus, applying it sufficiently long at each point to produce an eschar. If, instead of this escharotic effect, we are desirous of producing electrolysis of the mass *in toto*, we should use the negative pole within the uterine canal. By this means we are enabled to secure the benefit of much higher powers than with the positive pole, which chars the tissues more deeply, so as to produce sloughing. Use the positive pole within the uterus, then, to affect the mucous membrane especially and to arrest hemorrhage, the negative for electrolytic treatment. For the escharotic effect, thirty to fifty milliampères during ten minutes, repeated a few times, say five to eight, will do, or, if the patient tolerates the pain, employ a stronger current with fewer sittings.

For the electrolytic treatment we increase the power gradually up to the extreme limit which the patient will bear, and are to be guided by the current employed. The higher the intensity the shorter the sitting; from five to twenty minutes will be quite sufficient, the time for a repetition of the treatment being determined by the effect observed upon the tumor and the patient's general condition. Better effects are, I think, secured by extended treatment.

*Treatment of Ectopic Gestation.*—If we have a case of this character come under our observation, the question presents itself immediately, How shall we treat it?

I shall not enter upon the question of diagnosis, which has been fully discussed in another chapter of this work. Presuming now that the true nature of the case has been recognized, we must at once adopt a policy which shall insure our patient's safety and redound to our own credit.

Two different views are held as to its treatment, and the advocates of each support their position by numerous facts. Some will by preference, at all times and without delay, open the abdomen and remove the ovum. Others will without hesitation seek to arrest the development of the ovum by the use of electricity, provided that the pregnancy has not advanced beyond four months; but when it is of longer duration, if accidents have already occurred or if they occur subsequently, they also are ready to open the abdomen.

Both judge correctly from their own stand-point, and, as said above, both have had experiences which warrant the strong arguments which they use in defence of their position. Probably there is no one method of treatment in any line of surgery or medicine which will at all times be accepted by equally well equipped and right-thinking men, and the condition under consideration is not an exception. The importance of the question, the gravity of the situation, make the physician feel keenly the responsibility resting upon him, and it seems but justice to the patient and to one's self, under such circumstances, to seek the counsel of a respected confrère, so that they may weigh the facts together, and, these being duly considered, may make a deliberate choice, whether to use galvanism or to perform cœliotomy.

In cities, with every facility at our command and with competent aid to assist us at operations, we do not, perhaps, correctly estimate the perplexities of a physician in a small town or in the country, when placed in such a position. We must keep in mind that every family physician is not so sure of himself, either in regard to diagnosis or operative dexterity, as to be willing to expose his patient to a certain risk by opening the abdomen, in preference to exposing her to only a possible risk; many patients are entirely out of the reach of skilled surgery or of an expert opinion. I have therefore no hesitation whatever in saying to physicians so situated that I think they are eminently justified in using their batteries, even though their judgment may incline them to recommend the knife.

Having clearly made out that there is positively a gestation outside of the uterus, and that it has not proceeded beyond the fourth month, if the physician has the appliances for electrical work, is not a surgeon, has no confrère at hand upon whom he may rely to do a cœliotomy, and cannot well despatch the patient to a larger medical centre, he should take no chances by waiting, but should at once seek to arrest the pregnancy by destruction of the ovum.

Now, which current should he use, and in what manner should he apply it? He has the faradic at his command, also the galvanic, constant or interrupted. It has been thought that the faradic current might cause destruction of the fœtus through compression exerted upon it by the Fallopian tube, such a contraction being presupposed in view of the recognized action of this current elsewhere; and, on the other hand, that the effect of the galvanic current might be more directly destructive to the fœtus itself by chemical or electrolytic action. However one may be disposed to view this theory, it is a fact that our only reason for using the faradic current should be the faint hope of causing sufficient contraction of the Fallopian tube to force the ovum into the uterus. This seems plausible at times, of course being much more probable when the ovum is implanted near the uterine cornu. This same contraction may, it is true, be induced by the constant current, but the latter should not be used with any such purpose, as the force requisite for the one effect would also induce the death of the fœtus, and if one aims at the propulsion of the ovum into the cavity of the uterus it is as well to maintain such conditions as will allow it to continue to develop. This would be the ideal method in the very early stage.

As opposed to this mode of reasoning when choosing a method of destruction of the ovum, we should not lose sight of the very grave danger of establishing such contraction as I have just mentioned, in view of the possibility of our producing rupture of the tube and thus precipitating the alternative of a cœliotomy, probably immediate. The chances are many, as operations and post-mortem examinations show, that such rupture will take place within the folds of the broad ligament, and, as that is the usual locality, it may be considered the least harmful, and if that were the only result, no further disturbance might occur than is the case in a large number of unrecognized tubal gestations; but we must not disregard the probabilities of shock, of hemorrhage, and of peritonitis which such a mishap would entail if the rupture were intra-peritoneal.

As a matter of fact, we cannot tell what is the muscular development of the tube, how much expulsive force we may count upon, therefore, nor the direction in which any thinning may have taken place at any one portion of its wall; nor can we estimate the resistance which the tube may offer in any part of its circumference, due to adventitious thickening or to the fact that it may be resting against some resisting surface. We cannot know, either, if there exists a narrowing of the canal between the ovum and the uterus, which would naturally offer a resistance and allow any undue force applied to be directed towards the fimbriated extremity. We are able, on the other hand, to tell pretty accurately at what point in the tube the ovum is implanted, though many have been deceived by palpation, and thus we may estimate the chances of being able to direct the ovum into the uterine cavity; still, all due allowance being made for the occasional benefit which ensues, even though one's hopes should be realized, faradism is, all things considered, decidedly not the better agent to depend upon.

In one case which I treated with the galvanic current for the purpose of destroying the fœtus, I caused its propulsion into the uterine cavity; the galvanic current (fifty milliampères) caused the sac to rupture; the fœtus was expelled twenty-four hours later *per vias naturales,* and the rest of the product of conception in another forty-eight hours. A hæmatocele which formed later at the site of implantation (outer third of tube) seemed to warrant my interpretation. At the time I reported the case to the New York Obstetrical Society I thought that it was unique, and Mr. Tait, of Birmingham, on reading the Transactions in which it was published, wrote to the *Journal of Obstetrics* denying the possibility of such a thing; but other cases of a like nature have been observed by competent men, and in one the whole ovum was supposed to have been expelled into the uterus, where gestation proceeded to full term. I cannot conceive of the change of site of an ovum as it is constantly inferred and alluded to. Either such supposed cases represent errors in diagnosis as to the original site, or the fœtus must be expelled from the tube into the uterus, the placenta retaining its original implantation. The whole mass cannot thus be transferred without the death of the fœtus, if a nutritive basis has already been established.

In dealing with a case of ectopic gestation, the less it is disturbed the better. It is particularly harmful to examine it roughly, and for the same reason violence by the faradic current is injurious; it may produce rupture of the sac, and that is a sufficient argument. On that account, in choosing either one of these methods, the preponderance of testimony is in favor of the continued current. With it a less intense and unbroken contraction is established, there is a more marked and persistent effect, and it is presumable that with high dosage there is to some extent an electrolytic action produced, a beginning of normal disintegration; and surely a body which we may have succeeded in mummifying is much less a source of danger than is a mere dead body within an enclosed space.

The maintenance of a continuous current for a few minutes better meets our desired end in destroying life than does the interrupted current, which more particularly suspends animation.

The next question is, In case we decide to choose this agent instead of resorting to surgery, when and how shall we use it? There is no time for delay. The patient should be told the circumstances and what it is intended to accomplish. She should be at rest in her bed, and should have an aseptic vaginal douche. The current can be applied through the vagina and abdomen, through the rectum and abdomen, through the vagina and sacral region, or through the rectum and sacral region. These various positions are suggested by the many possibilities of location of the tube so treated. The positive pole may be placed over the abdomen or within the vagina, as desired. In this case the question of immediate local action does not arise; we merely wish the interpolar effect, and the strength of the current need not be such as to cause an eschar. It will be sufficient if, with one pole within the vagina or rectum and the other over the abdomen, we raise the strength of the current from thirty to forty or fifty milliampères, so as not to run the risk of producing contraction of the tube. This current, continued for ten minutes and repeated after a day's rest with the same strength and for the same length of time, will in all probability prove sufficient. To make sure, there is no harm in a third application after one more day's rest, and even a fourth if the low power has been used. No ill result has been known to occur from this repetition, and we may fairly assume that the desired electrolytic effect is only enhanced. When this has been accomplished, I can only add that the physician must await events and be prepared to act. The fœtus may be expelled, or it may mummify, or it may degenerate. He has done the best that he could under the circumstances; he has used good judgment; but he must be in readiness to act in the best manner possible, even at a moment's notice.

# CHAPTER IV.

## ANOMALIES OF DEVELOPMENT IN THE GENITAL TRACT.

BY BARTON COOKE HIRST, M.D.

THE whole genito-urinary tract of the female, from the ovaries to the vestibule of the vagina and to the bladder and urethra, may be absent, in part or wholly, or may be subject to more or less serious developmental anomalies, disturbing or entirely abrogating the functions of the affected organs.

### OVARIES.

The ovaries may be absent or so ill developed as to be incapable of performing their normal physiological functions. In the former case there is usually a deficient development of the whole genital tract.

The gland itself may be of nearly normal size and in a normal situation, but the gland-contents, the Graafian follicles and ovules, may be absent, or the egg-cords of the fœtal ovary may remain in their primitive condition. The opposite anomaly of development by excess is not uncommon. Accessory ovaries immediately adjoining a normal ovary and included usually within the same peritoneal envelope have been found by Winckel at postmortem examinations. The ovary may likewise be constricted so that it consists of two practically independent parts. A true supernumerary ovary far removed in situation from its fellows is extremely rare. Winckel reports a case in which the supernumerary ovary lay between the uterus and the bladder. The possibility of accessory and of supernumerary ovaries must be taken into account in the operation of oöphorectomy. The operator's intention to make the individual sterile may be defeated by the existence of an extra ovary or of accessory ovarian tissue that is not detected at the time of the operation.

### FALLOPIAN TUBES.

The tubes show a number of developmental anomalies of interest to the scientific student, but of little importance to the practical gynæcologist, except in the study of the etiology of tubal gestation. Accessory fimbriated extremities are not uncommon; there may be three or more on the end of a single tube. An accessory uterine orifice is also not extremely rare. The whole duct of the tube may be duplicated, one canal commonly lying beneath the other. In connection with imperfect development of the whole sexual apparatus the tubes may also be non-developed; they may possess an abnormally small calibre; they may be solid without any lumen at all, or they may be entirely absent. On the contrary, the tube may show an abnormally great development with an anomalous patency of the canal, allowing the easy passage of a sound or probe from the uterine cavity out towards the abdominal orifice of the tube, and likewise permitting the regurgitation of fluids into the abdominal cavity. This hyperplasia of the tubes is not very uncommon in connection with the development of the whole sexual apparatus under the stimulus of pregnancy. The writer has quite often seen the regurgitation of lochial discharge in small quantities into the peritoneal cavity, with a sharp, transitory, non-septic peritonitis as a result. The tubes may be congenitally displaced, usually backward and downward into Douglas's pouch, occasionally forward and outward in an inguinal hernia. They may be obstructed, possibly by a congenital angulation, perhaps interfering with impregnation, or more likely retarding the passage of the impregnated ovule towards the uterus, and thus causing extra-uterine pregnancy.

### UTERUS.

There is so great a variety in the manifestation of congenital defects of development in the uterus that for a long time it was thought that these were accidental and did not follow the well-defined lines which govern congenital deviations from the normal in the fœtal and infantile body as a whole. It is to Küssmaul and Fürst that we owe a full and clear explanation of the developmental anomalies affecting the uterus.

To understand these anomalies it is necessary to refer briefly to the embryogenesis of the uterus. It is formed by the junction and fusion of the ducts of Müller, which are accomplished in great part before the twelfth week of embryonal life. Up to the twentieth week of the embryo's existence, however, there still remain distinct traces of the fusion of the two ducts, the uterus in this period being still distinctly bicornate. After the twentieth week, and during early infancy, the uterus presents the peculiarities of the so-called fœtal uterus. The cervix is much more developed than the body of the womb, and the mucous

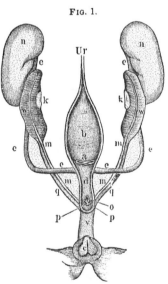

FIG. 1.

Development of the genito-urinary tract in the female.—*n, n,* kidneys; *e, e,* ureters; *a,* their orifices in the bladder; *w, w,* Wolffian bodies; *q, q,* their efferent ducts; *p, p,* their openings into the urethra; *k, k,* ovaries; *m, m,* ducts of Muller; *o,* their common orifice; *v,* uro-genital sinus; *Ur,* urachus; *c,* clitoris.

membrane of the cervical canal and of the uterine cavity is thrown into numerous folds. After the sixth year the fundus and body of the uterus have obviously attained considerable growth in comparison with the cervix, though there is nothing like the preponderance over the latter that occurs with puberty.

All the important developmental anomalies of the womb depend upon an arrest of development, and the nature of these anomalies depends in great part upon the time at which the development of the womb was arrested. If there is an arrest of the fusion of Müller's ducts before the twelfth week, a greater or less degree of duplicity in the womb must result. If the arrest of fusion in the two canals comes after the twelfth week, a bicornate or a septate uterus is the result. If the disturbance of development occurs at a later period, the womb retains a fœtal or an infantile character without longitudinal separation or distinct indication of the duplex manner of its formation. If the arrest of development affects the womb at a very early period, there may be simply a rudimentary bundle of muscle and connective-tissue fibres to indicate its situation, and in extraordinary cases there may be an entire absence of the organ.

Fig. 2.

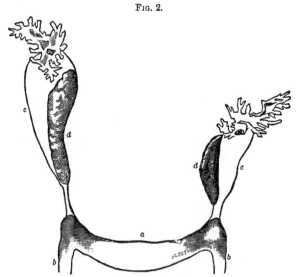

Rudimentary uterus.—*a*, ribbon-shaped rudiment of uterus; *b, b,* round ligaments; *c, c,* Fallopian tubes; *d, d,* ovaries.

*Absence or Rudimentary Development of the Uterus.*—Complete absence of the womb is an extremely rare occurrence, although an examination during life may fail to detect the slightest sign of its existence. After death there is commonly found an indication, at least, of the presence of the womb in a ribbon of muscle or connective tissue stretched across the pelvis

(Fig. 2), or, as in one case, in a mass of muscular substance on the posterior wall of the bladder (Fig. 3).

A rudimentary development of the uterus is not uncommon. There may be a solid muscular body of small size without a cavity, or a partial excavation with a shallow canal leading part way into the uterine substance. More commonly the uterus retains in adult life its fœtal or infantile char-

<table>
<tr><td align="center">Fig. 3.</td><td align="center">Fig. 4.</td></tr>
</table>

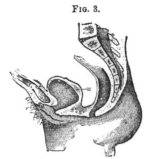
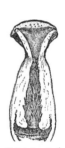

<table>
<tr><td align="center">Rudiment of uterus on posterior wall of bladder.—u, uterus.</td><td align="center">Fœtal, ill-developed uterus.</td></tr>
</table>

acter. The distinction is usually drawn between these two latter varieties of retarded growth in the womb, but for practical purposes this is entirely unnecessary.

Non-development of the uterus is commonly associated with acute anteflexion and with imperfect development of the nervous system. A large proportion of hysterical patients examined by the writer are found to have

Fig. 5

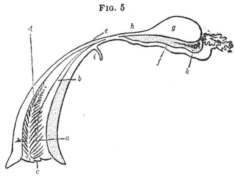

Ill-developed uterus unicornis.—<i>a</i>, cervix; <i>b</i>, fundus; <i>cd</i>, longitudinal axis of uterine body; <i>f</i>, tube; <i>g</i>, ovary; <i>h</i>, ovarian ligament; <i>i</i>, round ligament; <i>k</i>, parovarium.

this character of uterus. Usually the tubes and ovaries are likewise ill developed, but occasionally the ovaries are perfectly normal in anatomical development and physiological function; this is an unfortunate conjunction of conditions, for the periodical activity of the ovaries and the congestion of the pelvis are unrelieved by the menstrual discharge, and individuals thus affected suffer severely at each menstrual epoch. The writer has found it necessary in several well-marked cases of this kind to remove the ovaries, the individual having been entirely incapacitated for all occupation by the severity of the menstrual molimina. Women with non-developed uteri may show no indication of the defect in their general appearance and demeanor, but in the writer's experience it is more common to find ill

Fig. 6.

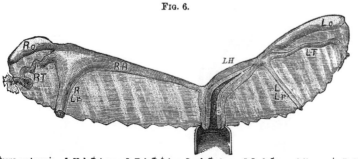

Uterus unicornis.—*L H*, left horn; *L T*, left tube; *L o*, left ovary; *L Lr*, left round ligament; *R H*, right horn; *R T*, right tube; *R o*, right ovary; *R Lr*, right round ligament.

development of the whole organism, a small stature, a slight frame, a feebly resisting nervous system, and a lack of mammary development.

The local treatment of arrested development of the uterus is extremely unsatisfactory. If, however, it is not too marked in degree, some advantage is occasionally derived from the use of the faradic current applied to the uterine cavity ; but in the majority of cases the sterility and the scanty

Fig. 7.

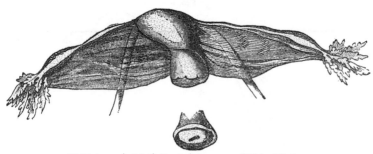

Ill development of right side of uterus; congenital lateral flexion.

menstruation for which the patient consults her physician must be pronounced incurable.

*Arrested Development of One of the Ducts of Müller ; Uterus Unicornis.*
—It occasionally happens that there is an arrest of development or a failure to appear on the part of one of Müller's ducts, with the consequent formation of but one side of the womb and a development of but one Fallopian tube. Both ovaries may be present. It is more common to see

an indication of an ill-developed Müllerian duct on one side in the shape of
a solid muscular band which runs outward to the insertion of the round
ligament. (Fig. 6.) The developed side of the uterus is situated entirely on
one side of the axis of the pelvic cavity, and it inclines quite strongly
towards the corresponding pelvic wall. There is no uterine fundus, and the
uterine body ends in a cone-shaped projection in which is inserted the
Fallopian tube. In slight degrees of arrested development on one side the
uterus may show rather sharp lateral flexion towards the undeveloped side.
These conditions do not call for gynæcological treatment. They are only
detected, if recognized at all, in the course of a pelvic examination for
suspected pregnancy in which there seems to be some abnormality. The
situation of the womb on one side of the pelvis may lead to the mistaken
diagnosis of tubal gestation.

FIG. 8.                                FIG. 9.

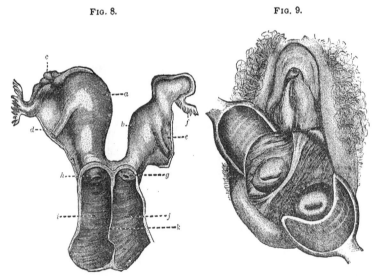

Uterus didelphys.—*a*, right segment; *b*, left segment; *c, d*, right ovary and round ligament; *f, e,*
left ovary and round ligament; *g, j*, left cervix and vagina; *k*, vaginal septum; *h, i*, right cervix and
vagina.

*Arrested Fusion of the Ducts of Müller; Uterus Didelphys; Double
Uterus.*—Occasionally the ducts of Müller remain entirely apart from each
other in the whole course of their development, the failure of union
resulting in the formation of two distinct uterine bodies, without even
external junction. There are two cervices and two distinct vaginal canals,
though the latter always lie in juxtaposition to each other. (Figs. 8 and
9.) It was thought at one time that this was an extremely rare variety
of duplex formation in the uterus, but by a more careful examination
of patients during life, and a more careful observation of specimens post
mortem, the number of these cases has lately grown considerably, and it is

a question if many of the examples of uterus bicornis should not be included under the heading of double uterus or uterus didelphys.

During life the diagnosis of complete separation of the two uterine bodies can be made by the introduction of the sound into each and the determination that one moves entirely independently of the other.

*Uterus Bicornis Duplex.*—In this variety of arrested fusion the two bodies of the uterus are in juxtaposition and are connected externally, but remain

FIG. 10.

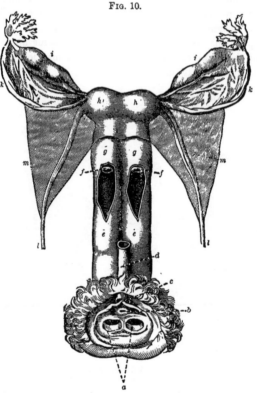

Uterus bicornis duplex.—*a*, double entrance to vagina; *b*, meatus urinarius; *c*, clitoris; *d*, urethra; *e, e*, double vagina; *f, f*, external orifices of uterus; *g, g*, double cervix; *h, h*, bodies and horns of uterus; *i, i*, ovaries; *k, k*, tubes; *l, l*, round ligaments; *m, m*, broad ligaments.

internally distinct and apart through their whole length, and are joined externally not so much by muscular tissue as by their peritoneal investment and connective tissue. There are, of course, two distinct uterine cavities, two cervices, and a double vagina.

*Uterus Bicornis Unicollis; Bifid Uterus.*—In this variety the junction of the two ducts is quite intimate below, so that there may be a single cervix without a dividing septum, but directly above this the two uterine halves diverge sharply from each other. It may not be easy to recognize

this variety of arrested fusion in the uterine body during life, but the writer
has been able to detect it in several instances by a careful bimanual exami-

Fig. 11.

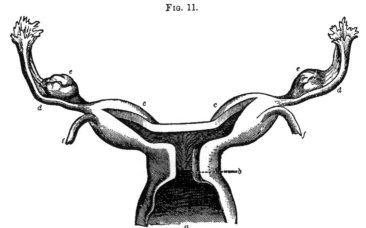

Uterus bicornis unicollis.—a, vagina; b, single neck; c, c, horns; d, d, tubes; e, e, ovaries; f, f, round
ligaments.

nation, followed by the use of the uterine sound, which detects the diver-
gence of the uterine canals. In one case a mistaken diagnosis was made

Fig. 12.

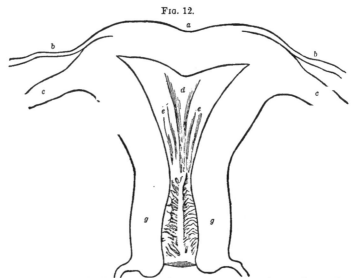

Uterus cordiformis.—a, indented fundus; b, b, tubes; c, c, round ligaments; d, central longitudinal
ridge on posterior wall of uterine cavity; e, e, lateral ridges of same; f, internal os; g, g, cervix.

that seemed scarcely avoidable: a bifid uterus was retroverted and firmly
fixed by inflammatory adhesions; it was taken for double pyosalpinx,

and it was only when the abdomen was opened that the true nature of the case was discovered. The adhesions were separated and the uterus was replaced.

*Uterus Cordiformis.*—In this variety of arrested development an indica-

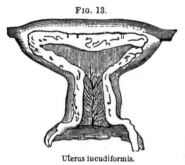

FIG. 13.

Uterus incudiformis.

tion externally of the imperfect fusion of the ducts is furnished by a depression in the middle of the fundus. The fundus is broad, and the uterus has a conventional heart shape. Associated with this external appearance there may or may not be a longitudinal septum within the uterine cavity.

*Uterus Incudiformis.*—This is an exaggeration of the uterus cordiformis without the median depression in the fundus. The upper portion of the uterus is stretched to either side, so that the whole organ has the shape somewhat of an anvil. These last two deformities are more important to

FIG. 14.

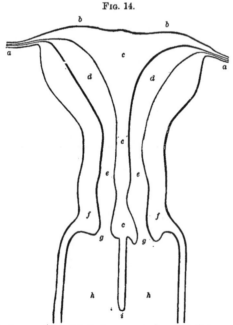

Uterus septus duplex.—*a, a,* tubes; *b, b,* fundus; *c, c, c,* septum; *d, d,* uterine cavities; *e, e,* internal orifices; *f, f,* external walls of cervix; *g, g,* external orifices; *h, h,* vaginal canals; *i,* septum dividing the upper third of the vagina.

the obstetrician than to the gynæcologist. They determine abnormalities in the position of the fœtus and in the mechanism of labor.

*Uterus Septus, Subseptus, Partitus, Semi-Partitus.*—With or without any external manifestation of imperfect fusion of Müller's ducts, there may be in the interior of the womb a longitudinal septum dividing the cavity in whole or in part.  The two divisions of the womb in a uterus septus are not commonly of equal size or development.  One is usually smaller and less developed than the other.  This condition has little interest, as a rule, for the gynæcologist, unless he should discover it as an accidental complication of some pathological condition of the genitalia.  Its main interest is for the obstetrician, as a complication of the childbearing process.

FIG. 15.

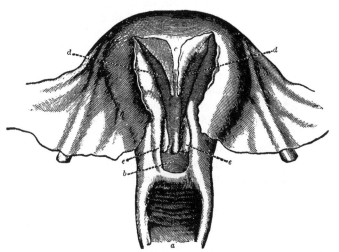

Uterus septus uniforis.—a, vagina; b, single os uteri; c, uterine septum; d, d, uterine cavities; e, e, ridges on the wall of the cervical canal.

The vagina is divided by a longitudinal septum in cases of uterus didelphys, uterus bicornis duplex, and sometimes in uterus subseptus.  The vagina and cervix (uterus biforis) may be divided longitudinally without division of the uterine cavity.

*Anomalies of Development in the Cervix.*—The commonest developmental anomaly in the cervix is a stenosis of the canal and of the external and internal os, associated frequently with a conical shape and small size of the cervix as a whole and often with an undersized and anteflexed uterus.  This condition of the cervical canal opposes a mechanical obstacle to the escape of blood at the menstrual period.  For the first few years after puberty, however, there may be very little trouble; but as time goes on and the menstrual flow becomes more profuse, there is greater difficulty in its discharge; the disturbance of the uterus, its distention, and the violent muscular action required to expel the blood irritate the lining membrane, which in time becomes chronically congested. This condition leads to a sudden onset, with a more profuse flow. This, of course, increases the difficulty, and so a vicious circle is established that causes greater suffering at each period, intermenstrual pain, and at length nervous break-down.

The clinical history of these cases is that at first the individual remains entirely free from pain in the intermenstrual period, the pain beginning only after the first hour or two of the flow, as a rule, and becoming more and more acute for the first twelve, fourteen, or even twenty-four hours, gradually passing off and entirely disappearing before the cessation of menstruation. The diagnosis of the condition is made by the foregoing clinical history and by a digital examination.

The treatment consists in the forcible dilatation of the cervical canal; on the whole, one of the most satisfactory of all gynæcological procedures. The technique of the operation is as follows. The woman is etherized and placed in the lithotomy position; the vagina is well scrubbed out with pledgets of cotton saturated with equal parts of tincture of green soap and hot water; a douche is given of bichloride of mercury solution (1 to 2000); the anterior lip of the cervix is seized with a double tenaculum and pulled down towards the vulvar orifice. A small two-branched dilator (the writer's preference being for Baer's) is inserted until the tip nearly reaches the fundus of the uterus; it is then withdrawn about a quarter of an inch and the branches are separated until the indicator marks about one inch, but, on account of the feathering of the blades, in reality only about half of this space is gained. This is followed by the insertion of one of the stronger and larger two-branched dilators, such as Wathen's; by this instrument the cervical canal is dilated in the course of twenty minutes up to an inch and one-quarter. The uterine cavity should be thoroughly curetted after the dilatation, for the irritation accompanying each menstrual period has led to an endometritis. The cavity is then swabbed out with a mixture of carbolic acid and glycerin, equal parts, and is thoroughly flushed with a good two-way catheter,—the best, in the writer's opinion, being Skene's reflex catheter for the urethra. No special device to secure drainage from the womb is necessary. The common fashion of packing the womb after this operation with a strip of iodoform gauze is reprehensible. It does no good, causes sometimes considerable pain, and perhaps prevents the escape of small fragments of uterine mucous membrane from the cavity.

In exceptional cases it may be necessary to begin the dilatation with a uterine probe, and to follow this with a very small two-branched instru-

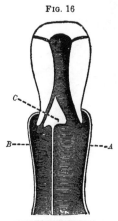

FIG. 16

Schematic drawing of double vagina and single uterus.—*A*, left vagina; *B*, right vagina; *C*, cervical septum.

ment, such as a Thomas's applicator, before it is possible to insert even as small a dilating instrument as Baer's. The best time for the operation is about a week before an expected period. The results of the operation are usually most satisfactory. The dysmenorrhœa is cured, the sterility in the case of a married woman is often obviated, and the reflex symptoms disappear. The writer has thus cured aggravated cases of vaginismus. Sometimes it may be necessary to repeat the dilatation. Rarely, in cases apparently most suitable, no relief is afforded by the operation, or not for some time afterwards. The nerves of the sexual apparatus have become accustomed to running riot at the menstrual period, and it may be a long time before they are calmed. The writer has seen the dysmenorrhœa continue for a year after dilatation, and then cease without other treatment being employed.

*Atresia of the Cervix, Congenital and Acquired.*—Congenital atresia of the cervix may have its seat at the internal or at the external os, or may affect the whole canal. It is not discovered until after puberty and the institution of menstruation. If there is no associated anomaly of the uterine body or ovaries, the menstrual molimina appear regularly and become more and more painful without the discharge of any blood from the genitalia. After a while, an examination being made, the physician will detect a spherical cystic tumor in the pelvis, occupying the position of this uterus. Exceptionally there is no attempt at menstruation in this anomaly, and occasionally the menstruation is vicarious.

Acquired atresia of the cervical canal is most frequently the result of cauterization of the cervix. It may be due to ulceration or to chronic inflammation from any cause, however, and occasionally its occurrence is absolutely inexplicable. The writer has seen this condition develop in a woman forty years of age who was approaching the menopause. There had been no operation nor local treatment, she had never borne a child, and there was absolutely nothing to explain it. In the course of eight years a very large collection of menstrual blood accumulated in the womb and in both tubes, necessitating a puncture of the cervix for the former and an abdominal section for the latter.

The diagnosis of atresia of the cervix, congenital or acquired, is easily made. It is impossible to pass a sound through the cervical canal. If there has been an accumulation of menstrual fluid or of mucus within the womb, the latter is converted into a cystic tumor with rather thick walls, and on both sides of it there are commonly very much enlarged and distended tubes. In the case of atresia at the internal os the external form of the cervix is well preserved. In the case of atresia at the external os the cervix is practically obliterated and becomes continuous with the vaginal vault. By digital examination it is impossible to detect any evidence of the existence of the cervix, but upon inspection through a speculum the cervix is indicated by a slightly projecting nipple in the middle of the vaginal vault and the seat of the external os is marked by a shallow dimple.

The treatment of atresia of the cervix, if associated with accumulation of fluid, is referred to under the head of Hæmatometra.

*Arrested Development of the Cervix.*—The cervix may be undeveloped in common with non-development of the uterus or of the whole genital apparatus. Occasionally it is the cervix alone that is affected, and in exceptional instances the whole vaginal portion may be lacking, while the rest of the genital apparatus is well developed. In these cases the vagina passes directly into the uterine cavity by a small constricted canal. It is easy to confound with this condition a congenital stenosis of the upper third of the vagina, in which the latter canal is suddenly reduced to a small sinus barely admitting the uterine sound. This condition is not usually demonstrated unless the woman becomes pregnant, or a vaginal examination is made for the detection of some other presupposed condition.

*Hypertrophy of the Cervix.*—The vaginal portion of the cervix occasionally shows very marked hypertrophy, presumably of congenital origin. There is no inversion of the vaginal mucous membrane, yet the cervix

FIG. 17.                          FIG. 18.

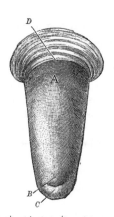

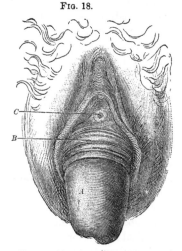

Hypertrophic elongation of the cervix.—*A*, cervix; *B, C,* anterior and posterior lips; *D*, uterine body.

Hypertrophic elongation of the cervix and prolapsus.—*A*, cervix; *B*, uterine body; *C*, meatus.

reaches to and projects beyond the vulva. It assumes in these cases a somewhat conical shape, but that portion of it which appears between the labia has a normal look as regards shape and size. There is no ulceration around the os, no marked increase in the transverse diameter ; in short, there are none of those changes which are common where the cervix is prolapsed in consequence of inversion of the vaginal walls and supra-vaginal hypertrophy of the cervix, the latter being always due to some of the injuries of childbirth, and having no place among the congenital anomalies of this region. It is a curious fact that hypertrophy of the infra-vaginal portion

PLATE I.

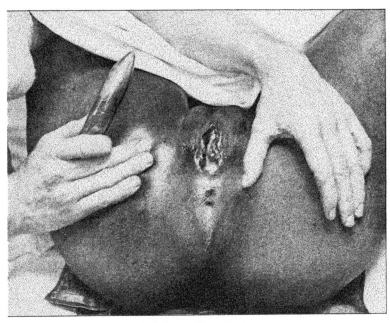

Atresia of the vagina. (Kelly.)

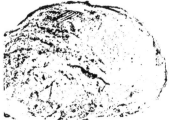 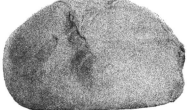

Double hæmatosalpinx associated with atresia of the cervix and hæmatometra.

of the cervix is much more common in negresses than in white women. The writer does not remember having seen a case in the latter, while in his dispensary service it is a common experience to have several marked instances every year of this hypertrophy in negresses. The treatment consists in the amputation of the cervix by Hegar's operation.

VAGINA.

The vagina may be absent, or may be indicated simply by a rudimentary cord of connective tissue. This condition may be associated with an absence of the whole internal genitalia, while the external genitals may possibly present a perfectly normal appearance, including the presence of a hymen. If the uterus and ovaries exist in a well-developed condition, the absence of the vagina will give rise to serious trouble as soon as menstruation begins. The menstrual fluid collects within the womb, causing more

FIG. 19.

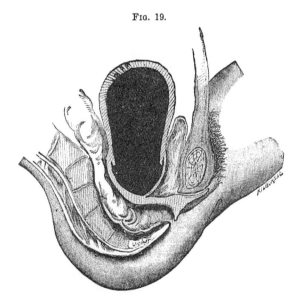

Atresia of the vagina.

and more pain, and accumulates also in the tubes, which before long threaten to rupture. On physical examination a cystic tumor is discovered, perhaps in the hypogastric region, while the examiner is unable to pass a finger or even a fine sound beyond the bottom of the vestibule. With a sound in the bladder and a digital examination of the rectum, the distended uterus and tubes can be detected high up in the pelvis. The thickness of the tissue representing the vagina, or the entire absence of such tissue, can be determined in the same manner. Such a condition demands radical treatment. A passage-way must be opened for the escape of the retained menstrual blood ; this is done by making a transverse incision in the perineum between the rectum and the urethra and then dissecting the tissue with the finger-tip or a blunt-pointed instrument, or, occasionally, the scissors, until the cervix is reached. The rectum and bladder are guarded from injury by a finger in one and a sound in the other. The uterus, when it is reached, is punctured, if necessary, with a large trocar, and the opening is at once further dilated by incisions with a blunt-pointed bistoury on either side of the trocar. The artificial vagina is kept open with great difficulty after such an operation. The best means, perhaps, is to transpose a flap of skin from the buttock into the vagina, sewing its ends, if possible, to the cervix. Persistent and frequent artificial dilatation with cylindrical dilators must follow. In spite of all efforts, however, the artificial opening may close again, or may become so contracted as to oppose a serious mechanical obstacle to the escape of the menstrual fluid. In one case, quoted by Pozzi, temporary success was attained after making the artificial vagina by electrolysis; but it is doubtful if the ultimate results of this treatment are any better than those that follow frequent and persistent mechanical dilatation.

FIG. 20.

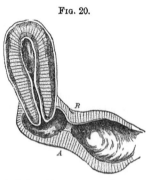

Occlusion of the vagina.—*A B*, transverse septum.

FIG. 21.

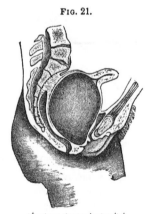

Atresia of the vaginal outlet.

FIG. 22.

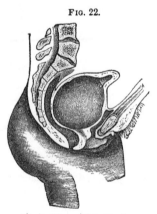

Atresia of lower third of vagina.

If there is absence or non-development of the uterus, so that menstruation does not occur, there is no excuse for resorting to the operation for making an artificial vagina. Should there be well-developed ovaries,

however, with absence of the vagina and uterus, so that there are menstrual
molimina, associated with great pain and nervous distress, oöphorectomy
may be called for.   In a few cases of absent vagina and uterus there has
been vicarious menstruation, the blood having been discharged from the
mucous membranes of the stomach and of the lungs, and in one case through
the skin of the extremities.

Occasionally the vagina is absent in only a part of its course, being
reduced to a solid fibrous cord, usually at about the middle.   The result
here is the same, of course, as though the entire canal were wanting.   The

Fig. 23.

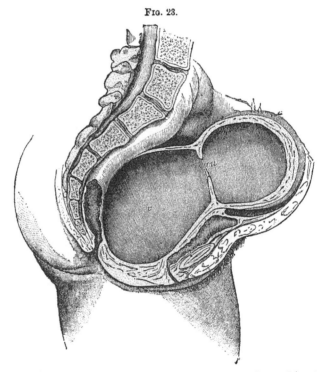

Atresia of the vaginal orifice; hæmatocolpos and hæmatometra.—*v*, vagina; *ou*, internal os.

menstrual fluid is dammed up, first distending the vaginal canal above the
point of atresia, then dilating the uterine cavity, and affecting also the
tubes.   This condition, however, is much more amenable to operative treatment than is a case of entire absence of the vagina.   Atresia of the vagina
may result if the depression at the vestibule fails to effect a union with the
vaginal canal.   The two passage-ways impinge upon each other, but the
barrier between them fails to melt away as it should normally.   In such
a case the vestibule is usually much deeper than common, but the accumulated fluid behind the barrier which prevents its escape is within easy reach

and its evacuation is attended with no special difficulties.    After making a
free opening or, if necessary, a dissection upward to reach the vaginal canal,

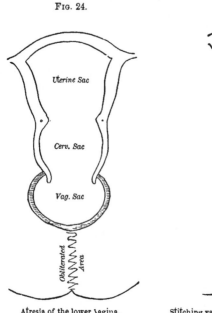

Fig. 24.

Atresia of the lower vagina.

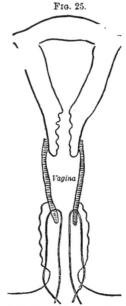

Fig. 25.

Stitching vaginal walls to external skin.    (Kelly.)

the mucous membrane of the vagina may be pulled down and stitched to
the skin of the vulva.

*Unilateral Vagina.*—It sometimes happens that one of the two Müller's

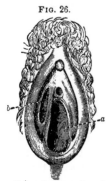

Fig. 26.

External appearance of
double vagina.—*a, b,* vaginal
orifices.

ducts which, when fused together, constitute the
normal vagina, fails to develop entirely, and the
vagina is formed by the growth of but a single
duct. This is seen in connection with a uterus
unicornis. It is doubtful whether it ever occurs
independently of this condition. In these cases
the canal is much narrower than common, and
may be situated to one side of the median line.

*Double Vagina.*—There may be a failure of
fusion on the part of the two Müller's ducts in their
lower portions, as there is a failure of fusion
above in the case of one of the different forms of
double or septate womb. The septum of the double
vagina is so arranged that one canal is somewhat
anterior to the other. The septum usually extends
the whole length of the vagina and is often associated with a double hymen.
In some cases, however, the septum may be lacking in part. The hymen

may be single, and there may be a considerable space between it and the commencement of the vaginal septum.  Occasionally the double vagina is asymmetrical, one of the canals being larger and better developed than the other.  In such a case the less developed canal is usually closed at its lower end.  After puberty this may result in a lateral hæmatocolpos if the undeveloped vaginal canal is connected with one side of a double uterus.

A double vagina is often overlooked, even in a gynæcological or obstetrical examination.  The two distinct orifices are often not detected, even in the course of a long labor and in spite of repeated examinations, or at any rate not until the presenting part finds an obstruction in the longitudinal septum.  In the case of lateral hæmatocolpos from atresia of one side of a double vagina, the diagnosis may present great difficulty, and is made only after a careful bimanual and rectal examination, and possibly only after a free incision has been made into the vaginal wall and the collection of fluid has been evacuated.

Fig. 27.

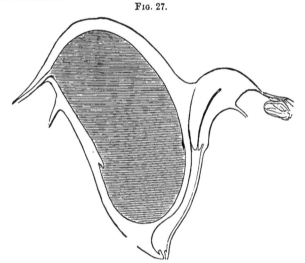

Unilateral hæmatocolpos and hæmatometra.  (Martin.)

*Stenosis of the Vagina.*—There may be narrowing of the whole vaginal canal in association with non development of the entire genital tract.  This, however, is not apt to be extreme, and it is of more interest to the obstetrician than to the gynæcologist.  Occasionally the vagina in one part of its course is reduced to a small tract no larger than the cervical canal.  This is most likely to be seen in the upper third of the canal, the vagina suddenly ending at a distance of an inch or more below the cervix.  The vagina may likewise be obstructed by transverse folds of mucous membrane and connective tissue, in some cases simulating a secondary hymen high up in the canal, in others taking the form of thick, fleshy, transverse bands.  Occasionally these bands run antero-posteriorly.  This condition is of little interest unless the patient becomes pregnant, when it may be necessary to cut the obstructing bands if they do not yield before the advance of the presenting part.

FIG. 28.

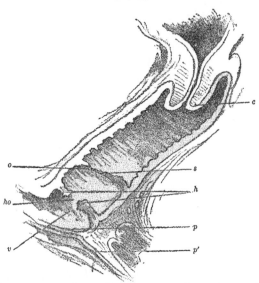

Transverse septum of the vagina, incomplete. (Heyder.)—c, cervix; s, septum; o, orifice of septum; h, hymen; ho, hymeneal orifice; v, vestibule; p, posterior commissure; p', perineum.

## VULVA.

At the end of the first month of the embryo's existence a depression is developed in the caudal region, growing deeper towards the allantois and opening into the latter and consequently into the intestines, to which it is joined, constituting the common opening, the so-called cloaca. A few days later the first indication of the sexual organs appears in the shape of a slight eminence above the cloaca, and on either side of this eminence appears a fold of skin. In the course of the next two weeks the wall partly separating the intestines and allantois grows downward into the cloaca, and, being met by a process from the external skin growing upward, forms the perineum and divides the genital from the intestinal canal. The genital eminence becomes later the clitoris, the folds of skin on either side the labia majora. Within these are later

FIG. 29.

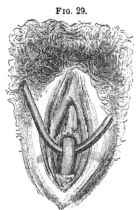

Longitudinal band dividing vaginal orifice.

developed the nymphæ or labia minora. Anteriorly the urethra is now
developed, and a septum divides the urinary from the genital tract. The
ducts of Müller descend more and more, making the uro-genital sinus,
as the common external opening is called, more and more shallow.

*Atresia of the Vulva.*—Very rarely there is an entire absence of the
successive steps in development by which the uro-genital sinus is formed,

Fig. 30.

Fig. 31.

Development of vulva.—*m*, Müller's ducts; *r*, rectum ; *all*, allantois; *b*, bladder; *v*, vagina; *u*, urethra;
*c*, clitoris; *s*, genito-urinary sinus.

and the skin is stretched evenly and unbroken from the pubes to the coccyx
and from one tuberosity of the ischium to the other. There is complete
atresia of the vulva. This is seen only in non-viable fœtuses.

*Arrested Development of the Uro-Genital Sinus.*—An arrest in the development of the uro-genital sinus occassionally results in a persistence of
the conditions that existed at the
stage of embryonal development
when the openings of the intestine,
bladder, and genital tract were
common and unseparated. There
may be thus hypospadias in the
female, which is, however, very
rare, or more commonly a persistent opening of the bowel into
the vestibule in front of the
hymen. To this condition the
name of atresia ano-vaginalis is
commonly given, a name not
strictly accurate, for there is, of
course, not a complete atresia of
the anus, but simply an abnormal position. Rarely there may
be, coincident with this abnormal
opening of the bowel into the
vestibule, a patent anus in the
normal situation, showing conclusively the growth inward of skin and

Fig. 32.

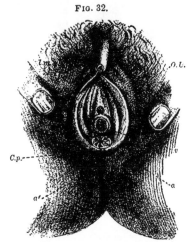

Anus vestibularis. (Himmelfarb) —*O.U.*, urethral
orifice; *l.m.*, labium minus; *v*, vaginal entrance and
hymen; *Cp.*, posterior commissure; *a*, anus; *a'*, perineum.

connective tissue to meet the downward growth of septum between the
genital and intestinal tracts. The failure on the part of these two processes
to unite may result in an opening at once into the vagina and externally
between the buttocks in the normal situation.

*Hyperplasia and Hypertrophy of the Vulva.*—Hypertrophy of the labia

16

majora is a very rare occurrence. The writer has seen but a single example, in which the labia projected an inch and a half from the surrounding skin and measured each one inch and three-quarters transversely. Supernumerary development of the labia minora is likewise extremely rare. Both these conditions are of interest to the scientific student, but call for no gynæcological treatment. Hypertrophy of the labia minora is a more common condition. It is found normally in certain races, as the Hottentots, and is occasionally seen in Caucasian women. If the hypertrophied nymphæ are irritated and inflamed, so that locomotion is difficult, or if they interfere with coition, they should be excised.

FIG. 33.

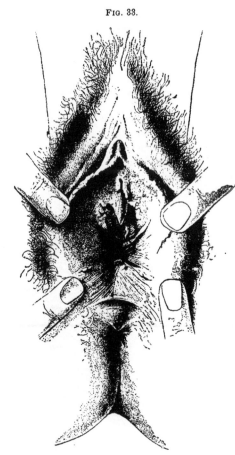

Anomalous openings of anus and urethra.

*Non-Development of the Vulva.*—If the internal genitalia are defective, the labia majora and minora may be small and flat, the vestibule shallow and narrow, the mons veneris not prominent and poorly provided with hair. On the other hand, with entire absence of the vagina and uterus, the external genitalia may be perfectly developed.

*Hypertrophy of the Clitoris.*—The clitoris is found hypertrophied in certain savage races, and (rarely) among prostitutes, to such an extent in some instances as to reach the size of a well-developed penis. If the overgrown organ interferes with coitus, or if it becomes easily inflamed or irritated and causes the individual decided discomfort, the redundant portion should be amputated. Nothing is gained by the amputation of the clitoris for nymphomania or for masturbation. To the discredit of gynæcology, this operation obtained considerable favor for a time by the enthusiastic advocacy of Baker Brown and a few indiscreet followers. It is now known to be useless.

*Anomalies of the Hymen.*—The hymen is normally a rather delicate annular membrane at the outlet of the vagina, with a central perforation into which the tip of the little finger can be inserted. There are, however, many variations from this rule of form and orifice. The latter may be crescentic, with the concavity embracing closely the urethra. There may be two symmetrical openings side by side, or the orifices may be punctate and numerous (cribriform hymen). The edge of the hymen may be dentated, looking as though it had been ruptured by coitus, or it may be apparently irregularly carved out of thickened tissue (sculptured hymen). The orifice may be exceedingly minute, or the membrane may be imperforate, causing, after puberty, hæmatocolpos and hæmatometra. The hymen is occasionally hypertrophied; it may project beyond the labia majora one to three centimetres. (Scanzoni.)

FIG. 34.

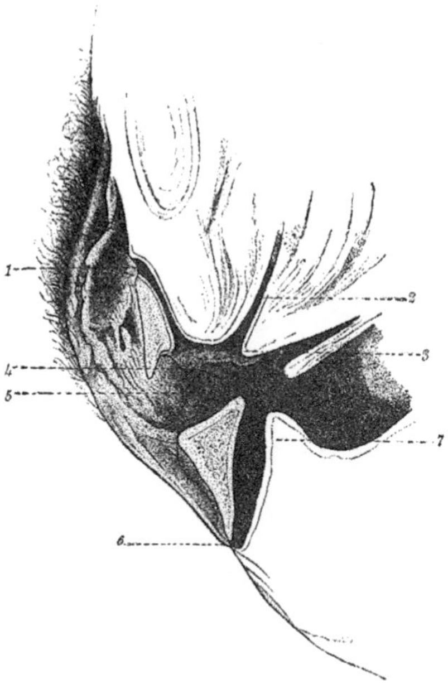

The same in vertical section.—1, cutaneous orifice of the urethra; 2, opening of the urethra into the vestibule; 3, urethra; 4, vagina; 5, anus vestibularis; 6, anus; 7, projection of posterior rectal wall.

FIG. 35.

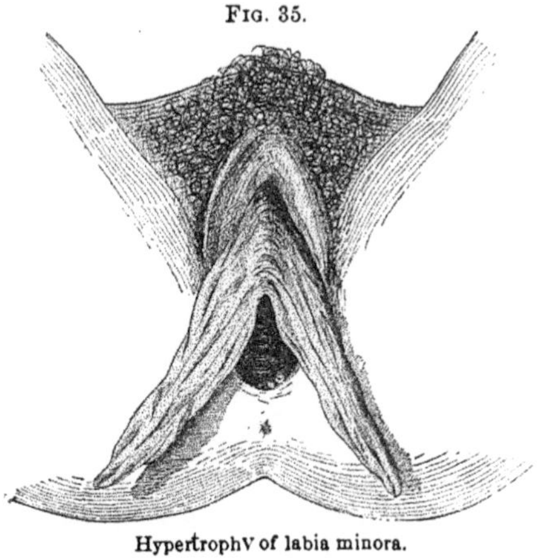

Hypertrophy of labia minora.

It is more commonly thickened, and opposes by its unnatural strength an insuperable barrier, perhaps, to coitus, but not to conception. The writer has attended two married women in confinement with unruptured hymens. It is this condition of the hymen that causes excessive bleeding on rupture in the first coitus. In one case the hemorrhage was fatal. (Winckel.) The force employed in coitus to rupture a resisting hymen may be so great as to separate it from its attachment posteriorly to the vagina, and even to perforate the floor of the vestibule into the

rectum, as in a case seen by the writer. In rare instances the hymen is
so elastic that coitus does not rupture it, nor even the birth of a pretty
well grown fœtus. The writer has seen an unruptured hymen in a

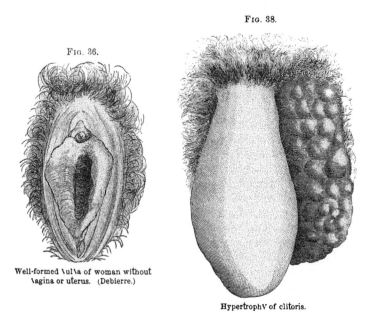

Fig. 36.

Well-formed vulva of woman without
vagina or uterus. (Debierre.)

Fig. 38.

Hypertrophy of clitoris.

prostitute who had plied her trade for years, and Winckel quotes a
case in which a five-months fœtus was born without laceration of the

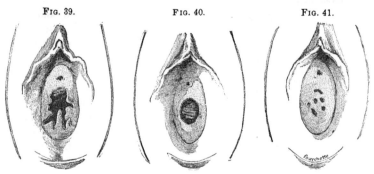

Fig. 39.    Fig. 40.    Fig. 41.

Different forms of hymens and their openings.

hymen. In a few instances complete absence of the hymen has been
noted, and it is occasionally represented merely by a few ill-developed
papillæ.

Fɪɢ. 37.

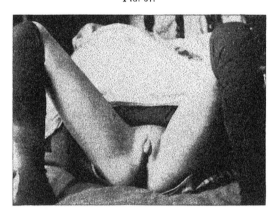

Enlarged clitoris.

FIG. 42.

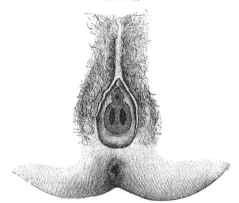

Hymen with double orifice.

FIG. 43.

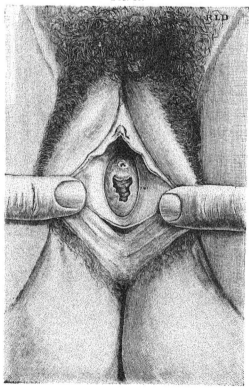

Hymen with irregularly shaped opening.

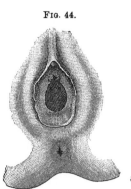

Fig. 44.

Hymen with two minute
perforations.

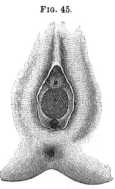

Fig. 45.

Hymen with minute central
perforation.

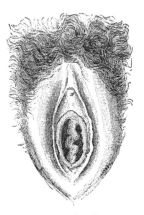

Fig. 46.

Hymeneal opening divided in
two by a vaginal septum.

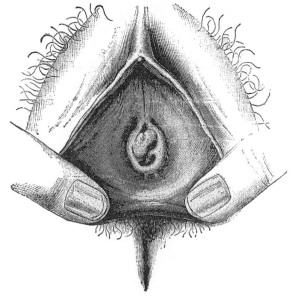

Fig 47.

Sculptured hymen.

Fig. 48.

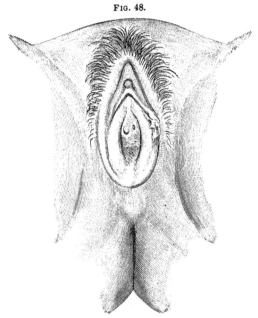

Imperforate hymen.

Fig. 49.

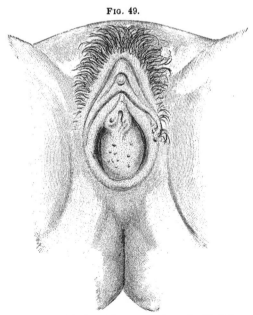

Imperforate hymen and distention of the vagina with menstrual fluid (hæmatocolpos).

*True Hermaphroditism.*—If one accepts Ahlfeld's definition of a true hermaphrodite,—an individual with functionally active glands of both sexes, provided with excretory ducts,—then a true hermaphrodite has not yet been discovered, and probably never will be. If, on the other hand, one allows an individual to be classed as a true hermaphrodite in whom there are sexual glands which histologically have the structure respectively of an ovary and a testicle, then there is a possibility of true hermaphroditism, for there have been several cases carefully observed that would appear to answer this description.

Klebs makes three divisions of true hermaphroditism, viz. :

I. Bilateral; on both sides an ovary and a testicle.

II. Unilateral; on one side an ovary and a testicle, on the other an ovary or a testicle.

III. Lateral; on one side an ovary, on the other a testicle.

This classification, it is needless to say, is as yet theoretical; there are no undoubted cases of the kinds described—with perfectly developed glands of both sexes—to justify it. In many instances true hermaphroditism has been claimed for an individual or a specimen, but very few indeed of these descriptions will bear scientific criticism.

Ahlfeld has collected quite a number of these cases from literature. Omitting all that are simply declared by the observer to be hermaphroditic without a histological examination of the glands, there remain :

The case described by Barkow, in which there was undoubtedly one testicle, without, however, a vas deferens, and another body described as an ovary, which histologically was made up mainly of fat, connective tissue, and blood-vessels.

The case of Berthold, in which there were a testicle in the right half of the scrotum, between the rectum and bladder a uterus unicornis, on the right side no adnexa, but on the left a round ligament, tube, and " ovary." The last lacked the characteristic histological elements of a normal ovary.

The case of Banon, in which on the left of the small uterus there were a tube and an ovary, on the right a testicle with vas deferens. The ovary again, in this case, showed no Graafian follicles ; it was made up principally of connective tissue.

The case of Cramer-Meyer-Klebs, in which there were a testicle in the left scrotal sac, a uterus with tubes, parovaria, and round ligaments, on the right side an ovary, on the left a testicle. The description of this case is faulty. The diagnosis was declared by one of the writers to rest upon careful macroscopic and microscopic examination. Another says nothing about the latter ; and Förster, in referring to the case, said that no Graafian follicles nor ovules could be discovered.

The cases of Gruber and of Klotz are too obscure to be of value. In one a cancerous mass was declared to be an ovary ; in the other a cyst was taken for an ovary. In both cases there was a testicle upon the opposite side.

The case described by Heppner was that of a two-months-old child. The external genitals were of the masculine type. The penis was imperforate. Internally, there was an infantile uterus with tubes and ovaries on either side. On each side also there was a testicle, separated from the ovary by the parovarium. While the microscopical examination demonstrated the nature of the ovaries, it could not be demonstrated clearly under the microscope that the neighboring glands were testicles. In addition to these cases collected by Ahlfeld, there has been described quite recently an interesting and important case of *hermaphroditismus verus lateralis*.[1]

Friedrich W., aged twenty-two years, art student from Berlin, sought admission to the surgical clinic in Leipsic for a congenital defect of the sexual organs, which proved to be hypospadias. He desired an operation in order that he might gain the power of procreation and "be able to urinate from the end of his penis like other men." A closer examination showed that the scrotum was rudimentary in development; it began immediately in front of the anus and was divided by a raphé. On the right side there was a small testicle; on the left, none. The penis was small, and drawn bow-like downward and inward. The glans was uncovered, well formed, but imperforate. On the under surface of the penis was a groove running backward three and two-tenths centimetres to a small slit about one-half centimetre long; directly back of this the raphé of the scrotum began. The operation to correct hypospadias was performed in two parts, first, to free the penis from its constrained position, second, to close the groove in it and to make a urethra. An attempt to pass a catheter after the first operation failed to evacuate the bladder. On injecting fluid a swelling was noticed in the left inguinal region; finally, the urine was drawn off by a Mercier catheter. After the second operation the same difficulty in catheterization was experienced, and again it was noticed that the left inguinal region became enlarged when fluid was injected into the catheter. Soon serious systemic symptoms developed, with swelling, redness, and pain in the left groin. The skin was incised in this region, and a body five centimetres long and two centimetres thick, with a hand like the vas deferens running into the abdomen, was exposed and removed. It was thought to be the left testicle. Shortly afterwards the patient died. The post-mortem examination resulted as follows. Face bearded, hairs about two centimetres long. Breasts undeveloped. Mons veneris had the hairy growth like a female, ending abruptly above. The penis, freed from its adhesions by the first operation, measured about five and one-half centimetres in length on the upper surface and had a circumference of eight centimetres. The glans was one and one-quarter centimetres long. At the sides of the penis were genital

---

[1] Ein Fall von Hermaphroditismus, G. Schmorl, Virchow's Archiv, Bd. cxiii. p. 229.

folds projecting above and grasping the penis between them. Internally, there was discovered an opening into the urethra three and one-half centimetres back of the external orifice, where the colliculis seminalis usually lies, into which a sound could be passed for fifteen centimetres. Further dissection discovered this canal to be a vagina and a uterus, the latter separated into cervical and corporeal portions. On the left side the tube ran into the inguinal canal and was continuous with the body removed at the operation, which was found to be mainly the distended and distorted fimbriated extremity. Microscopic examination of this body, however, showed in it the remains of a sexual gland having all the histological characteristics of a fœtal ovary without ovules. On the right side were a round ligament, tube, and ligament analogous to that of the ovary, all running down to the sexual gland in the right scrotal sac, which the microscope showed to be a testicle. There were no spermatozoa, nor was there a vas deferens. It really seems that this might be called an example of true lateral hermaphroditism.

There remains still another case to be referred to in this category. Schmorl (*loc. cit.*) mentions an example of true unilateral hermaphroditism described by Gast.[1] It was a still-born baby with exstrophy of the bladder. There was a rudimentary but well-developed penis, which was perforated by a urethra and lay between folds of skin. The internal genitalia were more of the female type. The uterus was bifid; on the right it was solid and had a sheath-like extension composed of fibrous tissue. From the body of this uterine division ran a tube three centimetres long with an abdominal ostium. The left half of the uterus, also solid, was hourglass-shaped, two and one-half centimetres long and three-quarters of a centimetre broad. From this side also ran a tube with fimbriated extremity. To this was adherent an ovary showing follicles and ovules with nucleus and nucleolus. On the same side there was a testicle the size of a pea, from which a ligament, the gubernaculum Hunteri, ran down to the base of the left scrotal sac. A microscopic examination showed this to be a testicle. On the right side no sexual gland could be found at all. This case can be called, therefore, one of true unilateral hermaphroditism,— that is, if the account of it can be trusted. In all these cases there were anomalies in the external genitalia which will be described under the head of pseudo-hermaphroditism.

*Pseudo-Hermaphroditism.*—Klebs classifies pseudo-hermaphrodites in the following manner :

Pseudo-hermaphrodites with double sexual formation of the external genitals, but with unisexual development of the reproductive glands (ovaries, testicles).

I. Male pseudo-hermaphrodites (with testicles).

1. Internal pseudo-hermaphrodites. Development of uterus masculinus.

---

[1] T. Gast, Beitrag zur Lehre von der Bauchblasengenitalspalte und vom Hermaphroditismus verus. Inaug. Dissert., Greifswald, 1884.

2. External pseudo-hermaphrodites.   External genitals approach female type; feminine appearance and build.

3. Complete pseudo-hermaphrodites (internal and external).   Uterus masculinus with tubes.   Separate efferent canals for bladder and uterus.

FIG. 50.

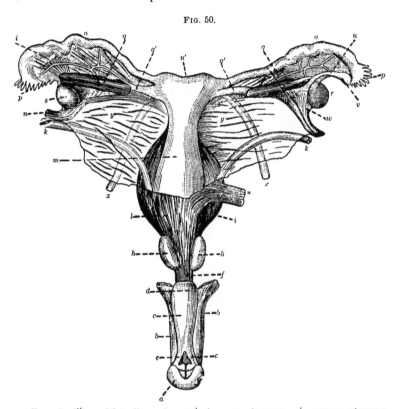

Hermaphroditismus bilateralis.—*a*, glans penis; *b*, corpus cavernosus penis; *c*, corpus cavernosus of uro-genital canal; *d*, its bulb; *e*, its anterior arm; *f*, membranous portion of uro-genital canal; *h*, prostate; *i*, bladder; *k*, ureters; *l*, vagina; *m*, uterus; *n'*, fundus uteri; *o, o*, tubes; *p, p*, their infundibula; *q, q*, ovaries; *q', q'*, their ligaments; *r*, right testicle; *s*, left testicle; *t*, left parovarium; *u*, right parovarium; *v*, hydatid of Morgagni; *n, w*, blood-vessels; *x, x*, round ligaments; *y, y*, broad ligaments; *\**, muscle-fibres from bladder and vagina.

II. Female pseudo-hermaphrodites (with ovaries).   Persistence of male sexual parts.

1. Internal hermaphrodites.   Formation of vas deferens and tubes.

2. External hermaphrodites.   Approach of external genitals to male type.

3. Complete hermaphrodites (external and internal).   Masculine formation of the external genitals and of a part of the sexual tract.

As may be seen in the classification, individuals of this class have the glands of one sex, but other sexual parts either intermediate or mixed.

They are in the vast majority of cases of the masculine sex, although this may be difficult to determine during life.   Numerous instances are recorded of mistakes as to sex which continued throughout a great part or the whole of life.   The writer has seen an individual don his first trousers at the age of nineteen.   He had been brought up as a girl, until his beard began to grow and he began to manifest sexual inclinations towards his female companions.

A masculine pseudo-hermaphrodite has in a number of instances married

FIG. 51.            FIG. 52.

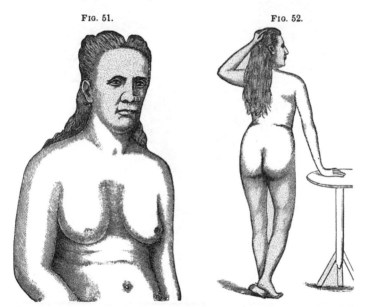

Carl Lohmann, masculine pseudo-hermaphrodite, who lived for forty-six years as a female.   He then assumed male attire and married as a man.

as a woman, and learned his true sex only on consulting a physician for sterility.   It is always better, in case of doubt, to regard the sex as masculine and to clothe and educate the individual as a male.

There are many degrees of masculine pseudo-hermaphroditism, from a simple enlargement of the vesicula prostatica, without abnormality of the external genitals, to the full development of a uterus masculinus, divided into corporeal and cervical portions, with perfect tubes and a vagina opening externally into a uro-genital cleft.   In the latter case the penis is rudimentary and there is hypospadias; the urethra opens by a separate canal at the uro-genital cleft; there is a rudimentary development of the scrotal halves, and the testicles may be in the abdominal cavity.   The vasa deferentia empty usually in the urethra, sometimes in the uro-genital cleft, and rarely in the cavity of the vesicula.   The character of the body approaches the female type closely in well-marked cases of masculine pseudo-

FIG. 53.

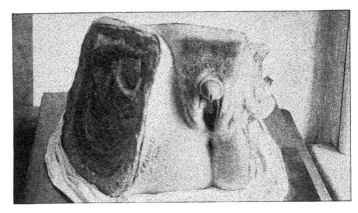

Pseudohermaphroditismus masculinus.

FIG. 54.

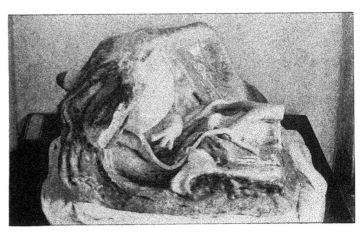

The same in profile section, showing uterus masculinus.

hermaphroditism.   The hair on the head grows long, the beard is very
scanty or fails to appear, the breasts are large and sometimes contain secretion, the waist is small, and
the hips are broad.   A regular monthly discharge of
blood and mucus from the
genitalia or the urethra has
been noted in several in-
stances.   It is not strange
that such creatures should be
regarded as females, for the
only true mark of their sex
may not be discoverable till
after death.   The best proofs
of sex during life are afforded
by the presence of spermatic
particles in the discharge accompanying sexual excite-
ment in the male and by impregnation in the female.   In
intermediate grades the external genitals may not be
much affected, and the uterus

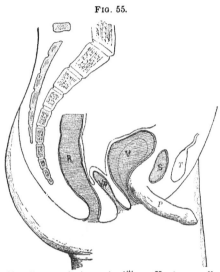

FIG. 55.

Masculine pseudo-hermaphroditism.—*Va*, vagina; *V*,
bladder; *R*, rectum; *P*, penis; *S*, symphysis; *T*, testicle.

masculinus and vagina may open into the urethral canal of a fairly well

FIG. 56.

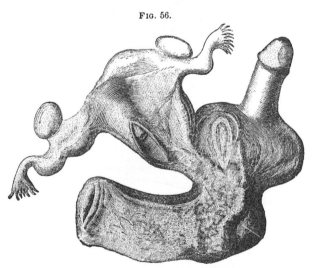

Masculine pseudo-hermaphroditism, with uterus masculinus and tubes.

formed penis.   The scrotum may show various grades of development:

one half may be pretty well formed and contain a testicle, while the other is rudimentary and empty. The testicle in such a case may be detected in the inguinal canal or may be altogether in the abdomen. However doubtful might be the sex of a masculine pseudo-hermaphrodite during life, an examination of the pelvic cavity after death should settle the matter

Fɪɢ. 57.

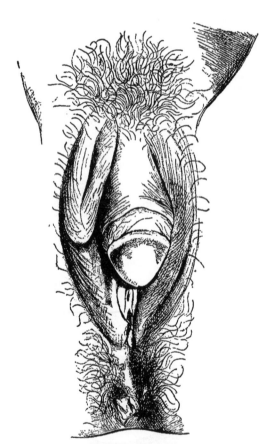

Feminine pseudo-hermaphroditism.—The right labium contained an ovary. (Fehling.)

definitely, and yet mistakes have been made in the description of post-mortem specimens. There was reported to the New York Obstetrical Society, March 1, 1887, a case of so-called true hermaphroditism, which was accepted unchallenged, and yet there was no microscopic examination of the sexual glands, and the bodies which were designated as ovaries are evidently nothing but convolutions of the tubes attached to the uterus masculinus.  This was undoubtedly a case of spurious hermaphroditism in the male.

Feminine pseudo-hermaphroditism is rare, and reported cases should always be regarded with a suspicion that the individual is really a man. An hypertrophied clitoris, perhaps a rudimentary vagina, ovaries prolapsed into the labia, the formation of the scrotum, and the existence of vasa deferentia are the characteristics of this class.

The following remarkable case was reported to the *New York Medical Journal*, November 22, 1890, by Dr. C. W. Fitch, at one time in charge of the sanitary service of Salvador, Central America:

"J. H. A., a house-servant, of masculine features and movements; aged twenty-eight years; height, five feet seven inches; weight, one hundred and thirty-nine pounds; was arrested by the police for violating the law governing prostitution.  On examination, both female and male organs of generation were found in a remarkably well developed condition.  The labia majora were of normal size, but flattened on their anterior surface. The labia minora and hymen were absent.  The vagina was capacious, four and one-half inches long anteriorly and six inches posteriorly. The os uteri was torn on the left side.  There was profuse leucorrhœa.  Seven years before she had given birth to a normal female infant.  In place of the clitoris there was a penis, which, when in erection, measured five inches and a quarter long by three and five-eighths inches in circumference. (?)   The glans penis and the urethra were perfectly formed.  The scrotum, which was two and one-eighth inches long, contained two testicles (?) about an inch in length and two inches and a half in circumference.  The mons veneris was sparsely covered with short, straight, black hair.  Both sets of organs were perfect in their functions, semen being ejected from the penis (?) and the ovaries being capable of

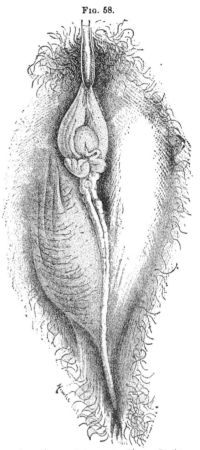

FIG. 58.

Masculine pseudo-hermaphroditism.  (Pozzi.)

producing eggs. Scanty menstruation occurred every three weeks and lasted but two days. Sexual gratification was said to be equally distributed between the two sets of organs." Stripped of inaccuracies, this is doubtless a description of a remarkable example of pseudo-hermaphroditismus feminus.

It seems to be a well-established fact that the external appearance of a masculine pseudo-hermaphrodite will correspond with the type of the

FIG. 59.

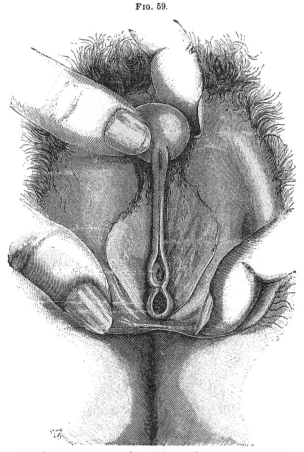

Masculine pseudo-hermaphroditism: perineo-scrotal hypospadias. (Pozzi.)

external genitals. This is well illustrated in the case of Carl Lohmann, and, negatively, in the case reported by Bonnet and Petit, of a man with pseudo-scrotal hypospadias, who was educated and clothed as a girl, but who had nothing feminine in his appearance except his long hair and his dresses. He was in the habit of copulating with his female companions,

Plate 11.

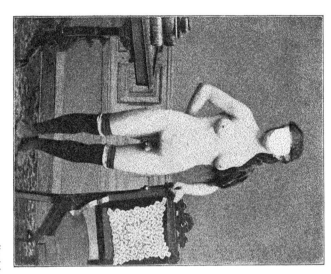

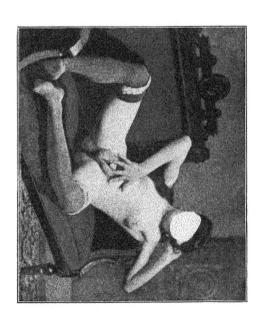

Feminine pseudo-hermaphroditism

and acquired in time a chancre.    In female hermaphrodites this rule does not seem to obtain : the feminine appearance is retained in spite of an

FIG. 61.

FIG. 60.

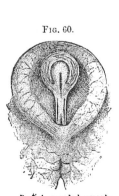

Partial pseudo-hermaph-
roditism, with hypertrophy of
clitoris. (Pozzi)

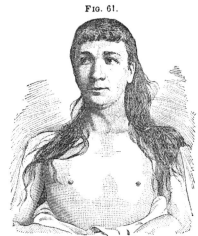

Masculine pseudo-hermaphroditism. (Bonnet and
Petit)

almost complete approximation of the male genitalia to the male type. This is shown in Plate II.

### RETENTION OF MUCUS AND BLOOD WITHIN THE GENITAL TRACT IN CONSEQUENCE OF ATRESIA.

As a result of atresia in any portion of the genital tract, either congenital or acquired, the secretion of the mucous membrane and the blood at the menstrual periods is unable to escape, and accumulates from time to time within the genitalia, in spite of a certain amount of absorption that goes on between the periods.

If the atresia is situated at the cervix, the mucus from the uterine mucous membrane and the blood of the menstrual period after puberty accumulate steadily, first dilating the cervical canal and in time the uterine cavity, until large quantities of blood may be contained within the womb, thinning the walls perhaps to the tenuity of paper, or possibly being accompanied by an eccentric hypertrophy of the uterus and thickening of the walls.    In the course of time there is always an accumulation within the tubes (hæmatosalpinx) as well as within the uterine cavity (hæmatometra). The fluid here is derived not so much from a backing up of uterine fluid into the tubes as from the exudation from the tubal mucous membrane itself.    All communication between the tube and the uterine cavity may be, and very likely is, shut off, proving conclusively the tubal origin of the accumulated blood.

The symptoms of hæmatometra or of hydrometra, hæmatosalpinx or

17

hydrosalpinx, as the fluid is mainly blood or mucus, appear only after puberty. There are at each menstrual epoch increasing pain of a cramp-like character and intense bearing-down efforts without the escape externally of blood. The patient herself or her friends will commonly recognize the fact that there is a mechanical obstruction to the escape of the menstrual fluid. After a little while, from irritation and congestion, an inflammation begins in the pelvis, and associated with the symptoms of retention of fluid within the uterus are the symptoms of pelvic peritonitis. Suppuration within the womb or within the tubes may occur, converting the case into one of pyometra or pyosalpinx.

The diagnosis of this condition has already been referred to. Its treatment consists in the puncture of the cervix with a trocar, and the free evacuation of the fluid, followed by dilatation of the cervical canal and a maintenance of the dilatation so as to permit free drainage. As already stated, the collection of fluid within the tubes may be entirely distinct from that within the uterus, and one must always be prepared to see a continuance of symptoms after the evacuation of the uterine accumulation, or perhaps the beginning of an infectious salpingitis following the evacuation of the fluid in the uterine cavity, and must hold himself prepared to open the abdomen before the septic inflammation of the tubes has progressed too far to permit of a cure by surgical means. This has occurred in the writer's practice, in spite of the utmost care in regard to the cleanliness of the operation in the puncture of the cervix and the evacuation of the uterine accumulations.

If the atresia is situated lower in the genital canal, at the middle third or outlet of the vagina, the fluid accumulates first within the vagina, and only after some time is there dilatation of the cervix, and at last of the uterine cavity, which very commonly preserves for a long period an hourglass form by the projection inward of the internal os. In examining such a case the uterus can be felt as a solid body perched upon the cystic tumor, consisting of the dilated vagina and cervix. The same treatment is demanded in this as in the former case,— free evacuation of the fluid by a good-sized opening at the site of atresia, dilatation of the opening, a thorough lavage of the genital canal, and the maintenance afterwards of free drainage. It has been stated that it is safer to make a small opening at the site of obstruction and to allow the fluid gradually to escape, so as to avoid rupture of the tubes; but Emmet's experience shows conclusively the advantages of the first-named plan, and it is doubtful if any precautions in regard to the evacuation of the fluid from the vagina and the uterus will avoid the danger of rupture of the tubal walls or of infection of the tubal contents in some cases. These accidents are likely to occur even when there is no communication between the tubes and the uterus. In neglected cases, or in those in which a correct diagnosis has not been made, there is occasionally a spontaneous evacuation of the fluid by a rupture at the seat of the atresia. These cases are very likely to end unfortunately; the fluid is

not freely evacuated, and the portion that remains behind is extremely likely
to become infected, the infection rapidly spreading to the tubes and thus to
the peritoneal cavity, or to the lymphatic and venous channels of the uterine
wall. Spontaneous rupture may likewise occur into the peritoneal cavity,

FIG. 62.

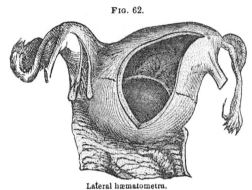

Lateral hæmatometra.

either by a laceration of the tubal walls or by rupture of the uterus above
its peritoneal attachment. This accident is followed by the rapid development of septic peritonitis. In cases of double uterus and vagina

FIG. 63.

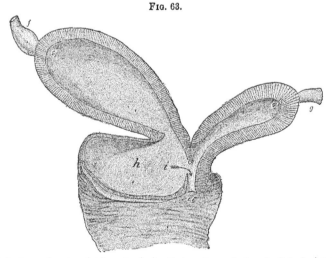

Lateral pyometra, evacuated through patent cervical canal.—e, c, fundus; f, g, Fallopian tubes;
h, cervical canal, dilated; i, opening into patent cervical canal; a, external os.

it is not uncommon to find atresia on one side, with a consequent lateral
hæmatometra or hæmatocolpos. Such cases are not so easy of recognition
as those already described, but a careful examination should almost always

avoid error. In the case of hæmatocolpos, a cystic tumor is found occupying one side of the vaginal canal, and a bimanual examination may reveal the body of a uterus above it, while on the unaffected side evidences of duplex formation in the womb may be apparent.

The treatment here is the same as that already outlined for other cases of accumulated fluids within the genital tract. A free opening should be made into the lateral vaginal wall, the fluid evacuated, the cavity washed out, and adequate drainage secured. The theoretical objection to this plan of treatment has been advanced that a large opening into a vaginal canal affected by atresia might permit impregnation, which a smaller orifice would prevent; but the rupture must be very small to prevent the entrance of a spermatozoön,—much too small, indeed, to allow the escape of the fluid which it is necessary to evacuate. If the atresia affects one side of the uterus only in a case of septate or double womb, a cystic tumor may be detected directly alongside the normal half of the uterus and obviously intimately connected with it. A history of periodicity in the pain caused by the accumulated fluids coincident with the menstrual period is also a help in the diagnosis. Finally, puncture of the obliterated half of the cervix will verify the presumptive diagnosis.

# CHAPTER V.

## TRAUMATIC LESIONS OF THE VULVA, VAGINA, AND CERVIX.

BY MATTHEW D. MANN, A.M., M D.

THREE classes of injuries are met with in the genital organs of women, differing according to their cause, whether this is external violence, coitus, or labor.

### WOUNDS DUE TO EXTERNAL VIOLENCE AND COITUS.

**Injuries of the Vulva.**—The vulva is so well protected by its situation that injuries are very uncommon. By a fall on some hard or sharp body the parts may be bruised, cut, or even deeply penetrated. In hospital experience it is not uncommon to meet with cases due to kicks with heavy boots. In this latter case there may be only a bruising of the parts, or the tissues may be cut as though by a knife.

Sometimes the skin is not broken, but the subjacent tissues are cut, allowing the blood to escape into the connective tissue, producing in this way enormous swellings. Several cases have occurred in the experience of the writer, an especially bad one having been met with in a pregnant woman.

If the skin is broken the hemorrhage may be very severe, as the parts are exceedingly vascular ; and should some of the large vessels be cut, the patient may easily bleed to death before help reaches her. Wounds around the clitoris are especially dangerous, owing to the greater vascularity of the tissues in this neighborhood.

The symptoms are pain and hemorrhage, followed by swelling, and in some instances, where there has been much bruising of the parts, by sloughing. In case the skin is not broken, the only symptoms will be pain and rapid swelling, due to the effusion of blood into the loose tissues. The tumor thus formed is known as a pudendal hæmatoma. The absence of valves in the veins of these parts allows of a rapid loss of blood. If the vagina is penetrated, the surrounding organs may be wounded and inflammation follow.

*Treatment.*—The treatment of injuries of this kind is generally simple, and the results are usually satisfactory. If the parts are merely bruised, cold applications may be made, or possibly a poultice applied. Should there be a hæmatoma, it is best not to open it, but to allow the blood to be absorbed, a result which will generally follow in a comparatively short time.

If the tissues show any tendency to slough or to suppurate, they should be freely incised, the clots removed, and the injured tissues thoroughly cleansed and dusted with iodoform, acetanilid, or some other similar dressing. Daily cleansing of the parts with peroxide of hydrogen, with the use of some antiseptic powder as a dressing, will probably result in rapid cure.

In case of hemorrhage, the application of pressure is generally easy, with the aid of a T-bandage. If the pressure does not stop the hemorrhage, or if it is very severe from the start, the bleeding vessels may be sought for and tied, or deep stitches may be taken under the bleeding parts and the bleeding tissues tied *en masse*. The greatest care should be taken to have the wounds thoroughly cleansed and dressed antiseptically.

**Injuries of the Vagina.**—The vagina, from its location, is rarely subject to injuries from external violence. There are a few recorded cases in which women have fallen upon stakes, that have deeply penetrated the parts, but such cases are very rare. The writer has never met with an instance of this kind.

A patient recently seen in the hospital service of the writer presented a serious laceration of the left side of the vagina, made by the fist of the husband which was forcibly thrust into it in a fit of anger. The tissues were deeply torn, and the hemorrhage was very severe. The flow had been stopped by a tampon when she was brought in. Deep stitches were placed, and recovery followed.

Some of the injuries met with in the vagina are due to coitus. Not long ago a patient was admitted to the hospital with a long rent in the recto-vaginal septum just above the perineal body. She stated that the injury had occurred from coitus, entrance having been effected from behind, though it was exceedingly difficult to believe it. She asserted that she was drunk at the time. She insisted upon that cause, and could, or would, give no other. The parts were ragged, torn, and bleeding, and there was evidently a fresh wound. After cicatrization had taken place the parts were denuded, and the opening, which had contracted down to the size of a twenty-five-cent piece, was closed from the vaginal surface. The patient recovered. Instances of vesico-vaginal fistulæ produced in this way have also been reported, and deep rents in the hymen and the edges of the vagina are of comparatively common occurrence. Several instances have been recorded in which newly-married women have nearly lost their lives from such accidents.

*Treatment.*—The cases are to be treated on general surgical principles, either by sewing up the wounds, or, if that be impossible, by applying a tampon if the wound lies well within the vaginal orifice.

**Injuries to the Cervix.**—The cervix is very rarely injured by external violence. The writer has never met with a case of this kind. The only injuries are those made by the surgeon's knife or those that occur in labor. The former class are so uncommon that they are hardly worth mentioning, while the latter will be treated of under another head.

INJURIES DURING PARTURITION.

**Injuries of the Vulva and Perineum.**—While injuries due to external violence are rare, those due to the passage of the child in labor are exceedingly common. These injuries make up a large class of cases in the practice of every gynæcologist; and while their importance is, I am sure, often overrated, still, in many instances they cause a great deal of trouble and inconvenience to the patient.

The importance of these lesions will best be understood by a careful consideration of the anatomy of the parts. That portion of the pelvic floor which intervenes between the anus and the outlet of the vagina, commonly known as the "perineum," has a very important function to fulfil. It is the centre in which a number of muscles are united and in which the fasciæ have their supporting point. While it can in no sense be called the key-stone of the arch, it is, nevertheless, the most important point in the pelvic floor. Should it be torn through, even though the sphincter ani be left, the loss of support to the parts above is so considerable that, though the results may not be felt at once, in the course of time trouble is very likely to occur.

While this is true, we cannot deny that a considerable number of women are seen in the consulting-room in whom the perineum is torn to an appreciable extent, but who do not seem to suffer in the slightest degree from this mishap. They come to us complaining of other troubles which have nothing to do with the perineum, and state that they have never suffered from this in the least. The writer has met with several instances where there was every reason to believe that the woman had gone through nearly the whole of her sexual life with a badly torn perineum and yet had never been inconvenienced by it.

These facts should be borne in mind when the question of diagnosis and the cause of the patient's ill health are under consideration. It certainly is not fair to attribute all the ills of which our patients complain to a slight tear in the perineum.

On the other hand, we see patients who are very greatly benefited by an operation, where the tear at first seemed to be almost trifling. Observation has taught the writer that the stretching and relaxation of the parts so frequently met with, generally associated with transverse tears, are of much more importance than actual median tears, provided that the sphincter is not involved.

The subjects of these relaxations of the pelvic outlet are generally of lax fibre, and often all the pelvic tissues seem to be affected to a greater or less degree in the same way. As a result, we find displacements of the vaginal walls and of the uterus,—conditions which seem to be due to the general relaxation rather than to the injury to the perineum alone.

This part of the subject will be again considered when we come to the question of treatment.

*Etiology.*—The consideration of the causes of rupture or relaxation of the perineum belongs properly to the subject of obstetrics. A few only of these causes, therefore, will be enumerated.

A relative disproportion between the head of the child and the vaginal outlet is sometimes met with. The writer was once consulted before the labor in a case of this kind. The woman, though large and well built, had so small a vulvar opening that it did not seem possible that the child could be born without serious laceration of the parts. The attending physician, a skilful accoucheur, was advised to make incisions in the parts and to deliver with the forceps. But the bad prognosis was fully realized, the woman being terribly torn, notwithstanding the greatest care and skill on the part of the physician.

As suits for malpractice have in a number of instances been brought for accidents of this kind, it is well that it should be distinctly stated and understood that lesions of the perineum are not always preventable.

Other causes are œdema of the vulva, very rapid labor, violent and uncontrollable pains just as the head is passing the perineum, and unusual size of the child. The writer has seen cases in which these causes were active, and in none of them did he think that rupture could have been prevented. One very bad laceration which he was called upon to sew up occurred in the hands of a careful man, who stated that just as the head was about to pass the perineum the woman threw herself violently across the bed, bore down with great force, and expelled the whole child in one pain. In this case the perineum was torn entirely through the sphincter, certainly without any fault of the accoucheur. A few stitches placed immediately after, fortunately, restored the parts entirely.

The proper management of the head in normal labor is now thoroughly taught in all text-books.

The causes here enumerated would seem to account for the cases of actual tear rather than for those of relaxation. In the latter it seems as if we must look for the cause to a certain extent in the natural constitution of the individual. All surgeons will recognize that the muscles, tendons, and other tissues of individuals differ very materially in elasticity and resisting power. Anybody who has had the opportunity of frequently opening the abdomen must have noticed the difference in the structures of the abdominal wall. If this is so, then we must admit that such differences would have an important influence in causing the relaxations, which are otherwise inexplicable.

*Varieties.*—Lacerations of the perineum have been divided according to their situation and degree. They may be in the median line, or they may be transverse.

Of those in the median line, the first degree includes those cases in which the tear extends less than half-way to the sphincter; the second degree, those which extend quite to, or around, the sphincter; and the third degree, those which pass through the sphincter and include more or less of the recto-vaginal septum. This division, while arbitrary, serves a good end for descriptive purposes.

The location of the tear is generally a little to one side of the median line, and may extend around the sphincter ani. Ruptures of the third degree seem to be always in the median line. Occasionally a tear is seen in which the sphincter and adjacent portions of the perineum are torn, while the fourchette remains intact. This is known as "central rupture." As the unruptured portion is of no use, the tear is practically the same as though it had been complete.

Besides the open lacerations above mentioned, we frequently meet with subcutaneous lacerations of the muscles and fascia in the median line. These may involve the transverse muscles and fascia, and occasionally, as Skene has pointed out, may involve the sphincter ani muscle. In these cases the integument and mucous membranes remain intact.

*Symptoms.*—The symptoms of laceration of the perineum depend entirely upon the degree. As already stated, many cases of the least degree of laceration are unattended by any symptoms. This is particularly true if there be no attendant relaxation. Even in lacerations of the second degree there may at first be very little trouble. But later, especially if the patient is of a constipated habit, the posterior vaginal wall, being deprived of its proper support, will begin to bulge forward during the act of defecation.

It must be remembered that the axis of the anus is nearly at a right angle to the axis of the rectum; and, although in certain positions of the body these axes are made more nearly parallel, still, it is necessary for the fæcal mass to turn quite a sharp angle before it is ejected. This it is enabled to do by the resisting power of the perineal body. If this is destroyed, then the posterior vaginal wall gives way under the continued pressure, and finally comes to pouch forward into the vaginal outlet and to form what is known as a "rectocele." As this rectocele arrests the fæcal mass upon its way down, a great amount of force must necessarily be used by the individual before it can be expelled. Thus the condition tends to grow continually worse.

The presence of a rectocele is also favored by a condition of subinvolution of the vagina, which is often found attending laceration and relaxation of the pelvic outlet. In some instances, for similar reasons, namely, loss of support, the anterior vaginal wall also bulges forward. This bulging gradually increases, until the base of the bladder may be contained in the pouching vaginal wall. With the formation of this cystocele, bladder-symptoms are often induced. Owing to the impossibility of thoroughly emptying the bladder, a portion of residual urine remains to decompose and set up a greater or less degree of irritation and inflammation. Although this is a recognized condition, it has very rarely occurred in the writer's experience.

In a recent hospital case, after the return of a badly prolapsed uterus, twenty-four uric-acid calculi the size of large peas were discharged from the bladder. The reason why vesical symptoms are not more frequently observed is that it is only in the very bad cases that the bladder is found in the so-called cystocele. Many of these are in fact merely cases of hypertrophy and prolapse of the anterior vaginal wall.

In the extreme degree of rectocele and cystocele the difficulty in emptying the rectum and bladder becomes very great. The writer has seen several patients who found it impossible to empty either of these organs without assuming the knee-chest position. It is not uncommon for women to be obliged to hold back the protruding viscera with their fingers before the evacuations can be secured. This they frequently learn by experience to do for themselves.

In some instances the lacerations of the perineum are accompanied by a sense of loss of support. The patients complain very much of bearing-down sensations in the pelvis, as if its contents were about to drop out. In other cases air enters the vagina in certain positions, and escapes when the position is changed, much to the annoyance of the patient.

Bad lacerations are commonly accompanied with displacements of the uterus, though this is more frequently associated with relaxation than with laceration alone. The writer has rarely observed a displacement in a case of laceration of the third degree. This would seem to show that the relaxation is of more importance than the laceration,—a point which has already been dwelt upon.

Some have attributed many reflex symptoms to lacerations and relaxations of the pelvic outlet. Thus, various neuralgic pains in the pelvis, gastric disturbances, and disturbances of other abdominal and thoracic organs have been referred to this cause. The writer must confess to being somewhat incredulous as to these results. If they occur they are certainly very uncommon, and are to be attributed to the attendant displacement, or to some inflammation or disease of the uterus, tubes, or ovaries, rather than to the laceration. Of course it cannot be denied that the laceration may in such cases be a serious complication, but that it should be the main cause the writer does not believe.

The symptoms of laceration in the third degree, whether the tear is open or is only subcutaneous, vary much from those already enumerated. Here the rupture of the sphincter entirely destroys the retentive power of the rectum. Hence the patient has no control over evacuations, fæces or gases, and is reduced thereby to a most deplorable condition. It is hard to imagine a more wretched object than a woman with a torn sphincter ani ; she is utterly debarred from most of the pleasures of life, is almost a prisoner in her own house, besides suffering more or less continually from pain and irritation in the rectum. In many of these cases there is often a considerable degree of catarrh of the rectum, perhaps due to the admission of air, or of dirt or dust from the outside. This catarrh is shown by frequent discharges of mucus, which keep the parts constantly moistened and irritated.

When constipation exists, the patient's state may be more endurable, but if she be troubled with looseness of the bowels, the condition is still more serious, and life comes to be almost not worth living. The wear and tear on the nervous system is so great that many of these women become practically invalids.

Transverse injuries have been described as internal lacerations, "which consist in laceration of the anterior fibres of the levator ani muscle and fascia, and this is usually attended with separation of the muscular layer of the vaginal wall from the pelvic floor. . . . In some cases the laceration is complete, involving the mucous membrane as well as the muscular coat of the vagina, and in very rare cases the laceration reaches upward and outward as far as the laceration of the levator ani muscle extends; but, as a rule, the laceration of the levator ani is subcutaneous,—that is to say, not attended with laceration of the mucous membrane of the vaginal wall."[1]

As a result of these transverse lacerations, there is a great sagging of the pelvic floor. No doubt many of the so-called cases of relaxation are due to this injury. Rectocele and cystocele may follow, though Skene holds that the rectocele and cystocele are more apparent than real, and are, in fact, a prolapse of the vaginal walls with dilatation of the veins. Under these circumstances the vaginal walls may be greatly hypertrophied, especially the anterior wall, the presence of the anterior column of the vagina giving it a greater normal thickness with more submucous connective tissue.

With this transverse laceration there may be more or less median laceration, or a subcutaneous sundering of the transverse muscles. A careful search for scars will often make clear the pathology of a case which otherwise is hard to understand. In one case the writer found a large rectocele coexisting with a laceration of the third degree, showing a rare combination of accidents. There still exists a good deal of difference of opinion regarding the nature of the various lesions around the pelvic outlet, but the above description may be accepted as at least practical.

*Treatment.*—Some of the symptoms of ruptured perineum may sometimes be ameliorated by properly adjusted pessaries, but anything like a cure can be sought only in surgery. The operation may be considered under two general heads, the immediate and the secondary operation.

*Immediate Operation.*— The history of the treatment of immediate ruptures of the perineum is comparatively recent. The first paper in American literature—one might almost say in English literature—calling attention to the importance of this subject is to be found in the *American Journal of Obstetrics* for 1873. This paper was followed by others by different authors, and from that time on a settled plan of procedure has been adopted. At present, the writer believes, all the authorities agree in saying that ruptures of the first and of the second degree should be closed by stitches as soon as practicable after the labor is completed.

---

[1] Skene, Transactions of the American Gynæcological Society, vol. xviii., 1893, p. 8.

Various plans of introducing the sutures have been suggested, but none seems to work so well as a stitch which goes in just above the lower angle of the rupture on one side, passes completely around, and comes out at a corresponding point on the other side, being buried through its entire course. This may be followed by one or more above[1] the first, according to the depth of the laceration. (See Fig. 1.)

Alloway has suggested a method of closing the rupture by one stitch. In my experience, however, this does not bring the deep and more posterior portions of the perineum together with sufficient firmness, and utterly fails in a transverse tear. The result is that the more superficial parts, that is, the parts nearer the skin, are firmly united, but the deeper perineal structures remain open. The resulting perineum is not good, and a rectocele may form, even though the skin surface may seem to be intact. By the plan first suggested, which is made clearer by the diagram, the perineal body is brought firmly together, and the resulting perineum is as good as it was before the tear.

The advisability of immediate suture of deep lacerations when the sphincter and certain portions of the rectum are involved is hardly settled yet. Some authors deprecate the plan, while others advocate it. The writer has had the opportunity of treating such cases in several instances, always with perfect cure: while such good results cannot always be expected, still, it seems as if it were but right to give the woman the chance to escape the pain and suffering of a secondary operation by closing the whole wound at once.

The immediate operation should usually be done within six hours after the accident, but may be successful if deferred even for twelve or twenty-four hours. One case has been reported in which forty-eight hours elapsed and yet perfect union resulted.

*Secondary Operation.*—From what has been said it will be evident that two distinct conditions are found in the perineum ; and although there may be a combination of accidents, most cases can be placed distinctly under one or the other head.

In the first class we place median tears, and in the second the transverse tears with relaxation. The first class includes two divisions, those which go to the sphincter and those which go through it.

If the tear is median, without involving the sphincter and without relaxation, we are rarely called upon to operate, as such tears seem to cause very little trouble. The tears involving the sphincter are rare, while the second class make up the greater bulk of operative cases.

*General Consideration of Operative Details.*—*Sutures.*—Different suture-materials are needed in different operations, or in different parts of the same operation. Silver wire has been generally discarded ; in its place

---

[1] The terms "above" and "below" are used with reference to the parts as the woman lies upon her back.

have been used silkworm-gut, silk, and catgut. All are good, and each has its place.

Silk should be prepared by boiling in beeswax. If not boiled too long, its strength is not impaired. Black silk is the easiest to see, and moderately coarse is best; sewing-machine silk answers a good purpose. The boiling in wax makes it aseptic and as impervious to fluids as silk-worm-gut, while it is softer and consequently less painful.

Catgut need not be chromicized, for if prepared by boiling in alcohol it is sufficiently strong and lasts long enough.

*Needles.*—The needles used should be straight and round, and some should have eyes large enough to hold good-sized catgut. No. 2 catgut is the size generally used.

*Instruments.*—Denudation can be done with scissors. The other instruments necessary are about the same as those used for the operation on the cervix.

*Operation for Simple Rupture.*—The patient being anæsthetized and placed on a table on her back, the thighs are flexed upon the body and held in place by Kelly's leg-holders. A Kelly pad is placed under the hips, with a suitable receptacle to receive the water.

The parts should be prepared by clipping the hair, followed by a thorough scrubbing with hot soapsuds. The vulva and vagina should then be irrigated with a sublimate solution (1 to 2000), or some other suitable antiseptic.

With a pair of small angular scissors the outline of the part to be denuded should be marked out. The line of incision should follow a line which would be made by continuing the hymen around to a corresponding point on the opposite side. It need not come as far outside as the four-chette. Usually some remnant of the hymen is visible to mark the spot. The upper border on each side should be only a short distance below the level of the anterior vaginal wall,—better too high than too low. The distance up the vaginal wall in the median line must be estimated for each case, but it need not go much farther than the internal edge of the internal anal sphincter. A finger in the rectum will easily determine this point. If there is a tendency to rectocele, it may go a little farther.

After the parts are all denuded (see Fig. 1) and the bleeding stopped, the stitches are placed, beginning with the lowest. A long needle, like a darning-needle,—the temper of which should not be too high, so that it will bend rather than break,—should be made to enter near the lower edge of the wound, and after passing through the recto-vaginal septum to come out at a corresponding point on the opposite side. The two upper stitches pass under the denuded surface on one side, then out across the vagina and under the denuded surface on the other side.

After the parts have been well douched, the stitches are tied, beginning at the lowest one. Care should be taken not to pull them too tight, so that they will not cut in. In order to have the edges of the wound within the vagina brought nicely together, superficial catgut stitches can be placed by simply pulling the newly-united perineum forward; or they can be put in one at a time alternately with the tying of the external stitches.

After the stitches are all placed, a drachm or two of iodoform should be placed in the vagina and more sprinkled over the outside of the wound.

*After-Treatment.*—The after-treatment is simple. The urine is drawn for a few days and the parts are kept well covered with iodoform. The bowels are moved on the second or third day by a cathartic, preceded by an enema, which is given some little time before the movement.

The stitches can be removed on the sixth or seventh day.

*Operation for Complete Rupture.*—When the laceration includes the sphincter, it oftens extends a greater or less distance up the recto-vaginal septum. If the tear of the septum is only slight, no special attention need be paid to it; but if it is a half-inch or more, then, in the experience of the writer, it is always better to close the septum by a preliminary operation.

In closing the septum the edges are denuded and brought together with silk stitches passing entirely through from the vaginal to the rectal mucous membrane, pretty near the edges, and back from the rectal surface to the vagina.

FIG. 1.                          FIG. 2.

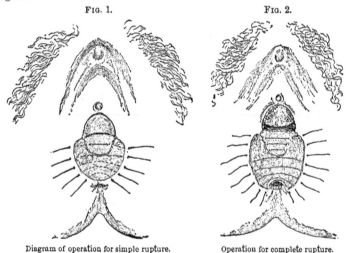

Diagram of operation for simple rupture.        Operation for complete rupture.

The patient need not stay in bed for more than a day. No pain follows, and in a week union is sufficiently strong to admit of the main operation being performed.

Unless the laceration be complicated with considerable relaxation, the general plan of the operation is the same as that previously described, the principal point of difference being the securing of the ends of the divided sphincter ani muscle. The ends of the muscle may be recognized by two dimples or depressions just at the end of the corrugated band which marks the outer margin of the anus. The sphincter muscle is spread out nearly straight. The ends must be denuded, and the stitches so placed as to bring them together. (Fig. 2.) It is to the ingenuity of Dr. Emmet that we owe the proper directions for the accomplishment of this.

The great difficulty is to understand the necessity of placing the first stitch near enough to the median line. A study of this diagram, which is drawn according to measurements, will show why this is so. (Fig. 3.) Unless the stitch $a$ is made to enter far enough back to include the end of the muscle at its upper part (c), and to come out at $b$ near enough to get the point $d$, the ends will not be brought together. Great care must be taken to go near enough to the median line.

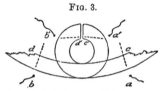

Fig. 3.

Method of placing the stitches so as to include the ends of the sphincter.

*After-Treatment.*—The after-treatment of this operation is of the utmost importance, and unless it is carefully followed out a failure will certainly result. The urine should be drawn for the first three or four days, and the parts kept well covered with iodoform, a considerable amount of iodoform having been placed in the vagina at the time of the operation.

On the evening of the third day a cathartic should be given,—the compound liquorice powder answers very well,—and in the morning before any action has occurred a teacupful of warm olive oil should be thrown into the rectum. The greatest precaution must be observed that the nozzle of the syringe passes behind the lowest stitches, otherwise the result of the whole operation may be destroyed. Care must also be taken that the patient does not strain and open the parts. If any large fæcal masses appear, they should be held back and broken before they come down. The best way of dissolving them, if the oil and cathartic have not accomplished this, is by an injection of a solution of inspissated bile. After the bowels have once been thoroughly moved, evacuations should occur daily, care being always taken that they are not hard and dry.

Sometimes large, hard, fæcal masses will descend as the result of long-standing accumulations in the colon; and it is well, unless the patient has been troubled with diarrhœa, to have the colon thoroughly flushed a number of days before the operation begins. This should be done in the knee-chest position, otherwise the injections will not run into the bowel.

It was formerly the plan to constipate the bowels for a number of days; but the collection of hard, dry fæcal matter thus made had almost as bad an influence on the newly-united perineum as the child's head had originally. The greatest care must be used to avoid this. If the first day or two there be an inclination for the bowels to move, it will be well to give an opiate to restrain them.

The accumulation of gas in the lower bowel may cause a great deal of pain. A soft-rubber catheter pushed into the rectum will draw this off and add much to the patient's comfort.

It is well to keep the patient in bed for about two weeks, and after that she may rise and gradually resume her ordinary duties.

*Operation for Transverse Lacerations with Relaxation.*—It is the belief of the writer that the plan of operation proposed by Dr. T. A. Emmet is the only one which effectually meets the conditions found in transverse lacerations with relaxation. The object of any operation must be to draw up the pelvic floor and to restore the vaginal outlet to its normal dimensions. This, as Dr. Emmet explains, is not a narrowing of the vagina, but a contraction of the over-distended tissues, so that the parts will be supported and held in place as before.

As in transverse tears the levator ani muscle and the fascia are separated from the perineum proper, any operation to effect relief must in some way reunite the torn muscle and fascia to the more external parts. This Emmet has succeeded in doing by his very ingenious operation.

The patient is placed in the same position as for the other operations. The line to be denuded is then marked out with a pair of sharp-pointed scissors, following the line of the hymen, or coming down a little outside of this line in the direction of the posterior commissure. It is always well to keep inside the mouths of the ducts of the vulvo-vaginal glands, so that they will not be obliterated by the operation. The line of denudation should run well up on the sides of the labium, just about on a level with the lower edge of the meatus, or very near to that point. It then runs along the side of the vagina well up into the sulcus on each side. By the sulcus is meant the depression between the centre and side of the vagina, a kind of groove which is normally found in this place. As there is always a rectocele in these cases, the denudation must run up the median line of the vagina as far as the top, or what Emmet calls "the crest of the rectocele."

The result of this plan is a denuded area shaped like the accompanying diagram (see Fig. 4), and it must be clearly understood that all this denuded surface is within the vagina.

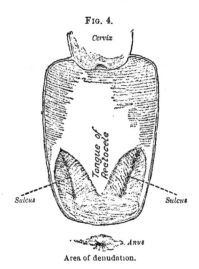

FIG. 4.

Cervix

Tongue of Rectocele

Sulcus    Sulcus

Anus

Area of denudation.

After the denudation is completed, the sutures are placed, beginning at the upper angle of the denuded surface in one sulcus. The stitch is passed from the outside towards the median line down to the middle of the sulcus, not straight across, but downward and at the same time inward to about the middle of the denuded area. (See Fig. 5.) It is then returned and passed up and out to the corresponding point in the tongue or flap of undenuded surface in the centre of the vagina.

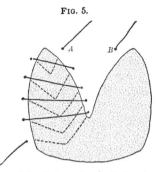

FIG. 5.

Area of denudation and method of placing stitches.

This suturing is done with the uninterrupted suture, catgut, in the experience of the writer, having given excellent results and presenting no difficulties in its removal.

After the point of the tongue on one side has been brought up to the centre of the vagina, the same process is continued on the other side. There is then left only a small area of raw surface, which is brought together by sutures placed very similarly to those in the operation for rupture of the second degree. (Fig. 6.)

The suture material for the outside stitches is silk or silkworm-gut; and it is to be remembered that the upper stitch—that is, the one nearest the urethra—must include the end of the tongue of undenuded surface on the posterior wall of the vagina. In this way the posterior vaginal wall is raised to the level of the new outlet of the vagina, and the whole vaginal floor is covered by normal mucous membrane.

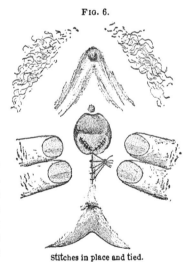

FIG. 6.

stitches in place and tied.

*After-Treatment.*—The after-treatment of this case is similar to that in the other instances.

*Other Operations.*—Besides the operations here described, there are a multitude of others having the same objects in view. The most popular at present is the so-called flap-splitting operation, designed by Dr. Jenks and Mr. Tait. This operation does not appear to the writer to fulfil the demands, and is in no way comparable to the operation here described. It has not been thought best to give an account of operations which cannot be recommended.

**Lacerations of the Cervix Uteri.**—*Etiology.*—By far the most common cause of lacerations of the cervix is parturition at, or near, full

18

term. It is quite possible that there should be a laceration in the early months of pregnancy, but it has never been the writer's experience to meet with a case where the laceration occurred before the fourth month.

A condition which somewhat approaches a bilateral laceration in appearance was formerly quite often met with as the result of bilateral incisions. But, operations of this kind having almost entirely passed out of use, such conditions are now seldom or never met with.

Any factor which causes a rapid delivery of the fœtus before the os externum is fully opened may cause a laceration, such as the improper use of forceps, the use of ergot, or undue activity on the part of the uterus from natural causes. Where instruments are not used, it is very doubtful whether much can be done in the way of prophylaxis, and therefore it may be said that these lacerations are generally unavoidable. This is still further proved by the fact that they occur more commonly in cases of dystocia and where there has been previous disease of the cervix. From this we must conclude that great care is demanded when the forceps are applied before the os is fully dilated.

It is stated by some authors that lacerations of sufficient importance to need attention occur in about one-third of all cases of labor. This would seem to the writer to be altogether too high an estimate, though without definite statistics to fall back upon nothing positive can be asserted in the matter. It does not appear that lacerations of the cervix are as common as they were formerly.

*Pathology.*—Lacerations may be partial or complete.

In partial laceration the cervical mucous membrane and the parts of the cervical canal between the outside of the cervix and the canal are torn, but the rent does not appear on the vaginal surface, except on each side of the os externum.

In complete lacerations the whole thickness of the cervix is torn, the tear extending more or less deeply into the cervical tissue, and sometimes almost to the internal os, so that the entire cervix is divided into two halves.

Complete lacerations may be unilateral, bilateral, and stellate.

The bilateral lacerations are by all means the most common; they almost always extend from side to side, and very rarely from before backward. The writer cannot remember having met with a single case of complete bilateral laceration where the rent was in the median line.

Unilateral lacerations may occur in any part of the cervix. They are said to be more common on the left side, owing to the frequency of the first position of the vertex. This is a mere assertion, without statistics to prove it.

Stellate lacerations, while sometimes not deep, are often of considerable extent, and constitute a condition which induces severe symptoms and presents great difficulties for the operator. Fortunately, they are rare.

It will thus be seen that the complete bilateral laceration is the one most commonly met with, and therefore demands the most attention.

Sometimes, after a deep laceration, a greater or less degree of healing will occur. The outside portions—that is, those near the vaginal surface, —may heal, leaving a large cavity within the cervical canal. This condition is almost as bad as though the parts were not healed at all, as secretions collect in this cavity and bad symptoms result. Sometimes there will be one or more fistulous openings leading into this cavity besides the true os.

The torn surfaces resulting from the laceration, being bathed in lochial discharge after confinement, rarely unite. They remain, however, as a source of irritation, often sufficient to prevent proper involution of the uterus. These raw, irritated surfaces tend to keep up a constant congestion of the uterus, which with the subinvolution causes great enlargement and eventually thickening of the uterine tissues.

Laceration of the cervix commonly causes a profuse discharge from the cervical glands; and these glands, from the growth of connective tissue, are often converted into cysts, their mouths being closed. These cysts grow to a considerable size, and seem to penetrate the cervix everywhere. They may finally become so large and numerous that an incision into the cervix will seem almost like cutting into a rather fine sponge filled with mucus. This cystic degeneration is one of the common results of laceration, but only a late condition. It may occur independently of laceration.

In some instances the two flaps, or portions of the cervix separated by the tear, become enormously hypertrophied by the formation of new connective tissue within their substance, so that they seem almost like small fibroid tumors, and the writer has more than once had cases referred to him for operation on the supposition that there were fibroid tumors present.

Occasionally, nature seems to make an effort to repair the laceration by the formation of a large amount of granulation tissue. The angles of the rent will thus be filled up nearly even with the surface. In process of time this granulation tissue becomes converted into a hard, almost cartilaginous, mass of connective tissue, and is by many, especially Emmet, thought to be a source of irritation, and one of the causes of the many reflex symptoms so commonly met with in these old bad cases.

It was formerly supposed that pelvic cellulitis was a common accompaniment of lacerations of the cervix. A truer pathology has shown us that pelvic cellulitis is a comparatively rare disease, and that the inflammatory exudations met with in the pelvis, accompanying lacerations of the cervix, are really inflammations of the tubes and ovaries, and may not have any direct connection with the laceration; but that they are very frequent accompaniments cannot be denied, and that they may have had their origin in septic processes occurring in labor is commonly admitted. These septic processes, in turn, may have had their origin in part in the lacerations. This is the only connection which can be admitted now between chronic pelvic inflammations and laceration of the cervix.

As a result of the loss of support attending a deep laceration,—the cervix being unable to hold any weight from above,—and also of the increased weight of the uterus and the relaxation of the uterine ligaments which always attends subinvolution, displacements are very commonly the accompaniments of lacerations of the cervix.

Lacerations of the perineum very frequently occur at the same time and materially aid in the production of displacements: thus it comes about that lacerations of the cervix, lacerations of the perineum, and uterine dis-displacements are often associated.

Sterility is a common result, as will be readily understood, the failure to conceive being due rather to the blocking up of the cervix by the cervical catarrh, or to the unhealthy condition of the endometrium, than to anything else. Abortions not infrequently occur in the case of deep laceration, the uterus being unable to hold the enlarging ovum.

It is undoubtedly a fact that a very large proportion of cases of cancer of the cervix are preceded by laceration. Some have asserted that all cases of malignant disease of the cervix result from laceration. This, however, is going too far, as the writer has himself seen a number of cases, both of carcinoma and sarcoma of the cervix, where the woman had never been pregnant. That these cases are decidedly the exception cannot be denied, but it must be maintained that they do exist. If cancer is so frequently preceded by laceration, it is but fair to look upon this lesion in the relation of cause to effect. How a laceration should produce cancer is one of the mysteries that we have not yet solved.

In a few instances the laceration is so deep as to involve a ureter or the bladder. We may then have a vesico-uterine or a uretero-uterine fistula as a complication. The writer has met with a single case of each of these varieties. Others have been described in the books.

*Symptoms.*—In some instances there is a great deal of tenderness in and about the seat of the laceration. This is manifested at the time of sexual intercourse, and becomes a fruitful source of trouble. The surface, remaining eroded, bleeds on the slightest mechanical interference, besides being sensitive. Usually the symptoms are mostly those of the complications. If there be a heavy uterus with displacement, the symptoms will be referable to the displacement rather than to the laceration. Leucorrhœa is an almost constant symptom, and disturbances of menstruation, especially menorrhagia due to the endometritis, are very common. The reflex neuroses are various. Pain over the sacrum is quite common, as well as pain under the left breast, due to intercostal neuralgia. Neuroses of the eyes, head, stomach, and bowels are also frequently met with, and these not of a distinctively hysterical type. Hysterical symptoms may be superadded, and are not infrequently seen.

*Physical Signs.*—Laceration of the cervix is best recognized by the sense of touch. In passing the finger into the vagina the laceration is usually easily recognizable. The finger passes between the flaps or segments of the cervix, and the fact that they are separable is quickly noted.

In some instances, however, the angle between the flaps has become so filled with connective tissue and large follicles that the space is nearly closed up and the tip of the cervix is nearly smooth. If now the finger be passed to the vaginal junction in front and behind the cervix, it will readily be felt that the lower end of the cervix is very much broader than the portion at the vaginal junction; in other words, that the cervix is club-shaped. This is an almost sure sign of laceration.

If, in such a case, a Sims speculum is introduced and the two outer edges of the cervix are pulled together, the fact that there has been a laceration will be more readily recognized. The surface often feels rough and granular from the large follicles; in other instances it feels velvety and soft from erosion, and is generally covered by a mucous discharge, which may be clear like the white of egg, or green or yellowish in character. Linear cicatrices may be felt, extending a considerable distance along the vault of the vagina, showing that the laceration has originally been deeper than it now is, the portions within the vaginal walls having healed by granulation.

In cases where the laceration is only partial, the finger may be admitted within the external os and passed up the cervical canal for a considerable distance. One not understanding the true nature of the case might suppose that the cervix was simply dilated or patulous, as we may find it soon after an abortion; but, as such a condition (dilatation) never exists for any length of time, a second examination showing the existence of the same condition will prove that there is a laceration. If one trusts to sight alone to diagnose lacerations, he will often be deceived, especially if a tubular or bivalve speculum be used. Undoubtedly the finger gives us the clearest information, and our suspicions may be confirmed by the use of the Sims speculum and tenacula.

In making bimanual palpation, if the fundus lies in front, so that the uterus can be pushed down upon the finger, the laceration may be spread forcibly apart and be more readily recognized in this way. The position of the uterus and the condition of the tubes and ovaries will also be best recognized by the aid of the bimanual or conjoined manipulation.

*Immediate Treatment.*—The treatment of lacerations immediately after their occurrence is now strongly advocated by some. Soon after labor the cervix hangs down in soft folds, and the recognition of the point at which the vagina ends and the cervix begins is exceedingly difficult. Any one who has had to sew up a laceration under these circumstances will appreciate the difficulties of the situation. It can be done, however, and, if the laceration is recognized and there is nothing to prevent, it may be a wise procedure. The continuous catgut suture should be used, the seam being made from the inside and the sewed part left to take care of itself. Of course if wire or silk were used, their removal would be almost impossible after the cervix had contracted. The writer has performed this operation several times, with what seemed to be satisfactory results; but the difficulty of understanding the relations of the parts and of bringing them together properly can hardly be overestimated. The mere placing of the stitches is exceedingly easy. The operation can best be performed with the patient on her back and with a Simon's speculum. In this way the cervix can be brought almost outside of the body.

*Secondary Treatment.*—The question at once arises, if we reject this immediate treatment, how soon after labor is it admissible to operate? Lately it has been proposed that the operation should be done before the woman leaves the lying-in room, say at the end of ten or twelve days. It is maintained that by doing the operation at this time no cutting is necessary; the granulating surface can be freshened by simply scraping it, and the parts can then be brought together very easily, not sufficient time having elapsed for indurations and hypertrophies to occur.

While the writer has had no experience with this method, it seems to show certain advantages, and should the opportunity arise he would undoubtedly advise its trial. The greater part of the process of involution is practically complete at the end of ten days; the remainder of the process would doubtless be better and more thoroughly completed after such an operation than if the rent were left to heal slowly.

In practice, however, very few cases will be brought to the notice of the gynæcologist at so early a date. Few physicians examine their patients after labor to know whether there have been lacerations of the cervix or not; consequently the lesion is not discovered until the patient begins to suffer from its effects. Then an examination is made and the first intimation is given that a laceration has occurred. Many are unrecognized even at this late date, and some pass from one physician to another until somebody appreciates the true cause of the woman's sufferings and employs the proper remedies. A case once occurred in the practice of the writer in which eighteen physicians had treated the woman during a period of ten years without any relief, the cause of her sufferings all the time being an unrecognized partial, but very deep and extensive, laceration.

One of the first questions to be decided is, How deep should a laceration be to require operation? Unfortunately, no definite answer can be given to this question. We sometimes see women with very slight lacerations who are apparently incurable except by the restoration of the cervix. In other instances deep lacerations will exist for years without, to all appearance, causing much trouble. The degree of eversion or erosion may be the determining factor, or the idiosyncrasy of the individual or some peculiar susceptibility of the nervous system must account for the difference of these two classes of cases. The writer can only say that some of his most satisfactory cases have been those in which the degree of laceration was comparatively slight.

*Preliminary Treatment.*—The advisability of correcting backward displacements before doing the operation for laceration has been disputed. It has always seemed best to the writer to do the operation first and to replace the displaced organ afterwards, for the reason that the flaps of the torn cervix would be pressed farther apart by bringing the uterus into a right angle with the posterior vaginal wall. As long as the uterus is retroverted, the flaps are kept together by the pressure of the vaginal walls, the uterus lying approximately in the same axis as the vagina.

Some have thought it advisable to cure the erosion of the cervix before operating. This has never seemed to the writer to be necessary. If there is extensive cystic degeneration of the cervix, this had better be treated for a time by incisions and painting with iodine, so that at least a strip of mucous membrane in the centre of each flap will be quite healthy and clear of cysts. Cysts on the side are not of much importance, as they can be cut out when the denudation is done.

Surrounding inflammatory troubles are mentioned by some writers as absolute bars to operation. Unless these inflammatory exudations contain pus, the writer fails to see how an operation can do any harm, provided, of course, that too great traction be not made upon the cervix. In several instances where patients have refused cœliotomy, or where cœliotomy did not seem to be clearly indicated, the writer has operated upon the cervix notwithstanding the presence of old extensive inflammatory masses. This inflammatory trouble seems in each case to have been greatly benefited by the operation. Great care was taken not only not to pull down the cervix, but also not to pass any instruments into the uterus at the time of the operation on the cervix.

Many cases of non-suppurative pelvic inflammation it is believed may be benefited by a careful operation on the cervix. The writer is perfectly well aware that this is quite contrary to common doctrine, but the knowledge that such inflammations affect the tubes and ovaries and not the cellular tissue has led to this change of opinion. Of course in the case of a pus-tube, or even where the presence of pus is strongly suspected, no such operation should be done unless it is proposed to open the abdomen immediately afterwards and to remove the products of inflammation.

Preparatory curettage of the uterine cavity has also been advised when endometritis exists; but the writer has always preferred to do this operation at the same sitting, dilating the cervix and curetting and then mopping out the cavity with Churchill's tincture of iodine before beginning the denudation. This he has done repeatedly, and has never seen any harm result, but, on the contrary, has witnessed a great deal of good.

*Operation.*—The instruments needed for an operation for laceration of the cervix are not many. They may be named as follows: a Sims speculum with a broad, short blade; two pairs of Emmet's curved scissors and a pair of long scissors, curved on the flat, for cutting wire or ligatures; a needle-holder, that devised by Dr. Bache Emmet being one of the best; two uterine tenacula, one of them with a heavy shank, as devised by Emmet for counter-pressure; a pair of double tenacula, or bullet-forceps;

if silver wire be used, a wire twister and shield; if shotted silkworm-gut be thought desirable, then a shot-compressor will be serviceable; two or more needles. Some use a peculiar pair of scissors devised by Dr. Skene, and known as the "hawk-bill" scissors, for taking out the hard mass of connective tissue sometimes found at the angle of the laceration. A dozen sponge-holders will also be needed, and a fountain syringe filled with an antiseptic solution.

The instruments chosen are those used when the operation is done through the Sims speculum and in the Sims position. Some prefer operating with the patient on the back, using Simon's speculum and a knife rather than scissors in denuding. The writer's custom has been always to use the Sims position, as it seems to give much more room for manipulation than the other, and the passage of the needle seems to be very much easier than when the patient is lying on the back. The only advantage of the dorsal position is that constant irrigation of the vagina can be kept up and sponges are done away with. But in the Sims position the parts can be frequently washed with a stream of water, if desired, and if the patient be placed on a Kelly pad, the water is conducted away almost as well as if she were lying on her back. The choice of position and speculum is largely a matter of education and habit.

The best needles to employ are straight needles with triangular points, of fairly good size, and not too highly tempered. It is better to have them bend than break, and in some cases it is very difficult to introduce them through the hard and hypertrophied tissues resulting from a long-standing laceration. In such cases there is great danger of breaking them. A triangular-pointed needle will go through any tissue easily, whereas a round-pointed needle could hardly be forced through an indurated cervix. A straight needle is better than a curved one, as we can always tell where the point is, which it is sometimes difficult to do with a curved one. With the patient lying on the back, the ordinary surgical half-curved needle is more commonly used.

The suture material is largely a matter of indifference. Custom and habit will probably decide the operator as to whether he will use silver wire, silkworm-gut, silk, or catgut. The writer has used all of them in turn, and gives his preference to either silver wire or catgut.[1] Where an operation on the perineum is not to be done at the same time, wire is generally preferred. If the perineum is to be closed at the same sitting, then catgut—which will be absorbed in the course of ten days— will be the best. Silk in the cervix is very difficult to find and remove afterwards.

The needle should not be threaded directly with the wire or with the catgut, but should be threaded with silk, doubled and tied, a loop of at least a foot being left, in which the end of the wire is fastened and drawn

---

[1] Silver-plated copper wire will do just as well, and is much cheaper.

through the tissue by the silk, which has previously been drawn partly through. The gut can be treated in the same way.

The silver wire is usually twisted, but silk, catgut, and silkworm-gut can be tied, or a shot with a large hole can be passed over both strands and then compressed after the parts have been drawn together. It is easier to adjust the parts with the shot than it is to tie, and the catgut is less likely to slip when treated in this way.

The question of the necessity of giving anæsthetics for this operation frequently arises. In small lacerations, when it is not necessary to do a great deal of cutting, and when the operation can be done quickly, an anæsthetic may be dispensed with,—provided, of course, that the patient is willing to endure the pain, which is not very great. The writer has operated a number of times in this way. Cocaine may also be used to deaden the pain, the parts being rendered almost insensitive by several injections of the four-per-cent. solution introduced well into the cervical tissue with a hypodermic syringe. Complete surgical anæsthesia is generally best, and most patients will prefer it.

The patient being anæsthetized and placed in the Sims position upon a Kelly pad, a large-sized Sims speculum is introduced. The mucus from the cervix is then carefully cleared away by balls of dry absorbent cotton. After this the entire vagina and cervix are thoroughly washed with an antiseptic douche, either sublimate or hydronaphthol, or with whatever the operator may deem best. The water is then carefully mopped out of the vagina and the parts are thoroughly dried. (Fig. 7.)

FIG. 7.

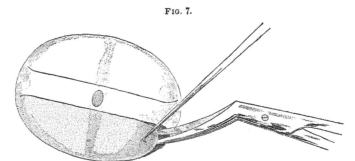

The area to be denuded cleansed. and denudation begun.

The next step is the marking out of the line of denudation. This may be done with a knife or scissors, a clear strip being left in the centre for the formation of the cervical canal. After this has been done, the left edge of the anterior lip is seized with a tenaculum; and the mucous membrane, with a sufficient thickness of submucous tissue, is raised from the surrounding tissue with the scissors. The cutting process is continued until the angle is reached. Here it may be necessary to go quite deeply in order to remove all the cicatricial tissue. This may be done by the hawk-bill scissors as the first step in the operation, if it be so desired, and the writer believes that for beginners this may be of great assistance. After the angle has been passed, the denudation is continued on to the posterior lip until the whole of the left-hand side of the torn surface has been denuded. The upper or left-hand side of the cervix is then denuded in like manner.

It is necessary to avoid going too far out on the vaginal wall, for when the cervix is pushed back into the vagina too much tension might be made by the sutures. Hemorrhage during this stage of the operation is often quite severe: an assistant must at all times sponge away the blood so as to keep the field of operation clear. In the dorsal position constant irrigation will accomplish the same thing.

After the parts have been thoroughly denuded, and all arterial hemorrhage checked by the application, if necessary, of hæmostatic forceps or deep suture, we may proceed to the placing of the sutures. The first suture to be introduced is that nearest the angle on the left-hand side. The needle is made to enter as in Fig. 8, and to emerge in the undenuded strip in the centre of the flap. It then is made to enter the opposite flap at a corresponding distance from the angle, and to emerge on the vaginal surface of the cervix at the same distance from the angle as the point of entrance on the opposite lip.

FIG. 8.

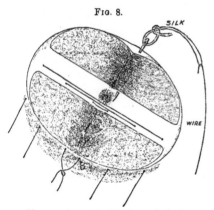

Stitches in place on the left side, needle in place on the right side.

The second stitch is placed near the middle of the flap, but in the same general way, —that is, through the anterior lip over to the posterior flap and out on the vaginal surface. The third stitch—and three on a side are generally enough —will be quite near the external os, and may possibly be passed through both flaps at once.

After the sutures have been placed on one side, the ends are gathered together and seized with a hæmostatic forceps and left loose until the opposite side has been sutured. This is done in the same way, only the direction of the needle is reversed.

The stitches being all inserted, the parts are carefully sponged and then douched with an antiseptic solution, and the wound is closed by either twisting the wire, or tying, or shotting the other ligature-material, whatever it may be. If the stitches have not been placed close enough together to bring the edges nicely into apposition, a few catgut stitches can be introduced afterwards to bring them into this relation. (Fig. 9.)

All the hemorrhage will now have ceased from the pressure of the sutures, and, after the vagina is thoroughly dried, about two or three drachms of iodoform should be scattered around the cervix. This will do away with the necessity for irrigation or any other after-treatment, and it will remain in place for a period of at least a week, retaining a perfectly aseptic condition.

*After - Treatment.* — The after-treatment of these cases is exceedingly simple. While it is not absolutely necessary that the patient should remain in bed, it is better, as a rule, that she should do so. Un-

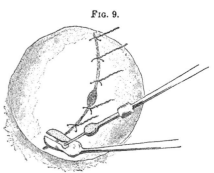

FIG. 9.

Twisting the last stitches.

doubtedly the rest in bed and the freedom from care and anxiety which this entails do a great deal of good in some of these cases. As there is very little pain or annoyance connected with the operation, the patients often get up from their rest of a week or ten days feeling very much stronger, better, and freer from pain than they were before the operation. After about a week the patient may be allowed to sit up in bed, and at the end of two weeks may be walking about as usual.

The stitches can be removed about the tenth day. If removed earlier, there is danger of tearing the flaps apart and spoiling the result. As they cause no pain and do no harm, it will not make any difference if they are left even longer than ten days. Emmet reports a case in which a woman went to Europe and was gone a long time with the silver-wire stitches in place: no harm resulted. I have myself several times overlooked a stitch, and have found it after a period of months, or even years, the patient not having been conscious of its presence.

*Complicated Operations.*—The operation as thus far described is that of a simple bilateral laceration.

In the case of incomplete lacerations, the best plan is to cut through the portion of the cervical wall which remains intact, and thus to convert the laceration into the complete bilateral form. Only in this way can the deep portions of the laceration be denuded. After this has been done, the operation is carried on as heretofore described.

When the laceration is stellate, in some instances the portion intervening between two lacerations, if they happen to be very near together, can be entirely removed, thus converting the double laceration into a single one. When a bilateral laceration is joined with a laceration of the anterior or of the posterior lip, it is best first to denude and close this latter tear entirely, leaving only the bilateral laceration, which then can be proceeded with according to the usual method.

In some instances we meet with a great disproportion between the size of the two lips or flaps. Usually the anterior is much the larger, and when denuded and brought into apposition with the posterior lip will greatly overlap it. A number of plans have been devised for overcoming this difficulty. One is to amputate the overlapping portion of the anterior lip. Another is to take out a wedge-shaped piece from the anterior lip, cutting from side to side. This incision does not extend through to the vaginal surface, but begins on the inside of the cervix, or on the cervical mucous membrane. After this wedge-shaped piece has been removed, the incision is closed and the usual operation for bilateral laceration is completed.

When there is great hypertrophy of one lip with atrophy of the other, the writer has several times cut the anterior lip down to a size proportionate to the posterior lip, denuding the entire torn surface. A strip broader than usual is then left undenuded on the posterior flap, so that there may be plenty of room for the cervical canal, due allowance being made for contraction. After having performed this operation a number of times without seeing any bad result, the writer has no hesitation in recommending it.

In several instances in which there has been an extensive cystic degeneration of both lips, the writer has entirely denuded both surfaces, cutting away all the degenerated tissue. Then, in order to preserve a canal, he has placed a small section of a rubber drainage-tube between the flaps and sewed it with silver wire, the wire passing entirely through the anterior lip and being twisted in front. This was left for two weeks or more, until the parts were healed, and then, the wire being cut, the rubber could be readily removed. A patient who was operated upon as much as ten years ago has been heard from occasionally, and is known to have experienced great benefit and no harm from this method of procedure.

*Results.*—Operations for laceration of the cervix are almost always successful. The writer recalls but one case of death directly traceable to the operation. In this instance it was the operator's first case, and the operation was long. There may have been some pre-existing inflammatory trouble in the tubes or pelvic peritoneum; but of this the writer cannot speak with certainty, not having seen the woman until she was moribund.

Failure of union, if the operation be carefully done and the after-treatment be carried out in the way indicated, will not occur in more than two or three per cent. of the cases. In fact, the writer cannot remember a single failure in a very large number of recent cases, mounting well up into the hundreds.

The relief to the general symptoms is very great; and, although we sometimes see a failure in this way, still, the results are in the main eminently satisfactory. Hundreds—yes, thousands—of women have in the last twenty years been rescued from chronic invalidism and have been made useful members of society by this simple procedure.

The question is often asked whether there will be danger of a repetition of the laceration in case of another labor. The almost universal verdict is that a cervix which has been repaired will dilate better than one which is the seat of hypertrophy or cystic degeneration. A tear, of course, may occur a second time, but this is not usually the case. The writer has seen a considerable number of women who have gone through their second and subsequent labors without any reproduction of the laceration.

the excretions of the uterus, fluids which may come from the non-infected uterus; but, since these are at times an appropriate culture medium, the pathogenetic germs already present may quickly multiply and set up inflammations. Then, again, injury inflicted directly upon the vagina may in itself be enough to induce such an outflow of secretion as to furnish directly the needed culture fluid. In the virginal state the orifice is guarded by a special membrane, so that the entrance of germs, under the ordinary conditions of atmospheric pressure, is hindered, but after parturition the orifice is often so widened that air may have easy access, especially with the individual in the recumbent posture.

The lowering of the general systemic powers plays some part in predisposition to all inflammation, but, apart from this agency, other general conditions, with a predisposition to implications of the vaginal along with other mucous tracts, have a more direct bearing here, such, for instance, as measles and scarlet fever, in which epithelial exfoliation leaves a surface readily infected.

These general considerations are enough to account for the frequency of vaginitis, and as a fact, in some form, acute or chronic, it is a very common ailment. The congestion of the vagina associated with menstruation, the menopause, and pregnancy renders this canal, as might naturally be expected, more vulnerable to causative agencies. And, lastly, the atrophic changes of old age, while hardly in the nature of inflammation, may deprive the mucous membrane of its epithelium, and thus present a surface easily infected.

These agencies may be enumerated as follows: exposure to cold; excessive coitus; irritant injections and applications; the pressure of a pessary; masturbation; oxyurides; the contact of the vesical or rectal contents, as in fistulæ; irritating discharges from the direction of the uterus, as in simple or septic metritis or carcinoma; the extension of a vulvitis, as in children with acid urine, or in women with diabetes. Struma, uncleanliness, and the traumatisms and infections attendant upon parturition or abortion are other causes; but perhaps the most important of all is gonorrhœa. Owing to the virulence of this cause, its tendency to wide extension, its ability to lie latent in various parts of the genital canal for extensive periods and then reappear in force, gonorrhœa is the most interesting of the etiological factors. Its virility seems to be due to a specific germ (gonococcus), whose *rôle* (according to Pozzi) "was long undisputed, the facts proving its preponderating agency appearing to be easily demonstrated." "Most numerous in the acute stage," continues the same author, "rarer in the chronic forms, they multiply or diminish in number according as the disease is active or latent. They are found in gonorrhœal discharges from the urethra, the glands of Bartholini, the rectum, in gonorrhœal salpingitis, and in purulent ophthalmia. They have even been discovered in the blood and in the articular synovial fluid of patients suffering from gonorrhœal rheumatism.

"Succeeding to this period of certainty has come a time of doubt and criticism. The specific value of the gonococcus has been denied on account of its extreme resemblance to the non-pathogenic diplococci. These microbes, or pseudo-gonococci, so to speak, are found in intestinal, pulmonary, and buccal ulcerations, according to Eklund; according to Amicis, in simple experimental urethritis; and according to Steinberg, in urine, which he considers their normal habitat (*Micrococcus ureæ*). Is, then, the gonococcus but an indifferent saprophyte, capable of taking on pathogenic characters under peculiar conditions? or is it a distinct species, having definite pathogenic properties and susceptible of attenuation and of preserving in a latent state the noxious properties to which it reverts in a favorable medium? This is the hypothesis which appears most probable; but, on the other hand, direct experiments by means of cultures and inoculations have not given a decisive result. Sometimes they produce gonorrhœa, but more often not. Besides the presence of the microbe itself, there are other necessary factors which can be inferred, but have not yet been demonstrated."

*Pathological Anatomy.*—Following C. Ruge, we find this disease commonly presenting itself under three forms,—simple, granular, and senile vaginitis. A third form, present in pregnancy, is added, called emphysematous. It is rare for the entire surface to be involved, the disease presenting itself usually in patches or zones, healthy tissue intervening. If, however, the whole surface be involved, it is in the acute stage of a gonorrhœal, exanthematous, septic, or traumatic inflammation, dependent, under the last head, upon caustic or scalding hot injections. In the simple form the surface is smooth, but here and there patches of thickened tissue are seen. In these spots the papillæ are swollen and the neighboring tissue is infiltrated with small cells, the epithelial layers alone partaking in the proliferation. In the granular form, the more common variety, the papillæ are infiltrated with small cells, and so enlarged that they greatly encroach upon the intervening spaces. Ultimately, the surface has a granular appearance, which is due in part to the fusing of the papillæ and in part to the thinning of the overlying epithelial reflections.

In senile vaginitis the patches of diseased tissue are in places cechymotous, in others denuded of epithelium, leaving raw surfaces, which may, when opposed, adhere, tending to obliterate the canal.

The emphysematous, or gaseous, form belongs to pregnancy, but it may be present without it. The gas is probably situated in the meshes of the connective tissue, though the lymphatic capillaries are said to be the place of its development.

Diphtheritic vaginitis is merely the local expression of a general condition, and is marked by a greatly swollen mucous membrane, which is more or less covered with necrotic tissue. It belongs to the puerperal state and to such infectious disorders as measles, small-pox, and typhus fever; it is mostly an intense septic process engrafted upon a simple inflammation, which may result in extensive loss of tissue. Wide-spread exfoliation of the epithelial coat and deep-seated inflammatory changes in the subjacent coat are seen in consequence of the action of caustic or scalding-hot douches (accidental events, as a rule), and localized deep-seated ulcerative changes may be present in consequence of a neglected pessary. Abscess, the result either of inflammation of a cyst of the wall, of traumatism in forceps delivery, or of a development in the course of grave febrile states, may also be present.

*Symptoms.*—Acute vaginitis is indicated by dull pain and a sense of fulness in the lower pelvic regions. The discomfort is increased by micturition, by defecation, and by walking. There is discharge, which tends to increase rather than diminish, especially if the case be one of gonorrhœal origin. The fact that urethral and vesical symptoms, such as a burning pain in urination and vesical tenesmus, are added, indicates with fair certainty the causative agency of gonorrhœa, and the same may be said of the presence of inguinal pain and tenderness, due to the implication of the inguinal glands. Digital examination shows the vaginal orifice to be sensitive, the canal to be hot and swollen, and at a later period roughened. If the urethra be involved, it will be found thickened and tender, and pressure along its course from within outward may drive a drop of pus from the meatus. Pus from this quarter is said to be conclusive evidence of gonorrhœa, and as the gonococci thrive best upon this mucous membrane, their presence here may be said to complete the evidence in favor of the specific nature of the attack. If the bladder be infected, pressure upon the anterior vaginal wall will quickly reveal the fact by the marked increase in pain which is produced. Inspection may show the presence of acute vulvitis, and, if so, the orifice of the vagina, the orifices of the vulvo-vaginal glands (especially in gonorrhœa), the vestibule, and the meatus are the parts chiefly involved : all will be covered by a muco-purulent or purulent discharge. If the vagina can be inspected, its walls will be found covered with a similar secretion, beneath which, as in the vulva, the tissue is seen to be swollen and of a deepened red color.

An acute may pass into a chronic vaginitis if the conditions be neglected, if the patient be of enfeebled constitution, or if the disease be gonorrhœal. If the latter, it may be latent in its places of retreat, the posterior and anterior fornices of the vagina, ready, however, to resume an acute form whenever adequate irritation is forthcoming.

Chronic vaginitis presents no special local symptoms other than discharge (leucorrhœa). It may follow the acute stage, but more often is from the first a subacute or a chronic process ; such, for instance, as develops in consequence of discharges from the direction of the uterus, or as the result of senile changes, etc.

Leucorrhœa, therefore, while the usual expression of a chronic vaginitis, may comprise a discharge of uterine origin. Of this we shall speak more fully later. Originating in the vagina, it may be thin and whitish (mucoid) or thick and yellowish (purulent), the former indicative of the milder grades of the lesion under discussion, the latter showing the more severe ones.

In senile vaginitis this discharge is sero-purulent and yellowish, but occasionally it is brownish from the admixture of blood. Apart from any change obvious to the naked eye, the most striking development of leucorrhœa is seen in fat lithæmic women and in strumous subjects, and, as might be expected, such forms prove most rebellious to treatment. In the presence of a foreign body, such as a dirty or ill-fitting pessary, the discharge will be indicative of the kind of lesion produced, for in the event of ulceration of the wall a purulent or even blood-stained flow may appear; and just here it is well to mention that, following the use of douches which are too hot, or those which contain an excess of caustic ingredients, such as carbolic acid, and following also certain septic and exanthematous disorders, the discharges, which under such circumstances soon become purulent and perhaps bloody, may also contain shreds of the exfoliated epithelial covering of the vagina. (See Pathology.) As might be inferred, the more acrid and abundant the discharges of a chronic vaginitis become, the more likely are they to produce " vulvitis," with " pruritus vulvæ." Touch and sight reveal the roughened surfaces of a chronic vaginitis, and after gonorrhœa and in a pregnancy vegetations are not uncommon.

The swollen crepitating walls presented in the rare emphysematous form of the disease are characteristic of this variety, as are also the dark-red, swollen, and perhaps (in places) necrotic walls of the so-called diphtheritic form.

A simple vaginitis rarely involves the general health, but one that causes profuse and long-continued discharge of any kind, especially if it be purulent, will surely depress the general health. This will be manifested by loss of energy, by gastric disturbances, and perhaps by constipation and loss of nerve-control.

*Diagnosis.*—A vaginitis should not be confounded with any other lesion, a close inspection of the parts with the speculum sufficing to reveal the lesion. But it is not always easy to distinguish one form of vaginitis from another, and yet the fact that one variety is infectious is enough to render a distinction important. The presence of the gonococcus is no doubt sufficient to establish the presence of this form, but its absence does not appear now to be adequate proof of the absence of the disease. Corroborative evidence in its favor is found, however, in other directions; for instance, in the sudden onset, the virulence and course of the disease, as well as in the prompt implication of the urethra, perhaps of the bladder, the involvement of the vulvo-vaginal ducts and glands, and later by the tendency of the disease to invade the uterus and to extend to the adnexa. The fact that a woman with a vaginitis develops a conjunctivitis also points to its gonorrhœal nature, and, in the absence of pregnancy, the appearance of vegetations in the vagina is additional proof in the same direction. Lastly, if the examiner is so fortunate as to have the opportunity to inspect the " party of the first part" with whom the unfortunate woman has cohabited, and finds a gonorrhœa in him, the combined evidence may be said to be conclusive. The importance of all this search is more pressing in the event of medico-legal complications, such as may arise in consequence of actions for rape, for damages, or perhaps for divorce; but under ordinary circumstances the differentiation need not be deferred because of the absence of many of these proofs.

*Prognosis.*—In simple vaginitis it is very good in all directions, but not so in gonorrhœal. First, because of its obstinacy, its tendency to hide away in the urethra, in the vagina, and in the cervix, and its ability to reappear in response to the action of such common causes as coition, a check of menstruation, or parturition; second, because of its capacity for widespread extension, such as to the uterus, the adnexa, and even to the peritoneum, with the effects upon the health, the childbearing function, and even the life of the individual which are involved in such inflammations of these organs; its evil influence upon the puerperium, in which it appears competent to initiate septic peritonitis, and its ability to complicate the fruits of parturition by setting up ophthalmia in the new-born.

For all these reasons the prognosis in gonorrhœal vaginitis is grave and complicated. But here, as elsewhere in disease, the prognosis is largely influenced for the better by treatment.

*Treatment.*—Simple acute vaginitis is readily controlled and cured by keeping the patient at rest, by freeing the bowels with mild cathartics, and by the copious use of douches. These douches should consist of a saturated solution of biborate of sodium in water, the temperature should be about 110° F., and at least a gallon of the fluid should be used three times in twenty-four hours. The patient should take the douche lying on the back, the appropriate apparatus—viz., a fountain syringe and a bed-pan—being employed. In the gonorrhœal form, rest and a free state of the bowels are even more imperative, and the fluid used for the douching should contain, in place of the borax, bichloride of mercury in the strength of 1 to 10,000. The douche nozzle—glass or hard rubber—should be cleansed after use, and should be kept in a solution of carbolic acid (1 to 40). It is probable that the introduction of the nozzle may be very painful; in that event, oleate of cocaine may be first applied to the ostium vaginæ.

As soon as the acute symptoms subside the practitioner should institute energetic local measures. The surfaces should be gently cleansed with warm water and soap, the finger or, if possible, a sponge upon a holder being used to reach the inequalities of the vaginal surface, cocaine being used to lessen pain, if necessary. Then introduce a Ferguson's speculum, and, beginning at the cervix, paint over the entire surface (as the speculum is slowly withdrawn) with a solution of bichloride of mercury (1 to 1000). Then wash out with warm water, reintroduce the speculum, and place in position a piece of sterilized gauze of three or four thicknesses, the gauze to reach from the posterior fornix to the ostium vaginæ. By this measure the vaginal walls are kept apart and free drainage is provided. This treatment should be repeated daily until the disease is conquered. If at a later period the tissues should need stimulation, then paint the surfaces with tincture of iodine.

In the chronic forms, seek for the cause, whether local, as in discharges from above, or from oxyurides, or general, as in struma, and as far as possible remove or control them; wash out the vagina with soap and water, as already described, then, using the speculum as above, paint the entire surface freely with nitrate of silver (1 to 10 or 20), or even with full strength, if a decided reaction is needed. The strip of gauze is also needed here. This treatment may be given every day or every other day, as is required, the patient being directed to remove the gauze and take a warm, cleansing douche of a saturated aqueous solution of borax night and morning.

Reverting to the urethritis which occurs as a part of the gonorrhœal form, we find that it is best treated as follows : First inject a four-per-cent. solution of cocaine; then, making pressure upon the vesical end of the urethra, introduce a small glass nozzle and irrigate the canal with a 1 to 20,000 solution of bichloride of mercury. This should be repeated every day, if necessary. The administration of diluents is necessary, also a non-irritating diet, one free from stimulants especially, and frequently the use of salicylate of sodium or salol may prove beneficial in keeping the urine in a favorable condition.

In the deep-seated inflammations of the vaginal wall, such, for instance, as result in exfoliations of the epithelial coat, the primary indication is the promotion of the decline of the process and the relief of pain. The first is met by the warm biborate of sodium douches; the second, by the use of anodynes, either locally in the shape of vaginal or rectal suppositories, or by the mouth, as is deemed appropriate. With the subsidence of the inflammation comes the need for measures to prevent adhesion between the walls, or, where deeper sloughs have occurred, to prevent atresia. The first indication is met by carefully watching the healing process, keeping the surfaces apart by gauze strips soaked in mild astringent solutions, and promoting the reparative action by application of nitrate of silver or tincture of iodine. The same rule applies in the deeper losses of tissue, but here it may be necessary ultimately to use a glass vaginal plug upon which the vagina must heal, in order to prevent the contraction which otherwise might occur. In all these forms the case should be closely watched until the completion of the healing process.

Abscesses of the vaginal wall are to be treated by free incision and subsequent douchings of the canal. It is obvious that the graver forms of vaginitis must react unfavorably upon the general system. If such be the case, the condition must be met by appropriate tonics and by a close supervision of the digestive and assimilative functions.

### INFLAMMATION OF THE UTERUS.

*Etiology of Metritis and Endometritis.*—No more fitting place than this can be found at which to consider the agency of bacteria in causing inflammations of the genital tract. We have already shown the relation of the gonococcus to vaginitis, etc., and now state that it is potent to cause similar inflammations in the uterus. A favorite resting-place is the cervical canal, whose irregularities of surface afford easy harbor for these and other microbes. The fornices of the vagina likewise afford refuge for such products, so that we find a part of this genital tract (the cervical canal and upper portion of the vagina) which we may view as a dangerous zone, the habitat of pathogenic germs.

The statements made touching the causes of vaginitis show how easily germs gain access to this region, and as a fact, even in health, the different bacteria supposed to be the active agents in the phenomena of inflammation are present here; their attenuation is such that they are for the time harmless; how long they are to remain so, however, probably depends upon the possibility of finding a proper culture-medium. This may be found in the condition of the fluids of the body—a state as yet undetermined—or in the products of decomposition of retained blood or decidual material. The infection growing out of a combination of conditions here outlined is called "auto-infection," and auto-infection plays a prominent part in helping careless doctors and negligent nurses to escape responsibility. But, while we must admit such an origin for sepsis, it is established that auto-infection in the face of antiseptic or aseptic precautions is very rare, and if developed is of the milder type. Infection from without overshadows all other sources of sepsis, a fact which cannot be gainsaid, nor can its importance be overstated. Our present knowledge permits us to believe that in the absence of certain germs, introduced in general from without, the so-called causes of endometritis and metritis would be inoperative, or at most would produce simple destruction of tissue. This is in keeping with observations upon the surface and within its cavities, as illustrated in modern surgery. The agency of the gonococcus has been already indicated. Of greater importance, however, because more common and perhaps more virulent, are the microbes common to inflammations elsewhere, such as in the surgical infections in erysipelas, diphtheria, and in certain exanthems, as scarlet fever and measles. Bearing upon this subject are the very valuable deductions of S. W. Lambert and H. McM. Painter, to be found in their conjoint article on "Fever in the Puerperal Woman" (Report of the New York Lying-in Hospital, 1894). Under the head of so-called Surgical Infection (page 51), they say,—

"The nomenclature of wound-infection has become quite complicated, and various authors have designated distinct pathological processes by the same name. There are two grand divisions of this class of cases, according as there is simply an absorption of the chemical products of bacterial growth from the local seat of infection into the general system, or as there is added an invasion of the living tissues by living germs. These two conditions have been variously styled putrid intoxication and septic infection; wound intoxication and wound infection; sapræmia and septicæmia; but these terms are not precise enough. Instead of two divisions, there are four which the labors of Bumm prove to be possible, if not probable. Each of the above conditions may be caused by the germs of putrefaction or the pyogenic bacteria. We may therefore have a putrid or saprous absorption or a putrid or saprous invasion, and either would be sapræmia. The same is true of septicæmic processes. Either an absorption alone or in addition an invasion of the living tissues may result from a septic infection.

"Sapræmia may be caused by more than one species of bacterium. Rosenbach has described several, and Bumm has separated a distinct form which decomposes albuminous substances with the production of strong poisons and without the synchronous formation of odorous bodies.

"Sapræmia of puerperal origin uncomplicated by septicæmia is rarely met with. However, Braun von Fernwald found in a series of seven thousand six hundred labors one hundred and one cases which he describes under the name of endometritis puerperalis, but some few of these were evidently complicated by a general septicæmic invasion. Bumm, in eleven cases of putrid endometritis which appeared clinically to be uncomplicated by septic infection, failed to find pathogenic germs only three times, and he himself doubts the accuracy of his three negative observations. The most recent publication that has come to our notice, that of Von Franqué, also leads to the same conclusion. This author has investigated cases of post-partum fever with special reference to the etiology of mild cases. He found in eleven cases of mild fever pyogenic germs six times, gonococcus and *bacterium coli commune* each once, and had three negative results. In his six pyogenic cases, *streptococcus pyogenes*, either alone or in combination, occurred five times.

"Puerperal septicæmia also can be caused by a number of different germs. All of the pyogenic micrococci, acting separately or in various combinations with one another, have been proved to have caused puerperal sepsis. Of these, the *streptococcus*, styled *pyogenes* by Rosenbach, has been more lately christened, in view of its manifold manifestations, the *streptococcus septicus* by Bumm, and is certainly the most commonly present and the most virulent. This germ has been isolated from such cases by Pasteur and Doléris, and later by Döderlein, Haushalter, Widal, Bumm, Gärtner, and many others.

"The *staphylococcus pyogenes aureus* has been isolated by Steffeck from a fatal case of septicæmia, and the white variety has been proved by the same author to have been the causative agent in two similar cases. He describes two double infections also, one by *aureus* and *albus* together, and the other by *albus* combined with *streptococcus septicus*. Döderlein gives an account of an epidemic of three cases in which there was an infection by two germs, the *streptococcus septicus* and the *staphylococcus aureus*.

"Chantemesse has described an interesting case of fatal septic infection, originating from an attempt to produce abortion in a presumably pregnant, but really non-pregnant, uterus. *Streptococcus septicus* was found post mortem in pure culture throughout the tissues."

The *streptococcus pyogenes* or *septicus* being, then, the common agent in septic infection, it is interesting in this connection to note that the identity and interchangeability of the germ of erysipelas and this germ have been established. (Marboix.) The same may be said of the germ of croupous inflammation. Marboix says, " A varying virulence in the germ itself is at present assumed as a working hypothesis to account for the fact that a germ apparently the same will cause different pathological processes."

In accordance with this theory, it must be conceded that the *streptococcus pyogenes* in a state of extreme virulence will cause an erysipelas of the skin or a metritis, according as the infection takes place through the skin or through the endometrium. Touching diphtheria as a source, it appears that it has not been proved that its bacillus—"the Klebs-Loeffler"—has ever infected a puerperal wound; its associate germ, however, is indistinguishable, except by its action, from the other pathogenic streptococcus. The relation, therefore, appears to be similar to that of erysipelas; but, like erysipelas, it may—as in the throat, for instance—run its course as a local lesion, the puerperal wound escaping infection. The presence of the streptococcus as a constant element in the complications of scarlet fever and measles (the angina, the rhinitis, etc.) sufficiently explains the agency of these disorders as conveyers of septic infection.

Bearing in mind, then, the place held by these germs in the initiation of metritis and endometritis, we enumerate the conditions commonly viewed as primary causative agents, but which in reality should be viewed as subordinate factors, as predisposing causes rather. Violent congestion of the uterus, such as occurs in acute suppression of menstruation, and the prolonged congestion growing out of flexions and versions, especially when these malformations and malpositions are insured by the action of adhesions, are prominent factors in these lesions. The irritation of the organ incident to the action of stenosis in retarding the escape of purulent blood is another. The irritation of excessive copulation at the time of menstrual congestion may also be named. But potent for evil are accidents which may be classed under the head of traumatism.

Of these, the injuries inseparable from abortion and labor stand first in order of frequency and gravity. Close observations upon the agency of operations upon the cervix, which are presumably lacking in precautions against sepsis, are conclusive as to their influence, to which may be added the use of sounds improperly cleansed, and occasionally the action of excessively hot or cold douches, especially if taken at the time of menstruation.

The inflammation about the cervix due to ill-fitting or neglected pessaries may readily involve the deeper parts of the uterus, as, in fact, may any inflammation of the vagina, no matter how induced. Apart from the influence of agents associated with the exanthemata, already noticed in connection with the bacteriology of the subject, the specific germ of these diseases appears to be capable of inducing mild inflammatory changes upon the mucous membrane of the entire uterus.  These changes seem to be similar to those set up in other mucous tracts (the conjunctivæ, for instance, in measles), and, like them, tend to disappear with the subsidence of the disease. Lastly, we may refer to the action of diathesis and enfeebled states of the general health from any cause.  It corresponds here to their actions upon the body at large.  In scrofula, constitutional syphilis, extreme lithæmia, chlorosis, anæmic and scorbutic states, the resistance of the mucous tracts in general is lowered, so that agents of disease easily resisted under better conditions are here potent for evil.  The influence of such conditions in retarding cure is equally evident, impressing upon the practitioner the imperative necessity for constitutional as well as local measures of treatment.

Acute Endometritis.—*Pathology.*—The extent of the lesion is dependent upon the virulence and activity of the infecting element, and varies

FIG. 1.

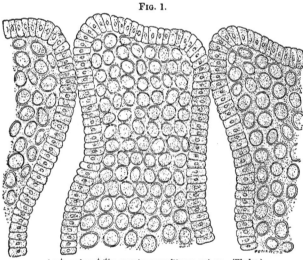

Acute endometritis; membranous dysmenorrhœa.  (Wyder.)

from a mild injection of the endometrium to a deep and wide-spread infiltration with the products of inflammation.  The material bathing the infected surface is likewise dependent upon the same kind of influence, being in mild cases merely a mucous or muco-purulent fluid, and in others purulent and even bloody.

The normal red color is deepened proportionately, till in severe cases it may be almost livid in hue.  The endometrium is thickened, softened, even pulpy at times.  The interglandular spaces show an increase of round cells, which in extreme cases are so abundant as to obliterate all the homogeneous intercellular substance, the whole having a resemblance to granulation tissue.  The epithelium of the glands is swollen, which fact, together with

the pressure of the surrounding densely-packed cells upon the glands themselves, serves to lessen and even obliterate the lumen of these organs in
many places.  The epithelial covering of the endometrium is infiltrated
and even destroyed in certain spaces, and the cilia in general may be said
to have shared a like fate.  The thickened mucous membrane is easily torn
from its attachment to the muscular wall, which, in turn, is swollen and
softened, the degree and depth of this change being again dependent upon
the nature and intensity of the infection.

Acute Metritis.—The implication of the muscular coat is slight,
except in some cases of gonorrhœal infection, in which a superficial serous
infiltration is witnessed.  The microscope reveals the usual swelling of the
muscular fibres and the increase of cell formation in the interspaces.  The
changes indicative of acute inflammation of the uterine wall are, however,

FIG. 2.

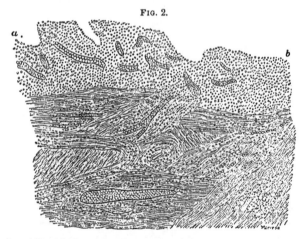

Acute septic metritis.  Slightly enlarged view of entire uterine wall.—a, b, surface of mucous membrane.  Below are seen sections of muscular bundles.  (Pozzi.)

most strikingly shown in uteri recently pregnant, as after abortion or labor
at term.  The inner surface is bathed with decidual detritus, which appears
as a thick, sanious material; the surface is ragged, especially at the serotina,
the ragged aspect being the more general prior to the formation of the
placenta.  The entire thickness of the uterine wall is more or less involved
in the inflammatory changes.  It is softened throughout, infiltrated with
serous or sero-purulent fluid, the muscular fibres show granular degenerative changes, the connective tissue is swollen, and the lymphatics and
lymph-spaces are filled with opaque, purulent fluid, containing micrococci.
The blood-vessels, especially in advanced states of pregnant development,
contain thrombi, which may be more or less infected with the micrococci
present in the lymphatics.  As bearing upon the question of the extension
of the inflammatory process, it is well in this connection to recall the extent

and distribution of the lymphatic supply of the uterus and its appendages. As is known, it is most abundant extending from the lateral surfaces of the uterus along two lines of connection to reach the general system. One chain departing from the cervix and lower part of the organ leaves the uterus at the lower half of the broad ligament; the other—the more important—leaves it along the upper border, where it freely connects with the lymphatic supply of the Fallopian tubes and ovaries. The intimate connection of the lymph-vessels of the tubes and ovaries, particularly the latter, with the chain of vessels coming from the uterus is especially worthy of note, in view of the frequent infection of the ovarian stroma, in these cases an infection often resulting in abscess-formation, and undoubtedly originating from absorption along these channels direct from the uterus, as well as from the more evident pathway, an inflamed Fallopian tube.

*Symptoms of Acute Endometritis and Metritis.*—Of necessity, the symptoms increase with the depth and extent of the lesion. In simple acute endometritis they may be comparatively insignificant. There will be a sense of fulness in the pelvis, which is more pronounced if there be arrest of the menstrual flow, but which is relieved should this flow come on; frequency of micturition, with some rectal tenesmus, may be present. There are no constitutional reactions beyond a slight malaise and want of appetite.

In more severe cases the above symptoms are pronounced, and in addition there are dull, deep-seated pelvic pain, backache referred to the upper sacral region, and aching pains down the inside of the thighs. All these local symptoms are increased by motion, by micturition, and by movement of the bowels. Slight febrile reaction will be present, with loss of appetite and a tendency to constipation.

*Septic cases,* such as may occur after improperly performed operations, or more especially after abortions and labors, present most aggravated and pronounced symptoms. The local symptomatic indications above noted are present, but are liable to be confounded with those of similar character dependent upon the unavoidable violence to which the organ may have been subjected; but no such confusion enters into the picture presented by the constitutional symptoms. Here a chill more or less pronounced ushers in the general disturbance. This is accompanied and followed by a rapid and decided rise in temperature, which lasts for a few hours, and then falls, to rise again at a later period. No absolute regularity pertains to the subsequent elevations of temperature, but, as a general thing, elevations are more frequent in the later hours of the day. If the inflammation extends to the peritoneal covering through the uterus, the phenomena of local peritonitis are directly added; if through the Fallopian tubes, the evidences of tubal disease appear, to be followed or accompanied by those of local peritonitis. General peritonitis with characteristic evidences may supervene, or this may not occur, and yet extreme symptoms indicative of septic absorption and constitutional infection may develop, such as would come from absorption of the poison through the lymphatics, or the scattering of infected thrombi through the body.  The ravages dependent upon an extension of disease through these channels of propagation belong to a subsequent portion of this subject, but are mentioned in order that their connection with the area of inflammation here treated of may not be overlooked.  The extension of a septic endometritis and metritis in cases of abortion and labor, in all the ways just indicated, is a common event in consequence of neglect, but in the non-pregnant uterus even a septic inflammation travels onward, as a rule, more easily by way of the tubes than through other channels, so that in such cases the phenomena of salpingitis and peritonitis are more pronounced than those of septic absorption alone.

Fortunately, these extreme symptoms do not belong to the history of the usual lesion of acute endometritis and metritis met with in the non-pregnant uterus.  Salpingitis and local peritonitis, with their particular evidences, may be said to represent the extreme of extension in such cases, the poison of gonorrhœa being responsible for the larger proportion of these.

*Signs.*—In the milder forms of this lesion touch reveals but slight change in the cervix.  If the disease begins within the organ, there may be none; if it be the extension of a vaginitis, the outer face of the cervix will have lost its velvety feeling, and be even roughened in the advanced stages of the disease.  Pressure upward upon the cervix causes pain, which is even more pronounced when the body of the organ is brought under conjoined palpation.  As a rule, the tenderness of the pelvic region is such that the uterus cannot be satisfactorily mapped out, but if it can be it will be found slightly enlarged.  In some instances the tenderness can be shown to be limited to the uterus proper, but this refinement need not be expected, because the tenderness is diffused over pretty much the entire pelvic area, lessening, however, as the examining finger leaves the uterus.  Inspection is of service only so far as the cervix is concerned.  The picture will differ with the point of origin of the disease.  When dependent upon vaginitis, the outer surface of the cervix will be deep red and covered with muco-purulent or purulent discharge.  This surface will ultimately present a granular appearance, made evident by wiping away the discharge.  It may bleed easily on touch.  The os externum will be patulous and its covering membrane œdematous and pouting.  Projecting from the canal will be a tough, glairy, opaque secretion, the product of the Nabothian glands.  When the disease starts in the uterine canal, the portio will present a nearly normal appearance.

In septic inflammations, especially such as follow operations, abortions, or labor, in addition to the traumatisms incident to such conditions, the cervix is much softened, enlarged, and of a deep red, even livid, color.  Flowing from it may be a thick, ichorous, bloody discharge which may or may not have the odor of decomposition.  These are especially pronounced features after abortion or labor.  In these latter conditions more particularly gray patches of necrosed tissue may sometimes be seen, the necrosed spots corresponding to the tears in the cervix. This is the so-called diphtheritic type of inflammation already noticed.

*Diagnosis.*—Proper inquiry into the symptoms and signs will always reveal this lesion in the non-pregnant uterus, and, with few exceptions, the same statement is true of the uterus after labors and abortions. Occasionally it begins so insidiously and with such a resemblance to malarial infection that one may be lulled into a sense of security; and if, as is often the case, no pain, no tenderness, and no odor of decomposition in the discharges be present, the deception may be complete. As a rule, such cases are of late development, but, early or late, they are dangerous. The free action of quinine should make the differentiation; but the writer prefers to view all these cases as evidences of uterine or of mammary inflammation, and if careful examination of the breasts fails to reveal the cause, then the uterus should be subjected to careful examination of its interior, and treatment. The mere absence of lochia from the vagina is a suspicious event in these cases, for it generally means retention, by reason of obstruction from flexure or other causes; but if it be present, its freedom from odor of decomposition is not a safe guide. The condition of the uterus as a whole is of some service, because arrest of involution is an accompaniment of all these lesions. Look, then, to the comparative dimensions and density of the uterus in all suspicious cases, and in view of the comparative innocuousness of proper antiseptic treatment of the interior of the uterus, it is safer in all such cases to take the risks of interference rather than those of delay. For reasons dependent upon the depth, the degree, and the rate of infection, twenty-four hours should be the outside limit of delay of this treatment.

*Prognosis.*—This presents itself under the twofold head of danger to life and danger to the integrity of the organ. In simple acute endometritis and metritis life is rarely endangered, but in the septic forms of the disease it commonly is, either through general peritonitis or through general septic infection.

The integrity of the organ is always endangered, but, of course, the danger is in proportion to the severity of the inflammatory process. Slight, if any, in the milder forms, it is pronounced in the graver. This results in part from the chronic changes in the uterus itself, the offspring of the severe acute processes, and in part from the implication of the adnexa and surroundings of the uterus,—implications (in the shape of tubal and ovarian disease and peritoneal adhesion) which may render impossible the return of the uterus to its normal state so long as they exist.

The bearing of all this upon menstruation and childbearing is self-evident. And it may be said in brief that the prognosis as regards life in the milder forms of this lesion is good, in the graver forms it is serious and may be very bad. As regards recovery of normal function and structure, it is largely dependent upon the resultant complications.

But here, as elsewhere, the question of prognosis turns as much upon treatment as upon the original nature of the disease, if not indeed more. Thanks to the principles of antisepsis, prompt and intelligent treatment improves to a wonderful degree the prognosis in all cases, no matter how grave the outset.   Delay is fatal.

Chronic Endometritis.—To the naked eye the mucous membrane is swollen and soft; in color it resembles quince jelly, with here and there lighter areas, and again spots even darker.   It is easily stripped from its attachment, after which it is seen that the muscular coat partakes of the congestion.   This may be marked through the entire organ; so much so, in fact, that upon section of the wall perpendicularly to the mucous surface it may be difficult to distinguish muscle from mucous membrane. But the softening of the mucous membrane so much exceeds that of the subjacent muscular tissue that it can be easily scraped off, leaving the latter comparatively intact.   The bearing of this fact upon the therapeutic use of the curette will be noted in the appropriate place.   The surface of the mucous membrane is irregular, presenting alternate projections and depressions.   These projections or fungosities may be quite large, of a round and elongated form, and may be veritable polypi, sessile or pedunculated.   In other cases there are small cysts resembling similar bodies met with in the cervix, having the same glandular origin, but containing a less viscid fluid.   This cystic formation is more frequent in aged subjects than in the young.

In cases where atrophy of the mucous membrane has resulted, the appearance of this membrane is similar to that which is seen as the result of senile atrophy.   Such surfaces are smooth and glistening, with here and there slight depressions.   The membrane is evidently very thin and transparent, indicating extreme atrophic change.

Microscopically, chronic endometritis presents itself as three types, which may appear separately or be combined in one and the same subject.   They are the interstitial, the glandular, and the polypoid.   In the interstitial form the interglandular tissue is transformed into cicatricial tissue, and as a result the glands are so compressed that in many places complete obliteration occurs (Fig. 3); in other places they are converted into cysts, a few appearing here and there, proportioned in number to the degree of the connective-tissue development.   Over the whole surface in extreme cases, and in spots in cases in which the process has reached its ultimate stage, such is the destruction of the mucous membrane that in its place little remains beyond a thin layer of sclerosed connective tissue, and this, in turn, is now covered by pavement epithelium, the general aspect of the surface being that noted above as occurring in senile atrophy.   Embedded in this sclerosed tissue, here and there, are cystic cavities, evidently the remains of constricted and degenerated glands.

In the glandular type of chronic endometritis the glands, without losing their normal structure, act the chief part.   There are two forms of this variety, one in which the glands are increased in their dimensions (hypertrophic), another in which there is an actual increase in the quantity of gland tissue (hyperplastic). In the former the glands no longer appear as a series of straight tubes, but are twisted, elongated, and arranged spirally. In the second form not only does one find an increase in the number of the glands, but they are distorted, and here and there present lateral prolongations or diverticulæ. It is probable that all cases of glandular endometritis present a combination, in varying proportion, of these two forms of degeneration.

FIG. 3.

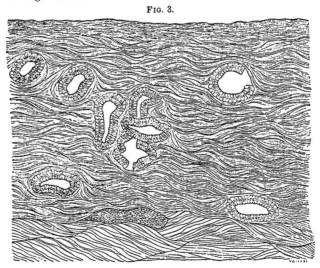

Interstitial endometritis, with partial atrophy of the glands. (Wyder.)

The third type of this lesion—chronic polypoid endometritis—is that in which the mucous membrane presents the villous projections or vegetations already noted. Histologically, it is a combination of the interstitial and glandular varieties, with marked cystic formation, together with great increase of the vessels, both in number and in dimensions, and of the interglandular structure. The cysts, as in the interstitial variety, are the remains of occluded and degenerated glands, and are present in greater numbers at the surface of the membrane than in its deeper portions; here they are more nearly normal in structure, but yet are deflected so that they run obliquely or even parallel to the subjacent muscular structure. They may even extend beyond their usual limitations and dip down between the muscular fibres. In some parts of the field it will be noted around the cysts and around the intact glands, deep down in the mucous membrane, that the normal interglandular substance is replaced by a homogeneous tissue. The marked increase of the vascular area in this variety is of consequence in connection with its clinical behavior, hemorrhage (menorrhagia) being the striking symptomatic feature of such cases. (Fig. 4.)

In connection with this last variety of chronic endometritis is a form resulting from the retention of portions of the decidua (vera or serotina), after abortion chiefly, but occasionally after labor at term.   The retained tissue presents itself as a projection or projections from the general surface of the mucous membrane, of deeper hue than the surrounding surface; it is soft, and is easily detached from the subjacent muscular structure.   Microscopically, it is distinguishable by the presence of decidual tissue which has undergone degenerative change and is surrounded with a mass of small cells.   In general, it may be said to approach in type the interstitial variety of chronic endometritis, but clinically it presents a tendency to the polypoid form, in that it is generally indicated by profuse menstrual flow.

FIG. 4.

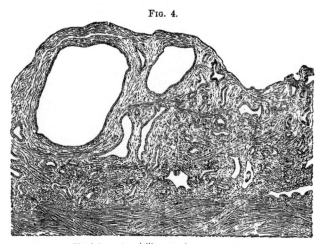

Glandular endometritis, polypoid form.   (Wyder.)

Diphtheritic endometritis, like its prototype in the vagina, is really the result of a gangrenous change, and is found in connection with septicæmia, or after severe local injury, or as a result of ordinary inflammation in old people.

Chronic Metritis.—It is clearly impossible for changes such as we have just depicted to continue for any length of time without more or less implication of the deeper portions of the uterine wall; but, apart from such influences, the uterus derives chronic and wide-spread alteration from the remaining influences of a prior acute process, which has its origin in the septic inflammations, abortions, and labors.   We have already called attention to these, so that we are in position to present a picture of chronic metritis, no matter whether it be secondary to a chronic inflammation of the endometrium or to the more extended influence of a prior septic acute metritis or endometritis.   Speaking first of the form which appears to spring from, or is perhaps the companion of, chronic endometritis, we find that there is neither infiltration nor induration. In the first, the uterus is softened, the vessels are dilated, encroaching upon the adjacent tissues, so that on section an areolar appearance is presented, embryonal nuclei abound, but above all there is a marked increase in the connective tissue of the organ. It is doubtful if there is any increase of muscular tissue in this form,—such, for instance, as exists in subinvolution, to be mentioned later. In other cases dilatation of the lymph-spaces has been observed, and marked increase of the perivascular connective tissue, with consequent thickening of the walls of the blood-vessels and diminution of their calibre, the net result being sclerosis of a special kind. (Fig. 5.)

FIG. 5.

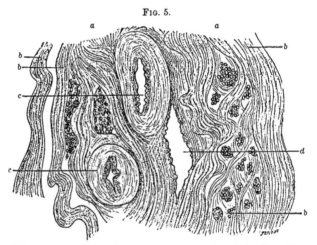

Chronic metritis.—*a, a*, muscular tissue traversed by bands of smooth connective tissue; *b, b*, connective tissue; *c, c*, vessels with thickened walls; *d*, lymph-space. (Pozzi.)

As might be inferred, the stage of induration is marked by thickening of the walls, due to a new formation of connective tissue which displaces the muscular structure. This latter structure is pale, and is crossed by opaque lines which are thickened and sclerotic arterioles undergoing similar degeneration. The connective-tissue formation is most marked about the vessels, veins as well as arteries, and the hardening of the structure is due not so much to cicatricial contraction of the connective tissue as to an actual increase in its volume.

The changes in the mucous membrane which accompany these alterations in the walls of the uterus are some one or more of the forms already noted.

From what has been said under the heads of pathology and etiology, it is evident that metritis may be complicated and aggravated by such conditions as inflammation of the adnexa, peritonitis, displacements, with or without adhesions, and stenosis of the canal; and it is improbable that many cases would long remain free from these attendants, though without such complications at the outset of the process.

Returning now to that state of the uterus which is the outcome of a production of involution by septic inflammation especially, but which is also due at times to more serious causes, we find that there is a transition from the state of normal fatty degeneration of the tissues, with its accompanying softness of structure, to one of induration, due to the presence of an abnormal amount of connective tissue. This indicates that for a time a double process is going on in the uterus,—fatty degeneration of the superabundant tissues, especially of the muscular and vascular structures, and the creation of new connective-tissue elements, the ultimate result being, as in the more clearly defined lesion of chronic metritis, a diminution of the muscular structure, a large increase of connective tissue, an hypertrophy of the endometrium, induration of the organ as a whole, and an arrest of its return to normal dimensions.

Although the pathological process is thus seen to differ in some essential particulars from that seen in ordinary chronic metritis, yet the ultimate outcome, especially in the face of complicating inflammations of adjacent structures (tubes, ovaries, and peritoneum), will be much the same. The clinical and therapeutic bearings of this lesion (subinvolution) being also similar to those in chronic metritis *per se*, a consideration of the condition in this connection seems appropriate; and it would also seem to be a proper place in which to speak of hyperinvolution,—a rare occurrence, but one which is seen as a result of normal involution carried beyond the physiological limit; a condition likewise seen in cases of chronic metritis which have been subjected to the depletion incident to curettage and extreme distention of the cavity with gauze packing. It is generally temporary, the loss of tissue being usually soon regained, but cases following parturition have been reported in which the condition became permanent. The uterus is decidedly reduced in size, and its walls are hardened, the condition being, in all probability, dependent upon cicatricial contraction of connective tissue.

Just here we may say that the causes are obscure, and that its permanent form is one which is very difficult to treat successfully.

**Cervicitis and Endocervicitis.**—Inflammations of the cervix exist independently of like lesions in the body of the uterus, the position of the cervix exposing it to disease to a far greater extent than the deeper portions of the organ; yet the two parts of the organ are so often involved that at first it would seem unnecessary to consider the lesions of the two sections of the organ separately. This applies with special force to the acute processes, especially those derived from gonorrhœa, as septic infection. It does not apply, however, to the chronic forms of the disease, because in the milder forms the cervix is frequently involved, and yet there is no implication of the deeper parts of the uterus. The appearance presented by the cervix in acute inflammation depends upon the direction from which the infecting element acts. In gonorrhœal infection we have already noted the appearance of the vaginal face of this structure: the mucous membrane of the canal is swollen and softened, and its cavity is filled with a viscid, muco-purulent secretion. This secretion protrudes from the os externum, from which it is difficult to remove it, owing to its glue-like tendency to adhere to the surface from which it is derived. The deeper portions of the cervical structure, if involved at all, show serous infiltration of the connective-tissue spaces, softening of the connective and muscular tissues, and an increase in the calibre of the vessels. In cases of septic infection due to the introduction of dirty instruments a similar appearance will be found.

These observations apply to the uninjured cervix. Where this tissue has been bruised and lacerated, as in abortions and labors, or where it has been incised, as in operations, the exudate in the canal, while partaking of the viscidity above mentioned, is somewhat fluid and is tinged with blood.

The appearance presented by the deeper portions of the cervix, in the conditions just mentioned, is in all respects similar to that met with under corresponding conditions in the body of the uterus. Where the septic process is extreme in its destructive action, the cut or torn places in this structure may be covered by the usual whitish coating, due to superficial necrosis.

When one bears in mind the arrangement of the mucous membrane of the cervix, and the number and depth of its folds, it is easy to realize the frequency of chronic infection here. It is especially easy to realize the ease with which gonorrhœa here finds a hiding-place, so that long after the subsidence of the process in the region below its poison remains here, keeping up the phenomena of a chronic inflammation which, in some respects, has been compared to gleet in the opposite sex. The cervix may be the seat of a superficial chronic inflammation of its lining membrane; it may be enlarged from chronic congestion, or from hypertrophy; it may be torn, as in childbirth; and, when torn, the entire lacerated cervix, together with the mucous membrane of the canal, may be everted, and covered with what may seem to be a granulating surface, but which is really epithelium, derived from an extension of that which belongs to the canal. Cystic formations upon all the surfaces of the cervix are common. The cysts are found to be distended glands of Naboth, filled with the characteristic colloid secretion; these becoming inflamed, the wall breaks down, the contents are discharged, and a deep, inflamed excavation remains. In chronic endocervicitis there will be a viscid, white-of-egg discharge at the os externum. The mucous membrane is everted at the os externum. It is deep red, forming a marked contrast with the adjacent surrounding and external face of the cervix. At first this everted structure is smooth, but soon it assumes a granular appearance. Microscopically, it is an infiltrated, congested tissue upon which the cylindrical epithelium has given place to pavement epithelium.

This brings us to the consideration of the so-called ulcers or erosions of the cervix. True ulcers of the cervix are rare, being found principally in connection with syphilitic disease, but occasionally there may be an entire disappearance of the epithelium. What is usually spoken of as "ulceration" is in reality a deep-red surface of varying dimensions, covered by a single layer of long, narrow epithelial cells, so transparent as to permit the subjacent vascular tissue, which is largely increased, to show through: hence the red and in some cases even cock's-comb appearance of this structure. This surface is thrown into numerous folds, the result being the creation of recesses which, because of the epithelial lining, become

FIG. 6.

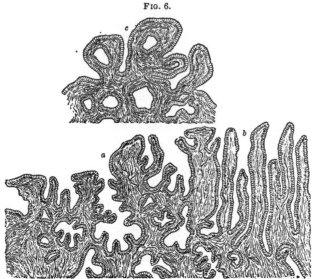

Erosion of the cervix.—*a*, *b*, simple papillary erosion; *c*, follicular, slightly enlarged. (Pozzi.)

of a glandular nature. The convexities of the folds stand out as processes, producing the glandular or papillary appearance of the surface. The processes are not merely upheavals of epithelial tissue, but have a connective-tissue basis, and are in time provided with a radical vessel. The deeper and more narrow the recesses are, the more clearly differentiated become the processes, so that in certain cases the latter figure as papillæ, giving us the papillary erosion, which is merely an exaggeration of the granular erosion. (Fig. 6.) In such cases the recesses become virtually racemose glands, the epithelium furnishing the secreting surface. In some cases these processes coalesce near the outer extremity, thus obliterating what has become the opening of the gland. The secretion continuing, a retention cyst is produced, which may increase in size, approach the surface, and, bursting, leave an eroded, follicular depression, giving us the follicular erosion.  This red papillary or granular surface is, then, really a newly-formed glandular secreting surface resembling somewhat the cervical mucous membrane.

In connection with the above superficial changes there is an increase in the connective tissue of the deeper parts of the cervix, and, as a result, a general enlargement of this body.  The secretions in obstructed glands may become inspissated.  These glands are then felt as hard nodules scattered throughout the superficial portions of the cervix.  In pregnancy the glands of the cervix are so enormously increased that catarrh developing after that process is more prone to glandular implication, with the resulting production of nodules and follicular ulcerations, than under other circumstances.  Large single cysts in the cervix are uncommon, but when present are due to an obstruction of a mucous gland.

FIG. 7.

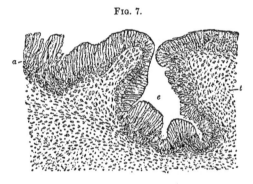

Chronic inflammation of the mucous membrane of the portio, × 200 diam.—a, superficial epithelial laver, formed of cylindrical cells much elongated; e, interpapillary depression; t, connective tissue. (Cornil.)

Lacerations of the cervix exercise a potent influence upon cervical disease, but this, after all, is largely dependent upon the degree of infection which is present.

In the absence of infection, here as elsewhere, it is possible for such repair to occur as will leave the tissues free from disease.  Such good union may take place between the surfaces as greatly to obliterate even extreme tears, or the surfaces, remaining apart, may receive so good a covering of pavement epithelium as to approach in appearance very nearly to the standard of the vaginal cervical surface.  In consequence of infection after the subsidence of the acute process, even the slighter tears will present a true granulating surface, similar in appearance and anatomy to that presented in the so-called erosions above described.  Cylindrical epithelium, the product of the adjacent glands of the lining membrane of the cervix, will extend over the surface; this surface, thrown into folds, will present the papillary appearance and structure already mentioned.  This development may be so exuberant as to give a veritable cock's-comb appearance, suggesting even epithelioma, but the comparative softness of the growth is usually sufficient to permit a clinical differentiation. Eversion of the torn surfaces is generally present, and now and then, in the case of extreme tears, the ectropion is so great as to evert almost the whole surface. The condition is largely dependent upon the degree of inflammatory infiltration of the subjacent cervical structure.

These observations relate to lacerations which involve the entire thick-ness of the cervical wall, from canal to vaginal face; but there are tears which, involving the entire length of the cervix, stop short of the outer coat; these may present, from like causes, changes similar to those so evident when eversion exists. The eversion is prevented in these cases by the restraining action of this external coat. The os externum is of course enlarged, and the cervix as a whole is increased in its circumference; the rents with intervening ridges may be traced by touch, and even by sight in some cases, well into the depths of the canal. As has been intimated, the result of these tears is dependent upon the degree of infection to which they may be subjected. When infection is controlled or avoided, they may heal throughout, the integrity of the cervix being in large measure restored; but when infected, especially if it be seriously, the resulting infiltration and subsequent development of cicatricial contraction will exercise a bad influence upon the cervix and even upon the body of the organ. Take for instance an infected tear extending into the vaginal wall or even to the cervico-vaginal junction: first there is arrest of involution in the cervix and body; then come the after-effects, which in the cervix are summed up in the after-contraction of the connective tissue, causing sclerosis of tissue, occlusion of glands with subsequent formation of cysts, and the development of sensitive cicatrices in the angles of the wound. When the laceration extends to the vagina, the subsequent contraction of the line of the tear will displace the cervix to that side, and, by putting a check upon the mobility of the uterus, lead to injury by dragging upon it when it is moved by any of the influences commonly acting. Finally, the fact that these torn surfaces are not only exposed to all the vicious elements which may gain access to the vagina or come from the uterus, but, through rupture of the perineum, may be directly exposed to the air, explains the frequent development upon these surfaces of the extreme granular changes described.

*Symptoms of Chronic Metritis and Endometritis.—Leucorrhœa.*—When the lesion is confined to the cervix (especially to the lining membrane) and is of short duration, the case may be free of all symptoms except a vaginal discharge. This, however, is in some degree characteristic. In the first place, it is not continuous, nor, in the absence of vaginal implications, is it abundant. It is viscid and jelly-like, and is transparent, opaque, or yellowish, according to the amount of purulent admixture.

In the presence of cervical laceration together with the erosions already described, this secretion is accompanied and mixed with a more abundant muco-purulent discharge, the leucorrhœa, under such circumstances, being a more constant quantity. The viscid discharge is the product of the Nabothian glands, and the muco-purulent one comes from mucous glands and from the eroded surfaces. The effect of long continuance of these discharges, especially in fat women, may be the induction of a simple but annoying vulvitis, and in time the draught upon the system at large may, in any case, evince itself by some deterioration of the general health, a matter to be explained more in detail as we unfold the symptoms of the graver forms of these chronic inflammations of the uterus.

In the deeper-seated implications of the cervix, such as congestion and enlargement, even though there be but little discharge, distinct, though not characteristic, symptoms will be present; they are dull lumbo-sacral pain and perhaps reflex nervous symptoms, such as neuralgias and even mild hysteria. These neuroses are said to be present in marked degree in such cases of laceration of the cervix as present dense cicatrices in the angles of the tear.

The conditions of the cervix which act as causes of a more extended symptomatology than has been given are so intermixed with the lesions of chronic metritis and endometritis that it is difficult, if not impossible, to say where the influence of the one begins and that of the other stops. As most, if not all, of these symptoms may spring from the body of the organ, and as they are present even though the cervix be but little involved, it is surely better to give them as indicative of disorders of the body rather than of the neck alone. With this understood, we present the following as indicative of chronic inflammations of the uterus:

The leucorrhœal discharge is practically the same as that noticed just above. In senile cases, and sometimes in younger subjects, the "white-of-egg" Nabothian secretion is absent, or is present in very small amount; the discharge in senile cases may be free and purulent. In the most common cases, however,—that is, in cases developed during the years of greatest menstrual activity,—the discharge is a mixture of viscid and muco-purulent secretion, the major portion of the latter coming from the uterus.

In the atrophic metritis which so often follows removal of the adnexa, a muco-purulent discharge, sometimes profuse, is common; it is constant for a year or more; then, again, it may occur at intervals of days and sometimes of as much as two weeks, lasting three, four, and five hours, or a day or two, and then ceasing. These latter cases differ from the forms complicated with salpingitis, in which there may be a sudden intermittent discharge of a quantity of purulent or watery fluid.

These last are instances of pyo- or hydrosalpinx discharging their contents through the uterine end of the tube, but may represent cases already operated upon in which considerable portions of tube have been improperly left behind, the stumps becoming sacculated.

*Pain.*—The lumbo-sacral pain, already noted, is a prominent feature in metritis, and it may radiate down the thighs. Dull, persistent, deep-seated pelvic pain is also present, or rather a sense of deep-seated pelvic fulness, extending perhaps even to the perineum. The patient feels as though some heavy body was located here, and that it would be a relief to expel it. If the organ be weighty and anteverted, there is frequency in micturition and perhaps even vesical distress, such as is felt early in pregnancy. If the uterus be retroverted, there may be mechanical constipation, the result of pressure upon the rectum, and pain along the sciatic nerves, the result of pressure upon the sciatic plexus. Stair-climbing, prolonged standing, continuous walking, and especially the joltings of a rough ride, increase the pain. It is also increased during the premenstrual congestion and lessened after the flow. To these local discomforts distant neuralgic pains may be added ; for instance, occipital headache, as in the metritis accompanying retroversion. Occasionally we also find intercostal and lumbo-abdominal neuralgias, coccygodynia, and even facial neuralgias.

*Menstruation.*—This function is not necessarily affected, but it usually is, the departure from the normal consisting in pain (dysmenorrhœa), in excessive flow (menorrhagia, metrorrhagia), in an altered flow (blood-clots or an endometrial exfoliation), and sometimes in diminished flow. Dysmenorrhœa is found in connection with cervical stenosis or flexure ; also as an accompaniment of excessive flow (menorrhagia) and in conjunction with exfoliation of the endometrium (membranous dysmenorrhœa). In all these conditions the pain is an expression of the uterine effort to free its cavity of the blood, or, as in exfoliative endometritis, of the membrane. In stenosis the flow is retarded by obstruction in the cervical canal, usually at its upper third, and this obstruction may be a congenital narrowing quite independent of such as may result from a flexion, or it may be the result of a flexion or of a version. When present in connection with menorrhagia, the condition underlying the pain is less a state of menstrual obstruction than one of rapid overfilling of the inflamed cavity with blood, which, undergoing coagulation, presents itself as a solid body that must be forced out by uterine contractions, the result being, after all, similar to actual stenosis.

The pain of membranous exfoliation is practically the same as this last, but generally it is more severe, resembling more nearly that which prevails in early abortions, with which it has been, through carelessness, confounded, the uterus in both cases casting off and forcibly expelling a membrane.

Menorrhagia and metrorrhagia are generally expressions of the vegetative or polypoid forms of chronic endometritis, or of that which accompanies the retention of bits of decidual tissue. Menorrhagia is common about the menopause, and occasionally occurs also in conjunction with the establishment of menstruation in the young.

A striking development of metrorrhagia, as a part of the clinical picture of chronic changes in the cervix, is found in conjunction with polypi springing from the cervical canal, these bodies having a tendency to a constant oozing of blood. Intermittent bleedings are frequently present as an expression of the changes set up in the uterus by removal of the appendages ; but the flow, under these circumstances, is no longer the menstrual exudation, but is virtually a hemorrhage. The most striking development of a menorrhagia, however, is in conjunction with the endometritis of submucous fibroid growths.

The changes in the character and in the amount of the menstrual flow, above noted, are those commonly met with, but another feature is occasionally added, and that is the presence of shreds of hypertrophic mucous membrane. There may even be a complete cast of the inner surface of the uterine body, the entire thickened structure being cast off, as a part of the phenomena of menstruation. These are instances of exfoliative endometritis, already noted in connection with dysmenorrhœa.

The hemorrhages which may thus result from a chronic endometritis sometimes end in such continual losses that the patient may be brought to an extreme degree of anæmia, with all the accompanying results of anæmia to the nervous, circulatory, and digestive systems. Amenorrhœa can hardly be said to result from the lesion under discussion, but in certain rare cases, where extensive atrophy of the mucous membrane prevails, the flow is apt to be scanty.

Sterility is a common accompaniment of the chronic inflammations of the uterus, a fact easily comprehended when we remember the several obstacles, first, to impregnation, and then to proper decidual growth, presented in its lesions. The devitalizing and obstructive influences of morbid cervical secretions upon the spermatozoa seem to be fairly established, and though the fecundated ovum may plant itself successfully upon the endometrium, the pathological processes there at work often prevent the formation of a proper decidua, leading to imperfect development, death, and ultimate expulsion (abortion).

The relation existing between the uterus and the stomach, through the nervous system, is so clearly displayed in pregnancy that it should not be surprising that we find digestive disturbance a common factor in the symptomatology of prolonged inflammation of this organ. In fact, so pronounced is the influence of the uterus upon the stomach that dilatation of this latter organ is said to be a sequela of prolonged metritis. Loss of appetite, nausea, chronic flatulence, and constipation are common, the result being, even in the absence of other drains, a decided loss to the general health.

In speaking of symptoms which appear to relate to cervical tears, allusion was made to neuralgias and hysteria. Such manifestations, confined usually to women of sensitive, nervous organization, are even more pronounced in advanced chronic metritis, taking on many different forms. Globus hystericus, a persistent, metallic cough without expectoration, and sometimes even hystero-epilepsy, may be present, and chorea and even pure epilepsy have been said to spring from chronic metritis.

A review of the symptoms of chronic metritis which we have given will be seen to contain nothing distinctive of the condition, unless it be found in those which pertain to the menstrual function. Aside from these, the symptoms might be the exponents of other chronic disorders, but the grouping of the whole is fairly characteristic. And if we add the physical signs, a diagnosis can always be made.

*Physical Signs.* — *Palpation; Lesions of the Cervix.* — These may be summarized as follows: enlargement, erosions, and cysts without lacerations, and the same conditions with lacerations.

The enlargements are recognized by the apparent shortening of the cervix. Instead of the length of this structure being as great as or greater than the diameter, we find what seems to be a change in this relation, the diameter even at the lower portion being as great as or greater than the length. The conoidal shape of the structure is consequently, in general, lost.

If erosions be present, they are revealed by soft inequalities in a surface which normally is smooth. The external os is patulous, and in the event of a polypoid projection from the canal this will be felt as a small rounded body filling the external os or projecting from it. Where cysts are present, they can be felt as small, hard, round nodules embedded in the softer cervical tissue.

The tears in the cervix are easily appreciated, and their extent can be determined better by touch than by any other means; and the indurations belonging to the lacerated surfaces are discovered by the relatively hard, gristly resistance met with. The irregularities of the eroded surfaces are here even more apparent than where lacerations are wanting, and the deep-seated cysts are also plainly revealed as the round, hard nodules already mentioned.

The sensitive spots in the angles of the tears are brought out by direct pressure, and the remains of the lacerations extending outward from the cervix are marked by the rigid band of cicatricial tissue which the healing process generally leaves behind in the vault of the vagina.

*Lesions of the Uterus.* — Touch shows nothing but a general enlargement of the uterus, an exception being in superinvolution, where it is found to be small. Generally the organ, as a whole, is tender on pressure. Pressure upward upon the cervix is especially painful, and the same symptom is brought out by rocking the uterus from side to side by alternate quick pressure upon the two sides of the cervix.

In the absence of complicating disease of the adnexa, the utero-sacral ligaments, and the peritoneal surroundings, the organ is freely movable, but it may be lower in the pelvis as the patient stands, and may fall forward (anteverted) if the enlargement be pronounced. On the contrary, in the recumbent posture the fundus of the organ may sink back towards the sacrum. In subinvolution and sometimes in conjunction with retroversion and retroflexion the organ is softer than normal, in superinvolution and in chronic metritis of long standing it is harder.

These alterations in the dimensions and perhaps in the density of the organ may be made out by conjoined vaginal palpation; but if not, then conjoined rectal palpation will reveal them, the uterus in this form of examination being caught at the cervix with a tenaculum and drawn well downward so as to permit easy access to its posterior surface.

*Inspection.*—This is made upon the back by means of a bivalve speculum, or upon the side by means of a Sims speculum, the latter affording the better view. It reveals but little relating to the body of the organ, as might be inferred, but upon the condition of the cervix it throws much light. The enlargement filling the depths of the vagina is apparent, also the loss of the conical form. The red erosions are shown, and the patulous os, with the transparent, or more often opaque or even purulent, string of ropy discharge protruding from the canal. The lacerations are revealed, though less clearly defined than by touch, even though the lips be separated by tenacula, and the wide extent of red, exuberant erosions which is sometimes present in such cases comes plainly into view. The yellowish cysts showing through the eroded surface will give it a spotted appearance. Here and there where a cyst has discharged its contents a deep excoriation appears (folliculitis). As to the general appearance of the cervix, that depends upon the existence or non-existence of erosions and upon the state of its circulation. The eroded surfaces are redder than the normal tissue, and vary from deep pink to deep red. The secretion present upon the vaginal aspect, which may be whitish or yellowish, according to the degree of inflammatory change present, will obscure the face of the cervix in proportion to its amount, but after wiping it away the appearances above noted will be revealed.

Information concerning the condition of the interior of the uterus is obtained by means of the sound. This instrument should be introduced into the uterus only after careful antiseptic precautions. The outer face of the cervix and the cervical canal should be carefully cleansed, and then a thoroughly disinfected sound may be passed into the organ. By means of this instrument we acquire information as to the general dimension of the uterine canal, and, consequently, of the organ as a whole. The canal may measure as much as three and three-fourths or four inches. Care should be taken in this measurement to place the point of the sound about midway between the cornua, so as to avoid an oblique measurement of the canal. This can be done by fixing the uterus with a tenaculum, and then locating the cornual depressions, a feat easily accomplished. In cases of metritis characterized by menorrhagia, those dependent upon retained decidua being generally an exception, the internal os is apt to be contracted and perhaps even indurated; in other forms the entire cervical canal is, as a rule, enlarged, the exceptions here being in cases of congenital stenosis and in flexions. In most cases a sensitive spot is met with at the internal os, particularly in congenital stenosis, and occasionally the fundus is markedly sensitive. As a rule, the sound conveys but little information as to the state of the endometrium, unless it be by the induction of bleeding in the decidual and other hemorrhagic forms; sometimes the inequalities of the surface present, for instance, in a variety of the polypoid form in which more than the usual amount of induration of the sessile growths has occurred, can be appreciated.

**Acute Endometritis and Metritis.**—*Diagnosis.*—In the non-pregnant uterus this lesion is indicated by the tenderness of the organ, by the discharge from the cervix, taken in conjunction with the comparative suddenness of an attack developed in connection with an acute suppression of menstruation, with a prior vaginitis, or with some such cause as an operation upon the cervix or the introduction of a sound.

After an abortion or labor it is commonly indicated by a chill or chilly sensations, followed by rise of temperature, and a temporary arrest of the lochia, with its subsequent reappearance, at which time it may have an odor of decomposition. Tenderness of the organ is rarely present at first, but it generally appears in a few hours, or perhaps not for a day or two. Subsequently the organ loses its firmness, becoming soft. But, in view of the insidious nature of this lesion, it cannot be too often repeated that cases of septic endometritis and metritis after abortion and labor may develop to an extreme degree,—to a point, in fact, at which a fatal termination is almost certain, no matter what treatment may be adopted,—and yet neither unusual pain, nor tenderness in or about the uterus, nor the odor of decomposition in the discharges be present. Under such circumstances the diagnosis must rest upon the antecedent condition and the symptoms, taken in conjunction with the loss of firmness which the uterus suffers.

Such cases may be confounded with typhoid or malarial fevers. In view of the absolute necessity for the most prompt treatment, early diagnosis is imperative. If the case be one of pure malarial type, quinine will control it absolutely; but if not, and especially if it belong to typhoid infection, quinine will not. The differences in the rise and fall of temperature in the two conditions may not be so well marked at the outset as materially to aid differentiation, and, as every other diagnostic characteristic may be absent, it is always wiser to assume the presence of septic infection and act accordingly.

Localized mastitis is another source of error, but careful examination of the breasts will suffice for the diagnosis.

Lastly, the sudden onset of an acute cystitis has been known as a source of error. This condition, however, can be so easily discovered by a proper examination of the bladder and urine that it need only be mentioned to insure its elimination as a source of error.

**Chronic Endometritis and Metritis.**—Pregnancy has been mentioned as a condition with which the lesions may be confounded, but this could never happen in the face of a proper examination; the essential differences in the symptoms and signs would quickly determine which condition was present. The only real embarrassment possible would be in the rare instance of chronic metritis with amenorrhœa. If the amenorrhœa be due to changes in the uterus, this organ would show atrophy, unless it be about the period of the menopause, when pregnancy is improbable. If the absence of menstruation be due to general causes, such as anæmia or obesity, these conditions will be evident; upon the other hand, if pregnancy be present, even though the stomach-symptoms be unreliable and the breast-changes uncertain, yet careful palpation of the uterus (by rectum, if necessary) will always reveal the globular outline of the uterine body and its peculiarly elastic resistance, a form of resistance which is in marked contrast with the state of the cervix, a contrast never present in metritis, where the resistance met with in the body is much the same as that met with in the cervix. After the eighth week of pregnancy every possibility of error disappears.

The condition presented by commencing fibroid disease in a uterus is one, however, which may easily confuse the observer, a confusion all the more possible in view of the constant presence of some form of endometritis in all such cases, generally the hemorrhagic variety. If the fibroid disease be interstitial, and more especially if it be subperitoneal, conjoined rectal examination, conducted with the uterus fixed and drawn down by a tenaculum or volsella, will reveal the inequalities of the outer surface, even though there be but little enlargement of the uterus as a whole, with but slight projection of the growths above the surface. But if the growths or growth be wholly submucous, such inequalities will not appear. The body of the organ, however, will still be as hard as or harder than in metritis, and more globular. The sound may detect the growth, provided it can be introduced, and, if it be introduced, provided it be manipulated in conjunction with a finger in the rectum, the uterus being fixed and drawn down, as above mentioned. Having the sound in the uterus, the points to be noted are these: in metritis the point of the instrument can be moved easily from cornu to cornu, where it can be readily and equally felt; such ease of motion to these points and equality of appreciation thereat will scarcely be found in the case of submucous fibroid. But if, after this examination, doubt should still exist, nothing remains but dilatation of the cervix by tents and digital exploration of the cavity. This will be conclusive.

Mucous polypi are discovered by the use of the sharp curette, or, better, by Emmet's double curette; and the same may be said of decidual débris or formations.

The hemorrhagic form of the lesion under discussion might be confounded with early abortion, especially if the former were presented in conjunction with membranous exfoliation (membranous dysmenorrhœa); but the antecedent history of the case, together with a careful examination of all the extruded membranes, will suffice for the differentiation.

The differentiation of certain forms of corporeal and cervical inflammatory lesions from carcinoma is a matter of pressing urgency, for the evident reason that prompt action is of vital importance in carcinoma, every day's delay only rendering doubtful so happy a result as cure in so terrible a disease. It is with the hemorrhagic forms of chronic metritis that perplexity most frequently arises, and of these the menorrhagiæ of the menopause are those about which doubt most often centres,—a fact well known to the profession, but, unfortunately, less clearly remembered by the laity, or perhaps less clearly applied to their own personality. As already intimated, the diagnosis, to be of service, must be made early. The clinical features of a severe case of hemorrhagic metritis and commencing carcinoma of the endometrium are insufficient for early diagnosis. Here the free use of the sharp curette and a careful microscopic examination of the scrapings are of service; but, even though this be inconclusive, the persistent return of the hemorrhages in anything like their original force, after two or more thorough curettings, cauterizing, and packing of the uterine cavity (see Treatment), should be ground sufficient to assume the presence of commencing carcinoma of the body (fibroid disease being excluded), and, in view of the comparative safety of vaginal hysterectomy, the uterus should be removed. The late differentiation of corporeal carcinoma is sufficiently easy to require no special mention here.

The inflammatory lesions of the cervix which simulate carcinoma are generally those which seem to stand in causative relation to that disease,— viz., lacerations of the cervix, with extensive erosions. The crucial test is to remove a piece of the tissue and examine a section under the microscope. This can always be done, and should never be omitted in doubtful cases. A profuse serous and blood-stained leucorrhœa is almost characteristic of cervical carcinoma, and so are the hard, exuberant, cauliflower excrescences springing from the vaginal aspect of the everted cervix. The hard and nodular base of some of these eroded, lacerated surfaces, which is due to the combined development of sclerosis and cysts, may deceive one at first, but puncture of the cysts and free incision of the surface will soon soften such tissue and reveal its true nature.

Where the carcinoma begins within a cervix whose canal, including the external os, is intact, doubt may exist for a time; but the serous and bloody character of the discharge and the relative hardness of the whole cervix should prompt one to excise a part of the lining membrane and submit it to the microscope. Such a course will always remove doubt.

The differentiation of the forms of metritis dependent upon or associated with disease of the adnexa or peritoneal adhesions can be best understood if presented in connection with those disorders. We therefore refer the reader to the part of this article which deals with them; and as to the confusion which may arise from disorders of the rectum or the bladder, this may exist if symptoms only be considered; if signs be consulted, however, no confusion need prevail. An examination of the several organs will quickly tell the true story.

Finally, as to the differentiation (one from the other) of the several forms of chronic metritis.

The polypoid form is generally characterized by menorrhagia and metrorrhagia, the other forms less by hemorrhage than by muco-purulent and purulent discharges. The differentiation of the hemorrhagic form due to the retention of pieces of decidua is dependent upon the antecedent fact of an abortion or a labor. Subinvolution dates back to an abortion or a labor, and the same may be said of the rare form known as superinvolution, which is further differentiated by the reduction in size below the normal standard, scanty and painful menstruation being also its usual accompaniments.

As to exfoliative endometritis, its commonly accepted name, membranous dysmenorrhœa, tells, in part, its story. It is characterized by painful menstruation, and along with the flow, which is excessive as a rule, a membranous cast of the cavity of the body of the uterus may appear, or at least shreds of such a membrane. Its differentiation from an abortion is made in part by the antecedent history, in part by the absence of any sign of a fœtus, and in part by the microscopic differences existing between it and fresh decidual tissue, the latter, however, being somewhat deceptive.

*Prognosis.*—As already stated, the acute forms of cervical and corporeal inflammation may subside entirely; on the contrary, however, they may end in the chronic forms, sepsis and gonorrhœa being mainly answerable for such an ending, as they are also chiefly chargeable for the extension of the acute process beyond the confines of the uterus, an event by no means uncommon. In the event of such extension, we may have a lesion limited to the adnexa and pelvic peritoneum; on the other hand, in the case of septic infection we may have general peritonitis or general sepsis and death.

The former dictum that all forms of chronic metritis are rebellious no longer holds good. Modern treatment, as with so many other chronic ailments, has wrought the change. Taken early, all forms yield readily, but after extensive sclerosis in the parenchyma of the organ, permanent cure is uncertain. But even in such cases, which, by the way, are not so common as might be supposed, we have still a chance of materially changing a prognosis which is based upon the incomplete measures of treatment antedating the aseptic period.

Chronic endometritis and metritis can be cured. Of all the forms, the polypoid (the hemorrhagic) is the most obstinate, and it also is the form which appears to tend most frequently to carcinomatous degeneration. The erosions developed in connection with cervical laceration likewise appear to tend in the same direction. So that, while we can positively assert that nearly every form of uncomplicated chronic endometritis and metritis is curable, rare forms are obstinate and perhaps incurable, and certain forms tend to the induction of cancer. All forms of the lesion tend towards the induction of inflammation of the adnexa and the peritoneum, these conditions, in turn, reacting unfavorably upon the irritating lesion; the acute septic forms being most pronounced in this action, the chronic forms next.

As to the prognosis touching the general health of the individual, this is so intimately connected with the local lesion that it may be assumed, in the absence of any serious development outside the uterus, that the health will be ultimately restored.

An important question in prognosis relates to the influence of these lesions upon pregnancy. All forms of inflammation in the cervical canal no doubt retard it, and one form seems to be almost prohibitive: it is that which is accompanied by the thick ropy secretions derived from the Nabothian glands. This viscid substance probably offers mainly a mechanical obstacle to the passage of the spermatozoa, but, in common with the other secretions, both from this surface, from the uterus, and from the vagina, it may possess pathological characteristics, as shown in part by its altered chemical reactions, which are destructive to the spermatozoa. But, even if the spermatozoa should escape these obstacles and reach the ovum, the conditions presented by the lining membrane of the body are not favorable to the development of a proper decidua. While, therefore, a pregnancy might be initiated, abortion would probably cut it short: so that it may be said in general that inflammations of the uterus tend·to sterility and abortions. But the restoration of the organ to its proper condition will restore this function: so that here the question of sterility depends upon the question of treatment. Proper treatment will in nearly all cases restore the organ to the full exercise of all its functions.

*Treatment.*—The milder forms of acute endometritis and metritis are best treated by rest in bed, together with free purgation by means of saline cathartics, to which measures copious hot vaginal douches (temperature 115° F.) should be added. At least four quarts should be used at a time; they should be taken in the recumbent posture, the patient lying on the back with a bed-pan beneath the buttocks, and they should be given once every three or four hours for at least twenty-four or thirty-six hours. A rapid depletion can be secured through free scarification of the cervix, which, if done in conjunction with a warm douche (temperature 106° F.), will insure sufficient bleeding to aid materially in the process of arrest. Perhaps the better plan is first to deplete by bleeding, and after this has secured the loss of an ounce or two of blood, then, after four or five hours, let the hot douches be commenced, continuing them at the interval above named. As soon as the acute symptoms have been controlled, cotton tampons soaked in glycerin should be placed against the cervix daily. By this means we still further aid resolution, and by the support offered add to the patient's comfort. The douching and perhaps the introduction of the tampons can be managed, in case of necessity, by the patient and her nurse, after some little instruction, but the scarification can be properly done only by the physician. To this end he exposes the cervix by means of a speculum, and then, after cleansing its surface carefully, he plunges a bistoury freely into its depths at half a dozen points. The bleeding which follows, as already noted, can be kept up by a flow of warm water. Should the blood-flow tend to a too long continuance, a hot douche (115° to 120° F.) will speedily control it. As a general thing, these measures, especially if they be supplemented with hot poultices over the hypogastrium, will control the pain sufficiently to render unnecessary the use of an opiate; but if they cannot be omitted, then use them as a rectal suppository, one or two doses being amply sufficient for any ordinary case.

The above measures of treatment are not wholly equal to the control of the more aggravated forms met with in gonorrhœa, therefore they should be supplemented with measures directed to the interior of the uterus.

As vaginitis is present, the treatment appropriate to the disease in this canal should form a part of the procedure, for so long as it remains here, reinfection of the uterus may take place.  The disease being in the uterus, the cavity of this organ should be attacked upon the same principle that governs the treatment of specific urethritis of the male.  As the internal os in all these cases of metritis is relaxed, and even somewhat open, the interior of the organ is easily reached, but not with the requisite freedom, unless in the presence of an anæsthetic, especially if the case be one of a woman who has not borne children; for the pain incident to the proper treatment of the uterus in acute gonorrhœal metritis and endometritis is generally greater than can be endured.  Therefore anæsthesia is to be preferred.  The cervix should be dilated, so as to admit the smaller-sized uterine speculum, through which the canal should then be copiously irrigated with a solution of bichloride of mercury (1 to 3000), a quart being run through, and then a strip of sterilized gauze (cheese-cloth) should be packed into the cavity, its free end protruding into the vagina.

The curette has been used by the writer in such cases, but in all,—four in number,—in spite of the utmost care and the most complete antisepsis, salpingitis followed; therefore he has adopted the less energetic course recommended above.  For the same reason he has avoided the use of caustics, his observations proving that careful cleansing, mild antisepsis, and thorough drainage give the best results.

At the end of twenty-four hours, or on the subsidence of symptoms, the irrigation may be repeated and the gauze renewed, this time without an anæsthetic, however, as the open state of the internal os will easily permit this, even without the aid of the speculum.  In this and in subsequent treatments, creolin, owing to its lubricity, will facilitate the introduction of the gauze drain better than bichloride; to this end, therefore, the gauze is soaked in a solution of that substance prior to introduction.  One, two, or three treatments of this kind may be needed, the symptoms and signs, as in other acute processes which we aim to abort, being our guide.

Turning next to septic endometritis and metritis occurring in the non-pregnant uterus after operations upon the cervix, for instance, it is proper to say, first, that such accidents happen as the result of negligence on the part of the operator, proper antisepsis having been omitted.  In the event of such a disaster, however, prompt and energetic measures are demanded. The cut surfaces upon the cervix should be exposed and freely cauterized with pure carbolic acid.  The internal os should be dilated, the cavity of the uterus freely irrigated with bichloride of mercury solution (1 to 3000), and the same cavity should then be packed with sterilized gauze, curettage rarely being required.  The wounded surfaces above mentioned should be kept apart by sterilized gauze freely packed between them, and this gauze, in turn, should be kept in place by the same kind of material packed in the vagina. If the symptoms subside, the packing in the vagina may be removed in forty-eight hours, but that in the uterus should not be disturbed for four or five days. It should then be withdrawn, if not already expelled, and the interior of the uterus need not be again entered. The vaginal douching should be commenced as soon as this canal has been emptied of its gauze, and it should be continued three times a day until the uterine packing is removed; then the glycerin tampons may be employed, as recommended above, to perfect the depletion. At a later period the cut surfaces may be dealt with by direct applications of astringents or cauterants, or by operations, as is deemed best. In the event of a persistence of unfavorable symptoms, the course to be followed is analogous to that to be mentioned in connection with the graver septic inflammations.

Coming now to the septic inflammations following abortions and labors, we find ourselves in the presence of not only the gravest form of the disorder under discussion, but a very common one,—so common, in fact, that it is hardly too much to say that most of the cases of uterine inflammation met with in practice spring from it. What has been said concerning its prognosis warrants the above statement, and points also to the urgent need for early recognition and prompt treatment. Prompt action means the arrest of the terrible disorder, the speedy cure of the patient, with the preservation of her fecundity; delayed action means the extension of the disorder, which in time means a general infection of the uterus and inflammation of the adnexa, with all that such a grade of inflammation therein implies. But, further than all this, delayed action means septic peritonitis or general septic infection through the lymphatics, or perhaps a pyæmia. Radical surgical measures should therefore be promptly applied. No time should be lost in attacking the uterus. Its cavity should be freely curetted, the sharp curette being employed, aided by the double curette or placental forceps, so that all débris may be scraped away and removed. In certain cases, where but little tenderness is present, the finger, or, if the uterus be large and flabby, two fingers, instead of the curette, may be used to remove the decidual débris. The method of procedure in these cases is of sufficient importance, however, to demand something more than a passing notice. The following detailed description is therefore submitted. As a rule, anæsthesia is advisable, because thoroughness is doubtful without it, and without thoroughness, failure may be expected. Cleanse the vulva, the vagina, the cervix, and the cervical canal carefully, using for this purpose the tincture of green soap and plenty of water. For the washing of these parts employ the fingers, aided by a wad of gauze in the jaws of a pair of long-handled forceps. Finishing this preliminary, irrigate the cavity of the uterus freely, first dilating the internal os, if it be not already sufficiently opened (it generally is, however) to permit this. If the uterus be large, the irrigation can be conducted suitably with only a glass tube (Chamberlain's); but if it be small, as after early abortions, some such provision should be made for the return flow of the fluid as is called for in the non-pregnant uterus, the uterine speculum and metallic nozzle tube being the preferable combination of instruments employed for this purpose (Fig. 14). The solution to be used is the 1 to 2000 of bichloride of mercury. Finishing this irrigation, the curettage should next be done, the fingers being introduced from time to time to make sure that all débris has been removed. It may be possible to do this last work with the fingers alone, as has been already intimated, but a combination of the sharp curette and the finger is useful, and, under anæsthesia, easily made. To facilitate the removal of the dislodged débris from the uterine cavity, the double curette forceps or the placental forceps is very useful. The sharp curette is to be preferred at all times to the dull, for the same reason that a sharp knife is preferable to a dull one. A minimum amount of pressure accomplishes our purpose here if a sharp instrument is used ; a maximum amount is needed with a dull instrument, and such pressure is far more likely to drive such an instrument through the softened uterine wall than the force requisite with the sharp instrument. Let the sharp curette, therefore, be used, employing a firm but light touch, checking its results by an occasional exploration with the finger to examine nodular regions which seem to call for the more energetic application of the instrument. A second copious irrigation with the bichloride solution above mentioned should immediately follow curettage, the solution being hot—115° or 120° F.—if there be excessive hemorrhage. There is always free bleeding in these cases, and occasionally it spurts forth as if from some large vessel. But little time need be given, however, to the checking of the bleeding by this method, for the reason that the succeeding step in the treatment will do so promptly. This consists in packing the uterus fully and firmly with sterilized gauze. In a large uterus, having a well-opened canal, this can be quickly done by using the curette forceps as a dresser. By means of it a long strip of the gauze, folded lengthwise half a dozen times, is passed in length by length, carefully packing it away, first in one cornu, then in the other, then at the fundus, and so on down to the external os, through which into the vagina the free end is finally brought. The vagina is then packed loosely, first around the cervix and then down to the ostium. If the uterus be small, as in the earlier abortions, the irrigation and the packing can be best done through the uterine speculum, as in the inflammations of the non-pregnant uterus, the strips of gauze in such cases being of about four thicknesses, folded to the width of the index finger, and of sufficient length to enable one piece to fill completely the uterine cavity.

In all septic cases one may expect a chill and febrile reaction to follow the above treatment, but the temperature quickly falls, and the subsequent progress of the case, provided it be attacked early, is generally towards a prompt and complete recovery. The packing of the vagina should be removed at the end of twenty-four hours, warm cleansing douches of a saturated solution of boracic acid being given twice in twenty-four hours.

At the end of from forty-eight to seventy-two hours the uterine packing may be removed in all these septic cases, and if no fever be present, the cavity of the uterus need not be again entered; but if the temperature is still elevated, then remove the packing at the end of twenty-four hours, irrigate the cavity again, and apply fresh gauze. This may be done at the above intervals as often as may be necessary.

In certain rare cases where the poison is of intense virulence, the condition of the patient, in spite of the above treatment, may approximate that in which the interior of the uterus has been too long neglected; in which, therefore, general infection with possibly a peritonitis has supervened. One should not despair, however. The cleansing and drainage should be continued. In the event that one approaches the case for the first time, after even general infection, salpingitis, and peritonitis have supervened, the directions for curettage and packing already mentioned should be carried out, seemingly desperate cases not infrequently yielding to these measures.

The gravest perplexity in surgery arises, however, in connection with all cases of general septic infection and peritonitis, the perplexity occurring in consequence of the possibilities of further and more extended operative procedures. The removal of the infected uterus either through the vagina or by cœliotomy would offer the surest relief, could the shock of so grave an operation be controlled. But patients infected with a general sepsis rarely withstand any grave abdominal or even pelvic operation; therefore, if further operative measures be determined upon, they should be confined to removal of the adnexa where they are the clearly defined channels of the peritoneal infection, to irrigation of the infected peritoneal surfaces, and to subsequent free drainage by the open method, as mentioned below. In the event of a general infection through the lymphatics, as shown by the condition of these vessels in the broad ligaments, the steps after cœliotomy should be confined to an attempt at further diversion of the poison by packing sterilized gauze about the uterus, bringing the free ends out through the opening in the abdominal wall, thus establishing drainage by means of what is known as the "open abdominal method,"—the method of Mikulicz, —as an addition to that already instituted from the cavity of the uterus, as given above. Theoretically, it might be permissible to ligate the ovarian vessels and broad ligaments, such a step adding but little to the shock; but all measures depending upon invasion of the peritoneal cavity are, in the presence of such cases, desperate resorts, and permissible only in view of the desperate conditions which one aims to circumvent. If pyæmia be already present, cœliotomy can offer no possible hope.

Turning now to the general measures of treatment called for in septic cases, they consist in mild purgation with salines, the relief of pain by opiates, the careful and frequent administration of easily digested food, preferably milk and its preparations, such as koumys and matzoon, or other forms of concentrated food, and the free administration of stimulants, such as champagne, brandy, or whiskey, aided by strychnine. Prolonged convalescence may be expected in all severe cases which are fortunate enough to recover. This appears to be due to the changes developed in the lymphatic system and in the blood-making glands. Malnutrition and anæmia are common results, and the obstinacy with which such states are frequently maintained calls for a constant supervision as to food, tonics, and hygiene, extending in some cases over several years.

*Chronic Endometritis and Metritis.*—Commencing with the cervix, we shall first present the treatment appropriate to this section of the uterus. Erosions of the vaginal face of an untorn cervix, depending as they usually do upon a vaginitis of some kind, should be treated with a view to this fact; therefore the vaginitis should be treated along the lines already laid out. At the same time the eroded surface should be painted daily with Churchill's tincture of iodine, and if cysts be present they should be evacuated and the remaining excavations cleaned out and cauterized, the treatment being continued until cure is effected.

Another condition presented by the untorn cervix is a thickening or general enlargement, with the characteristic tough, gelatinous discharge already noted. This combination means a general implication of the mucous membrane, of the Nabothian glands, and of the deeper cervical structures. To cure it promptly, the cervix should be laid open by a free incision from side to side as high as the vaginal junction. The entire mucous surface, from the internal os down, should be carefully and thoroughly scraped with a sharp curette as deep as the submucous structure. The surface, after being carefully dried, should be painted with Churchill's tincture of iodine, the cut surfaces being then reunited with catgut. If the canal be the seat of old tears, and the surrounding tissue be sclerosed and cystic, it is best to cut away all this diseased tissue. (Fig. 8.) For this purpose lay open the cervix from side to side as high as the vaginal junction, turn back the posterior flap, and then make a transverse incision through the cervical tissue at the angle of the original cut; this transverse cut must extend across the entire face of this new surface, and it must also be made so deep as to pass beyond the limits of the diseased tissue. Its general direction in the depths of the tissue is obliquely towards the outer surface and lower segment of the cervix. Commencing next at the lower part of this flap, all tissue is cut away from below upward, until finally the depths of the transverse incision are reached; in this way all diseased tissue is removed, and the flap of the cervix is so thinned that it can be folded inward upon itself in such a manner as to bring the mucous membrane of the lower outer face in relation with the angle of the original cut, from the centre of which angle the mucous membrane of the cervical canal protrudes. Mucous membrane is thus brought in touch with like structure, a feat necessary to the prevention of cicatricial contraction with obstruction of the cut end of the cervical canal. The anterior flap is next treated in the same manner. Catgut sutures being employed to keep the turned-in tissues in place, sutures of similar material are now placed in position on the outer aspects of the cervix at the vaginal junction, in order to prevent gaping at these points, two sutures upon each side being generally necessary for this purpose.

Where there is decided circumferential enlargement of the cervix, without special implication of the canal beyond dilatation, a V-shaped piece should be cut out from the entire thickness of the cervical wall upon each side, the apex of the extirpated tissue being taken from above. The flaps left should then be brought together from above downward, as in the repair of laceration, the contour of the cervix being thus preserved.

Fig. 8.

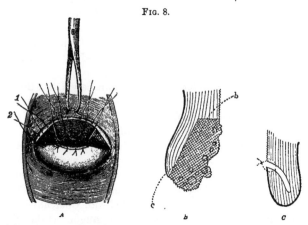

Amputation of the cervix by one flap, or excision of the mucosa (Schroeder's operation).—*A*, method of placing sutures; 1 and 2 are those uniting commissures; *B*, section showing shape of incisions and (*b, c*) line of sutures; *C*, position of lips after suturing. (Pozzi.)

Where this enlargement of the cervix takes the shape of an elongation as well as a thickening, amputation should be performed. This is accomplished in the following manner (Fig. 9):

Lay open the entire vaginal portion of the cervix from side to side, converting it into two flaps, as above described. Next remove the anterior flap, employing for this purpose two lines of transverse incision, which are commenced about a third of an inch below the level of the cervico-vaginal junction, one upon the outer face of the flap, the other upon the inner face. Cutting obliquely upward towards the supra-vaginal portion of the cervix, the two lines of incision are deepened so as to meet each other in the depths of the cervical tissue at a line about midway between the canal and the outer surface of the cervix. The two flaps thus formed are then stitched together. A similar operation is next performed upon the posterior lip or flap of the cervix. The mucous lining of the canal is thus brought in relation with that which covers the vaginal face of the cervix, and, as with the operative procedure (Schroeder's) described above, cicatricial stenosis is avoided.

In both of these operations the outer lines of the original incision, by which the cervix is first laid open, must be brought together from above downward, otherwise the two lips or flaps would gape as in a laceration. This is easily done, as mentioned in connection with the first, after which the operations stand completed. By employing catgut as the suture material in all these procedures, not only will a good result be obtained, but the patient will be spared the annoyance incident to the removal of sutures composed of other material.

Fɪɢ. 9.

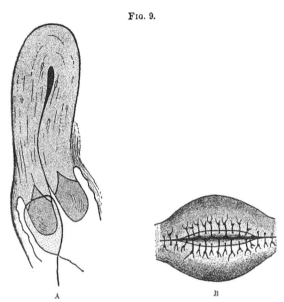

A            B

Amputation of the cervix with double flaps (Simon).—*A*, sectional view, showing lines of incision for formation of flaps and method of suture; *B*, front view of cervix, operation complete. (Pozzi.)

Turning our attention next to erosions connected with those lacerations which, by their extent, lead to eversion not only of the cervical canal, but of the surrounding tissue through which the tears extend, we will find that the operations devised by Emmet meet the requirements better than any other procedure yet devised. This statement presupposes, however, that the condition of the mucous lining of the canal is such as to warrant its retention. If it be so changed by cystic degeneration and sclerosis of the subjacent cervical tissue as to warrant the belief that it should be excised *in toto*, then one or the other of Schroeder's operations is to be preferred. In general, however, the state of the mucous lining in the class of cases under consideration will permit its retention, especially if it be treated by depletion and local alteration beforehand.

It should be thoroughly curetted, then all diseased tissue outside the line of the canal should be cut from the face of the everted tissue, the angles of the tear or tears should be freed from all cicatricial tissue, and the denuded surfaces should then be brought together with catgut.

There should be no question as to the benefits to be derived from treatment, short of operations, directed to the conditions of the cervix last considered. The congestions, the cystic degenerations, the scleroses, the erosions, and the accompanying enlargements are all favorably influenced by local depletion and local alterative applications. Depletion is best secured by means of scarification, aided by the action of hot douches and tamponades of cotton or wool soaked in a saturated solution of borax in glycerin. Indurated surfaces should be scarified, cysts should be evacuated and cauterized, and erosions should be destroyed by Churchill's tincture of iodine or even solutions of chromic acid. A daily use of the glycerin tampons, together with the hot douche (115° F.), need not extend beyond two or three weeks, especially if aided by scarification and the local applications above mentioned. Then, if further treatment be needed, it had better take the form of some one of the operative measures mentioned above as appropriate.

Wherever possible, the integrity of the cervix should be restored, and this precaution is especially called for in the face of posterior displacements of the uterus, for without a good cervical projection into the vagina the leverage necessary to the proper action of a pessary is difficult to obtain.

The writer forbears to enter into any detailed account of the different steps needful in the application of Emmet's operation to the different forms of lacerated cervix, as the subject belongs properly to another chapter in this work.

We shall now consider the treatment of chronic inflammation of the corpus uteri.

During the stage of infiltration, all cases of this form of the lesion yield to treatment. After the stage of induration has become fixed from long continuance, every case is stubborn; but, as already intimated, even the larger number of these can be cured, leaving the cases of this lesion which are absolutely incurable greatly in the minority.

The cases which respond most readily to treatment are those classed as "subinvolution." This condition being largely an arrest of a normal process, rather than a pathological change *per se*, one can easily see why it should furnish the best results. As a part of this state, we have the cases of the hemorrhagic form in which decidual remnants are the focus of the endometrial change. For convenience of reference we shall designate all this class under the head Class A.

In contrast to this latter condition, we have the pure hemorrhagic types associated with the stage of induration, and particularly such cases as develop in connection with the menopause or present membranous exfoliations. We also have that rare condition, superinvolution. All these conditions are prone to stubbornness. All this class we designate Class B.

Between the two we have cases associated with stenosis, with flexions and versions, in which mechanical problems are presented as a part of the therapeutic question to be solved, and cases long in the stage of infiltration, in which the glandular form of endometritis predominates, a muco-purulent discharge, with perhaps a lessening of the menstrual discharge, characterizing them. These we designate as Class C.

Standing apart from these, we have cases associated with chronic disease of the adnexa or peritoneal adhesions, especially where the adhesions have fixed the uterus in an abnormal position,—retroversion, for instance; but consideration of such cases belongs rather to the subject of salpingitis, etc., to which the reader is therefore referred. We shall include them under Class D.

A proper conception of the appropriate treatment of a chronically inflamed uterus can only be had when we bring ourselves to that point which views this organ as a hollow structure having communication with the exterior. It will then be seen that it is amenable only to the kind of treatment whose principles prevail in the treatment of other cavities similarly situated.

It is needless to say that the sooner treatment is inaugurated the better, because when the stage of induration is accomplished, such is the condition of the mucous membrane and walls, owing to connective-tissue sclerosis, that a cure is difficult, and in some rare instances impossible. Taken during the stage of infiltration, however, and treated in accordance with the principle above indicated, results will be brilliant.

The appropriate measures are cleansing the uterine cavity, removing exuberant and diseased tissue, and checking its reproduction by direct application of reagents, aided by enforced depletion and efficient drainage.

All this is best accomplished by irrigations, by curettage, by direct use of iodine or some similar reagent, and finally by forcibly distending the entire cavity with sterilized gauze, bringing, for the purposes of drainage, the ends of the gauze through the cervical canal into the vagina. The principle is identical with that already enunciated in conjunction with the treatment of acute metritis, but there are certain minor differences rendering necessary a reconsideration of the matter in connection with chronic metritis.

As might be inferred, such treatment ranks with the minor pelvic operations, and should always be so considered, because, unless it is carried out with as much regard to cleanliness as prevails in a vaginal hysterectomy, it may do harm in place of good, the harm being the creation of a salpingitis and peritonitis. When done in accordance with the rules laid down, nothing but good can come of it, for it may even be used beneficially in the face of these last-named conditions, as has been proved in hundreds of cases.

Having indicated above the order which obtains among cases of chronic endometritis and metritis in yielding to treatment, we shall proceed to the treatment appropriate to all, designating as we progress exceptional steps which peculiarities of type demand.

*Curettage, Alterative or Caustic Applications, Depletion, Drainage.*—This combination of measures demands anæsthesia. Some women can undergo the ordeal without it, but for perfection of method and consequent freedom from subsequent complications anæsthesia is essential. This being secured,

Fig. 10.

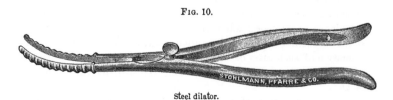

Steel dilator.

the vulva, the vagina, and the cervical canal are cleansed most thoroughly, exceeding, if possible, the suggestions already given in connection with the acute disorders. Dilatation of the cervix is the next step; this is followed by the introduction of the uterine cylindrical speculum (Fig. 14), through which the cavity of the uterus is now copiously flushed, using a warm

Fig. 11.

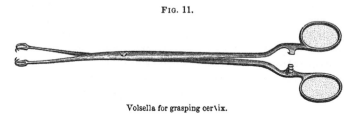

Volsella for grasping cervix.

bichloride of mercury solution (1 to 2000), to the amount of one or two pints.

Curettage is the next step. This is performed with the sharp curette (Sims), aided by the double curette-forceps of Emmet. (Figs. 12, 13.) With the first the entire cavity is scraped, the persistence and vigor with

Fig. 12.

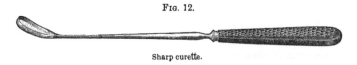

Sharp curette.

which this is done being governed by the conditions present, the hemorrhagic forms calling for greater persistence and vigor than recent subinvolution and the endometritis of simple stenosis, as in anteflexion. The anterior wall, the posterior wall, the lateral sulci where these two come together, the fundus, and the recesses of the cornua are scraped in turn. Pay special attention to the fundus and cornua, and call to aid the double curette-forceps, using this instrument to pinch or bite off all excrescences.

Then use them finally to clean out all débris from the cavity as a whole. During curettage the uterus is fixed with a tenaculum or volsella, so that thorough work may be done with the curette. One need have no fear of penetrating the walls, if the vigor with which the curette is applied is in proportion to the resistance offered by the tissues; but even if the wall

FIG. 13.

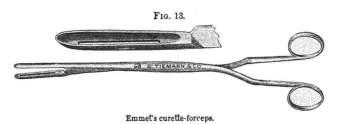

Emmet's curette-forceps.

should be penetrated, while such an accident is very undesirable, yet, in the presence of such antiseptic precautions as now universally prevail, it would be of small consequence. After completing the curettage, reintroduce the uterine speculum and again copiously irrigate the cavity with warm bichloride of mercury solution of the same strength as that first

FIG. 14.

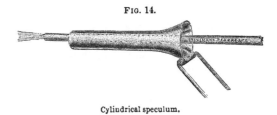

Cylindrical speculum.

employed. At the outset of the operation the surgeon places his gauze in a bichloride of mercury solution (1 to 500); a strip about four feet in length, folded four times, so as to present a width throughout about equal to that of the index finger, is that which has been prepared for the cavity. Catching an end upon a Sims tampon screw, it is passed into the uterus

FIG. 15.

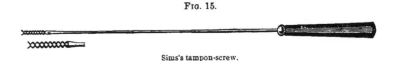

Sims's tampon-screw.

through the speculum length by length, packing it away first in one cornu, then in the other, then at the fundus, then down step by step until the cervix is reached. To this end the speculum is gradually withdrawn as the packing encroaches upon it. Reaching the internal os, the packing ceases, the free end of the gauze being then brought out through the cervix into the vagina; the excess is now either cut off or coiled up against the cervix. The vagina is now loosely filled with larger pieces of gauze, this step completing the operation. At the end of forty-eight hours the vaginal packing is removed, the vagina being after this douched twice daily until the uterine packing is removed. This should be done on the sixth day, a final vaginal douche being then given, unless the douches be continued from time to time

FIG. 16.

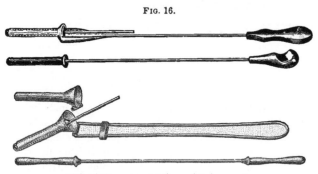

Cylindrical specula and instrument for tamponade.

as a means of cleanliness. In some cases the uterus expels the packing in part on the second or third day; but as some of it always remains, and by so doing insures the patency of the cervix, and therefore drainage, it should not be disturbed until the day specified. The premenstrual period—six or seven days before—is the time of election for this operation, it being that at which the greatest amount of depletion can be secured; and, as depletion is the essence of this treatment, nothing should be omitted which will insure it. The fact that menstruation may begin while the gauze is in place constitutes no objection to the selection of this time, for the gauze will do no harm, many patients having carried it throughout a period without an unusual symptom or sequence.

All cases belonging to Class A yield promptly to the above treatment, and the same may be said of Class C, with certain limitations, however, which I shall now state. Cases with stenosis, flexions, or versions require correction of these defects, otherwise the endometritis and metritis will be reproduced. The flexions and versions must be cured either by pessary or by operation, and the stenosis by operation and the prolonged wearing of the cervical or uterine stem, all of which may be done in conjunction with the dilatation, curettage, and packing, as those measures consume very little time. The remaining cases of Class C may relapse several months after the first operation; but if the patients are once thoroughly curetted, and the uterine cavity then treated with Churchill's tincture of iodine, and finally packed as above, a relapse is very improbable. All cases belonging to Class B are stubborn, and if they are those of commencing malignant disease of the endometrium or of fibroid disease with a sub-mucous growth, the treatment will fail to do more than alleviate the hemorrhages.  It may be stated as a rule that all cases of Class B re-quire the most thorough curettage and then the application of caustics to the endometrium, exfoliative endometritis calling especially for this combination of measures.  If the uterine speculum is used, there is no

FIG. 17.

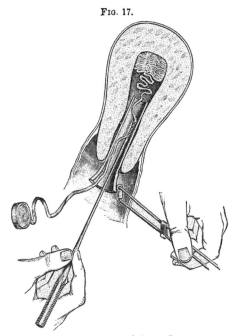

Tamponade of the uterine cavity.

fear of undue action upon the internal os, with subsequent stenosis.  The method to be employed is as follows.  After curettage, pack the uterine cavity firmly with gauze, as above described, leave this in place about ten or twenty minutes, then withdraw it and irrigate the cavity with *hot* bichloride solution (1 to 2000), as above.  These measures will stop the bleeding and free the cavity of clots.  The next step is to apply the caustic by means of cotton wrapped about the tampon screw.  The writer's prefer-ence is for carbolic or chromic acid, and in the more obstinate cases nitric acid or the galvano-cautery, using a glass tube in the application of nitric acid.  After a few moments the canal should be again irrigated, plain water being now used ; and finally the packing should be replaced and the vagina filled with gauze, as already described.

Temporary expedients may be required to arrest a too profuse hemorrhage from the uterus. When prompt action is needed, the copious hot douche (120° F.) may suffice; if not, then the vagina should be tamponed with sterilized cotton pledgets, which should be soaked in a solution of alum before being applied. For the less urgent bleedings, ergot and hydrastis, aided by the hot douches, may be employed; but if, in spite of all, the bleedings persist, then ligation of the uterine arteries, or even vaginal hysterectomy, will be demanded.

A few words will suffice as to superinvolution. It is a rare condition. When the uterus is yet soft, the faradic current will be serviceable; but when induration has supervened, the treatment is mainly symptomatic. Dysmenorrhœa is to be controlled by hot applications and perhaps dilatation, and the general health is to be cared for.

Cases belonging to Class D are treated much as are cases belonging to Class A or C, but other measures are needed, which can be presented only in connection with diseases of the adnexa: we refer the reader, therefore, for additional consideration of such cases, to the division of this article devoted to salpingitis and peritonitis. It remains only to say a word concerning the use of electricity and abdomino-vaginal massage (Thure Brandt's method) as agents of cure in the chronic inflammation of the uterus. The first is of doubtful efficacy, and the second is unnecessary. A good abdominal supporter will, however, give comfort to many of these people, especially when relaxation of the abdominal muscle prevails. The pelvic, lumbosacral, and crural pains which are so annoying to many of these patients, and which are most pronounced towards the close of the day, are best treated by hot sitz-baths taken just before the patient retires to bed.

From what was said concerning the general health of these subjects under the head of symptoms, it is evident that some treatment of the general system, and particularly of the digestive system, will be called for. These measures may be briefly summarized as follows:

Obstinate dyspepsia associated with dilatation of the stomach is best treated by "lavage," the washing of the stomach being conducted under the ordinary rules governing this process. Less pronounced cases of stomachic disorder call simply for regulation of the diet, for stomachic tonics, and for regulation of the bowels. Where ordinary exercise cannot be taken, general massage aided by general faradization will prove useful. Tonics directed to the improvement of the blood state and those bearing upon the nervous system may be indicated. Finally, freedom from the marital relation, freedom from the cares of the housewife, and a judicious employment of out-door exercise will render essential service wherever indicated or permissible. For such as can afford it, the disease of the uterus being obstinate, much good may be obtained by the use of such courses of treatment as can be had at Kreutznach or Schwalbach, or, in the event of the rheumatic complications which may appear as a sequence of gonorrhœa, at such places as the Hot Springs of Virginia, or of Arkansas, or of Aix-les-Bains in France. As to the use of such specific drugs as iodide of potassium or the mercurials, they are of little service, except in cases that have syphilis as a complication.

A concluding word should now be said touching the effect of treatment as above outlined upon the matter of sterility. No treatment can be said to be entirely successful in the diseases of a uterus still within the period of full menstrual activity unless this blight be overcome. Measures of local treatment are those about which this problem mainly revolves, and the writer can only say that the measure of treatment which has yielded the best results in his hands is that which has been described under the head of curettage, with subsequent depletion by means of packing and drainage.

### INFLAMMATIONS OF THE UTERINE APPENDAGES AND THE PERITONEUM (PELVIC INFLAMMATION).

The intimate relation existing between the Fallopian tubes, the ovaries, and the peritoneum compels the almost constant association which is characteristic of the lesions of inflammations affecting them, and this association is so close that, while it may be possible to determine clinically which structure presents the prominent lesion, it is generally impossible to determine by symptoms and signs alone the presence or absence of minor changes in the others. In view, then, of the close anatomical, pathological, and clinical association, we shall consider the subject so that the student shall never lose sight of the intermingling of lesion and outward expression, and yet shall be given a clear insight to the individuality of each structure, first as to its specific lesion, next as to the clinical expression of this lesion, and finally as to such difference of treatment as may be called for.

The causes which underlie the inflammation of these structures are so nearly the same for all that we shall depart somewhat from our plan in dealing with this phase of the subject. Etiology will, therefore, be considered, in the main, under a single head.

*Causes.*—With few exceptions, the causes of salpingitis, oöphoritis, cellulitis, lymphangitis, and pelvic peritonitis spring from the uterus. Endometritis and metritis may then be said, speaking broadly, to be the cause of the lesions under discussion. The exceptions are found in a peritonitis developed in connection with the growth of *certain ovarian tumors* whose origin is supposed to depend upon conditions within the ovary itself, as, for instance, hæmatomas of the ovary, dermoid cysts, and even the simpler ovarian cysts; and yet the fact already noted in connection with the causation of endometritis and metritis should not be forgotten,—namely, that the pressure of such growths upon the uterus sometimes provokes chronic inflammations of this organ, so that the peritonitis may not be the direct result of changes originating in the ovary, but rather an indirect sequence, coming, after all, from the uterus, the source which more than every other stands responsible for this lesion. *Acute suppression of menstruation* is another extra-uterine cause which has been named, and the writer, in common with other observers, can cite an instance, the case being that of a girl of fourteen, in whom, in the light of an autopsy, the phenomena of a fatal acute general peritonitis could be traced to no other cause than acute suppression of menstruation. But the absence of any bacteriological examination in this case and, so far as the writer is aware, in all similar cases leaves the question of possible infection from the uterus unsettled, this organ, as has been already stated, being, even in the most chaste (to which the writer's case certainly belonged), the habitat of pathogenic germs, which, in the presence of a constitutional state furnishing fluids efficient as a culture medium, might initiate a peritonitis, even of the widest extent. Nevertheless, until a proper pathological differentiation is made in all such cases, we must accept acute suppression of the menstrual flow as one cause, particularly of oöphoritis and peritonitis, which acts without the interior of the uterus figuring as a direct intermediary.

It is hardly proper to specify fibroid tumors as a cause of inflammatory disease of the structures under discussion, unless we speak of them as indirect rather than direct agents. These growths provoke endometritis, and this, in turn, produces the lesion of the tubes, ovaries, and peritoneum. It is, then, to endometritis rather than to the neoplasm that we should attribute the inflammation.

Coming to the prime source of the lesions under discussion, we reach the inflammatory diseases of the uterus and of its lining membrane, and the conditions which lie back of both. If one grasps fully the causes of endometritis and metritis, he will comprehend their relation to the lesions before us.

Bearing in mind all that has been said concerning the causation of the inflammations of the uterus and the endometrium, we find that while it is possible for any one of them to act so as to produce inflammation in the tubes, ovaries, cellular tissue, and peritoneum, yet, as a fact, it is the septic and specific poisons which produce these lesions most frequently.

In the non-pregnant uterus the premenstrual period is the one of greatest susceptibility, while in the uterus recently pregnant the first three days occupy this position. Observation proves that the inflammations set up in this latter type of uterus are responsible for a larger proportion of the lesions under discussion than all other causes combined, and that, of these, such as are dependent upon criminal interference with the pregnant uterus rank highest in point of infecting capacity, as they generally represent the extremes of septic infection. To all of the above causes may be added such as occur in the non-pregnant uterus in connection with any traumatism inflicted without due regard to antiseptic precautions, such as operations upon the cervix, curettage, or even the use of a dirty sound.

The rôle played by gonorrhœa in the inflammations of the lower genital tract is freely admitted by all observers, but question has arisen as to its potency in the production of the lesions before us. So far as the writer is concerned, he can only say that in one case he has by direct inspection successfully followed a gonorrhœa from its appearance at the ostium vaginæ to its appearance at the fimbriæ of both tubes, all within the space of six weeks. Less doubt pertains to the *rôle* of an acute and virulent gonorrhœa than to that of the chronic cases, the so-called gleet of the male; but even here clinical evidence strongly favors the generally accepted idea as to its potency in the production of the inflammations in question.

In that part of this article which deals with the causation of endometritis and metritis we have given a sufficient statement concerning the pathogenic germs which underlie all septic infections. We have shown the sources of origin, and have alluded to the lines which they follow in the invasion of the deeper tissues. We therefore refer the reader to that paragraph for information upon these points; excepting, however, the statements relating to the lines of propagation. Upon this matter something further needs to be said.

Conceding the contention that the inflammations, with the exceptions already named, of the tubes, ovaries, pelvic peritoneum, etc., are derivatives of similar processes in the uterus, the question at issue is as to the channel of communication. Our space forbids any notice of the many arguments upon this question. The writer's observations and conclusions were succinctly stated before the Society of Physicians and Pathologists in June, 1886,[1] and he can add that his experiences in abdomino-pelvic operations since that date have served to confirm in his mind what he then stated. This, in effect, was that the Fallopian tubes were the principal channels of intercommunication in all those cases which presented clinically the physical evidences of periuterine inflammation.

There can be no question as to the participation of the lymphatics and veins in the propagation of sepsis. In pyæmia, for instance, the presence of infected thrombi in distant parts proves the participation of the veins, while the presence of pus in the lymph-spaces of the uterine wall and the lymph-vessels of the broad ligaments shows the position of the lymphatics as channels of infection. While this may be inconclusive as to the changes wrought in the tubes, it certainly is not so as to those in the ovaries and peritoneum, because the writer, in common with other observers, has witnessed the phenomena of the development of a peritonitis from a septic metritis, and on opening the abdomen has found the peritoneal coat of the uterus covered with recent lymph, the ovaries greatly enlarged from acute interstitial congestion, and the whole length of the upper part of the broad ligaments thickened from intra-ligamentous serous exudate; and yet, aside from some injection of the vessels upon the peritoneal coat of the tubes, these structures were practically unaffected, thus showing that they had not been the channels of infection. The retroactive influence upon a tube of a peritonitis or an oöphoritis thus induced is so insignificant compared to that which prevails consequent upon a direct extension of inflammation to its

---

[1] New York Medical Record, September 18, 1886, p. 1.

mucous surface from the same membrane in the uterus (the one being merely an extension of the other), that it may be largely, if not entirely, ignored as a factor in the production of the chronic changes in the tube. In the sepsis of recently pregnant uteri, the extension to the ovaries and peritoneum is by way of the tubes and also through the lymphatics, but the extension most destructive to the integrity of the ovary and peritoneum is that through the tube. In a few cases of this latter class (the sepsis of recently pregnant uteri) the extension to the ovaries and peritoneum is wholly through the lymphatics, and the extension through the veins and the so-called direct extension are subordinated to this lymphatic extension, being chiefly witnessed after these vessels have been choked with pathogenic germs.

As to cases of inflammation of the appendages which occur in connection with the non-pregnant uterus, the weight of testimony agrees with the writer's observations, which are to the effect that such extensions take place along the lining membrane of the tube, he never having observed such thickenings in the broad ligaments in acute cases as would warrant the inference that the lymphatics had played any part in the induction of the lesions presented.

Upon the whole, then, it may be said that, where the uterus is the starting or intermediary point of the inflammation, the peritoneum and appendages are infected, as a rule, by way of the canal of the tubes, in some by way of the lymphatics and the tubes, and in a few by way of the lymphatics alone, the ovaries, the cellular tissue, and the peritoneum being here the chief sufferers.

It seems but natural that any writer dealing with inflammations of the uterine appendages should include tuberculosis among the etiological factors. The subject, however, is of such importance, and bears so close a relation to the general consideration of the disease, that the editor has wisely classed this subject separately. The writer, therefore, refers the reader to the article upon tuberculosis in another part of this volume.

Reference should be made to scarlet fever, measles, and small-pox as possible etiological factors. Whether their agency is an indirect one, through the medium of the vagina and uterus, as already discussed, or a direct one, as manifested by a direct action of the specific poison of the diseases in question upon the structures under consideration, is as yet unsettled. The weight of testimony, however, is in favor of an indirect action, the inflammation set up in the lower genital tract extending to the appendages. Mumps, however, appears to be a disease which can create an oöphoritis by direct action of its specific poison, the action in women being similar to that witnessed so often in men, where orchitis is not infrequently one of the manifestations of this disease. Syphilis is undoubtedly a cause, the tertiary formation simulating, at least, the condition seen in pelvic inflammation.

Another cause is *extra-uterine pregnancy.* Here we have not only marked degenerative changes left in the tubes, but also peritoneal adhesions and associated changes in the adjacent ovary. It is true that these changes, at their outset, represent actual new growth rather than inflammatory changes; yet the results, particularly to the tube, and to the ovary and peritoneum as well, are in so many ways analogous to those depending upon inflammation that extra-uterine pregnancy should at least have mention as a cause of tubal, ovarian, and peritoneal lesion alongside of those dependent upon pure inflammation.

A further excuse for this mention may also be found in the fact that, after all, an inflammatory lesion probably lies at the bottom of extra-uterine pregnancy, the changes in the tubes resulting therefrom causing the arrest of the ovum at its unnatural position. In addition to all this, inflammatory changes are added not infrequently to such as may be associated with the rupture of an extra-uterine fœtation, as witness the development of a pelvic abscess therefrom, the infection in such cases originating in the uterus, it being immaterial, in this connection, whether it come through the implicated tube or its fellow.

*Pathology.*—Following the suggestion made at the outset of this portion of our subject, we now present a statement of the lesions peculiar to each one of the structures under consideration, which will be succeeded by a picture of the combined effects of inflammation upon these structures as a whole. Under each head we shall endeavor to present every grade of inflammatory change, from the simplest to the gravest. The description is based, in the main, upon the writer's observations at the operating and post-mortem tables, these observations being verified, where necessary, by the many statements recently published upon this subject.

**Acute Salpingitis.**—In the milder grades of a recent inflammation but little is noticed beyond changes in the mucous lining of the tubes and their fimbriæ, the shape and dimensions of the tubes being unaltered. The condition is really an endosalpingitis, and is commonly classed as a variety of catarrhal salpingitis. The lining of the tube is injected, having a grayish-blue appearance, is swollen and its surface is covered with a mucous or muco-purulent exudate; the same condition is witnessed at the fimbriæ. The changes are best marked in the ampulla. With the microscope, the folds of the mucous membrane are found swollen from infiltrations with embryonic cells; the surface shows the beginning formation of vegetations which, having a vasculo-cellular basis, may assume extended proportions in chronic forms of the lesion; but little implication of the deeper structure of the tube will be present, and the outer end of the tube remains open.

This degree of lesion represents the mildest form of salpingitis, and is generally found in but one tube, the other being healthy. Resolution is the rule.

In a more severe form of recent inflammation the appearances upon the mucous membrane, noted above, are intensified. The surface exudate is decidedly purulent, the color is the grayish-blue above noted, the epithelium is softened and robbed of its cilia, the swelling of the mucous membrane is most pronounced, and the entire wall is thickened, this thickening being due in part to ordinary inflammatory infiltration of the muscular coat and in part to a similar condition in the subserous cellular coat. The tube, as a whole, is enlarged, the increase reaching sometimes the dimensions of the adult middle finger or thumb. If the fimbriated end be closed, the increase in size, owing to distention of the ampulla, may be even greater; but the closure of the outer end of a tube which is of sufficient firmness to permit distention of the ampulla beyond its normal limit is a late result of an acute process rather than an early expression, such a closure representing, in fact, an organization of the exudate, and belonging, therefore, to the chronic rather than to the acute stage of inflammations. The condition of the tube under discussion is best seen in conjunction with an acute peritonitis, the structure of the tube being then attacked from without as well as from within. As a rule, the fimbriated end of all such tubes is closed by recent exudate, but occasionally it remains partially open, giving exit to the muco-purulent exudate from the cavity of the tube.

In place of actual closure by adhesion of the fimbriæ to each other, this condition may result from a fixation of the open mouth of the tube against some one of the adjacent viscera; the ovary is the organ against which the free end of the tube is most frequently fixed in this manner, but the end may be found in contact with some part of the pelvic floor or wall, with the back of the broad ligament, or of the uterus, or in front of these latter structures in connection with the bladder; and again, though but rarely, it may rest at some point in the iliac fossa. In all the cases of marked interstitial infiltration the condition, as already stated, is in part a parenchymatous process in the muscular coat and in part a sero-cellular infiltration of the subperitoneal connective tissue. The tissue is commonly very friable, unless it be an instance of an acute process superimposed upon tissue already changed by prior chronic changes; then it may retain some of its resistance. Resolution may take place in this condition, but the tendency is towards the chronic forms. Both tubes are, as a rule, attacked, one, however, to a greater degree than the other, the left being the one most often implicated.

In the more virulent septic inflammations following labors and abortions the process may move forward so rapidly to a fatal termination as to afford few evidences of infiltration and thickening of the tubes, but such changes as are presented belong to the class above mentioned. The infiltrated tissues are much softened, and the tube-cavity is filled with a watery, purulent exudate, similar to that found upon the adjacent surfaces of the peritoneum. These cases are seen most frequently upon the post-mortem table, and always show the widest possible extension of a suppurative inflammatory process.

**Chronic Salpingitis.**—In chronic salpingitis both tubes are commonly involved, one to a greater extent than the other. The mucous membrane is covered to a greater or less extent with vegetations, and presents a grayish-purple appearance; the vegetations are covered with a mueo-purulent or purulent secretion, and, when they can be isolated, stand out as club-shaped projections. As the lesions progress, the tendency of the vegetations is to coalesce at the extremity, and, secondary formations developing there-from, a mass of reticulated tissue is produced in the tube, made up of a connective-tissue and vascular basis, the whole infiltrated with embryonic cells and containing innumerable sinuses and even cavities.

Upon the surface of this exuberant formation the normal ciliated epithe-lium gives place to the flat and cubical varieties into which, after losing its all-essential cilia, the epithelium is transformed. In the sinuses and cavi-ties formed within this vegetation tissue the epithelial cells in many places retain the columnar form, giving to the recesses the appearance of secondary glandular formations.

In conjunction with these changes in the mucous membrane there is involvement to a greater or less extent of all the structures of the wall of the tube, so that, as a whole, the tube is enlarged. In the absence of occlu-sion of the fimbriated end, this enlargement rarely exceeds the dimensions of the thumb. With complete closure of this opening, however, a saccular enlargement may be developed, consequent upon the encysting of a secre-tion, which will far exceed the above dimensions, as will appear when this phase of development is described.

The thickening of the wall of the tube may be mainly confined to the inner half of the structure, the wall of the ampulla suffering relatively but little; on the other hand, however, this arrangement may suffer a reversal, or, at any rate, the wall of the ampulla may be so much more affected that the naturally wide cavity may be almost obliterated. This thickening of the tube is mainly interstitial, an inflammation of the entire thickness of the wall,—an interstitial or parenchymatous salpingitis in which all the elements participate, but chiefly the connective tissue,—the changes, in fact, being analogous to those met with under similar conditions in the wall of the uterus. This interstitial process is most pronounced when peritonitis is superadded, because then the tube is attacked both from within and from without. Naturally, the greater the encroachment upon the cavity of the tube the less evident become the changes in the mucous lining; but these changes, though overshadowed, are none the less present, as is evident upon close inspection.

In the presence of acute exacerbations of the inflammatory process extending to its outer as well as to its inner face (exacerbations, by the way, very common in the earlier phases of all cases of chronic salpingitis), the tube, as a whole, is much softened, resembling in this particular the structure of the uterus when it suffers a similar extension of the acute process to its peritoneal aspect. In the absence of such exacerbations, the tissue of the tube is hard and generally brittle, though it may be tough, the cut surface resembling in appearance and consistency infiltrated carti-laginous tissue. Now and then nodules as large even as a pea are formed upon the surface of the tube, such features being located, as a rule, near the uterus, generally at about the cornua. They are found most frequently in conjunction with the acute exacerbations above mentioned, and contain pus, being, in fact, little more than real abscesses in the wall of the tube. It might be inferred that the abdominal end of the tube would be closed in all cases of marked chronic salpingitis, especially in the interstitial forms; but such is not the case, for many times the abdominal end, though fixed by adhesions, is partly, if not entirely, open. A constriction of the opening at the base of the fimbriæ, however, is common in such cases.

Confining ourselves to the subsequent changes in such tubes as above described, we find that there is reason to believe, judging from similar conditions in other organs, that resolution may occur, and that, in the absence of constricting peritoneal adhesions, the abdominal end remaining open, there may be a restoration of function. Repeated and prolonged inflammatory action, however, may prevent this,—a circumstance all the more likely if peritoneal adhesions confine and constrict the tube as a whole or close its end. It is possible that a closed tube may regain its patency in whole or in part by resolution and absorption of the inflammatory exudate; but should it fail to do so, its function, in the absence of outside aid, is destroyed. An interesting question connected with tubes which, although open at both ends, have suffered from inflammation is the subject of extra-uterine pregnancy. The weight of evidence indicates that the changes in the calibre of the tube and in the character of the mucous membrane—particularly the destruction of the cilia which such mucous membranes suffer—are causes of arrest of the fecundated ova at points outside the uterus. When resolution fails in interstitial salpingitis, connective-tissue sclerosis takes place, leading ultimately to conversion of the tube into a mere cord of indurated tissue with obliteration of its canal. Peritoneal adhesions play an important part in this process of destruction, and in the presence of such alterations are rarely, if ever, absent.

We now come to the changes which take place in tubes whose outer ends are closed. As already said, such closures may disappear by resolution; but if the closure remains, the ampulla of the tube is converted into a sac or cyst. Firm and lasting closure may take place in any kind of chronic salpingitis, the changes in form which such tubes undergo being most striking. (See Plates I., II., III., IV.)

**Pyosalpinx.**—The most common is the pus-sac, or "pyosalpinx." It is merely a tube whose walls show interstitial inflammation, and whose outer and perhaps inner end is closed, the closure of the outer being the result either of agglutination of the fimbriæ (the common condition), or of fixation of this end against the ovary or some adjacent structure; the contraction of the inner end being the result of inflammatory adhesion of the opposed inner surfaces of the tube, this closure being most common near the cornua, but possible at any point of the narrower stretches of the canal. The contractions in question account for the retention of secretions and ex-

PLATE I.

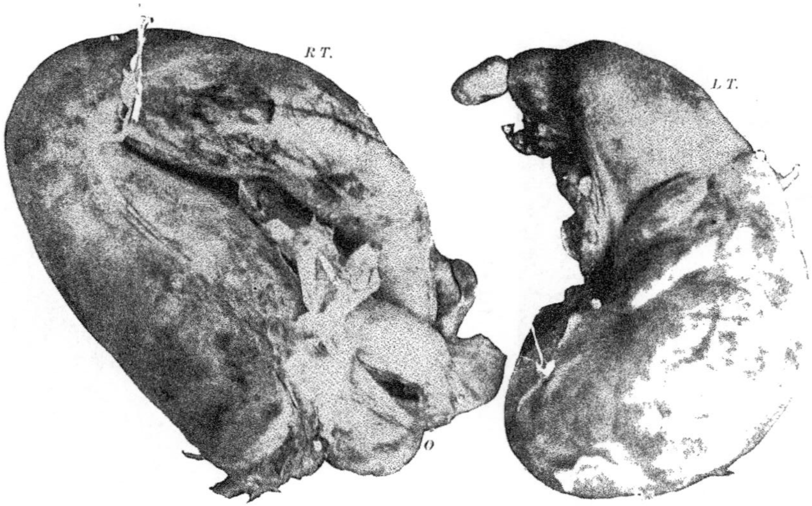

Pyosalpinx.—*L. T.* left tube; *R. T.* right tube; *O.* ovary with surface adhesions.

PLATE II.

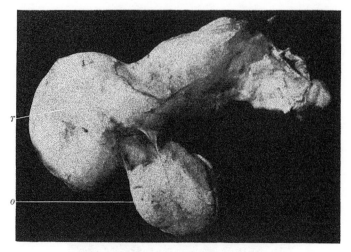

Pyosalpinx.—*T*, tube; *O*, ovary with surface adhesions.

PLATE III.

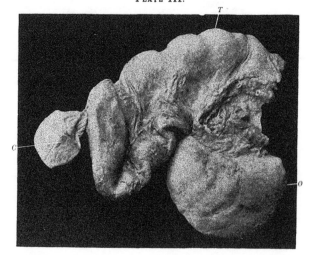

Pyosalpinx.—*T*, tube with ampulla empty, in order to show constrictions;
*O*, ovary; *C*, small cyst.

udates within the tube, and the accumulation of such substances accounts for the enlargement which the ampulla of the tube undergoes.   The greater enlargements occur as the result of closure of both ends of the tube, the lesser are found in conjunction with a free uterine end, the contents of the tube thus having opportunity for escape into the uterus; this escape is either a constant leakage, or more likely an intermittent discharge, brought on either by direct contraction of the tube or by such pressure as may be developed in efforts such as defecation.   It is certain that direct pressure with the finger will cause the partial evacuation of some of these pus-sacs.

Pyosalpinx may be bilateral or unilateral, generally the latter; but it is uncommon for this condition to exist in one tube without some grade of salpingitis existing in its fellow.

The condition presents itself in various shapes and sizes.   The common form is a general enlargement of the tube, club-shaped at the outer end, tapering gradually towards the uterus, or more or less convoluted, the convolutions depending upon the restraining action of what may be called the mesosalpinx, the peritoneal attachment to the broad ligament, and to its connection with the ovary.   (See Plate II.)   The tube may be doubled upon itself (see Plate I.), or it may show constrictions, a condition of sacculation prevailing, such constrictions being dependent upon peritoneal adhesions and bands.   (See Plate III.)

The diameter of such tubes may reach an inch or more.   The greatest development is generally seen in tubes measurably free from constrictions; they then assume the appearance of pear-shaped cysts, and in general attain to about the size of the average normal uterus; rarely they may be much larger, reaching even the dimension of the average fœtal head.

The position occupied by an inflamed tube depends somewhat upon the position of the uterus; if this be an approximation to that held normally by the non-pregnant organ, the general course of the tube is an approximation to that which it normally holds,—that is, with its outer end turned inward, downward, and backward, the fimbriæ usually resting against or near to the ovary.   (Plate IV.)   With an increase of the weight of the tube, the enlarged end sinks so that it will rest in the lateral fossa of Douglas, or even in the depths of the cul-de-sac itself.   If the uterus be retroverted, the tubes resting as above will be overcapped by the upper parts of the broad ligament.   In cases following labor at term or associated with a uterus enlarged from any cause, the tubes may occupy a higher position, not infrequently resting in the iliac fossa.   The writer has seen one case in which the inflamed tube filled the whole of the central, upper, and outer portions of the left iliac fossa, resting beneath the sigmoid flexure, which practically formed a covering for all of the inflamed mass.   A statement has been already made touching the eccentric positions which the inflamed tubes may occupy, and if we add it to what we have just said, we shall be in a position to follow to a conclusion what we now propose to say concerning the further behavior of pyosalpinx.

While we speak of the collection under consideration as pus, as a fact there is always a large admixture of mucus, and it may be of blood, so that the collections do not commonly present the active tendencies of collections of pure pus, witnessed, for instance, in the connective tissue or muscular spaces. Collections of pus in a tube will often remain relatively quiescent for considerable periods of time, and occasionally, in common with similar collections elsewhere, may suffer partial absorption and inspissation, appearing ultimately as a pultaceous mass. The tendency, however, is towards escape; the direction of escape being probably most often along the canal of the uterus; next, through the abdominal end of the tube, the fluid forcing its way between the agglutinated fimbriæ; and, lastly, by the combination of stretching and degeneration, an opening is made in the tube-wall, through which escape occurs. The part of the dilated wall through which such discharge takes place most often is at the upper posterior face, about the middle of the ampulla; another point is at the line of union of the layers of the broad ligament,—that is, upon the under face of the tube. An opening at the first point would mean a discharge of the tube-contents into the peritoneal cavity, with all that such an accident implies, if it were not that, as a rule, such discharges take place so slowly that ample time is given the adjacent peritoneum to throw out enough lymph to continue the incapsulation of the fluid, and thus save the general peritoneal surface from infection. In the event of a discharge downward between the layers of the broad ligament, the pus reaches the subperitoneal cellular tissue, where its further incapsulation is largely provided for.

The frequent discharge of the contents of a pyosalpinx through the canal into the uterus explains, in part, the not uncommon fact that such cases are for a time free from dangerous symptoms. The tendency is for the tube to refill, and, thus alternately emptying and refilling, the condition may exist for a long time, either ending in atrophy of the tube or, by closure of the channel of escape, resulting in a complete pus-sac. Resolution with restoration of function of such a structure is probably impossible; the best that can be hoped for is some form of atrophic change. In the absence of this change we may expect the contents of such sacs to escape outward.

Returning now to the developments which follow the escape of pus towards the peritoneal surface, we find that leakage from the abdominal end of pus-tubes is fairly common, each escape being accompanied and followed, as already said, by the phenomena of a local peritonitis proportional to the amount and specific virulence of the fluid.

Leakage through the wall of the tube is less common, but where it takes place towards the peritoneal surfaces the phenomena above noted appear. It is a rare circumstance to find a pyosalpinx without such an implication of its covering peritoneum and the adjacent surfaces of this structure as will insure a wall of reinforcing false membrane (see Plate VI.), such sacs being adherent to adjacent structure in whole or in part. Where, however, a pyosalpinx is uncovered by peritoneal adhesions, especially if such nakedness pertains to its entire circumference, it is a doubly dangerous product. Sudden rupture of such sacs is very possible, and such ruptures are apt to lead to so free an escape of the contents into the general peritoneal cavity as to render impossible any attempt at limitation by lymph-formation; a general peritonitis may thus be induced. It is even possible for such a wide-extended rupture to take place in the wall of a tube surrounded by adhesions as will permit free escape into the general peritoneal cavity, the result being similar to that above mentioned. Fortunately, however, most cases of pyosalpinx beget such an amount of local peritonitis about them as will insure a strong protecting environment of peritoneal adhesions; and, as already stated, the occasional leakages only add to and extend the adhesions, so that even though secondary foci of pus develop outside the tube they are again held in check. It is in this way that pelvic abscesses are formed, for, whether they originate in the tube or in the ovary, the constant effort of the peritoneum is to circumscribe and hedge them in.

The further consideration of the behavior of pus-collections originating in pyosalpinx belongs to pelvic abscess, to which subdivision of this chapter we refer the reader. We shall add, however, a word just here as to the different degrees of virulence possessed by the contents of pus-tubes. These differences account for the stormy course pursued by some and the mild behavior of others, allusion to which has already been made. The naked eye cannot detect the variations, but it may be said that the source of the infection points to a differentiation, cases originating in septic abortions or labors presenting the most virulent pus, those originating in gonorrhœal infection ranking next, and all other cases producing, as a rule, the less virulent forms of pus, the presence of the streptococcus and staphylococcus marking the most virulent forms.

Hydrosalpinx is a cystic enlargement of the tube in which the general outlines and dimensions of the organ are in the main similar to those found in pyosalpinx. (Plate V.) There are radical differences, however. In the first place, the contents are serous, not purulent, and in many cases as limpid as water. The walls of such sacs have generally lost their original anatomical structure, connective tissue taking the place of all others. This change is most pronounced in the mucous and muscular structures. The wall may be so thin in places as to be transparent. It is probably a late result of a pyosalpinx, and it represents a practical destruction of the tube. It is found as a bilateral rather than a unilateral disease, and is rarely without the association of strong, well-organized adhesions. It is free from the aggressive action characterizing pyosalpinx, tending to quiescence, sometimes to intermittent discharge through the canal into the uterus, and finally to absorption and general atrophy (more particularly) of the outer parts of the tube.

Hæmatosalpinx is the remaining cystic development in the tube. Like pyo- and hydrosalpinx, its seat is in the ampulla, and in form and dimensions it resembles those enlargements. It is covered with peritoneal adhesions in most cases, though the lesser forms may be comparatively free from such association, save at the outer end of the tube. Like pyo- and hydrosalpinx, it depends upon closure of the abdominal as well as of the uterine end of the tube, and, like them, it may occasionally discharge itself through the canal into the uterus.

There are two general types. The milder presents itself as a moderate dilatation of the tube,—to about the size of the middle finger, for instance. The contents are fluid blood. The tube-wall is moderately thickened from infiltration. The blood is, no doubt, menstrual, and is retained in the tube because of arrest growing out of the closure of the abdominal end by some prior mild inflammation. It is probable that in this type the uterine end of the tube is open, which would account for some of the obstinate cases of metrorrhagia found to be an associate of certain cases of tubal enlargement. The disorder may be bilateral, but in general it is single.

The remaining type of hæmatosalpinx represents a graver condition than the above. Here we find even extreme dilatation of the tube, reaching sometimes, as in pyosalpinx, the dimensions of a fœtal head. The tube-wall is greatly thickened by infiltration ; the outer surface is covered with adhesions, and may be closely bound to adjacent structures ; and, finally, it may rupture, with some escape of blood into the peritoneal cavity. The bleeding, however, is rarely sufficient to produce alarming symptoms, the condition differing, in this respect, from one with which it may be confounded,—extra-uterine pregnancy.

Opening the tube, we find it filled with a stratified blood-clot, the centre of the mass presenting a cavity of greater or less extent, filled with broken-down blood-products. The process of formation and disintegration of this clot is as follows :

There is originally disease of the inner surface of the tube ; from this a true hemorrhage occurs, probably at a menstrual epoch. This blood coagulates, filling the ampulla ; a subsequent hemorrhage occurs, with coagulation of the blood about the original clot. This process is repeated until finally a large mass is produced, which is made up of successive strata of coagulated blood. In time softening begins at the centre, and this may lead finally to the conversion of the entire mass into a collection of blood débris. This may be ultimately absorbed, but, again, it may receive infection from the uterus and, becoming purulent, take on the behavior of a pyosalpinx. This form always leads to destruction of the tube.

A word should now be said concerning changes which take place in tubes that are ligated, as in the operation for removal of the appendages as now commonly performed. Often the ligation is made half an inch or more from the tube, this fault being more than probable with the employment of the "Staffordshire knot." Under such circumstances, the portion of the tube between the uterus and the ligature is liable to dilate, blood or muco-purulent fluid accumulating therein. These formations resemble conditions presented in pyosalpinx and hæmatosalpinx. They may persist for years, and although free from pressing dangers, the uterine end of the tube being usually patent, they cause distressing symptoms, such as pain and reflex nervous disturbance, together with a troublesome purulent or bloody discharge, all of which is not only vexatious to the patient, but a reflection upon the operator. Where tubes are removed *in toto*, such conditions are avoided.

### INFLAMMATION OF THE OVARIES.

**Acute Oöphoritis.**—As a rule, both organs are involved. The proximity of the ovary to the abdominal end of the tube insures an almost constant implication of the former in the inflammations of the latter, perioöphoritis being here the form first presented. The relations of the lymphatics leading from the uterus must not be forgotten, however, and it should be borne in mind in this connection that the lymphatics leading from the ovary connect in the meshes of the broad ligament with those coming from the upper parts of the uterus. We know the office of these vessels as carriers of infection, and we also know that the streptococcus and staphylococcus frequent these vessels in bad forms of septic inflammation. It is easy for such pathogenic germs to reach the ovary through the channels in question, which no doubt accounts for the frequency with which oöphoritis accompanies puerperal septic infection, even in the absence of salpingitis. (The writer has seen several such cases.) Oöphoritis, therefore, while mainly a sequence of salpingitis, occurs quite independently of this latter disorder. Interstitial oöphoritis is the form here first presented. But whether the initial ovarian lesion begins within or without the organ, the ultimate result will generally be the same, because outside implication will extend to the interior, and inside will generally find its way to the exterior, the lymphatics in both instances being the route of intercommunication. Primary interstitial development is, no doubt, the rule in all cases arising from causes acting directly upon the ovary, such as acute suppression of menstruation.

Where the disease begins as a perioöphoritis, we find the surface covered with a serous, plastic, or purulent exudate, in accordance with the grade of inflammatory action present. It is enlarged as a whole, and in the plastic and serous types the interior (chiefly the cortex) is more or less infiltrated with the small round cells common to inflammatory processes in other organs. If the type of inflammation be purulent, pus-cells will predominate. Along with all are the usual inflammatory hyperæmia and œdema. Beginning as an interstitial process, the same elements pervade the organ, the predominance of the simpler inflammatory elements upon the one hand or those indicative of suppuration upon the other being governed by the presence or absence of the so-called septic element in the causation. The Graafian follicles in all these cases suffer changes kindred to those going on around them. There is turbidity of the liquor folliculi, with softening and disintegration of the membrana granulosa and the ovum.

In the absence of purulent infiltration, resolution may occur, or, on the other hand, connective-tissue sclerosis may take place, leading to atrophy. Another change is the conversion of the follicles into cysts, the ova and membrana granulosa undergoing fatty degeneration. These cysts will be again noticed in conjunction with the chronic changes.

Purulent infiltration leads to the development of abscesses, coalescence of which may convert the ovary into a complete pus-sac, nothing remaining but the tunica albuginea. These collections of pus may be transformed into cheesy masses and become encysted, but the rule is a continuance of suppuration until the pus finally makes its way through the tunic, after which its course is analogous to similar escapes from the tube. Should it be a mere leakage, the peritoneum will furnish incapsulation for these secondary formations, loculi of pus being thus formed in what, but for the incapsulation, would be the free cavity. Should it be a free escape, then general peritonitis may supervene. The direction taken in such migrations is therefore towards the peritoneal surface, but it is permissible to believe that it may be along the line of the vessels between the folds of attachment to the broad ligaments, in which event a condition of things in keeping with similar migrations from the tube into the broad ligaments will prevail.

It may be said in general that suppuration in an ovary presents two extremes. In conjunction with the more virulent forms of puerperal septic poisoning, it quickly destroys the organ, and may speedily cause rupture, an event eminently disastrous, were it not that in such cases there is generally a wide-spread peritoneal infection to the mortality of which rupture of an ovarian abscess can add but little. The other extreme is one of long continuance and slow progression. As a rule, the adjacent peritoneal surfaces add layer after layer of adhesions, which, together with the thickened albuginea, serve to keep it within its original bounds, even for several years. The dimensions of such sacs may ultimately exceed those of a normal fœtal head at term, surpassing those of the tube. (Plate VI.) But violence may at any time rupture such abscesses, and if it be towards the peritoneal surface a quick and disastrous result will follow. It is clear, therefore, that here, as with the tube, the patient depends greatly for safety upon the action of the peritoneum.

The tendency of all enlarged ovaries is downward, so that collections of pus of ovarian origin are more commonly confined to the posterior portions of the true pelvis than those of tubal origin, the greater latitude in movement enjoyed by the end of the tube accounting for this difference. The pus in an ovary which is disintegrated by a rapidly progressive septic process possesses the watery characteristics of all pus developed in consequence of such processes. That formed in the sacs of slow development is thick, greenish yellow, or brownish from blood admixture, and, owing to the common proximity of the rectum, especially if the left ovary be the sufferer, is frequently very offensive.

**Chronic Oöphoritis.**—This disorder presents itself either as a chronic process from the outset or as a sequence of the acute processes. The common changes are atrophy and cystic degeneration. Atrophy is best marked in conjunction with adhesions, which, by compressing the organ, further the sclerotic changes set in motion by the acute interstitial process. The whole organ may be converted into a small mass of connective tissue, with almost entire, if not entire, disappearance of distinctive formation. Atrophy may occur independently of outside inflammation, the organ then being free from adhesions, much reduced in size, with a shrivelled, white, greatly thickened albuginea, its interior presenting changes similar to those just mentioned. In the cystic form the albuginea is thickened, and the organ is filled with cysts intermixed with comparatively normal follicles. The cysts are transformed follicles with thickened walls surrounded by indurated tissue; the ova and membrana granulosa undergo fatty degeneration and absorption, leaving merely a limpid fluid. In other cases the cysts contain a gelatinous or colloid material. Corpora lutea may degenerate into such cysts. Some of these cysts may be so large as to occupy nearly the whole of the ovary, and no doubt represent the beginning of an ovarian tumor. The stroma of all such ovaries shows some degree of connective-tissue increase leading to more or less induration, but whether this formation is a cause of the follicular changes or a result does not clearly appear. It may be said, however, that, in the absence of decided thickening of the albuginea, these ovaries continue their function, a sufficient amount of normal tissue being present to permit this.

Chronic hyperplasia is best seen in conjunction with prolapse of an ovary, the faulty position being no doubt largely responsible for this; but the improvement witnessed as a result of permanent reposition of these structures warrants the statement that such hyperplasiæ disappear to such a degree as to permit normal action on the part of the ovaries.

**Lymphangitis.**—Some implication of the lymphatics is a factor in all inflammations, and the more abundant the supply of these vessels the more pronounced the implication. The most potent influence, however, lies in the nature of the infecting element. This is made evident by contrasting the condition of the lymphatics in the two extremes of the inflammatory process, the so-called simple and the septic. In the former the implication is quite limited, in the latter it is very extensive. In the inflammations of the non-pregnant uterus and its appendages this implication is so subordinated to the lesions which beget it that close inspection is needed to recognize it. In the septic inflammations of the recently pregnant uterus we find the lymph-spaces and lymph-vessels of the uterus, of the appendages, and of the broad ligaments filled with purulent fluid; the more advanced the pregnancy and the more virulent the poison the more pronounced are these evidences of lymphangitis. The vessels and spaces are more or less crowded with the bacteria of sepsis, this crowding being so great in the worst cases as practically to choke up these vessels.

We have already, under the head of etiology, spoken of the *rôle* played by the lymphatics as channels of infection, and shown how this is subordinated to the state of the uterus and the degree of virulence of the infecting agent : as those statements agree with the phenomena of inflammation as developed in other tissues of the body, we must conclude that a distinctly septic element must be present in order that a lymphangitis may produce a metritis, a salpingitis, an oöphoritis, a cellulitis, or a peritonitis.

**Cellulitis.**—The part borne by this disorder was until recently so much exaggerated that its *rôle* was made to overshadow that of all other inflammatory processes about the uterus. The observations at the operating-table have so far corrected this that it now holds a position in keeping with that which it plays in other regions of the body. It is dependent on lymphangitis, and consequently may appear as an associate of an inflammation in any part of the genital tract. The writer is disposed to ignore the initiation of this disorder by the so-called direct extension of the infecting element to the cellular tissue, and also that through the veins, as both are subordinate to lymphatic extension occurring after these vessels have become choked with infecting elements.

Cellulitis belongs essentially to septic processes, those in which putrefactive germs figure; and the facts already noted—first, as to the frequent presence of these agents in the inflammations of the recently pregnant uterus, and, next, as to the abundant supply of lymphatics in such uteri—readily account for the additional fact that cellulitis is a more common and a more pronounced associate of the inflammation of abortions and labors than of that developed in the non-pregnant uterus.

Anatomically, it consists of a serous exudate in the meshes of the connective tissue, which is accompanied by active cell-proliferation. This process may resolve, may pass into the suppurative stage, or may lead to organization of new connective tissue, with subsequent contraction, leading to shrinkage and sclerosis in the affected region. It is generally a circumscribed process. If the initiating inflammation be of the virulent type, the process will be purulent from the outset; it will not be circumscribed, but will tend, on the contrary, to wide-spread extension, with necrosis of tissue.

*Chronic cellulitis* presents itself either as the organized, sclerosed, and shrunken remnant of an acute process, or as an adjunct of a similar process going on in an adjacent organ. Should the process in the adjacent organ become purulent, and the route of evacuation be towards the area of cellulitis, this area, assuming the purulent type, will become a circumscribed abscess. This change is witnessed in conjunction with the migration of pus from a tube, from an ovary, or from a loculus of pus encysted within the peritoneal cavity. Such abscesses are, therefore, indirect rather than direct formations, and are present in all cases in which pus from the sources above named makes its way into the broad ligaments or through the pelvic wall or floor. Cellulitis presents itself far more frequently as an associate and dependent of salpingitis and oöphoritis than of metritis, but its gravest, its extended forms come from metritis,—from the metritis of abortions and labors. Under these circumstances it is not infrequently present when both tubes and ovaries have been practically free from inflammatory implication. The broad ligaments are the common seat of cellulitis, but, it being an accompaniment, to some degree, of inflammation wherever seated, it is to be found beneath every focus of inflammation which rests near the connective-tissue plane of the pelvis. We thus find it in the utero-sacral ligaments and around and about the lower segment of the uterus. In the latter situation the cellular inflammation is so much a part of that going on in the structure or upon the surface on which it begins, that it very rarely presents itself as a clinical entity, being rather a part of the process as a whole. This statement also applies to cellulitis when it appears in the broad ligaments as a dependant of salpingitis and oöphoritis; but such is not the case when it is clearly a dependant of metritis, implication of the appendages being wanting, or at least trivial. Under these circumstances it is generally a double process. It commonly appears as a diffuse infiltration extended along the upper borders of the broad ligaments, following the lines of the lymphatic vessels coming from the body of the uterus. It rarely attains large dimensions, unless it should form an abscess, its tendency being to resolution. Its conversion into an abscess is possible, the change being a common accompaniment of puerperal septic inflammations which end fatally; but with recovery the rule is resolution, or, at most, some organization of the exudate, with subsequent contraction. Abscess-formation is so rare that the writer, in his entire experience with coeliotomy, has met with but one case, all other cases being clearly instances in which the pus was merely migrating from an ovary, a tube, or a loculus encysted within the peritoneal cavity. Cellulitis ending in diffluent pus-formation in the meshes of the pelvic connective tissue is an accompaniment of the virulent forms of septic metritis, etc., but opportunity for investigating such conditions belongs to the post-mortem rather than to the operating table.

A word must now be said concerning cellulitis as it occurs in conjunction with lesions of the cervix and upper vagina. It may lead to suppuration, as after the traumatisms of forced delivery, or it may result in connective-tissue increase, with a subsequent organization and sclerosis, the condition extending widely through the lower areas of the pelvic connective tissue. A slight degree of this condition is not infrequently seen in close relation with those cervical lacerations which, involving the vaginal roof, have extended into the contiguous connective-tissue areas, and which, owing to improper asepsis, are infected and heal slowly. The wide-extended induration and thickening of this area of connective tissue, which have been mentioned above, constitute a rare condition. It was formerly the custom to view the indurations about the uterus which were met with clinically as expressions of cellulitis. Coeliotomy has shown this to be a fallacy, for we now know that in nearly every instance such induration represents the thickened and adherent appendages; and, while some of it may be due to thickening of the cellular tissue, it is a thickening so wholly dependent upon the state of the appendages that clinically as well as pathologically it can be viewed only as a subordinate element.

Peritonitis.—The changes witnessed here are in keeping with those common to other serous cavities which may be similarly infected, the pleural cavities affording conditions more nearly illustrative of what we find in the peritoneum. The sources of infection are the cavities of the uterus and the tubes, and occasionally the ovary. Mere rupture of a physiological cyst (Graafian follicle), with even some contact of blood, will not cause peritonitis, as is proved by the phenomena of ovulation; but morbid processes within an ovary will sooner or later infect the peritoneum, as is abundantly shown in the conduct of even the milder varieties of ovarian cysts.

The phenomena of peritonitis are presented in three general types,—the serous, the fibrinous, and the suppurative. The simplest (the serous) appears as a clear serous transudation following upon the initial infection, which is the starting-point for all. It is possible, no doubt, for such a transudation to be unaccompanied by any exudation of lymph,—to be free, therefore, from any associated adhesions or bands of new tissue; but, as a fact, some degree of lymph-formation may be expected. This exudate—serum and lymph— may be absorbed, leaving scarcely a trace; on the other hand, the lymph may undergo organization, presenting itself then as adhesions, as bands, or even as a kind of membranous formation which in some places is thick, in others filmy and transparent, forming sacs or pockets which imprison more or less of the serous exudate. Considerable portions of the peritoneal cavity may thus be cut off and sacculated or encysted. These accumulations of serous fluid may disappear with the subsidence of the slight inflammation provoking them, leaving the false membrane, which by subsequent contraction may become a serious hinderance to the organs to which they are attached. On the other hand, any serous exudate, through the influence of an additional inflammatory impulse, may assume the characteristics of a sero-purulent exudate, in which event its membranous incapsulation is increased in thickness and density, the combination of the two tending to the production of an encysted abscess.

The fibrinous variety of this ailment may form a part of the serous, as already indicated; but a fibrinous exudate may be the predominating feature from the first. We here find the peritoneal surface covered to a greater or less extent with a coating of lymph, the serous exudate being a subordinate feature. The tendency of such conditions is towards organization, with the creation of strong and well-formed areas of new connective tissue, which serve to bind together the apposed faces of the organs or tissues involved.

From this source we may have an imprisonment of every affected organ. This condition of affairs is best seen in the fastening of the appendages in their several abnormal positions, already noted, in the fixation of the uterus

PLATE IV.

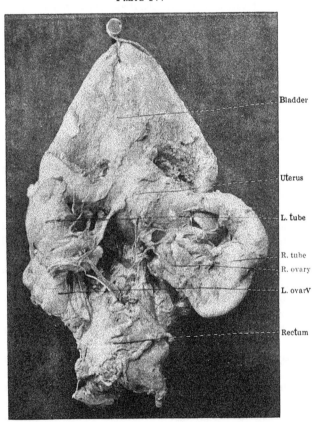

Bladder

Uterus

L. tube

R. tube
R. ovary
L. ovarv

Rectum

Bladder, uterus and appendages, and rectum all united bv adhesions.

generally a direct development from an exudation upon the peritoneal surface in conjunction with a salpingitis or an oöphoritis, it is also a formation
secondary to ovarian abscesses, to pyosalpinx, to a ruptured extra-uterine
fœtation, to peritoneal hæmatocele, and perhaps to a cellulitis.  When secondary to pyosalpinx, ovarian abscess, and cellulitis, it results from the
migration of pus from these sources, the peritoneum, as already pointed out,
furnishing limiting adhesions as the migration progresses.  When secondary
to extra-uterine fœtation or hæmatocele, it appears merely to represent the
transformation of the extravasated material into pus, the transformation
being the result of infection from some such source as associated salpingitis.[1]

**Pelvic Abscess.**—Reference to what has been said upon the subject of
suppurative inflammation in the various organs and structures of the female
pelvis will clearly indicate the sources of pelvic abscess.  It springs from a
pyosalpinx, an ovarian abscess, suppurative inflammation of the peritoneal
surface, or the same process as a sequence with intra-peritoneal extravasations of extra-uterine pregnancy or hæmatocele.  Very rarely it may spring
from cellulitis.  These origins account for the common location of these
collections of pus, which are in the posterior and lower portions of the true
pelvis, but pelvic abscess may be found wherever the end of an inflamed
Fallopian tube may lie; therefore it sometimes occurs in the iliac fossa,
particularly in puerperal cases and in conjunction with fibroid tumors,
because in such cases the tubes are higher than in other conditions with
which salpingitis is associated.  In rare cases the abscess may develop
anteriorly to the uterus, but when found here.it is generally the product of
a migration from elsewhere.

The common form of pelvic abscess is that derived from and associated
with pyosalpinx.  It is therefore met with most frequently in the region
of the cul-de-sac and that of the lateral fossa.  Its tendency is to discharge
itself either into the vagina or into the rectum.  It may make its way
externally by way of the obturator or sciatic foramina, discharging itself
alternately upon the inner or posterior face of the thigh.  On the contrary, it may perforate the broad ligaments and discharge into the bladder.
Collections of pus anterior to the uterus tend towards the bladder;
those situated high up tend towards the iliac fossa, and empty themselves
through the abdominal wall above Poupart's ligament.  Occasionally an
abscess will make its way through the iliac fossa and discharge itself below
Poupart's ligament upon the inner anterior aspect of the thigh.  From
what has been written concerning the behavior of the peritoneum in connection with these collections of pus, it is plain that its tendency is towards
the construction of a strong limiting layer of adhesions around and about all

---

[1] Although the subject of inflammation of the pelvic peritoneum and connective tissue
is thoroughly discussed in a separate chapter, it is deemed proper to allow another author
to present his own views from a somewhat different stand-point.  The reader will note
that peritonitis and cellulitis are here regarded as sequelæ, rather than as distinct affections.—ED.

## PLATE V.

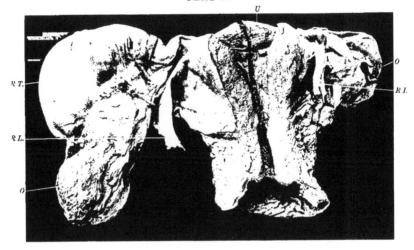

Hydrosalpinx.—*U*, uterus; *R T*, left tube; *O, O*, ovaries; *R L*, round ligaments

## PLATE VI.

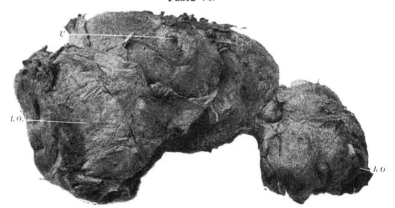

Ovarian abscess.—*U*, uterus, *L O*, left ovary; *R O*, right ovary, universal adhesions

such collections, no matter what their seat. It is in this way that bad cases of pyosalpinx and ovarian abscess receive dense coats of false membrane, and that all collections of pus in the pelvis are cut off from the free peritoneal cavity, being roofed over, as it were, by the same formation of false membrane. We wish to draw special attention to this formation, for upon it depends the possibility of escape of pus from a pelvic abscess into the free peritoneal cavity. Such an escape is possible, but it is a very rare occurrence, and, in the absence of violence, is always preceded by an abundant series of warnings. There are instances of suddenly developed pyosalpinx which, in the absence of well-organized adhesions, might rupture; but any collection of pus, no matter where located, which has been present for some weeks, will be provided with an ample environment of new limiting tissue, the exception to this being in those bad cases so common as a sequence of grave puerperal septicæmia, and occasionally met with among the victims of constitutional syphilis or scrofulosis.

In the event of sudden rupture towards the general peritoneal cavity, the phenomena of acute general peritonitis may be expected, but the extent and virulence of such a peritonitis are more dependent upon the specific characteristics of the escaping pus than upon the mere fact that it is pus. Cases of pelvic abscess which have an antecedent history of puerperal sepsis, therefore, may be viewed as the most dangerous.

Taking now a general view of the pelvis as seen in extreme cases of pelvic inflammation, we may find adhesions throughout the hypogastric, iliac, and deep pelvic regions. The omentum is involved, the appendix may be implicated, filmy sacs of serous fluid may appear here and there, or there may be one large sac. These conditions are in the main superficial. In the true pelvis there may be a dense layer of adhesions matting the intestines into a kind of roof over the uterus and appendages. These organs are seemingly one single mass, so close is their union and so firm is the adhesion between them. Together they rest upon the floor of the pelvis, to which they are, as it were, glued.

The most striking picture of this kind which the writer has ever witnessed was a development of syphilis. The woman was the victim of the tertiary form, but had not been under treatment for some time. She was operated upon for double ovarian tumor. The pelvis was then wholly free from any evidence of peritonitis. Two weeks after the operation a tumor was found on the right side of the uterus; this steadily spread to the left side until the entire upper pelvis was filled with a hard mass. There was very slight general disturbance until the sixth week, when symptoms of intestinal obstruction began to appear. The abdomen was again opened, and the mass was found to consist of the sigmoid flexure, the rectum, the uterus, and the bladder. Thinking that the origin of the ailment might be infection of the ligatures, these were sought out and found to be free from any purulent formation; none was found elsewhere. The infiltrated sigmoid lay like a cake capping the pelvic brim. Wounding it accidentally, its walls were found to be nearly half an inch in thickness. The infiltration implicated all the coats except the mucous. This accounted for the obstruction. The uterus, the rectum, and the bladder showed an identical infiltration. Under antisyphilitic treatment the condition improved, and the mass is now steadily disappearing.

*Symptoms and Signs.*—The symptoms and even the signs of the several conditions which we have just described as separate pathological entities are—with a few exceptions to be mentioned later—so intermixed that any attempt to unravel them would lead to confusion. The practical outcome of such an attempt in the present state of our knowledge would be likewise questionable, because the treatment for all is so much along the same line. We shall therefore present the symptomatology as far as possible from the single stand-point of inflammation of the appendages and the adjacent peritoneum. We shall observe the distinction between the acute, the chronic, and the suppurative form of the inflammations as they are presented *en masse*, and in dealing with the signs and the question of differential diagnosis will endeavor to note distinctions where they exist.

*Acute Salpingitis, etc.*—The symptoms present in the milder, non-septic forms of the ailment are often so slight as to escape notice. They merely form a part of those already present as indications of an acute endometritis. If there be a decided increase of the area of pelvic pain and fulness, and if this increase be in the direction of the iliac region, it will be safe to infer that the appendages are implicated. The general constitutional disturbance suffers an increase along with the increase of local disturbance, but this may be insignificant, amounting to a temperature of little more than 101° F. or a pulse-rate of 110, the respiration suffering no change. Motion increases the pain, so that the patient prefers to remain at rest.

The picture presented thus far is the one generally found when the disease is a sequence of a simple acute endometritis or metritis. There is an exception, however, even in the milder cases, where, for instance, the lesions are the result of an acute suppression of the menstrual flow. Here the pelvic pain is apt to be violent from the outset ; to be widely extended over both the hypogastric and the iliac region ; to be accompanied by an oppressive sense of fulness in the same regions, with pain radiating to the back and down the thighs ; and to be accompanied by vesical irritation, by constipation, and by some meteorism. The patient cannot move without greatly adding to the pain, and the pulse, temperature, and respiration bear testimony to the shock to which the patient has been subjected. A pulse-rate of 120 may be reached, a temperature of 102° F., and a respiration of 26 or more. In other words, the evidences of a sharp attack of pelvic peritonitis may be present along with the suppression of the menstrual flow, this suppression, together with the cause producing it, indicating the source of the seizure. If the attack be uncomplicated by a prior endometritis or salpingitis, it may be expected to subside within a few days, but in proportion to its severity it may be counted upon as the forerunner of a chronic inflammation which may annoy the patient for many subsequent years. As a rule, the acute symptoms of the milder forms of pelvic inflammation prevail for a period varying from ten days to a month, after which, if they continue, they belong rather to the chronic manifestations of this complex disorder. The acute symptoms of the gonorrhœal forms of this disease may differ but little from those given above, but there are certain associations and peculiarities of development that are distinctive. The previous history of the case, together with a microscopic examination of the secretions from the vagina and from the urethra, will be of great value, and although in intensity the symptoms may ultimately rival those first mentioned as an associate of acute menstrual suppression, yet such an intensity is not reached so suddenly, but only after ample warning has been given by an endometritis and metritis, to say nothing of what may have appeared in the vagina and urethra.

The acute symptoms of the septic forms of the lesions in question differ somewhat, according to the soil upon which the poison is implanted. If it be a non-pregnant uterus upon which some traumatism has been inflicted, we have perhaps the history of such traumatism, following which we have a chill, with a sudden onset of high fever; following this we have first hypogastric and then iliac pain and fulness upon one or both sides, according as the ailment involves one or both sets of appendages. Contrary to the rule in the non-septic cases, a double involvement prevails here, so that general pelvic pain sooner or later predominates. The symptoms may now subside, but, in the absence of any attempt to strike at the root of the sepsis, they may be expected to persist and to pass within a few days into those of a well-marked attack of pelvic peritonitis, or perhaps, worse, into a general peritonitis, which speedily ends in death. The usual termination, however, is in a chronic pelvic inflammation, in which the tubes, ovaries, and peritoneum are involved to a greater or less degree.

If the soil presented be that of a recently pregnant uterus, we have the antecedent history, which, if it be a natural delivery at term, will excite less suspicion than if it be an abortion. But, whether it be one or the other, salpingitis and its associate inflammations are ushered in by symptoms which are akin to those just named. In most cases the symptoms of acute endometritis and metritis are so pronounced that ample warning is given; in others, however, the approach of this evil is veiled in an insidious development which demands the closest scrutiny of all puerperal cases, a fact to which we have called attention when treating of metritis. The initial chill and subsequent fever may be so slight as to cause but little apprehension; but pain, which may be absent over the uterus, soon appears upon one or both sides. Even this may be localized for several days, and if the case have a favorable tendency it may so remain. On the other hand, it may involve the entire pelvis, or may spread to the general abdominal cavity, the patient in the one case presenting the phenomena of pelvic peritonitis, in the other those of a general peritonitis.  If it assume this latter phase, death may be expected; but if the symptoms indicate restriction to the pelvis, they will end in those indicating chronic inflammation, passing not infrequently into those belonging to the development of an abscess.

In the more virulent forms of septic infection the symptoms may appear so suddenly, with such intensity, and be so wide-spread as to unite metritis and general pelvic inflammation in one vivid picture; and again, an even more virulent form may appear and may so benumb the sensoria as to annul any local discomfort, leaving only signs by which to estimate the conditions present.  In these two latter manifestations it is clear that pelvic inflammation is subordinated to a degree of general infection which renders futile any differentiation of condition, especially if it be undertaken with a view to operative or other treatment of the appendages of the uterus.

From what has been said, it is evident that while symptoms distinctive of inflammation of the appendages may be present, yet usually such is their complication with those belonging to inflammations of the uterus upon the one hand, or with those indicative of pelvic peritonitis upon the other, that they are apt, as a rule, to be shrouded.  However, when they do appear, they are referred to by the patient as pain and fulness in the regions on either side of the uterus, one or both, as the affection happens to involve one or both sets of the appendages.

*Physical Signs.*—These are sufficiently distinctive in nearly every case; for, no matter what may be the nature of the case, whether of the milder type or the more virulent, sooner or later the physical evidences are clear. Bimanual palpation generally suffices, but, if this fails, then recto-abdominal will be effectual.  The ease with which these examinations may be made depends somewhat upon the amount of tenderness which is present; then, too, the characteristic indurations to be mentioned are more pronounced the later the examinations are made.  Referring now once for all to the position of the patient which affords the best and quickest results, let it be said that she should be so placed that the examiner stands facing the buttocks.  If possible, the patient should be placed so that the buttocks rest at the edge of the bed, or, better, of an examining-table.  The thighs should be flexed and permitted to rotate well outward, the head and chest being slightly elevated.  With the finger or fingers of one hand in the vagina (the left hand being used to explore the left side of the patient's pelvis and the right for the right side), the free hand is used to make counter-pressure upon the hypogastric and iliac regions, as occasion requires.

Proceeding carefully, it will soon be found that the uterus is more or less fixed; that upon one side, or perhaps upon both, a mass of tissue can be felt.  If the uterus be small, as in the non-pregnant state, these masses will be low in the pelvis; if it be large, as in the puerperal state or with a fibroid, the masses will be higher, perhaps encroaching upon, or even within, the iliac fossa.  Supposing the case to be a double infection, that both sets of appendages are involved, and that the masses which they present are within the area of the true pelvis, particularly if they be near the pelvic floor, hardening in the region of the cul-de-sac will appear. This hardening may also appear as the result of implication of but one set of appendages, but it is more commonly present as an associate of the double infection. It merely represents the exudate resulting from the peritonitis which has been provoked, and belongs to the severe rather than to the milder cases. In general terms, it may be stated that the more pronounced the type of the infection the larger the resultant masses, because with such there is a greater tendency to implication not merely of the tubes, but also of the ovaries, the peritoneum, and the lymphatics and connective tissue of the broad ligaments. If the disease be confined in the main to the tube, the size of the mass relative to that of the uterus may be so small as to be difficult to appreciate, especially if there be much fat in the pelvis or in the abdominal walls. But little more than lateral tenderness may then be detected.

Referring again to the indurations as "masses about the uterus," it should be borne in mind that they are not an early feature of acute inflammation. They are preceded by a sense of resistance in the affected area, it is true, but the resistance is rather that of œdematous tissue, a boggy sensation, as it has been styled. The indurations appear later, and are then in direct proportion to the amount of solid exudate which may be present. This statement of the relation of the indurations to the amount of solid exudate has but one exception in this phase of the disease, and that pertains to accumulations in the tube. In certain cases, even when acute, in which the tube is abnormally developed, it may present its infundibulum as a dilated sac filled with muco-pus: while such a tube would probably be surrounded by more or less solid exudate, yet a portion of the indurated mass would then represent fluid exudate, a condition of affairs quite common in the chronic and suppurative forms of pelvic inflammation.

Owing to the tenderness which prevails in acute inflammations, it is doubtful whether, in the absence of anæsthesia, an examiner will be able to detect more than has been here mentioned; but should he be able to do so, it would relate to the dimensions, and the relation of the masses or indurations representing the inflamed appendages. This is a phase of the subject which can be best presented in conjunction with the chronic forms of the ailment. In order, therefore, to avoid repetition, the reader is referred to that section of this article for additional information. Summing up, then, the signs pertaining to acute pelvic inflammation, we find tenderness and resistance in the affected regions. Pressure upon the uterus by the examining finger in the vagina increases the pain, the mobility of the organ is sooner or later impaired, and, with much exudate present, may finally be absent. The sense of boggy resistance at the site of the inflamed organs generally increases until ultimately a well-defined mass is appreciated. This may be single, appearing upon one side of the uterus only, or there may be one upon each side. These masses are generally near the uterus, but they may be in one or both iliac fossæ, filling these regions more or less completely. If within the true pelvis, they may fill the entire interval between the uterus and the pelvic wall, displacing the uterus to the opposite side when single, but when double tending to push it forward. The forward displacement of the uterus is greatest when the mass or masses invade the cul-de-sac, and this development—the indurated mass in the cul-de-sac—is greatest when both ovaries and tubes are involved. Under such circumstances, the uterus may lie embedded in a mass of exudate, and, being pushed forward against the symphysis, the entire floor of the pelvis will present a hard surface to the examining finger. This extreme condition of affairs, while developed within the confines of the acute stage, is an indication that the process is passing either into the chronic or into the suppurative form; for while resolution may remove the smaller masses and cause the disappearance of a large portion of the more extended ones, yet with the latter a nucleus of indurated tissue will generally remain in and about the regions of the ovary and the end of the tube, constituting a variety of the chronic forms of the ailment. And again, in place of resolution, suppuration may soon supervene, a termination by no means rare in the septic types which follow abortions and labors. The symptoms and signs indicative of these changes will be presented as we proceed.

*Symptoms of Chronic Pelvic Inflammation.*—There may be a slow and apparently uneventful development of this ailment, as, for instance, its appearance in conjunction with a persistent retro-displacement of the uterus; but chronic inflammation is generally a sequence of a prior acute attack, gonorrhœa and the septic inflammations of abortions being the common causes, the latter largely predominating. With such a history we may expect every case of this affection to be associated with some degree of chronic endometritis and metritis, and consequently the symptoms and signs of chronic inflammation of the uterus are always commingled with those pertaining to the appendages and peritoneum; but there are certain additions which are dependent upon the condition of the latter which can be noticed. Chronic inflammation, as distinct from acute exacerbations, has no special effect upon the pulse or the temperature, but it has a decided influence upon the general nutrition and upon the nervous system; both are apt to suffer: so that such patients are the victims of digestive derangements, meteorism, and constipation. Neurasthenia, malnutrition, and muscular weakness may be expected, and yet there are some women who are so strong that they carry with comparative impunity an amount of lesion which in others would serve to render them bedridden invalids.

The special symptoms of this ailment can be best presented as peculiarities of pain, of menstruation, and of leucorrhœa. There is more or less pelvic pain and fulness; this feeling is increased prior to the menstrual flow, and sometimes reaches a point of great suffering during the flow. The pain is most marked upon one side of the uterus or upon both sides, in accordance with the single or the dual nature of the ailment. Any disturbance, such as motion or the sexual relation, will at any time increase the pelvic pain. A full bladder or rectum will likewise add to the discomfort; but, as the act of defecation and even that of micturition sometimes increases for the time the suffering, such patients not infrequently avoid both acts as much as possible, thereby incurring the additional vexations of constipation and vesical irritation.

There is no question that most patients suffer more pain when the left appendages are involved than when the affection is confined to the opposite side. This depends upon the proximity of the rectum and the sigmoid flexure, in which the motion of gases and fæcal matter is of such constant occurrence. The fact that the calibre of this intestine is not infrequently markedly diminished by the widely extended exudates is a sufficient explanation of this phenomenon. This pain, however, is a mixture of local pelvic suffering and intestinal griping. This griping is also a feature of those cases in which other intestinal coils have been implicated; but the latter variety of pain is not confined to the left iliac region, as is the case where merely the sigmoid or the rectum is involved, but is diffused somewhat widely over the entire lower abdominal region.

Recurrent attacks of local peritonitis constitute a feature of many cases of this chronic disorder. This means that every now and then—sometimes almost with every menstrual epoch—these patients are prostrated by an acute exacerbation presenting the symptoms of pelvic peritonitis, quite similar to those mentioned already as an accompaniment of the acute stage. The symptoms are apt to subside, but now and then they persist, the case then assuming the aspects of a more general peritonitis. On the other hand, however, it may pass at once into the suppurative stage, the symptoms of a pelvic abscess supervening.

There is yet another feature presented by some of these patients which is of interest: it relates to the pressure-effects of the masses of inflamed tissue. The effect upon the bladder and rectum has been already noted, but a word must be said as to the effects of pressure upon the sciatic plexus, the obturator and crural nerves, and the psoas and iliacus muscles. It is probable that the effects upon all these structures are caused by pressure, as said, but the irritant action of inflammation may enter into the phenomena. This is certainly the case with the suppurative phases of pelvic inflammation, for with this latter condition the effects to be noted are often greatly increased. The effects in question are represented by pain along the course of the involved nerve and by painful contraction of the implicated muscles: so that a crural neuralgia, together with pain in flexing the limb on the affected side, is a common feature of an iliac deposit, and sciatic pain is a feature of certain deposits in the pelvis.

While dysmenorrhœa is not a constant factor with these patients, yet some degree of menstrual disorder is rarely absent. It may be irregular, occurring too frequently, or being less frequent than normal. It may be excessive at any given period, and then, again, scanty. But there is little that is distinctive about the flow, unless it be in those cases where it assumes somewhat the features of a metrorrhagia, or in which by pressure upon the affected area we induce an increased flow of blood.   The tenor of these statements applies equally to the leucorrhœal discharges, for they can scarcely be distinguished from those which belong to an endometris; but occasionally cases are presented in which the discharge is suddenly increased, the increase lasting for some hours and being preceded by an increase of pain suggesting tubal and uterine contractions.   Pressure upon the affected area induces this same flow, so that it is fair to infer that the discharge comes from a diseased tube.   The quality of the discharge is either purulent or serous, according as the tube happens to be the seat of a pyo- or a hydrosalpinx.

*Physical Signs.*—Properly speaking, the phenomenon of a bloody, a purulent, or a serous discharge flowing from the uterus as the result of manipulation should be named as a sign, but for the sake of proper continuity it has been deemed best to name it along with symptoms, as has just been done.   The remaining signs are much the same as those already named as pertaining to the acute stages of this affection, but, owing to the usual lack of excessive tenderness, the conditions can be more easily appreciated in the chronic stage.   The uterus is generally enlarged, its mobility is lessened to a greater or less degree, upward pressure upon it causes pain, and it is displaced from its central position.   It may also be retroverted, or perhaps anteverted, the former condition being the more common.   The displacement of the uterus as a whole from its central position is at first in a direction opposite to that at which the mass of inflamed tissue rests, but as absorption, with subsequent contraction, takes place the uterus is drawn in the opposite direction : so that where in the early stages of inflammatory action it may be pushed well to the right, for instance, later, through the action of adhesions and a contraction of the tissues of the broad ligament, it will be drawn to the left.   This same action also explains the position forward (even against the symphysis, as it may be), and later the position backward, in which the uterus may be found when the mass or masses of inflamed tissue are formed throughout the posterior regions of the true pelvis.   In all of these extreme conditions there is always some downward displacement of the uterus.

Referring now more particularly to these indurated masses, they are in reality the distinctive sign of the affection.   We have already shown, under the head of pathology, the various positions in which they may develop, and it is evident that the area which they may present to the examining finger depends entirely upon the extent of tissue involved.   The induration may be bent upon one side, and be no longer than the end of one's thumb, or it may fill the interval between the uterus and the pelvic wall, even encroaching upon the corresponding iliac fossa.   Then, again, the induration may present itself upon both sides, or a small area may be found on one side and a larger one upon the other ; and, finally, not only both sides of the uterus may be occupied by such indurations, but the posterior regions as well, the uterus being, as already mentioned, literally embedded in a mass which, occupying the entire pelvic floor, has pushed the uterus forward against the symphysis. In certain cases the bulk of the mass may be found in one or other iliac fossa, but associated with it there will be found more or less induration within the corresponding side of the true pelvis, in greater or less proximity to the uterus. In fact, the mass may even extend quite down into the cul-de-sac, presenting thus an area of continuous induration extending from high up in the iliac fossa to the bottom of Douglas's cul-de-sac. In contrast with these extreme conditions, the examining finger may fail to find more than a small area of tenderness and resistance in the cul-de-sac, a state of things which is said to indicate inflammation of the utero-sacral ligaments. It is probable, however, that a rectal examination will reveal in such cases some evidence of disease in one or other of the appendages.

Touching now the element of tenderness, it is obvious that it is a constant factor; its degree, however, appears to depend largely upon the state of the process : where this is in a state of activity the tenderness is increased. But the disturbed state of the patient's nervous system is a factor not to be lost sight of here, because where this has developed a hyperæsthesia a comparatively small lesion may present an exaggerated tenderness. It is also probable that the condition of the ovary may have a bearing upon this question ; but, while this may be assumed, it can rarely be demonstrated. We have just said that the element of tenderness is a constant quantity, and yet one will sometimes meet with cases in which, in spite of the presence of even wide-spread indurations, very little pain or tenderness is complained of. It is not easy to account for this fact, especially as such indurations may be situated indifferently either at the pelvic floor or upon the wall, or be suspended upon the upper regions of the broad ligament.

Thus far we have confined our remarks to the results of conjoined palpation, but it is evident that percussion will furnish us some information. This will apply more particularly to the conditions presented above the pelvic brim, especially to such as develop in the iliac fossæ. Relative dulness marks the area of the masses, of course; but in the event of an encysted peritoneal accumulation—such, for instance, as a serous exudate—a lesser degree of relative dulness may extend far beyond the mere area of recognizable induration. Percussion becomes, under such circumstances, a valuable aid, seeing that the resistance in these accumulations brought out by palpation is frequently insufficient for purposes of accuracy.

Inspection is of service in revealing the more general distention which in the acute exacerbations may be present, or the localized distention which may mark the chronic interference with the sigmoid and the rectum, or even with the coils of the small intestine.

*Symptoms of Pelvic Abscess.*—If this description of pelvic inflammation has been followed thus far, it will be proper to begin the symptomatology of pelvic abscess at the point where that of acute pelvic inflammation, that of chronic inflammation, and that of pelvic hæmatocele—commonly intra-peritoneal, dependent upon extra-uterine pregnancy—cease. A reason for this is the fact that pelvic abscess, as a dependant upon the uterus or its appendages, is invariably an outcome of one or other of these processes. If it be from the first-named, the antecedent history will be comparatively short; if from the second, this history may be a long one, for it must be remembered that in some cases of pelvic inflammation suppuration quickly supervenes, while in others it may appear only after repeated exacerbations have been developed in the course of a chronic ailment. If abscess spring from the last-named of the above conditions, the antecedent history is suffi-ciently distinctive to need no more here than this allusion to it.

Reference to the pathology of the subject will show that abscesses begin in the tubes, in the ovary, upon the surface of the peritoneum, and in the cellular tissue, named in the order of frequency. Without attempting any differentiation here, it may be said in general terms that the sooner the implication of the peritoneum and cellular tissue the sooner the appearance of active symptoms, and the wider the area of suppuration the graver the symptoms. This statement is introduced to emphasize the fact that suppu-ration may be confined for a long time to a tube or an ovary and yet few urgent symptoms may appear. In fact, in some few cases, were it not for the recurrent attacks of local peritonitis induced, such patients may have but small warning of the seriousness of their ailment, the symptoms being otherwise little more than such as might belong to a limited chronic ailment. General symptoms are early indicators of suppuration. They take the shape of somewhat regular exacerbations of temperature, with which is associated an increase of the pulse- and respiration-rate; the three, keep-ing pace, will show a daily increase proportioned to the extent and activity of the suppurative process. In these daily exacerbations the three, gener-ally mounting to a higher plane with each exacerbation, may reach 105° F. for the temperature, 120 or 130 for the pulse, and 25 to 30 for the respira-tion. Short of disturbances indicative of a fatal termination, the above figures may be considered as marking an extreme case. Lower figures prevail in the less acute cases, and proper treatment may be counted upon to modify them favorably in nearly every instance. With the subsidence of the general symptoms—a subsidence which rarely reaches below 100° F. for the temperature, 90 for the pulse, and 20 for the respiration—there may be some perspiration. Free sweating, however, indicates a considerable degree of septic infection, and is, therefore, a symptom of some gravity. In the absence of proper treatment, these symptoms continue to prevail, appetite and digestion are seriously impaired, and the result of the combined influence of the disturbing factors is steady emaciation and loss of strength. It is needless to say that such patients are in great danger, for, apart from the dangers of rupture of the sac towards the general peritoneal cavity and those which pertain to pyæmia, there is always before one the steady decline of the vital powers incident to all forms of prolonged suppuration. A spontaneous favorable termination may possibly be reached by a discharge of the pus outward, especially if this be through the abdominal wall or through the vagina; but even here, the pus-sac remaining, it may continue to refill and discharge, perhaps through a tortuous sinus, and the evil effects of persistent absorption may exist. This is more apt to be the case should the sac discharge by way of the intestine, because in this instance fæcal gases and solid matter may enter the sac, and, keeping up the irritation, may not only aggravate the original lesion, but add to its malign influence that which pertains to the absorption of fæcal poisons. The local symptoms of pelvic abscess relate to an increase of pain and fulness in the affected region, with generally some increase of vesical and perhaps rectal irritation. Should the abscess point in the direction of either of these organs, there will always be increased irritation within them, and should it press upon the sciatic plexus or the crural or the obturator nerve, pain in the course of these nerves may be expected. An abscess located in the iliac fossa may be expected to cause some retraction of the thigh and leg of the affected side, and it rarely fails to induce pain with the motions of the thigh, all being dependent upon the implication of the surface of the psoas and iliacus muscles.

*Signs of Pelvic Abscess.*—As the indurated mass or masses already outlined in conjunction with the signs of chronic pelvic inflammation are invariably present in all cases of pelvic abscess, it is only necessary to add that the sign of suppuration in such masses is, first, the evidence furnished by aspiration, and, next, that which results from palpation. By the first we have the visual demonstration of the presence of pus; by the second, that which results from fluctuation. Pus may exist for some time in the depths of these masses, so that, beyond the fact of an increase in the area and in the tenderness, palpation may be negative. For such cases aspiration will suffice. As soon, however, as the pus approaches a surface that can be reached, such as the anterior abdominal wall, or the rectal or the vaginal walls, there will be first softening and then fluctuation within the affected area; the surface will steadily become more prominent, presenting from this time onward the characteristic appearances of a surface towards which pus is advancing. Percussion and inspection will aid us in outlining the upper limits of these accumulations, but beyond this they are of small service.

*Diagnosis of Pelvic Inflammation.*—In giving the differential diagnosis of pelvic inflammation we shall present the subject under two heads: first, the differentiation of pelvic inflammation as a whole from conditions which may simulate it; second, the differentiation, one from the other, of the conditions which enter into it.

The following diseased states may simulate pelvic inflammation: fæcal impaction, hæmatocele, cancer, fibroids, psoas abscess, and appendicitis.

*Fæcal Impaction.*—The catharsis which should precede all pelvic and abdominal examinations will generally remove fæcal masses; but, as there are cases in which this may not be quickly accomplished, or in which it has not been attempted, a word may be needed as to the diagnosis. Such masses may be painful, but careful pressure will always cause such an indentation, such a change in the outline of the tumor, that mistake is well-nigh impossible. An exception is to be made where the impaction is a part of organic constriction of the gut. Here there may be local peritonitis set up about the impacted mass, preventing the necessary manipulation; but anæsthesia will override this.

*Hæmatocele.*—The history of the case, especially that which marks the appearance of the tumor, is sufficiently different in the two conditions to warrant at least an approximation to a diagnosis. The sudden development of hæmatocele is quite unlike anything characteristic of pelvic inflammation. There is little difference in the signs, for an extensive development of inflammation may give appearances and effects quite like those pertaining to hæmatocele, and that, too, no matter at what stage of the two conditions the comparison is made. Both are soft at the inception, then hard, and later both may again soften. It should never be overlooked that the subsequent condition of the two is sooner or later identical,—that is to say, both are covered with peritoneal exudate : so that, after all, some degree of pelvic inflammation enters into every case of hæmatocele, whether it be intra- or extra-peritoneal. Signs, therefore, when taken alone, are unreliable, but when studied in conjunction with the history of the case they are of service.

In dealing with the pathology of pelvic abscess we spoke of the development of the condition as secondary to hæmatocele, intra-pelvic hæmatocele being the form the more likely to give it. Should, therefore, the symptoms and signs of pelvic abscess appear as a part of the history of a hæmatocele, the latter need not invalidate the diagnosis.

*Cancer.*—Cancer of the uterus can never be mistaken for pelvic inflammation, because, even though it may have as an associate more or less of the latter condition, the malignant development is sufficiently self-assertive to be always recognizable through some one of the channels of investigation at our command. Cancerous tumors of the sigmoid, of the rectum, and of the bladder are all indicated by symptoms closely connected with the organs involved : so that, although, in consequence of a perforating ulcerative process developed as a part of the malignant affection in any one of the situations mentioned, a localized peritonitis may occur, and although this peritonitis may lead to a considerable addition to the general area of the original tumor, yet the history of the case, together with the characteristic symptoms and signs of intestinal or vesical implication, will reveal the essential nature of the ailment. If the uterus and appendages could always remain free from any connection with such malignant developments, bimanual palpation would generally suffice to prove that they were not the seat of the disorder; but the localized peritonitis above mentioned sometimes implicates one or the other, making it appear that they are perhaps

the starting-point of the ailment.   Under such circumstances it is evident
that the history of the case, and the signs present, must together form the
basis of differential diagnosis.   It is possible that malignant disease of
some adjacent structure may be an associate of a pelvic inflammation which
belongs essentially to the uterus and its appendages, the conditions being
then independent as regards their origin, and yet so close one to the other
as to appear to spring from but one source.   A careful study of every
symptom and sign presented by the patient will always show the double
nature of the ailment, so that even here no confusion need arise.

There is, however, a cancerous development which may cause embarrassment; that is cancer of the ovary.   Owing to the fixation of such a mass
by surrounding peritonitis, one may find much the same kind of mass as
might be presented with pelvic inflammation.   The differentiation is made
by the development of abdominal ascites and by the gradual appearance of
the cancerous cachexia.

*Fibroid Tumors.*—There would never be any confusion in this field
were it not that occasionally a fibroid uterus small enough to remain in
the true pelvis becomes fixed therein by peritonitis, which is generally
provoked by salpingitis,—a not uncommon complication of fibroids.   The
appearances presented are then very similar to such as may result from a
combination of ovarian abscess or hæmatoma with salpingitis and peritonitis, both being, perhaps, nodular, both hard, and both giving a history
of recurrent attacks of peritonitis.   In such conditions the uterine sound
is of inestimable value, showing a marked increase in the depth of the
uterine canal in the case of fibroid and little or no increase in the other.
But it is needless to say that every resource of diagnostic method should
be brought to bear, if necessary, aspirations through the vagina being
beyond question the most serviceable of all.

We have deemed it unnecessary to dwell upon the difference between
pelvic inflammatory masses and uncomplicated fibroid disease, simply
because the mobility and outline of such structures coupled with the reve-
lations of the sound are sufficient for all purposes.

*Psoas Abscess.*—Pelvic inflammations which implicate the psoas and
iliacus muscles and the crural nerve may occasion symptoms and signs
referable to the lower limbs which simulate the above condition, but the
absence of spinal symptoms and signs, and the fact that a distinct line of
induration can be traced from the region of the uterus to the iliac fossa,
will determine the presence of pelvic inflammation.   It is only when the
two conditions occur in the same patient that confusion can arise.   One is
then liable to fall into error, and to infer that only pelvic inflammation is
present.   The exaggeration of the hip symptoms and signs should create
suspicion, however, and then further inquiry will not only reveal spinal
symptoms and signs, but will bring out the double history.

*Appendicitis.*—If the appendix were found only in the right iliac fossa,
the diagnosis of appendicitis from pelvic inflammation dependent upon

the uterus and its appendages would be comparatively easy; but we know that this body frequently extends across the pelvis down into its depths; we also know that it may even reach across the entire pelvis, so that its end, the point at which inflammation first commonly appears, may rest in the region of the left tube. Such being the fact, it is easy to see that confusion concerning the origin of the inflammation might arise. Then, again, the later history of appendicitis bears a resemblance to that of chronic pelvic inflammation, for in both recurrent exacerbations are characteristic. In spite of it all, however, close investigation will establish the distinction.

First, as to inflammation situated within the area of the iliac fossa. If this be dependent upon the appendages, there will almost certainly be an antecedent history of some condition giving an enlarged uterus,—such, for instance, as pregnancy, a fibroid uterus, a hæmato-, hydro-, or pyometra, because, as has already been stated, it is quite rare, aside from such conditions, for the appendages to rest upon the iliac fossa. The history of the case will show further that the exacerbations are connected with uterine disturbances, particularly with menstruation. Palpation will reveal a connecting induration between the uterus and the iliac mass, and also that the mobility of the uterus is impaired, as a whole.

If, on the contrary, the lesion depends upon appendicitis, the antecedent history will be that of intestinal derangement, the exacerbations will likewise be associated with intestinal symptoms, and binanual palpation will show that the seat of greatest tenderness is at McBurney's point, and that the uterus and appendages are free. When an appendicitis develops in conjunction with an enlarged uterus, confusion may be possible, for physical examination may show quite a close connection between such a uterus and the inflamed area; but a careful study of symptoms will suffice to establish the intestinal rather than uterine origin of the ailment.

Considering, next, inflammation within the area of the true pelvis, we can say as follows. If it be due to the appendages, an antecedent history of uterine disease will always be present; there will be a constant relation between the exacerbations and the uterine symptoms, as mentioned above; and if, as asserted by Edebohls, it be possible to palpate the normal appendix, this may be found within the area of the iliac fossa. If the lesion be due to the abnormally placed appendix, let it be noted that while the latter may stretch across the entire pelvis, yet it very rarely does so, resting commonly upon the right side, near the attachment of the broad ligament to the pelvic wall. The diseased organ would then be nearly always upon this same side, where it is to be distinguished from an inflammation of the right appendages. If the mass be small, palpation may enable one to detect the free tube and ovary; but if it be large, it may implicate these structures and may even encroach upon the uterus. Under such circumstances it is practically impossible to arrive at a diagnosis from the physical signs, unless we can trace the thickened appendix across the pelvic brim to its connection with the cæcum in the depths of the iliac fossa. With a more widely displaced appendix we have much the same kind of difficulty to deal with. In all cases where signs give but a negative result, we are thrown back upon symptoms; these, as already indicated, will, under the above circumstances, point more to an intestinal than to a pelvic origin. There is a source of error pertaining to the diagnosis of pelvic inflammations by physical signs as distinguished from intra-pelvic appendicitis which should never be lost sight of; it is the fact that a normal appendix will quite often be enveloped in a mass of inflammatory exudate belonging to the adnexa. The organ will be thickened from peripheral inflammation, so that a skilful palpator might recognize it as it left the mass and passed to its origin. From this he might readily infer that the appendix was responsible for the lesion. Symptoms, however, would enlighten him and perhaps clear up the diagnosis. Making a final reference to symptoms, much can be made out of the fact that the acute symptoms and those belonging to the exacerbations of appendicitis are more explosive than those associated with inflammations of the appendages, and they are commonly more severe, both in their local and in their general expressions. We have omitted mention of aspiration as an aid to the diagnosis, because its results are apt to be negative until suppuration occurs, but it may be used wherever the tumor is large enough to promise results. Should fæcal matter be obtained, it would be conclusive as to the presence of appendicitis, but pus with simply a fæcal odor would not be conclusive, as any purulent collection near a large intestine may possess this odor.

Turning now to the differentiation of the organs which are involved in the pelvic inflammations of the uterus and appendages, we find that in the milder grades of the affection this is comparatively easy, especially if one resorts to recto-abdominal palpation. The outline of the thickened tube can be followed from the cornua of the uterus to its bulbous or cystic enlargement at the infundibula, its convolutions may be recognized, and even its constrictions. The outline of the ovary may be felt, encircled, as it is apt to be, by the enlarged tube. A mere enlargement of the ovary may likewise be distinguished from that of the tube, the latter being traced to its connection at the cornua and found free from abnormal thickenings. The uterus under such conditions is so free that, no matter what may be its position, its outline can always be made out. Concerning the recognition of cellulitis the writer is sceptical, because every sign named as distinctive of it can be simulated so closely by allied conditions. The sign so often mentioned, that indurations located low down in the region of the broad ligament indicate cellulitis, is absolutely deceptive, for the reason that the end of the tube and the ovary may occupy just as low a position; in fact, with a thin pelvic floor, these structures may appear as if they were just beyond the vaginal roof, and, being fixed in this position by adhesions, may give the exact conditions claimed as distinctive of cellulitis. When there is induration anterior to the uterus it may be due to cellulitis, but

24

even this condition has been found dependent upon a thickened and adherent omentum.

The distinctive evidence of cellulitis consists in the development of a mass within the upper folds of the broad ligament, in connection with abortion or labor, when, by rectal palpation, one is able to distinguish free ovaries and tubes. That rare condition, chronic thickening of the cellular tissue about the lower circumference of the uterus, can be inferred from the fact that it extends between the uterus and the bladder.

Extreme cases of pelvic inflammation rarely permit recognition of separate organs. There is such an amount of peritoneal exudate that, beyond the uterus, the outlines of individual structures are hopelessly lost. With resolution they may reappear and may present the peculiarities above described, but in the absence of this favorable change we can recognize only the irregular hard masses heretofore described. Even the outlines of the uterus may be lost, but the sound will always locate this organ, from which, as a starting-point, we gain information as to the relative implication of the two sides.

The differentiation of pyo-, hæmato-, and hydrosalpinx will be aided by the copious and sudden discharges (sometimes as the result of direct pressure) from the uterus of the fluid characteristic of each; but if this fails, and a diagnosis is deemed essential, the aspirator may be used. A small ovarian cyst might be confounded with hydrosalpinx, but the latter condition would always present the antecedent history of chronic pelvic inflammation. Should the ovarian cyst develop subsequently to the tubal disease, careful palpation might enable one to distinguish the tube, and thus, by ascertaining its condition, to determine the question.

Coming now to pelvic abscess, it will be found that this condition is recognized by the appearance of the fever of suppuration, by a slight aggravation of the severity of the local symptoms, by increase in the size of the mass, and by fluctuation. In the quiescent cases of pelvic abscess pus is detected by the aspirator.

The aspirator has been frequently named as an aid to diagnosis; it is well, then, to caution the examiner here as to its use. Whenever employed, it should be the rule to empty as far as is possible any sac into which the needle is introduced, because if this be not done, and the sac be left tense with fluid, there may be escape through the opening made by the needle. As there are conditions in which this would be a serious accident, it is well to guard against it in all cases.

Before closing the subject of diagnosis it may be well to say that, while vagino-abdominal palpation may suffice, there are many cases in which the rectal method is indispensable. As this is a trying procedure when properly done, it may be well to employ anæsthesia.

Prognosis.—The prognosis in pelvic inflammation has been indicated in the description of the pathological changes which belong to it; some further mention is needed, however, here. The milder forms of salpingitis and ovaritis, etc., tend to recovery, the term recovery covering not merely the state of their anatomical structure, but function as well. Even though the fimbriated end should be closed, a re-establishment of its patency is possible. It cannot be said that this statement is based upon actual observation, but analogy fully sustains it, similar results having been observed in other canals where somewhat similar conditions have prevailed. The exact degree of closure and general disease of the tube which will resolve so that function may be restored is unknown; but, no matter what it may be, should palpation show a disappearance of thickening or enlargement of the tube and the ovary, as well as an approximate return to their normal mobility, satisfactory resolution may be inferred. Wherever the thickenings remain and fixation shows the persistence of adhesions, it is clear that the disease remains. The persistence of symptoms likewise suggests an unfavorable condition of affairs. The prognosis in all such cases is unfavorable from the stand-point of health and function, but treatment may modify this prognosis so as at least to improve health, if it does not restore function. The treatment here referred to is that which stops short of removal of the injured organs. The appearance of peritonitis is always a grave indication, and the more acute and wide-spread the evidences of this condition become the graver the prognosis. The same statement applies to sepsis. When either of these conditions is wide-spread, death usually closes the scene.

From these statements it is evident that the acute disease associated with the recently pregnant uterus is the most serious form of pelvic inflammation. The septic inflammations of the non-pregnant uterus are next in point of gravity; then come those dependent upon gonorrhœa. When the disease sinks into the chronic phases, the periods of gravity are those covered by the acute exacerbations. Any one of these accessions may lead to a general peritonitis or to an abscess. Whenever abscess appears, the patient is exposed to the dangers of a possible rupture towards the free peritoneal cavity on the one hand, and those pertaining to prolonged suppuration on the other. Touching such expressions of chronic inflammation as pyo-, hydro-, and hæmatosalpinx, the first and the last are the most serious, as they represent advancing phases of the disorder, whereas hydrosalpinx represents a quiescent and retrograde phase.

Wherever there are extensive adhesions, and these appear to be organized, the prognosis as regards recovery is very bad, but not so as regards life. Patients may even pass a fairly comfortable life, but the greater number of them are chronic sufferers. The influence of prolonged suffering upon some constitutions is, however, in itself a grave factor; so that although the patient may live, yet she lives at such a cost as to rob existence of much of its value. Then, too, the undermining which her constitution inevitably undergoes makes her an easy prey to intercurrent disorders.

In general terms it may be stated, then, that the mild acute forms of pelvic inflammation tend to recovery; the graver forms tend to become chronic, to terminate in pelvic abscess, and are sometimes rapidly fatal. The chronic forms tend rather to chronic invalidism, but may end in death, either by reason of an acute exacerbation, through the influence of prolonged suppuration, or from the slow depreciation of the vital forces by prolonged suffering and inaction.

Pelvic abscess is always a grave affection, first, because of the possibility of infection of the general peritoneal cavity, and, next, because of the possibility of prolonged suppuration and sepsis.

The question of sterility is a pressing one in many phases of this ailment, but it is one that cannot be readily answered in any but the graver forms of the chronic and suppurative manifestations. Here we may say positively that sterility will almost surely be present, but in all other conditions such are the possibilities of resolution and such the mystery of conception that no man can predict sterility. These patients should never be robbed of the hope of childbearing.

There is a phase of this question which should not be overlooked; it relates to the possibility of extra-uterine pregnancy. We have already alluded to the subject under the head of etiology, but will now speak more fully. The constrictions and other deformities produced in the tubes by inflammation appear to obstruct the passage of the fecundated ovum, so that an extra-uterine development may occur; this condition must therefore be taken into consideration in any prognosis that may be given. The exact relation between pelvic inflammation and the condition is as yet guesswork; while, therefore, the possibility is not to be lost sight of, it need not be held up as an imminent danger.

Prognosis so far has been presented as a subject aside from treatment, but treatment, fortunately, is capable of modifying favorably even a most unfavorable prognosis. This will appear as we proceed with our presentation of this the concluding subdivision of our subject.

Treatment of Pelvic Inflammation.—This subject will be presented along the lines adopted in our description of the symptoms and signs, adhering as far as possible to the subdivision adopted there. In describing the treatment which is appropriate to any given state, both the medical and the surgical treatment will be stated; but, in order to avoid repetition, the several surgical procedures will be described later, a mere reference being made to each as we proceed.

*Acute Pelvic Inflammation.*—The milder types of this affection require little beyond rest in bed, gentle saline catharsis, hot douches, and hot poultices over the hypogastrium,—the treatment, in fact, being about the same as that already named for the milder forms of acute metritis. If there be much pain, or if there be such shock as belongs to the acute suppression of menstruation, then opium must be added. As soon as the acute symptoms subside, vaginal tamponade, as already described, should be instituted. Should the pressure cause pain, however, then this measure must be omitted until such time as it can be used without adding annoying discomfort. The patient should be encouraged to move about leisurely, for there is such a thing as too much rest for these patients. The symptomatic effect of this kind of motion is the guide to its continuance. In the more severe forms, the above measures are indicated, but the care must be greater. Absolute confinement to the bed is imperative so long as the acute symptoms prevail; this necessitates a nurse to give proper attention to the emptying of the bowels and bladder, which must be done in the recumbent posture. Free saline catharsis is at first beneficial; after that a daily movement of the bowels suffices.

If the case be septic or gonorrhœal, the attentions to the interior of the uterus already noted must be resorted to, if they have been previously omitted. The mischief which an early treatment of the uterine cavity would have prevented is here present, but its course can be modified for the better by freeing the uterus of débris, and then providing for drainage by means of the gauze, as already described. A sharp eye must be directed to the development of peritonitis and sepsis, for these are the indications for operative measures. Some peritonitis is always present, but it is a question of extent rather than presence. In septic cases, sepsis goes hand in hand with peritonitis, much as it does in appendicitis; but, unfortunately, the seat of the sepsis is in one instance an organ of small moment, with no vital connection, whereas in the other its seat is the uterus, an organ of such wide-spread and intricate anatomical connections that it cannot be dealt with in the prompt and radical fashion found so serviceable in the case of the appendix. This being the fact, it remains a problem as to how far surgical interference should be carried in the condition before us. The more general the implication the more hopeless is surgical interference. Therefore, the moment symptoms and signs appear which indicate the coming of general peritonitis or the advent of sepsis, operation should be done. The most radical procedure permissible is the removal of the appendages; but should the state of the patient forbid even this operation, or the firm fixation of the appendages involve too much shock in their removal, then one must be content with a free opening into the centre and depths of the inflamed mass and subsequent free drainage. The line of approach to such masses depends upon their location. If high up in the pelvis or within an iliac fossa, abdominal section should be the operation; if low in the pelvis, an opening through the vaginal roof is indicated. But, no matter which route is taken, after carefully washing out the affected area, sterilized gauze should be packed into the cavity formed, the free ends of the gauze to be brought out at the opening. Should a favorable result be obtained, the gauze may be removed at the end of three or four days. Care should be exercised in its removal, so as to avoid breaking through the adhesions which are always thrown out around the gauze. By packing the gauze after the manner of Mikulicz this step can be executed with least risk. Should further drainage be deemed necessary, a fresh packing of gauze may be made. If the opening has been made through the abdominal wall, some attention will be needed at the opening to lessen the chances of hernia; but this subject will be dealt with later. The vaginal opening can be left to care for itself, as hernia will not develop here.

Many patients will go to the verge of what might easily prove a fatal peritonitis and yet recover, and yet no one can foretell such a result. Should operation be declined, it only remains to support the powers of the patient by food and stimulation, and to ease pain by opium and fomentations. Catharsis will add to the comfort of the patient, but whether in such cases it has any eliminative effect worthy of mention is doubtful.

*Chronic Pelvic Inflammation.*—The treatment for this condition varies with its duration. In recent cases, especially if the uterus be in the early stages of endometritis and metritis, much good can be obtained by addressing treatment to this organ. The dependence of chronic pelvic inflammation upon the state of the uterus has been sufficiently explained, so that it is easy to see how its improvement will lead to improvement in the inflammation about it. In all such cases the uterus should be curetted and packed with sterilized gauze, as already explained under the head of chronic uterine inflammation. While the improvement will not extend so far as to include a complete disappearance of the results of pelvic inflammation, it will in the majority of such cases cause enough improvement to warrant the prediction of a speedy restoration to efficient health. The action of the uterine tamponade may be supplemented by the use of the vaginal tampon, the latter being continued, at intervals of two days, for a period of a month or more. The hot vaginal douche will also exercise a favorable influence in all these cases. It may be used in conjunction with the vaginal or uterine tampon. The rules governing its use are much the same as those already mentioned in connection with chronic disease of the uterus.

Pelvic massage after the method of Thure Brandt has of late been introduced as an associate treatment of pelvic inflammation. It is peculiarly applicable to chronic cases, and particularly to such as present non-suppurative indurations with fixation of the uterus and appendages. There can be no question of its efficacy; but as it is a somewhat objectionable procedure, and is hardly superior to other measures capable of reaching the same end, its employment is by no means urgent. So far as the treatment of mere fixation of the uterus and appendages by adhesions is concerned, the forcible disruption of such adhesions under anæsthesia by the method of Schultze will generally suffice; but even this procedure should be undertaken with caution, particularly if there be such enlargement of the tubes or the ovaries as would suggest infectious accumulations in either.

If the case of chronic pelvic inflammation be of long standing; if the uterus be in a state of induration, such as belongs to the latter stages of chronic metritis; if the tubes under such circumstances show a decided enlargement, such as pertains to pyo-, hydro-, or hæmatosalpinx; if there be reason to believe that the ovary is causing the persistence of symptoms; if recurrent attacks of peritonitis persist in spite of the treatment of the interior of the uterus; and, finally, if suffering and invalidism continue in spite of treatment, the only resource left is the removal of the offending organs.

There are certain rules of action governing operations upon the appendages which the writer has applied satisfactorily to his own work in this field, and which he will now present.

1. As a rule, women are better mentally and physically for the maintenance of menstruation and ovulation up to the period of nature's menopause; the further they are from the menopause, the more forcible is this rule.

2. The minor discomforts which pertain to the function, even though they be clearly dependent upon the ovary and tube, do not require removal of these organs.

3. The appendages may be operated upon to the promotion of child-bearing.

4. Disease of the appendages does not always demand complete removal, certain conditions permitting partial removal.

5. The condition of the ovary should be the chief factor in determining the question of procedure.

6. If the ovary contains pus, it and the associated tube should be removed, it being the rule that whenever an ovary is removed the tube must accompany it.

7. If the tube contains pus, the ovary being free from pus or disseminated degeneration, the operator is at liberty to amputate the tube and leave the ovary; the same rule may apply in cases of hydrosalpinx and hæmatosalpinx.

8. Cysts of the ovary do not demand its removal, provided they are not general throughout the organ and can be enucleated, hæmatoma of the ovary being a possible exception.

9. Tubes with open infundibula, even though adherent and affected with parenchymatous inflammation and endosalpingitis, do not demand removal, except when one opens into a pus-cavity.

10. A tube the outer end of which is closed, but which is otherwise in good condition, may be opened, cleansed, and its inner and outer coats coaptated, and then be returned to the abdominal cavity, provided that it does not contain pus or old blood.

11. Adhesions do not demand the removal of the tubes and ovaries, unless they be so dense that in breaking them the appendages are seriously injured. This presupposes that the appendages themselves are not sufficiently diseased to demand removal.

12. In all cases of subacute or chronic tubal disease it is of the first importance to treat the interior of the uterus, curetting it with the sharp curette and then firmly packing it with gauze being the best method of treatment.

In all forms of chronic pelvic inflammation close attention must be given to the general health. Diet and exercise must be regulated, and the alimentary canal must be placed in the best possible condition. Ferruginous tonics are always indicated, and the same may be said of cod liver oil in very many instances. Certain of the less urgent cases can be benefited by such a course of treatment as can be had at Kreuznach, or at the hot springs in our own country; daily general massage and a mild Turkish bath once or twice a week will also serve a good purpose.

*Pelvic Abscess.*—The treatment of this condition is essentially surgical, such medical treatment as may be indicated relating rather to the general state of the patient. This is largely symptomatic at first, but in the period of convalescence it is upon the same lines as relate to any slowly exhausting ailment. The general directions just mentioned under the head of chronic inflammation will therefore apply here.

The seat of the abscess and the state of the patient will indicate the kind of operation which should be performed. If the patient be in a state of exhaustion, it is unwise to attempt anything beyond mere evacuation and drainage. This will annul the urgent symptoms and afford time for sufficient recovery to permit of a more extended operation, should one be necessary. In some cases evacuation and drainage will be all that is required, the sac closing down and healing by granulation. This is more apt to be the case when the seat of the abscess is the peritoneal surface. When it is a tube or an ovary, the sac generally continues to form pus, so that a suppurating sinus and sac are apt to oppress the patient. Nothing short of complete enucleation and removal of such sacs will suffice to secure complete recovery. Therefore, if this cannot be accomplished at the initial operation, it should be done as soon thereafter as possible, the indication being then the persistence of the suppuration.

In evacuating such abscesses the rule is to open at the point nearest to it; therefore an abscess located low in the pelvis should be opened from the vagina, and one high up from the direction of the abdominal wall. In the radical treatment of these abscesses we have a choice between removal from above by cœliotomy and removal from below by morcellation. When the element of shock must be considered, the latter method is to be preferred, but it must be borne in mind that the uterus will then be sacrificed. The layer of protecting lymph which generally unites the coils of intestine above such deposits need not be disturbed in morcellation, whereas with cœliotomy it is sacrificed, thereby increasing the risks of peritonitis. In spite of all this, however, cœliotomy may prove the better method, and undoubtedly it will whenever the abscess is high up in the pelvis. Morcellation, in fact, is contra-indicated in most of these cases, and in all where the accumulation is in either of the iliac fossæ. Wherever an abscess has already opened into the intestine, more than usual care is required in removing its sac. The opening in the gut should be closed at the time of operation, if possible; but should this be impossible from any cause, then ample drainage must be provided for.

The question of hysterectomy in connection with the lesions of pelvic inflammation is one which is not infrequently forced upon the operator. This arises most often in consequence of the damage sustained by the uterus, first, in consequence of the adjacent and surrounding lesions in which it must take part, and, second, in consequence of the necessary surgical measures addressed to the removal of these lesions. In morcellation the uterus is placed upon the same footing as the appendages and is removed along with them, the operation being practically vaginal hysterectomy. When operating from above, however, hysterectomy may be avoided, and apart from any question of sentiment, but wholly in the immediate interests of the patient (if the case be one of pelvic abscess), this is as it should be here, because there are not many cases of pelvic abscess which are in sufficiently good condition to permit hysterectomy by the supra-pubic method. Should the conditions be favorable, however, to a radical operation, and the relations of the uterus to the suppurating sac and the damaged appendages be such as to compel in the removal of them serious injury (even if it be merely to the external coat of the uterus), then the latter organ should be included in the removal.

Our space does not permit any extended notice of this subject, but it may be stated that the rule of practice already accepted by operators is this : the condition of the patient permitting, the uterus should be removed in every case of pelvic inflammation in which there is such a close connection between it and the diseased appendages as to make it easier to remove the entire mass than to remove a part ; the uterus should also be removed in cases in which removal of the appendages or pus-sac compels extensive denudation of its surface or serious interference with its blood-supply.

It is perhaps best to say just here that if the operator concludes that one set of appendages or an ovary can be left, then the uterus must be left, it being, metaphorically, the mouth-piece of the appendages.

Our remarks so far have related to hysterectomy as applied to conditions which prevail with pelvic abscess ; we shall now speak of it in its relation to the general question of removal of the ovaries and tubes.

Every operator must regard not merely the immediate relief of his patient, but her future condition as well. While, therefore, immediate relief of symptoms and dangers may be obtained by the ablation of the appendages only, the writer believes that with very few exceptions the future condition of all such patients is best served by simultaneous removal of the uterus. This presupposes, of course, that both ovaries are removed,—a sacrifice, as will be seen by reference to the rules just given in connection with chronic pelvic inflammation, which the writer avoids in many cases in which they were heretofore condemned.

The basis for this advocacy of hysterectomy as a logical sequence of double ablation of the appendages is the clinical observation of the relatively better after-condition of the one class of patients as compared with the other, the annoying sequences of the enforced menopause being far less after cases of hysterectomy. It is evident, however, that the addition of hysterectomy increases the dangers of this operation, particularly if it be done as a cœliotomy; it therefore is always a question whether the patient should submit to the increased risk at the outset or face the chances of less complete relief. This is a matter for her decision.

*Surgical Operations.—Abdominal.*—All operations upon the abdominal contents demand the most scrupulous attention to the details of antisepsis, because sepsis here means not merely a prolonged convalescence, but generally the death of the patient. So far as the details of the preparation of the abdominal surface go, it is the same for all cœliotomies, and the same may be said touching the passage through the wall into the cavity of the peritoneum. The vagina should always be prepared as for vaginal hysterectomy, since hysterectomy may be necessary. When once within the cavity, the conditions possible in pelvic inflammations are sufficiently varied to demand special description of the steps needed to meet them. The difficulties revolve mainly around the presence or absence of adhesions, the state of these adhesions as regards the degree of organization which they have undergone, the extent to which the intestines are involved in the adhesions, and, lastly, the presence or absence of pus or other infecting fluids. Injury to the intestines can be avoided by proper care in operating; but, as accidents may happen, no cœliotomy should be planned without provision being made for such an accident. The question of drainage is ever present, but, in the absence of infecting fluids within the field of the operation, it is unnecessary. Whenever such fluids are present, if they be so encapsulated that capsule and fluid can be removed intact, drainage may be unnecessary. This applies, of course, to cases of pyo-, hydro-, and hæmatosalpinx, and to ovarian abscess. I have said that under the above circumstances drainage *may* be unnecessary. The word "may" is used advisedly, because, in the event of numerous adhesions or of extensive injury to the bed from which the pus-sac is removed, there may be much oozing of blood. Under such circumstances the writer prefers drainage. He also prefers strips of sterilized gauze instead of glass tubes as channels of drainage; but with intestinal fistulæ, if the drainage be supra-pubic, the addition of a glass tube to the gauze is preferable, the tube being surrounded with the gauze with a view to the creation of an outlying area of protective lymph as soon as possible. A single strip of gauze folded three or four times to the width of the thumb, carried down to the bottom of the diseased area or to the bottom of the cul-de-sac, will generally suffice; but if all the drainage possible be needed, and especially if at the same time it be desired to check by pressure such multiform bleedings as come from innumerable oozing points, then the gauze drain or packing after the method of Mikulicz is to be employed. The gauze should be removed as soon as it ceases to drain, say about the third or fourth day; but judgment must be exercised in its removal, for if its removal be strongly resisted, then the traction may so disrupt the adhesions which are formed about it as to set up a peritonitis which may prove fatal. Under such circumstances it is better to wait until by a more gentle teasing process the drain can be extracted. This suggestion is of special value when the surface has been infected. The question of irrigation is one as yet somewhat open, at least for the writer, his rule being to employ it for all infected cases, but for none other. Touching the length of the incision to be made into the abdominal wall, the rule is to gain as free access to the diseased area as is demanded for a good operation, and a good operation means the employment of sight upon the field of the operation should the operator doubt the efficiency of touch alone. With firm adhesions and an infecting fluid present, a free opening is best.

As regards the position in which the patient should be placed, there can be no doubt as to the advantages of the Trendelenburg posture in all difficult cases; in fact, it is a necessity in all such, and can be used in every case if so desired. The respiration and cardiac action of some patients are embarrassed by the posture, however, so that it is necessary that the assistant in charge of the anæsthetic should be on his guard to a greater extent than usual. In the simple forms of pelvic inflammation which call for operation the surgeon has an easy task. After opening the abdomen, he passes his fingers at once to the region of the uterus; locating this organ, he maps out the diseased area upon one or both sides, or behind, as it may be; he then determines the presence of adhesions. If none be present, the diseased appendages are lifted carefully to the surface for examination. If their removal be expedient, it is carried out in the following manner. Using silk or catgut as one may elect, the ovarian vessels are ligated *en masse* just outside the ovary and fimbriated end of the tube. The tube is then dissected out as far as the cornu of the uterus, bleeding points being caught up and ligated as one proceeds, with catgut or fine silk. The ovary is next cut away, the bleeding points being treated in the same manner. As in all abdominal operations it is a prime object to present as few raw surfaces as possible, the raw surface left by the removal of the tube and ovary should be covered up, if possible, by stitching back the round ligament to the line of the broad ligament, immediately below that just occupied by the tube; the tube should be amputated at the cornu by an oblique incision from behind forward and inward, thus leaving a surface which can be apposed to the round ligament. This simple precaution may not be possible in cases in which much distortion or contraction of the tissues has occurred, but when possible it should always be observed, because every raw surface left means the possibility of an omental or intestinal adhesion which may mar the results of the operation.

If the case be one coming under the head of the rules of procedure named in connection with chronic inflammations,—rules for what has been called "conservative operations" upon the appendages,—we proceed accordingly. For instance, if it be determined to sacrifice the tube but to retain the ovary, as in certain cases of pyo-, hydro-, or hæmatosalpinx, the tube should be cut away as far back as the commencement of its dilatation, the bleeding points being ligated as above described. The mesosalpinx may be ligated *en masse* between the tube and the ovary, care being taken to avoid the ovarian artery and vein, and then the tube may be cut away. Small cysts in the ovary may be treated by ignipuncture, and larger ones by enucleation or even by resection of a portion of the ovary, the outer edges left being drawn together by the Lembert suture. The conditions permitting the retention of a tube the outer end of which has been closed have been mentioned, so that it only remains to say that when the ends of such tubes are opened the freed borders should be turned back and stitched to the outer coat of the tube, catgut being always used for this purpose.

It will have been noticed that even in the radical removal of the appendages ligation of the tube is avoided. This is a measure to which the writer attaches great importance, because he believes that many of the recurrent symptoms to which patients are often subjected are due to the presence of the ligature upon the tube. They become so often infected through the stump of the tube that, in place of being innocuous, they become a source of irritation and inflammation, leading to many vexatious symptoms. This statement holds good even though the ligature be applied at the cornu, as the writer has found to his cost.

Coming next to the management of appendages embedded in adhesions, we reach a difficult operation. In all such cases the position of Trendelenburg is invaluable, for one's best powers may be needed to insure a good operation. Naturally, the stronger and more numerous the adhesions the greater the difficulties, but care and patience will surmount them all, so that none of these cases can be said to be inoperable. The fingers and the scissors are our means of disposing of adhesions; with one or both the appendages can be freed and finally brought to the surface. In dealing with this complication one must keep close to the appendages in the dissection, avoiding by this plan injury to the coats of any structure to which they may be attached. This is of urgent importance when the attached surface happens to be an intestine or the pelvic wall; it is of less moment when it happens to be the pelvic floor, the broad ligament, or the uterus. Still, as mutilation of even these structures is to be avoided, the rule applies in all cases. If the adhesions are imperfectly organized or are softened from recent inflammation, the separation, even though the adhesions be of wide extent, is often easier than would at first be inferred. The fingers then suffice. Pressing the ends of the fingers upon the inflamed mass, sulci are sought out; then, gently but firmly advancing, the thumb and forefinger are made to do most of the separation. Points of least resistance are sought out, and, pressing here and pinching there, the formed anatomical structures are gradually recognized and separated, until finally the offending structures are laid bare and brought to the surface.

If we are dealing with a pus-sac, ovarian or tubal, a cyst, or a hydro- or hæmatosalpinx, it is best to try to separate them intact from their attachments; but should the strength of the resistance suggest rupture, one had better avoid the chance by first aspirating. The difficulty of removal is thus increased, but the danger of peritoneal infection is avoided.

Should hysterectomy be deemed necessary, the operator should pass as quickly to it as possible. The ovarian vessels and broad ligaments are ligated and cut away, the uterus, meanwhile, being drawn well up, both to control hemorrhage from the uterine end of the cut vessels and to lift up the lower attachments of the organ; the uterine arteries are secured close to the uterus, so as to avoid injury of the ureters. Beginning then just above the utero-vesical fold, a circular incision is made about the organ and it is peeled out of its outer coat down to the vagina; the few bleeding points coming from vaginal anastomosis are ligated, the raw surfaces are turned in, and the outer coat left, with its peritoneal covering, is turned down into the vagina. A gauze drain is placed at the opening into the vagina, being carried down into that canal, which is then packed with gauze.

We have stated that there may be cases of pelvic abscess in which, owing to the low state of vitality, nothing beyond incision and drainage is permissible primarily, the radical operation being a measure for the future. The location of such of these abscesses as come within the domain of cœliotomy has been already noted. Being then high up in the pelvis, generally near the surface, and adherent, it may be possible to open them without entering the free peritoneal cavity. Free incision and drainage are all that will be immediately called for. It may be possible in the case of iliac abscesses to cut so near to Poupart's ligament as to evacuate the pus beneath the reflection of the peritoneum along the face of the iliac fascia. If the conditions above suggested be absent, then we face the necessity of draining such cavities along a channel which is simply a part of the free peritoneal cavity; this means the certainty of some infection of that cavity, no matter how carefully we evacuate and irrigate. Could one always promptly determine the degree of infecting power of such collections, he might with the comparatively benign forms risk the introduction of an abundance of gauze as a drain; though upon the whole, all things considered, the chances of such patients are best secured by enucleation. There is an exception, however, and that pertains to the possibility of stitching the sac-wall to the abdominal opening. If this can be done, the shock of enucleation may be avoided.

In reference to final closure of the abdominal wall after cœliotomy, the better method is to close it layer by layer, using catgut, silkworm-gut, or even silver wire, as the operator prefers. The writer has had satisfactory results with catgut.

*Vaginal Operation.*—For the purpose of merely opening a pelvic abscess pointing towards the pelvic floor, the vagina must be carefully cleansed and rendered thoroughly aseptic in the manner recommended in hysterectomy. The location at which the abscess tends to point having been determined, an exploring-needle is entered, care being taken to avoid vessels of any size which may be detected in the vaginal roof overlying the abscess-sac. A pair of scissors may then be passed into the sac, the needle being used as a guide. The blades being separated and withdrawn, a free opening is made into the abscess-cavity. The finger should then be passed into the sac with an irrigating tube and its cavity thoroughly cleansed by manipulation and free washing. The abscess-cavity is then closely packed with a long strip of sterilized gauze, the end of the gauze being brought through the incision into the vagina, this being also filled lightly with sterilized gauze. At the end of three or four days this dressing should be removed, the abscess-cavity irrigated with sterilized water, followed by peroxide of hydrogen, and the gauze packing renewed. This procedure should be repeated every second day until the abscess-cavity is obliterated.

If morcellation be decided upon, it is practically vaginal hysterectomy with the addition of removal of the pus-sac from below. The rules already laid down for the preparation of the vagina for hysterectomy should be carefully observed. Ligatures or clamps may be used to control hemorrhage. The uterus having been removed as in vaginal hysterectomy, the abscess-sac is carefully enucleated by the fingers, the same caution being used here as has been suggested under the head of cœliotomy. The adhesions in these cases between the abscess-sac and the intestines are numerous and intimate, and too much care cannot be exercised in the removal of the pus-sac, with the uterus and its appendages, to avoid injury to the adherent intestines. The cavity thus left should be filled with sterilized gauze, a free opening being left through which the gauze is carried into the vagina. The after-treatment of these cases is identical with that to be pursued in vaginal hysterectomy.

# CHAPTER VII.

## GENITAL TUBERCULOSIS.

BY J. WHITRIDGE WILLIAMS, M D.

WHILE tuberculosis of the female generative organs has long been well known to pathologists, it is only recently that it has attracted the attention of practical gynæcologists ; for previously it was known only as a concomitant of advanced phthisis, and it was not until cœliotomy demonstrated its frequent occurrence, either alone or in combination with tubercular peritonitis, that its clinical importance began to be appreciated. In this article I shall attempt to deal with the subject from a practical stand-point, referring those who desire more minute information as to its pathological anatomy, etiology, history, etc., to my monograph, "Tuberculosis of the Female Generative Organs," Johns Hopkins Hospital Reports, vol. iii., 1892.

Genital tuberculosis is usually secondary to tuberculosis elsewhere in the body, though in a considerable number of cases it may be primary and may represent the sole localization of the disease. It may involve any or all of the various parts of the genital tract, though some portions are far more frequently affected than others, the order of frequency being the tubes, uterus, ovaries, vagina, cervix, and vulva. The disease may present numerous variations, according to the organ affected, and I believe that it will be more clearly understood if we consider each organ separately.

**Vulva.**—Of all portions of the generative tract the vulva is least frequently affected by tuberculosis. There is no doubt that some of the cases described by Huguier and others as esthiomène and lupus of the vulva were of tuberculous origin ; but, on the other hand, it is certain that the great majority of the cases described by the various observers as tuberculosis, or lupus, had nothing to do with that affection, but were elephantiasis, carcinoma, or syphilis. Such being the fact, we shall consider as tuberculous only those vulvar affections in which tubercle-bacilli have been demonstrated or inoculation experiments have given positive results.

Measured by this standard, tuberculosis of the vulva appears to occur very rarely, cases having been described only by Deschamps, Chiari, Zweigbaum, and Viatte.

From the reported cases it would appear that vulvar tuberculosis is not usually associated with tuberculosis of other portions of the genital tract, and that it is due either to blood infection or to direct infection of wounds about the vulva.

Tuberculous ulcers of the vulva may attain a considerable size, and are usually shallow; their margins are irregular, sharply cut, slightly raised above the general surface, and of a more or less granular appearance. When the secretion is removed, their bases are seen to be studded by a greater or less number of granulations, some of which are grayish and semi-transparent, while others are bright yellow in color, usually not exceeding a millet-seed in size.

**Vagina.**—Tuberculosis of the vagina occurs much more frequently than tuberculosis of the vulva, and is usually secondary to tuberculosis affecting the higher portions of the genital tract, though it may occasionally occur independently of any other affection of the genitalia.

It occurs either in the form of miliary tubercles or as tuberculous ulcers arising from their caseation and breaking down, or as a combination of both forms. The miliary tubercles may be of various sizes, the largest not exceeding the size of a millet-seed, and may vary in color from gray to opaque yellow. By their caseation and breaking down, tuberculous ulcerations are produced, which present several characteristics which in most instances serve to distinguish them from ulcerations of other origin. Their outlines are irregular and their margins sharply cut and perpendicular; the base is shallow, studded by granulations of varying size and color, and covered by a more or less thick layer of caseous material; and about the circumference is a reddish areola in which many miliary tubercles may be found.

Tuberculosis of the vagina is usually limited to the posterior wall or to the cul-de-sac, and does not ordinarily extend below the upper third. Its location is readily explained by its mode of origin; for it is commonly due to infection by secretions from the tuberculous uterus or tubes, which trickle down the posterior vaginal wall. It appears that its comparatively infrequent occurrence is entirely due to the resistant structure of the vaginal mucous membrane.

Tuberculous ulcers of the vagina, by their extension, may perforate the wall upon which they are situated, and, according to their location, may lead to the formation of vesico-vaginal or recto-vaginal fistulæ, or may extend downward to the vulva.

Vaginal tuberculosis is not always the result of tuberculosis of the uterus or tubes, but in some instances may be due to extension from other organs. For example, cases have been described by Virchow and Menetria in which the vaginal affection was due to tuberculosis of the urinary organs; in other cases tuberculous ulcers of the bladder or rectum or even peri-rectal abscesses may perforate the vagina and so lead to its infection. In some instances miliary tuberculosis of the vagina may be secondary to phthisis, and may represent the sole lesion in the genital tract. Particular attention was directed to such cases by Lancereaux.

**Uterus.**—Tuberculosis of the uterus is not a rare affection, and is familiar to all who have witnessed a considerable number of autopsies upon phthisical women. It is generally associated with tuberculosis of the tubes, from which it has usually originated, and is frequently secondary to phthisis, or occurs as part of a general infection; and in some instances it may represent the only focus of tuberculosis in the body.

It is nearly always limited to the corpus uteri, rarely extending beyond the os internum to involve the cervix; when tuberculosis of the cervix occurs, it is usually without any involvement of the rest of the uterus.

The tuberculosis is at first limited to the endometrium, and it is only at a later period that the muscularis becomes involved; so that in most cases we have to deal simply with tubercular endometritis, which may occur in three forms: 1, miliary tuberculosis, with or without the formation of ulcerations; 2, chronic diffuse tuberculosis (caseous endometritis); 3, chronic fibroid tuberculosis.

Miliary tuberculosis of the endometrium is no doubt the initial lesion in nearly all cases of tuberculosis of the uterus, but it is rarely observed except at autopsy upon cases of general miliary tuberculosis; for in most other instances it has advanced beyond this stage and occurs either in the form of ulcerations, involving a larger or smaller portion of the endometrium, or as the typical caseous endometritis. The formation of the miliary tubercles occurs just beneath the epithelium of the endometrium, and may or may not be combined with inflammatory changes. The appearance of the tubercles and of the ulcerations resulting from them does not differ essentially from that observed in tuberculosis of other mucous membranes.

Chronic diffuse tuberculosis occurs much more frequently; it is the variety usually met with at autopsies, and is what is generally understood when one speaks of tuberculosis of the uterus.

In this form, the entire interior of the body of the uterus is filled with caseous material, which forms a thicker or thinner layer over its inner surface. On scraping it off, one sees that the subjacent tissue is very jagged and irregular and studded with tubercles in all stages of development, from the typical grayish, semi-transparent nodule to the irregularly shaped ulcer. This process is usually limited by the internal os, and the cervical canal remains perfectly intact. As the disease progresses, tubercles are gradually formed in the muscularis, which thus undergoes hypertrophy, and leads to a considerable enlargement of the uterus. Caseation and softening may go on to such an extent as to lead to rupture of the uterus, as occurred in a case reported by H. Cooper.

Microscopic sections of chronic diffuse tuberculous endometritis show the mucous membrane almost, if not entirely, destroyed, and its place taken by a new formation of diffuse tuberculous tissue, which contains numerous well-marked tubercles and here and there areas of caseation, which increase in amount as the cavity of the uterus is approached, the most superficial layers consisting wholly of caseous material.

Chronic fibroid tuberculosis of the endometrium has not yet been described, but, as a similar process occurs in the tubes, it is more than likely that it also occurs in the uterus.

By the obliteration or clogging up of the cervical canal, the uterine secretions become unable to escape into the vagina, and so lead to the formation of a pyometra. This condition is frequently noted, cases having been described at the extreme ages of five and eighty-one years by Silcock and Krzywicki.

In contradistinction to tuberculosis of the corpus uteri, tuberculosis of the cervix occurs but rarely. Both Rokitansky and Lebert have, indeed, stated that it does not occur. Later observations, however, have demonstrated that it does occur, and several cases are recorded in the literature. In these cases, as stated above, the cervix is usually the only portion of the uterus affected, but it is frequently involved in connection with tuberculosis of the vagina. In a considerable number of cases it may be the sole localization of tuberculosis in the genitals of phthisical women, and in rare instances it may be the only focus of the disease in the entire body, as in cases mentioned by Friedländer and Péan.

It occurs either in the form of miliary tubercles or of tuberculous ulcerations, or as a combination of both forms. The ulcerative form has sometimes been mistaken for carcinoma and operated upon under that supposition.

**Tubes.**—The Fallopian tubes are far more frequently affected by tuberculosis than any other portion of the genital tract, and in the great majority of cases either the uterus or the ovaries or both are likewise affected, and in some instances every portion of the genital tract may be involved in the process. In most cases the tubal affection is secondary to tuberculosis elsewhere, but in nearly all these cases it is the first manifestation of the tuberculous process, so far as the genitals are concerned. On the other hand, in a not inconsiderable number of cases the tubes are the seat of primary tuberculosis. This fact has long been known, but it is only recently that the frequency of this condition has been appreciated, and I believe that I was the first to demonstrate that it occurred oftener than has generally been suspected.

Like tuberculosis of the uterus, the tubal affection may occur in three forms: 1, miliary tuberculosis; 2, chronic diffuse tuberculosis; 3, chronic fibroid tuberculosis.

It is generally stated that the first form is rarely met with except in cases of general miliary tuberculosis, and some authors, as Daurios, completely deny its occurrence. But I have shown that it not infrequently occurs, especially in the cases to which I have applied the term "unsuspected genital tuberculosis," in which the process would have escaped detection were it not for a careful microscopic examination of all tubes and ovaries removed.

Miliary tuberculosis of the tubes presents the general characteristics of miliary tuberculosis of other mucous membranes, but, owing to the peculiar structure of the tubes, it readily escapes observation unless very well marked.

Chronic diffuse tuberculosis of the tubes is the form with which we are all familiar under the name of caseous-pus tubes, and corresponds to the like-named process in the uterus.

The gross appearance of the tubes in these cases varies according to the severity of the disease, and according as the peritoneum is likewise involved. In advanced cases the tube is greatly enlarged, and, according as the peritoneum is involved or not, its external surface is studded with tubercles in various stages of development, and occasionally covered by a layer of caseous material. In many instances the tube is densely adherent to the surrounding structures, and in some cases presents an almost stony hardness. In most instances the fimbriated extremity has become occluded, but when still patulous a mass of caseous material may often be seen protruding from it into the abdominal cavity. On cutting open the tube, its lumen is found more or less dilated and filled with typical yellowish caseous material, which varies greatly in consistency, sometimes being fluid, sometimes forming a soft mass, and in other cases being dry and almost solid, and occasionally even partially calcified. The normal appearance of the mucosa has disappeared, and on removing the caseous material we come upon a ragged ulcerated surface, over which are strewn tubercles in all stages of development. This process is usually limited to the mucosa, and it is only rarely that the muscularis is affected; but in most cases there is marked hypertrophy of the tube walls.

In some instances, instead of the typical caseous-pus tubes, we may have the formation of pus sacs, which occasionally attain a very large size. In one case I found the tuberculosis limited to a very circumscribed area, when it gave rise to a single nodular enlargement of the median end of the tube, about one centimetre in diameter, which bore a marked resemblance to the nodular enlargements described by Chiari and Schauta as resulting from catarrhal salpingitis.

Chronic fibroid tuberculosis of the tubes was first described by me, and differs from the other varieties in the excessive formation of fibrous tissue in and between the tubercles. In this form of tubal tuberculosis the lumen of the tube is distorted, and may or may not be the seat of the ordinary inflammatory affections. There is but slight tendency to caseation in these cases, and their most marked feature appears to be their chronicity; and no doubt in some instances it may indicate the spontaneous healing of the affection, just as occurs in other organs.

Ovary.—Most of the older writers stated that tuberculosis of the ovary rarely, if ever, occurred; but according to my experience, it occurs in a considerable number of cases, though not with the same frequency as in the tubes or the uterus.

It is usually met with in combination with other forms of genital tuberculosis, but in some cases of tubercular peritonitis and phthisis the ovary may be the only portion of the genital tract affected, though as yet no one has described a case of primary tuberculosis of the ovary.

In ovarian tuberculosis the process may be limited to the surface of the ovary or may invade the entire organ. Macroscopically, it occurs in the form of miliary tubercles, caseous masses, or tubercular abscesses.

Of the four cases which I have observed, in one the process was limited to the surface of the ovary, which was covered by miliary tubercles and small ulcers; in another, on section, the entire organ was seen to be studded with miliary tubercles; and in the two other cases the ovaries were converted into abscess-cavities.

### FREQUENCY.

The statements as to the frequency of genital tuberculosis present the greatest possible variations: my own observation places me among those who consider it a not infrequent affection.

According to Pollock, Schramm, and Winckel, it is found about once in every one hundred autopsies upon women. The following statement will serve to indicate the very divergent frequency with which it was observed by various writers at autopsies upon phthisical women. Courty found one case in every one hundred autopsies, Louis one in sixty-six, Cornil one in from fifty to sixty, Kiwisch one in forty, Mosler one in forty, Schramm one in twenty-four, and Nomias and Christoforis one in twelve. In other words, genital tuberculosis has been observed in from one to eight and a half per cent. of all autopsies upon phthisical women; leaving out of consideration the figures of Nomias and Christoforis, in from one to four per cent.

The statistics from operative sources also vary considerably. Thus, Edebohls observed it in four per cent. of all his cœliotomies, Martin in three per cent., and in one hundred and sixty-nine cœliotomies performed at the Johns Hopkins Hospital it was noted in two cases, or one and a quarter per cent.

These figures apply only to the well-known and readily recognized forms of the disease, and do not include any of the cases of "unsuspected tuberculosis." Beside the two cases in which the condition was recognized at the time of operation, careful microscopic examination of all tubes and ovaries removed for all causes demonstrated that "unsuspected tuberculosis" occurred in six other cases, thus making in all eight cases of genital tuberculosis, or four and three-quarters per cent.

In a considerable proportion of the one hundred and sixty-nine cœliotomies the tubes and ovaries were perfectly normal, having been removed for various causes, or were converted into cystomata and presented no other lesion. But in ninety-six cases they were removed on account of past or present inflammatory disease, and it is only in this class of cases that we meet with tuberculosis. Accordingly, of the ninety-six cases coming within this category, genital tuberculosis was noted in eight, or eight and one-fifth per cent. In other words, in our material, we have found tuberculosis of the tubes and ovaries in about every twelfth case operated upon for past or present inflammatory disease. Only two of the eight cases (twenty-five per cent.) were recognized at the time of operation, and it is evident that the other seventy-five per cent. would have escaped observation had it not been for the routine microscopic examination.

Consequently, in my experience three cases of "unsuspected genital tuberculosis" occur to one in which the diagnosis is made at the time of operation, and, should this ratio hold good, it becomes evident that we must multiply the figures of other observers by three in order to obtain the actual frequency of the affection. Whether our relative figures are correct or not, the discovery that so large a number of cases may readily escape observation proves that the affection is considerably more frequent than is generally supposed, and consequently renders it more worthy of attention on the part of practical gynæcologists.

As to the relative frequency with which the various organs are affected, I would say that the tubes are involved in nearly every case, the uterus in from sixty-five to seventy-five per cent., and the ovaries in forty per cent. of all cases.

### ETIOLOGY.

It is quite probable that the usual inflammatory diseases may predispose the genital tract to tuberculous infection; and the fact that I demonstrated gonococci in a tuberculous pus tube renders it quite likely that the gonorrhœal process prepared the way for the tuberculosis.

The actual cause of all cases of genital tuberculosis is the tubercle-bacillus, and in considering the etiology of the affection it is necessary to consider how the bacilli gain access to the genital tract. In general, they may be said to be derived from two sources,—from areas of tuberculosis within the patient, and from the outside world.

As a large number of cases are met with at autopsies upon phthisical patients in whose bodies there is no trace of peritoneal or intestinal tuberculosis, it is probable that the infection occurred through the blood. This mode of infection is rendered absolutely certain in the cases of general miliary tuberculosis in puerperal women, in which the disease is most marked at the placental site. For the production of blood infection, the presence of a large tuberculous focus is not necessary; and in this connection we need only to recall some of the cases of isolated tuberculosis, in which one is unable to discover any primary lesion, but at the same time would hesitate to regard the process as primary.

One of the most frequent sources of genital tuberculosis is tuberculous peritonitis. The fact that the distal end of the tube is usually most affected led the earlier observers to conclude that infection from the peritoneum was the most common mode of origin for these cases; tuberculosis of the tubes is far more frequently the result than the cause of tuberculous peritonitis.

Tubercle-bacilli from the surface of intestinal ulcers or from other tuberculous abdominal organs may find their way into the peritoneal cavity and fall to its lowest part, the pelvic cavity, without giving rise to tuberculous peritonitis; and from there they may be wafted into the tubes by the currents produced by the action of their cilia, and, if they meet with suitable conditions, may lead to their infection. The possibility of this mode of infection was demonstrated by Pinner by means of powdered cinnabar and other foreign bodies.

Bacilli may also gain access to the genitalia from other organs, which are the seat of tuberculosis, by the perforation of tuberculous ulcers and the formation of fistulæ between the diseased structure and various portions of the genital tract. Thus, the intestines may become adherent to the uterus or tubes, and the subsequent perforation of a tuberculous ulcer may lead to the production of a fistulous tract, by which bacilli may gain access to the genitalia. Cases of this character have been reported by Kaufmann and Mosler. Tuberculous ulcers of the rectum or bladder may perforate the vagina and thus afford an opportunity for infection, as may also peri-rectal abscesses. It is evident to any one who considers the almost universal distribution of the tubercle-bacilli that they not infrequently gain access to the vagina from the outside world. They may be introduced by the examining finger, by dirty instruments and syringes, from soiled linen, and in a multitude of other ways, and particularly by coitus with persons affected with the various forms of genito-urinary tuberculosis.

As it is evident that bacilli are frequently introduced into the vagina, it becomes important to ascertain whether they are capable of thus giving rise to the disease. Infection by coitus is, of course, the most interesting of these various modes of infection, and its consideration will serve as a type for all other modes of infection from the outside world.

The possibility of this mode of infection was first suggested by Cohnheim, was more thoroughly developed by Verneuil, and has received considerable attention, particularly at the hands of French writers.

The not infrequent occurrence of the various forms of genito-urinary tuberculosis in the male, and the presence of tubercle-bacilli in the testes and prostate glands of phthisical men presenting no sign of tuberculosis, as found by Jani, certainly afford a means for the introduction of bacilli into the vagina. The question is, do bacilli so introduced give rise to genital tuberculosis in the female? Owing to the resistant structure of the vagina and cervix, we would expect to find that they are not frequently affected, and that infection results only after the bacilli have gained access to the uterus or tubes.

In most cases it is not probable that bacilli introduced into the vagina enter the uterus, and consequently they cannot be expected to give rise to infection; on the other hand, even should a miliary tuberculosis of the endometrium follow their introduction, it is probable that the exfoliation of the superficial layers of the mucosa at each menstrual period would in most cases lead to the destruction of the newly-formed tubercles. So it would appear that infection would not be likely to follow their introduction, except in rare instances, unless the bacilli entered the tubes, where they could multiply unmolested. If this theory should hold good, it will explain why the tubes are more frequently affected than the uterus, even in primary cases. When there are areas of the vagina or cervix denuded of their epithelium, it is possible that bacilli may be taken up by the lymphatics and by their aid may reach the internal genitals.

Numerous observers have busied themselves with the question of infection by coitus; while all agree that it probably does occur, most of them state that its occurrence has not yet been scientifically demonstrated. The most conclusive work upon the subject is that of Derville, who in eight cases of genital tuberculosis in women found bacilli in the vaginal secretions from five, and on examining their husbands or lovers found that all of them had hard masses in their epididymes which he considers were of tuberculous origin. Derville's observation makes infection by coitus practically certain, but it does not afford scientific proof, because he did not demonstrate that the affections in the men were undoubtedly tuberculous.

Cornil and Dobrolowsky state that they have been able to produce tuberculous endometritis by injecting pure cultures of tubercle-bacilli into the vaginæ of rabbits; but later work by Oncarani and ourselves failed to verify their statements.

From my own work upon the subject and from the statements of others, I do not consider that infection by coitus has yet been proved. Nevertheless, I am inclined to believe that it does occur in some cases. It is evident, however, that the great majority of cases of tuberculosis of the female generative organs are of secondary and not primary origin.

Primary cases do undoubtedly occur, but we are not justified in regarding any case as primary if it be possible to find any other focus of tuberculosis in the body; and we may add that Sauger and Borschke in their recent articles take a similar view.

### CLINICAL HISTORY.

No period of life is exempt from genital tuberculosis, cases having occurred at every age between the extremes of ten weeks (Brouardel) and eighty-three years (Krzywicki); but the period of life in which its occurrence is most frequent is that of the greatest sexual activity, or between the ages of twenty and forty years. It is during this period that the cases of primary genital tuberculosis have been observed, while the cases occurring at the extremes of age have been due, almost without exception, to secondary infection.

Unfortunately, the clinical history of genital tuberculosis, like that of tuberculous peritonitis, does not present the clear-cut characteristics which are so necessary to the early recognition of a disease, its symptoms being only too often so masked by those of the primary affection that the involvement of the genitals is not suspected and is only found accidentally at the autopsy.  Even in the rarer cases of primary infection of the genitals, the symptoms are frequently so obscure that not only is the tuberculous nature of the malady not suspected, but its discovery at operation or autopsy is a matter of surprise.

Of course, tuberculosis of the vulva and lower portions of the vagina gives rise to the symptoms common to all ulcerative processes and soon leads the patient to seek medical aid.  In these instances simple inspection is frequently all that is required to direct one's attention to the true nature of the affection, but a perfectly positive diagnosis can be made only by means of the microscope.  In this variety of genital tuberculosis there are two points that should always be borne in mind, the chronicity of the affection and its ready amenability to treatment; the latter, however, is only apparent, for the ulcerations are particularly prone to recurrence.

In several instances of tuberculous ulcerations of the cervix (Péan, Zweifel), profuse hemorrhage and suppuration were the symptoms which led the patient to consult a physician, and in each instance a diagnosis of carcinoma was made; but in Zweifel's case, after the microscopic examination of curetted portions of the ulceration, the diagnosis was changed to that of tuberculosis.

In many instances, to tuberculosis of the internal genitals is assigned a prominent part in the production of symptoms which in reality are due to tuberculosis of other organs.  This is particularly true of the cases of general miliary tuberculosis associated with tuberculosis of the genitals, which have been reported by Rokitansky, Schellong, Heimbs, and others. On the other hand, in the cases occurring during phthisis the symptoms on the part of the genital tract are either entirely overshadowed by those due to the pulmonary process, or considered as the result of an ordinary endometritis or salpingitis.  It is in the primary cases and in those secondary cases in which the pulmonary process has not attained a great headway that symptoms are occasionally observed which serve to direct one's attention to the tuberculous nature of the genital affection.

In the cases in which the uterus is affected there is frequently a very profuse leucorrhœa, which in some instances consists of a mixture of the caseous material and the usual secretions of the uterus.  I, however, do not believe, as did Madame Boivin and others, that it is possible from the macroscopic appearance of the leucorrhœal secretions to reach a definite conclusion as to a tuberculous affection of the uterus.  As the disease progresses there is frequently a considerable hypertrophy of the uterus, but neither of these signs, nor both combined, would direct one's attention to a possible tuberculous affection, unless some point in the history of the patient or her husband (as a genito-urinary tuberculosis on his part) or the development of pulmonary symptoms were to suggest such a possibility.

Spath and Derville lay great stress upon the occurrence of menstrual disturbances as important symptoms in the early periods of the disease, but, as I shall demonstrate further on, no great value should be attached to them.

The symptoms produced by tuberculous disease of the ovaries and tubes, whether associated with tuberculosis of the uterus or not, vary greatly according as the process is limited to them or has involved the peritoneum. Of course the symptoms may be merged with those of phthisis or tuberculous peritonitis, and the genital affection may be entirely overlooked; on the other hand, primary tuberculosis limited to the tubes may produce no symptoms at all, and the fact that there is any disease of the genitals may be discovered only at autopsy after death from some other cause, as in the cases of Thompson and Tomlinson. As long as the process is limited to the tubes and ovaries and has not led to the production of diseases elsewhere, the symptoms may vary from those of a simple salpingitis to those of the most severe forms of pelvic abscess, and in spite of careful examination nothing will be found to indicate the tuberculous nature of the affection. Thus, in none of our cases was a diagnosis made previous to operation, and in each instance it was thought that we had to deal with either an ordinary case of "adherent tubes and ovaries" (perisalpingo-oöphoritis) or a pus-tube. In some instances the first sign of disease is the discovery by the patient of tumor-masses occupying the lower portion of the abdomen, as in a case reported by Munster and Orthmann.

Amenorrhœa, as stated by the older writers, is not necessarily an accompaniment of genital tuberculosis, but if it occurs it is usually due to the coincident phthisis. An analysis of six of our cases, in which we have notes concerning the menstruation, demonstrates that the menstrual disturbances attending tuberculous disease of the genitals do not vary from those accompanying other inflammatory diseases of the tubes and ovaries; and, as in them, we find no menstrual derangement in some instances, while in others menstruation may be very irregular and scanty or even completely suppressed, and in still others there may be marked menorrhagia, in some instances the loss of blood being almost constant. Thus, in two of our cases there was no change; in two, menorrhagia; in one, scanty, irregular menstruation; and in another, amenorrhœa. Strange to say, in the two cases in which the disease was most advanced there was absolutely no menstrual disturbance, even though one of them exhibited signs of phthisis.

That our experience is not isolated is shown by the fact that Daurios makes the same statement; and in reviewing the literature we met with cases described by Boivin, Kiwisch, Brouardel, and Gardner, in which the occurrence of menorrhagia was also noted.

It would thus appear that tuberculosis, so long as it is limited to the tubes and ovaries, does not give rise to any symptoms which would of themselves cause us to suspect its occurrence, and accordingly its physical diagnosis becomes impossible in most instances. Not so, however, when the disease is associated with pulmonary or peritoneal tuberculosis, for in these instances the discovery of tumor-masses involving the tubes and ovaries should at once lead us to suspect tuberculosis.

It would lead us too far, however, to attempt to discuss the protean clinical pictures which may be presented by this affection when combined with tuberculosis of the peritoneum, and I would refer the reader to the articles by Kaulich, König, and Osler in this connection.

Tuberculosis of the genitals, when primary, may lead to the secondary infection of other organs and may produce tuberculous peritonitis, phthisis, or general miliary tuberculosis, and thus indirectly cause the death of the patient. In other instances, whether the genital affection is primary or secondary, it may lead to death by marasmus and hectic fever, or, by the rupture of tubal or ovarian abscesses into the peritoneal cavity, to the production of a septic peritonitis from secondary infection. Rupture of a pregnant tuberculous uterus, with the production of peritonitis and death, has been reported by H. Cooper, but the tuberculous nature of the affection is open to doubt.

### DIAGNOSIS.

When we consider the clinical history of the affection it becomes evident that prior to the discovery of the tubercle-bacillus a positive diagnosis of genital tuberculosis could not be made *intra vitam*, and even a probable one only in very rare instances.

The difficulty of diagnosis varies considerably according to the portion of the genital tract involved by the process, it being much easier when the more readily accessible portions are affected, as the vulva, vagina, and uterus.

Tuberculosis affecting the vulva and vagina may be confounded with a number of affections to which it bears a superficial resemblance ; but in all doubtful cases the microscope will be able to render a final decision. Thus, miliary tubercles occurring in the vagina should be distinguished from the granulations due to a granular vaginitis. The frequency of the latter, compared with the great rarity of vaginal tuberculosis, is of itself almost sufficient for diagnosis, but, when one considers that tuberculosis of the vagina occurs nearly always in phthisical women whose internal genitals usually present marked changes, while granular vaginitis is frequently associated with pregnancy or gonorrhœa, a mistake should not occur. Tubercles should also be diagnosed from the papular and ulcerative syphilides by the history, by the entire absence of pain, and principally by the total disappearance of the latter under anti-syphilitic treatment. Herpetic eruptions about the vulva and entrance to the vagina may occasionally be a source of confusion. Their anatomical character, occurring as small cysts filled with clear fluid, should be evidence of their nature, and this, in connection with the fact that they usually appear about the menstrual period and disappear soon after it, should make their recognition certain.

Tuberculous ulcers might be mistaken for either hard or soft chancres, but the well-known characteristics of both these varieties of ulcerations and their history should not leave the diagnosis doubtful for any great length of time. Lastly, they may be mistaken for carcinoma. If in any case the diagnosis appears doubtful, the microscopic examination of a small portion of the suspected area will conclusively settle the question.

That tuberculous ulcerations of the cervix have been mistaken and operated upon for carcinoma has already been mentioned, and no doubt this mistake has frequently occurred. It shows the necessity for the microscopic examination of an excised portion of the cervix previous to any radical operation, for, while such examination will but rarely result in the discovery of a tuberculous ulcer, it will demonstrate in many instances that the growth is benign and will spare the patient a serious operation.

In any case in which there is the slightest suspicion of genital tuberculosis, the vaginal and uterine secretions should be inspected with the greatest care for tubercle-bacilli. The secretion should be removed by a platinum wire loop, previously sterilized over a flame, and spread in a thin layer on a cover-glass and stained with carbol-fuchsin, just as if it were sputum. If this inspection proves negative, the uterus should be curetted and the scrapings hardened in alcohol and submitted to microscopic examination; if tuberculosis exists, its histological characteristics will be amply sufficient for diagnosis.

To Babes (1883) belongs the credit of being the first to demonstrate tubercle-bacilli in vaginal secretions, and the method has now passed into routine practice. By this means Derville, Jouin, and others have been able to diagnose with certainty cases of tuberculosis of the uterus in which there was apparently no trace of tuberculosis elsewhere; and Derville states that Nocard diagnosed tuberculosis of a cow's uterus by finding tubercle-bacilli in the vaginal secretion, and that the diagnosis was verified at the autopsy.

In suspected cases in which bacilli are not found in the secretions and the histological examination of the uterine scrapings is not satisfactory, the peritoneal cavity of rabbits or guinea-pigs should be inoculated with small portions of the endometrium, when the production of tuberculosis would confirm the diagnosis.

I would recommend the examination of the secretions and curetted portions of the endometrium not only in suspected cases of genital tuberculosis, but also in every intractable case of endometritis for which a perfectly definite cause cannot be assigned, and I feel confident that by this means we shall not infrequently meet with and diagnose cases of this variety.

The diagnosis of tuberculous disease of the tubes and ovaries is more difficult than that of tuberculous disease of the uterus, for the reason that their secretion is not so readily obtained for examination.

I consider that it is impossible to diagnose tuberculosis of the tubes and ovaries by bimanual palpation alone, and do not regard as of any significance the thickened and nodular condition of the uterine end of the tube, to which Hegar attaches so much importance; for a thickening of the uterine end of the tube is met with in many cases of pyosalpinx in which there is absolutely no trace of tuberculosis. The nodular condition of the tubes is likewise of no diagnostic value, for, while it was present in one of our cases, Chiari and Schauta have described a similar condition resulting from catarrhal salpingitis, and it is evident that small myomata of the tube may give rise to a similar condition. Various observers have called attention to the hardness of tuberculous tubal tumors; as, however, hardness is occasionally noted in ordinary cases of pyosalpinx, it cannot be considered as at all pathognomonic of tuberculosis. In cases in which the process has extended to the peritoneum, if the pelvic organs are not too much matted together by adhesions, tuberculous granulations may sometimes be felt on the posterior surface of the uterus and broad ligaments; this, however, is possible only in the rarest instances. A probable diagnosis of tuberculosis of the tubes may be made in any case when in addition to distinct tubo-ovarian masses we are able to diagnose tubercular peritonitis; or, as Osler expresses it, "the association of a tubal tumor with an ill-defined anomalous mass (tubercular tumor) in the abdominal cavity should arouse suspicion at once."

Edebohls, in his excellent article on the subject, lays the greatest stress on the value of plaque-like thickenings of the subperitoneal tissues of the abdominal wall in the diagnosis of tubercular peritonitis, and says, "The coexistence of a tubal tumor or tumors with plaque-like thickenings of the subperitoneal tissues points with the greatest distinctness to tuberculosis. The tuberculosis under these conditions may fairly be assumed to be primary in the tube or tubes if no other deep-seated tumors can be palpated in the abdominal cavity."

If, on the other hand, the tubal tumor occurs in a phthisical woman who presents no trace of tuberculous peritonitis, we shall not even be able to make a probable diagnosis, but in these cases we should always bear in mind the possibility that the affection is of a tuberculous nature.

And lastly, if the tuberculosis is limited to the tubes and ovaries, without any pulmonary or peritoneal involvement, I do not believe that it will be possible to diagnose the affection merely by the physical examination of the patient. In some instances, no doubt, the examination of the vaginal secretions might reveal the presence of tubercle-bacilli, but in the vast majority of cases it would yield negative results. In one case of pyosalpinx which was suspected of being tuberculous, a positive diagnosis was made by Edebohls, by the vaginal puncture of the pus-sac, under the guidance of careful bimanual palpation, and the examination of the fluid removed for tubercle-bacilli. While it is possible that the method may enable us to make a diagnosis in some instances in which the process has gone on to abscess-formation, it is evident that the diagnosis of a large proportion of primary cases becomes practically impossible.

Even though this outlook does not appear especially promising, we cannot lay too much stress on the frequent examination of the uterine secretions, and I am confident that its more general adoption will lead to the recognition of not a few cases which now pass unrecognized.

### PROGNOSIS.

Generally speaking, the prognosis of genital tuberculosis is grave, whether it be of primary or of secondary origin. Primary tuberculosis of the genitals is always to be regarded as a serious affection; for, even if it remains limited, it always presents the possibility, as does any other focus of tuberculosis, of a general infection, with its uniformly fatal termination.

Tuberculosis of the tubes and ovaries, as previously indicated, has a marked tendency to lead to the production of tuberculous peritonitis. And even if the process remains limited to the genitals, it is always possible that it may go on to suppuration, with the formation of abscesses in the tubes or ovaries, which in turn may lead to a fatal termination by marasmus and hectic fever, or, by their rupture, to peritonitis. If, on the other hand, the genital tuberculosis is secondary to tuberculosis of the lungs or of the peritoneum, the above-mentioned possibilities will be added to the already serious primary affection of the other organs.

Genital tuberculosis may undergo conservative fibroid changes, and it is possible that healing by calcification may occur, as mentioned by the older writers. But it must be admitted that these conservative processes occur but rarely, and that the usual course of the affection is one of progressive advancement.

The results of operative treatment, however, tend to a considerable extent to brighten the grave prognosis of the affection when left to itself. If the tuberculosis is limited to the tubes and ovaries, or even if it has led to tuberculous peritonitis, but without involving other organs, the prognosis after their removal by cœliotomy will be hardly more grave than if they were removed for the usual inflammatory affection.

### TREATMENT.

As in some instances it appears quite probable that infection of the genital tract has occurred from without, the necessity for prophylaxis becomes apparent. Of course, possible infection by the physician and attendants should be carefully guarded against by attention to the well-known rules of cleanliness. This should be borne in mind particularly in the conduct of obstetrical cases.

The danger of infection by coitus being more than theoretical, we should attempt to impress upon persons afflicted with genital tuberculosis, whether male or female, the dangers of the situation and the advisability of abstaining from coitus.

The ideas as to the treatment of genital tuberculosis have undergone great changes during the past ten years; for it was only in 1881 that Gehle stated that the removal of the tubes and ovaries for tuberculosis was absolutely unjustifiable, even if a diagnosis could be made, while now in many instances operative treatment is urgently advocated. It is particularly to Hegar that credit is due for insisting upon the value of cœliotomy and the removal of the tubes and ovaries, and his monograph on genital tuberculosis may justly be regarded as marking the turning-point in the sentiment of the profession as to the treatment of these cases.

Of course the treatment varies according as different portions of the genital tract are affected, and whether the affection is primary or secondary ; it is also greatly influenced by the condition of the patient and the various complications which individual cases may present.

Tuberculous ulcers of the vagina and vulva are in the vast majority of cases secondary to tuberculosis elsewhere. It was pointed out by Cornil, Verneuil, and Derville that these ulcers are very amenable to treatment : the application to them of the tincture of iodine is frequently followed by their rapid disappearance. But, unfortunately, they have a marked tendency to recurrence, and frequently before one ulcer is quite healed another will make its appearance alongside of it. In some instances, however, the application of tincture of iodine, iodoform, or lactic acid will lead to the total healing of the ulcer by granulation. In the few instances in which the ulceration is isolated and resists the more palliative methods of treatment, it should be excised and the edges of the incision brought together by sutures.

If a tuberculous ulcer of the cervix is recognized and fails to respond to conservative treatment, we should not hesitate to amputate the cervix by one of the recognized methods, if we feel reasonably sure that the rest of the uterus is not also affected.

If we have to deal with tuberculous endometritis we should first satisfy ourselves that the tubes are intact. Any apparent inflammatory disease of the tubes along with tuberculosis of the uterus would indicate that they are likewise involved. If the process is limited to the uterus, we should at once curette it thoroughly and then introduce suppositories of iodoform, as recommended by Hegar and Derville; and if after this there is the slightest recurrence of the affection, there should be no question as to the propriety of vaginal extirpation of the uterus (Zweifel). In all such cases it is best to remove the tubes and ovaries at the same time, as it is impossible to tell whether they are perfectly healthy or not, especially in view of the great frequency of "unsuspected tuberculosis."

The question as to the removal of the tubes and ovaries when they are the seat of tuberculosis becomes very complicated in many instances. On account of the great difficulty of diagnosis of primary tuberculosis limited to the tubes and ovaries, it is very rarely that one has to face the question of their removal, except in cases of cœliotomy undertaken for other indications, when their condition is a matter of surprise. Of course, in these instances there can be no hesitation as to the propriety of their removal. But when, on the other hand, the process is secondary and associated with phthisis or tuberculous peritonitis, the question as to the propriety of operating becomes a grave one, and can be decided by the operator only after a careful survey of the general condition of the patient.

Generally speaking, in advanced cases of phthisis there should be no thought of operating, but in the early stages of the disease the general condition of the patient should be our guide; certainly, so long as the condition of the lungs holds out any hope of recovery, the operation should be undertaken, with the view of preventing the complications which might arise from the disease of the genitals.

In cases associated with tubercular peritonitis, we should not hesitate to perform cœliotomy and remove the tubes and ovaries, if possible, unless the general condition of the patient is particularly unfavorable (advanced phthisis), for we should bear in mind the curative influence which this operation frequently exerts in tuberculous peritonitis and the possibility of the affection having originated in the tubes.

In the cases in which both the tubes and ovaries and the uterus are involved, the problem becomes very complicated; it is doubtful whether many operators will adopt Hegar's suggestion of a supra-vaginal amputation of the uterus. It appears more rational to remove the entire uterus, as well as the tubes and ovaries, by either the vaginal or the abdominal method; though others advocate the removal of the tubes and ovaries, and the subsequent treatment of the uterus by curettage and iodoform. It is hardly necessary to state that the patient should be put upon general treatment, cod liver oil, guaiacol, etc., and placed in the best hygienic surroundings both before and after the operation.

The results after operations for this class of cases certainly afford encouragement enough for us to continue to advocate operative treatment. In a number of instances the women have been perfectly well four or five years after the operation. In our own practice the results have not been unsatisfactory: of the four patients from whom we have heard since their departure from the hospital, three were greatly improved, while the fourth, who had dulness at the apex of one lung, states that she is better than before the operation. All of these patients were, however, operated upon too recently to justify any definite statement as to their ultimate recovery.

# CHAPTER VIII.

## INFLAMMATORY LESIONS OF THE PELVIC PERITONEUM AND CONNECTIVE TISSUE.

BY HENRY T. BYFORD, M.D.

THE peritoneum is composed of vascular connective tissue covered with endothelium and filled with a net-work of lymphatic vessels, the countless open mouths of which communicate directly with the peritoneal cavity. The endothelium clings closely to the abdominal and upper pelvic viscera by means of a small amount of fibrous connective tissue, but is separated from the walls of the abdomen and pelvic cavity by an abundance of fatty connective tissue. This tissue is particularly abundant behind the kidneys and colon and in the pelvis, under the reflections of the peritoneal surfaces that form the broad, the sacro-uterine, and the vesico-uterine ligaments. Around the cervix and vagina, extending along the vesico-vaginal septum, under the sacro-uterine ligaments, and in the broad ligaments as far as the ureters, it contains but little, if any, fat, and is exceedingly compressible and contractile. These latter qualities are undoubtedly increased by the extension of muscular fibres from the uterus into it in nearly all directions.

Inflammation commencing in the pelvic peritoneum nearly always involves more or less of the connective tissue, and *vice versa;* yet the abundance of connective tissue that lies entirely below the peritoneal surfaces makes it possible for inflammation of such tissue to exist with the participation of but little of the endothelial surface. Hence we shall consider pelvic cellulitis separately.

## PELVIC PERITONITIS.

Peritonitis occurs under many forms and in many places, and a large part of the literature upon the subject leaves the impression upon the mind of a vast pseudo-scientific jumble. In order to escape vagueness of description, I shall make three divisions of peritonitis. The first I shall call *primary,* or *idiopathic,* including only such cases as commence on the epithelial side, or within the peritoneal cavity; the second, *secondary,* or *symptomatic,* including all cases that commence on the connective-tissue side. The third will include cases that are caused by certain specific diseases.

400

*Etiology and Nomenclature.*—*Primary or idiopathic peritonitis* has not necessarily any direct etiological connection with disease of the abdominal or pelvic viscera, since it must be caused by an irritant applied directly to the endothelial side. A typical example of this kind has often been produced by the entrance of a foreign body into the cavity by way of the Fallopian tube after intra-uterine injections. Rupture of the gall-bladder or urinary bladder, or of an ulcerated intestine or appendix vermiformis, or of a parturient uterus, pregnant Fallopian tube, pyosalpinx, ovarian abscess, or even of a blood-vessel, may allow irritating or septic materials to enter the abdominal cavity and cause a primary or what I have also called an idiopathic peritonitis.

The disease would take its name from the region attacked rather than from the organ from which the irritating material came. Thus, a ruptured gall-bladder or appendix may cause a pelvic peritonitis; a dripping Fallopian tube may cause a peritonitis of the iliac region, spreading upward *from* the tube instead of *around* the tube towards the uterus.

*Secondary or symptomatic peritonitis*, on the other hand, develops by extension from the inflamed connective tissue, or more frequently from an inflamed organ. The inflammatory action extends through the walls of the organ or by way of its lymphatics, and affects the peritoneal coat or covering secondarily. The peritonitis is not the primary disease, but a part of the disease of the organ or tissue which it covers. Thus, a purulent inflammation of the Fallopian tube may affect first the mucous membrane, then the muscular walls, and finally the peritoneum, so as to give rise to adhesions without any pus having escaped through the ostium abdominale. But, on the other hand, the pus may find its way through the ostium into the free abdominal cavity before the tubal wall has had time to become extensively infiltrated, and we have peritonitis in the iliac region, commencing on the endothelial side, that is as much a primary peritonitis as if we injected pus or some chemical agent through the healthy uterus and tube. Secondary peritonitis includes the forms designated by the prefix *peri :* thus, perimetritis is an extension of a metritis to the peritoneal investment of the uterus; perisalpingitis, an extension of a salpingitis to the peritoneal coat; perityphlitis or periappendicitis, an extension of the inflammation through the unruptured walls of the cæcum or appendix. Perforation of the appendix or cæcum would cause a primary peritonitis which might be pelvic, general, or localized in the iliac region, but would not, in the sense above mentioned, be a periappendicitis or perityphlitis.

*Specific Peritonitis.*—Certain forms of peritonitis are due to the action of specific poisons or germs, such as tuberculous, papillomatous, and malignant forms. The first-named is treated at length in works on general medicine, to which the reader is referred.

*Peritonitis after abdominal section* may be either primary or secondary, and will be considered briefly under a separate heading.

We might then make the following classification of peritonitis:

ACUTE. {
  Primary or idiopathic. { Simple.
                                 Septic.
  Secondary or symptomatic. { Simple.
                                         Septic.
}

CHRONIC. { Primary or idiopathic.
           Secondary or symptomatic.

SPECIFIC. { Tuberculous.
          Rheumatic.
          Malignant.

POST-OPERATIVE.

In the male, the peritoneum surrounds a closed cavity which is widely separated from the organs of generation. In the female, the generative organs are to a great extent covered by peritoneum, and form a canal that leads from the external world directly into the cavity. We are here concerned mainly with the peritoneal inflammations that arise in consequence of this latter arrangement.

### ACUTE PRIMARY PELVIC PERITONITIS, SIMPLE AND SEPTIC.

We shall make use of the above classification, and take up first the two forms of acute primary or idiopathic pelvic peritonitis, viz., simple and septic. Clinically speaking, nearly all forms of primary pelvic peritonitis are due to septic causes, yet we shall reserve the term septic for those in which the more distinctly septic germs, such as the staphylococci and the streptococci, penetrate to the cavity.

*Acute Primary Simple Peritonitis.*—*Etiology.*—Hemorrhage into the peritoneal cavity from rupture of a pregnant tube, or rupture of a vessel of the ovary or tube in consequence of suppression of the menses, or of undue sexual excitement, or from expulsion of menstrual fluid into the abdominal cavity in case of stenosis or contraction of the cervix, gives rise to transient peritonitis. Fluids from vaginal douches and intra-uterine injections have many times found their way through the Fallopian tubes and been followed by sharp attacks. In cases of infantile or stenotic cervix with catarrhal endometritis or salpingitis, the mucus may find its way through the ostium abdominale and cause a mild, localized, simple peritonitis. Thus, the relationship between cervical erosion and salpingitis has been mentioned by Bland Sutton and others. Masturbation, by the introduction of saprophytic germs into the vagina, may start a catarrhal inflammation on its way to the peritoneum. Rupture of the uterus by attempts at dilatation and curetting are occasional causes. I have twice opened the peritoneal cavity while curetting the cancerous cervix. In both cases I disinfected the parts and had mild, insignificant cases of localized primary peritonitis to deal with. I once saw a case of simple peritonitis result from the introduction of a lead-pencil into the uterus for the purpose of interrupting a supposed pregnancy ; the uterine walls were probably penetrated.

Rupture of an ovarian cyst or cystic fibroma, or escape of the fluid after an imperfect tapping, may be enumerated among occasional causes. Abdominal growth, by pressure, may produce local irritation and interference of function that will result in inflammation of the peritoneum.

The changes produced by some of the above enumerated causes are often called reparative processes by pathologists, rather than inflammation, yet from a clinical point of view it is convenient to classify them with the transient forms of inflammation whenever they produce appreciable disturbances in the system of the patient.

*Pathological Anatomy.*—As death seldom results from simple primary pelvic peritonitis, it is difficult to give an exact description of the pathological conditions in the human being. Reasoning from the evidence afforded by the physical examination of patients, secondary peritoneal sections, and autopsies after peritoneal sections, and by analogy from experiments upon animals, we may arrive at a very satisfactory knowledge of these conditions.

After an effusion of blood, or of a mildly irritating fluid like simple mucus, we have a sudden increase of vascularity of the peritoneum, followed in a few hours by transudation or exudation of serum both in the peritoneal cavity and in the contiguous connective tissue, containing leucocytes and new endothelial cells. The serum in the cavity mixes as far as it can with the foreign substances, while the leucocytes and cells are entangled on the surface around it by the fibrin that is formed from the blood-ferments. Partial organization of the fibrinous exudate occurs within forty-eight hours, forming a capsule to which intestines, omentum, and pelvic organs adhere, while absorption of such of the blood, water, or mucus as is absorbable, or is rendered so by admixture with the serum, takes place. These changes are confined largely to the leucocytes and new embryonic tissue, so that the exudate may be completely absorbed and the peritoneum return to its original state; or a solid organized residuum may remain, surrounded by newly-formed connective tissue forming peritoneal adhesions. The exudate in the connective tissue hardens quickly and is rapidly absorbed. In case the foreign body possesses a certain kind of irritating quality, or becomes affected by the occurrence of a second attack, or by secondary infection, a collection of serum or sero-purulent fluid may remain encapsulated for an indefinite period of time. The disease then passes into a chronic or residuary form.

*Acute Primary Septic Peritonitis.*—*Etiology.*—Probably the most frequent cause of acute primary septic peritonitis is infection directly from the fimbriæ of an infected Fallopian tube, or by escape of pus or mucopus by way of the ostium abdominale. In this manner arise many of the recurrent attacks of peritonitis that follow violent exertion or sexual excesses in those already affected with tubal disease.

The gonorrhœal poison may travel through the uterus and Fallopian tubes until it reaches the peritoneum. Septic poison developed in the puerperal state, whether after abortion or labor, is a great rival of gonorrhœa in producing first or original attacks. Unclean gynæcological operations, stem pessaries, sea-tangle and other tents, may act in a similar way. Rupture of the uterus, with infection, during labor, abortion, or operations upon the uterus, may act even more directly. In fact, all the causes given for the simple cases may, if infection be added, cause this form. Rupture of a pyosalpinx or pelvic abscess into the peritoneal cavity causes a severe local, or more often a fatal general, peritonitis.

*Pathological Anatomy.*—In case the peritoneum is previously healthy and the infection is of a mild character, the pathological changes may be the same as in simple cases. Usually, however, instead of remaining localized about the area of primary irritation, the changes involve the tissues for some distance, so that the whole pelvic peritoneum and a large portion of the pelvic connective tissue often become involved in an exudate. Sometimes the exudate extends high up in one or both iliac regions, and in some cases to a large part of the abdominal cavity, gluing the distended intestines together. This is especially apt to happen in cases occurring during the puerperal state.

The transudate or exudate may become absorbed within a week or two (that in the connective tissue even earlier), so that nothing but a false membrane of fibrinous character may remain, gluing the peritoneal surfaces together. This usually becomes fibrillated and organized to a greater or less extent into connective tissue, with destruction of some of the involved muscular fibres, and may unite the viscera so firmly that they cannot be separated without laceration into or through their weakened walls; or the union may be slighter, the connective tissue being drawn out into fibrinous bands covered with endothelium and resembling normal peritoneum. The first result of the exudation, contraction, absorption, and stretching may be distortion and displacement of the diseased pelvic viscera, with numerous bands of adhesions passing in all directions, fixing everything as firmly as if plaster of Paris had been poured into the pelvis.

In other cases the exudate is not readily absorbed. The fluid becomes turbid from the rapid development of pus, and localized pus-accumulations form, which may become encapsulated, particularly in the cul-de-sac of Douglas, or may ulcerate into the rectum, bladder, or intestines. Thus relief and partial recovery, or chronic abscesses, with the danger of general sepsis, pyæmia, and exhaustion, may ensue.

In old cases, collections of serum, bloody serum, altered blood, cheesy substance, and even calcareous deposits, may be found between the false membranes and the distorted viscera. Infiltrations, degenerations, and cicatrizations of portions of the pelvic organs naturally follow.

When a large abscess ruptures into the peritoneal cavity, the whole pelvic peritoneal and a portion of the general peritoneal surface assume a bright red color, and rapid proliferation of embryonic cells takes place on the surfaces. Death usually results within forty-eight hours, from shock or rapidly developing sepsis. The effused pus, and, if life be sufficiently prolonged, some turbid or bloody serum and a few flakes of fibrin, will be found. About and above this the reddened peritoneal surfaces are extensively, although in the beginning not firmly, glued together, the same as in simple peritonitis.

*Signs, Symptoms, and Course of Simple Peritonitis.*—These vary from almost nothing to those of the greatest intensity. The onset is usually announced by sudden, severe, and continuous pain, with exacerbations produced by peristalsis, bodily movements, coughing, etc. Distinct rigors are not usually experienced, being in all probability suppressed by the vascular and nervous excitement resulting from the pains. Owing to shock, the temperature is often low or subnormal at the onset of pain, but ordinarily it goes up in a few hours to between 101° and 104° F., with dry skin, headache, and restlessness. The pulse soon becomes full and bounding. Tympanites comes on promptly, and local tenderness is marked. Nausea may or may not be prominent. The symptoms may subside in a day or two, or continue for a week or more, or run into a chronic form.

In cases resulting from effusion of blood into the peritoneal cavity, the inflammation frequently subsides so rapidly as to be entirely overlooked. The patient experiences sudden pain in the lower abdomen, becomes faint from loss of blood or shock, or both, has cold feet, is nauseated, and probably vomits. The pulse is rapid and weak and the pupils are dilated. Some gaseous distention and tenderness of the lower abdomen are noticed. The temperature rises to 100° F., or possibly to 102° F., the next day, with a pulse of 100 to 120, while the pain, tenderness, and nausea subside. During the next twenty-four hours the temperature declines almost to normal, and at the end of three or four days the patient may want to get up. In the mean time, the physician will have discovered a large lump in or over the recto-uterine space, displacing the uterus more or less forward, will pronounce the case one of hæmatocele, and will forget all about the peritonitis. If the patient gets up too soon, however, the symptoms of peritonitis will come on again : she will go to bed, and the symptoms will again pass off. Constipation is, as a rule, quite obstinate, partly due to pressure of the effused blood upon the rectum.

Rupture of a parovarian or simple serous cyst of the broad ligament gives rise to mild symptoms of the same character, that disappear rapidly. The shock and nausea and frequent pulse are less marked if the cyst be small. Rupture of an ordinary ovarian or papillomatous cystoma gives rise to the same pains, temperature, and tenderness; but the elevation of temperature, dry skin, fulness of pulse, and abdominal tenderness may persist for a number of days. The prominence of the abdomen is at first diminished when a large cyst bursts, but increases again with the accumulation of gas in the intestine. There is more resonance in the upper abdomen and less definitely defined dulness below. Rupture of a papillomatous cyst may not cause much appreciable change in the abdomen, nor any symptom other than a slight rise in temperature and some tenderness; but the temperature may remain a degree or two above normal for weeks, and may be attended by moderate but gradually increasing ascites, with local and reflex disturbances such as accompany chronic serous peritonitis.

Attacks dependent upon the effusion of larger quantities of more irritating fluid present similar signs and symptoms and run a similar course, but the symptoms are of the character of those mentioned at the beginning of this section.

If a few drops of mucus or only a small quantity of blood be effused from the cavity, the symptoms may be even less pronounced. The pain, tenderness, and tympanites may be confined to one iliac region, the temperature may not exceed 100° or 101° F., and may subside quickly, and the pulse, although a little too full and hard, may not exceed eighty or ninety beats per minute. Nausea may not be felt. Nothing, at first, but fulness and tenderness may be observable to the vaginal touch, although there are apt to be signs of pre-existing tubal disease, such as tender spots of induration beside and behind the uterus, with or without fixation or displacement of the corpus uteri. An afternoon temperature of 99° F. will often persist for a week or so, with some iliac tenderness and pain upon moving the limb of the affected side or upon using the bed-pan or vessel. The bowels will seldom move of their own accord, may require considerable prompting by laxatives, and the pain may return with greater intensity with the first evacuation. The bimanual examination will show some induration at the roof of the pelvis on one side restricting the mobility of the fundus uteri and making all attempts at pushing up the uterus, or deep pressure into the side of the pelvis, acutely painful. Later, all signs of the disease may pass off, except those of the chronic salpingitis or ovaritis.

*Symptoms of Septic Peritonitis.*—These vary with the amount of traumatism and the amount and intensity of the infection. A hæmatocele, or rupture of a pregnant tube, or even laceration of the uterus, or an overflow from a Fallopian tube, may present symptoms similar to those already described for simple peritonitis, but remain in a mild form for days or weeks, and sooner or later be followed by a sudden increase of pain, temperature, pulse-frequency, night-sweats, tenderness in the lower abdomen or the vagina, and perhaps by tympanites. The temperature creeps up daily by degrees or half-degrees, registering from one to three or four degrees higher in the afternoon, until it gets up to 103° or 104° F., when an abscess bursts into the vagina, rectum, or bladder, or externally in the iliac or inguinal region. The pulse keeps pace with the temperature, and is very full and frequent when the temperature is high. In other cases the temperature jumps from 99.5° or 100° to 103° F. quite suddenly, often preceded by a chill or chilly sensations. Softening and the ordinary signs of a pointing abscess will of course be observed at the place of suppuration, with concentration of pain or tenderness in the viscus or region invaded by the advancing pus. Complete discharge with adequate drainage may bring about a cure, or the abscess-cavity may refill, the symptoms return, and another evacuation follow.  This process of relief and recurrence may take place a few times, with final recovery, or may go on almost indefinitely until it undermines the patient's constitution and even results in death.

The escape of a large quantity of septic pus from a Fallopian tube, or the bursting of a pyosalpinx or an ovarian or a pelvic abscess into the peritoneal cavity, gives rise to the symptoms of extensive pelvic, merging into general, peritonitis.  Shock, sudden lancinating and grinding pain in the lower abdomen, often extending to the epigastric region, nausea, followed by a rapid rise in the temperature to 103° or 104° F., a dry skin, headache, a full, bounding pulse of 100 to 110, or, in more severe attacks, a rapid, hard, rather than full, pulse of 120 to 140, great tympany, and extreme tenderness spreading from the iliac regions, are the ordinary early symptoms. The patient assumes the dorsal decubitus with knees drawn up, exhibits great anxiety and restlessness, vomits nearly everything that is taken, refuses food, shows a dry, coated tongue, and sleeps but little.  She resists motion or manipulation, and breathes only with the chest muscles, to avoid the pain accompanying movements of the diaphragm.  The face assumes a sunken, drawn appearance, the lips become dry, and occasional mental aberration is observed.  After ten days or two weeks the stomach becomes gradually more retentive, the tympanites less, the temperature falls, and, in fact, all the symptoms improve, and the case may go on to a complete, or apparently complete, recovery, so far as the peritonitis is concerned, and the patient may be able to leave the bed in from two to six weeks; or the symptoms may persist, and the patient pass into a state of collapse and die.

In some cases the septic symptoms predominate over those of inflammation, or the endothelium has been destroyed and permanent adhesions formed by previous attacks, and there may be a puzzling irregularity of manifestations.  Thus, a case may run its course with scarcely any rise of temperature, or the pains may subside spontaneously in a few hours, or but little acute pain may be felt.  The pulse, with a high temperature, may not exceed seventy beats per minute, or more often there is rapid pulse with a slight rise of temperature.  Vomiting may be absent, or there may be diarrhœa.  The patient may feel unusually well and her mind may be clear, or she may be unusually talkative throughout a fatal attack, or she may be almost comatose from the beginning.  As a rule, a very rapid pulse and an irregular temperature indicate the predominance of sepsis, while a steady high temperature and a full, bounding, but not very rapid pulse are the registers of inflammatory action.

The effusion of a large amount of pus into the pelvis may also cause a sudden general peritonitis.  The symptoms commence in the same way as in a septic pelvic peritonitis just described, but run a more rapid course. The temperature rises rapidly to 103°, 104°, and 105° F.; the pulse quickly becomes small, hard, and thready, beating from 120 to 160 times per minute. The whole abdomen distends rapidly, until the skin is tense and the body barrel-shaped and resonant as a drum. The respiration is thoracic and labored. The expression is anxious, the eyes sunken and surrounded by leaden areas, the cheek-bones prominent, the tongue dry and coated, the extremities cool, and the skin changed from dryness to clamminess. The hands move tremulously. The mind, clear at first, grows confused. Often the patient becomes delirious and tries to get up, or lies in a stupor. The stomach ejects a mouthful of dark-green fluid every few minutes. The secretion of urine is suppressed. The respiration is shallow, gasping, irregular, and greatly accelerated. The pulse is finally lost at the wrist, and unconsciousness supervenes. The temperature, if not already high, goes up rapidly to 106° or 107° F. (by rectum), and death relieves the sufferer.

The escape of a large amount of pus into an already inflamed pelvic peritoneum, particularly in the puerperal state, may cause death in a few hours or in a day, the symptoms of shock and acute sepsis supplanting those of peritonitis.

*Diagnosis.—(a) Pelvic Cellulitis.*—The onset of acute primary pelvic peritonitis is quite characteristic in that it is sudden and severe and is rapidly followed by febrile reaction. The acute, constant pain in the iliac region or whole lower abdomen is accompanied by great tenderness on superficial pressure and the rapid development of local tympanites with tension of the abdominal muscles. Disinclination to move and recurrent exacerbations of pain are characteristic. The exudates do not form quite so rapidly as in pelvic cellulitis, and are usually found either in the recto-uterine cul-de-sac, on the posterior surface of the broad ligament surrounding the uterine appendages, so as to leave a sulcus between them and the uterus, or high up, forming palpable lumps in the lower abdomen. These lumps are hard and more or less resonant, the resonance varying with the amount of gas in the intestines adherent in them. A finger in the rectum can feel that the hard masses do not extend along the sacro-uterine ligaments or the base of the broad ligaments, where the cellular tissue abounds, but that they are in the peritoneal spaces between, behind, and above these. Cellulitis can nearly always be traced to recent traumatism of the genital tract. (See Diagnosis of Primary Pelvic Cellulitis, page 443.)

*(b) Appendicitis with Peritonitis.*—This can be differentiated by the location of the pain entirely above the pelvis, centring near McBurney's point, two inches from the anterior superior spine of the ilium, in the direction of the umbilicus, or above or posterior to this. Recurrent attacks of pain in the same region are characteristic, and alternating constipation and diarrhœa may be noticeable. A temperature below 100° F. for a few days, and tenderness over the appendix, followed by a sudden acute pain and rise of temperature to 100°, 101°, or 102° F., then by a diminution of pain and temperature for two or three days, represent a very common commencement of peritonitis following appendicitis. In this case the focus of infection is small, and is rapidly followed by a strictly localized peritonitis with protective exudation. A dull area with induration may be felt near McBurney's

point, surrounded by resonance, developing into a local abscess. In primary pelvic peritonitis, similar symptoms follow previous disease of the appendages, but the local symptoms are lower down, and the exudates are in or over the pelvis and can be recognized per vaginam. In case the peritonitis is more general, with high temperature, nausea, thoracic respiration, anxious countenance, rapid pulse, etc., the symptoms of previous disease of the appendages are still more pronounced, or else there will be a distinctly recognizable cause, such as intra-vaginal or intra-uterine manipulation or operations, puerperality, etc. Peritonitis from appendicitis is usually, although not always, less stormy in the beginning, and is followed by the somewhat gradual development of the symptoms of perforative peritonitis; while primary pelvic peritonitis, unless of the most severe character at the onset, tends after a short time to improve gradually. Peritonitis from typhlitis, that commences with the stormy symptoms noticeable in primary peritonitis, usually proves rapidly fatal. Vaginal examination gives negative results in one case and more or less positive information in the other.

(c) *Acute metritis* may be ushered in with a chill and high temperature, but, unless there is more than the ordinary involvement of the peritoneum, there is an absence of the tympanites and abdominal tenderness to moderate pressure. The pain is more in the vesical and sacral regions, particularly in the latter, and the cervix is more sensitive to a slight touch. In peritonitis the pain becomes severe only when the cervix is pressed hard enough to stir the uterus in its surroundings. The cervix is much softer in metritis.

(d) *Acute salpingitis* without peritonitis has not the acute pain and active symptoms of the latter. The lower abdomen is not hard and tympanitic, nor so tender to moderate pressure. The temperature seldom rises as high, particularly in the beginning.

(e) In *acute enteritis* the onset is either more gradual or less severe so far as abdominal and pelvic pains are concerned. The centre of pain is near the umbilicus, instead of being in or over the pelvis. The tenderness is not so great. There are characteristic alvine discharges, instead of constipation. The pelvic examination is negative.

(f) From *colic* we distinguish peritonitis by the temperature, the persistence of pain between the severer paroxysms, the tenderness on slight pressure and pain upon motion in the former, and the absence of discoverable cause in the pelvis by vaginal indagation. *Hepatic* and *renal colic* may be similarly differentiated. They are also characterized by extreme paroxysms of pain in the upper abdomen with sudden complete intervals of ease, and by the products discovered in the urine and stools.

(g) *Pelvic pains* or chronic pelvic disease with *hysteria* may closely simulate peritonitis, but there is an irregularity of symptoms that makes the diagnosis easy to the careful observer. A patient may be distended, restless, in pain, and may complain of great tenderness upon pressure, yet the temperature, instead of being very high, as it is in peritonitis with these symptoms, is almost normal. The patient can move without pain, and deep pressure, gradually made, causes no more pain than a slight touch. The pulse, when the patient is quiet, is about normal. There are apt to be tender spots about the spine or the ovarian region, and a history of previous attacks of hysteria.

(*h*) *Intestinal obstruction*, when fully developed, may simulate or even develop into peritonitis. The symptoms, however, develop in an inverse order. Acute idiopathic pelvic peritonitis begins with the severest symptoms and then pursues a regressive course, the pain and temperature developing in a couple of days and then gradually subsiding. If there be fæcal or duodenal vomiting, it will be near the beginning. In intestinal obstruction the symptoms are progressive: there are preceding constipation, intestinal disorder, colic, etc., without tympanites or marked tenderness. These latter symptoms, with elevation of temperature, accelerated pulse, and vomiting, develop later and somewhat gradually. Fæcal vomiting comes on near the fatal termination. The mind is usually clear until near death. The pain-centre will be in the region of the cæcum or the true abdominal cavity instead of in the pelvis, and the examination will exclude pelvic peritonitis.

A sudden, complete obstruction of the bowels may commence in a stormy way, but the temperature, pulse, and tenderness will not correspond with the other symptoms until later.

*Prognosis.*—In all but the severer septic cases, such as those resulting from the effusion of a large amount of pus in the pelvis, the prognosis is favorable with regard to life; but, as a rule, some damage is done to the pelvic organs that is never perfectly relieved. (See Chronic Pelvic Peritonitis.) In the more severe cases just mentioned the prognosis is unfavorable, death frequently resulting from general peritonitis. When, after a slight run of fever with symptoms of salpingitis or ovaritis, we find a sudden onset of acute pain, a rise of temperature from 100° to 103° or 104° F., rapid pulse, thoracic respiration, general tympanites, frequent vomiting, and extreme anxiety and restlessness, we may know that a general peritonitis is setting in, which will probably result fatally unless relieved by operative measures.

A comatose state beginning early and persisting, unusual and constant talkativeness, gasping respiration, a pulse above 130, bilious vomiting, and persistent delirium, with attempts to leave the bed, may be considered as unfavorable symptoms.

The pulse is a more reliable guide to the condition of the patient than the temperature. The more rapid and thready the pulse, the worse the prognosis. A rapid increase in pulse-frequency, with diminution in volume, is often the first sign that the patient will not recover. The temperature sometimes gives no indication of the gravity of the disease until a few hours before dissolution. A secondary gradual rise in temperature without apparent cause, after a subsidence of symptoms, usually denotes a localized septic condition with an unfavorable tendency.

*Treatment.*—Mild cases of simple peritonitis, due to the effusion of blood, ovarian fluid, or simple mucus and the like, require but little treatment beyond rest in bed. Hot fomentations kept constantly applied to the abdomen during the acute painful stage, and later counter-irritation, such as turpentine stupes or chloroform liniment embrocations, are of material benefit. The bowels should be moved on the second or third day, preferably by repeated small doses of salines,—viz., six grammes (two drachms) of the granular citrate of magnesium every two or three hours, or fifty grammes (about two ounces) of the liquid citrate, or three grammes (one drachm) of salts. When the bowels begin to move, an enema of plain water or weak soapsuds will assist the movement.

The symptoms are treated as they arise. Pain not relieved by hot fomentations may call for an opiate, and this should preferably be given hypodermatically, with a little atropine to prevent nausea. Morphine, from one-fourth to one-third of a grain, with atropine, one-seventy-fifth of a grain, may be given, and the morphine, without the atropine, may be repeated every hour until the pain is relieved or decidedly mitigated. An ice-bag, if applied in the beginning, sometimes acts both as anodyne and local sedative, and may diminish the severity of the disease.

Excessive vascular excitement may be tempered by a few doses of aconite or veratrum in persons of a plethoric habit. A yellowish, furred tongue may be considered an indication for a mercurial laxative.

Nausea is to be treated by different remedies. Small repeated doses of morphine are often helpful for the early vomiting. One drop of carbolic acid may be given in two tablespoonfuls of warm water. A mild aromatic draught—three or four drops of the essence of peppermint with six grains of carbonate of magnesium every hour or two in a little acacia and water —sometimes relieves the flatulence. From two to four grammes of the granular citrate of magnesium in thirty grammes of water may be tried in those cases in which there is not much febrile reaction, or after that has subsided. Bits of ice rubbed on the lips or placed on the tongue have a sedative action, diminishing the nausea, which is largely nervous. Large quantities of ice, on the contrary, are apt to do more harm than good. Small drinks of diluted ginger ale, alkaline carbonated waters, or hot water may be given for thirst.

One or two tablespoonfuls of koumys, milk and lime water, rice water, or barley water, every hour, may be tried for nourishment, and increased tentatively as the stomach regains its equilibrium.

The patient should be kept in bed until the temperature, tenderness, and tympanites have subsided. The bowels should be kept soluble throughout by salines, and the diet carefully regulated.

In more severe and septic cases an ice-bag or cold-water coil should be placed on the lower abdomen, over two or three layers of flannel, and kept there from twenty-four to forty-eight hours, according to the intensity of the symptoms or the tolerance of the patient. After that, hot fomentations or counter-irritants are advisable. In plethoric patients twenty or thirty leeches may be placed over the seat of the pain, but only during the first few hours.

The remainder of the treatment should be such as is described above for milder cases. During convalescence, alcoholic stimulants, quinine, iron, strychnine, digestive ferments, general massage, electricity, etc., are valuable.

In cases due to an escape of a large quantity of pus or of septic matter into the free abdominal cavity, with decided symptoms, the abdomen should be promptly opened, the cavity washed out, any offending pus-tube or ovary removed, and the parts drained. After general peritonitis has set in, the time for successful surgery is usually past, and the only treatment left is an unavailing medical one. At the very onset of general peritonitis, however, an operation is occasionally successful.

## ACUTE SECONDARY PELVIC PERITONITIS.

*Acute Secondary Pelvic Peritonitis.—Etiology.*—Secondary peritonitis is in its nature an extension of inflammation from the connective tissue surrounding the peritoneum, or from contiguous organs, to its endothelial lining. Traumatism over the lower abdomen, or in the vagina, uterus, rectum, or bladder, by producing lesions in the subperitoneal connective tissue, may originate a secondary peritonitis.

Septic inflammation of the uterus or Fallopian tubes, whether from parturition, abortion, or operative procedures, may give rise to a simple peritonitis, for the septic germs may not traverse the entire thickness of the uterine or tubal walls. Pelvic cellulitis frequently extends to the pelvic peritoneum. Ovaritis involves the peritoneal covering in most instances.

Recurrent attacks in women who have old disease of the appendages, with adhesions, constitute the most common variety. They are generally reproduced by traumatic influences, such as active or prolonged bodily exercise, coitus, etc.

Acute inflammation arising in abdominal tumors from blows, twisting of the pedicle, impaction, septic absorption, etc., affects the peritoneal covering and to a certain extent the peritoneal surfaces lying in contact with it. Ovarian tumors with long pedicles and old dermoid tumors are frequent starting-points.

*Pathological Anatomy.*—Inflammation of the organ or tissue from which the peritonitis proceeds, with either active or passive congestion, according to the cause, are the first changes. Then the changes peculiar to adhesive peritonitis occur,—viz., moderate exudation with rapid fibrinization, absorption, adhesions between opposed peritoneal surfaces, and organization. Sometimes sufficient effusion will be present to form a large exudate, but when this takes place the peritonitis is liable to become septic. The pathological changes may begin over a small area and gradually extend all about the tissues from which they proceed, or even beyond, resulting in extensive peritonitis with adhesions. The disease is apt to occur after previous attacks and adhesions, and to lead to increase and extension of exudate and adhesion until the entire pelvic peritoneum and pelvic organs, with a part of the omentum, may participate in the inflammation and aggluti- nation.   In such cases peritoneal transudates may become encysted in a peritoneal pouch or cul-de-sac, more often in the recto-uterine.

Peritonitis originating in an ovarian tumor with twisted pedicle will be accompanied by extravasation of venous blood and serum within one or more of the sacs, passive congestion over these sacs, and a serous exudate, a part of which will remain in the free abdominal cavity, and a part will fibrinize on the surface and glue it to the abdominal parietes, omentum, or intestines lying against it.   The adhesions usually organize and the serum becomes absorbed.

Peritonitis surrounding an infected tumor or abscess usually produces similar adhesions around the whole mass, or is apt to persist in a subacute or chronic form, with ecchymosis and extensive changes in the tumor or abscess-wall.

*Symptoms.*—Simple secondary peritonitis occurring as an extension of acute inflammation of the uterine appendages or of the uterus is preceded, of course, by the symptoms of these diseases.   The peritonitis is ushered in by acute pain in the iliac regions or across the lower abdomen, which is seldom as acute and extensive as in primary pelvic peritonitis ; or, if so at the beginning, it soon assumes a milder character, with more soreness in proportion to the sharp lancinating pains.   The temperature either does not go so high during the first twenty-four hours, or it drops to within a degree or two of where it was before, sooner than is the case in primary peritonitis following acute inflammation of the uterus and appendages.   It is apt to remain moderately elevated for a longer time, often for weeks. The pulse corresponds quite closely with the temperature.   The tympanites, nausea, constipation, and, in fact, nearly all the symptoms, are less marked than in the primary form, as if toned down by the association with the disease from which it originates.   Constipation is the rule, and nausea is not uncommon.

In connection with pelvic cellulitis, sharp abdominal pains and tym- panites, and perhaps nausea and abdominal pains, are added to the symp- toms of that disease.

Recurrent attacks occur in connection with chronic disease of the append- ages, being ushered in quite rapidly or even suddenly, although in many cases there has been premonitory pain for a few days.   The pain is apt to be on one side, strictly localized, or radiates from a localized spot over the Fallopian tube.   It subsides rapidly when the patient keeps quiet, and returns when she gets up, somewhat as it does in acute peritonitis due to hæmatocele.   But the temperature does not subside so quickly and com- pletely, remaining one or two degrees above normal for several days or a week or two.   The tympanites is circumscribed and soon subsides, so that often a distinct peritoneal exudate gluing the intestines to the appendages may be felt. This is tympanitic on percussion, although hard and board-like on palpation. The pulse, at first full, becomes normal in a day or two, and may be softer and weaker than in health. The pain subsides completely, but some tenderness remains. The patient soon becomes quite comfortable while lying down, but the tendency to a return upon sitting up persists and is characteristic. Sometimes the movement of the bowels and the evacuation of the bladder are painful.

Peritonitis due to twisting of the pedicle in an ovarian tumor is preceded by a rapid enlargement of the tumor, particularly if it is a cystic or a vascular tumor, and by dull pain and tenderness in some parts of it or all over it. Some sharp pain is usually felt at the same place, but there is often but little pain or tympanites in the neighboring abdominal regions. The temperature rises to 101° or even to 103° or 104° F. within two, three, or four days. The pulse shows reaction, going up to from 80 to 100, being somewhat full and resistant unless profuse hemorrhage has taken place into the tumor, when it will be rapid and feeble. Certain positions may be associated with more pain than others. The tenderness remains for some days and then gradually passes away with the other symptoms. Occasionally some tenderness and slight elevation of temperature remain, symptomatic of adhesions that interfere with the functions of the abdominal organs. When the hemorrhage into the tumor has been considerable, the peritonitis may become general. Twisting of the pedicle during pregnancy or after labor is apt to be followed by serious symptoms : the temperature runs high, the pulse is rapid, and the pain and tympanites are marked.

*Diagnosis.*—From primary peritonitis the secondary form is chiefly distinguishable by the connection of the symptoms with the disease of the pelvic organs with which it is associated. The onset and subsidence are apt to be more gradual, the symptoms less accentuated and extreme, and the area affected more limited. Severe septic cases, whether primary or secondary, are frequently the same in their manifestations, except in the manner of beginning.

*Acute Secondary Septic Peritonitis.*—*Etiology.*—The most frequent cause of secondary as well as of primary septic peritonitis is infection from the Fallopian tube, not by way of the fimbriæ, but by spread of the septic poison through the inflamed tubal walls. Pyosalpinx, ovarian abscess, pelvic abscess, under the influence of traumatism, whether from external violence, parturition, abortion, coitus, prolonged or violent physical exertion, fæcal impaction, or surgical manipulations, may be the starting-point.

Secondary infection of peritoneal exudates and encysted transudates may convert a simple peritonitis into a septic, or cause a recurrence of an apparently cured simple form in the shape of a septic one.

Nearly all the causes given for simple secondary peritonitis may, under favoring influences, cause the septic variety.

*Pathological Anatomy.*—Secondary septic peritonitis commences in the same way as the simple kind. The infiltration of the subperitoneal tissue is much greater, the exudate more abundant, but seldom copious. Absorption and fibrinization are less complete, or may be absent altogether. The exudate becomes rapidly more and more turbid about the diseased organs as the leucocytes and enlarged cells become converted into pus-corpuscles. But the pus may be shut off from the general peritoneal cavity by adhesions farther away, and thus we have a septic peritonitis in one place and simple peritonitis surrounding it and constituting the first step towards a cure. In other cases the infection will spread, the fibrin will disintegrate into pus and fibrinous flakes, and general peritonitis will result. In many cases the peritoneum has suffered from previous attacks that have diminished its powers of protecting itself. (See Chronic Peritonitis.)

*Signs, Symptoms, and Course.*—Either just before the attack or some time previous, some symptoms of pelvic or peritoneal inflammation will have been noticed, in connection with inflammation of the uterus and appendages, a uterine or ovarian tumor, or pelvic abscess. As a result of exposure, fatigue, traumatism, an attack of indigestion, or without discoverable cause, a sudden or rapid onset or exacerbation of symptoms will come on, with acute pelvic peritoneal pain, increase of temperature and pulse-rate, tympanites and tenderness of the lower abdomen, and, in fact, about all the symptoms of primary pelvic peritonitis. The temperature, however, does not usually rise so rapidly nor so high. The pulse, full at first, becomes daily more rapid and loses in fulness, even after the temperature ceases to advance. The temperature is unequal, often having a daily afternoon rise, say, to 102° or 103° F. and a daily fall down to 100° or 101° F., or the rise and fall may recur oftener, or irregularly. The pulse, although somewhat similarly variable, is more consistent, increasing in rapidity and diminishing in fulness and force as the disease advances. The tympanites usually spreads, although pain and tenderness upon slight pressure may diminish. As a rule, nausea and vomiting become prominent in grave eases, often characterized by frequently repeated bilious vomiting. Restlessness may become extreme, or somnolence may be present, or they may alternate, or restlessness may give way to somnolence. In the latter stages the symptoms coincide with those of primary septic peritonitis.

In milder cases the pain subsides after the first few days, but some tenderness, high temperature, and tympanites, with a weak pulse, remain for a variable period, gradually subsiding, and leaving the patient with a chronic inflammation, or with septic symptoms, such as irregular temperature, hectic fever, anorexia, etc., that culminate in a pyocele. Not infrequently some localized pelvic pain will remain for weeks or months, with a slight elevation of temperature, and will finally subside, or will be subject to exacerbations upon the slightest provocation.

*Pelvic Cellulitis, Salpingitis, Metritis, Appendicitis, Colic, Hysteria, and Intestinal Obstruction.*—If developed secondary to cellulitis, the acute peritoneal pains in the lower abdomen, with tenderness, tympanites, nausea, following those of cellulitis, will be noticed. The local signs present the same points of difference as in primary peritonitis.

Except the sudden onset, the symptoms given in the diagnosis of primary peritonitis will serve to differentiate the secondary form from salpingitis, metritis, appendicitis, colic, hysteria, and intestinal obstruction. (See Diagnosis of Acute Primary Peritonitis.)

*Prognosis.*—The prognosis is affected by the conditions mentioned in the prognosis of the primary forms. The extent of the pelvic inflammation (usually septic) upon which the secondary peritonitis depends is an important factor, and is apt to make the prognosis more unfavorable than that of primary peritonitis of equal severity of symptoms. Peritonitis from a twisted pedicle may be associated with danger from the abundance of the hemorrhage into the cyst, or when the accident occurs in the puerperal state.

*Treatment.*—In the way of prophylaxis, the strict observance of aseptic and antiseptic precautions, and the avoidance of undue traumatism in the management of labor at term, abortions, gynæcological operations, manipulations, and examinations, are of first importance. The same may be said of all forms of traumatism arising from carelessness on the part of a patient suffering with pelvic tumors and diseases, such as over-exertion, exposure to inclemency of weather, venereal excesses, blows, etc.

Some surgeons use an ice-bag over the abdomen after all pelvic operations of any magnitude; others always administer an opiate as soon as the influence of the anæsthetic begins to wear off. A properly performed operation in an appropriate case should not require such routine treatment; but absolute quiet and rest in bed after labor, abortion, and gynæcological operations should always be enforced as a means of preventing further traumatism.

It need hardly be mentioned that prompt and efficient treatment of all the severer forms of pelvic inflammation should be instituted as a preventive of extension to the peritoneum.

In addition to the treatment of the inflammation that has extended to the peritoneum, energetic measures should be taken at the onset of peritoneal symptoms to limit the amount of peritoneal congestion and exudate. Except in plethoric patients, leeching is hardly as applicable as in primary cases, in which the onset is more often so extremely aggressive. An ice-bag should be applied for twenty-four or thirty-six hours, followed by hot fomentations; in milder cases, or for patients who do not bear cold applications well, hot fomentations or poultices are indicated from the beginning. Later, counter-irritants over the abdomen, saline or mercurial laxatives, or enemata of soapsuds should be used.

Those suffering with chronic disease of the appendages will often recover from recurrent acute attacks by going to bed for a few days or weeks until the temperature becomes normal and the exudate, which is so often felt in the iliac region, disappears. Hot poultices until the pain subsides, and then counter-irritation, laxatives, and tonics, constitute all that may be needed. Some patients learn to go to bed and to use poultices upon the first recurrence of symptoms, and thus manage to live in some sort of comfort until the tendency to recurrence wears off, as it often does after the Fallopian tube and ovary have lost their septic qualities and only adhesions remain to embarrass them.

In severe septic cases, with the formation of pus in the free peritoneal cavity, peritoneal section for the removal of the pus and diseased structures is the only rational treatment; but the extent of disease usually found would seem to render it less hopeful than in primary peritonitis. A pyocele in the cul-de-sac of Douglas calls for evacuation per vaginam. If situated elsewhere, with symptoms threatening general peritonitis, an abdominal section should not be shunned.

On account of the pre-existing adhesions so often found in old cases of secondary peritonitis, the general peritoneal cavity is protected, and many patients with purulent secondary peritonitis make a partial recovery under expectant treatment, and live to be operated upon later, or even to enjoy a tolerable state of health for long periods.

*Symptomatic.*—The symptomatic treatment is, in the main, the same as that for acute primary pelvic peritonitis (*q. v.*).

### CHRONIC PRIMARY PELVIC PERITONITIS.

*Etiology.*—Acute primary pelvic peritonitis may result in the chronic or subacute form when an irritating body or material remains in the pelvic cavity as a foreign substance, when irritation is frequently renewed by the entrance of more offending matter, or when the trauma is constantly repeated by the functional activity of the organs about the diseased tissue, by other local pathological conditions, or by external violence. Thus, a quantity of pus from a Fallopian tube, a foetus from a ruptured tube, a septic ligature left after an abdominal section, etc., may remain for a long time a source of inflammatory action before terminating in absorption, elimination, or encapsulation. Again, repeated drippings from the Fallopian tubes, or frequent escape of gas or fæces from a perforated appendix, may light up a case of subsiding or latent peritonitis; or the pathological changes brought about by a previous pelvic peritonitis (exudates, adhesions, effusions) may be of such a character that violent peristalsis, blows upon the abdomen, prolonged or laborious muscular action, menstruation, abortions, labor at term, gynæcological manipulations or operations, growing tumors, etc., may produce such frequent, constant, or severe trauma that the peritonitis is renewed or perpetuated.

*Pathological Anatomy.*—Leaving out of consideration the diseased conditions of the pelvic and abdominal viscera that precede acute primary pelvic peritonitis, there are certain pathological conditions of an inflammatory nature or origin that persist after the acute attack.

In the first place, there may result an organized exudate about the effused pus, or other foreign substance, uniting the neighboring tissues or

27

viscera around it so as to give rise to large agglutinated masses of infiltrated tissue. Thus, the indurated Fallopian tube may be curled over the cystic or infected ovary, with infiltration and thickening of the mesosalpinx. This club-shaped mass may, in turn, be adherent to the posterior surface of the broad ligament, or to the sacro-uterine ligament, with more or less subperitoneal infiltration in the ligament. Over this the omentum is usually adherent, and may by infiltration become opaque and thickened (in some cases as thick as the hand), reddened and friable. Again, the rectum, colon, appendix vermiformis, or loops of small intestine may be adherent to the pelvic mass. When the affection is bilateral and severe, the whole pelvic cavity may be filled as with a solid mass, over which the thickened omentum adheres like the top to a tight cask. The pelvic organs can be reached only by breaking through it. The upper portions of the broad ligaments then extend across the pelvis, forming a mass as hard as if carved of wood, from which the adherent organs cannot be separated without tearing into their vascular substance or leaving portions of the organs attached. Fatty degeneration and absorption of the intestinal walls may occur to such an extent that their separation from the mass either ruptures them immediately or leaves them incapable of enduring the strain of normal function. These more severe forms are usually of long standing, and connected with repeated septic invasions of the peritoneal cavity or a septic invasion followed by repeated traumatic influences.

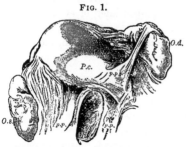

FIG. 1.

Peritoneal adhesions displacing uterus, view from behind.—*O.d.*, right ovary; *O.s.*, left ovary; *P.c.*, Douglas's cul-de-sac; *P.p.*, peritoneal folds. The dark space between the *p.p*'s is the severed rectum. (Bandl.)

In the acute, the subacute, and even the early chronic stages the exudates are soft, imperfectly organized, and their vascularity mainly of a capillary kind, so that adhesions are easily separated and bleed only a few minutes. In the later chronic stages the exudates are firm, the adhesions are separated with difficulty, and the vessels are so large that the bleeding persists for some time and may be fatal from the tearing of the visceral walls that often results.

When the disease results from the presence of growing tumors, with septic infection, the pathological changes may be even more extensive than those already mentioned.

In these old cases, particularly those in which there has been a prolonged septic influence, the degenerative changes in the heart, kidney, liver, and spleen, such as occur in general septic conditions, are found to a greater or less extent.

The pathological conditions are constantly varying in the progress of the same case. In an acute attack almost the entire pelvis may seem to

be filled with an inflammatory exudate, which a few days afterwards may be almost entirely dissipated. When, in a chronic case, the source of irrita-
tion disappears, the parts often return to their natural state in a surprisingly short time, as is observed after the evacuation of an accumulation of pus or the removal of a septic ligature.

In many cases the irritating body remains a long time or almost indefinitely encapsulated, as when aseptic ligatures are left: a certain amount of organized exudate remains around them, but the adhesions are absorbed. When the foreign body is finally removed the exudate around it also disappears. When the irritation about the adhesions is kept up for

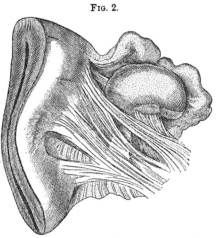

FIG. 2.

Organized peritoneal exudate displacing uterus. Uterus bisected, tube embracing ovary above. Peritoneal bands below. (Heitzmann.)

a long time and traction is made upon them before their absorption, as by visceral motions, they become drawn out into false membranes composed of fibrous tissue and even covered by endothelium. Such adhesions may remain almost indefinitely.

*Course and Symptoms.*—Many patients with chronic pelvic peritonitis complain but little and give no history of an acute attack. The acute attacks have been mild and have been confounded with other conditions. Other cases can be traced to an acute attack connected with the menses, an abortion, or labor, with subsequent attacks at longer or shorter intervals. Sometimes the first attack will be a severe one, confining the patient to bed for several weeks, and will be followed at longer intervals by milder attacks; at other times the first attack will be a mild one, followed at intervals of a few weeks by attacks of increasing severity, until the patient is bedridden much of the time. Exposure and over-exertion, particularly during the menstrual periods, precipitate attacks, while physical quiet and care are followed by long intervals of comparative health, and may result in a symptomatic, if not a complete, cure.

The symptoms are similar to those of an acute attack, but of less severity, and are more enduring. Persistent pain over the site of the disease or radiating from it is quite common,—*i.e.*, pain near the anterior superior iliac spine, sometimes extending up over the crest of the ilium, or to the groin or the nates, or down the thigh. The patient soon learns that she feels worse when she exercises freely and is better when quiet. Backache is frequently complained of, and is due to the accompanying endometritis. When there are intestinal adhesions, some tympanites and local tenderness are observable. Lying on the affected side generally causes discomfort or pain.

Perhaps one of the most constant symptoms is a slight afternoon rise in temperature of one or two degrees, with a normal, or nearly normal, morning temperature.

Menstruation is usually attended with more pain and a little higher temperature. The flow is sometimes increased in amount, but is more apt to drag along beyond the usual length of time, and may recur at irregular intervals. Coitus is usually painful, and defecation and micturition may be so. Laxative enemata sometimes cause great distress, as indeed may an ordinary evacuation of the bowels.

As a result of the enforced quiet, mental worry, loss of sleep, and want of exercise, the general health becomes impaired. Indigestion, constipation, cephalalgia, palpitation of the heart, etc., help to add to the misery of the patient.

Sterility is the ordinary condition, and when pregnancy occurs it is liable to be of the extra-uterine variety.

*Diagnosis.*—The diagnosis is based upon the symptoms just mentioned and upon the physical signs that are elicited by the bimanual examination. These are much the same as those of acute peritonitis, but with less tenderness. The finger in the vagina will feel a hardness and tender area behind or beside the uterus; this induration may be on one or both sides and so high up that it can scarcely be reached, or may be felt as a roundish or oval body lying behind the uterus or upon the broad ligament. Pressure over the pubes forces the uterus and tissues lower down, so that they are palpated better, and enables us to get the parts between the fingers of the two hands, so as to judge of the extent of the exudate and of the mobility of the uterus. The uterus may be firmly fixed in the exudate or may be only slightly restricted in mobility. Pressure that moves the uterus generally causes pain in the affected area; the organ is often felt to be out of place, either retroverted, or displaced laterally, or forward and laterally.

*Prognosis.*—When the disease has passed to the chronic form it seldom results fatally, except under very unfavorable conditions. When the septic influence is great, fresh attacks may result in general peritonitis and death; but even in such cases the patient often lingers along for years in a septic condition, and finally dies of exhaustion, or is carried away by some intercurrent affection. In the great majority of cases she learns to take care of herself, and gradually regains a tolerable condition of health. Some adhesions and permanent impairment of function of the pelvic organs remain to remind the patient of her former invalidism.

*Treatment.*—When acute symptoms arise in the course of the chronic inflammation the patient should be treated as already recommended in acute primary pelvic peritonitis. She should be kept in bed for some days, or even weeks, as may be necessary for a complete subsidence of the pain, tenderness, and febrile reaction. An enforcement of this rule will often be followed by a complete cure of the acute attacks and put the patient on the road to a recovery from the chronic symptoms.

But the case should not be abandoned as soon as the symptoms subside, or the patient will be apt to conduct herself so as to develop acute attacks or to perpetuate the chronic condition. She should for many weeks, or even months, keep her bed during the menstrual period, lie down two hours in the middle of each day between periods, avoid over-exertion, sexual excesses, all sources of intestinal irritation,—in short, everything that brings back any of her old symptoms,—and should receive such local treatment as will be recommended below.

A patient who continues to have an afternoon rise of temperature and still complains of pains upon taking exercise should at first be allowed to sit up for a short time each day, and be guided in rising and going about by the effect upon her symptoms. When the pain returns she should lie down. If the pain gets worse day by day, she should understand that she is getting up too fast and must spend more time in bed. In such cases, massage administered every morning and general electrization every evening will do much to maintain the vigor of the circulation and to secure sleep at night. The diet should be simple, but nourishing, and the bowels should be prompted as necessary by mild laxatives, in order to promote nutrition and to avoid irritation from the alimentary canal. A pill containing three or four grains of blue mass, at bedtime, every third or fourth night, followed the next morning by a Seidlitz powder, acts well as alterative, laxative, and tonic to digestion. Iron, nerve tonics, and the digestive ferments are needed in some cases. Counter-irritation over the iliac regions should, as a rule, be maintained. The skin may be kept tender by the application of the tincture of iodine. Blisters are useful in severe cases. When the manipulations are not harmful, copious hot-water douches give some relief. The application two or three times weekly of tincture of iodine to the cervix and vaginal fornices and the use of glycerin wool tampons in the vagina are beneficial in many cases, but the latter should not be used when they cause distress. A ten-per-cent. solution of ichthyol in glycerin on the tampons is a good application.

When an offending foreign body lies within the peritoneal cavity, steps should be taken to effect its removal. Abdominal fistulæ should be kept dilated with gauze packing, with drainage-tubes, or by periodical dilatation. After a reasonable delay the abdominal opening should be enlarged and the sinus explored with the finger, and when the offending body is felt it should be extracted. If the fistula be first disinfected, this procedure is quite safe, for even though the peritoneal cavity be opened its infection can be avoided.

When no external fistula exists, the abdomen should, in bad cases, be opened and the pelvis cleared of foreign matter, including the removal of seriously diseased appendages, whether they be dripping pus or not.

### CHRONIC SECONDARY PELVIC PERITONITIS.

*Etiology.*—Chronic secondary pelvic peritonitis may result from an acute attack, or may develop during the course of disease of the pelvic organs without having passed through any recognized acute stage.

The most common causes are salpingitis, pyosalpinx, ovaritis, and pelvic abscess. Metritis, ulcerative rectitis and cystitis, appendicitis, and pelvic cellulitis are occasional causes.

Ovarian abscess is probably due in most instances to infection from an overflowing tube, as I have demonstrated at the operating-table, and this overflow is attended by a primary peritonitis; yet a subsequent chronic peritonitis may be produced and perpetuated by the condition of the diseased ovary and tube without any subsequent overflow, and is then secondary.

FIG. 3.

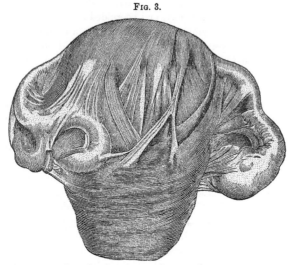

Adnexa imprisoned in adhesions. (Heitzmann.)

The various fixed malpositions in which the pelvic organs are held by the adhesions, due either to preceding acute primary peritonitis with contraction of exudates, or to misplacements occurring at the time of the acute attack, have much to do with the persistence of the inflammation both in the diseased organs and in the peritoneum. The ovary may be bound by adhesions to the rectum or beside the uterus, and kept in a state of irritation by their interference with the proper performance of the ovarian function. The uterus may be retroflexed or displaced laterally and kept in a state of chronic inflammation or congestion, and thus may react badly, more especially during the menstrual period, upon the ovaritis and peritonitis. The discharge of the contents of a septic tube is sooner or later interfered with by the changes in the uterus and the thickening of the walls of the tube at the uterine horn. If, as has been known to occur in connection with pathological conditions of the uterus, blood be effused from the tubal mucous membrane during menstruation, the swelling of the imprisoned or pinioned tube and the pressure upon the surrounding tissues add to the general inflammation.

*Pathology.*—The pathological conditions consist of the various diseases of the pelvic organs with adhesions. The adhesions may involve changes in the omentum and intestines similar to those observed in chronic primary pelvic peritonitis (*q. v.*). Organized exudates usually exist in the connective tissue contiguous to the diseased viscus and on the peritoneal covering, gluing it to the neighboring peritoneal surfaces that envelop other viscera,

Fig. 4.

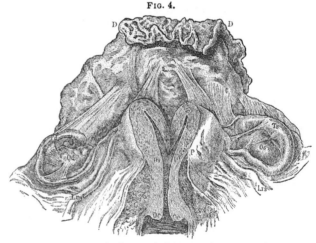

Adhesions due to secondary peritonitis.—*D*, intestine; *P*, peritoneum; *Oi*, internal os; *Oe*, external os; *Td*, right tube; *Ts*, left tube; *Od*, right ovary; *Os*, left ovary; *Lrd*, right round ligament; *Lrs*, left round ligament; *Par*, parovarium. (Bandl.)

spread over the pelvic connective tissue, or line the pelvic walls. Changes due to antecedent acute primary inflammation are often present.

Pus-tubes or suppurating ovaries are generally surrounded by extensive and firm adhesions, with an abundance of exudate in the immediate vicinity and greatly increased vascularity of the pelvic organs. In very old cases, however, the pus may lose its virulent character and become an inoffending mass of granular débris. Rupture of a pyosalpinx or suppurating ovary into the rectum, into the posterior vaginal fornix, or externally in the iliac or inguinal region may be followed for a long time by a fistula that closes and breaks out periodically. If efficient drainage is maintained, the cavity gradually becomes obliterated by granulation and cicatrization.

There is a class of cases in which active disease in the sexual organs has subsided. The ovaries are sclerotic or atrophied, the tube collapsed and hardened, the uterus anæmic or atrophic, and the adhesions thoroughly organized, often membranous. This represents the last stage of extensive but moderate inflammation.

· Recurrent attacks are apt to be accompanied by temporary exudates of wide extent between the viscera, which can be felt through the abdominal walls, and in the pelvic connective tissue so as temporarily to fill one or both sides of the pelvis. These may arise suddenly and may be absorbed with surprising rapidity, or they may come on slowly and be still more slowly absorbed. Some remains are generally left for a considerable period of time.

*Signs and Symptoms.*—The symptoms are largely those of the disease of the affected pelvic viscera, pain in one or both iliac regions, often radiating to the iliac, sacral, or lumbar region, being perhaps the most common one. There are, however, more acute pain, greater local sensitiveness, and a greater tendency to exacerbations from over-exertion, traumatism, exposure to changes of temperature, etc. All grades of symptoms are found in different cases, from those that make a patient permanently bedridden to those that are only of occasional inconvenience.

Most cases give a history of exacerbations and remissions, from a succession of frequently occurring acute attacks to an alternation of periods of pelvic pains and comparative health. There is usually a limit with regard to exercise, exposure, etc., within which the patient can live with comfort, but beyond which she cannot go without a return of the symptoms.

The prolonged invalidism involved not infrequently results in an exaggerated notion of symptoms and the various forms of hysteria. Transient and unimportant pains produced by exertion will be considered as indications for keeping the bed, and in time the patient may become bedridden, and may remain so for years after the necessity for it has passed. Three years ago I performed an abdominal section upon a woman who for several years had been unable to sit up except in bed. I found an agglutination of the omentum over the old site of a pyosalpinx that had discharged into the rectum and become obliterated. I merely separated the adhesions sufficiently to determine the condition, and then closed the abdomen. The patient, believing that the operation was to cure her, got on her feet as rapidly as is usual after a peritoneal section, was soon doing her own housework, and has been well ever since. The rapidity with which bedridden patients with the remains of pelvic peritonitis recover after going through a course of the Weir Mitchell treatment is another warning to us to be on our guard with reference to their complaints of pains, aches, and ingenious combinations of symptoms.

One of the most constant classes of symptoms is that connected with menstruation. It is quite common for some pain or discomfort to be felt for several days before the menstrual period, with relief upon the establishment of the flow. The relief felt at the appearance of the flow often leads the patient to say that she feels best while menstruating. The pain is usually felt in one or both iliac regions, but a dull ache across the pelvis, or aching in the limbs, or nausea with sick headache, may take the place of acute pain.  The character of the flow is also changed in many instances. It will appear at the right time, or a little late, and dribble for a few days before getting started, and then continue the usual time.  Or it may begin normally, but dribble along for a week or more after the proper time for it to stop.  Again, it may be much more scanty than normally, and last only a day or two, or may recur only once in two or three months, or may appear with less and less frequency until a premature menopause supervenes.

Endometritis usually exists with secondary pelvic peritonitis, and may cause backache and other pains throughout the menstrual period, and keep up a menorrhagia rather than a scanty menstruation.  The backache so prominent in some cases is usually due to endometritis, but it may be caused by adhesions of the uterus and appendages posteriorly.  The profuse leucorrhœa, with occasional gushes of mucous or muco-purulent discharge, sometimes accompanied by shooting pains through the pelvis, is often thought to come from a dilated tube; it is, however, nearly always a uterine discharge which occasionally accumulates in the uterine cavity as the result of a temporarily increased flexion, or of a contraction at the internal os. Pelvic peritonitis or salpingitis may even be absent altogether.  The failure of local treatment to benefit the endometritis, and the intolerance of the endometrium to any local applications, are often due to existing pelvic peritonitis secondary to tubal or ovarian disease.

Painful and difficult defecation, a tendency to the accumulation of hardened fæces above the plane of the adhesions and exudate, and the occasional or frequent passage of lumps of mucus are sometimes observed.

Dysuria, vesical tenesmus, and vesical catarrh are prominent symptoms in some cases.

As in the primary forms of peritonitis, sterility is the rule.  When impregnation does take place it is liable to be followed by an early abortion or by the ectopic form.  Old adhesions and exudates may be loosened and absorbed so as to allow the pregnancy to go to term.  Parturition is, however, more liable to be complicated, and may even be fraught with danger from rupture of an old pus-sac.

In case of adherent retroversion or adhesions of the appendages in the recto-uterine cul-de-sac, coition and gynæcological examinations are apt to be painful.

*Diagnosis.*—The uterus and appendages, whether displaced or not, are generally fixed.  The uterus is not usually tender, but any attempt to move it is painful, except in those cases of long standing in which all pelvic sensitiveness has subsided.  The appendages, as a rule, enlarged and hardened, remain sensitive for a long time, particularly when they are moved so as to produce traction upon the adhesions.  In some cases the pelvis feels to the examining finger as if filled by a hard exudate that immobilizes the uterus; in others, rounded or oblong masses are felt beside or behind the uterus, displacing it and restricting its mobility. Rectal palpation detects adhesions of the appendages to the rectum, or to the broad or sacro-uterine ligaments, even after the uterus has regained a limited degree of mobility and when the vaginal examination is almost negative. Bimanual examination, undertaken after a thorough evacuation of the bowels, enables us to press the parts down within easier reach from the vagina or rectum, and reveals exudates that could not be palpated from below.

*Treatment.*—The treatment recommended for chronic primary peritonitis (*q. v.*) may be considered as applicable to the chronic secondary form, as may also the treatment recommended elsewhere for diseased uterine appendages. In fact, the treatment consists largely in remedying these diseases.

The accompanying endometritis should also receive attention, for the uterus is commonly the avenue of infection, and a catarrhal endometritis is a constant source of danger. If the cervix is not sufficiently patulous to allow of an unrestricted outflow of mucus or pus, it should be gradually dilated with bougies or sounds until large enough to admit of a No. 10 or No. 12 urethral sound, and kept so dilated by passing the sound once or twice weekly. Before dilatation, the mucus should be wiped from the cervix and fornices and the parts thoroughly swabbed out with a five-per-cent. solution of carbolic acid. If this precaution is not observed, the uterine cavity will become infected and fresh attacks will sooner or later be produced. After passing the sound, a twenty-per-cent. solution of ichthyol in boiled glycerin should be passed on an applicator to the fundus, and also applied to the cervix on a tampon. Strong intra-uterine applications are harmful, and even the mild one mentioned may not always be well borne. The tampons should be left in place from twenty-four to thirty-six hours. Dilatation and curettage of the uterus (Polk) and drainage of the Fallopian tubes by Veuillet's method of uterine tamponade with gauze often act beneficially. Extreme antiseptic precautions should be observed in all these manipulations.

There is a class of cases in which the active signs and symptoms of inflammation have so far subsided that the patient complains only after unusual exertion or exposure or during menstrual periods. The uterus or ovaries are held in abnormal positions and prevent a complete return of health. Uterine massage or manipulations for the purpose of moving the organs towards their normal positions, and thus stretching the adhesions, have succeeded in removing the disability of the patient, although not always in restoring the normal relationship of the parts.

When adhesions with impaired functions and distressing symptoms remain, we are sometimes justified in opening the peritoneal cavity either by incision through the posterior vaginal fornix or through the linea alba, and breaking up the adhesions. Diseased ovaries and tubes may be treated by the excision of portions of them, or the injection of enlarged follicles with tincture of iodine, etc., as recommended by Polk and A. Martin.

In a certain proportion of cases all palliative treatment fails to afford relief, and the only remedy is to remove the diseased ovaries, the tubes, and even the uterus.  In the very worst class of cases vaginal hysterectomy has been advocated with the removal of as much of the conglomerated and suppurating appendages as may be, and the opening and drainage of all pus-centres from below.  Intestinal adhesions above are, by preference, left undisturbed.

### SPECIFIC PERITONITIS.

Of the varieties of so-called " specific" peritonitis, we shall consider here only the rheumatic and malignant forms.

*Rheumatic Peritonitis.*—Rheumatism sometimes affects the peritoneum as it does other serous membranes.  The peritonitis either precedes, accompanies, or follows the arthritic or muscular symptoms, or may even exist without them.  The symptoms usually come on suddenly, and may depart or change suddenly to be referred to other parts of the peritoneum or other serous membranes.  The character of the pains and the temperature are about the same as in simple non-specific peritonitis.  The pulse is usually full, hard, and accelerated.

The diagnosis is based mainly upon the presence of rheumatism elsewhere, the shifting character of the pain, the absence of other cause, and the relief afforded by anti-rheumatic remedies.

The treatment consists in hot applications and counter-irritation over the abdomen and the administration of anodynes for the pain, and the salicylates, antacids, mercurials, colchicum, cimicifuga, guaiacum, etc., for the rheumatic condition.

*Malignant Peritonitis.*—In the course of malignant disease of the pelvic viscera the peritoneum suffers from secondary inflammation and presents the usual changes and symptoms of secondary peritonitis.  Metastatic or primary deposits in the subperitoneal connective tissue may be the starting-point.  It usually assumes a subacute character, and may be of either a serous or an exudative variety.

The serous variety is found in cases of malignant tumors that project into the free abdominal cavity.  The inflammation develops gradually, and is accompanied by an effusion of serum that may prevent adhesions for a longer or shorter period of time.  The pain is usually slight, and may be said to exist in an inverse ratio to the amount of ascites.  When, however, the tumor becomes large enough to press firmly against the abdominal walls or viscera, adhesions form.  The peritoneum retains its glistening, endothelial character for a long time.  The inflammation is confined to the peritoneum covering the diseased organ as long as the ascitic fluid protects the surrounding serous surfaces from pressure or friction.

The diagnosis is based mainly upon the signs and symptoms of the malignant tumor or diseased organ, the presence of ascites, and sometimes of enlarged lymphatic glands in the pelvis, in the mesentery, or under the skin.  The pulse is weaker and more rapid than would be the case in simple chronic peritonitis, and the appearances of anæmia are often marked.

The treatment consists, of course, in the early removal of the malignant tumor or diseased organ.  Tapping may afford temporary relief by removing the pressure of the ascitic fluid.

In the exudative form there are repeated attacks of secondary peritonitis over the site of the diseased organs from which it proceeds.  These are mild at first, but progressive.  The attacks become more severe and the pain more constant, and exudates and adhesions form which unite the abdominal or pelvic viscera in large, hard masses.  The temperature is elevated and the pulse very much accelerated, as in attacks of ordinary secondary peritonitis, but the pulse is weaker and the anæmia greater.  The specific nature of the peritonitis depends upon the diagnosis of the original malignant disease.  The treatment is palliative, and consists mainly in the use of anodynes.

Papillomatous tumors projecting into the abdominal cavity give rise to the same kind of serous peritonitis as the more malignant ones.  Papillomatous ovarian tumors, just before the papillæ break through the capsule, may cause a serous secondary peritonitis with effusion, or, if that part of the tumor lies against another serous surface, may cause an adhesive peritonitis.  In some cases there is an abundance of fluid, with papillomatous masses projecting into the free abdominal cavity, or there may be but little ascites and general affection of the connective tissue and adhesions.  When there is extensive effusion we nearly always find perforation of the capsule.  When perforation occurs, if not before, an attack of primary peritonitis may be lighted up.  Projecting papillomatous particles become detached and disseminated in the peritoneal cavity and give rise to scattered metastatic deposits and primary peritonitis of moderate severity, with serous effusion.

The diagnosis is made by the discovery of ascites and hard masses about the site of the original disease, with a slight elevation of temperature and a somewhat accelerated pulse.  From carcinoma papilloma may be known by the fact that pain, anæmia, and depression of the vital powers are much less in proportion to the duration and amount of disease discovered.  Papillomatous ovarian tumors are often developed in the pelvic connective tissue and present hard, immovable masses about the uterus, sometimes displacing the latter.

The treatment consists in the removal of the originally diseased structures and the larger metastatic deposits.  The smaller deposits sometimes disappear, and with them the evidences of peritonitis.

Peritonitis in connection with ovarian tumors has been included in the description of primary and secondary pelvic peritonitis.

### POST-OPERATIVE PERITONITIS.

The conditions attending the development of peritonitis after the peritoneal cavity has been laid open and subjected to the manipulations necessary for the relief of intra-peritoneal pathological conditions are somewhat different from those attending other forms.  The difference is more of a clinical than of a pathological nature.  In ordinary cases of peritonitis the character and extent of the disease depend largely upon what goes into the peritoneal cavity.  In post-operative peritonitis it does not so much matter what enters—for that can be taken out—as what is left there.

The disease may be classified as follows :

$$
\text{LOCAL.} \left\{ \begin{array}{l} \text{Exudative or adhesive.} \\ \text{Suppurative.} \end{array} \right.
$$

$$
\text{GENERAL.} \left\{ \begin{array}{l} \text{Serous.} \\ \text{Exudative.} \\ \text{Suppurative.} \end{array} \right.
$$

*Etiology.*—The predisposing causes are the disease for which the operation is performed, and septic conditions about the patient's body, particularly of the alimentary canal and the skin.

The immediate causes are: (1) prolonged exposure of the peritoneum to the atmosphere; (2) destruction or injury of the peritoneal endothelium by the manipulations of the surgeon (whether by mechanical or by chemical action) or in the separation of adhesions; (3) foreign bodies or dead matter left in the cavity; (4) the unhealthy condition of tissues that are left; (5) direct infection by the introduction of septic microbes; (6) infection through the drainage-tube; (7) the ulceration or bursting of purulent or septic extra-peritoneal accumulations into the abdominal cavity; and (8) the separation of the abdominal wound from violence.

Among aggravating causes may be mentioned shock, prolonged anæsthesia, acute anæmia, and toxæmia from suppressed secretions.

By way of illustrating the immediate causes of peritonitis we might say that the first two mentioned—viz., prolonged exposure and injury of endothelium—exist when long abdominal incisions are made, when the intestines are eventrated, when prolonged efforts are made to bring up adherent intra-pelvic tumors or diseased organs, or when disinfectants are poured into the cavity or applied to the peritoneal surfaces.

Foreign bodies or dead matter left in the cavity consist of numerous or large ligatures, gauze, forgotten sponges and instruments, fluids from ruptured tumors and organs, blood, tissue-débris, and the like.  Even fatty particles from the abdominal incision may get into the cavity and cause peritonitis.

Among diseased tissues which cannot be removed, yet which have been subjected to sufficient manipulation to produce inflammation in them or to destroy their vitality, may be mentioned the denuded or mutilated organs from which the removed structures have been separated, such as lacerated or denuded intestines, uterus, or bladder, diseased uterine appendages, an adherent vermiform appendix, inflamed or malignant tumors with inseparable adhesions, a fibroid uterus from which some, but not all, of the tumors have been enucleated, also obscure pathological conditions, such as abscesses, displaced or distorted intestinal folds, etc.

Direct infection may come from germs on the assistant's hand, those underneath the invisible and temporary crust formed on the cuticle by the disinfectant, or from the handling by nurses and assistants of things about the room or operating-table without subsequent adequate disinfection, and in general from a want of proper disinfection of all the surroundings. The fact that infection occurs in so many prolonged manipulations is proof of the presence of germs about the field of many operations.

Under (7) may be mentioned bruised and infected abdominal wounds, vaginal openings imperfectly closed or drained, rupture of an intestine, kidney, bladder, abscess, etc.

*Pathology.*—(See also Pathological Anatomy of Chronic Primary Pelvic Peritonitis, page 417.)  When the peritoneum covering the intestines is exposed to the air, even without being brought in contact with any other substance, some irritation occurs, which usually results in reflex atony of the intestinal muscular system,—tympanites.  When rough substances, even the fingers of the operator, are brought in contact with any considerable surface of the intestinal peritoneum, more or less congestion and sensitiveness follow, which, as a rule, render the subsequent peristalsis painful. When the friction between the sterilized finger and the intestines is continued for a long time, or a chemical irritant is applied, an inflammation with fibrinous exudate forms, which rapidly agglutinates the surfaces and suppresses peristalsis in the affected area.

If, in addition to such irritation, foreign substances such as small blood-clots or débris are left, even in small quantities, an exudation forms which, on account of the impaired absorbent powers of the peritoneum, readily undergoes septic changes and forms an abscess commensurate with the extent of the injury and the soiling of surface.  Whether the omnipresent saprophytic germs in the atmosphere are sufficient to induce the septic changes or not may be questioned. . They act more slowly than inoculated pus-germs, but, as suppuration is the final outcome, pus-germs must in some way get there.  Direct infection by an abundance of pus-germs leads to a rapid formation of pus, which tends to produce a general septic peritonitis.

When, with a small degree of traumatism and a minimum quantity of serum or bloody serum, the peritoneal cavity is infected, a general septic peritonitis of serous character is lighted up.  If the patient dies within two or three days, the general peritoneum is deep red and vascular, with some exfoliation of endothelium, and a variable, though seldom large, amount of more or less bloody serum is found in the pelvis.  If life be prolonged, suppurative peritonitis develops.

When the endothelium is completely destroyed over a limited area by excessive manipulations or the separation of adhesions, exudative inflammation and new adhesions occur; when, in addition to this, blood-clots or débris are allowed to remain, the exudative peritonitis is sooner or later converted into the purulent variety. When the injured area is small and the infection but slight, a local abscess forms; when the injured area is large or the infection considerable, extensive or general purulent peritonitis results, unless the amount of poison inoculated is such that the patient dies of sepsis before the local changes have had time to develop. When both a large injured area with débris is left and direct infection with an abundance of pus-germs occurs, death may occur from acute sepsis during the serous stage. Bloody serum about the site of the injury and a general congestion of the peritoneal covering will be found. If life be prolonged, some fibrinous flakes will be found scattered on the neighboring peritoneal surface and a commencing formation of pus in the serum. If death be delayed, general purulent peritonitis ensues, with pus scattered over the peritoneum, or accumulations in separate pockets.

In some cases the peritoneal surfaces have been but little exposed to the air or to manipulations, but pus-sacs have been enucleated or abscesses opened and cleaned, and the tissues are already infiltrated with septic matters and the patient more or less poisoned by them. Under these conditions complete removal of the diseased tissues will be followed by a localized reparative inflammation of the exudative or adhesive variety; but an incomplete removal of the septic tissues will sometimes be followed by so rapid a development of sepsis and such rapid absorption that death from acute sepsis results without any manifestation of peritonitis either to a clinical or to a post-mortem examination.

Infection of the abdominal wound without infection of the peritoneum may result in local abscesses of greater or less extent on the connective-tissue side of the peritoneum without involving the cavity. The peritonitis is secondary and of the exudative variety, and is confined to the neighboring peritoneal surface and the contiguous surface of omentum or intestine. Death may result from the accompanying systemic infection.

In more severe cases a part or the whole of the abdominal incision is opened up by the invading germs and a primary suppurating peritonitis is set up. If this is not quickly checked, the barriers of exudate are soon broken down and a general septic peritonitis supervenes, which proves fatal within two or three days. If subject to proper local treatment, the inflammation may remain localized over the adherent omentum or a few intestinal coils, or may gradually spread from one coil of intestine to another until a large surface is affected and ulceration and even perforation of the gut may occur. Death always takes place before the entire peritoneal membrane is thus affected, although I treated a case in which life was prolonged for six weeks and the whole anterior portion of the abdominal cavity and the entire pelvic peritoneal cavity were suppurating. A fæcal fistula formed a short time before death.

When the abdominal incision is burst open by violence and is not promptly closed, general septic peritonitis ensues. If previous adhesions have been formed, a local peritonitis follows, which soon becomes purulent and pursues about the same course as in the case when the edges of the wound are parted by ulceration from an extra-peritoneal parietal abscess.

When operations are accompanied by profuse hemorrhage, or are prolonged in cases of anæmia and septicæmia, or when oozing masses of adherent, degenerated issue of malignant or septic character are left, the patient may succumb during the second twenty-four hours from shock or exhaustion, with only a general or local redness of the peritoneal membrane and the effusion of bloody serum.

Occasionally a localized peritonitis with exudate and adhesions will be perpetuated about a stump in which some active ovarian tissue has been left. Suppuration seldom occurs, but there is a succession of slight effusions, followed by partial absorption.

Obstruction to the passage of the contents of the bowels may be due to the paralysis following a general peritonitis or to the adhesion of intestinal coils attending localized attacks. Extensive adhesions, however, do not cause obstruction unless the intestines are compressed, twisted, or kinked to some extent. I once removed a fibro-cystic tumor reaching high above the umbilicus from a patient who enjoyed good health, yet in whom I made an incision reaching above the umbilicus and could not find the free abdominal cavity on account of the universal adhesions of the intestines to each other and to the tumor over its entire posterior and part of its lateral surface. It seemed as if all the intestinal coils were adherent to one another and yet had caused no symptoms. At a post-mortem upon another patient whom I had treated many times for peritonitis, and who had finally died, without operation, of purulent peritonitis, the intestines were united everywhere with old adhesions, yet there had always been during the attacks a tendency to looseness of the bowels. But when the intestines have been much disturbed through an abdominal incision, adhesive peritonitis, even of small extent, is very liable to be accompanied by obstruction. In fact, such is the most common cause, particularly when the adhesions are about the abdominal incision, where the intestines have been the most disturbed. Sometimes the adhesion of one or more displaced loops or of the mesentery to the stump, without much surrounding inflammation, will interfere, by traction, pressure, or twisting, with the passage of the fæces. In other cases cicatricial bands or narrow spaces between displaced tissues or organs may imprison and compress a fold of intestine, which often occurred formerly when the ovarian stump was fixed in the wound and drew the broad ligament up to the anterior abdominal wall.

The accumulation of septic matter in the distended intestine above the obstruction leads to invasion of the walls of the gut, and finally of the general peritoneal cavity, by the microbes. Profound congestion and discoloration, with progressive exfoliation of endothelium and the formation of fibrinous exudate, are found over the affected bowel, but life is seldom sufficiently prolonged for the formation of pus, except at the site of the original adhesions, where commencing suppuration is observed.

Obstruction occurring after some weeks is usually due to a localized post-operative peritonitis leaving permanent adhesions of the bowel to some neighboring organ or tissue. Twisting, knotting, or compression occurs as the result of peristalsis or changes in the surrounding parts.

*Symptoms and Course.*—After all peritoneal sections a reparative process takes place, with symptoms, more or less pronounced, of inflammation. In the so-called normal cases the temperature, after the first depression attending the shock, goes up to $99\frac{1}{2}°$ F. the second day, and often reaches 100° on the afternoon of the second or third day. It, however, quickly subsides below 99° in the forenoon and within a fraction of that in the afternoon. Towards the end of the week it generally sinks permanently below 99°. The pulse is fuller than normal on the second day and sometimes on the third day. In abdominal sections acute peritoneal pain is usually observed after the first few hours, coincident with peristaltic action, and may be a favorable symptom, in that it indicates an absence of complete paralysis of the intestines. It is probably produced by the rubbing of congested peritoneal surfaces together. Absence of pain does not necessarily denote the absence of such congestion, but may indicate complete intestinal paralysis and consequent absence of peristaltic action.

· A rise of the temperature to 101° to 102° F. during the first day, with corresponding fulness and frequency of the pulse, is apt to be due to reaction from nervous influences connected with the mental condition of the patient, or to irritation arising from an imperfectly prepared state of the secretions and excretions. The temperature usually begins to subside after a few hours, and no bad effects follow.

After ordinary vaginal sections there is less shock than after abdominal section for pelvic disease; there is also less reaction and but little peritoneal pain.

The amount of nausea or the intensity of the vomiting during the first twenty-four hours has but little to do with the severity of the operation or with the amount of inflammation that may be expected. After prolonged or mutilating intra-peritoneal manipulations there is often no nausea, while after a rapid and simple operation there may be excessive vomiting for two or three days, followed by a smooth recovery. This nausea is produced by the anæsthetic, and depends upon the condition and idiosyncrasy of the patient. Occasional attacks of vomiting, becoming less frequent and subsiding during the second day, may be said to be the rule. Vomiting lasting for three or four days, with excessive nausea and straining, may be called nervous vomiting, and is not an unfavorable symptom. When the nausea and straining diminish or cease during the second day, and are replaced by regurgitations of fluid without much nausea, we have indications of intestinal paralysis or peritonitis. Frequent vomiting of small quantities of a dark fluid almost from the beginning, without very much straining, is a symptom of peritonitis. Regurgitation, or easy vomiting of increasing amounts of fluid after long intervals of gastric quiet, denotes intestinal paralysis or obstruction.

Mild attacks of peritonitis, unless it is situated high up in the abdominal cavity, seldom occasion any nausea that is distinguishable from that connected with the anæsthetic. Constipation is the rule. The abdominal tenderness and peristaltic pain are usually marked; the temperature reaches 101°, or 102°, or even 103° F. on the second or third day, while the pulse becomes full and bounding, ranging from 80 to 100 or more. When there is no decided septic element the temperature subsides somewhat within twenty-four hours, and remains in the neighborhood of 100° or 101° F. for a day or two, usually a degree higher in the afternoon than in the morning, and during the second week becomes normal. If an exudate be so situated as to interfere with the circulation or function of any of the viscera, or if it be subject to disturbance by visceral motion, some local tenderness and elevation of temperature may continue during the third or fourth week, or even longer. Degenerative changes in the stump may cause a temperature of 99° or 100° F. for many months, or until the cause is removed by surgical means. Nausea, tympany, and acute pain subside with the temperature, more rapidly if the bowels are evacuated and flatus is freely passed per rectum. Abundant eructations of gas, with slight temporary relief, are frequently observed even in the mildest cases.

In case there be a small septic focus left, there will be a partial but not complete subsidence of pain and fever, followed in a few hours or days, according to the amount and extent of infection, by a steady and often rapid rise in temperature and pulse-rate, with return of pain and increase of the tympanites over the infected area. The pulse, instead of remaining full and firm, becomes rapid, small, and wiry ; vomiting returns, the bowels sometimes run off and become offensive, and, unless evacuation of the pus takes place, the ordinary symptoms of septic peritonitis, described elsewhere, are developed (q. v.). In some cases these symptoms will remain of a comparatively mild character for several weeks until an abscess is discovered or discharges.

In more severe cases the pains, tympanites, nausea, temperature, and pulse-rate increase from the first, the pulse becomes thready and weak, the patient extremely restless, and the symptoms rapidly develop into those of a fatal septic peritonitis.

In other cases the symptoms of moderate peritonitis already mentioned will come on rapidly and partly subside. The pain, however, is either inconsiderable or disappears within a few hours ; but the temperature hovers between 99½° and 101° F., and a localized area of tympanites at one side of or near the abdominal incision is noticeable, in which the intestinal coils can often be distinguished. There is a localized adhesive peritonitis. The bowels are obstinately constipated, and cannot be moved by cathartics or by enema. The patient is comfortable, and at first takes nourishment quite well; but after a few days the stomach begins to reject food, the pulse becomes weaker, the patient's mind is somewhat dull, and the temperature creeps up a little higher every afternoon. A week or ten days after the operation, or possibly a little later, decided symptoms of intestinal obstruction develop, and the patient dies of septic exhaustion. The progress is insidious and slow, and no medical treatment seems to have any effect. Towards the end the temperature often rises to 105° or 106° F.

In other cases the inflammation is more extensive, and the patient succumbs in a few days with symptoms of peritonitis and without a movement of the bowels, in spite of active cathartics.

In still other cases in which the intestines have been exposed for some time, or have been subjected to considerable manipulation, tympanites will be marked and general from the beginning, especially if the intestinal canal has not been previously well evacuated and disinfected. The pains are sometimes severe, but seldom excessive. The stomach tolerates but little food, and the constipation is obstinate. Considerable gas is belched and but little passed : yet the temperature does not rise above 102° F., nor does the pulse exceed 120 beats per minute. After a week, or even sooner, the temperature begins to subside, the pulse improves, gas passes per rectum, the bowels respond to laxatives or enemata, food is tolerated in large quantities, and convalescence is finally established. These cases cause the surgeon much anxiety, for the fatal effects of intestinal paralysis are to be feared.

Sometimes a case will pursue a similar course after a severe operation in which many ligatures have been left, or many adhesions separated, or irritating fluids spilled into the peritoneal cavity. The tympanites will be less prompt, but will be progressive, the temperature and pulse will show a little more reaction each afternoon, the symptoms of general or extensive peritonitis will develop gradually, and the case will end fatally after several weeks. In such cases one or more abscesses will develop, and then spontaneous or artificial evacuation is the only hope for the patient. This is apt to be the course when an instrument or a sponge is left, although the tympanites is more or less localized or is more prominent over the source of the inflammation.

When a drainage-tube or several tubes are used, the peritoneal symptoms are more often mild during the first two or three days, or partially subside. When the tube is removed, they increase rapidly and go on steadily to a fatal issue unless the tube is reintroduced or the opening is dilated either artificially from without or by the pressure of pus from within. In other cases, whether the tube is removed or not, progressive peritoneal symptoms arise after two or three days, due to inefficient drainage, and end fatally unless the wound is promptly reopened and the undrained pocket is emptied. After vaginal section in which a drainage-tube has been left for two or three days, the following peritonitis is usually relieved after the temperature has gone up to 103° or 104° F., with a bounding pulse, by spontaneous evacuation through the drainage-tube. The peritonitis is local ;

the cavity above, having been subjected to no manipulation, is quickly shut off by adhesions, and the pus finds least resistance by way of the drainage-track.

When a large gauze drain has been introduced through the abdominal incision, or has projected into the peritoneal cavity through a vaginal incision, the peritonitis is usually accompanied by symptoms of obstruction of the bowels, due to adhesions and kinking or compression of intestinal coils about the gauze. As the gauze rapidly removes the serum, the adhesions are quickly formed and symptoms of obstruction develop early. The symptoms of general peritonitis following peritoneal section are described under septic peritonitis.

*Prognosis.*—The prognosis depends less upon the severity of the early symptoms than upon their course. Severe symptoms at the outset that begin to subside in forty-eight hours are seldom serious. Such symptoms commencing after four or five days, or a week, generally denote a septic focus that will induce fatal results unless followed by evacuation. The pulse is a more reliable guide than the temperature, for the latter is influenced by many things and may be erratic and unreliable. A soft, slow pulse remaining the same for several days is one of the most comforting phenomena in otherwise puzzling cases; a rapid, irregular, thready pulse points to danger ahead. The absence of intestinal flatus for several days, in spite of saline cathartics and enemata, constitutes a danger-signal. Regurgitation of large quantities of fluids after intervals of gastric quietude gives warning of obstruction of the bowels. The vomiting of blackish-green fluid indicates a serious but not necessarily fatal form of peritonitis. When the vomited substance assumes a fæcal odor a fatal issue may be expected, and the time for successful surgical interference is, or will soon be, past.

The importance of particular symptoms is given above in the description of the symptoms and course.

*Treatment.*—The prophylactic treatment of post-operative peritonitis consists in good operating. It is beyond the province of this article to go into the details of peritoneal section, and I shall content myself with mentioning four things that should ever be kept in the mind of the operator. First, the operation should be a scrupulously aseptic one. Asepsis covers nearly all operative sins; but, as perfect asepsis is not always attainable, even under the most favorable circumstances, we should always operate as if we had some sepsis to combat. We must, therefore, secondly, avoid as far as possible all traumatism of the organs and tissues to be left in the peritoneal cavity, for fear that they will undergo septic inflammation. Thirdly, we should leave the peritoneal cavity clean and free from foreign material that might develop sepsis, such as blood-clot, débris, fluids, etc. Fourthly, if we find it impossible to cleanse the peritoneal cavity perfectly or to prevent extensive oozing of blood, we should choose the least of two evils and use drainage. Many are opposed to drainage of the peritoneal cavity; but even though we recognize the fact that there is danger in drainage, and that the peritoneum can to a certain extent drain itself, yet this part of the body forms no exception to the rest. Drainage cannot always be dispensed with.

To limit as far as possible the natural reaction from the traumatism of the operation, we should keep the patient very quiet during the first thirty-six hours. She should turn in bed only when necessary, and then be assisted. She should be cautioned to avoid moaning, talking, tossing of her limbs, etc., as such exertions and motions increase the pains and restlessness and tend to produce or increase inflammation. The atony of the intestines and consequent distention should deter us from allowing large quantities of cold water or of food difficult of digestion. Small, frequently repeated hot drinks, one or two tablespoonfuls of hot water or weak tea, or of cold drinks rendered stimulating by brandy, ginger, or some aromatic, are preferable. No food should be given for twenty-four hours, and then only small quantities of liquid nourishment for forty-eight hours longer, or until the intestines have regained their tone.

An enema composed of an ounce each of glycerin, water, and sulphate of magnesium acts beneficially in securing an evacuation of irritating gases when the ineffectual but painful intestinal contractions seem to act preju-dicially or cannot be tolerated. The relief afforded is often great.

When flatulence is persistently troublesome, saline laxatives often add materially to the comfort of the patient and remove symptoms that seem to threaten inflammation. If she cannot retain an ordinary dose, a tea-spoonful of the sulphate or granular citrate of magnesium may be given every hour until gas commences to pass per rectum, and then be aided by an enema of glycerin or soapsuds.

Opiates should be avoided, as they cause retention of intestinal gases and thereby favor inflammation. Extreme restlessness or protracted spells of nervous vomiting, with excessive straining, can be moderated by chloral enemata of twenty-five grains of the drug in a cupful of water, repeated once or twice, two or three hours apart, according to the urgency.

It may be said, however, that medical treatment is almost entirely pal-liative or accessory in character, for the outcome is usually determined by the character of the operative manœuvres, and in cases progressing towards a fatal issue there is usually no help except by surgical procedures or some equivalent aid on the part of nature.

Mild attacks of peritonitis usually need no further treatment than that mentioned. Attacks following prolonged operations involving acute anæmia and shock may require subcutaneous or intra-venous transfusions of one or two pints of a six-tenths-per-cent. saline solution, with or without a large dose of brandy, strychnine, and digitalis dissolved in each, or copious rectal enemata of the same character, to tide the patient over the dangerous stage. Severe attacks of local or general peritonitis, whether septic or not, may require such a stimulating or supporting treatment before, during, or after the operative procedures. But the necessity of a complicated course of treatment is of itself almost a sure indication that it alone will prove inadequate.

In some cases an early secondary operation is required.

When the attack follows the removal of a drainage-tube, the tube should be reintroduced, or a probe passed down its track to let out the offending fluid. Sometimes the finger must be introduced to search for a pocket in the hollows of the sacrum.

If symptoms of intestinal obstruction follow the use of a Mikulicz drain, then much time must not be lost in dallying with enemata and cathartics, but the gauze must be partially or entirely removed and a smaller gauze drain or a tube must be introduced. If this does not help, the adherent intestinal coils about the drain must be separated; and to be successful, these, as well as nearly all other operative manœuvres, must be done before the pulse becomes weak and thready.

When there is a moderate, slightly progressive, local peritonitis without symptoms of ileus, the treatment must be supporting, while the surgeon, by examinations and watchfulness, determines the time and place for interference in order to let out the offending matter.

When there is localized adhesive peritonitis with intestinal paralysis persisting in spite of laxatives and enemata, there is usually nothing to do but to reopen the wound and separate the adhesions or to establish an artificial anus above them. Large doses of saline cathartics and stimulating rectal enemata should, however, be tried first.

Rapidly developing general peritonitis calls for early reopening of the wound, cleansing of the field of operation, and drainage.

When there is obstruction of the bowel, with either local or general peritonitis, and the patient's strength is such as no longer to admit of such intra-peritoneal manipulation as would be necessary for the separation of extensive adhesions, a small abdominal incision may be made over the site of an intestinal coil above the seat of obstruction, a longitudinal incision made into the bowel, its contents evacuated or washed out as thoroughly as practicable, and the edges stitched into the abdominal wound so as to form an artificial anus. Either at the same time or subsequently, according to the condition of the patient, it may be desirable to open the incision and separate as many adhesions as is necessary to clean out any septic pockets or areas, and drain. A combination of these procedures has been employed in cases of appendicitis by Henrotin, with brilliant results. (*American Journal of Obstetrics*, August, 1893.)

Wide experience is nowhere so valuable as in determining the propriety and character of secondary operations. As a rule, the young operator, trusting to Providence for an amelioration of symptoms, allows the disease to progress too far before venturing. On the other hand, there is danger that he will operate unnecessarily and kill his patient in those cases in which stormy symptoms immediately follow the operation and are due to inflammation of short duration. In such cases, if flatus can be made to escape from the rectum and the pulse is strong and bounding and not beyond 120 nor the temperature above 104° F., it may be well to wait for the first reaction to subside. If, however, the symptoms after thirty-six or forty-eight hours are progressive, instead of being stationary or retrogressive, the advisability of operative interference ought to be considered.

Colliquative diarrhœa calls for evacuation of the pus, if its location can be determined before the vital powers have become too much depressed. The stomach is usually unable to digest sufficient food to keep up the strength, and rapid exhaustion may be expected.

## PELVIC CELLULITIS (PARAMETRITIS, PARACOLPITIS, PARAPROCTITIS, PARACYSTITIS, PARASALPINGITIS).

Connective tissue exists in all parts of the body; it surrounds the abdominal and pelvic viscera, and constitutes the framework upon and in

FIG. 5.

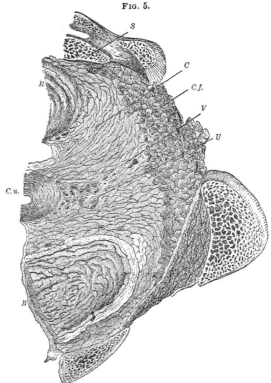

Pelvic connective tissue.—*S*, sacrum; *B*, bladder; *R*, rectum; *C u*, cervix uteri; *C*, connective tissue; *C.f.*, connective tissue bearing fat; *V*, blood-vessels; *U*, ureter. (Freund.)

which the peritoneal endothelium and glandular structure are developed; hence all cases of peritonitis are, to a certain extent, also cases of cellulitis, particularly that which we have called the secondary form, in which the inflammation starts in the viscera and extends through the connective tissue to the peritoneal surface. But there are certain pelvic organs, such as the lower rectum, urethra, bladder, vagina, and cervix uteri, which have little or no peritoneal covering; inflammation in these organs may involve the surrounding connective tissue without reaching the peritoneum, or may involve the peritoneum to a limited extent only: hence the term peritonitis would be an inadequate one.

The connective tissue has no function except the passive one of supporting and protecting the organs and tissues. It may be affected by inflam-

FIG. 6.

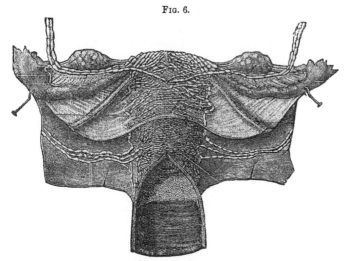

Lymphatics of the uterus. (Poirier.)

mation due to direct traumatism, by extension from the neighboring organs and tissues, and by the introduction of septic agents. Cellulitis depending upon traumatism is of transient duration, and as an acute affection is unimportant unless connected with other pelvic disease or complicated by the introduction or supervention of sepsis. Cellulitis may also extend from an inflamed Fallopian tube, uterus, vagina, bladder, rectum, etc. These forms are called parasalpingitis, parametritis, paracolpitis, paracystitis, paraproctitis (W. A. Freund), but are more commonly included under the term parametritis (Virchow). The most important forms, clinically, are those dependent upon the invasion of the connective tissue by septic agents, and are called septic phlegmon, diffuse suppurative cellulitis, pelvic abscess, etc.

The numerous lymphatic vessels about the uterus extending through the base and upper part of the broad ligament to the pelvic walls play an important part in the transmission of sepsis.

We may therefore make the following classification : acute primary or traumatic cellulitis; acute secondary cellulitis, or acute parametritis; chronic cellulitis, or chronic parametritis ; septic cellulitis, and pelvic abscess.

## ACUTE PRIMARY OR TRAUMATIC CELLULITIS.

*Etiology.*—This disease, as its name indicates, is the result of traumatism. In every case of difficult or prolonged labor some cellulitis is produced. A striking example is that seen and felt about the tissues at the vaginal entrance after labor. The tissues about the cervix and vagina are similarly, although often much less profoundly, affected. Prolonged manipulations during operations upon the pelvic organs are a frequent cause. Forcible dilatation of an anteflexed uterus has been known to cause a rupture through the anterior cervical wall, cellulitis between the uterus and the bladder, and subsequent abscess that had to be evacuated by a supra-pubic incision. Long-continued and oft-repeated bodily exertions at the time of the menstrual congestion, or during the course of other forms of pelvic inflammation, may lead to it.

*Pathology.*—The tissues about the perineum and vaginal entrance are perhaps most frequently affected in a traumatic way, as the scars, deficiencies, and displacements of tissue about the vaginal entrance of multiparæ will testify. But these inflammations are unimportant as compared with those of the parametrium proper, and belong more to the subject of perineal lacerations. The pathological changes are, however, similar to those of primary pelvic cellulitis, or parametritis.

The first changes that follow the traumatism are the same as would be found in connective tissue elsewhere. If there be no extensive lesion of tissue the changes seldom pass to the full development of inflammation. After difficult enucleation of an intra-mural uterine fibroid per vaginam, or after a labor in which a large head presses for a long time on the pelvic tissue, there will be some general pelvic hyperæmia with sufficient lesion of the capillary system to cause in a few hours a slight transudation of serum and leucocytes in the connective tissue about the cervix and vagina, at the same time that some exudate occurs in the uterine or vaginal walls. After twenty-four or thirty-six hours, absorption of the fluid and repair of the capillary vessels commence, so that in from two to six days the parts have recovered their integrity.

In case the injury be sufficient to produce much lesion of tissue, such as rupture of capillaries and cell-destruction, there will be, in addition to any minute or extensive extravasations of blood that may occur, a surrounding exudate consisting of the blood-serum, leucocytes, and some blood-corpuscles. This exudate is sometimes rapidly absorbed ; at other times the vitality of the connective-tissue cells is interfered with. The fluid in the latter case becomes absorbed and leaves a solid exudate to be removed gradually and to be followed by cicatricial contraction of tissue. Such inflammations are often found about the lower end of the vagina and urethra after first labors in old primiparæ, keeping the parts swelled and sensitive for many days and rendering urination and coition painful. The connective tissue about the cervix is seldom primarily affected by traumatism, except anteriorly, because of its elasticity and the absence of hard tissues against which it can be pressed and bruised.

Direct lacerations into the connective tissue occurring during labor are, on account of the difficulty of aseptic treatment, liable to develop rapidly into the septic variety. If the lesion occur during an operation, and antiseptic precautions be employed, there will be a localized hyperæmia with transudation of serum and leucocytes for a few hours, followed by adhesion of the raw surfaces or else by complete cicatrization.

The process is often one of regeneration rather than of inflammation. When the lesion is extensive and the exudate proportionately large, an abundant formation of embryonal tissue takes place, and, by subsequent infection with bacteria or pus-microbes, also some suppuration. Cicatricial contraction goes on in the granulation-tissue beneath the surface until the wound-surface is obliterated. Without antiseptic treatment the embryonal tissue is all converted into pus and the deeper tissue is invaded until all, or nearly all, of the pelvic connective tissue becomes converted into one or more abscesses. After recovery, the sites of the original lesions are represented by cicatricial bands that may distort the parts. We have examples of these in the bands that are so often found to extend from a lacerated cervix through the vaginal fornices to the pelvic wall or down the vaginal walls. Cicatrices in the perineum afford analogous illustrations.

Traumatism in the form of prolonged pressure of the head during labor, or of other foreign bodies, is followed by a transudation and exudation sufficient to produce a stasis in the circulation and death of the parts by strangulation. Thus, necrosis may open up tracks through the vesico-vaginal septum which, with the addition of lacerations of the vagina and perineum posteriorly, may convert the bladder, vagina, and rectum into one cavity. If sepsis comes in to complicate the conditions, as it usually does, destruction of large portions of the vagina and cervix may occur, and by subsequent cicatricial contraction lead to their partial or complete obliteration.[1]

*Signs, Symptoms, and Course.*—Traumatic cellulitis is not followed by very active symptoms. There is but little pain, except that connected with the other parts injured at the same time. Often no pain is felt, except upon motion of the body or manipulation. Pain and tenderness are more marked when a solid exudate is formed, and may become acute if the overlying peritoneum be affected. The position of the pain is over the seat of the disease, extending sometimes along the nerve-trunks.

The temperature in severer cases goes up to 100° or 102° F., but sub-

---

[1] The author once made an artificial vagina in a case in which the uterus all but the fundus, the entire cervix and vagina, and nearly all of the perineum had disappeared after labor as if they had never existed.

sides in two or three days almost to the normal.   If there be a wound that becomes infected there will usually be an afternoon rise of temperature corresponding in degree to the amount of septic absorption.   The pulse, corresponding to the temperature, is full and rapid, usually from 80 to 100 beats per minute.   If sepsis develops, the pulse will be full and frequent in the afternoon, and rather weak, but not so much accelerated, in the forenoon.   Colliquative diarrhœa and tympanites frequently supervene.   (See Septic Cellulitis.)

The examining finger will find the vagina during the first days warmer than natural.   If the inflammation be about the lower portion of the vagina, the vaginal entrance will be found tender and the tissues tumefied. Disease deeper in the pelvis gives to the finger a diminished sense of elasticity and an increased fulness about the vaginal fornices and cervix.   The tissues are all tender, and, although the cervix be mobile, any displacing pressure upon it causes pain.   The abdomen will be found to be soft and not tender to slight pressure, unless distended from functional intestinal disease, which may be removed by a laxative or an efficient enema.   In case of direct laceration into the connective tissue there will at first be felt a soft cavity, small and circumscribed if through the anterior vaginal wall or lower end of the vagina, but large and indefinite if into tissues about the cervix. After from twenty-four to forty-eight hours an area of induration will be found about the vaginal wound and also about the connective-tissue pocket or pockets ; if the connective tissue about the cervix becomes broken down by suppuration, there will be a large cavity on one or even both sides, reaching to the walls and floor of the pelvis and to the reflections of the peritoneum.

When the inflammation is such as to lead to necrosis, the temperature becomes elevated to 103° or 105° F., the pulse to 120 or 130, and the soreness and sensitiveness within the pelvis are extreme.   The parts in the vagina are so tumefied and tender to the touch that a thorough examination without an anæsthetic is almost impossible.   In a few days infection by saprophytes occurs, extensive suppuration and sloughing follow, and for two weeks the patient runs a course of general sepsis, with foul-smelling and purulent vaginal discharges.   The sloughs become separated during the second and third weeks, the odor passes off, suppuration diminishes, and cicatrization takes place with or without vesical or rectal fistula and destruction of the vaginal lumen.

*Diagnosis.*—The rapid onset of the attack following traumatism, with elevation of temperature, pelvic tenderness, and exudate in the connective tissue of the pelvis, is characteristic.   A laceration directly into the connective tissue is easily felt by the examining finger, which penetrates the soft tissues beside the vagina or cervix and easily palpates the whole pelvic space on the injured side.   The pelvic walls and soft resistance of the broad ligaments are recognized, and, if there be a rupture into the peritoneal cavity, the intestines and uterine appendages also.   Deep lacerations of the cervix posteriorly are apt to penetrate the peritoneal cavity.

Pelvic peritonitis with salpingitis produces more acute pelvic pain and tenderness of the lower abdomen, with distention or hardening. The exudate can sometimes be felt over Poupart's ligament. The examining finger finds the connective tissue about the vagina and cervix free, but feels a hard mass either in the recto-uterine peritoneal pouch or on the posterior surface of the broad ligament, touching, perhaps, the upper end of the cervix posteriorly and at one side or possibly on both sides, or a mass beside the uterus, higher up, sometimes easily and sometimes not easily reached. The peritoneal and parametric exudates have a further distinguishing characteristic, viz., the manner of attachment to the uterus. In the former case (Fig. 7) the exudate is distinct from the uterus and is as if attached to it, with an acute angle extending up a short distance between them. In the latter case (Fig. 8) the exudate is as if it had grown out of the uterus

FIG. 7.

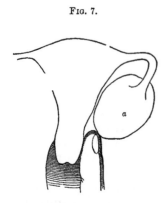

Manner of attachment of a pyosalpinx or ovarian abscess to the uterus.—a, diseased appendage.

FIG. 8.

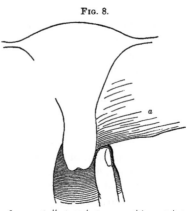

Manner of attachment of a parametric exudate to the uterus.—a, parametric exudate.

and is directly continuous with it, and meets the uterus lower down. Rectal indagation often reveals this difference more distinctly, and we can trace the parametric exudate to the sides of the pelvis or under the sacro-uterine peritoneal folds around the rectum. If the exudate extend into both sacro-uterine ligaments, the rectum will be surrounded by a hard ring touching the sacrum posteriorly, which may so diminish its calibre that the finger cannot pass it. In peritonitis unaccompanied by extensive cellulitis the exudate never forms this ring, and bodies corresponding to the swollen uterine appendages can usually be made out quite satisfactorily. Bimanually, the peritoneal exudate can often be detected above the pubes or Poupart's ligament, the parametric exudate only exceptionally. When the latter can be felt above, it is dull on percussion, not far from the median line, and can be palpated below through the anterior vaginal wall, along the anterior layer of the broad ligament beside the uterus, or fused with it;

the former usually extends more to one side and is more resonant on its abdominal aspect, and is felt bimanually to be connected below with the lateral wall of the uterus farther back and higher up above the cervix, or to the posterior surface of the broad ligament.

Pelvic hæmatoma, or hemorrhage into the pelvic connective tissue, might be mistaken for parametritis. The onset is sudden, often accompanied with pain and a temporary rise of temperature to 101° or even 102° F.; but the temperature, tenderness, and pain subside more quickly,—often within a few hours. There is a larger mass, with firmer elastic resistance in the beginning and a slower hardening. The hemorrhage usually displaces the cervix more to one side and forward, as it passes behind the uterus into the sacro-uterine ligaments and causes some bulging of the vaginal fornices. After hardening it is more easily recognized by deep abdominal pressure during the bimanual examination. The rectal examination often shows the mass surrounding the rectum so closely as almost to obliterate its lumen and cause obstinate constipation. The tenderness after two or three days is usually almost entirely gone.

Fibroid tumors of the lower portion of the uterus may extend into the broad ligament and simulate an exudate. They have not the tenderness of the parametric exudate, are usually somewhat elastic, and do not fix the uterus unless large enough to fill the pelvis. They do not attach themselves to the wall of the pelvis as the exudate does, but, if they reach to it, form an acute angle or sulcus with it, instead of running straight into it. The uterus is usually larger when tumors are present.

*Prognosis.*—The prognosis is favorable unless the traumatism has caused complete necrosis of tissue or unless sepsis supervenes. In the first place, fistulæ or destruction of organs may occur; in the latter, death. In these aseptic and antiseptic days we seldom expect death to occur from traumatic cellulitis.

*Treatment.*—When injury has occurred and cellulitis is to be expected or has already commenced, an ice-bag kept continuously on the lower abdomen for from thirty-six to forty-eight hours is one of the most useful remedies in arresting the progress of the disease. Vaginal, and in some puerperal cases uterine, antiseptic douches should be employed to prevent or limit, if possible, the infection that usually occurs. Absolute rest in bed is, of course, of the same value as rest for traumatism elsewhere. Intestinal gas or rectal fæces should be removed by laxatives, preferably salines and enemata. The diet should be a light one. After the first forty-eight hours hot fomentations to the abdomen may be substituted for the cold, as being less liable to do harm and more potent in favoring absorption of deposits. Anodynes and antipyretics are seldom called for, except to procure rest during the height of the attack.

When lacerations of the cervix and vagina extend deeply into the connective tissue, the rent should, within three or four hours, be partly or entirely sewed up with stitches that close the deeper parts. The connective-tissue cavity left should be disinfected with a 1 to 2000 bichloride solution and packed loosely with iodoform gauze; vaginal retractors or a Sims speculum will usually expose the parts sufficiently for these manœuvres. The gauze should be removed in about thirty hours, by which time the bloody oozing will have stopped, and the vagina douched out with a six-tenths-per-cent. solution of chloride of sodium in boiled water. The patient should then lie on the side opposite to the tear, so that the lochia will not flow into the wound. After three or four days, or sooner if a septic temperature develops, the vagina should be douched with a 1 to 2000 bichloride solution and afterwards with a one- or two-per-cent. carbolic acid solution every eight or twelve hours. If this proves insufficient to prevent general sepsis, an attempt may be made to pack the wound daily, or even twice daily, with iodoform gauze. Stimulants, quinine in tonic doses, and concentrated nourishment should constitute the general treatment.

### ACUTE SECONDARY CELLULITIS, OR ACUTE PARAMETRITIS.

Under this heading we propose to consider inflammation of the pelvic connective tissue consequent upon a primary or previous inflammation of one or more of the organs surrounded by it or contiguous to it.

*Etiology.*—The immediate cause of the disease is the inflammation of the diseased pelvic organ; the remote cause is that which produced the inflammation of the organ. Thus, many of the causes given for traumatic cellulitis, such as labor at term, abortion, gynæcological operations, etc., may produce injury or laceration of the genital tract with temporary surrounding inflammation of the connective tissue. Ordinarily, the wound becomes secondarily infected by saprophytic or other germs, and the inflammation becomes a prolonged septic one, spreading either gradually or rapidly to the connective tissue of the inflamed organ,—from a lacerated cervix, for instance, to the tissue surrounding it. Gonorrhœal, purulent, or tuberculous salpingitis often gives rise to a secondary cellulitis in the upper and outer portions of the broad ligaments.

*Pathology.*—It is a well-known fact that a septic inflammation in a viscus surrounded by connective tissue may give rise to a non-septic inflammation in the surrounding tissue; *i.e.*, the septic microbes contained in the viscus either cannot be detected in this surrounding tissue or extend but a short distance. Thus, a pyosalpinx may occasion an exudate in the mesosalpinx, which extends along the upper border of the broad ligament to the pelvic wall, and gives to the finger that examines it from the inside of the peritoneal cavity, either post mortem or by abdominal section, the feeling of a thick fleshy mass. This exudate may last for a long time in a subacute stage without showing any decided septic changes. After laceration of the cervix there is sometimes found extending from the cervix laterally to the pelvic wall an exudate, which is gradually removed by absorption. Less frequently a small exudate has been felt curving around the cervix posteriorly and extending a short distance under the sacro-uterine ligaments;

or a flat exudate may be found anteriorly. These are at first fluid, and form about and against the diseased organ. As a rule, the fluid is absorbed within forty-eight hours and the solid embryonic tissue remains for a longer or shorter period, according to the intensity of the inflammatory process. If the lesion of the viscus be a deep one and the septic influence be strong or uncontrolled, the exudate remains for some time, or the embryonic tissue is invaded by more germs than it can destroy, and abscess-formation is the result.

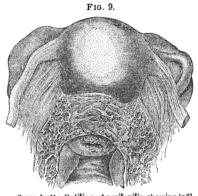

FIG. 9.

Secondary cellulitis and peritonitis, showing infiltrated connective tissue about cervix. (Heitzmann.)

The cellulitis beginning at the diseased viscus extends in the direction of least resistance to the microbes. In case of a primarily infected wound the direct infection may proceed by way of the lymphatics which surround the cervix (periuterine adenitis), and may also extend in abundance towards the ovary and pelvic wall. In the first case we find enlarged glands from the size of a millet-seed to that of a walnut; in the second, a mass of exudate. A wound that is secondarily infected will usually be surrounded by a limiting exudate of moderate size. When there has been considerable bruising of the neighboring connective tissue the exudate extends most quickly over the injured area, is more abundant there, remains fluid longer, and is more readily broken down by the invading microbes.

In a general way it may be said that the direction of least resistance to the progress of the inflammation is from the sides of the cervix towards the pelvic wall under the infundibulo-pelvic ligaments, where the fatty connective tissue and lymphatics are abundant. From the posterior wall of the cervix it extends under the sacro-uterine peritoneal folds. From the anterior wall of the cervix it extends towards the inguinal rings, along the round ligament, and under the anterior fold of the broad ligament. The inflammation is generally unilateral, and, even when distinctly septic, seldom crosses the vesico-vaginal septum or extends under the rectum, although I have seen it do so. The connective tissue between the recto-vaginal junction posteriorly and the cul-de-sac of Douglas does not possess so much resistance, and often allows the inflammation to pass across. When the inflammation exists on both sides there are usually two foci from which it proceeds.

Just how much the lymphatics are concerned in the extension of the disease is difficult to determine accurately, yet I have no doubt that in those cases in which a long exudate extends out in a particular direction the lymphatics play an important part. In the more severe septic cases all the tissue is undoubtedly affected alike.

*Signs and Symptoms.*—The symptoms of secondary cellulitis are those of the traumatic form plus those of the disease from which it proceeds.

There is pain in the pelvis and back, or lower abdomen, proceeding from the inflamed uterus, Fallopian tube, or peritoneum, as the case may be. The temperature often rises to 102°, 103°, or 104° F. during the first days, and remains at or above 100° F. for a few days or weeks, according to the condition. The pulse shows reaction, being either unusually full or frequent. There is apt to be some additional tenderness and gaseous fulness in the lower abdomen. Rectal and vesical distress and dysuria are often present.

When the disease is developed in connection with the tubes and peritoneum, the symptoms will be those of pelvic peritonitis (*q. v.*). When the uterus is the starting-point, backache and sometimes colicky pains in the lower abdomen will be noticeable. When the vagina is primarily affected, a soreness and burning in the vagina and dysuria attract attention, without much or any abdominal tenderness. When the bladder, or urethra, or rectum is the starting-point, the main distress is referable to the organ affected.

Vaginal indagation in the beginning of the attack reveals tenderness and swelling of the vagina, uterus or uterine appendages, urethra, or rectum, according to the situation, usually with general pelvic tenderness and a boggy instead of soft elastic resistance about the vagina or cervix. After two or three days a hard, tender area will be developed about some portion or portions of the vaginal wall, perhaps on one side of the urethra, or along the anterior vaginal wall, or about the cervix, as, for instance, at the side of the cervix, extending towards the side of the pelvis under and into the broad ligament, or under the broad and sacro-uterine ligaments, around the posterior wall of the cervix like a bow, or on both sides of the uterus. These exudates immobilize the tissues about them. Or the hard area may be higher up and be about the diseased and adherent appendages. We may leave out of consideration, at present, those cases which are secondary to diseases of the appendages, as non-suppurative cellulitis in such cases is but a small part of the pelvic peritonitis.

*Diagnosis.*—The signs and symptoms of injury or inflammation of one or more of the pelvic organs, with exudate such as has been described, usually fixing the uterus, ordinarily establish the diagnosis. Peritonitis is connected with exudates above or behind the connective-tissue area, or in the lower abdomen, and more acute pain and greater tenderness and fulness over the pubes and groins. Pelvic peritonitis immobilizes the corpus uteri, while cellulitis fixes the cervix and vaginal fornices. (See Diagnosis of Acute Primary Pelvic Cellulitis.)

*Prognosis.*—The prognosis is, as a rule, favorable, unless the disease becomes converted into the septic form.

*Treatment.*—The inflammation of the pelvic organ primarily affected should be treated in the usual manner. As the cellulitis is secondary, the time for an ice-bag is usually past, and hot fomentations over the lower abdomen are to be preferred. When the cervix or vagina is the starting-point, vaginal douches to prevent or cure infection are indicated ; but, if the primary inflammation be beyond the parts that can be reached by the water injected, such as the uterine appendages, the douches are less useful, and should not be used during the first few days, for fear of increasing the inflammation by traumatism. If a septic focus exists within the uterus, intra-uterine douches and, if possible, curettage should be employed, the latter under anæsthesia. Fixation of the uterus by exudate may, however, render such treatment impracticable. Bodily quiet is of prime importance. Pain may be relieved by anodynes. The bowels should be moved daily, or at least every other day, by salines, aided, if necessary, by unirritating enemata. As soon as the condition of the patient will admit of the manipulation, counter-irritation over the pubes and Poupart's ligament may be expected to be of some benefit. Stimulating liniments and, later, tincture of iodine are useful. Alteratives, other than a mercurial laxative every two or three days, I seldom employ. Tonics, such as the digestive ferments, quinine, strychnine, and particularly iron, are, I think, more useful during the stage of convalescence.

The patient should not be allowed to walk about to any extent until the temperature has subsided and the principal part of the exudate is absorbed. To render the absorption more complete and to restore elasticity to the tissues, intra-pelvic massage may be employed after all sensitiveness has subsided.

Any remaining disease of the pelvic organs should be treated, in order to make the recovery as perfect and as permanent as possible. Tincture of iodine to the cervix and the vaginal vault. and glycerin wool tampons, used two or three times weekly, often do much towards completing the cure.

### CHRONIC SECONDARY CELLULITIS, OR CHRONIC PARAMETRITIS.

Like acute symptomatic cellulitis, the chronic form is an extension of an inflammation of one of the pelvic viscera to the surrounding connective tissue. It is kept up by the continued inflammation of the viscus, and usually subsides with it, although the connective tissue may not recover its former elasticity.

*Etiology.*—The causes are similar to those of the acute form, but are more lasting and less active in their influence. A pyosalpinx may keep up an inflammation in the mesosalpinx so long as the pus remains to cause irritation, but the cases are more often called peritonitis, on account of the predominance of the peritoneal inflammation. Urethritis and cystitis, with or without ulceration, may give rise to chronic cellulitis around the vesico-vaginal septum. Ulceration about the vaginal fornices, chronic endometritis, particularly in the cervix and lower portions of the corpus uteri, and rectitis with ulceration (Freund) give rise to inflammation in the broad and sacro-uterine ligaments. Dysentery, constipation, catheterization, masturbation, inflammation extending from the vulva and vagina in children,

suppression of menstruation, excessive labor during the menstrual congestion, stenosis of the cervix, etc., are ordinary causes leading up to it.  Miscarriages and abnormal labors more frequently cause the acute than the
chronic forms.  A previous acute stage has usually existed, but when mild
has been unrecognized or forgotten.

*Pathological Anatomy.*—The pathological changes are not easily traced,
for the disease is not fatal, and originates in a gradual and unsuspected
manner.  The irritation from the diseased viscus occasions but a small
amount of effusion at a time, and this condenses slowly by absorption of
its fluid portion, so as to compress the tissue gradually and in places.  As
the exudate becomes organized, there is a contraction in the fibrous tissue
which compresses some of the veins, nerves, and muscular fibres, causing
their atrophy, and draws some of the others apart, dilating veins and
separating muscular fibres and nervous ganglia.  We thus have a mass of
finely striated scar-tissue radiating from the point of origin to the cervix,
bladder, or rectum.  In some cases these changes are general throughout
the tissues, but ordinarily only a portion is affected.  Under the latter conditions the contraction usually draws the cervix towards the part (*parametritis chronica atrophicans circumscripta* of Freund).  Thus, in a case of
inflammation of the sacro-uterine ligaments the cervix may be drawn
against the rectum so as to interfere somewhat with the passage of solid
fæces and cause a decided anteflexion or anteversion ; or inflammation in
the vesico-vaginal septum may draw the cervix forward and throw the
uterus into retroflexion ; or inflammation in a broad ligament may draw
the cervix or whole uterus towards the lateral pelvic wall, producing latero-
version or latero-position ; or the cervix may be drawn backward or to one
side and rotated on its long axis by inflammation in one sacro-uterine ligament alone, or in a sacro-uterine ligament and the broad ligament of the
same side.  In long-continued cases of retraction of the cervix in young
girls, the development of the cervix may be interfered with so that it
remains small and conical.

When the whole pelvic cellular tissue is affected (*parametritis chronica
atrophicans diffusa* of Freund) the changes are more marked.  The tissue
around the cervix is traversed in all directions by these fine scars, displacing the cervix slightly in the direction of the place where the inflammation began, more often backward and to the left.  Higher up, the peritoneal surfaces of the broad ligament are held rigidly together and the
mesovarium and mesosalpinx are so shortened as to draw those organs more
into the edge of the broad ligament.  The interference with the circulation
leads in nearly all cases to a passive hyperæmia about the lower portion of
the rectum and vagina, the vulva, and the neck of the bladder.  Hemorrhoids and vesical irritation are common.  The vulva is flabby.  The vaginal
mucous membrane is smooth, the walls of the vagina being inelastic and
atrophic.  The cervix and uterus are hyperæmic at first, with an abnormal
catarrhal secretion, but later become progressively atrophic, with a narrow-

ing of the uterine canal.   The pelvic ganglia and nerve-fibres likewise atrophy.   The condition is similar to that of senile atrophy.

*Symptoms.*—Perhaps the most characteristic symptom is an almost constant pain in one iliac region or in the back, according as the disease is located in one of the broad, or in the sacro-uterine, ligaments.   Dysuria and ischuria are in many cases persistent and troublesome.   Vaginal hyperæsthesia and coccygodynia are occasional accompaniments, and seem to be caused by it.   Cystitis, endometritis, and hemorrhoids, with their particular symptoms, usually help to complete the clinical history.   Pain of a colicky kind just before and during the first day or two of the menstrual period is often produced by the malposition of the cervix and flexion of the uterus dependent upon the retraction of the sacro-uterine ligaments.   Cervical endometritis is nearly always found, and often a conical or an imperfectly developed cervix.

There are also many general symptoms dependent upon chronic secondary cellulitis which are similar to those dependent upon other kinds of pelvic disease.   Among these may be mentioned intercostal pains, cephalalgia, mastodynia, dyspepsia, sudden abdominal bloating, constipation, various neuroses, and hysterical manifestations.

*Diagnosis.*—The diagnosis is based upon the positions in which the pelvic organs, particularly the uterus, are displaced, the condition of the pelvic organs, and the palpability per vaginam and per rectum of the retracted scar-tissue.

In the circumscribed form the cervix is drawn in the direction of the disease.   When the disease is in the sacro-uterine ligaments, the vagina is long and the cervix far back in the pelvis, from three to four inches from the pubic arch, and the uterus is in a state of anteflexion or anteversion.   When in the vesico-vaginal septum, the anterior vaginal wall is contracted and the cervix is drawn forward within one or two inches of the pubic bone, and the uterus is sometimes retroverted.   When in a broad ligament, the cervix is felt at one side, sometimes against the lateral wall of the pelvis.   The cervix is often drawn backward and to one side.   The uterus is somewhat movable about, but not from, the constricted area: it swings or sways around it.   An attempt to pull the cervix away from its abnormal position is nearly always accompanied by pain in the contracted ligament.   In cases of pelvic peritonitis with adhesions the fixation is higher up about the body of the uterus and the mobility is more restricted.   In displacement from pelvic peritonitis the corpus uteri is apt to be displaced farther from the centre of the pelvis than the cervix, or the whole organ is displaced together; while in pelvic cellulitis the cervix is usually farther from the normal position than the fundus.   In the former case displacement of the cervix or uterus in almost any direction is painful.

The condition of inflammation or ulceration of the uterus, bladder, or rectum, lacerated cervix, etc., aid in the diagnosis.   The premature senile changes that are found in cases of general chronic cellulitis are characteristic and noticeable. (See Pathological Anatomy.)

The resistance felt in the vaginal fornix nearest the affected part may be mistaken for a peritoneal or parametric exudate, but by pushing gently but firmly against the resistance some yielding, and no definite exudate, will be noticed. The fornix remains concave, whereas in peritonitis there is no yielding, and there is a definite mass that is flat or often convex. The finger in the rectum feels distinctly the rigid connective-tissue fibres passing from the cervix to the pelvic wall, and finds no hard exudate.

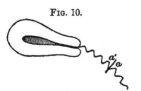

FIG. 10.

Incision of vaginal scar and suturing of wound.—The zigzag line represents the scar extending from laceration in cervix; a, a', line of incision.

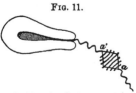

FIG. 11.

Incision of vaginal scar and suturing of wound.—a, a', sides of incision; sutures introduced parallel to line of incision.

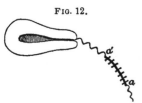

FIG. 12.

Incision of vaginal scar and suturing of wound.—a, a', sutures tied, closing wound at right angles to incision and parallel with scar, separating the cut ends of the scar.

*Prognosis.*—The disease is scarcely ever fatal. Perfect cures are seldom obtained, but symptomatic cures usually may be. The contractions in the tissues remain, but after the cure of other pelvic disease they seldom give trouble. Pregnancy may take place and exert a beneficial influence upon the condition. The accompanying uterine disease may, however, be a permanent cause of sterility.

*Treatment.* — This consists mainly in measures directed to the cure of the accompanying disease of the pelvic organs, the bladder, urethra, uterus, vagina, and rectum, —whichever may be affected.

Endometritis should be treated faithfully. A diseased and lacerated cervix should receive proper attention. A scar extending from the lacerated cervix and drawing the parts out of place may be incised at right angles to its centre and the contracted parametric tissue stretched by the fingers and by traction of the cervix towards the opposite side. The wound should then be sutured so as to form a line at right angles to the incision. This brings the two ends of the incision together in the line of union and places the cut ends of the scar-tissue far apart. I have made use of this procedure with the most satisfactory results.

Vaginal tamponade employed for many months is of marked benefit in the majority of cases. I usually apply a small pledget of commercial (not absorbent) cotton, saturated in boiled glycerin, under the cervix, and then a large dry wool tampon to fill the vagina. These are applied three times a week in the forenoon, and left for the patient to remove on the evening of the next day, the main object being to deplete the pelvic circulation and to support the uterus high up in the pelvis.   If the cervix be denuded of epithelium I use a fifty-per-cent. solution of boroglyceride in glycerin upon the cotton, or, if an alterative be required for inflammation of the uterus or its adnexa, a ten-per-cent. solution of ichthyol in glycerin.

Ferruginous and nerve tonics often have a decided effect upon both the local and the general symptoms.   Digestives, laxatives, abundant exercise in the morning and afternoon, with a rest of two hours in the recumbent position during the middle of the day, massage, sponge-baths, etc., will not infrequently be indicated for the accompanying general condition.   Many cases are associated with neurasthenia which may persist after the disappearance of the active local trouble.   In such instances the Weir Mitchell plan of treatment will lead to a complete recovery, so far as the symptoms are concerned.

Intra-pelvic massage, consisting mainly of vaginal and bimanual manipulation applied so as forcibly to stretch the contracted parts, would, if employed frequently, exert a beneficial influence ; but I have usually preferred the intelligent use of the vaginal tamponade.

Vaginal douches of a temperature from 110° to 120° F., taken while lying on the back, and kept up for half an hour just before the noonday rest of two hours, and at bedtime, have an alleviating, but not very powerful, influence upon the disease.

### SEPTIC CELLULITIS AND PELVIC ABSCESS.

Under the term septic cellulitis we shall include those cases that go on to suppuration.

*Pathology.*—At the outset the congestion and transudation occur as in ordinary cases, but either the effused fluid becomes rapidly purulent without coagulation, or the exudate, instead of being absorbed, breaks down into pus.   When there is an external lesion directly involving the connective tissue, suppuration commences on the surface of the exposed tissue and liquefies the surrounding exudate to a greater or less extent, giving rise to a large suppurating surface.   Sometimes the intensity of the disease is so great that death occurs during the stage of serous effusion.

The uterus and Fallopian tubes, ovaries, and peritoneum may be affected primarily or secondarily, according as the inflammation commences as a primary or a secondary affection.

In the puerperal state the effusion sometimes spreads from the uterus in the same way as erysipelas spreads through superficial connective tissue, and may be considered as identical in character with it. (Virchow.)

The exudates may start from several lesions and result in multiple abscesses ; or pus may burrow about the uterus from a ruptured pyosalpinx or abscess and form multiple abscesses, with or without sinuses, extending along the hollow viscera or along the muscular sheaths and peritoneal surfaces into the lumbar, iliac, or pubic region ; or ulceration may even extend through the levator ani muscle into the ischio-rectal fossa, or through the pelvic foramina. Skene has recorded cases in which the pus of pelvic abscesses has reached and perforated the diaphragm. When the abscess is

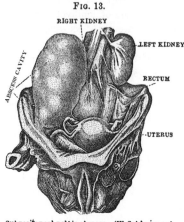

Fig. 13.

the result of an infected blood-clot (hæmatoma), it is usually in the shape of a pus-sac with a smooth layer of exudate below forming a capsule, and an indurated, more or less irregular mass of exudate on the peritoneal side above.

If the pus be not evacuated it may lose its active qualities and become encysted and inoffensive, or it may retain a certain degree of virulence without progressing beyond its capsule for a long period of time, but ever ready to resume activity as the result of renewed congestion or inflammation about it. In the majority of instances, however, the ulcerative process goes on and the pus discharges into the vagina, rectum, upper intestines, bladder, or peritoneal cavity, or externally in the iliac, inguinal, pubic, vulval, anal, or gluteal region. Rupture into the vagina is one of the most frequent and favorable terminations, and is often followed by a rapid contraction of the cavity and a cure. Rupture externally in the iliac, inguinal, or pubic region also frequently allows of free drainage and rapid contraction. Rupture into the bladder and rectum ordinarily occurs after more or less burrowing along the walls of the viscus, so that the outlet is sinuous or valvular and the evacuation is incomplete. The cavity refills and discharges, gradually becoming smaller until obliterated, or the pus may go on burrowing until another outlet is made. In old cases the cavity becomes more or less filled and divided by growths of unhealthy granulation-tissue, so that complete evacuation and contraction cannot take place. Rupture into the peritoneal cavity gives rise to septic peritonitis, but is a very rare occurrence.

About these abscesses and sinuses are found masses of indurated tissue, fixing the pelvic viscera in abnormal positions. As the abscess cavity or cavities contract and become obliterated, the viscera, particularly the uterus and adnexa, are drawn out of place to fill the space formerly occupied by the pus-cavity. Thus, the uterus may be drawn against the rectum and hollow of the sacrum, the base of the bladder be stretched antero-posteriorly across the pelvis, the rectal walls be held widely apart, so as to form a long, hollow cavity incapable of collapsing, and the uterine appendages be drawn towards the bottom of the pelvis. After the discharge of the pus due to infected hæmatoma, the capsule may be absorbed and the broad ligaments become collapsed, so as to leave the pelvic organs in an approximately normal condition.

The amount of general infection connected with pelvic cellulitis is variable. In acute puerperal cases it is great, and rapidly deteriorates the vital powers of the patient. After early abortions and operations it may be equally great, or it may be but slight, owing to the extent and completeness of the surrounding protecting exudate. Secondary infection and abscesses occupying the seat of hæmatomata often affect the general system to a slight degree only. In chronic cases the general infection is usually slight, but may be serious from its long continuance.

Periuterine adenitis, or inflammation of the lymphatic glands about the uterus, may, as the result of specific venereal infection, lead to localized parametric abscesses; but such is probably not often the case, except as a part of septic salpingitis and peritonitis.

*Etiology.*—All causes of parametritis with the addition of infection may be put down as causes of the septic form. The infection may occur during the action of the primary cause, viz., by unclean hands or instruments during labor and gynæcological operations, or it may occur at a later period. Thus, when a wound after labor or a gynæcological operation is left to granulate, the secretions may become infected at the vaginal outlet and the infection be communicated to retained or stagnant secretions about the wound higher up. Sometimes a benign cellulitis is converted into a purulent one by a succession of acute attacks due to violence or other cause, and infection from the pelvic viscera, which sooner or later takes place in the parts whose resistance to infection has been reduced to a minimum.

*Signs, Symptoms, and Course.*—In addition to the ordinary signs and symptoms already described as peculiar to acute, or traumatic, and secondary cellulitis, there are those due to the general infection. The temperature runs higher, particularly in the afternoon, or sometimes twice during twenty-four hours, and may reach 105° or even 106° F., with a corresponding reaction in the pulse. The latter may reach 130 or 140 beats a minute, with increased fulness and force until, from heart-failure, it becomes weak and thready. One or more chills often precede the septic reaction, and may or may not precede each rise of temperature. The respiration becomes rapid and labored, the countenance assumes an anxious expression, the mind wanders, the motions of the limbs become unsteady or tremulous, and the patient loses the power even to turn in bed. In other cases the delirium may be more active and accompanied by vigorous spasmodic movements of the body, due, apparently, to both mental and physical distress.

On the other hand, the general infection may from the very start outrun the local inflammatory changes, and the system may become so profoundly depressed that no symptoms of reaction appear. The pulse is rapid and weak, the mental condition one of somnolence or mild delirium, or perhaps of normal clearness and comfort. The temperature may be high, but is often normal or subnormal. The respiration is rapid and sighing, and is either labored or becomes so upon the least disturbance. The disease may run its fatal course in forty-eight hours, and colliquative diarrhœa may be added to the other symptoms, to hasten the fatal termination.

In case the primary infection has been slight or has occurred secondarily, there will be a moderate reaction in the pulse and temperature during the first two days, which, instead of subsiding, increases day by day until the symptoms of a fully-developed septic cellulitis have taken possession of the patient. Or an offensive diarrhœa and loathing of food may complicate or even supplement them, and may be almost the only symptom noticeable, the temperature being normal or subnormal, the pulse without reaction, and the pains conspicuous only by their absence, or by their presence just before a stool.

Again, the pains may be severe during the first two or three days and then abate or be completely relieved by anodynes, with partial, but not complete, subsidence of the temperature and pelvic reaction, so as to lead the patient or careless medical attendant to believe that all danger is past. But in two, three, or four days the pain returns, with reaction in the pulse and temperature. Sometimes the pain may again subside or may be relieved by anodynes or local applications, with, however, only a slight reduction of temperature and pulse-reaction. Such exacerbations may occur two, three, or more times, until finally they become more severe than ever, and an abscess evacuates itself, or is evacuated by the surgeon, in one of the regions already mentioned. The symptoms then subside more or less completely, and the patient may go on to recovery; or the pus may reaccumulate for want of adequate drainage, and the symptoms recur until relieved by another evacuation. Some cases may thus go on for weeks, months, or even years. In these cases a septic diarrhœa may come and go with the exacerbations, and is sometimes the most reliable guide to the amount of pus accumulated.

In a few cases there will be slight symptoms of cellulitis, with an afternoon temperature of 99° to 100° F., for one, two, or three weeks, and the disease may seem to be subsiding; but the pelvic induration does not clear up and the general condition does not improve, although the patient may be able to sit up awhile each day. Suddenly, without warning, she has a chill, and the temperature goes up to 101° or 102° F. The next day it is up again in the afternoon, and perhaps reaches 103° F. Other chills may occur, but often they do not. More soreness and pain are felt in some portions of the pelvis. A careful examination discovers a softening in the pelvic exudate. If this is not evacuated, the septic symptoms become fully developed, with increasing pain, loss of appetite, and perhaps diarrhœa, until relieved by the escape of the pus.

Pyæmia with abscess in the lungs or liver is occasionally observed.

(The signs and symptoms of septic cellulitis due to necrosis of tissue after labor are included with those of traumatic primary cellulitis.)

*Diagnosis.*—In the severer cases, which result fatally in a few days, we must depend upon the general symptoms of great systemic depression and our knowledge of the conditions that are acting as causes of such intoxica-tion.   Labor, abortion, operations, etc., with injury of the lower portion of the uterus or vagina, are factors that point to the place of infection.   On vaginal examination we may discover fluid infiltration of the pelvic con-nective tissue, encroaching upon the vaginal walls and giving a doughy sensation to the examining finger.

The diagnosis of the less severe forms is similar to that of primary and secondary cellulitis, already described, with the addition of the septic signs and symptoms.   Septic cellulitis does not usually get well rapidly, except by the evacuation of pus.   Exacerbations of pain and temperature every few days or weeks, the persistence of the exudate, and the formation of abscess are characteristic.   As felt per vaginam, the exudate is against the vagina or lower part of the cervix, connecting the cervical walls with the pelvic walls laterally or anteriorly, or extending across the recto-vaginal septum in front of the recto uterine cul-de-sac.   This exudate is slightly rounded, and feels as if it were a solid exudate or tumor in the cul-de-sac. A finger introduced into the rectum, however, discovers the mass to be a comparatively thin layer of exudate over the rectum, under which the rectum remains expanded or ballooned, incapable of collapsing.   Some-where in the rectum, against this hard mass and below the sacro-uterine ligaments, will often be found a dimple of cicatricial tissue, which may or may not be surrounded by a small boggy area, showing where the pus has discharged.   When the dimple and boggy area are on the anterior or lateral rectal wall, just above the sacro-uterine fold, we have usually to deal with a pyosalpinx or an ovarian abscess that has discharged into the rectum. From the number of such cases which I have observed, I would say that a rupture of a pyosalpinx or an ovarian abscess into the rectum is a much more common occurrence than the escape of pus from the connective tissue into the rectum.   Pus in the connective tissue more often finds its way out through the vaginal walls; pus in a tube or an ovary, unless adherent in the cul-de-sac of Douglas, seldom escapes externally without first discharg-ing into the connective tissue.   A pelvic cellular abscess usually bulges into the vaginal space, pressing the cervix forward or to one side, and is soft, increases rapidly in size, and generally becomes quite large before bursting. Pyosalpinx and ovarian abscess push the body of the uterus farther out of place than the cervix, and seldom form large masses low down, unless from a suppurating hæmatocele in the cul-de-sac of Douglas.   As felt per rectum, the cellulitic abscesses present low down below the sacro-uterine folds, while the intra-peritoneal accumulation is usually felt on one side or the other of a sacro-uterine ligament, or still farther up.   The former often extends down beside the rectum against the coccyx or the ischium, so as to push the lower part of the rectum somewhat to one side, or it may burrow along the rectal wall almost to the anus.

*Prognosis.*—The prognosis in the severer forms, with great depression and few or no physical signs, is unfavorable.   Death usually results in from two to four days.  In other forms death seldom results, unless from other coexisting pathological conditions, because the pus discharges into the vagina or low down in the rectum, or finds its way to the skin.  In the exceptional cases in which the pus burrows upward towards the lumbar region, the result may, however, be serious and even fatal.

Unless a free outlet for the pus is secured it may reaccumulate many times, destroy almost the entire pelvic connective tissue, infect the system, undermine the constitution, and prove disastrous.  It is quite common for writers to say that the pelvis may become honey-combed from multiple cellular abscesses.  When such is the case there is usually a pyosalpinx or an ovarian abscess, discharging little by little into the pelvic connective tissue.  I have been able to put my finger from the rectum into a cellulitic abscess, and from this, through an opening just large enough for the finger, into a pus-tube.

An abscess discharging into the bladder may get well after one evacuation, but usually does not until after several accumulations and evacuations. The irritation of the bladder is often excessive, and the effect upon the patient quite serious.

*Treatment.*—The treatment of septic cellulitis due to a laceration of the cervix has been considered in the treatment of traumatic cellulitis (*q. v.*).

The treatment of acute septic puerperal cellulitis, with rapid general infection, usually consists in general stimulation and supporting food, for the disease proves serious and even fatal before there are any local signs that warrant interference.  The proper conduct of labor and the complete evacuation of the uterus at the end of labor, combined with intra-uterine disinfection, belong to the prophylactic treatment, and should be studied in works upon obstetrics.  The administration of large quantities of stimulants—viz., an ounce of brandy every two or four hours, or double that quantity of Tokay or sherry, port wine or champagne, or even more—has been attended with remarkable benefit; but such quantities cannot always be borne by the stomach.  Quinine in moderate doses, from fifteen to thirty grains a day, particularly in malarial districts, is occasionally found to do good.  In a few cases large doses of the tincture of chloride of iron have had a decidedly favorable influence.  Small quantities of liquid and concentrated nourishment should be administered at frequent intervals. Raw eggs, beef peptones, peptonized milk, koumys, or matzoon may be given, according to the patient's preference.  Unfortunately, the condition of the patient's stomach, particularly when septic diarrhœa is present, is such that she cannot be well nourished.  An occasional opiate, predigested food, and the stronger aromatics and local stimulants, such as piperin, menthol, oil of sassafras, etc., help to restrain excessive diarrhœa and give tone to the stomach.  When the disease is somewhat protracted, strychnine and digitalis are most useful remedies.

After the formation of pus it should be our aim to secure its evacuation, but at the same time we should beware of hasty interference.  We should not open through a hard mass of exudate, nor penetrate the pelvic tissues blindly with an exploring needle, unless the most urgent symptoms call for it. There is but little probability of the abscess opening into the peritoneal cavity, and hence but little danger to life.

As soon, however, as the pus can be located and reached without passing through intervening structures containing large vessels, ureters, or portions of viscera that might be wounded, it should be evacuated. When the pus has burrowed upward and points in the inguinal, iliac, or lumbar region, it should be evacuated where it points, and the cavity washed out with a six-tenths-per-cent. solution of chloride of sodium and drained with a drainage-tube or gauze. When the accumulation can be easily reached per vaginam, it should be opened there, care being taken to avoid wounding the uterine arteries, ureters, or rectum. An aspirating needle should first be introduced, and, as soon as the pus is found, a sharp-pointed pair of scissors pushed in along the needle until they have entered the abscess-cavity, and then be partly opened and withdrawn, so that the dull sides of the scissor blades may enlarge the opening ; or a knife may be introduced in the same manner, and, after cutting a small opening, the finger inserted to guide the knife. Any masses of granular tissue or septa that impede the outflow of pus should be freely broken down by the finger and the cavity thoroughly irrigated and drained. Sometimes the vaginal wall can be slit down towards the vulva far enough to allow daily irrigation and packing with gauze by the nurse. When the opening is deep in the vagina it is well to stitch a double rubber tube to the vaginal edges with deep silkworm sutures. The sutures usually hold for a couple of weeks, during which time the cavity may be irrigated twice daily with a saturated solution of boric acid, or, if well borne, by a one-per-cent. solution of carbolic acid. After the rubber tube comes out, I always insert a small self-retaining drainage-tube and employ one-per-cent. carbolic vaginal douches. The accompanying cut (Fig. 14) shows a semicircular form of tube that

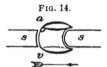

Fig. 14.

Semicircular drainage-tube for pelvic abscess.—a, abscess-cavity ; s s, septum between abscess-cavity and vagina or rectum; v, vagina or rectum.

I employ. It has the advantage that it projects but little either into the vagina or into the abscess, and is not liable to become displaced or to cause irritation. When the cavity becomes obliterated it is usually pushed out. It should not be introduced until the opening is sufficiently contracted for the tube to go in under slight pressure. If the hole is too large it will fall out in a few moments. In that case it should be reintroduced in a few days, after the opening has contracted.

When the abscess has already broken into the vagina, but does not heal, the opening should be enlarged and the case treated in the same way.

When the abscess bulges into the rectum below the sacro-uterine ligaments it may sometimes be treated through the vagina, but at other times there is a considerable depth of tissue to traverse from the vagina in order to reach the pus.  In such cases I have repeatedly opened per rectum and obtained a speedy cure.  I feel carefully, to be sure that no pulsating vessel is over the bulging portion, and, after widely dilating the sphincter, plunge a pair of sharp-pointed scissors into the lower portion of the abscess at the median line and withdraw them partly open.  The opening is enlarged with the fingers and the cavity washed out.  The rectum is washed out three or four times daily with the boric-acid solution, and when the opening has become too small to admit the finger it is either torn open again or the semicircular drainage-tube above described (Fig. 14) is introduced in such a position that the fæces will pass the tube in the direction of the arrow and not be forced into it, and the injections from the anus will pass in the opposite direction and tend to enter it.  The fæces have but little effect in preventing cicatrization so long as drainage is maintained.

When the abscess has already discharged into the rectum, I enlarge the opening by tearing, and tear down towards the anus as far as any pockets extend.  In one case I tore a distance of three inches, coming down almost to the internal sphincter, and I never saw an abscess anywhere heal more quickly and leave fewer signs of its former existence.  In this case a vaginal incision could not have laid open and obliterated the abscess-track (which lay against the rectal mucous membrane) so quickly.  If the sphincter be dilated widely, so that it will take it four or five days to recover its tone, the drainage will be better.

When the abscess has broken into the bladder and does not heal, the opening and abscess can sometimes be found by making a vaginal incision in front of the cervix and separating the bladder from the uterus as far as the peritoneal reflection, and drainage can then be established into the vagina (Buckmaster).  In some cases it is more feasible to make an artificial vesico-vaginal fistula and through it to dilate the old opening of the abscess into the bladder.

# CHAPTER IX.

## DISPLACEMENTS OF THE UTERUS.

BY PAUL F. MUNDÉ, M.D.

**Definition.**—By displacement of the uterus is implied a more or less permanent deviation of that organ from the position which it naturally holds in perfect health.

### NORMAL ANATOMY AND TOPOGRAPHY OF THE PELVIC ORGANS.

Under normal conditions the uterus occupies a position between the bladder in front and the rectum behind, the general abdominal cavity above

FIG. 1.

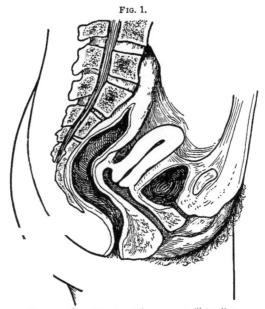

Normal position of female pelvic organs,—sagittal section.

and the vagina below. The attachments between the uterus and the bladder consist partly of a slight amount of cellular tissue and chiefly of a fold of peritoneum which dips down from the anterior abdominal wall to the fundus of the bladder, then slightly between the bladder and the uterus, and is reflected upon the upper portion of the body of the uterus, thence extends down along the posterior surface of that organ nearly to its inferior orifice, and then again on the anterior surface of the rectum. The attachment of the peritoneum to the body of the uterus from the point where it touches the anterior aspect of the organ down to a spot corresponding to the junction of the cervix and the body is so close that only very careful dissection will succeed in separating the uterus from its enveloping peritoneum. This point is of importance in understanding the method of suspension of the uterus in the pelvic cavity.

As a rule, the shallow excavation between the bladder and the uterus

FIG. 2.

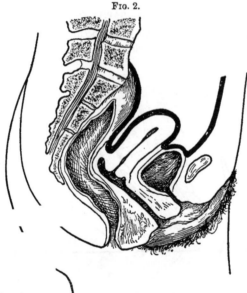

Sagittal section of female pelvic organs, showing relations of pelvic peritoneum.

is either empty or occupied temporarily by coils of small intestine. The much deeper pouch known as Douglas's pouch, situated between the uterus and the rectum, is usually empty, the posterior uterine and the anterior rectal wall being in apposition in the normal erect position of the woman. If a coil of small intestine is found in Douglas's pouch, it may be considered a pathological condition due to accidental complications or to inflammatory adhesions of the intestine at that particular spot.

The uterus is composed of body and neck, or, in the Latin terms, corpus and cervix. The body of the uterus comprises two-thirds of the bulk of the whole organ; the neck or cervix composes the remaining third. The upper portion of the uterine body is known as the fundus, and is situated above the exit of the Fallopian tubes and round ligaments. The body of the uterus is situated within the peritoneal cavity. One-half of the cervix is included within the broad ligaments and the cellular tissue, the other

FIG. 3.

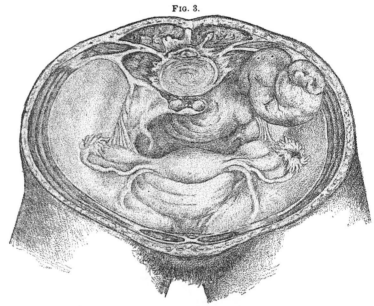

Transverse section of body, showing uterine ligaments and Douglas's pouch. (Savage.)

half projects into the vagina. The length of the normal uterus, as measured by a sound passed into the uterine cavity, is two and a half inches. In

FIG. 4.

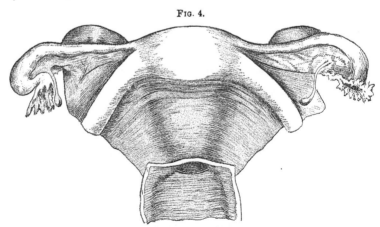

Uterus and appendages, front view. (Beigel.)

shape the uterus resembles a pear flattened antero-posteriorly. The slen-

derest spot of the uterus is the point at which the cervix joins the body, and it is at this point that flexions of the organ most frequently occur. It may further be remarked that the body of the uterus is most prone to enlargement in consequence of inflammatory deposits or neoplasms (fibroids), and, moreover, that the most common diseases of the cervix are catarrh occurring at any time and laceration produced during parturition.

**Supports of the Uterus.**—The uterus is supported in its normal position by the following agencies: 1, ligaments; 2, supports.

1. *Ligaments.*—There are eight ligaments which serve to keep the uterus in its normal position, four on each side.

A. *The Broad Ligaments.*—These are folds of peritoneum which extend laterally on either side from the peritoneal membrane which firmly invests the body of the uterus to each pelvic wall. These folds of peritoneum are closely adherent and ordinarily do not admit of physiological separation;

Fig. 5.

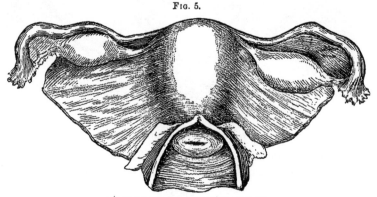

Uterus and appendages, rear view. (Beigel.)

but between them nestle portions of the ovaries with their blood-vessels, nerves, and lymphatics, and between them are very frequently developed effusions of blood, fibroid tumors of the uterus, and ovarian tumors, as well as collections of plastic lymph and subsequent pus, which separate very widely the otherwise closely connected anterior and posterior layers of the broad ligaments. Normally the broad ligaments also contain a certain number of smooth muscular fibres continued into them from the uterine tissue. The object of these muscular fibres is undoubtedly to aid the normal resilience of the peritoneal folds in keeping the uterus in its proper suspension. Posteriorly the broad ligaments are reflected upward on the rectum and posterior aspect of the pelvic cavity, anteriorly on the bladder and anterior aspect of the pelvic cavity. I think that to these ligaments—that is, the two broad ligaments—is to be ascribed the greatest influence in the retention of the uterus in its normal position, hereafter to be described.

B. *Vesico-Uterine Ligaments.*—Of very much less importance are two folds of peritoneum which stretch from the anterior surface of the body of the uterus to the fundus of the bladder and thence to the anterior abdominal wall. The connection between bladder and uterus being so much less close than between rectum and uterus, of course much less can be expected from the suspensory powers of these ligaments.

C. *Round Ligaments.*—From the anterior superior portion of each side of the uterine body spread two round strands of about the thickness of a goose-quill, which, diverging laterally between the layers of the broad ligaments, find their way through the internal inguinal ring into the Nuckian canal and finally are implanted near the spine of the pubes on each side of the pubic symphysis. These are the round ligaments. Unlike the other ligaments supporting the uterus, they contain striated muscular fibres,—that is to say, muscular fibres subject to the influence of the will. Their object is obviously to prevent the body of the uterus from tipping backward; but it is supposed that the striated muscular fibre has the purpose of permitting contraction of the ligaments at certain times,—that is to say, during sexual connection; the intention being, by drawing the body of the uterus forward and downward, to press the neck of the uterus deeper into the vagina and thus bring it in closer contact with the male organ and the seminal fluid. This is, of course, merely a supposition or theory, but it is a very plausible one.

D. *Utero-Recto-Sacral Ligaments.*—These are folds of peritoneal membrane which extend from the posterior attachment of the vagina to the uterine cervix to the reflection of the peritoneum on the face of the sacrum on either side, including between them the rectal tube. These folds of peritoneum also contain smooth muscular fibres derived from the uterus. Between them is situated a pocket of peritoneum which extends down to the very roof of the vagina behind the cervix, and which is known as Douglas's pouch. On either side a similar but less deep pouch exists, deeper on the left than on the right, owing to the peculiar course of the rectum, and each of these pouches is known by the name of the right and left Douglas's pouch. Between the broad ligaments and wherever two serous membranes or organic bodies come in apposition is to be found a certain amount of cellular or areolar tissue, through which run the arteries, veins, nerves, and lymphatics which supply the various organs. This cellular tissue also undoubtedly plays an important *rôle* in the cohesion of the different organs and the support afforded to the uterus. The above eight ligaments are the proper and true ligaments of the uterus.

2. *Supports of the Uterus.*—But there are other supports of the uterus which are not ligaments, and of these must be mentioned first the vagina,—a strong, tubular, muscular canal attached in front to the bladder and behind to the rectum, which in its normal conditions undoubtedly helps to keep the uterus in its natural position. The vagina is supported below by a strong muscular body called the perineum, which forms a barrier between

the rectum and the vaginal orifice. Anteriorly unquestionably the body of the uterus is more or less supported by the bladder, which in its conditions of varying fulness acts as a water-cushion to that organ. Posteriorly the rectum, curving forward in its lower segment, also acts as a cushion to the lower portion of the uterus.

3. Besides, there are two areas of pelvic fascia which help to keep the organs in their proper relations: one conforming to a line drawn from the middle of the sacrum to the lower border of the symphysis pubis and therefore corresponding to the vaginal roof and base of the bladder, the second drawn from the tip of the coccyx also to the lower border of the symphysis pubis corresponding with the perineum and pubic attachment of the bladder. Between all these organs there is, as has already been stated, in the normal condition, sufficient cellular tissue to secure correct approximation and return to the normal positions after temporary displacement, in healthy subjects.

Finally, it must be remembered that the movable condition of the abdominal viscera produces a certain amount of tension upon all these uterine ligaments and supports which temporarily changes their relations: thus with each inspiration and expiration the pelvic organs descend and remount.

**Normal Position of the Uterus.**—Strange to say, there is still a diversity of opinion among authorities as to the normal position of the uterus. Some authors describe and depict the organ as lying with its whole anterior surface in close contact with the upper border of the bladder and forming a sharply acute angle with the vaginal canal. Others, again, have drawn the

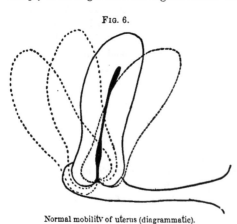

Fig. 6.

Normal mobility of uterus (diagrammatic).

uterus suspended midway between the distended bladder and the dilated rectum, the angle between the uterine and vaginal axes being more a right or an obtuse angle. To me, the normal position of the uterus has seemed to lie between these two extremes, the uterine axis being at an angle of about 45° with that of the vagina. I, for my part, have never seen a uterus in what I considered to be the normal position, tipped so far forward as to bring its axis to an angle of 30° with that of the vagina, which would practically place the fundus uteri against the symphysis pubis and crowd the bladder downward or out of the way. The reason why, in my estimation, these different opinions have been advanced is that some authors have not taken into account the fact that in its physiological condition the uterus is a movable organ subject to all the variations of position which are dependent upon the different degrees of fulness of the bladder and of the rectum and the movements of expiration and inspiration and of increased or diminished intra-abdominal pressure. The other reason why authors differ or have differed in their description of the normal position of the uterus is that they have drawn their inferences from the examinations of uteri which were not in the normal position, since it stands to reason that the large majority of women who submit to an examination of their sexual organs do so because they have or suspect some disease of those organs, and therefore very frequently the uterus is found in an abnormal position.

There is really, therefore, no absolute normal position of the uterus,

Fig. 7.

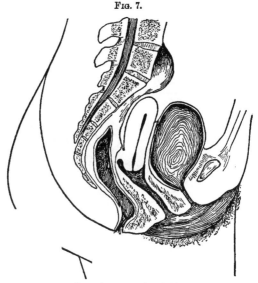

Uterus displaced by full bladder.

since a certain degree of mobility forward, backward, downward, and to either side is consistent with health and normal physiological conditions. For the sake of convenience I have adopted and for many years taught the assumption that the uterus may be temporarily displaced forward to an angle of 40° or even 35° with the vagina, and backward to an angle of 135°, without the position of the organ being considered pathological. When once the uterus has become permanently deflected forward to an angle of 30° or backward to an angle of 150° to 180°, the deviation may be said to be a positive displacement and one which probably requires treatment for its relief.

In the average normal position of the uterus, therefore, a line drawn through the longitudinal uterine axis should, as a rule, extend from the junction between the second and third bone of the sacrum to a point about two inches above the upper border of the symphysis pubis. A line drawn through the longitudinal axis of the vagina should meet the uterine line at the external os at an angle of about 45°. Bimanual examination—that is, with one finger in the vagina and the fingers of the other hand pressing through the abdominal wall—should always find the body of the uterus occupying this position. If it cannot be reached in this manner,—that is to say, if it is situated so close to the symphysis pubis that the outer fingers cannot pass between it and the symphysis,—the uterus must be anteverted. If, on the other hand, the outer fingers do not find the body of the

FIG. 8.

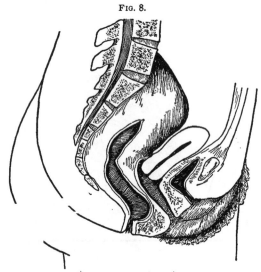

Uterus displaced by full rectum.

uterus in front when feeling at this spot, the uterus must be considered to be displaced backward. It should further be remarked that the uterine axis is not entirely straight, but assumes a slight forward curvature, the beginning of the curve being situated at the junction of the cervix and the body, at the point which is known as the internal os. An increased weight of the uterus by temporary congestion such as immediately precedes the menstrual flow or as is present in the early weeks of pregnancy will naturally augment the tendency of the organ to either a physiological or a pathological displacement.

### GENERAL REMARKS ON DISPLACEMENTS.

**Varieties of Displacements.**—First, forward,—anteversion and anteflexion; second, backward,—retroversion and retroflexion; third, sideways,—latero-version and latero-flexion; fourth, downward,—prolapsus; and fifth, inversion. Each of these varieties will be described in detail in its proper place.

**Relative Frequency of Versions and Flexions.**—As a general rule, it may be stated that anteflexions by far exceed in frequency anteversions; anteflexion being to a certain extent merely an exaggeration of the normal position of the virgin uterus, whereas anteversion is usually the result of changes following parturition. In backward displacements retroversion, on the other hand, is by far the more frequent, it being usually found as a consequence of the increase in weight of the organ and relaxation of the ligaments following childbirth. Retroflexion, or the formation of an angle at the internal os, is commonly a secondary condition dependent upon the downward pressure of a loaded rectum and intra-abdominal atmospheric influences. Anteflexion may therefore be said to be more frequent in the unmarried and in the nulliparous woman, whereas retroversion and retroflexion occur more frequently in the woman who has borne children. That both displacements may be found under reverse conditions can, however, not be denied. It is scarcely worth while to attempt to formulate statistics as to the relative frequency of anterior and posterior displacements, since, as I have just stated, the anterior occur more frequently in nulliparous and the posterior in parous women. Latero-version and latero-flexion are very much less common than either of the other two mentioned varieties. Prolapsus of the uterus in its various degrees, from that of mere sagging or dropping of the organ to complete extrusion, occurs with rare exceptions in parous women, chiefly in those who have borne a large number of children. Inversion does not really belong in the category of displacements of the uterus, since it is caused by factors entirely different from those which produce the dislocations of the organ to which we have already referred. As a matter of completeness and because the organ is of course displaced,—that is, turned inside out,—it is usually placed in this category, and as such I shall here consider it. Fortunately, it is not very common.

**Relative Significance of Displacements.**—I shall not attempt to anticipate now what I will describe in greater detail later on, but will merely say that on general principles anteversion is a condition of no particular significance; neither is anteflexion, unless it is of the higher degrees, when it may produce either dysmenorrhœa or sterility. Retroversion or retroflexion, in itself, may not cause any symptoms whatever; but in consequence of the interference with the circulation in the organ, the production of uterine catarrh, the frequently accompanying displacement of the ovaries and tubes, with possible adhesion of the uterus and appendages to the adjacent peritoneum; further, through interference with the calibre of the rectum, in course of time backward displacements of the uterus, if of the major degrees, usually do produce symptoms which call for relief. Prolapsus uteri, even in the minor degrees known as simple descensus, is seldom

without significance, because women thus affected usually feel the dragging
and dropping sensations which prevent their being long in the erect position.
Lateral displacements possess a very slight significance and are usually
merely interesting on account of their tendency to produce sterility. Inversion of the uterus, of course, is always a serious condition, in fact, the only
one of all these varieties of displacement which may be dangerous to life.

Causes of Displacement.—Some displacements of the uterus are
congenital. Thus, new-born children have been found at post-mortem to
have the uterus either sharply anteflexed or sharply retroflexed or retroverted; but these are exceptional cases, and probably very few children
grow to puberty and come into the hands of the gynæcologist with a displacement which has existed from birth. The normal antecurved position
of the uterus, as I have already stated, naturally tends to facilitate the
bending forward of the body of the uterus from its point of attachment
with the cervix, which is the weakest spot in the whole uterine anatomy.
There is no question in my mind that the habits of dress which obtain
with our present women, which in fact have existed for many generations,
are responsible to a very great extent for the anterior and downward displacement of the uterus, chiefly for the anteflexion which we so frequently
find in young unmarried or childless married women. The compression of
the thorax and mainly of the upper portion of the abdominal cavity by the
corset, and largely the pressure of the skirts upon the yielding abdominal
walls,—a pressure which is by no means counterbalanced by the support
the skirts are supposed to derive from the hip bones,—this pressure, I am
confident, by forcing the abdominal viscera downward and forward, does
in course of time produce many an anteflexion and moderate prolapsus.
Of course, if there is a tendency for the uterus to tip backward originally,
as may have been the case from childhood, this pressure will increase the
backward displacement, and the cases of retroversion and retroflexion
which we find in virgins and nulliparous women are easily explained. To
understand the peculiar effect of intra-abdominal pressure faultily or excessively exerted upon the movable pelvic organs, all we have to do is to
look at the accompanying diagram of a woman in the erect position. The
line drawn from her vertex to the upper border of her symphysis pubis
strikes just in front of the fundus uteri. Now let the small intestines
which normally lie in front of the fundus uteri and against the anterior
abdominal wall be forced still farther down and forward by compression
around the waist, room is given for the fundus uteri to tip forward; the
superincumbent intestines then press the body of the uterus still farther
down until it occupies the position believed by some to be the normal one,
—namely, at an angle of 35° with the vagina. It only requires time and
a continuance of this abnormal pressure to increase the angle of flexion at
the internal os and produce a truly pathological condition.

Constipation is undoubtedly also a fruitful factor of displacement forward, backward, and downward. The full bowel resting upon the body

FIG. 9.

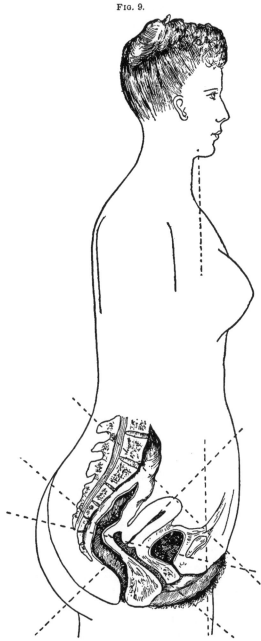

Longitudinal sagittal section of woman in erect position, showing the various axes of the uterine and vaginal canals and pelvic brim and vaginal roof.

of the uterus will tend to displace it in the position to which it naturally inclines, and the straining of a constipated stool will, of course, help to force the uterus down and relax its ligaments. The habit of allowing the bladder to fill to over-distention may also be held responsible for a certain number of backward displacements. Apart from the causes already mentioned, which hold good in unmarried, married, and parous women, childbirth is, in my opinion, by far the most frequent factor in the causation of uterine displacements. Relaxation of the uterine ligaments and supports, injury—that is, laceration—of the perineum and its component muscles, laceration of the cervix uteri with subinvolution and consequent increase in weight of the uterus, prolapse of the vaginal walls with bladder and rectum, inflammatory conditions affecting the uterine ligaments and the pelvic peritoneum,—all are more or less frequent causes of displacements of the uterus, and of these displacements those backward and downward are by far the most common as a result of parturition. Occasionally a sudden downward strain or a violent shock produced by a fall may cause a displacement of the uterus even in the virgin. Thus, I have seen a complete prolapsus of the uterus and vagina in an unmarried woman produced by lifting a heavy wash-tub, and a sharp retroflexion brought about by a fall down-stairs.

General Symptoms.—According to the form and degree of the displacement the symptoms produced by it will vary and be more or less pronounced. Anterior displacements may cause pressure on the bladder, frequent desire to urinate, bearing-down sensation of weight and "dropping." Dysmenorrhœa is not uncommon in anteflexion, as is also sterility. Retroversion and retroflexion, when they eventually cause discomfort, do so by pressure on the rectum, sacralgia or pain in the lower part of the back, interference with evacuation of the fæces, bearing-down and "dropping" sensations. Both anterior and posterior displacements may in some mysterious way cause reflex disturbances in other portions of the body which at first sight seem to be entirely disassociated with the pelvic organs. We can only explain these peculiar nervous relations by the undoubted sympathy which exists between the sexual organs and the general nervous system of the patient. In prolapsus, of course, the greater its degree the more decided its local symptoms. In a general way it can hardly be said to cause special inconvenience except as its existence produces discomfort. In inversion, associated as it is with more or less constant metrorrhagia, the resulting anæmia and general depression of the patient's health are the main symptoms.

General Therapeutics.—Displacements of the uterus being practically of a mechanical nature, it stands to reason that only local measures of a mechanical character adapted to each individual form are the proper means for relief and cure. I do not mean to say that in a generally dehilitated condition of the system a relaxation of the uterine ligaments and supports may not be benefited by tonic and invigorating remedies, and it is in such cases that the use of *local* massage may be beneficial; but so far as my experience goes I have seen few cases of well-marked uterine displacement which were cured by any other than by properly applied mechanical or operative means. The details of these measures must be reserved for the respective sections.

**Mechanical Supports.**—I wish to say a few words here as to the use of mechanical supports for the displaced uterus after it has been replaced. I know that there is a great deal of difference of opinion as to the value and as to the uses of mechanical supporters, or pessaries as they are generally called, in the treatment of uterine displacements. Some authors, whose experience cannot be denied and whose opinions must be respected, utterly denounce them and never employ them. Others, again, of equal eminence and experience, do not see how they can do without them, and use them daily. I have heard gentlemen of the former class declare that they had removed more pessaries than they had ever introduced, and one gentleman told me that his habit was to throw every such instrument removed by him into the back yard. I could simply deplore the ignorance of these gentlemen, who, having removed so many instruments introduced by others, and apparently having the opportunity, should not have taken the trouble to learn how to introduce them properly themselves. Disagreeable and in many ways obnoxious as all forms of uterine supporters undoubtedly are, it seems to me that the question is simply, in a large proportion of displacements of the uterus, notably of the backward varieties, whether we shall allow the displacement to remain untreated and the patient unrelieved or subjected to frequent and annoying manipulations, or whether, on the other hand, we shall replace the organ, keep it in position by a properly fitting supporter, and give the patient complete relief, the only drawback being an occasional visit to the office for the purpose of supervision and cleansing of the instrument. One might just as well refuse to use crutches or a cane for a cripple and thus confine him to his bed or chair, simply because one does not like crutches or a cane, as to deprive a woman with a badly retroverted or retroflexed uterus of the comfort and relief which she derives from a well-fitting vaginal pessary. As regards anterior displacements, both flexions and versions, I am by no means of the same opinion, believing as I do that these conditions but seldom require mechanical support. Prolapsus, of course, does require mechanical support, but the results are by no means as satisfactory as in retrodisplacements. Not every patient who has a displacement of the uterus wishes to be operated on for its permanent cure, and for such cases I think mechanical support by pessaries of the replaced organ is indispensable wherever it can be safely employed.

*Curability.*—I do not wish to be understood, through my earnest advocacy of mechanical supports, as claiming that they *cure* displacements. They relieve, they keep the uterus in position, they give the ligaments a chance to regain their tone; they may, in recent cases where the relaxation has not been severe and where the displacement is not of the most aggra-

vated variety, in the course of a few months or a year or two enable the
ligaments and supports to become so strong that when the pessary is removed the uterus remains in its normal position ; but I grieve to say that
in my experience this result is the exception and not the rule.   In 1881 I
read a paper before the International Medical Congress in London on " The
Curability of Uterine Displacements," in which, basing on a material of
over a thousand cases of displacement, I was able to report scarcely a dozen
instances in which a permanent cure had been effected by the wearing of
vaginal pessaries.   I have had no reason, in the thirteen years which have
since expired, to change my opinion on this subject, and hence I have in
these past years employed many times operative procedures for the cure
of prolapse and retrodisplacements where formerly I was in the habit of
trusting to vaginal supports.   And still I feel honestly and conscientiously
that if I were debarred from the use of vaginal pessaries—and I refer here
almost entirely to cases of backward displacement—I should wish either
to give up the practice of gynæcology or refuse to treat such cases.   No
tampons, no astringents, no massage, no electricity, no posture, no baths,
no vaginal douches, will, in my experience, take the place of a properly
fitted vaginal pessary, introduced only after the uterus has been returned
to its normal position and carefully watched from time to time.

## ANTEVERSION.

**Definition.**—The uterus is said to be anteverted when its position is
so changed from the normal one that the fundus approaches the symphysis
pubis and the cervix points towards the upper portion of the sacrum ; the
cervix and fundus being on the same horizontal line, or, in extreme cases,
the fundus lying lower than the cervix.   The literal translation of the word
means tipping forward of the uterus,—that is to say, an exaggeration of the
normal, slightly antecurved position.

**Degrees.**—There are accepted two degrees of anteversion,—the first in
which the uterine axis is at an angle of 30° with the vagina, and the second
in which the uterine angle is still further
lessened, until it and that of the vagina are
parallel.   I myself do not remember ever
having seen an anteversion of so pronounced
a degree as that last mentioned.   Beigel,
in his classical work on sterility, depicts a
uterus anteverted to that degree.   Anteversion and anteflexion may exist at the
same time, as may also anteversion and a
moderate degree of prolapsus.

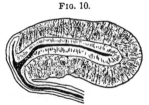

FIG. 10.

Extreme anteversion of uterus. (Beigel.)

**Causes.**—The causes of anteversion of the uterus are usually increased
weight of the organ, produced by subinvolution, hypertrophy, fibroid tumors
of the anterior uterine wall, and pregnancy, and are generally accompanied
by other factors which allow the anteverted uterus to sink down in the

cavity of the pelvis,—namely, relaxation of the ligaments and supports. Thus, a heavy uterus with relaxed broad ligaments and flabby vaginal walls will, if it naturally inclines rather forward, have a tendency to antevert and sag into the pelvic cavity. A pendulous abdomen with increased superincumbent abdominal pressure will increase this tendency to anteversion and prolapsus.

**Frequency.**—In my experience, anteversion is by no means as frequent as anteflexion; indeed, I see comparatively few cases in which I can, from my stand-point of the normal position, consider the uterus to be anteverted, and when I do so find it, as I have already said, a minor degree of prolapsus is usually associated with it. I confess that in recent years my views on this subject have changed somewhat, and that I now find anteversion less frequently than I formerly did; and, as I have already stated, it occurs most commonly as the result of one or other consequence of parturition, and hence is most frequently found in women who have borne children.

**Significance.**—As regards the significance of anteversion,—that is, of its injurious effect upon the female system,—my views also have materially changed within recent years. While formerly I followed the precepts taught in most of the works on diseases of women and attributed to anteversion a very marked influence upon the complaints peculiar to the female sex, I have of late years grown to look upon it as of very secondary importance. In fact, I quite agree with the view enunciated by Dr. Thomas Addis Emmet, that whenever an anteversion produces decided symptoms, these symptoms may be attributed quite as much to the coexisting downward displacement of the uterus as to the anteversion. But rarely does the pressure on the bladder produced by an anteverted uterus alone induce the patient to consult a physician. So far as the production of sterility is concerned, which was formerly considered to be one of the important results of anteversion, I do not deny that this may be the case; but I think that it is comparatively rare, since the degrees of anteversion in which an actual obstacle to conception is produced by the displacement—namely, those of the second or aggravated degree—are very seldom met with.

**Symptoms.**—The symptoms of anteversion have already been touched upon in the preceding remarks. I will merely emphasize them by stating that pressure on the bladder, bearing-down sensation in the erect and sitting postures, and a certain uncomfortable dragging feeling in the pelvis when walking are the most prominent. Except in the very aggravated forms of anteversion, no such complications as are almost invariably found in the backward displacements, such as chronic uterine catarrh and congestion of the organ, occur.

**Diagnosis.**—The diagnosis of anteversion is very easy: one has but to find the body and fundus of the uterus close to or touching the symphysis pubis, or even below it,—that is, the uterine axis parallel to the vaginal canal and the cervix pointing towards the middle or upper portion of the sacral excavation,—in order to determine the existence of an anteversion. Bimanual palpation, of course, is essential to the formation of the diagnosis, as it is to that of the majority of uterine displacements. If, of course, one inclines to the view of Schultze, Fritsch, and some other more or less prominent gynæcologists, that the normal position of the uterus is

FIG. 11.

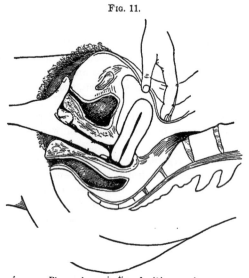

Bimanual examination of pelvic organs.[1]

really that given by me as the first degree of anteversion, the frequency of anteversion will be very materially diminished. Indeed, did my views permit me to agree with the gentlemen just mentioned, I should probably be almost inclined to omit anteversion, so far as my experience goes, from the list of uterine displacements. That this is not the case, however, I have already stated.

Complications.—Besides the almost invariable presence of prolapsus in the first degree, together with enlargement of the body of the uterus, I have only to record the presence of an interstitial or subperitoneal fibroid tumor in the anterior wall of the uterus as a not very rare complication of this displacement. Adhesion of the body of the uterus to the peritoneum covering the bladder, which Fritsch speaks of as not uncommon, I do not remember ever to have seen. Anteflexion may be present at the same time with anteversion, but will, as a rule, not materially alter the description and symptoms already given.

---

[1] The diagrams of uterine displacements which are recognized by a digital and bimanual examination in the usual dorsal recumbent position represent the subject lying in that position. Herein they differ from similar illustrations in other works, where the subject is usually shown in the erect posture.

**Treatment.**—I must here again confess that recent experiences—that is to say, experiences of the past ten years—have led me to discard to a very great extent the numerous methods and appliances which, copying from the older text-books, I then thought necessary for this displacement, since the symptoms produced by anteversion, except as it is complicated by the other conditions mentioned, are so trifling that I cannot of recent years remember more than a few cases where I have found it necessary and advisable to resort to local treatment. Of course, the complications, if possible, should be removed, but only exceptionally do I find it necessary to use a mechanical support, either vaginal or abdominal or both, for the rectification of an anteversion. If I do so, it is usually the prolapsus and

FIG. 12.

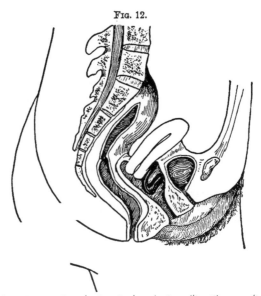

Gehrung's pessary for cystocele and anteversion in position (diagrammatic).

not the anteversion which produces the symptoms and which leads me to apply the relief. The old text-books, even those published within the last few years, still show a number of illustrations of supports (pessaries) for anteversion. I myself plead guilty to having retained a few of these in the revision which I made of Dr. Thomas's book in 1891. I did this partly because the author of the work did not feel disposed to agree with me that anteversions were of so little pathological significance as I am convinced they are, and partly because there are certain cases where pessaries are useful and indispensable. But I can honestly say that in the last five or six years I have never found it necessary to apply to an anteverted uterus any other than one of two supports : the first being that of Gehrung, of St. Louis, which is a double horseshoe (see Fig. 12), and the other the

Hitchcock, which is a flexible ring with a cross-bar to support the body of
the uterus. (Fig. 13.) The introduction of the latter instrument is exceedingly simple, it being necessary only to say that it is compressed with
the fingers and slipped into the vagina so that the cervix rests in the ring,

FIG. 13.

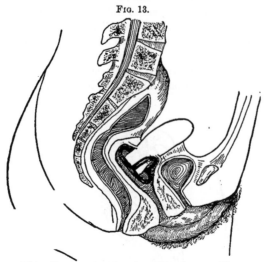

Hitchcock's pessary for anteversion and descensus in position.

while the body is supported by the elevated cross-bar. The insertion of the
Gehrung is not so simple, and requires some experience. Suffice it to say
that it is slipped sideways into the vagina and then turned so that both
bars rest between the symphysis pubis and the anterior aspect of the uterus.
In this way the anterior vaginal wall with the bladder, and indirectly
the body of the uterus, are elevated and prevented from sagging down
towards the pelvic cavity and the symphysis pubis. The rules which govern
the use of pessaries in general must, of course, apply to both these instruments. As regards the Gehrung, I must emphasize that, as it sustains all
the downward pressure of the abdominal viscera when the woman is in the
erect position, the strain upon it is much greater than upon any other
form of pessary, and therefore it is more liable to indent the anterior
vaginal wall as well as those points on the posterior vaginal wall where
the posterior curve rests. It is, therefore, necessary to watch it more
carefully and remove it more frequently than the pessaries used for retroversion. In fresh cases the packing of the vagina with wool tampons
dipped in iodoform and tannin powder (equal parts), the woman at the time
occupying the knee-chest position, may succeed in restoring tone to the
anterior vaginal wall and the attachment of the bladder and in thus curing
the anteversion, particularly if a prolapse of the anterior vaginal wall with
the posterior wall of the bladder (so-called cystocele) is present at the same

time. I am not familiar with any operative measures for the cure of ante-version which have more than a theoretical value. Shortening the anterior vaginal wall by a plastic operation has been proposed, but has not, so far as I know, become popular, since its results are both uncertain as to healing and, if successful, a retroversion is quite as likely to take the place of the former anteversion.

### ANTEFLEXION.

**Definition.**—By anteflexion of the uterus is meant a more or less sharp bending of the body of the organ upon the cervix, or the reverse,—that is to say, the body of the uterus may be bent down upon the cervix, and this is called anteflexion of the body, or the cervix of the uterus may be bent upward towards the body, and this is called anteflexion of the cervix.

FIG. 14.

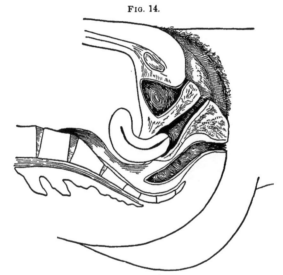

Anteflexion, first degree.

**Anatomy.**—In anteflexion, either of body or cervix, the uterus is usually thin and slender, the thinnest portion being, in anteflexion of the body, at the internal os; in anteflexion of the cervix, at the junction of the cervix and vagina. In well-marked cases of anteflexion of the body the point corresponding to the internal os may be so thin that it seems to be almost like a hinge between the body and the cervix. In anteflexion of the cervix that part is usually long and slender, particularly the portion protruding into the vagina. In the majority of cases of anteflexion both the external and internal orifices are abnormally small. In some cases the body of the uterus, instead of being unusually movable upon the cervix, is immovably fixed, the cause of this being either congenital or inflammatory rigidity of the tissues. Usually, however, the anteflexed uterus, no matter how marked the degree of flexion, can easily be straightened out with the fingers or the sound.

**Degrees.**—The majority of authorities accept three degrees of ante-flexion, the first being the least marked, the third the most severe. In the first degree the angle of flexion is about 90°, or a right angle; the second, 45°; and the third, 40°. Of course this is entirely approximate, there being numerous variations between these three degrees. In these forms of ante-flexion of the body of the uterus let it be understood that the direction of the cervix is usually normal,—that is, pointing either slightly towards the excavation of the sacrum or towards the axis of the vagina. In anteflexion of the cervix, on the other hand, the body of the uterus occupies the normal position, while the cervix is curled upward and forward, more or less.

FIG. 15.

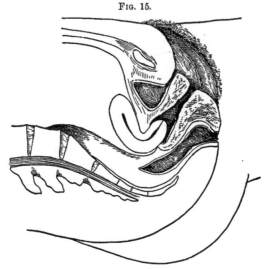

Anteflexion, second degree.

There are no fixed degrees for this anteflexion of the cervix, which I shall consider separately at the close of this section.

**Causes.**—As I have already stated under general remarks, an ante-flexion of the uterus is but an exaggeration of the normal antecurved position of the organ. The tendency to this exaggeration undoubtedly is congenital,—that is to say, the child is born and develops with a weak spot in her uterus, and that is the junction of the body and the cervix. Either she has the anteflexion at birth or it is developed in the course of growth under the influences of dress, posture, constipation, etc., which I have already touched upon under general remarks. The one displacement of the uterus which is met with in young unmarried and married childless women with the greatest frequency is anteflexion. It is hardly necessary to enter into any great detail on this question, because what I have already said, and common sense, will lead to the natural inference as to how this statement is correct. Occasionally there may be an inflammatory contraction of the anterior uterine wall which produces an anteflexion, but I think this is comparatively quite a rare occurrence, and I cannot remember finding an adhesion of the fundus of the anteflexed uterus which I could conscientiously look upon as the cause of the anteflexion and not the result. The causes of anteflexion may, therefore, be briefly stated to be either congenital —probably the minority—or acquired,—undoubtedly the majority,—but the latter depending mostly upon a congenital predisposition. An anteflexion acquired as the result of parturition is to me an improbability. A fibroid tumor, however, developing in the anterior or posterior wall of the body of the uterus may produce an anteflexion by its weight.

Fig. 16.

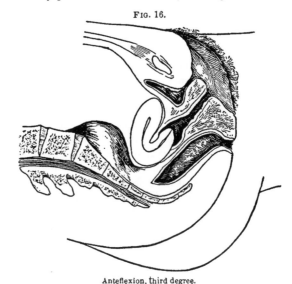

Anteflexion, third degree.

**Frequency.**—In unmarried and sterile women anteflexion is by far the most common form of displacement.

**Significance.**—As with anteversion, so to a much greater extent with anteflexion, our views—that is to say, mine—have materially changed during the last ten years. Pages upon pages and chapter upon chapter have been written upon the pathology and significance of anteflexion, and bushels upon bushels of pessaries have been devised for the cure of this displacement: the old books are full of diagrams of such instruments. But recent investigations and a calmer deliberation have shown us that anteflexion in its minor degrees is practically of no importance whatever, neither causing pain nor preventing conception nor in any way inconveniencing the woman, and that anteflexions of more marked character produce only two possible bad results,—namely, dysmenorrhœa and sterility. It is only these last

31

cases of a marked degree that, therefore, I nowadays consider worthy of notice and of treatment. An anteflexion of the second and third degrees may—I do not say necessarily does, but may—produce both of these results just mentioned, and if this is the case requires treatment; but if neither dysmenorrhœa exists nor—the patient being unmarried—sterility is present, certainly the anteflexion in itself requires no treatment. And I can honestly say that in recent years, with the exception of these two varieties, I have found no occasion to employ operative means or mechanical supports. As regards the causation of dysmenorrhœa and sterility by these flexions of marked degree, I would add that even in very decided flexions there is often no dysmenorrhœa, and that many a woman has conceived whose uterine canal was flexed to an angle of 30° ; but still, if women with these degrees of flexion were found to be suffering from either one of these two symptoms, it would be fair to assume that this was the cause and that the removal of the cause would be the proper indication.

Diagnosis.—Bimanual examination will very easily enable the physician to make the diagnosis of the flexion in any one of the degrees mentioned. It must be remembered that a small fibroid tumor situated in the anterior uterine wall may simulate an anteflexion, and that only a very careful examination, together with the use of the sound, will enable the examiner to make the diagnosis. An increase in size of the body of the uterus will naturally contribute to a correct understanding of the case. The calibre of the external and internal orifices of the uterine canal can, of course, only be ascertained by the introduction of the uterine sound. Let it be distinctly understood that the differential diagnosis between a version and a flexion consists therein, that in a version the uterine canal is straight, no matter how much it may be deviated from the vaginal axis; but that in a flexion there is a more or less sharp angle in the canal at a point corresponding to the internal os.

Symptoms.—As I have already said that only the most aggravated forms of anteflexion produce disturbance of any kind, it is obvious that the symptoms of this displacement are not very marked. Aside from dysmenorrhœa and sterility, an uncomplicated flexion produces no symptoms. But there are certain complications which may be present even in the minor degrees of flexion which do produce symptoms, and such complications are a chronic catarrh of the uterine mucous membrane, so-called chronic endometritis, and a spasmodic contraction of the circular fibres at the internal os. The first of these conditions will produce dysmenorrhœa of the congestive variety, the second dysmenorrhœa of the obstructive or neuralgic variety, both being possibly associated in the same case. Only very aggravated forms of anteflexion will produce pressure on the bladder, since the uterus in those cases is usually so small that its body exerts but very little influence upon the elastic bladder.

Treatment.—The minor degrees of anteflexion require no treatment. If complications exist, they should be attended to. Catarrh of the endometrium, engorgement of the uterus, congestion of the ovaries and tubes, if present, should be treated on accepted principles. Having already stated that the main symptoms of aggravated degrees of anteflexion are either dysmenorrhœa or sterility, I have but to say that all our treatment must be directed towards the relief of these two conditions. Substantially the treatment consists in, first, thoroughly dilating and straightening the uterine canal, and, secondly, in keeping it straight until either symptom is relieved, —that is to say, the dysmenorrhœa is cured or conception takes place. For the relief of the dysmenorrhœa I have for many years satisfactorily employed the dilatation of the uterus with the modified Ellinger's dilator (steel two-branched), Palmer's being the instrument I employ ; dilating the uterine orifices to the width of a quarter to a third of an inch once a week during several intermenstrual periods. I have usually employed this treatment in my office, and sent the patients home with direc-tions to keep quiet during the rest of that day and avoid exposure to cold which might

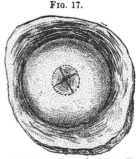

Fig. 17.

Crucial incision of external os. The dotted lines show the four flaps to be trimmed off.

possibly produce an inflammatory reaction ; but I confess that with each succeeding year I am becoming less and less disposed to subject my patients to risks of any kind, and I do not deny that the dilatation of the uterine canal to this extent in the office or out-door clinic is attended with a certain amount of danger. I would, therefore, where it is practicable, advise that this dilatation be performed at the patient's house or in a locality where she can be put in bed, at least for the rest of that day. Such moderate dilata-tion as this has, in my experience, usually relieved, temporarily if not always permanently, mild forms of dysmenorrhœa. It has not, however,—and that

Fig. 18.

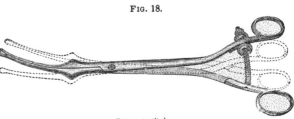

Palmer's dilator.

I did not expect from or claim for it,—resulted in keeping the uterine canal permanently straight. Temporarily straightening it, and keeping it patulous and straight, are two quite different things. Since, after all, the majority of patients who consult us are married women, those in whom I found a sharp anteflexion came to me sometimes for dysmenorrhœa, but usually for sterility ; and in these I found it worth my while to advise and perform a much more decided operative course than mere superficial dilatation. In these women, where it was not only my object thoroughly to dilate but also to keep open the uterine canal with a view to conception, I have adopted the following plan :

I have placed them where they could stay in bed for at least a week, have, under an anæsthetic and with all proper antiseptic precautions, incised the external os in four directions,—so-called crucial incisions,—trimmed off the little flaps thus made with scissors, passed a blunt, slender, straight bistoury through the internal os, slit the circular fibres very slightly in four directions, have then introduced the two-branched dilator, separated its blades gently to half an inch internal diameter, and have then packed the uterine canal lightly with iodoform gauze, as well as the vagina, for drainage and to guard against any possible secondary hemorrhage. The patients were then put to bed with an ice-bag on the abdomen for at least forty-eight hours, after which time the gauze was removed through the speculum and reintroduced if there was any bleeding. After another forty-eight hours the gauze was removed again, and if no bleeding was present, a hard-rubber stem, not more than two and a quarter inches in length, was inserted into the uterus under proper antiseptic precautions and retained in

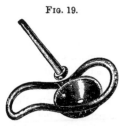

Fig. 19.

Thomas's cup pessary and stem.

place by iodoform gauze packing, and the patient allowed to leave her bed on the next day, provided she had no pain. If there was pain to any marked degree, the gauze and stem were immediately removed. Before returning home or before leaving my immediate care, the gauze was removed from the vagina and replaced by a Thomas's cup pessary, made for the purpose of retaining the stem in position. Daily carbolized vaginal douches were then ordered and the patient allowed to go about her ordinary affairs, with the distinct and strict caution, however, that any pain of more than a momentary duration in the lower part of the abdomen called for an immediate removal of the stem and pessary, whether by the first physician at hand or by me if I were attainable. The danger of a pelvic peritonitis with its sequelæ was thoroughly and pointedly explained to her in case she failed to obey these directions. Within a day or two before every menstrual period the stem and pessary were to be removed and reintroduced immediately afterwards, provided it seemed that the canal still required their presence to remain straight and patulous. As a rule, not less than three, and probably not more than six, months' wearing of the stem and pessary is required in order to effect a greater or lesser permanency of the result. Sexual intercourse during this time is strictly forbidden. According to the severity of the case, after from three to six months the stem and pessary may be dispensed with and a month's time be given to see whether the canal remains straight and open or bends and contracts again. In the mean time coition may be permitted, and should even be enjoined.

I will say that nothing, in my experience, but this operation and the wearing of a straight stem in the uterine cavity for a certain number of months will ever cure a well-marked anteflexion of the uterus. The risks of this treatment will naturally render the operator exceedingly careful as to when and how he advises and employs it. The very slightest sign of a previous inflammatory condition in the uterine appendages or the pelvic peritoneum would counterindicate this treatment in the majority of cases. Still, I have, well knowing the risks, seen some excellent results as regards the relief of dysmenorrhœa, and even the cure of the sterility in several cases of subacute salpingitis. The operator must be careful never to promise the

Fig. 20.

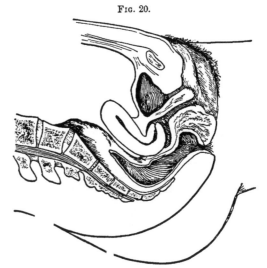

Anteflexion of the cervix.

patient any positive benefit from his treatment, since nothing is more uncertain than the cure of sterility. In some cases the stem will absolutely not be borne, producing so much pain, so much uterine colic, and such severe nervous symptoms, that it has to be removed almost as soon as introduced. In these cases, packing the uterine cavity with iodoform gauze may, to a certain extent, act as a substitute, particularly if there is a chronic endometritis also present. Frequently the curetting of the uterine canal after dilatation and its cauterization with chloride of zinc (fifty-per-cent. solution), or iodized phenol, equal parts, for the cure of a chronic endometritis, may have to be employed immediately after discission and dilatation. In such cases the iodoform gauze packing would have to be continued for a week or more, until the uterine mucous membrane assumes a healthy condition, before the stem can be introduced.

**Curability.**—I need but repeat what I have just stated, that the mechanical treatment described in the preceding section is, to my mind, the only possible means of curing an aggravated form of anteflexion, with the sole exception of nature's cure,—namely, pregnancy and parturition, which, unfortunately, in extreme cases, do not often take place, since it is exactly to attain that happy event that such patients usually consult us.

### ANTEFLEXION OF THE CERVIX.

This condition is congenital, and is a very frequent cause of sterility; otherwise it produces no symptoms whatever, not even that of dysmen-orrhœa. A short or long slender cervix curled upward against the anterior vaginal wall is an almost insuperable obstacle to conception. The only treatment which I know for it is to enlarge the external os by the crucial incisions above referred to, thoroughly dilate the uterine canal, and treat it just as in anteflexion of the body. The posterior division of the cervix to the vaginal insertion, with the excision of a wedge, so as to enlarge the external os in that direction,—an operation devised by Sims,—has not proved a practical success.

### ANTEFLEXION WITH RETROPOSITION.

This peculiar position of the uterus is always congenital. It may be described as though an anteflexed uterus were hung on a pivot passed

FIG. 21.

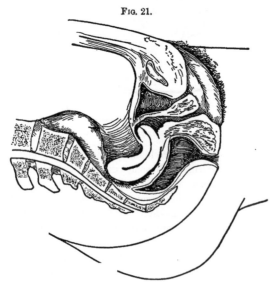

Anteflexion with retroposition.

through a point corresponding with the junction of the vagina and cervix. The body of the uterus is now tipped backward, the cervix upward, and we have a retroposed uterus with an anteflexed body. The vaginal vault is usually shallow and the broad ligaments are tense in this condition; the external os looks upward towards the anterior vaginal wall, and the fundus uteri forward towards the bladder. The sound passes through the uterine canal with anterior curvature forward. This position of the uterus was not recognized, or at least is not mentioned, in the older books. So far as I know, J. Marion Sims first described it and figured it in the American Gynæcological Transactions for 1876.

The symptoms of this position of the uterus are entirely negative, except in so far as it produces sterility; and while I have seen some women with the uterus in this position who had borne children, I am not able to say whether the position existed before or after parturition; but I have seen very many more who were sterile for no other obvious reason than this position of the uterus.

The treatment is by no means satisfactory or simple. It consists in straightening the uterine canal by discission and dilatation and a stem as above described, and then, if the posterior vaginal vault is sufficiently deep, introducing a retroversion pessary, so as to place the straightened uterus in its normal relation to the vagina; but usually the posterior vaginal vault is so shallow that the pessary can exert no leverage and fails to effect its object. We are then left to the device of deepening the posterior vaginal vault by tamponade with cotton pledgets or to using an abdomino-vaginal pessary known as Cutter's retroversion stem. I cannot say that my own results have been very satisfactory in the treatment of this form of uterine displacement.

### RETROVERSION AND RETROFLEXION.

**Definition.**—A uterus is said to be retroverted when the body of the organ is turned backward and rests in the excavation of the sacrum, in exact opposition to the normal position of the uterus. The axis of the uterus in retroversion is straight; when there is an angle at the junction of the cervix and the body the condition of retroflexion exists.

**Degrees.**—For practical purposes there are accepted three degrees of retroversion and three of retroflexion. In the first degree of retroversion the axis of the vagina and that of the uterus are substantially on the same plane, in the second degree of retroversion the axis of the uterus occupies an angle of 130° to that of the vagina, and in the third degree of 90° to that of the vagina, or a right angle. As in anterior displacements, a number of minor degrees may be present. The three degrees of retroflexion can be easily understood by simply imagining the body of the uterus bent backward from the internal os to an extent proportionate to the degree of the retroversion.

**Complications.**—There are usually a number of conditions complicating retroversions and retroflexions which must not be overlooked. Such are, *first*, a prolapsus of the uterus of a moderate degree, due to the same causes which produce retroversion,—namely, relaxation of the supports.

Indeed, I believe that a prolapsus of the first degree is a very usual prece-
dent of retroversion, since it is only after the fundus uteri sinks below the

FIG. 22.

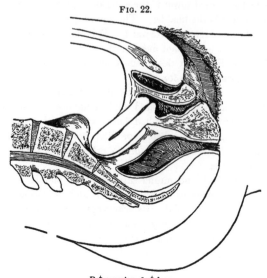

Retroversion, first degree.

level of the promontory of the sacrum that it has room to tip back into
the excavation of that bone. *Second.* The body of the uterus resting in

FIG. 23.

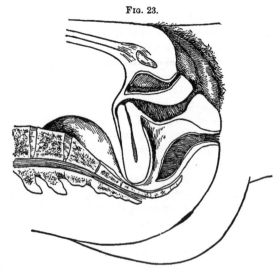

Retroversion, second degree.

Douglas's pouch, and therefore in close and constant apposition to a sensitive peritoneal membrane, is very liable to produce irritation by friction, and adhesion will result; the fundus uteri is then attached to the bottom of Douglas's pouch and not replaceable. *Third.* The ovaries and tubes, following the backward displacement of the body of the uterus, drop into either lateral half of Douglas's pouch, and also, by a process peculiar to

FIG. 24.

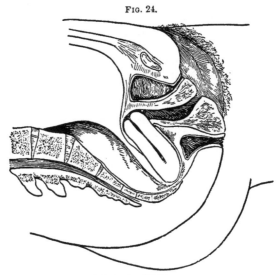

Retroversion, third degree.

adjacent serous surfaces, may become adherent. Thus, whether the fundus of the uterus and the appendages are adherent in Douglas's pouch or not, a prolapsus of the appendages is a very common accompaniment of the higher degrees of backward displacement of the uterus. *Fourth.*

Compression of the rectum by the body of the uterus and consequent interference with free action of that part of the bowel is one of the complications of the aggravated forms of retroversion and retroflexion. *Fifth.* Chronic endometritis, both of body and cervix, is also liable to result from interference of circulation produced by this displacement. *Sixth.* At times the pressure of the cervix against the base of the bladder produces irritation of that organ, and may on rare occasions (early pregnancy and impaction of the body of the uterus) even cause temporary obstruction to the escape of the urine. *Seventh.* If pregnancy in the early months should be present, the enlargement of the body of the uterus will produce more decided symptoms of pressure in the pelvis,

FIG. 25.

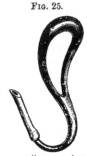

Cutter's vaginal stem pessary for retroversion, modified by Thomas.

and the inability of the organ to develop on account of its limited space will, unless the displacement is reduced, result in a miscarriage, usually before the fourth month. A fibrous tumor in the posterior wall of the uterus may simulate a retroversion or retroflexion, if the uterus has a tendency to drop backward.

A very frequent combination of complications of retrodisplacements of the uterus is the following: 1. Laceration of the cervix. 2. Subinvolution. 3. Intra-uterine catarrh. 4. Intra-uterine vegetations. 5. Retroversion or retroflexion. 6. Prolapse, first degree. Each one of these conditions is more or less dependent upon parturition, and one follows the other in a more or less direct sequence. The treatment of this series of pathological changes is in the inverse ratio of their occurrence. Thus, we will first replace the uterus to its normal position, then curette the endometrium for the vegetations or the chronic endometritis, treat the endometrium until it is restored to a healthy condition by the proper intra-uterine applications, of course retaining the uterus in its normal position by tampons or a properly fitting pessary while this treatment is going on; then finally restore the lacerated cervix by the well-known plastic operation. A pessary may have to be worn for some time until the uterine supports have regained their tone, or indefinitely perhaps; but the symptoms of which the patient complains are permanently removed by this systematic course of treatment. It may be well to remark here that intra-uterine vegetations—that is to say, multiple adenomata of the mucous membrane of the body of the uterus—and the resulting menorrhagia are not at all infrequent consequences of chronic backward displacements of the uterus.

Causes.—I have already stated that backward displacements of the uterus occur most frequently in women who have borne children, the natural inference being that the relaxation of the uterine ligaments and supports and the increased weight of the uterus so commonly following parturition are the chief factors in the production of this displacement. Prolonged and difficult labors, laceration of the neck of the womb with subsequent subinvolution of the organ,—that is to say, a more or less permanent increase in its size and weight; further, subinvolution of the suspensory ligaments of the uterus and very often of the inferior supports, vagina and perineum, —these are among the most common and potent factors in this displacement. It is not necessary that the perineum should be torn in order that the vagina may be relaxed and prolapsed, and thus one of the inferior supports of the uterus be removed; a mere want of involution of the perineum—that is to say, a failure of the organ to regain its normal tone and strength—is equivalent to an absolute loss of the part. If the bladder and rectum also prolapse there is still less support for the uterus from below, and once a descent of the organ into the cavity of the pelvis having taken place, a backward tipping of its body is an almost inevitable result.

But not every retroversion or retroflexion occurs in a parous woman or is due to the injuries accompanying and the conditions resulting from parturition: in a very fair number of cases retroversion and retroflexion are found in women who have never borne children and who are even virgins.

The explanation for the occurrence of the displacement in these cases must be that either the woman grew up with the displacement,—in which case a congenital shortening of the utero-recto-sacral ligaments may be supposed,—or else that some sudden physical shock, such as a sharp fall on the buttocks, may have caused the backward displacement. Besides, I do not doubt that in some cases a congenital tendency to retroversion existed as an embryonal malformation, and that the downward pressure of the abdominal viscera during the development of the girl gradually increased this tendency until a full-fledged retroversion or retroflexion was accomplished. The development of a fibrous tumor in the posterior wall of the uterus may produce a backward displacement, and so also may the pressure of an ovarian tumor force the body of the uterus backward.

**Frequency.**—Of all the displacements of the uterus which may be considered truly pathological, retroversion and retroflexion are by all means the most common. I do not consider anteflexion in the first degree to be really pathological; otherwise it would probably, as being the nearest the normal position, be the most frequent. Certainly, in women who have borne children backward displacement of the uterus by far exceeds any of the other deviations. Thus, out of eight hundred and ninety-five cases of displacement of the uterus collected by me (see my article before the International Medical Congress in 1881), there were three hundred and forty-eight cases of retroversion and fifty-five of retroflexion, only five of which occurred in single women. There were, it is true, three hundred and ninety-seven cases of anteflexion and anteversion, but of these only a very small proportion were pathological and productive of any symptoms or required any treatment. This proportion, therefore, bears out the statement I have just made, that anteflexion in the minor degrees is the most common displacement; still, retroversion and retroflexion much more frequently require treatment.

**Significance.**—There is still some difference of opinion as to whether a backward displacement of the uterus, in itself, has any particular significance in the production of local pain or reflex symptoms. I will admit that a retroversion or retroflexion of the first degree in all probability is of no particular consequence and in no decided way inconveniences the woman, except possibly in the production of sterility; and I am also willing to allow that a backward displacement of the second or third degree, either version or flexion, may, if the uterus is small and movable and the ovaries are not prolapsed with it, exist for years without in any way attracting the attention of the patient; but as regards this last class of cases I must insist that it is the exception for a uterus to be retroverted or retroflexed in the second or third degree without, in course of time, an adhesion of the fundus or a prolapsus and adhesion of the appendages to occur or a uterine catarrh to supervene, in consequence of the changes of circulation produced by the displacement, and then inevitably come the symptoms peculiar to the aggravated forms of this displacement. It is not, therefore, the displacement alone which produces pain, local and general, and the other symptoms peculiar to the displacement, but the complications produced by and naturally following the condition. Should a uterus retrovert during the first two months of pregnancy, or should a retroverted or retroflexed uterus become pregnant, as occasionally does occur, the significance of the displacement very soon becomes decidedly marked. The growing organ soon finds the pelvic cavity too limited, and, being prevented by the promontory of the sacrum from rising into the abdominal cavity, begins to rebel. Incarceration of the pregnant uterus has taken place, and uterine contractions, hemorrhage, and abortion are the inevitable results, unless the displacement is speedily rectified and the uterus kept in place by a properly fitting supporter. Besides the usual symptoms produced by backward displacement, sterility may be considered a very frequent result. At least it is fair to assume if, in a woman who has been sterile for years, the uterus is found to be retroverted or retroflexed even in the first degree, that the sterility—no other cause for it being apparent—is due to this displacement. Of course the influence of possible prolapse of the ovaries and of uterine catarrh should be taken into consideration as additional factors in the production of sterility.

In an unmarried woman the presence of a backward displacement of the uterus which produces no symptoms whatever is of no special significance, since if she remains unmarried the chances are largely in favor of the displacement never giving her any inconvenience. Such displacements are often discovered unexpectedly during a vaginal examination made for some supposed pelvic disease. It has always been questionable with me whether, under such circumstances, it was worth while to rupture the hymen, replace the uterus, and insert a supporter. It is only when the discomforts complained of undoubtedly depended upon the displacement that I have felt myself justified in instituting active treatment.

**Symptoms.**—Whenever a uterus is retroverted or retroflexed in the second or third degree, and the displacement has persisted for some months or years, the probability is that the patient will complain of the following symptoms: bearing down, a dropping sensation in the pelvis during standing or walking, pain in the lower part of the sacrum and coccyx, perhaps extending down the back of either thigh along the sciatic nerve, an inability to walk any distance or stand for any length of time, leucorrhœa, often profuse menstruation. Besides, if the ovaries are prolapsed at the same time, there will be a more acute pain than is common in retrodisplacement alone in the region of each sacro-ischiatic notch. These are the local symptoms. The reflex symptoms are exceedingly varied and diffuse, and may be classified under the heading of general neuroses or disturbances of the nervous system; not neuralgia or pains, because the disturbances are not always actually painful. Thus, a woman with an aggravated retroversion or retroflexion may have hemicrania, frontal, vertical, or occipital headache, intercostal neuralgia, gastralgia, nausea and vomiting, or may feel generally

depressed and nervous without any special localized pain.   There is really
no one distinct symptom which positively points to the presence of a backward displacement of the uterus, for even the one symptom which one
would suppose to be inevitable, the pain in the sacrum and coccyx, may be
due entirely to so-called "spinal irritation" found during neurasthenia, the
uterus being in a perfectly normal position.

Diagnosis.—The diagnosis can only be made by a vaginal examination.   The examining finger will find the body of the uterus either horizontal on a line with the axis of the vagina (first degree) or tipped backward
more or less into the excavation of the sacrum, with the cervix pointing
upward towards the anterior wall of the vagina in retroversion, or in the
axis of the vagina with an angle at the junction of the cervix and body in

Fig. 26.

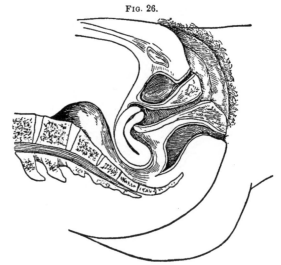

Retroflexion, second degree.

retroflexion.   The acuteness of the angle will designate the degree of the
flexion.   The immediate continuance of the cervix into the body will show
that the round elastic mass which is felt through the posterior vaginal vault
is the body of the uterus and not some other organ.   Bimanual palpation will show that the body of the uterus is absent in the position which
it should naturally occupy.   In case of doubt the sound or probe will
verify the diagnosis of backward displacement.   If the uterus is not adherent, the examining finger will be able to lift up the body of the organ
and possibly even restore it to its normal position by the aid of the other
hand pressing through the abdominal walls.   If the ovaries and tubes are
prolapsed at the same time, they will be found lying to either side or immediately behind the body of the uterus; the left appendages usually lying
deeper than the right, owing to the normally greater depth of Douglas's

pouch on the left side. If the uterus is adherent or impacted between the utero-recto-sacral ligaments, it is not replaceable, and the diagnosis may become doubtful. To beginners it is necessary to emphasize that bimanual palpation is absolutely essential to the diagnosis of retroversion and retroflexion, as, indeed, it is to nearly all the other displacements of the uterus.

*Differential Diagnosis.*—There are other bodies besides the corpus uteri which may occupy Douglas's pouch and simulate a backward displacement. These are fibroids, small ovarian tumors, plastic exudations, effusions of blood, and abscesses. In such cases the sounding of the uterus may be necessary to make the diagnosis, and even then the most experienced touch may be at fault.

FIG. 27.

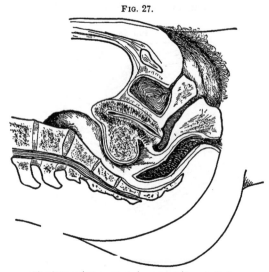

Fibroid in posterior wall of uterus simulating retroflexion.

**Treatment.**—The question as to whether a retrodisplacement of the uterus requires treatment will depend largely upon the symptoms it produces. The treatment comprises simply and concisely two main points: first, the restoration of the displaced organ to its normal position, and, second, its retention therein.

*First.* The elevation of the retrodisplaced uterus may be accomplished by the fingers, posture, and instruments (sound and repositor). With a woman in the dorsal recumbent position, one or two fingers in the vagina may elevate the uterus until the fingers of the other hand can grasp the fundus through the abdominal walls and tilt it forward. This is possible only in very thin and lax abdominal walls. (Fig. 28.) The usual method of replacing a retrodisplaced uterus is by putting the patient in the left latero-abdominal position (Sims's), inserting the index and middle finger of the right hand into the vagina, and, standing well behind the patient, pressing the body of the uterus upward until it is so far elevated that the fingers can barely touch the fundus. Then the index finger is passed in front of the cervix and draws that part backward, while the middle finger still remains in the posterior pouch. By thus gradually drawing the cervix backward and pushing the fundus upward the body of the uterus is slowly tipped forward into the normal anteverted position. (Figs. 29, 30, and 31.) Should this manipulation fail, the woman may be put in the genu-pectoral position and efforts made to dislodge the body of the uterus from the sacral excavation by means of the fingers passed into the vagina, or, in extreme cases, into the rectum, or a Sims depressor or sponge or cotton on a holder may be used as a means of exerting pressure on the retroverted organ. At times the elevation of

FIG. 28.

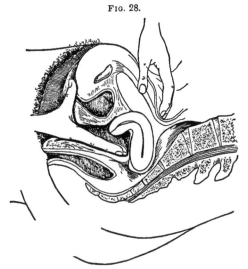

Reposition of retroflexed uterus in dorsal position. The outer hand is supposed to grasp the fundus as it is elevated by the internal fingers. Only possible in very relaxed abdominal walls.

the perineum by a Sims speculum and the drawing down of the cervix by a tenaculum hooked into it may succeed in dislodging the fundus from its impacted position in the sacral cavity, and then the pressure of air exerted with special force on the vaginal vault with the woman in this position will aid in replacing the uterus. This position and manipulation are specially applicable to cases of impaction of the retrodisplaced gravid uterus. Finally, if these manual and postural methods fail or it appears from the beginning that the displacement is too aggravated to render its rectification by them probable in experienced hands, the reposition of the uterus may be attempted with a large blunt sound or, what is much better, the Sims or Emmet repositor. This can be done either on the back through guidance of the finger or on the side through Sims's speculum. The sound, be it understood, exerts its pressure entirely on the sensitive fundus uteri, and a perforation of the organ at that point might easily be produced by

Fig. 29.

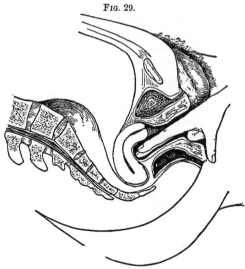

Reposition of retroflexed uterus in left lateral position, first step.

careless and rough manipulation. The repositor, on the other hand, has for a fulcrum a broad flange which presses against the lips of the external

Fig. 30.

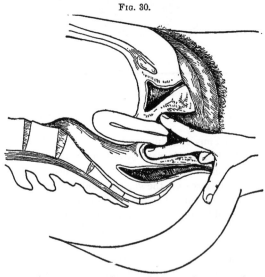

Reposition of retroflexed uterus in left lateral position, second step.

os, the intra-uterine part not touching the fundus at all. There is, therefore, no danger of injuring the organ by this instrument, for which reason I prefer it.

The uterus having been replaced by any one of these methods, should be at once retained in its now normal position by a properly-fitting support, or, if it does not seem advisable to use such a one at once, by balls of cotton or the common substitute nowadays, iodoform gauze packing.

Should the uterus be found unreplaceable by any of these measures, it may safely be inferred that it is adherent and that nothing short of operative interference will succeed in replacing it. Pessaries are, therefore, not indicated unless the organ has been restored to its normal position.

At times it may be impossible to replace a uterus at the first attempt or to keep it in that position after it has been replaced. In that case repeated

FIG. 31.

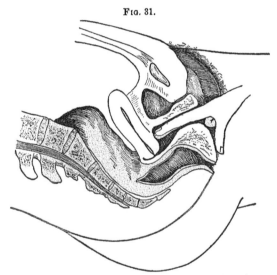

Reposition of retroflexed uterus in left lateral position, third step.

attempts must be made, the vagina being in the interval well tamponed with cotton or gauze in order to retain the advantage which has been gained at each sitting. Excessive tenderness or impaction of the uterus, or great relaxation of the vagina, may be the reason for failure in such cases.

*Pessaries.*—There is such a diversity of opinion on the use of pessaries in the treatment of backward displacements of the uterus that I think it worth while to devote a special section to their discussion.

In the first place, let it be understood that in my opinion a pessary is a necessary evil, so to speak. If we could do without pessaries no one would be better pleased than I; but, as I have already said under general remarks, if I were compelled to give them up I should feel almost powerless in the treatment of a very large proportion of backward displacements of

the uterus. I have already stated that in anterior displacements I make
very little use of pessaries because I do not think they are needed. I shall
hereafter mention that in prolapsus pessaries also do not in my experience
produce the beneficial results which I would like to see in that form of
displacement. The remedy has there to be sought rather in operative procedures. But in retrodisplacements of the uterus I do not see how I can

FIG. 32.

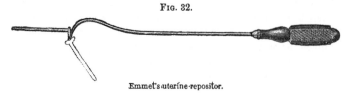

Emmet's uterine-repositor.

possibly do without pessaries. Two indispensable conditions to the proper
use of these instruments and to the beneficial results to be obtained therefrom are, first, that the uterus should be returned to its normal position, and,
second, that the pessary should be properly fitted and should, without injury
or discomfort to its wearer, retain the uterus in the position which it normally occupies.

*Varieties.*—The cardinal principle upon which pessaries for retrodisplacements of the uterus are constructed is that of leverage, first introduced
by Dr. Hugh L. Hodge, of Philadelphia. Before his time pessaries were
nothing but crude, often exceedingly complicated and more or less dangerous, contrivances, mostly intended to act by distention of the vagina and
by their bulk. Dr. Hodge's instrument, however, acts on the easily under-
standable principle of the pushing down of a short anterior lever and the
consequent tilting upward of a long posterior lever. All the pessaries
which are now used in retrodisplacements, with a few unpractical exceptions, are based on this idea, which has undergone many variations at the

FIG. 33.

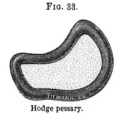

Hodge pessary.

FIG. 34.

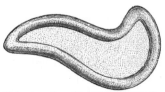

Hodge pessary, modified by Albert H. Smith.

hands of different gynæcologists. The first instrument devised by Hodge
was of equal width at both its lower and upper extremities and had only
one longitudinal curve; later on two curves were added, and Dr. Albert
H. Smith made a still further modification by narrowing and pointing
the lower extremity in order to enable it to rest under the symphysis
pubis. This last innovation has proved a permanent one, and nearly
all pessaries for backward displacement are now constructed after this

plan. According to the length and width of the vagina, according to the depth and width of the posterior vaginal pouch, according to the firmness or relaxation of the posterior vaginal wall and perineum, a pessary will have to be broader, longer, or more or less curved. In fact, it is only after the uterus has been replaced that the physician can estimate what exact shape and variety of pessary will be required for each given case. If there is a retroflexion with considerable relaxation of the posterior

FIG. 35.

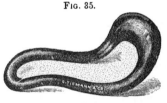

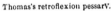

Thomas's retroflexion pessary.

FIG. 36.

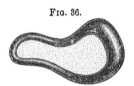

Munde's retroflexion pessary.

vaginal wall and uterine ligaments, a pessary with a sharp posterior curve will usually be required, and for this very form of displacement an improvement has been added by Dr. T. G. Thomas, which consists in a bulbous enlargement of the posterior cross-bar of the pessary, whereby the body of the uterus is prevented from tipping and bending backward. I have modified this supporter by shortening and broadening it somewhat, so that the posterior vaginal vault is put more on a lateral stretch and the pessary is

FIG. 37.

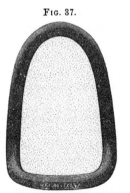

Front view of usual Albert Smith pessary.

FIG. 38.

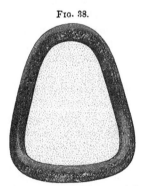

Front view of same pessary spread bilaterally
(Mundé).

more easily retained than when it is long and slender, as Dr. Thomas recommended it. As I have indicated, it is necessary to fit a particular pessary to every particular vagina, therefore the assortment to be kept on hand should be varied not only in size, but also in difference of curve. I have found it useful for some cases to spread the lateral diameter of the ordinary retroversion pessaries somewhat, so as to increase their power of retention. My experience, extending over more than twenty years, has taught me that there is nothing more difficult in mechanical gynæcology than to fit a pessary to a bad case of retroflexed and prolapsed uterus. If, therefore, one or two trials do not succeed, the attempt should not be given up so long as the uterus is movable and the patient bears the manipulation. In those cases in which, after repeated trials, the extent of displacement and the relaxation of the ligaments and supports, added to perhaps a laceration of the perineum, render the successful fitting and wearing of a supporter improbable, the operative measures hereafter to be described will naturally suggest themselves.

*Indications.*—A backward displacement of the uterus which in the opinion of gynæcologists requires replacement should also, *cæteris paribus*, call for the insertion of a pessary to insure the permanency of the replacement. I have already stated that retroversions and retroflexions of the first degree, except in cases where sterility seems to be produced by this displacement, do not require reposition and a support; but I maintain that all backward displacements of a more aggravated degree than the first should be rectified and the uterus kept in place by a pessary as soon as discovered, whether they produce direct symptoms or not. The only exception to this rule might be the cases of virgins in whom such displacement is accidentally discovered, of women beyond the menopause, or of old maids, in none of whom the displacement produces positive symptoms, and in all of whom the reposition of the uterus, and the introduction and wearing of a support, would entail more inconvenience than the doubtful possibility of future trouble from the displacement. This means that I would consider every backward displacement of the uterus of the second and third degrees in a young *married* woman to warrant replacement and introduction of a pessary. In a virgin, or in a married woman beyond the menopause, I should be guided in this respect entirely by the direct discomfort produced by the displacement. Before proceeding to perform an operation for the relief of displacement I should certainly always give the pessary a chance.

*Counterindications.*—An immovable, non-replaceable uterus is always an absolute counterindication to the use of a pessary, whether the cause of the adhesion—pelvic peritonitis—is recent or remote. Retrodisplacements produced by the presence of fibroid or ovarian tumors would likewise counterindicate the use of a support, since it is scarcely probable that the instrument would be able to keep the uterus in place.

*Dangers.*—If a pessary has been properly fitted it should produce neither pain nor discomfort of any kind, nor any more than a slight increase of the ordinary leucorrhœal discharge common to the majority of women. But women are not all alike, and some do not bear the constant pressure of the support as well as others, and after a month or two, more or less, an abrasion is formed, usually behind the cervix, by the pressure of the instrument. I have even seen, in neglected cases, a pessary entirely embedded in the vaginal walls, the discharge being so foul as to simulate malignant disease. In former days the cutting of one of the old-fashioned supports into the bladder or the rectum was a not very infrequent occurrence. Only the grossest negligence could, with the supporters we are now in the habit of using, result in such an accident. A very large, ill-fitting pessary may produce an inflammation with exudate into the cellular tissue at some point in the pelvic cavity, or it may press upon the bladder or the rectum so much as to interfere with the functions of these organs.

*Precautions.*—The following rules may be laid down for the guidance of the practitioner in the use of pessaries. *First.* Always replace the uterus before choosing and introducing the pessary. *Second.* Never insert a pessary which is so large that it is not freely movable in the vagina and does not allow the examining finger to pass easily between it and the vaginal wall.

Fig. 39.

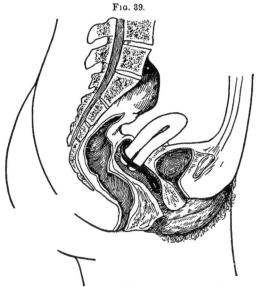

Retroversion pessary in position: woman in erect position.

*Third.* Always adapt the pessary to the individual case. *Fourth.* Examine the woman in the standing posture before allowing her to depart, in order to see whether the pessary remains in place in that position. *Fifth.* Tell the woman that she is wearing a pessary, and that it must give her no pain and inconvenience whatever, so that, if it does, she may know that it is not right and may at once call to have it rectified or may, in a case of emergency, remove it herself; and show her how to do so. *Sixth.* Tell her to call again in about a week, so that you may see whether the pessary is doing its duty. *Seventh.* Tell her to use a tepid vaginal douche every day as a matter of cleanliness, for all pessaries produce more or less leucorrhœa. Use no alum or other salt in the douches, as rough incrustations on the pessary are produced thereby. *Eighth.* Do not omit to tell her that she will have to wear a pessary for a number of months, perhaps years, and that the cure of the displacement can be ascertained only by her not wearing the instrument for a short time.  *Ninth.*  Finally, caution her to be sure to come to see you in case she should become pregnant while wearing the pessary, which of course means that connection is not to be refrained from during that time.  Should she become pregnant while wearing the pessary, it will be necessary to remove it at about the end of the third month.

*Modes of Insertion.*—I usually replace a retrodisplaced uterus with my fingers, the woman occupying the left semi-prone position.  When the uterus is replaced and I have satisfied myself by my measurements of the vagina what kind of a pessary will suit her, I select it, wash and anoint it with vaseline, and pass it into the vagina upside down, so as to place the upper curve in front of the cervix ; with the index finger of my right hand passed into the lumen of the pessary I pull the upper curve back over the cervix, and twist the instrument so as to place it in the longitudinal axis of the vagina.  It takes some little skill to perform this manœuvre, but it is comparatively simple when once learned.  I then settle the pessary in its place by pulling the lower extremity gently backward.  I prefer this method to the one very commonly used by the general practitioner, of slipping the pessary in position with the patient on her back, because, as I have already said, the reposition of the organ is easier on the side and the insertion of the pessary still more easy.  In some cases of very difficult replacement, particularly of the pregnant uterus, I replace the organ and insert the pessary in the knee-chest position.  It is almost impossible to convey the exact details of these manœuvres in a few words.  A lesson at the bedside will in a few moments express more than pages of description.

I think the wearing of skirt supporters which will prevent the abdominal viscera from pressing down upon the displaced or replaced uterus will give very much relief and assist the efforts of nature in retaining the organ in its normal position.  The assumption by the patient of the genu-pectoral position for a few minutes several times a day, with entirely relaxed abdominal muscles (absence of corsets and skirts), will undoubtedly aid very much in restoring tone to the uterine ligaments and supports by removing the strain which is constantly upon them when the patient is in the erect position.

Following the lead of Thure Brandt, a Swedish officer who exchanged the sword for the, to him, more congenial employment of manual massage, Profanter, Schultze, and a number of other enthusiastic gynæcologists have adopted and endeavored to introduce into general practice the treatment of uterine displacements by massage of the relaxed ligaments and supports.  There can be no doubt that in cases not too ancient such manipulations may restore the normal tone to the organs.  The massage is conducted on entirely sound scientific and mechanical principles, the ligaments being separately kneaded and manipulated so as to induce them to regain their healthy tone.  The vagina, the perineum, and the uterus itself are also

subjected to the same systematic manipulations, and this treatment is practised daily for weeks and months, together with other mechanical details
which I cannot here describe. In Sweden, where Turkish baths are given
to men by women, such manipulations of the female sexual organs by males
do not seem to excite any particular objection. In this country, however,
ladies have not as yet become accustomed to the idea of having men,
even their physicians, manipulate their sexual organs by the hour. If
female massage operators could be taught the anatomy of the female sexual
organs and the rationale of this treatment, I dare say it would not be so
difficult to introduce it into this country, for I really believe that it would
be of great benefit.

*Adhesion of the Retrodisplaced Uterus.*—When the fundus and body
of the uterus are adherent in Douglas's pouch, manual and instrumental
attempts to replace the organ will usually fail, although once in a while
a slightly adherent uterus may be peeled loose by repeated firm pressure
with the fingers in the vagina. If the appendages are adherent at the
same time, however, such attempts will scarcely ever succeed. Such
patients do not always complain of pain or particular discomfort depending upon the displacement; hence, if we do not succeed in replacing the
organ easily, it may at times be advisable to let well enough alone, pend-
ing the occurrence of symptoms which warrant more decided interference.
But usually when patients complain of the backache, etc., which backward displacements so frequently produce, we are obliged to do something for their relief. We can endeavor to soften and gradually detach
the adhesions, if they are not too old and firm, by packing the vagina as
tightly as the patient can stand with pledgets of lamb's wool impregnated
with iodoform powder to keep them sweet, the resiliency of the wool.
exerting more pressure upon the parts which it touches than cotton. This
manipulation can be done either in the Sims or, better, in the knee-chest
position. The tampons can be allowed to remain for three or four days or
even longer if properly iodoformized, and the treatment will have to be continued for months, except during the menstrual epoch, in order to secure a
result. I have repeatedly seen an apparently immovable adherent uterus
in time become movable and replaceable after months of this treatment.
Efforts can be made at the same time, at each visit, with the fingers or the
repositor, to elevate the uterus. Care must be taken not to mistake an
impaction of the body of the uterus between the two utero-recto-sacral ligaments for an adhesion : it will take some little experience to be able to distinguish between these two conditions. An impacted uterus will after a
certain amount of manipulation suddenly snap up and be replaced, when
the error in diagnosis will be at once recognized. In cases where the adhesions of the uterus to the adjacent peritoneum do not seem to be very firm
and where the appendages are loose, the plan of B. S. Schultze, of Jena,
may be followed,—namely, to endeavor by bimanual manipulation under
anæsthesia to peel loose the adherent uterus and replace it. I have several

times been enabled to do this with perfect satisfaction. One must always remember that such manipulations, if at all forcible, incur the risk of a possible return of pelvic peritonitis.

### OPERATIVE TREATMENT.

In cases where our most persistent endeavors have failed to retain the uterus in its normal position by pessaries or by astringent cotton tampons, where the uterus and its appendages are entirely movable,—indeed, by far too movable,—where the ligaments and supports are both excessively relaxed, where the patient wishes to be rid of the annoyance of the displacement as well as of the constant local treatment,—in fact, wishes to be *cured* as speedily as possible,—it is our duty to place before

FIG. 40.

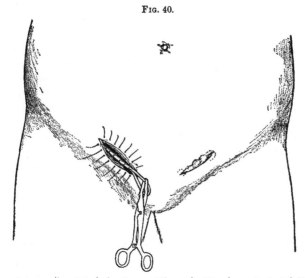

Alexander's operation of shortening the round ligaments of the uterus. On the left side is shown the knuckle of fat which protrudes as soon as the fascia covering the external ring is nicked. This knuckle of fat contains the diffuse and vague terminal fibres of the ligament where they are attached over the pubic spine. The right side shows the ligament drawn out to its full extent, still attached to the pubic spine, and pierced by the sutures.

her the means by which such a cure can be effected, other than those already fruitlessly employed. They are the following:

1. *Alexander's Operation for Shortening the Round Ligaments of the Uterus.*—This consists in making an incision over the external inguinal ring on each side, dissecting out, picking up, and drawing out the round ligament until the fundus uteri points towards the anterior abdominal wall, then sewing the ligament into the wound by sutures which pass through the pillars of the ring and the ligament, and then cutting off the excess of the ligament. In my opinion, this is by far the most successful, the most logical, and the least dangerous operation for the permanent cure

of an otherwise incurable retroversion or retroflexion. I should scarcely ever employ it unless I failed to keep the uterus in place with a pessary; but as this latter occurrence is not so very uncommon, the opportunity is frequently offered to perform this operation. I have thus far, during the past ten years, performed it sixty-five times, with such success both as to the immediate and permanent results as to render me more and more enthusiastic in its favor. I have not only succeeded in lifting up and keeping the uterus in its normal position for years after the operation, but I have seen probably as many as a dozen of the cases conceive, go to term, be normally delivered, and the uterus retain the position in which I placed it. In one case I saw the patient in consultation after her fifth confinement following the operation, and found the uterus in its normal position. She was dying of puerperal septicæmia, to be sure; but the operation had nothing to do with that. A few cases have been failures, I must admit; but they were either badly chosen, the uterus being too large and again

Fig. 41.

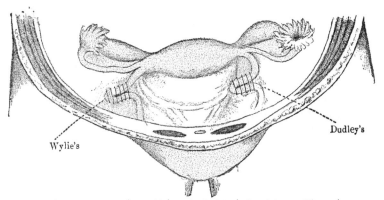

Wylie's

Dudley's

Wylie's and Dudley's methods of intra-abdominal shortening of the round ligaments.

dragging down the shortened ligaments, or the ligaments were too thin and broke during the operation, and therefore did not give the support which they properly should.

There are several objections to this operation, and they are: That it is an uncertain one, for one never knows when one will find thick, strong, easily tractable ligaments, or ligaments which are thin, adherent, readily broken, and can then no longer be recovered. This may be at times the fault of the operator, but also at times of the anatomical structures themselves, and no man can tell before he has opened the inguinal canal and found the ligaments whether they will be thick or thin, weak or strong, easily sliding in their sheaths or adherent along the whole track. Besides, the operator has to keep his wits about him, or he will easily miss the pubic attachment of the ligament and then pronounce the operation a fraud. But I can safely say that a failure to find the ligaments is *always* the fault of the operator; the other accidents he is not responsible for. I have had no evil results from this operation; in a few cases the wounds have suppurated and union has been gained by second intention, but I have had no deaths or anything to give more than passing apprehension; and I repeat that the results, particularly as to permanency, so far as I have been able to trace the cases, have been beyond all my expectations.

It should be stated that this operation, while named after Dr. William Alexander, of Liverpool, who first scientifically described it and secured its adoption, was hinted at by a Frenchman named Alquié and by an Englishman called Adams before Dr. Alexander revived it; hence the Germans designate this operation as the Alquié-Adams-Alexander operation.

2. Another method of shortening the round ligaments has been devised (I believe Wylie claims the priority), and consists in opening the abdominal cavity, drawing up the fundus uteri, doubling each round ligament upon itself, and sewing the doubled surfaces together and to the peritoneal covering of the uterus with catgut. I believe Polk, Palmer Dudley, and Mann have practised this operation also, with minor modifications of their own; all speak highly of it. I have had but one experience with it, of quite recent occurrence, in which I peeled the adherent tubes and ovaries loose, restored the calibre of the tubes by probing, and doubled the round ligaments upon themselves and sewed them with triple sutures of catgut. For some reason or other, suppuration developed along the line of the round ligaments, adhesion of the anterior surface of the uterus to the abdominal wall occurred, and, fortunately, the pus broke through the abdominal wound. While the patient made a good recovery, the case for a time seemed doubtful and gave me considerable anxiety. I am afraid that possibly I may have constricted the ligaments too much and produced their sloughing. The position of the uterus after sewing together the ligaments was absolutely ideal, as demonstrated in the Trendelenburg position, and I think, therefore, that I shall repeat this operation; but I shall limit it to cases where I am obliged to open the abdominal cavity for adherent tubes and ovaries and where I do not feel disposed to remove the appendages or am prohibited by the patient from doing so.

3. *Ventral Fixation.*—This means the stitching of the fundus uteri to the anterior abdominal wall. Saenger, Howard Kelly, Leopold, Klotz, and some others were the first to carry out this practice in cases of retro-displacement with normal appendages. The stitching of the pedicles into the abdominal wound after removal of the diseased appendages, in order to cure a backward displacement of the uterus, has been practised for years by the majority of abdominal operators, myself included. It is, of course, a comparatively simple matter to open the abdominal cavity, seize the fundus uteri with a volsellum or have it lifted up by the fingers of an assistant in the vagina, and pass several stitches through it and through the abdominal walls and thus attach it to the anterior abdominal wall; having also, to

insure thorough adhesion, abraded the fundus with a scalpel. But there are two objections to this plan: one is the danger that will always be inseparable from an abdominal section, no matter how skilfully and carefully it is done and no matter who does it; the other is that an organ the body of which should be naturally movable is immovably attached to the anterior abdominal wall. This would, perhaps, be of little consequence under ordinary circumstances; but if the woman should chance to become pregnant, the attachment of the fundus would interfere with the upward enlargement of the organ as the pregnancy advanced, and an interruption of the pregnancy before term would, therefore, be a very probable result. I have performed this operation about a dozen times, partly for backward displacement, partly for prolapsus. I have had only one death· from it, but I have had the experience of seeing one woman abort in the fifth month after several weeks of severe uterine pain, and in a case of prolapsus I have seen the abdominal walls with the adherent fundus sink down and allow the prolapsus to return. I confess that the operation does not in any way appeal to my sympathies, and that I very much doubt whether I shall ever repeat it. It seems to me an illogical and mechanically incorrect operation. I can admit it only in cases where the appendages and the uterus also are adherent, and where it is necessary anyway to open the abdominal cavity in order to detach these adhesions. Then it is the question whether ventral fixation, internal duplication of the round ligaments, or Alexander's operation should be performed, and the individual predilection of each operator will probably have to settle the matter. In my opinion, there can be no question of choice between Alexander's operation and ventral fixation, since Alexander's operation should be performed only and exclusively when the uterus and appendages are freely movable and in no way adherent. In such a case I certainly would never open the abdominal cavity for the cure of the displacement; it is only when the uterus and appendages are adherent that I consider the operation of abdominal section possibly justifiable.

Schücking has devised an ingenious but utterly illogical operation for the cure of retroflexion, which consists in passing a hollow probe containing a needle into the uterus, anteflexing the organ, and then shooting the needle through the anterior vaginal fornix into the vagina, of course avoiding the bladder (if possible). A thread is then passed through the eye of the needle and the instrument withdrawn. One end of the thread then passes through the anterior fornix vaginæ and the fundus, the other out of the cervix. The two ends being tied together, of course the uterus is placed in an anteflexed position. The thread is removed in due time, and the anteflexed uterus is supposed to replace satisfactorily the retroflexed organ.

Mackinrodt, of Berlin, has recently suggested a similar illogical operation,—namely, to make a longitudinal incision through the anterior vaginal fornix, push up the bladder with the fingers, anteflex the uterus with the sound, and sew the fundus to the vagina. Here again an immovable anteflexion is substituted for a movable retroflexion. It scarcely seems necessary to describe these two operations, except for the purpose of condemning them. They will probably hardly live as long as the publication of this work.

The late Dr. James B. Hunter suggested sewing the cervix to the posterior vaginal fornix and in this way keeping the fundus anteverted. Possibly this operation might be of use in retroversion; in retroflexion it evidently would do nothing but increase the angle of flexion, since the posterior attachment of the cervix would by no means result in anteverting the body. The operation has not, I believe, been accepted.

In conclusion, I will merely repeat that to my mind the most logical and successful operation is that devised by Alexander, and I see no reason for experimenting and risking our patients' lives by dangerous and questionable procedures. In fact, I do not think that we have a right to inflict upon our patients an operation from which they may possibly die, simply for the purpose of curing them of a condition which merely renders them uncomfortable, but in no way threatens their lives.

### LATERO-VERSION AND LATERO-FLEXION.

**Definition.**—A uterus is said to be latero-verted or latero-flexed when its body is tipped or bent to one side or the other of the median line.

**Causes.**—These displacements are either congenital or acquired, in either case through a shortening of the broad ligament of the side towards which the body tips. The reasons for congenital shortening of the broad ligaments are, of course, not known; those of acquired shortening are simply the contraction following an inflammation involving the affected broad ligament.

**Significance.**—The only real importance which these displacements assume is the usual production of sterility. If the cervix is tipped towards the opposite side from where the fundus is directed, it is naturally out of the axis of the vaginal canal and therefore not so accessible to the spermatozoa as nature intended it should be. If a flexion is present, of course the chances are still less for conception. There is no pain produced by these displacements, and in all probability they would not be discovered except when an examination is made to ascertain the cause of sterility.

The diagnosis is, of course, easy, being made by bimanual examination, aided if necessary by the sound.

The treatment is practically *nil*, since we have no means of lengthening congenital or artificially acquired contractions of the broad ligaments. Numerous pessaries have been devised for the purpose, but they have not proved efficient. Persistent tamponade of the vagina, so as to stretch the contracted ligament, and massage, would seem to offer the only reasonable chances of success.

### ASCENT OF THE UTERUS.

This condition is always secondary to disease of some neighboring organ, and I mention it only for completeness' sake. It is not properly a displacement of the uterus in itself. The uterus may be pushed up by a fibroid tumor which develops downward into the pelvic cavity, or by a large intra-pelvic plastic exudate or effusion of blood, or by an ovarian tumor growing downward into the pelvic cavity; or it may be drawn up by an intra-ligamentous ovarian cyst which grows upward towards the diaphragm. There are, of course, no other special symptoms produced by this secondary displacement of the uterus, and there is no relief except the removal of the cause, when the uterus will probably return of itself to its normal position.

## PROLAPSUS UTERI.

**Definition.**—By prolapsus of the uterus is meant a sinking or falling of that organ into the pelvic cavity and even outside of the vulva. The

FIG. 42.

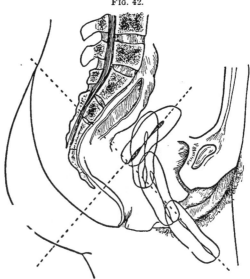

Degrees of prolapsus uteri (diagrammatic). The first uterus shows the normal position with correct uterine and vaginal axes.

popular name for this condition is " falling of the womb," which may mean any of the various degrees of the displacement. Other terms are : descensus and procidentia.

**Degrees.**—For all practical purposes three degrees suffice. 1. The cervix touches the floor of the pelvis. 2. The cervix reaches the vaginal introitus. 3. The cervix passes the vaginal introitus and more or less of the whole body of the uterus is extruded beyond the vulva. Of course there are innumerable minor degrees between these three chief divisions.

**Anatomy.**—In prolapsus of the first degree the cervix touches the floor of the pelvis, the fundus uteri is proportionately below its normal

level, and the uterine axis inclines slightly backward.   The suspensory
ligaments of the uterus, chiefly the broad ligaments, are more or less relaxed, otherwise this sinking of the organ could not take place.   Neither
the bladder, the rectum, nor the vagina is necessarily involved in this first
degree of prolapsus.   In the second degree the external os approaches the
vaginal orifice, the body of the uterus is retroverted and lies in the sacral
excavation, the suspensory ligaments are proportionately relaxed and drawn
down, and usually the anterior vaginal wall and the posterior wall of the
bladder accompany, if they do not precede, the prolapse of the uterus.
The posterior vaginal wall and the rectum are as yet usually in their normal position.   In the third degree the cervix protrudes from the vulva
more or less, even to the extent of the entire extrusion of the uterus.   The

FIG. 43.

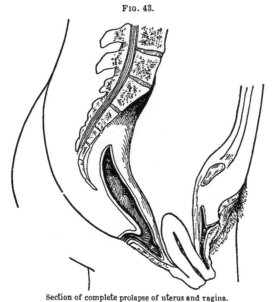

Section of complete prolapse of uterus and vagina.

anterior vaginal wall, and the posterior wall of the bladder down to the
meatus urinarius, protrude from the pelvic cavity, and in a very large
proportion of cases the posterior vaginal wall and the anterior wall of
the rectum are prolapsed to the same extent.   The sound passed into the
bladder through the urethra and the finger introduced into the rectum
will at their lowest points be on a level with the external os, showing a
complete prolapsus of the anterior and posterior vaginal walls with the corresponding walls of the bladder and the rectum.   Almost invariably in
prolapsus uteri of the second and third degrees the organ is found retroverted or retroflexed.   This is due to the tendency of the uterus to drop
backward when its fundus falls below the excavation of the sacrum.   In

consequence of the downward traction of the adherent vaginal walls and a certain amount of pathological hypertrophy of the supra-vaginal portion of the cervix, a uterus prolapsed in the third degree is almost always elongated, so that instead of measuring two and a half inches in depth it often attains a length of from four to seven inches. A curious feature of this elongation of the uterus is that when the uterus is replaced, together with the prolapsed vagina, its length diminishes, and the sound, which before entered six inches, we will say, now reaches the fundus at a depth of only three inches. This peculiar phenomenon has been explained by Emmet on the principle of the drawing out of a cone of putty and its shortening when it is pushed together. A truly hypertrophied uterus could not, of course, be

FIG. 44.

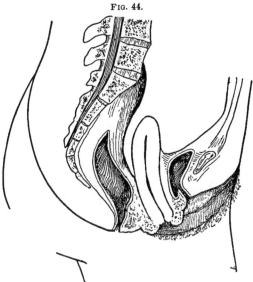

Section of prolapsus uteri et vaginæ with hypertrophic elongation of supra-vaginal portion of cervix.

reduced in length by being replaced. We must, therefore, assume that the downward traction of the attached prolapsed vagina draws out the uterine tissue, and on reposition the same tissue shrinks. There are a few instances on record in which an anteflexed or retroflexed uterus of perfectly normal size was found prolapsed outside of the vaginal orifice, surrounded by the completely prolapsed vaginal walls with bladder and rectum. These latter cases are very rare, and can only be explained on the principle that a very small uterus, either anteflexed or retroflexed, was gradually or forcibly drawn down by the prolapsing vaginal walls. This, however, is by no means the usual mode of formation of prolapse of the uterus and vagina. It should be stated that these rare forms of prolapse of the normal retroflexed or anteflexed uterus occurred in virgins of advanced years, in whom the natural relaxation of the pelvic connective tissue permitted a vaginal and uterine prolapse.

To recapitulate : complete prolapse of the uterus is usually associated with complete prolapse of the anterior and posterior vaginal walls, together with the corresponding portions of the bladder and rectum. When only one vaginal wall is prolapsed, it is usually the anterior with the corresponding portion of the rectum, and in the large majority of cases this is the way in which a uterine prolapse first begins,—namely, prolapse of the anterior vaginal wall and bladder; second, dragging down of the heavy uterus; and, third, prolapse of the posterior vaginal wall and rectum.

FIG. 45.

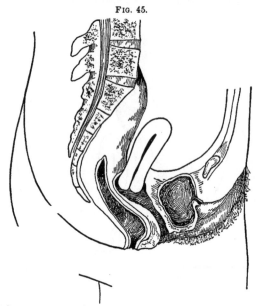

Section of prolapse of anterior vaginal wall and bladder.  Slight rectocele.

**Causes.**—The causes of prolapse of the uterus are twofold: 1. A heavy uterus dragging down the suspensory ligaments, chiefly the broad ligaments, and gradually sinking deeper and deeper into the pelvic cavity until it finally draws down with it the anterior vaginal wall with the bladder and then the posterior vaginal wall with the rectum. 2. Prolapse of the anterior vaginal wall with the bladder, dragging down of the uterus, probably also more or less enlarged, and, finally, prolapse of the posterior vaginal wall with the rectum. In the first instance it is the heavy uterus which primarily causes the prolapsus; in the second, it is the relaxed and descending vaginal walls which drag down after them the heavy uterus.

As indirect causes of prolapsus uteri must be mentioned the laceration or equivalent relaxation of the perineum and the pelvic floor, whereby prolapsus of the vaginal walls is facilitated ; and, furthermore, the multitudinous, more or less constantly acting, influences which force down the abdominal viscera towards the pelvic roof and help to produce the other forms of displacement as well as the one under present consideration, such as dress, overwork, too much exercise in the erect position, too long standing, constipation, and overdistended bladder. Undoubtedly, one of the most common causes of prolapsus uteri is too frequent and too rapidly repeated parturition. By far the large majority of cases of prolapsus uteri et vaginæ occur in women who after one or more severe childbirths are unable to remain at rest for a sufficient length of time to allow the pelvic organs to regain their normal tone. A very slight strain, such as lifting a heavy

FIG. 46.

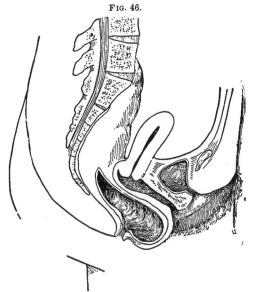

Section of prolapse of posterior vaginal wall and rectum.

weight or forcing at stool, will in such cases either produce an immediate prolapsus of the uterus or a repetition of those causes will effect that displacement in course of time. Complete prolapsus of the uterus is, therefore, far more common in women of the working-classes, who cannot give themselves the proper attention after childbirth, than it is among the wealthy. But even in the virgin and nulliparous woman prolapsus of the uterus may occur, partly from a generally debilitated condition of the system which causes a want of tone of the uterine ligaments and supports, and partly from accidental forcible causes, such as lifting heavy weights or sudden physical shocks and strains. I have seen several cases of complete prolapsus uteri et vaginæ in virgins produced by the lifting of a heavy weight, such as, in one instance, a wash-tub full of wet clothes. In two such cases the prolapsed vagina was so œdematous that it required compression by the elastic bandage for several days before it could be replaced.[1]

**Complications.**—As already mentioned, besides the uterus, the anterior and posterior vaginal walls and the corresponding portion of the bladder and rectum are prolapsed in extreme cases. Of course the ovaries will descend into the pelvic cavity to the depth of Douglas's pouch, together with the prolapsed uterus. One of the most common complications of prolapsus uteri is a laceration and eversion of the lips of the cervix, which condition, indeed, probably was the first step in the chain of events which ultimately resulted in the prolapsus,—namely, laceration of the cervix, consequent subinvolution, heavy uterus, relaxation of uterine ligaments, prolapse of the uterus and vagina, etc. Together with the laceration of the cervix, a laceration of the perineum is a very frequent occurrence, which, as I have already mentioned, predisposes to weakening and prolapsus of the vaginal walls. A hypertrophy of the cervix is also a common occurrence in consequence of the irritation produced by the laceration ; this hypertrophy may be both longitudinal and transverse. It is not only subinvolution of the uterus which may render the organ heavy and liable to prolapse, but also tumors, chiefly fibroids. For instance, I have recently seen such a case in which the whole uterus was firmly wedged into the pelvic cavity, obstructing both bladder and rectum, the cause of the obstruction being subperitoneal fibroids. Occasionally pregnancy may cause prolapsus of the uterus when the ligaments and supports are very much relaxed and some sudden strain forces the enlarged organ down into the pelvic cavity. As a rule, however, pregnancy helps to elevate the uterus out of the pelvic cavity as gestation advances. Occasionally a deep location of the uterus is congenital, being associated with a comparatively short vagina.

**Frequency.**—I will not attempt to give any figures as to the relative frequency of prolapsus compared with the other displacements. This is not a matter of any importance, and is at best merely a statistical formality. Suffice it to say that prolapsus uteri in the minor degrees, associated with both anteversion and retrodisplacement, is one of the most common forms of malposition of the uterus. In its second and third degrees it is also very common, being confined almost exclusively to the parous woman.

**Significance.**—It stands to reason that the greater the degree of prolapsus the greater its influence upon the comfort of the woman. Prolapsus of the first degree will probably produce but very slight discomfort, except in the feeling of weight and bearing down which it entails. The inconvenience of prolapsus of the second degree is greater in proportion, and that of the third degree need merely be mentioned to be appreciated. A woman with a uterus and vagina hanging between her thighs; with the

---

[1] I was amused to see a recent article by a Frenchman with a Russian name (which I do not remember) in which the writer reported as a novel and most excellent device this same elastic compression of a prolapsed uterus. It never even occurred to me to report so simple a method.

external os lacerated, eroded, bleeding, discharging; with the prolapsed vaginal walls toughened and ulcerated in places; and with the constant sensation of losing all her "insides," so to speak, cannot be considered to be in a very comfortable position. It is not that such women are going to die from their ailment; but the greater its degree the less real comfort will they derive from life so long as they are on their feet and the downward dragging of the displaced organ exerts its pernicious influence. Really dangerous results do not accompany or follow prolapsus uteri. Malignant disease of the uterus is no more commonly found in prolapsus than when the uterus is in its normal position. Sterility, even, is not always the result, since women have been known to become pregnant in whom the uterus was entirely prolapsed. But we must not forget that, besides the uterus, the bladder and rectum are also prolapsed, and it is the bladder chiefly which gives rise to decided symptoms. The stagnation of the urine in the prolapsed portion of the bladder causes decomposition of that fluid, irritation of the vesical mucous membrane, and in time cystitis, which is in itself quite sufficient to render the patient miserable, irrespective of the prolapsus of the uterus and rectum. Further, accumulation of fæces in the prolapsed portion of the rectum may also give rise to more or less inconvenience. In short, a woman with a completely prolapsed uterus must be considered to be more or less a chronic invalid.

Diagnosis.—The diagnosis of prolapsus of the uterus is, of course, exceedingly easy. It requires merely a practised finger to be enabled to determine that the cervix uteri is lower in the pelvic cavity than it should be; and even a layman can recognize in the large ovoid, glistening, more or less eroded body lying outside of the vulva a complete prolapse of the uterus and vagina. A sound passed into the uterus will verify the fact that it is the uterus which is prolapsed. Still, there may be an opportunity for error as regards the presence of a true prolapse, in that, as already mentioned, the supra-vaginal portion of the cervix may be hypertrophied, and, having grown downward together with the attached anterior and posterior vaginal walls, may simulate a real prolapse of the uterus, whereas the condition is one of hypertrophy of the cervix and prolapse of the vagina, the body of the uterus remaining about at its normal altitude in the pelvis. The sound introduced to the fundus uteri will reveal the correct diagnosis, since it will be found that two-thirds of this seemingly prolapsed organ is cervix and only one-third body, and that the fundus retains its normal elevation in the pelvic cavity.

Prognosis.—Taken as a rule, prolapsus uteri of the first and second degrees, unless relieved by proper mechanical and operative procedures, will eventually result in a prolapse of the organ to the third degree. A cure of the displacement is scarcely to be expected by natural means,—that is to say, by a spontaneous restoration to the normal position,—with one exception,—namely, the possibility that the processes of involution which follow parturition may, under proper precautions, restore the uterus and its ligaments to their normal position and tone. A prolapsus of the third degree will probably never be cured by the efforts of nature alone. As I have already said, there is nothing necessarily prejudicial to life in prolapsus uteri of any degree, and a woman with her uterus and vagina dangling between her thighs may thus attain the age of a hundred years, so far as this pathological condition is concerned.

**Treatment.**—The treatment of prolapsus uteri is either palliative or radical. Among the palliative measures for the minor degrees of prolapsus are, in the recent cases, astringent injections, tampons applied to the vagina, chiefly in the genu-pectoral position, with the view to contracting the parts and restoring them to their normal tone. As prolapsus in the minor degrees is associated with anteversion and retrodisplacement, so will the pessaries which have been described as adapted to these conditions also be useful for these forms of prolapsus. When it comes to a prolapsus of the second degree and, finally, of the third degree, I confess that mechanical and palliative means have had but very poor success in my hands. Undoubtedly, in the more recent cases, when there is still a possibility of the relaxed ligaments and supports regaining their tone, a systematic contraction of the vaginal walls by astringent tampons *may* in the course of time result in cure. If one could keep such women in the genu-pectoral position, or with their hips so elevated that the vaginal vault would be on a deeper level than the vaginal orifice for a sufficient length of time to allow the organs to regain their tone, one might cure such cases simply by posture. I understand from Emmet that among the Southern negroes it was customary in old times to suspend women with prolapsus uteri et vaginæ in hammocks with their hips elevated in the manner described, and then to fill their vaginæ with a decoction of oak bark, which was left there for several weeks, the object of this treatment being to produce contraction of the vaginal walls and a cure of the prolapsus. I doubt whether our society ladies would be willing to subject themselves to such heroic treatment, however effectual it might be. Electricity in the shape of the faradic current applied to the vaginal walls and uterine ligaments, and systematic massage, have many advocates and seem to have a certain measure of plausibility in their favor. I confess that I have never had the patience to submit my patients to so protracted and uncertain a course of treatment. I have already referred to pregnancy as a possible cure of prolapsus, owing to the return of the organs to their normal tone during puerperal involution.

*Pessaries.*—There has been no form of displacement which has evolved so many varieties of mechanical supports for its relief and cure as prolapsus uteri. From time immemorial the text-books and instrument-makers' shops have been full of these contrivances, many of them of the most fantastic and barbarous description. A collection of the instruments of torture of an old chamber of inquisition could scarcely surpass in horror the implements which human ingenuity has devised for the cure of prolapsus uteri, and some of the modern text-books still reproduce a few of the less horrible relics. Thus, Zwanck's pessary is still found here and there; but nothing is said, if I remember aright, of the cases in which it gradually worked its way through the vaginal wall into the bladder or rectum, although it undoubtedly kept up very well the prolapsed uterus. Our medical journals teem with the advertisements and pictures of complicated vagino-abdominal supporters for prolapsus; cups of different shapes and rings more or less ingeniously constructed and supported, attached to vaginal stems which again connect with belts, are seen daily, even at present. And still I regret to say that I am obliged to consider each and all of these contrivances to be absolutely useless and injurious. I do not know one of them which will permanently keep up a totally prolapsed uterus and vagina with comfort and without injury to the patient. They all, in course of time, produce excoriation and ulceration of the vaginal wall where they exert their pressure, and have to be removed until the wound is healed. None of them, it is certain, ever produces a cure. I cannot, therefore, conscientiously recommend any one of these numerous supports. Indeed, I know nothing better for the retention of a completely prolapsed uterus and vagina than a large

FIG. 48.　　　　　　　　　FIG. 49.

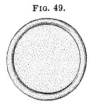

Ring pessary for prolapsus (inflated rubber).　　Peaslee's ring pessary.

hard-rubber, glass, or wooden ring (aluminum is a good metal for this purpose) which retains the uterus in the pelvic cavity simply by its size, and which can easily be removed and replaced by the patient every night or several times a week. If this is not done, ulceration of the vagina is pretty sure to result. A well-fitting vulvar pad, retained in place by a T-bandage, will materially aid in keeping the vaginal disk in position. I do not advise these makeshifts, because they certainly do not cure; but I know no other form of pessary which, to my mind, is equally simple, satisfactory, and safe.

There is one exception, however, and that applies solely to the cases of prolapsus where cystocele or prolapsus of the anterior vaginal wall and bladder is the main feature besides the prolapse of the uterus. In these cases a Gehrung pessary of larger size, such as I have described in speaking of anteversion and anteflexion, will retain easily, permanently, and without pain the anterior vaginal wall and bladder and with it the uterus. This is by all odds the simplest and most effectual support for prolapsus with which I am acquainted. If the patient can be induced to introduce every morning into her vagina, while she occupies the recumbent position, a large cotton wad covered with vaseline and rolled in a mixture of iodoform and tannin, equal parts, pressing this well up into the pelvic cavity and retaining it in position by a T-bandage, she will probably derive as much satisfaction and comfort, with the possible chance of a return of tone of the vaginal walls, as she can from any other form of support. The trouble is that I have been unable to induce patients to carry even this simple plan out with any degree of system, regularity, or perseverance. They want to be relieved by some easy, less troublesome plan.

For mild forms of descensus, with or without retroversion, the simple elastic ring of wire strands devised by Peaslee answers very well, or the Hitchcock pessary. (See Figs. 49 and 13.)

*Operative Treatment.*—Our object in carrying out the operative cure of prolapsus uteri et vaginæ must be based on three cardinal principles: 1, the diminution in size of the uterus; 2, the restoration of the tone of the uterine ligaments; and, 3, the repair of the uterine supports,—that is, vagina and perineum.

1. The diminution in size of the uterus can be attained by two measures, —namely, amputation of the cervix, and repair of the laceration of the cervix. If a uterus measures, instead of two and a half, five or six inches or more, and that increase is due mostly to hypertrophy of the supra-vaginal portion of the cervix, it stands to reason that that is the part of the organ from which the reduction should be made. This condition is found only in cases of prolapsus of the second and chiefly of the third degree, and it is, therefore, to these degrees that this operation is applicable. I have been in the habit, in such cases, of making a circular incision around the cervix, just above the junction of the vaginal wall to the cervical mucous membrane, pushing up the bladder in front and the rectum or the vaginal wall alone behind with the finger, until as much of the cervix was exposed as I thought necessary to remove, and have then amputated the cervix at that point with the galvano-cautery wire, pushed the stump up into the vaginal vault, passed a strip of iodoform gauze into the cervical canal so as to prevent its complete closure, and packed the vagina with iodoform gauze. The result of this operation was that in the course of cicatricial contraction the cervix and adjacent portions of the vagina remained high up in the pelvic cavity and thus a cure of the prolapsus was attained. Of course I was careful to aid this cure by supporting the vaginal roof for a number of weeks with iodoform gauze, introduced twice a week or thereabouts, or with a soft ring pessary. Recently I have been adopting a different plan, where I was afraid that cicatrization from the cautery might produce closure of the external os,—that is, in women below the menopause,—namely, amputating the exposed portion of the cervix with the knife or scissors, and sewing the vaginal walls over and to the cervix at each side with deep catgut sutures which were so passed as to keep the external os open. The advantage of the extensive cicatricial contraction following the galvano-cautery was lost in these cases, but the possibility of their conceiving was

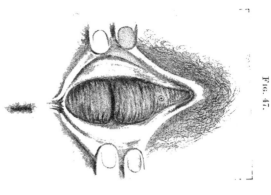

Fig. 47.

Front view of cystocele and rectocele.

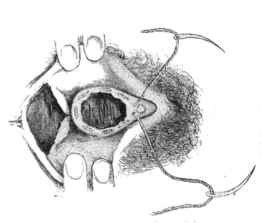

Fig. 50.

Front view of Stoltz's operation for cystocele, with circular suture inserted, and of Hegar's operation for rectocele and lacerated perineum.

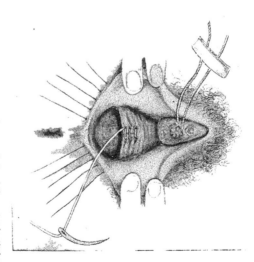

Fig. 51.

The same, with the cystocele-suture tied and the rectocele stitches partly introduced, showing method of running suture of the denudation on the posterior wall.

still left open to them, which, I admit, may be considered a doubtful advantage after all, in view of the probable future return of the prolapsus after a subsequent confinement. In addition to this latter operation,—that is, where the galvano-cautery was not used,—I have constricted both the anterior and posterior walls by plastic operations in order to make the retention of the uterus trebly sure.

The closure of the laceration of the cervix should be practised in every case of prolapsus, no matter of what degree. Its object is not only to restore the cervix to its normal condition and cure such uterine catarrh as may be present, but also to stimulate the organ to a diminution in size, —a result which is well known to follow this operation. As these remarks are intended to cover mainly the results of my own experience, I will here state that my usual practice for a number of years, in cases of prolapsus uteri of the second and third degrees where there was a lacerated cervix, a prolapsus uteri, a prolapse of the anterior and posterior vaginal walls, and laceration of the perineum, has been to perform at one sitting the following operations, in the order given : first, trachelorrhaphy ; second, Alexander's for shortening the round ligaments ; third, Stoltz's for narrowing the anterior wall of the vagina (circular denudation, tobacco-pouch suture) ; fourth, Hegar's for rectocele and ruptured perineum (triangular denudation, upper angle near the cervix, two lower angles on respective labia). In these operations I have used catgut for the cervix, silkworm-gut for the Alexander, silk for the Stoltz, catgut running suture for the intra-vaginal portion, and silkworm-gut for the perineal portion of Hegar's operation. This combination of operations, of course, takes some time, say from one to two hours, but the results have been in my hands so good, particularly if I was careful to keep the patients for a long time on their backs, say three to four weeks until solid cicatrization had taken place, that I have seen no occasion to adopt any other form of operation for complete prolapsus uteri. Fritsch, Freund, Martin, Bischof, Thomas Addis Emmet, and other operators too numerous to mention have each devised some modification and some new method of denudation and suture for retaining the prolapsed uterus in position. Their operations are all based more or less upon the same principle of narrowing the anterior and posterior walls of the vagina and closing the vaginal orifice so as to prevent the vagina from relaxing and the uterus from prolapsing again. The operations are too complicated for me to detail here. From a very extensive experience I have really never found it necessary to practise any of them, except merely as an experiment, and have been quite satisfied with the combination of operations which I have above detailed. It goes without saying that an absolute and scrupulous attention to antiseptic details is indispensable to the success of these as of all plastic operations.

There is one great objection to all plastic operations, no matter by whom devised, for the cure of prolapsus uteri et vaginæ, and that is, if the patient subjects herself again within a year or two to the same influences which originally produced the prolapsus,—namely, parturition, carrying heavy weights, straining, and similar factors,—the prolapse is liable to return. I do not, therefore, feel that the ideal operation for prolapsus uteri et vaginæ has yet been discovered,—namely, one which will restore the organs to such firmness and stability that they are able to withstand all the strains which should naturally be put upon the virginal pelvic organs.

The above operations are not of a dangerous character under proper precautions; but another class of operative procedures for prolapsus uteri has been devised of which the same cannot be said. Two operations are comprised in this category: the one is, sewing the fundus uteri to the abdominal walls, to which may be added restoration of the vagina and perineum; and the second is hysterectomy or extirpation of the prolapsed uterus. Neither operation need necessarily be said to be absolutely dangerous to life; still, I have lost one patient from tympanites and consequent heart-failure after ventral fixation for prolapsus, who, so far as I know, would be alive to-day if I had not operated on her; and vaginal hysterectomy for prolapsus cannot either be considered to be entirely without its risks. I certainly shall never again employ ventral fixation of a prolapsed uterus, because usually in such cases the abdominal walls are so relaxed that even if the fundus uteri remains attached it will gradually drag down its abdominal attachment, producing a funnel-shaped depression, and the cervix will again protrude from the vulva. Vaginal hysterectomy, however, I think has a future before it, which is limited mostly to old cases in which the relaxation of the tissues seems to offer very slight hope of a permanent cure by the plastic operations above mentioned. As a general rule, I should not advocate plastic operations of any kind for the restoration of the parts to their normal condition in women long beyond the menopause, for the simple reason that such senile tissues are not very favorable for permanent results.

A very ingenious operation has recently been recommended by Herman Freund, which consists in constricting the vagina from above downward by a series of circular sutures of silkworm-gut, which are entirely buried. The ends are cut short and the sutures left for good. It is, of course, applicable only to old women beyond the menopause in whom the vagina has ceased to be of practical use. I have performed the operation once on a woman sixty-seven years of age, using strong silver wire. I found it quite easy of execution and exceedingly effective so far as retention of uterus and vagina goes. I left a narrow passage for the escape of possible utero-vaginal secretions.

### INVERSION OF THE UTERUS.

**Definition.**—By inversion of the uterus is meant a more or less complete turning inside out of the body of the organ, so that in the complete degree the fundus uteri occupies a position lower than that of the cervix.

**Degrees.**—There are generally accepted but two degrees of inversion, —namely, the incomplete and the complete: the incomplete representing all the various degrees from that of a slight denting inward of a portion of the body down to an inversion where the fundus touches the internal os; the complete implying the passage of the entirely inverted organ through the cervical canal into the vagina.

**Causes.**—These are either acute or chronic. The chief cause of *acute* inversion of the uterus of the complete variety is puerperal, the fundus uteri either being forced through the cervix into the vagina by spontaneous contractions of the uterus or by traction on the cord of the adherent placenta by the obstetric attendant. The chief cause of *chronic* inversion of the uterus, either of the incomplete or the complete variety, is the forcing downward by uterine contractions of a fibroid tumor situated near the fundus uteri (usually incomplete inversion) and the drawing through the cervical canal of the tumor and the fundus by instruments in the hands of the operator (complete inversion). When a fibroid tumor inverts the uterus, so long as the inversion is incomplete, it usually starts from one side of the uterus where the tumor happens to be attached. It is only when the efforts of nature alone force the tumor down into the vagina or the operator draws it down that the inversion becomes complete. Chronic inversion of the uterus, either partial or complete, may occupy a number of months in its accomplishment.

FIG. 52.

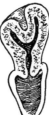

FIG. 53.

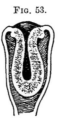

Incomplete inversion of uterus.    Complete inversion of uterus.

**Frequency.**—Puerperal inversion is not so commonly met with by the gynæcologist, because at the present day general practitioners are more apt to make a physical examination if anything unexpected occurs, and therefore, discovering the inversion, proceed at once to rectify it. Still, in a practice of twenty-five years I remember having met with seven such cases in which the condition had been entirely overlooked by the obstetric physician and subsequent attendants. Inversion of the chronic variety, particularly of the partial degree, is very much more common, since fibroid tumors situated at or near the fundus uteri and projecting into the uterine cavity are very frequent. I have certainly seen dozens of such cases, and make it a universal rule when I find a fibroid tumor projecting into the uterine cavity or from the external os, to carefully examine the fundus uteri in order to make out whether an inversion of the body of the organ exists or not. Complete inversion of the chronic variety is frequent in proportion to the forcing or drawing down of the tumor into the vagina, either before or during the operation for its removal.

**Significance.**—Inversion of the complete variety, when of puerperal origin, is of supreme importance, since the symptoms which it produces—

that is, chiefly prolonged and violent hemorrhage—weaken the patient so much that she will eventually succumb to the strain if not relieved. Inversion of the non-puerperal variety is in itself of little consequence, since it is but the result of another, more serious, causative element,—namely, the fibroid tumor,—which, to be sure, produces the same symptoms,—namely, hemorrhage; but on removal of the tumor, if this can be done without injuring the uterine wall, the reposition of the inversion is easily effected and the displacement in itself loses all significance.

**Symptoms.**—As I have just stated, the symptoms of inversion are comprised in one word,—hemorrhage,—whether the hemorrhage comes from the simple inverted uterus or from the fibroid tumor complicating and producing the inversion. Bearing down, feeling of weight, "dropping" sensation in the pelvis, are of course natural symptoms.

**Diagnosis.**—The patient presents herself for vaginal hemorrhage, and examination reveals a pear-shaped, oblong body more or less filling the vaginal canal and terminating above in the circle of the cervix uteri. This body bleeds on manipulation, is soft, semi-elastic to the touch, more or less painful. Bimanual palpation, if it can be thoroughly carried out, shows an absence of the uterine body in its normal position above the pubis. A sound passed into the groove within the cervical circle fails to enter the uterine cavity. The peculiarly shaped body in the vagina, the absence of the body of the uterus above the pubis, the failure of the sound to enter into the uterine cavity,—these three points combined make the positive diagnosis of inversion of the uterus. A rectal examination can, if necessary, be made to confirm the absence of the body of the uterus in its normal position. In incomplete inversion a more or less irregular body is felt in the vaginal canal; on bimanual examination an irregular mass corresponding to the body of the uterus, but indented on one side, is felt above the symphysis pubis, and the sound enters to a limited depth,—that is, instead of two and a half inches, only one and a half or two inches. Pulling down by the fingers or volsellum the body felt in the vagina, this depression of the mass felt above the symphysis is increased. The sound will enter to the opposite side from where the depression is, perhaps to its normal depth, showing that the depth of the uterine cavity on the side of the depression is diminished. This would naturally point towards a partial inversion.

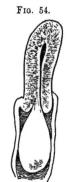

Fig. 54.

Polypus simulating complete inversion of uterus.

**Differential Diagnosis.**—A tumor corresponding exactly in shape and size to the inverted uterus may be found in the vaginal canal; the relations of it to the cervix and its ring are exactly similar to those of inversion, and the uterine sound does not pass into the canal. The thick or rigid abdominal walls prevent thorough bimanual palpation, even under an anæsthetic. The thick walls may not allow the examiner to clearly map out the body of the uterus, supposing it to be in its normal position. The vaginal tumor is not particularly sensitive, whereas the inverted uterus usually is quite tender to the touch; but it bleeds, and the patient's history does not give any distinct information as to the occurrence of this condition. Now, how is the examiner to ascertain what he has before him; whether it is a complete inversion of the uterus, or a uterine polypus which has forced its way into the vagina and more or less inverted the body of the uterus? This question is often exceedingly difficult of decision. I have seen men as prominent as Emmet, Barker, Isaac E. Taylor, Lusk, and Scanzoni at fault as to the exact nature of the case until an attempt at removal revealed the true facts. The explanation for the failure of the sound to pass up into the uterine canal in case of a polypus is that agglutination of the pedicle of the polypus may take place to the adjacent wall of the cervix and thus close the uterine canal entirely. I have myself had a very close escape from attempting to replace a uterine polypus in a case of this kind, and was finally saved the discomfiture of a mistaken diagnosis by fortunately, under repeated anæsthesia, being able to map out the rudimentary body of the uterus above the symphysis pubis. Feeling sure of this, I then, of course, forced my way into the uterine cavity through the adhesions at the side of the pedicle of the polypus. When one is in doubt in such cases it is a safe plan not to attempt to remove the supposed polypus, but to submit the patient to another examination (as I once saw Emmet do a week after his first unsatisfactory exploration), and then with a calm, judicial mind endeavor to arrive at a true conclusion and proceed accordingly. To amputate the inverted uterus would be a great and almost criminal error; and to attempt to replace a uterine polypus would be about as grave an error, certainly a very ridiculous one.

Prognosis.—Very little need be said on this subject, since, with scarcely an exception, a completely inverted uterus never of its own accord returns to its normal position; therefore, so long as the inversion continues and it proves to be unreplaceable, the prognosis as regards cure is bad, although the patient may live for a length of time,—that is to say, so long as her strength can resist the loss of blood. I say, with scarcely an exception, because there are several—not more than two or three—curious cases on record in which a puerperally inverted uterus was spontaneously reduced during straining efforts made by the patient at stool and otherwise. Spiegelberg reports such a case. The prognosis of partial inversion accompanying uterine polypus is, of course, dependent entirely upon the removal of the tumor.

Treatment.—An acute inversion of puerperal origin does not properly come within our province. I may, of course, state that its immediate return is the only proper treatment, and that a neglect to do so is a grave error on the part of the practitioner. Chronic complete inversion should, of course, be reduced as soon as recognized.

The methods for such reduction are manual, instrumental, and opera-

tive. The *manual* methods consist in placing the patient under an anæsthetic and with the hand in the vagina compressing the body of the uterus,
either pushing the fundus upward or first attempting to return one horn or
the other, while the fingers of the other hand exert counter-pressure through
the abdominal walls and attempt to dilate the ring at the cervix, which
forms the great obstacle to the reposition of the organ. Emmet and Sims
recommended pushing the fundus uteri straight up; Noeggerath first advised
pressing up one of the horns of the uterus. The object is, of course, to
dilate with the outer fingers the infundibulum or ring of the cervix sufficiently to enable the vaginal fingers to press the inverted body through it.
Once the ring being passed by a certain portion of the body of the uterus,

FIG. 55.

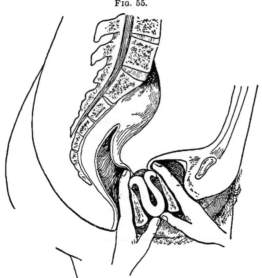

Tate's method of reducing an inverted uterus.

its complete reposition is easily effected. This manipulation, however, is
by no means as easy as it seems to be. I have never met with an obstacle
in surgery so difficult to overcome as the constricted ring of an inverted
uterus. Hence, Tate, of Cincinnati, recommended passing one index finger
into the rectum, the other index finger through the dilated urethra into the
bladder, both these fingers to meet in the ring of the cervix and both
thumbs pressing against the fundus uteri in the vagina. By conjoined
stretching of the cervical ring and upward pushing of the thumbs in the
vagina the fundus uteri is to be forced through the dilated ring and restored
to its normal position. Tate succeeded, if I remember right, in replacing
a uterus which had been inverted for forty years. No operator must be
disappointed if he fails in the manual reduction of an inverted uterus at

the first attempt, but he must try and try again until he is satisfied that efforts of this kind are positively ineffectual.

*Instrumental.*—Finding that manual reposition was often ineffectual, a number of ingenious minds have devised instruments by which a steady pressure could be effected upon the inverted fundus uteri, while a dilating counter-pressure was exercised upon the cervical ring, the steady pressure being exerted, not by the hand of the operator in the vagina, but by a cup-shaped instrument which received the body of the uterus and which was connected with a spring placed against the chest of the operator. Instruments of this kind were devised by White, of Buffalo, and Byrne, of Brooklyn, and have each been successful. Wing, of Boston, succeeded with a very ingenious device represented by a conical plug surmounted by a thick rubber ring which was passed into the vagina over and against the fundus, and to the outer end of which were attached stout rubber tubes which were again fixed to the posterior surface of a bandage passed around the waist of the patient. The steady pressure exerted by the elastic traction of these tubes upon the plug in the vagina succeeded after twenty-four hours or more in gradually overcoming the resistance of the cervical ring against the return of the uterus, and the reposition of the inverted organ was thus effected. Packing the vagina with wool or cotton wads or iodoform gauze has also, I believe, been effectual in gradually reducing an inverted uterus.

*Operative.*—The only operative measure which has been proposed for the reduction of the inverted uterus is one carried out by Thomas many years ago, which consisted in opening the abdominal cavity, stretching the cervical ring with a glove-stretcher, while at the same time the intra-vaginal hand forced the fundus uteri through the ring and into its normal place. Thomas operated on two such cases, I believe, with success; but the dangers of the operation, which I should imagine at the time he performed it must have consisted mostly in the abdominal section itself, seem to have deterred the majority of surgeons from following his example. At the present day the fact that the abdominal cavity has to be opened in order to permit this manoeuvre should certainly not deter us from its adoption, if we fail by the other more common methods. I myself have had the opportunity to attempt this method of Thomas in a case which baffled all other efforts at reduction. The inversion had been subjected to repeated attempts by other operators before I saw the patient. I made two attempts under anæsthesia and failed, and finally, having become completely worn out and feeling sure that the body of the uterus would not stand any more manipulation without the risk of perforation, opened the abdominal cavity, dilated the ring with two glove-stretchers, and tried to push the fundus through the thus dilated ring; but it proved impossible. As soon as the glove-stretchers were removed in order to allow the uterus to pass through, the ring contracted like a vice, and I was obliged to give up the attempt. I then passed a Peaslee's needle through the abdominal incision into the inverted uterus and out of the

fundus into the vagina, attached a strong silk ligature to the needle, armed
with a button of lead to act as a fulcrum upon the fundus and enable me
to draw it through the cervical ring; but on attempting traction the uterine
tissue at the fundus, rendered soft by the many manipulations, gave way,
and the button was pulled through and out of the abdominal incision.
Nothing else remained for me then but to remove the ovaries, close the
abdominal incision, and apply an elastic ligature around the body of the
uterus as near the external os as was possible. The patient made a perfectly uneventful recovery, the uterus sloughing off on the thirteenth day.
I cannot exactly recommend this procedure, but under the circumstances I
do not see what else I could have done.

Amputation of the inverted uterus should always be considered as a
last resort, to be performed only when all other measures have failed. If
amputation is to be done, I think that, for my part, the elastic ligature is
superior to any other method, because it gradually by adhesive agglutination closes the peritoneal cavity, and when the stump sloughs away there is
no danger of infection of the peritoneum.

### HERNIA UTERI.

Merely as a matter of completeness I will refer to a very peculiar and,
fortunately, very rare accident which must be logically classed under the
head of uterine displacements,—namely, a displacement of the uterus into
the sac of an inguinal hernia. There are only five such cases on record,
one of which it was my fortune to see when assistant to Professor Scanzoni
at Würzburg in 1868. An additional interest was added to the case by
the fact that the woman was four months pregnant, having probably become
so before the uterus was thus displaced. In consequence of the danger of
rupture of the pregnant uterus, together with its hernial sac and skin, by
advice of Scanzoni an abortion was induced by me by means of a catheter,
which I with much difficulty succeeded in passing into the uterine cavity.
The uterus, of course, rapidly diminished in size and practically lost its
importance to us and to the patient, with whose further career I am
unacquainted. Winckel performed Porro's operation on a woman for a
similar indication, with recovery.

# CHAPTER X.

## NEOPLASMS OF THE VULVA AND VAGINA.

BY HERMANN J. BOLDT, M.D.

### CONDYLOMATA.

THE most frequent new growths on the vulva are the condylomata, often called papillomata. They may be divided into two varieties: 1. Simple papillomata, or ordinary warts, which are non-specific, and cause no annoyance, except, very rarely, by their size. No particular cause is known for their occurrence. Their usual site is on the labia majora and the mons veneris. 2. Pointed condylomata, or condylomata acuminata.

.FIG. 1.

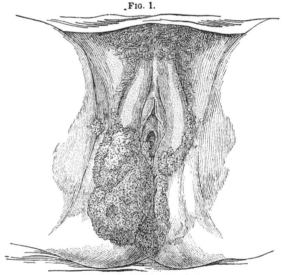

Condyloma of vulva. (Tarnier.)

In structure the simple papillomata resemble ordinary warts; they vary in size from that of a pin-head to that of a fœtal head, and when isolated they project so prominently that the name "cock's comb" has been applied to them. When a number of condylomata coalesce, they resemble in shape a head of cauliflower.

527

They are most frequently situated upon the vulva and around the anus, but they also occur on the perineum, and occasionally in the vagina. Fowlerton reports a case in which the papillomata blocked up the vagina, causing obstruction to coitus. Their color is usually a very pale pink, but the vegetations may assume a dark and occasionally a turgid hue.

The flat condylomata (*plaques muqueuses*), which are not tumors in the proper sense of the word, are invariably caused by syphilis; and in women they not infrequently represent the primary form of the disease.

The condylomata acuminata, or pointed condylomata, it is taught, may occur independently of gonorrhœal infection. The correctness of this teaching is doubtful: I have never seen a case in which a specific source could not be traced with reasonable certainty. The argument brought forward as conclusive evidence that these growths do occur without venereal infection is, that they occur occasionally in chaste women during pregnancy, usually disappearing spontaneously after labor. Though the woman be chaste, that does not make the husband so. Observation has shown their occurrence even in children, although bacteriologists have not yet succeeded in proving the presence of gonococci in pointed condylomata. The case reported by Marshall as papilloma in a child two years old admits of some doubt as to the exact nature of the neoplasm.

Their spontaneous disappearance after parturition is accounted for by the changes which take place in the circulation of the parts, but such disappearance is not the rule, neither is it advisable to wait for it, on account of the danger of ophthalmia in the new-born infant, resulting from infection. The prognosis is favorable.

In the treatment of these condylomata cleanliness must be observed. Locally, pure tannic acid is one of the best astringents. Any astringent, however, will act beneficially. The preferable treatment is surgical. It is best to cut them off with scissors and to touch the base of the wound with nitrate of silver, perchloride of iron, or the actual cautery, to control the usually rather profuse hemorrhage.

We must also employ other local treatment to allay the vaginal discharge. I prefer for this purpose a solution of nitrate of silver 1 : 20 to 1 : 30, used locally with an absorbent cotton swab over the vaginal mucosa, or to fill the vagina with subnitrate of bismuth every second day, using a douche of 1 : 2000 hot sublimate solution prior to the insufflation.

### LIPOMA.

Fatty tumors have their origin either in the labium majus or in the mons veneris; they sometimes attain large dimensions, causing inconvenience to the patient. Thus, Strigele removed one weighing ten pounds; Deekens reports a lipoma the size of a lemon which underwent an ulcerative process and caused dangerous hemorrhage. I have removed one weighing ten ounces, which was attached to the left labium majus by a pedicle two inches long. (See Fig. 2.) In this case the tumor was not altogether of fat tissue, the lobules of the latter being enveloped with a fibrous connective tissue: hence the designation fibro-lipoma.

These tumors may be mistaken for fibromata and elephantiasis. From the former they are distinguished by their elasticity, which is quite characteristic on palpation; from the latter, by being circumscribed and usually pedunculated, which is rare in elephantiasis. The derma at the base of the tumor is changed in elephantiasis and is normal in lipoma.

FIG. 2.

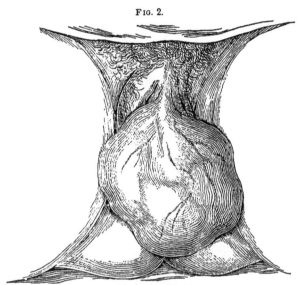

Lipoma of vulva.

The treatment is surgical; they are readily removed. If attached by a thin pedicle, as in my case, a ligature is placed around this and the tumor is snipped off. If there is a broad base, the growth must be excised and its bed stitched, preferably with a continuous catgut suture.

### MYOMA, FIBROMA, MYO-FIBROMA, MYXOMA, AND MIXED GROWTHS.

These tumors have their origin ordinarily in the labium majus, although they are not limited to this part, being sometimes situated on the nymphæ. They are composed mainly of fibrous connective tissue, with some muscular structure; the latter is presumably derived from fibres of the round ligament or the numerous muscle-bundles of the derma. In appearance they do not differ from the lipomata previously described.

Myxomata occur occasionally in the same locality, and are so designated on account of the preponderance of myxomatous tissue.

Mixed varieties occur, as myxo-lipoma and myo-fibroma.

These tumors have a tendency to increase slightly in size during pregnancy and menstruation, but usually diminish to their former volume after the subsidence of these processes, unless, as occasionally happens, a hemorrhage takes place into their interior, when the increase in size is sudden and permanent; otherwise their growth is slow.

FIG. 3.

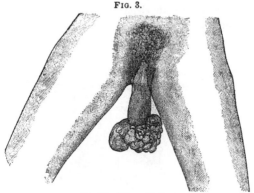

Fibroid polypus of vulva.

Inasmuch as their tendency is to grow in the direction of least resistance, it is not unusual for them to become pedunculated; they sometimes reach as low as the knees: under such circumstances it is not uncommon for inflammation and ulceration of the surfaces to occur, as the result of friction. They are benign, and their treatment is surgical, being the same as for lipoma. The removal of the growths, if done with ordinary care, is devoid of danger.

### ELEPHANTIASIS VULVÆ.

The disease may affect the entire vulva, or only a part of it: if the growth is limited, which is usually the case, its location is generally the labia majora, next the clitoris; the labia minora are rarely affected. In our climate we seldom see the affection, but in the tropics it is not infrequent. Sometimes these tumors attain an enormous size, reaching in weight from twenty to thirty or more pounds, and extending down to the knees. As a rule, they are attached by a broad base, but they may be pedunculated. Several cases are reported of congenital elephantiasis, but this is exceptional. Nahde's case showed a few red spots on the labia majora at the time of birth. When the infant was six weeks old the growth was as large as a pear, and at fifteen weeks it was as large as a child's head. The most frequent period of development of acquired elephantiasis is between the ages of twenty and thirty years, but the disease may occur at any time.

Pathology.—Histologically several varieties of this disease occur, but they all have one element in common,—namely, a change in the lymphatic circulation. The lymph-vessels are dilated and indurated from the beginning. There are repeated attacks of lymphangitis, which ultimately result in a hyperplasia of the entire derma and subcutaneous connective tissue. In some cases (L. Heitzmann) microscopical examination does not reveal enlargement of the papillæ nor increase of epithelium. In so-called soft elephantiasis the superficial structures are prominently myxomatous; the deeper layers are myxo-fibrous, with various stages of transition from one tissue-form to the other. The lymphatics are very numerous and dilated and at places cyst-like, so that one might speak of them as lymph-angiomata. They are partly empty and partly filled with

FIG. 4.

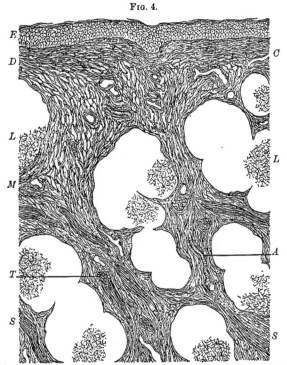

Elephantiasis of labium majus, or mvxo-lvmph-angioma, × 100.—*E*, stratified epithelium on surface; *D*, dense mvxo-fibrous tissue beneath epithelium; *M*, mvxo-fibrous connective tissue; *S, S*, smooth muscle-bundles, in longitudinal section; *T*, bundle of smooth muscle-fibres, in transverse section; *A*, arterv; *C*, capillarv blood-vessel; *L, L*, lvmph-vessels, partlv filled with coagulated fibrin.

lymph-corpuscles, between which a delicate net-work of coagulated fibrin and varying quantities of coagulated, finely granular albumen are recognizable.

The myxomatous and myxo-fibrous structure is largely saturated with a sero-albuminous fluid, which exudes in large quantity when the tumor is cut into. The blood-vessels consist principally of much enlarged capillaries, and are scarce. Their endothelia, as well as those lining the walls of the lymphatics, are unusually large.

In the hard tumors, delicate fibrillated connective tissue predominates and muscle tissue is scanty, whereas the latter is abundant in the myxomatous variety. The lymphatics, although dilated, are not increased, but the blood-vessels are numerous, especially the arterioles. The capillaries are not dilated; numerous nests of inflammatory corpuscles are conspicuous, especially around the arterioles. There exist combinations of tissues. When inflammatory changes with new formations occur first in the superficial layers predominating in the papillæ, that form of tumor is produced which strongly resembles the large coalescing condylomata sometimes found in pregnant women.

The large tumors are liable to extensive ulceration from local irritation, so that they may occasionally give rise to difficulty in diagnosis. The warty form, besides being a source of great annoyance from the accumulation of repulsive secretions, may undergo malignant degeneration.

Fig. 5.

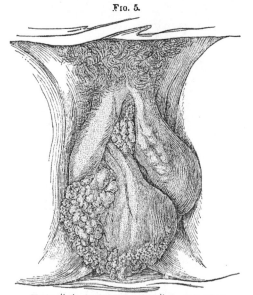

Elephantiasis of vulva, before operation. (Schroeder.)

**Etiology.**—The causative factors are quite numerous, but all hinge on the same principle,—a local irritation. Thus, syphilis, traumatism, local inflammation, as pruritus, eczema, or recurrent attacks of dermatitis, may be enumerated; but any of these conditions must produce an inflammation and obstruction of the lymphatics in order to give rise to elephantiasis. The direct cause is considered to be the presence of a parasite, the filaria sanguinis hominis, in the blood and lymphatics of the parts affected.

**Symptoms.**—The invasion of the disease is marked by local inflammation, which ceases later, when the tumor has attained a moderate size.

The growth does not annoy the patient until it has reached a size sufficient to produce inconvenience and pain by reason of its weight. Tumors which reach to the base of the urethra usually produce incontinence of urine. Verrucose or papillary tumors are especially annoying because of secretions accumulating between the projections of the papillæ. Ulcerations, although not infrequent, have a tendency to heal spontaneously if the parts are kept clean. In some cases very large quantities of sero-albuminous fluid exude from the neoplasm, necessitating frequent changes of clothing and the wearing of napkins. Eventually the general health of the patient will become more or less undermined, according to the amount and kind of discomfort caused by the tumor.

The prognosis as to longevity is good, although the tumors, when once established, never disappear spontaneously. They seldom recur if excised. The inguinal glands are always enlarged.

FIG. 6.

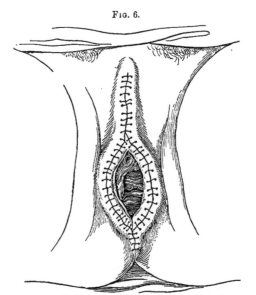

Elephantiasis of vulva, after operation. (Schroeder.)

Diagnosis.—If the pathology is borne in mind the diagnosis can readily be made. As stated under the head of etiology, frequent attacks of local inflammation mark the beginning, which cause the derma to be very much thickened, and consequently large condylomatous tumors which might otherwise be mistaken for the products of elephantiasis are distinguished from them by the presence of normal skin around the base of the condyloma. Ulcerated tumors may be mistaken for malignant growths and hypertrophic lupus. The microscope will aid in deciding the question if the clinical history alone is not satisfactory. The characteristic forms of the latter diseases as compared with elephantiasis should be sufficient. We must not forget, however, that one variety of elephantiasis may become carcinomatous: hence when we find a warty tumor ulcerating it is well to be on our guard.

Treatment.—All medicinal treatment has thus far proved futile. The same may be said of the galvanic current, which has nevertheless been favorably mentioned by some authors. The only rational treatment is surgical, and the operation is neither difficult nor dangerous.

With a sessile growth it is best to proceed as was done in the case illustrated,—to incise all around the base of the growth, then to cut it out step by step, uniting the wound immediately with deep sutures.

## VULVO-VAGINAL CYSTS, CYSTS OF BARTHOLIN'S OR DUVERNEY'S GLAND.

The Bartholinian glands belong to the racemose variety, and are analogous to Cowper's glands in the male. They are situated on either side of the introitus vaginæ, one on each labium majus. They are about the size of á bean, are shaped like an almond, of a yellowish-red color, and are plentifully surrounded by fibrous connective tissue. Their excretory ducts are about two centimetres long, open immediately in front of the hymen or carunculæ myrtiformes, and admit a very fine probe. They secrete a mucoid fluid, which during sexual excitement is increased and is thrown out in small jets by the action of the constrictor vaginæ.

Cysts of the ducts and cysts of the gland proper may exist; the tumors of the former variety are usually smaller than those of the gland and are of an ovoid shape. The duct-cysts, when they have attained the size of a hazel-nut or larger, cause much inconvenience. Sometimes some of the contents of the cysts may escape through the opening of the duct, if this is pervious, but it soon fills again.

The retention-cysts of the gland proper are similar to the duct-cysts. I have seen one as large as a duck's egg, rendering coitus impossible and the attempt painful. It is, however, not unusual for an active inflammation and suppuration of the cysts to take place subsequently. As a rule, the affection is unilateral, and in my experience one side is just as liable to be affected as the other, although the majority of writers state that these tumors are most frequently found on the left side. The contents of these cysts may vary, in different cases, from a thin limpid fluid to one of viscous character, which at times may have a chocolate hue, due to the presence of blood.

These cysts may be caused by unclean habits in the patient, or by the closure of the duct by inflammatory processes about the introitus, especially gonorrheal inflammation; and in the course of the latter affection it is not uncommon to find small pointed condylomata protruding into the duct. The gonorrheal poison may remain in the mouth of the duct for a long time and be a source of infection. This is readily ascertained by examining a case of vaginitis, cleaning off the secretion with a little absorbent cotton, and noticing the mouth of the gland, which is surrounded by a small red zone of inflammation: upon making gentle pressure upward along the course of the gland, a small drop of pus will usually be found to exude.

Vulvo-vaginal abscess may also be caused by excessive indulgence in coitus, especially during menstruation, when the staphylococci have easy access to the hyperæmic gland.

The inflammation of the duct may be continuous with that of the gland and so intense as to enhance suppuration. Primary inflammation of the gland is, in my experience, more frequently due to traumatism than to an extension of vaginitis. Should suppuration follow inflammation, the pus may be absorbed and a cystic cavity be left, with viscid contents.

Diagnosis.—Pudendal hernia and hydrocele of the round ligament are the two important conditions from which vulvo-vaginal cysts must be distinguished.

Hernia is reducible, and gives a distinct impulse when the patient is requested to cough: its feel to the examining finger is not so elastic as is the case in cysts. Hydrocele of the round ligament is also partially reducible, gives no impulse on coughing, to the touch has rather a doughy feel, and causes a more diffuse swelling. Cysts are distinctly elastic to the touch, are irreducible, circumscribed, and of ovoid form. They cause no pain unless inflammation sets in, grow slowly, and the percussion-sound is dull; whereas the appearance of a hernia is sudden, and, if an enterocele, resonance on percussion is elicited. We must, however, bear in mind the possibility of there being fluid in the hernial sac: should this be the case the diagnosis is rendered more difficult. When suppuration has taken place, either primarily or supervening upon the inflammation of a cyst, the symptoms are those of an ordinary abscess,—increase in volume of the tumor, intense pain, redness, œdema, fluctuation, etc.

Treatment.—As previously noted, cysts, when emptied, rapidly refill, so that a more radical course must be adopted. They may be incised at the junction of the skin and the mucous surface within the free edge of the labium, and, after evacuation of the contents, the sac wiped out with tincture of iodine or a ten-per-cent. solution of chloride of zinc, then packed with iodoform gauze. The cavity is to be cleansed with a mild solution of carbolic acid every day and lightly repacked. It is desirable to remove a portion of the sac wall after having incised the cyst. This procedure is absolutely certain in its results, and, although somewhat tedious, is the best to follow, provided the cyst cannot be enucleated in toto, which is usually a difficult undertaking, because it is generally adherent and ruptures before completion. To facilitate the total extirpation of the sac wall, Pozzi punctures the cyst with a trocar, as in hydrocele, after having incised the integument, washes it out with hot water, and then fills the cavity with liquid paraffin at a low temperature. When the cavity is distended, a cold application is applied to harden the paraffin, and after the lapse of a few minutes the enucleation may be undertaken. If the extirpation has been completely made, the cavity should be closed entirely with deep sutures. Catgut or silk may be used. I prefer superimposed silkworm-gut sutures in two rows. Both rows are brought out on the skin. The first row is placed at the bottom of the cavity, and the ends are not tied until the second row has been placed at half the depth between the previous stitches; when all have been inserted the sutures are tied, the deep row first. Care must be taken not to insert the sutures too close together, so as to avoid strangulation. A little flexible collodion is applied over the wound. The sutures are removed after five days, when the wound will be found healed. Another form of treatment in vogue is to empty the cyst with a fine aspirating needle, and then to inject the cavity with tincture of iodine or ten-per-cent. solution of chloride of zinc, so as to cause adhesive inflammation. This is bad treatment, and should not be resorted to. When suppuration has occurred, the abscess must be widely opened, washed out with full-strength peroxide of hydrogen, and lightly packed with gauze. This cleansing and packing are to be repeated daily until the cavity has become obliterated. One should not waste time with cataplasms and waiting for spontaneous opening.

Besides the cysts of Bartholin's gland, we meet with sebaceous cysts in the labia majora: these are superficial, and in every respect resemble the ordinary wen. Other cysts which have no connection with Bartholin's gland may occur on different portions of the vulva: their contents are usually clear serum. Dermoid tumors have been encountered, and Taylor described a pedunculated cholesterin tumor. The diagnosis is somewhat difficult as soon as the tumor becomes tense; in some cases the insertion of a hypodermic needle will be necessary to aid in the diagnosis.

The treatment must be on the same plan as that described for the cysts of Bartholin's gland.

*Chondromata* are exceedingly rare. Schneevogt describes such a cartilaginous tumor (pedunculated) of the clitoris, as large as the fist, in a woman fifty-six years old. Bartholin cites the singular case of a prostitute who had on the clitoris a growth of this nature, which was ossified to such an extent that men who had coitus with her had abrasions produced on the penis.

*Neuromata* are even more rare. Simpson reported the only case which is not open to doubt. It was a small painful nodule near the meatus urinarius.

### VARICOSE TUMORS—VARICES.

Such tumors may occur as the result of pressure of a pathological or a physiological growth in the pelvis; pregnancy is the usual cause. I have seen a bunch of distended veins, as large as the two fists, on the right labium majus, in a woman in the fourth month of gestation. The patient died subsequently from sepsis the result of a suppurating hæmatoma. The distended veins are readily recognized, and can hardly be mistaken for any other condition. As a rule, they cause very little inconvenience except that consequent upon physical exertion; but they are nevertheless no inconsiderable source of danger in consequence of their great distention during parturition, especially if, during the passage of the head, the varix ruptures externally or subcutaneously. Traumatism or unusual physical exertion may cause the rupture of a varix at any time, and, if exteriorly, such profuse hemorrhage may occur as to cause death. Varicose veins on the thighs and legs generally are associated with varices of the vulva.

The treatment, if the varicose tumor is due to pregnancy and is large, consists in keeping the patient in the horizontal position as much as possible, and in having her wear a well-fitting abdominal supporter to take the pressure off the pelvic vessels. If the tumor has attained an unusual size, as in a case reported by Holden, in which it was as large as an infant's head, the production of abortion should be taken into consideration. If pelvic tumors cause the venous dilatation, they should be removed.

*Hæmatoma* usually results from the subcutaneous rupture of a varix. Outside of pregnancy, vulvar hæmatoma occurs only as the result of traumatism. That resulting from parturition sometimes attains a very large size. It must be considered a grave complication of the parturient state if the hæmatoma is large or even of medium size. Small hæmatomata, as a rule, become absorbed, and even with large blood tumors it is advisable to let nature take her course and give them a chance to disappear; but should suppuration take place and the symptoms of septicæmia manifest themselves, the tumor should at once be widely opened, evacuated, and the cavity packed with iodoform gauze. Hæmatoma cannot be mistaken for any other enlargement: its characteristic violet color, with the history of sudden appearance, is sufficient to establish the diagnosis.

### POLYPI.

Polypoid growths of the meatus urinarius are not of rare occurrence: they are usually pedunculated, and are very vascular, and hence appear crimson or purplish-red to the eye. Their vessels are not greatly dilated, nor their walls thickened, as in telangiectasis; nevertheless, they sometimes bleed repeatedly and profusely. The growths vary in size from that of a pin-head to that of a hazel-nut; being of a myxomatous or myxo-fibrous structure, they are usually soft to the touch. They are very painful, and cause much trouble in micturition, so that their symptoms strongly resemble those of cystitis: hence it is necessary to examine the urethra in cases presenting such symptoms by making pressure upon it in a forward direction, towards the orifice of the meatus, with a finger in the vagina, when the small growth hidden within will generally be brought to view. If the growth is pedunculated, so that a catgut ligature can be thrown around it, it may be cut off above the ligature, or it may be at once excised and the bleeding stopped with a fine suture of catgut. A five- or ten-per-cent. solution of cocaine should be used as a local anæsthetic.

### LUPUS.

Guibourt and Huguier first described this affection, under the name of *esthiomène*. It is rare, and its occurrence is usually between the ages of twenty and thirty years. Clinically we distinguish two forms, the hypertrophic and the ulcerative, and the latter has been subdivided into several varieties.

The disease is of very slow growth and is difficult to cure. The patient from whom the photograph was taken was finally cured after complete excision of the neoplasm, all other treatment having failed.

Fig. 7.

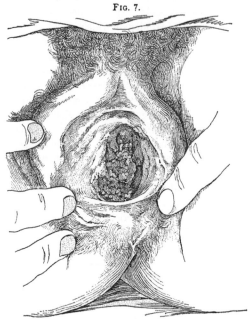

Ulcerated form of lupus, four months after the beginning of the disease.

The cause of the disease is, as demonstrated by the discovery of A. Pfeiffer and Pagenstecher, a local infection with tubercle-bacilli. Clinicians long ago suspected tuberculosis of being an etiological factor in the production of the disease. A peculiarity of lupus is that some parts after having ulcerated begin to cicatrize; this forms one of the distinguishing features from dermoid cancer of the vulva, with which it may possibly be confounded. Pain is seldom present, whereas it nearly always accompanies cancer. Lupus also differs from epithelioma by the absence, as a rule, of enlarged lymphatics in the former.

Microscopical examination (Fig. 8) reveals either considerable hypertrophy of the superficial layers of connective tissue and their papillæ, together with an acute infiltration with inflammatory corpuscles in scattered nests, constituting hypertrophic lupus, or loss of substance in both the epithelial and subjacent connective-tissue layers, together with considerable infiltration with inflammatory corpuscles,—ulcerative lupus. The essential feature is, however, the lupus nodule, an aggregation of inflammatory corpuscles in cheesy or colloid degeneration. Nests of such corpuscles completely lack blood-vessels, which are abundant both around the nodule and

FIG. 8.

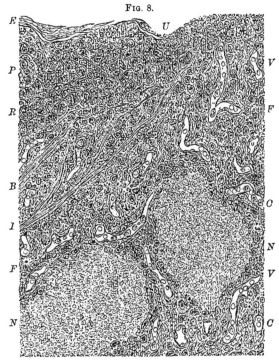

Lupus of vulva, × 250.—*E*, epidermis; *P*, inflamed papillæ in transverse section; *R*, rete mucosum, inflamed; *U*, ulcer on surface; *F*, *F*, fibrous connective tissue in inflammatory infiltration; *B*, *B*, remnants of bundles of fibrous connective tissue; *C*, *C*, blood-vessels, mostly dilated; *N*, *N*, lupus nodules, non-vascular.

in the hyperplastic tissue some distance away from the nodule. Tubercle-bacilli are always scanty in the lupus nodule.

**Treatment.**—If possible, the growth should be completely excised with curved scissors. When this is not feasible, gouging with a sharp curette must be resorted to, with subsequent application of the actual cautery or strong caustics.

### CANCER OF THE VULVA.

Primary cancer of the vulva is a great rarity, the majority of cases being instances complicated with malignant disease of the vagina or of the uterus, or of both. Martin reports a primary cancer of Bartholin's glands in a patient seventy years old. Cancer of these glands may be of very slow progress, as in Schweizer's case of three years' standing, the patient being alive at the time of the report. The most prevalent form is dermoid cancer or epithelioma (Fig. 9), and the inner and lower part of the labium majus is its predominating situation : it may, however, also originate from the clitoris, selecting its prepuce for the primary seat, or from the urethral orifice.

**Pathology.**—The most characteristic feature of dermoid cancer under the microscope is the thickening of the epithelial layers, with a pronounced growth into the depth, whereby the papillæ are likewise enlarged. The epithelia produce ingrowths, which frequently are interconnected, resulting in a plexiform arrangement. In the interior of these, as well as independently, the epithelia become arranged in concentric layers, retaining their flat form. Thus onion-like layers are produced, which are termed cancernests. In the midst of these nests the epithelia coalesce, forming masses of high refraction, owing to a colloid degeneration,—the so-called cancer pearls. Aside from these new epithelial formations, the subjacent connective tissue is found transformed into globules closely resembling those of inflammatory infiltration. Virchow terms this condition the small cellular infiltration ; Waldeyer, the inflammatory reaction. C. Heitzmann considers this infiltration the incipient stage of cancer, since he has proved that from the globules new epithelia will arise. The more pronounced this infiltration, the more malignant is the type of cancer.

**Etiology.**—There is nothing definitely known as to the causation. Advanced age predisposes towards the formation, so that it is most frequently met with between the ages of forty and sixty years; but it may occur at any time of life, even during childhood or very old age. Mundé reports an epithelioma of the vaginal fornix at twenty-four years, but it has been found as early as five years and as late as beyond seventy. Traumatism and frequently recurring attacks of vulvitis may lead to it. Chronic eczema leading to a thickening of the mucosa of the labia in scattered patches, the so-called kraurosis of Breisky, is a predisposing cause of epithelioma.

**Symptoms.**—It begins in the form of small, hard, round, irregular nodules slightly elevated above the skin, which are covered with thick layers of scaly epithelium ; these in the early stage are of slow growth and occasionally produce no symptoms; usually, however, pruritus vulvæ of greater or less intensity is present. This stage may last several months. Later, when these nodules have attained a larger size, they begin to secernate, owing to a greater blood-supply in their vicinity. Soon the epithelium becomes denuded, and superficial ulceration is the result ; now the growth is more rapid, and the inguinal glands become involved, these sometimes attaining an enormous size, as in the case reported by Schuh, in which the conglomeration was as large as an infant's head. Pain, which in

Fig. 9.

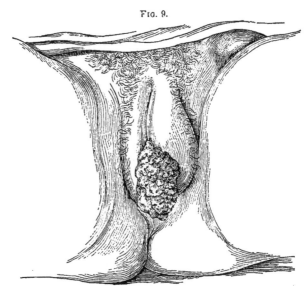

Dermoid cancer or epithelioma of left labium majus   (Kaposi.)

Fig. 10.

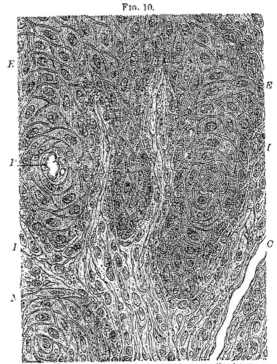

Dermoid cancer or epithelioma of labium majus, × 500.—E, E, epithelial plugs, penetrating into the derma; N, epithelial nest; P, cancer pearl; I, I, connective tissue crowded with protoplasmic bodies; C, capillary blood-vessel.

the beginning was absent, now frequently becomes a prominent symptom, although some patients complain very little. The borders and base of the ulceration are uneven, hard, and livid. The usually sero-purulent secretion has a very disagreeable odor. Upon pressure, small plugs will appear at the base, which are the epithelia in fatty and colloid degeneration and should not be mistaken for pus. Pressure, however, should always be exerted gently, since Gerster has enunciated the plausible view that by pressure the cancer epithelia are detached and driven into the lymphatics, thus causing a more rapid propagation of the disease, especially in the adjacent lymph ganglia. Hemorrhages are infrequent and seldom of large quantity. It is as unusual for the disease to pass to the other labium by contiguity as it is for it to occur simultaneously on both labia, but the epithelioma does spread to the perineum, and even to the thighs, the vagina, the bladder, and the rectum.

The patients finally die of marasmus, superinduced by a low but continuous septic infection, in from two to five years after the initiatory nodules are noticed.

Medullary cancer and scirrhous cancer are of still greater rarity as primary neoplasms in this locality, and are of decidedly graver prognosis. The symptoms noted for epithelioma also occur in these forms of malignant diseases, only in more rapid succession and with greater intensity.

Diagnosis.—The microscope will settle the diagnosis in all cases, and it should be invariably called in as an aid. Syphilis and ulcerating lupus may be mistaken for epithelioma, but the history is so very different, and the symptoms are so unlike, that with a little care such errors should be avoided.

### SARCOMA.

Sarcoma (or myeloma) is the least prevalent of the malignant diseases of the vulva, and occurs as melanotic sarcoma. (Fig. 11.) The symptoms are similar to those of other varieties of malignant disease, with the exception that sarcomata very rarely ulcerate, whereas ulceration is an essential feature of cancer. The adjacent lymph ganglia are only exceptionally affected in sarcoma, whereas in cancer they almost invariably become enlarged and infiltrated.

Pathology of Sarcoma (Myeloma) (Fig. 12). — This type of tumor, before Virchow's time, was termed encephaloid, the same term being also applied to rapidly growing medullary cancer. Virchow was the first to call attention to the fact that cancer is mainly an epithelial growth, and sarcoma a connective-tissue growth, this tissue being in an embryonal or medullary condition. Such tumors are made up either of lobular or of spindle-shaped elements, often of the two intermixed, and either white or more or less saturated with a brown or black granular or diffuse pigment. The structure of sarcoma is uniform, and, as Billroth has shown, may exhibit an alveolar structure somewhat resembling that of cancer, though lacking epithelia; the blood-vessels are always scanty. In melanotic sarcoma deposits of a dark granular pigment may be seen in the layer of epithelia covering the tumor, or in the thin framework of fibrous connective tissue surrounding the alveoli, or in the multiform bodies filling the alveoli.

The prognosis is still more serious than in cancer, since it destroys life usually within two years. The microscope alone can determine with certainty with which form of disease we have to deal.

**Treatment.**—The diagnosis having been made with certainty, there is but one method to pursue in either of these forms of malignant neoplasm which will offer any chance for the life of the patient, provided that the disease has not already progressed too far for its adoption. The new growth must be completely removed. The only question is which method should be employed, the knife or the galvano-cautery. It is asserted that

FIG 11.

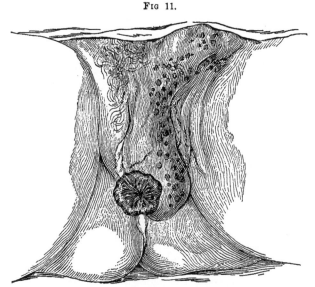

Melanotic sarcoma of left labium majus. (Kaposi).

with the latter there is less danger of hemorrhage; but any one who undertakes such work must be competent to manage a bleeding surface, and if the operation is done with dexterity and rapidity with the knife and scissors the hemorrhage should not be very great; while the advantage is that we are likely to obtain union by first intention. Care should be used to operate sufficiently far in healthy tissue to insure annihilation of the disease, since it has been proved that the slightest trace of the so-called inflammatory infiltration of the connective tissue left at the cut surface is enough to produce a recurrence. The entire chain of lymphatics on the corresponding side should also be removed on the slightest evidence of enlargement. Great care must be taken in restoring the meatus urinarius if the neoplasm has originated in that locality. In a patient of mine with melanotic sarcoma, all the lymphatics, though very little enlarged, were removed at the time of operation upon the tumors, and there has been no recurrence up to the present time, three years since the operation. The use of caustic pastes, or other caustics, after the use of the knife, with the idea of more deeply destroying the neoplasm, is to be deprecated. If palliative treatment becomes necessary on account of too great advancement, recourse must be had to some method which will stop the ichorous discharge from

Fig. 12.

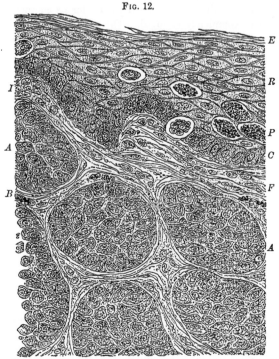

Melanotic alveolar sarcoma of the skin, × 500.—E, epidermis; R, rete mucosum with compressed epithelia; P, pigmented clusters of living matter sprung from epithelia; C, row of short pigmented columnar epithelia; F, fibrous connective tissue; I, infiltration of fibrous connective tissue with proto-plasmic bodies; B, black pigment clusters; A, A, alveoli filled with multiform pigmented corpuscles.

the ulcerating surface. First remove all soft, broken-down tissue with a sharp curette, and then use the actual cautery. As a dressing, powdered charcoal, or one part of aristol mixed with three parts of bismuth, may be employed. Lotions of lysol, creolin, or carbolic acid solution are advantageous, and to prevent the clothing from becoming soiled by the secretions an occlusion pad should be worn. If the pain becomes very severe, narcotics must be used.

The use of pyoktanin blue will be referred to under cancer of the uterus.

## CYSTS.

A variety of cystic formation occasionally found during pregnancy has been carefully studied by Winckel and termed by him *kolpohyperplasia cystica*. Zweifel gives the name *vaginitis emphysematosa* to the same condition, and in my opinion this is a better term. The cysts are very small, usually not larger than a millet-seed, and are filled with gas; they produce no symptoms except leucorrhœa, and are therefore of no great importance. What the origin of the gas is we do not know. Their lining is composed of endothelium.

Another form of true cysts is, in my experience, not infrequently found, about the origin of which diversity of opinion exists. As a rule, they occur singly, but several have been found in a row. I have seen two beside each other. Their seat is generally on either the anterior or the posterior vaginal wall, but I have been unable to notice any predilection as to which one, or as to which portion of the vagina, whether the upper, middle, or lower third. They sometimes occur on the lateral walls, but I have seen only two instances in this situation. The tumors vary in size from that of a pea to that of a hen's egg or more, and the mucous membrane covering the cysts often retains its normal appearance; generally, however, it becomes smooth and glossy, owing to the distention of the cyst. Often it is so thin that the cyst looks like a miniature rubber balloon attached to the vaginal mucosa. The growth of these cysts is very slow, and they may require many years to attain the size of a hen's egg. But exceptions occur to this rule, as in a case reported by Hörder, in which the cyst grew rapidly in six months. Their tendency is to grow first towards the lumen of the vagina; when situated in the lower portion, they bulge towards the exit after having attained a certain size. They are sessile, but may become somewhat pedunculated if the base is lax. Their contents vary: sometimes the contained fluid is a clear serum, in other cases it is thick and tenacious, and in still others it is dark red, or rather chocolate-colored, showing the presence of blood.

Microscopically we find fat, epithelium, granular corpuscles, blood, and pus, some of which may be occasionally absent. The cyst wall is composed of connective tissue, sometimes containing muscle elements, and is lined with epithelium which belongs to either the cylindrical, the pavement, or the ciliated variety, the first mentioned being the most common.

If we follow the histology and give the literature of careful observers due attention, we must come to the conclusion that the origin is not always the same. I lean towards the opinion expressed by von Preuschen, that most cysts originate from glands exceptionally present in the vagina, rendering them retention-cysts. It is also thought by some that they have their origin from the remnants of the Wolffian canal, or canal of Gärtner. This view, enunciated by Veit, is very plausible, and undoubtedly must be accepted for some cases. Retention in dilated lymph-vessels, and, according to Winckel, traumatism, may be mentioned among the causes.

**Symptoms.**—Unless the growths are larger than a hazel-nut, they are not likely to cause any symptoms; and if symptoms are present they will depend greatly upon the situation of the cyst, as well as its size. When the cyst becomes inflamed and suppuration takes place, considerable pain will be felt, as in any other inflamed part. The larger cysts, when situated on the anterior wall and in the middle or lower third of the vagina, cause vesical disturbance, a dragging sensation, sometimes descent of the vaginal wall, impressing the patient with the feeling of having prolapsus uteri, leucorrhœa, discomfort in walking, hinderance to coition, and if situated in the upper third they may be a cause of sterility. On the other hand, a case is known in which a vaginal cyst in a virgin was ruptured on first intercourse after marriage, a great part of the ruptured cyst wall being torn off and discharged. If on the upper part of the posterior wall, these cysts may cause antedisplacement, thus giving rise to the usual train of symptoms caused by anteflexion or version. Some of these symptoms may be absent, or in some aggravated cases all may be present. Cysts of unusually large size may cause an obstruction to parturition. Veit's case is probably the largest cyst ever observed,—viz., the size of an infant's head.

The prognosis is favorable for cure if they are properly treated. They do not endanger life if left alone, but expectant treatment should not be adopted if they are of sufficient size to cause symptoms and if the patient will submit to an operation.

**Diagnosis.**—This should never cause any difficulty, but some very amusing errors have occurred; for instance, they have been mistaken for prolapsus, and so treated. Rectocele and cystocele are readily differentiated, if not at once by the appearance and character of the tumor, by touch, certainly by a rectal examination in the former instance, and in the latter by the introduction of a catheter into the bladder. The same point of distinction holds good for peri-urethral cysts.

Vulvo-vaginal cysts are recognized by their location. Incomplete closure of Müller's ducts may give rise to an error only on superficial examination without operation; the bifidity of the vagina usually extends to the vulva, and produces a distention the peculiarity of which is that it can be palpated along the whole lateral wall of the vagina. Operation will of course at once dispel all errors.

Vaginal hernia will, on coughing, give an impulse to the finger; besides, a hernia can be reduced. It should be borne in mind that cysts are generally circumscribed, and have tense walls and an elastic feel. If one is in doubt, the introduction of a hypodermic syringe needle and withdrawal of some of the fluid will certainly dispel it, should the other diagnostic signs be insufficient.

**Treatment.**—Simple puncture or incision is useless, as the cysts always refill; and the injection of tincture of iodine or any other irritating fluid after puncture, although it may lead to a cure, should not be used for the purpose of causing adhesive inflammation and thus obliteration of the sac, since the gain is not worth the risk of producing a severe inflammatory reaction and suppuration, and in many such cases no cure results from this procedure. For small and medium-sized cysts I have always practised complete enucleation, and this can be done even with large cysts, or if a portion of the projecting part of the cyst be cut out with a pair of scissors and the cavity packed with a strip of iodoform gauze it will also invariably result in a cure. This is especially preferable in large cysts where there is reason to expect considerable hemorrhage, and also in cysts which are in the upper part of the vagina and in those which lie deep, near the urethra or the bladder. It is not necessary to unite the cyst wall and the vaginal mucous membrane, as Schroeder has advocated and as is now extensively practised. This procedure usually requires anæsthesia, whereas cutting out a small piece and packing the cavity can be quickly done without anæsthesia. Strict cleanliness must of course be observed.

### FIBRO-MYOMATA—POLYPI.

The latter are exceedingly rare, although a few cases have been observed. Martin has seen one in an infant one day old. In more than thirty thousand gynæcological cases examined by me I do not recall a single instance of fibrous polypus of the vagina.

No period of life is exempt from vaginal fibro-myomata, although they occur most frequently during the period of sexual activity. Their histology is similar to that of fibro-myomatous tumors of the uterus, and the reader is referred to the section on this subject for the description. Only one case of a tumor composed entirely of purely connective tissue is on record. In all other cases of vaginal polypi thus far observed the tumors have been composed of connective tissue with muscular structure. Their size varies from that of a pea to that of a mass ten pounds in weight, the majority of observed cases, however, being small. Their usual seat is on the upper and anterior wall. When the growths are larger, weighing a pound or more, they may ulcerate, and then strongly resemble sarcoma. This, however, is the only neoplasm with which they may pardonably be confounded, and the microscope alone will in some such instances give a solution. To diagnose sessile tumors from vaginal cysts may require an exploratory puncture.

The symptoms will vary with the location and size of the growth. Leucorrhœa will be the first noticeable. The larger tumors cause vesical and rectal disturbance, dragging sensations, and hemorrhage when the surface is ulcerated, and form obstacles to coition and parturition.

Treatment.—This can consist only of removal. In sessile tumors the vaginal mucosa should be cut nearly at the base of the growth and surrounding it, so as to get rid at the same time of superfluous structure. When the growth is enucleated, continuous catgut sutures are used to close the bed, care being observed to include the bed of the growth in the suture. Pedunculated growths are removed with the ligature and knife or scissors.

### CANCER OF THE VAGINA.

It is even more rare to find the primary seat of this neoplasm in the vagina than to encounter it on the vulva. It is generally found as a continuation of carcinoma of the portio vaginalis. In other instances it is associated with cancer of the vulva. It may occur at any period of life, even in childhood, as is shown by a specimen obtained from a child nine years old, in the pathological museum of Strasburg. The greater number of cases, however, occur between the thirtieth and the fortieth year.

It usually appears in one or other of two different forms. The broad-based papillary form generally has its origin on the posterior wall. These epitheliomata may attain such a size as to block up the vagina, and in the case of the child referred to above the epitheliomatous tumor was as large as a hen's egg. In other cases they occur as small isolated nodules or small ulcers with an indurated base, which rapidly become confluent and involve the whole vaginal circumference. This latter form varies in type histologically, sometimes being of the epitheliomatous, but usually of the medullary, and least frequently of the scirrhous variety.

We sometimes find it occurring as a complication of pregnancy, and it may then form an obstacle to delivery. The course of the disease is usually quite rapid, obviously owing to the fact that these tumors are generally recognized too late, whence the extremely bad prognosis as to cure. Unfortunately, the neoplasm in this situation seldom causes symptoms which attract the attention of the patient in its early stages. When the disease is discovered, disintegration has usually commenced, causing disagreeable vaginal discharges, and hemorrhage in greater or less amount, especially after coitus; in fact, the initiatory hemorrhage generally occurs subsequently to that act. Pain seldom is present until late, when the new growth has involved some deeper structures. Rectal and vesical symptoms appear according to the extent and situation of the disease. The most characteristic feature for clinical diagnosis is the induration surrounding the ulcer, provided one is already present; its indurated base can also readily be appreciated, as well as its ready bleeding under slight manipulation. If no ulcer is present, the peculiar induration alone should be sufficient. I have never met with any other pathological condition which simulated the unyielding induration of malignant disease. The only neoplasm which can be confounded with cancer is sarcoma: here the microscope must differentiate.

**Treatment.**—Extirpation of that part of the vagina involved is the only method which holds out a ray of hope; but even with this procedure I do not know of a case in which recurrence has not taken place, though unquestionably in some the incision was made in apparently perfectly healthy tissue; in most instances, however, the patients come under our care too late for radical operation. Why it is that cancerous infiltration of the vaginal walls contiguous to carcinoma of the cervix, after resection of the uterus and vagina, should give a better final prognosis than when the cancer has its origin in the vagina, I am unable to say, but clinically such seems to be the case.   I have resected the upper half of the vaginal pouch in two such instances, and a good portion in several others, with fair result ; in one, two years have elapsed without a recurrence.

Owing to the great laxity of the vagina, we can usually approximate the cut surface with a continuous catgut suture and thus obtain primary union.   The operation should be done under continuous irrigation, which keeps the field for work clearer and more antiseptic than sponging.   When the disease has advanced too far for the radical operation, the course of treatment advised for malignant disease of the vulva should be pursued.

## SARCOMATA.

These also occur in two varieties, as diffuse sarcomatous infiltration and as the circumscribed tumor sometimes clinically resembling a fibroid polypus. The differential diagnosis can, of course, be established only with the aid of the microscope.   Histologically, spindle-celled or fibro-sarcoma, round-celled, melanotic, and medullary sarcomata, have been reported.   No age is exempt, and the prognosis and treatment resemble those of the previously-discussed neoplasm.   Only one authenticated case is on record which was seemingly permanently cured, that of Spiegelberg, in which four years subsequent to the operation there had been no indication of recurrence.

# CHAPTER XI.

## BENIGN NEOPLASMS OF THE UTERUS.

BY HERMANN J. BOLDT, M.D.

### MYXOMA.

ALL so-called polypoid tumors of a jelly-like consistency and half translucent to the naked eye appear under the microscope to be made up mainly of myxomatous tissue. They originate in any portion of the uterine mucosa, most frequently in the cervix. They are analogous to the mucoid polypi of the nasal and pharyngeal cavities, their vascular supply being greater in the uterus than in the above-named localities. Originally the tumors are sessile, but with advancing growth they become pedunculated, frequently protruding through the os and there appearing as bluish or purplish-red lobules. Their clinical symptoms become apparent only after they have attained a certain size, and consist in leucorrhœa, due to endometritis, and hemorrhage, due to bursting of blood-vessels of the tumor or of the hyperæmic endometrium. Pain of a bearing-down character is frequently present. They may also be a cause of sterility.

Myxomatous tumors without complications with other tissues are exceptional. The most common complication is the presence of bundles of smooth muscle-fibres in the trabeculæ of the myxomatous tissue, the so-called myo-myxomata. Still more frequently we meet with a complication of glandular tissue, usually of the tubular type. Ciliated columnar epithelia make up the lining of such tubular glands. These tumors are most frequent in the cervical canal.

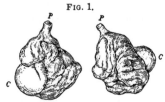

FIG. 1.

Cysto-myxo-adenoma of the cervical canal, or cervical polypi.—*P, P*, pedicles attached to mucosa; *C, C*, cysts.

The addition of the glandular element renders their surface lobulated or corrugated, whereas pure myxoma has a smooth surface. According as the myxomatous or the glandular tissue prevails, the tumors will be termed either adeno-myxoma or myxo-adenoma. Not infrequently myxomatous polypi contain cavities of varying sizes filled with a serous liquid. In pure myxoma such cavities result from partial liquefaction of the tissue, and then we term them hydro-myxoma.

If the cavities have originated from the glands and are lined with epithelium, the name of the tumor is cysto-myxoma or cysto-adeno-myxoma.

Treatment.—The removal of these tumors is readily accomplished with scissors and a sharp curette. Subsequent to their removal a local

Fig. 2.

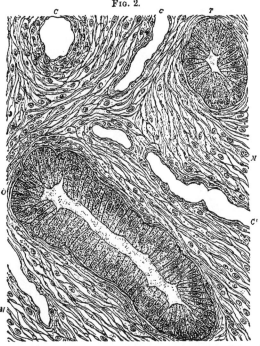

CYsto-mYxo-adenoma of cerVical mucosa, so-called polVpus, × 200.—*O*, oblique section of utricular gland: *T*, transVerse section of utricular gland; *M, M*, myxomatous and myxo-fibrous connectiVe tissue; *C, C*, wide capillarV blood-Vessels.

application of pure carbolic acid to the entire uterine mucosa should be made, on account of the coexisting endometritis. The patient should be kept in bed for the rest of the day of the operation.

## CYSTS.

Cysts in the cervical canal are of common occurrence, and are erroneously termed ovules of Naboth. Their clinical significance is but slight, and they require treatment—consisting in snipping the top off the cyst with scissors, or splitting it with a bistoury, with the subsequent local application of tincture of iodine to the interior of the sac—only in cases where endocervicitis or cervicitis is caused by them.

Like all other cysts lined with epithelium, they originate from glandular formations, with an increase in the size and number of the latter: therefore they have an adenomatous incipient stage. The lining of the cyst wall con-

sists, as a rule, of a single layer of columnar epithelium.   The contents
are in some cases liquid or semi-liquid, in others a jelly-like mass, in which

FIG. 3.

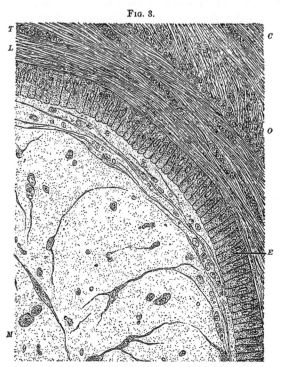

Cystic degeneration of a gland of the mucosa of the cervix uteri, so-called Naboth's ovulum, × 500.
—*E*, columnar epithelium lining cyst; *M*, contents of cyst; *C*, fibrous connective tissue: *L*, smooth
muscle-fibres in longitudinal section; *O*, smooth muscle-fibres in oblique section; *T*, smooth muscle-
fibres in transverse section.

are found embedded or scattered peculiar branching, nucleated protoplasmic
bodies, closely resembling those seen in myxomatous tissue.   To call these
cysts simply retention-cysts of the cervical glands is unquestionably erroneous; though their formation is not as yet fully understood.

### FIBRO-MYOMA OF THE UTERUS.

Myoma, myo-fibroma, fibro-myoma, fibroma, are the terms generally
adopted to designate neoplasms of the uterus which are composed of elements similar to those composing the normal wall of the uterus.   The
name ordinarily employed in this country is the last of the list, but this is
as erroneous as the first, unless in exceptionally rare cases.   The desig-
nations steatoma, leiomyoma, hysteroma, and tubercle have been abandoned
by recent authors.   The tumors are, as we shall see later, generally of
a mixed variety, composed of muscle and fibrous connective tissue: hence

the corresponding terms myo-fibroma or fibro-myoma, the prefix being applied according as one or the other of the two tissues is the more abundant. However, from a clinical stand-point this differentiation is immaterial, because the question as to the structure in many cases can be settled only by the microscope. This variety of neoplasm is benign: it is not, however, so harmless as older authors considered it to be, and consequently is of far greater importance than was taught by nearly all writers only a quarter of a century ago.

**Pathology.**—The rule is that these tumors grow slowly, but, as with so many other conditions, exceptions occur. They may be single, the so-called round uterine fibroid, or they may be multiple. If we examine a large number of extirpated uteri which have been the seat of fibro-myomatous tumors, we shall in the majority of cases be able to demonstrate that the latter condition is the rule. They vary in size from a microscopical point,

FIG. 4.

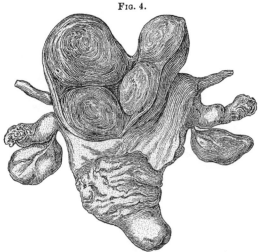

Section of subserous fibro-myoma, posterior surface of uterus.

or from a tumor the size of a pea, to a growth of immense proportions. I have seen one demonstrated by the late Dr. James B. Hunter, in the New York Obstetrical Society, weighing one hundred and forty pounds, which was fifty-five pounds more than the woman weighed after removal of the tumor. Their seat is also variable; the majority have their origin from the body of the uterus, and of these, again, the greater number are situated in the posterior wall; they least frequently spring from the cervix. The tumors are classified, according to the relative position which they maintain to their surroundings, into three principal varieties: (1) subperitoneal or subserous, (2) interstitial (or intra-parietal, or intra-muscular, or intra-mural), and (3) submucous fibro-myomata. Very often the growths belong to the category of mixed tumors; that is, when the growth in question belongs, on account of its anatomical relation, to two of the above divisions. The subserous variety is formed when the tumor develops near or directly beneath the peritoneal covering of the uterus; it then continues to grow towards the peritoneal cavity, because it there meets with the least resistance. The subperitoneal tumors have been designated peritoneal polypi by Virchow, but it is best to reserve the name polypi for tumors found in the interior of the uterus. The pedicle varies in length and in thickness. If it is thick and is intimately connected with the parenchyma of the uterus,

Fig. 5.

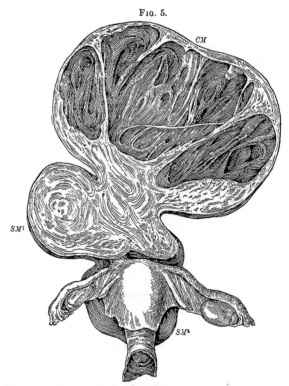

Trilobed fibro-myoma arising from fundus uteri with a thin pedicle.—*CM*, cystic part of tumor; *SM¹*, subperitoneal solid portion; *SM²*, subperitoneal solid fibro-myoma behind the uterus. (Schroeder.)

the growth of the tumor is more rapid than that of tumors connected with a thin pedicle, which sometimes are composed only of the peritoneum (derived from the uterus), subserous connective tissue, and blood-vessels of varying size. A short, thick pedicle at the fundus will draw the organ upward, so that, according to the size of the tumor, it may be difficult for the examining finger to reach the portio; the uterine cavity is often elongated in these cases, but remains of normal length in long-pedicled tumors. It is possible that the uterus may be so much drawn upward that the cervix becomes thinned out to a thin cord, and it may even happen that complete separation occurs. If for some reason the tumor causes a rotation in such an elongated cervix, hydrometra or hæmatometra is apt to occur; or the pedicle may be twisted the same as in an ovarian tumor and gangrene may set in, or it may be entirely separated from the uterus and may remain perfectly innocuous in the abdominal cavity. Localized peritonitis is not infrequently found, and the neoplasm forms attachments to the surrounding parts, as the abdominal walls, the intestines, or the bladder; the nutriment of the growth may be principally derived from vessels in the adhesions of the surroundings. If the pedunculated growth gravitates into the posterior cul-de-sac, symptoms referable to the bladder and rectum will occur. The

Fig. 6.

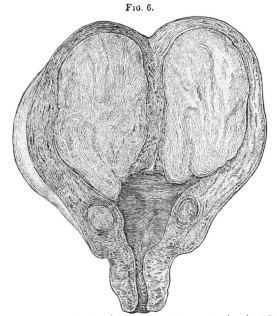

Large submucous and small intra-mural fibro-myoma, one-fourth natural size.

tumor may become adherent by an inflammatory process in the cul-de-sac and thus aggravate such symptoms; then the incarcerated tumor cannot be separated from the uterus. With the tumor on the anterior surface of the womb, that organ is soon retroposed, and we obtain the symptoms of retroflexion in addition to those of anteflexion. Intestinal obstruction may be caused by rotation of a pedunculated tumor adherent to a portion of intestine. The tumors of this class also develop into the folds of the broad ligament, but, fortunately, this is infrequent. The longer and thinner the pedicle the more independent are the movements of the tumor in the abdominal cavity and the greater are the chances that, as the result of local irritation, more or less ascitic fluid will accumulate in the peritoneal cavity.

*Submucous fibro-myomata* are generally entirely covered with mucous membrane, the mucosa being identical with the rest of the endometrium. They are formed by the neoplasm being forced by expulsory efforts towards the uterine cavity. The breadth of the base of the tumor varies; the very broad based growths, called by some submucous and by others intraparietal, usually belong to the mixed class, but for clinical reasons I class them as submucous tumors, and do not consider mixed tumors under a separate heading. They may become pedunculated, forming the fibroid polypus. The pedicle also varies in different cases. These polypoid growths are sometimes entirely devoid of a mucous membrane investment, and are then also without a muscular capsule, the pedicle consisting principally of connective tissue. The mucous membrane covering the large broad-based tumors is usually hypertrophied, but in some cases it is atrophied. The surrounding endometrium, sharing in the changes of circulation in the mucosa covering the tumor, also undergoes inflammatory changes. Sometimes the mucosa covering the growth, as the result of traumatism, will undergo more or less ulceration. As a rule, the submucous tumors contain less fibrous connective tissue and hence are softer than the other types. In the beginning the fibro-myomatous polypi are globular, but their contour sometimes changes to the shape of a pear, in conformity to the shape of the uterus, and sometimes they assume an hour-glass shape; this latter is due

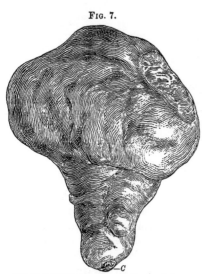

Fig. 7.

to a greater or less degree of imprisonment of a part of the growth by the internal or external os. It occasionally occurs that a submucous growth which has become pedunculated is entirely expelled and the pedicle detached, usually by the weight of the polypus. This may also take place with broad-based tumors, though more rarely. Cystic degeneration seldom occurs in this variety of tumor.

In this form of growths there is sometimes a formation of spaces, vascular lacunæ, due to a dilatation of blood-vessels, forming what has been described as myoma telangiectodes and myoma cavernosum, a condition not to be confounded with angioma cavernosum.

Myo-fibromatous polypus, one-half natural size.—
C, cut surface.

Interstitial fibro-myoma is the designation which we apply to tumors developed within the uterine wall and forming a part of it. Their natural tendency is to change into one of the previous varieties, even becoming pedunculated by uterine contractions. The uterine structure is nearly always hypertrophied, but there are cases in which the opposite condition is present. The mucous membrane of the uterus is almost invariably in a state of inflammation. The nearer the tumor is situated to the mucosa the more apt are we to find interstitial endometritis, and when farther away the glandular form predominates; but, just as occurs in chronic metritis, the same specimen may show various forms of inflammation. The ovaries are frequently the seat of inflammation, and occasionally also the Fallopian tubes. Of the gross lesions, I have most frequently found a suppurative condition of the tubes; hæmatosalpinx and hydrosalpinx less frequently. The adnexa may be displaced in various directions. Ordinarily the tumors are multiple, or a conglomeration of them is enclosed in the capsule which surrounds growths in this situation, and which is composed of muscular

FIG. 8.

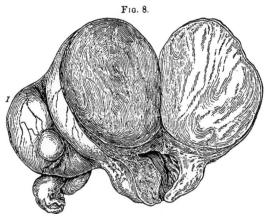

Interstitial fibro-myoma with an (*I*) intra-ligamentous fibro-myoma.

structure and loose connective tissue, so that when we cut through a uterus thus degenerated the neoplasm will protrude beyond the cut surface, rendering enucleation usually quite easy. In the so-called soft fibro-myomata, the connection with the bed of the tumor is generally quite intimate, and at the surface of adhesion the growth is nourished by blood-vessels of various sizes, whence the more rapid growth of this form.

The cavity of the uterus is invariably elongated, and at times is so tortuous, owing to the presence of several tumors in the organ, that a sound cannot be introduced into it. It is possible for a growth developed in the lower segment of the uterus to undergo a process of evolution into the cervix, as in Duchemin's case at the Strasburg clinic. The position of the uterus in the pelvis varies with the situation of the growth. It is generally displaced anteriorly, or posteriorly, or laterally; less often we find it elevated or low down in the pelvis. When the growth develops somewhat laterally in the lower segment of the posterior surface, with a

subperitoneal evolution, the pelvic contents are often seriously interfered
with and the uterus becomes displaced very markedly by the intra-ligamentous growth : usually the posterior fold of the broad ligament is first
bulged out.  There may be a complication of both varieties in one case.
From the pressure of large tumors, the abdominal muscles sometimes become thinned, and complete separation of the recti may take place, the fibro-
myomatous uterus protruding so that its covering consists of peritoneum
and skin only.

FIG. 9.

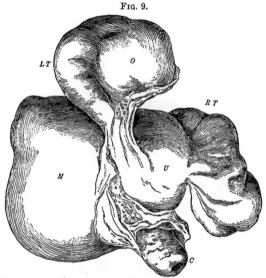

Subperitoneal fibro-myoma, with double suppurative salpingo-oöphoritis, posterior view.— *U*, uterus;
*C*, cervical portion; *RT*, right tube; *LT*, left tube; *O*, left ovary; *M*, fibro-myoma.

Fibro-myomata of the cervix are much more rare.  Anatomically they
are to be divided similarly to those of the body.  Clinically they should be
subdivided into those of the supra- and those of the infra-vaginal portion
of the cervix.  The subperitoneal tumors of the supra-vaginal portion
are of the utmost importance on account of the urgent symptoms produced
after they have attained sufficient size to fill the true pelvis, and also because of the difficulty of effectual treatment.  They generally develop either
into the folds of the broad ligament or between the layers of the pelvic
floor.  It is not rare to have renal lesions produced consequent to the neoplasm, but this is also the case in other varieties of pelvic tumors.  The
same may be said of the production of myocarditis, when the patients have
suffered much from metrorrhagia.  Pedunculated submucous fibro-myomata
of the cervix sometimes protrude from the vulva : they then may be mistaken for procidentia of the uterus, which condition can be caused by them.
They are also sometimes completely separated from their base : this may
happen especially when the neoplasm has attained some weight and the

pedicle is thin. The tumors developed in the infra-vaginal portion fill the vagina to a varying extent.

**Minute Anatomy of Fibro-Myomata.**—Tumors of great consistency exhibit under the microscope smooth muscle-fibres in excess of fibrous connective tissue. The smooth muscle-fibres are invariably arranged in bundles holding a number of spindles varying from four to a dozen, and are ensheathed by a delicate amount of connective tissue both around the bundles and around the individual fibres. It is almost im-

Fig. 10.

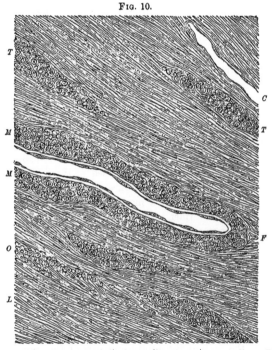

Fibro-myoma of uterus, × 500.—*L*, longitudinal section of smooth muscle-fibres; *T*, *T*, transverse sections of smooth muscle-fibres; *O*, oblique section of smooth muscle-fibres; *F*, fibrous connective tissue; *M*, *M*, muscle coat of artery, much thickened; *C*, capillary blood-vessel.

possible, in longitudinal sections of bundles, to distinguish between muscle and connective-tissue structure. This, however, is easy where the muscle-bundles are cut transversely. True fibro-myomata are composed of freely interlacing bundles of smooth muscles; their vascular supply is surprisingly scanty, and it is only in the broader track of connective tissue that we are able to trace scanty capillaries. Arteries, when met with, invariably show pronounced hyperplasia of the middle or muscular coat. Sometimes we meet with arteries in a state of waxy degeneration involving mainly the middle coat. Not infrequently we observe obliterated arteries still recognizable from the presence of the middle coat; and it is this feature which arouses the suspicion that the main source of growth of fibro-myoma is to be sought in endarteritis obliterans. Further researches are required in order to settle this important question.

Tumors of this type containing an excess of connective over muscle tissue are termed myo-fibroma, one of which is represented in Fig. 7. Here we notice a distinct amount of connective tissue both around the bundles and around the individual muscle-fibres. Again, the consistency of such tumors depends upon the nature of the connective tissue: if this is strictly fibrous, it renders the tumors hard; if, on the contrary, it is myxo-fibrous or myxomatous, the consistency is more or less soft. Lack of muscle-fibres will settle the diagnosis of fibroma or myxoma.

**Degeneration and Alteration.**—During sexual activity the growths usually undergo changes dependent upon physiological processes: thus, at the time of menstruation and during pregnancy a marked increase in size is sometimes noticed; this is especially true of tumors approaching the myxomatous type. Kiwisch has reported some as increasing to nearly double their volume in a few hours. The enlargement is due principally to changes in the circulation causing œdema of the growth. In the case of a patient with a large, soft, interstitial fibro-myoma, who consulted me for the first time during the menstrual flow, when electricity had just come into vogue, the tumor was so markedly diminished at the time of her next call that I anticipated complete disappearance of the growth from a continuance of the treatment. Within a month, however, I was undeceived by seeing it increase to its former size. In another case I have seen complete disappearance of the tumor within a few months after parturition. Œdema is frequently the forerunner of gangrene of the tumor. As in other parts of the body, so here, gangrene can take place only from circulatory changes, which may have various etiological factors. Among the most frequent causes in submucous tumors is undoubtedly traumatism of the mucosa covering the growth during treatment, or examination with the sound, which first produces ulceration at the injured point. Pedunculated sub-mucous tumors already partially expelled by nature undergo gangrene by constriction of the neck of the protruding part of the tumor. Electrical treatment undoubtedly gives rise occasionally to such disastrous results. Castration for the relief of symptoms caused by large soft tumors may have the same effect.

The majority of fibro-myomata undergo progressive induration at and after the menopause, when the tumor will diminish in volume. It is for this reason that calcified tumors are found so frequently in old women. Calcification is a very rare change: I have myself observed only one instance of it. Even calcified tumors are not exempt from the possibility of suppuration, which generally occurs in the myomatous tissue. The rule is that when the growth has become calcified it is practically innocuous. The process of calcification consists of an infiltration of the constituent elements with lime salts. The tumors were formerly described as osseous: this was undoubtedly an error, as is apparent under the microscope after treatment with solutions of chromic acid. Sometimes such tumors are expelled by the same process as pedunculated submucous growths. Such expelled neoplasms were called " uterine stones."

With regard to *fatty degeneration* causing diminution of the growth, I have serious doubts : pure fatty degeneration is certainly of very rare occurrence.

Myxomatous degeneration is said to have taken place when the interstitial tissue is infiltrated with a gelatinous or a mucous fluid.

Suppuration has purposely been omitted here, because the process generally so termed is really gangrene, although there are cases on record in which pus was present in the centre of the tumor. Mann's case of suppuration after parturition was of the fibro-cystic variety, and was preceded by fatty degeneration, as in Martin's case.

*Cystic Degeneration.*—In fibro-myoma we sometimes meet with a peculiar process of liquefaction invading both the muscle and the connective tissue. This process is allied to œdema, and finally leads to a disappearance of the constituent elements, which are replaced by serous liquid. Pathologists designate this process, though erroneously, cystic degeneration of the fibro-myoma. The designation hydro-myoma would be preferable, since the cavities filled with sero-albuminous liquid are never found lined with epithelium, which is the distinguishing characteristic of true cysts. A good illustration of such liquefaction of a fibro-myoma is shown in Schroeder's case. (Fig. 5.)

Primary *carcinomatous degeneration* of fibro-myxomatous tumors is of doubtful occurrence ; no authenticated case has yet been shown ; but the occurrence of cancer in connection with the neoplasm in question is not unusual, especially cancer of the portio vaginalis. The condition which has on several occasions been reported as carcinomatous degeneration of a fibro-myoma was apparently sarcomatous degeneration, the latter being somewhat common. Yet Schroeder cites a case in which, he asserts, the adenomatous mucosa, sending offshoots into the interior of the tumor, changed into adenoid cancer.

**Etiology.**—Although much attention has been paid to the causation of these neoplasms, we must admit that nothing is known ; not a single cause of the very many assigned has been proved with reasonable certainty. Winckel's careful study and that of others led, in my opinion, to no result. We usually see it noted that sterility is an etiological factor, but the correct statement would be that fibro-myomata are conducive to sterility. The theory that the tumors do not exist prior to puberty is disproved by the interesting case quoted by Sutton of a patient who had never menstruated or shown any evidence of ovulation, and yet had a large fibro-myoma of the uterus. I am convinced that they sometimes exist before puberty, but do not then produce any symptoms ; and their usually exceeding slow growth will account for the late presentation of the patients,—viz., at the time of

36

greatest sexual activity.  Our observation has only established that, in addition to age, race is an important factor: why it should be we cannot say; but it has been satisfactorily demonstrated that, whereas ovarian tumors and cancer of the uterus are rare in the negress, fibro-myomata are very common.

**Symptoms and Course.**—There is no disease or condition which is so simple histologically and yet presents such manifold symptoms as fibro-myoma of the uterus.  In order to appreciate this, the seat of the neoplasm of a typical case must be considered, and to some extent its histological construction.  Frequently small subserous tumors exist without causing any symptoms.  Hemorrhage, either menorrhagia or metrorrhagia, is common to nearly all the fibro-myomata; least frequent in the case of the subserous and most frequent in the submucous variety.  In pedunculated subserous tumors it is usually entirely absent; but if by their situation the circulation in the uterus is interfered with, causing changes in the uterine mucosa, this symptom manifests itself.  In the beginning the bleeding shows itself by prolonged and more profuse menstruation, but with submucous growths the loss of blood is occasionally atypical from the beginning.  The blood escapes from the tumor itself only under exceptional circumstances, as in a case reported by Duncan, in which death occurred from the rupture of a large uterine sinus.  The ordinary cause of bleeding is endometritis and stasis from mechanical causes.  More or less profuse leucorrhœa of variable character is also present in the majority of patients.

A symptom of equal importance with that of bleeding—often, indeed, of greater importance—is pain, at times of an intermittent character, most intense during menstruation, consisting of backache, bearing-down pain, and sensations similar to uterine colic: these are characteristic of interstitial and submucous tumors.  Growths filling the pelvis cause the most excruciating sciatica at times, also painful and difficult defecation, hemorrhoids, and vesical disturbance; but even very small tumors on the lower and anterior surface of the uterus will cause dysuria.  Suppression of urine can be produced by direct pressure on the ureters, with subsequent serious renal changes, as pyelo-nephritis.  Large subserous tumors sometimes cause local peritonitis from irritation, especially about the menstrual period, when the growths often increase in size temporarily from engorgement of the vessels; the patients may have marked pain from pressure on the serosa covering the tumor.  In exceptional cases, peritoneal adhesions form with the adjacent structures.  It is not unusual to meet with myocarditis if the tumor had given rise to irregular profuse hemorrhages: therefore a badly-acting heart is, contrary to the generally accepted view, an indication for early operation.  Displacements of the uterus depend on the position of the growth.  A tumor anterior to the uterus will cause it to be displaced posteriorly, as will also one in the posterior wall, or a pedunculated growth of the fundus sinking behind the uterus; later, however, the womb is pushed anteriorly and upward. Intra-ligamentous growths usually push the organ to a greater or less degree towards the opposite side. The uterus may also be dragged high up or pushed low down by fibro-myomata at the fundus.

Pedunculated subserous tumors falling behind the uterus in Douglas's cul-de-sac may, by inflammation of the serosa covering them, become firmly adherent, producing all the symptoms of incarcerated pelvic growths. Œdema of the lower extremities can thus be caused. Ascites also makes its appearance occasionally, as the result of the irritation produced by the subserous growths. Pedunculated submucous fibro-myomata may lead to complete inversion and procidentia of the uterus and vagina, and the bleeding caused by them, as long as they are intra-uterine, is occasionally alarming. This variety is exceedingly prone to undergo gangrene, when, in addition to pain and bleeding, sepsis of varying intensity and offensive discharge will be present. Interstitial myomata sometimes produce symptoms resembling those caused by subserous tumors; at other times the manifestations are like those of submucous growths. The more nearly the tumor approaches the uterine mucosa the more likely will be the presence of one of the forms of endometritis, which will cause bleeding and leucorrhœa.

To recapitulate, fibro-myomata cause as predominating symptoms menorrhagia or metrorrhagia, leucorrhœa, backache, abdominal pain of varying character; if intra-pelvic, bladder and bowel disorders, pain in the thighs, sometimes pain in the knees. Menstruation in patients with cervical, interstitial, and submucous tumors is usually painful. There may be numerous other symptoms in addition, such as cardiac palpitation, indigestion, headache, insomnia, etc., but the latter are inconstant, and, as stated previously, the first-named symptoms depend on the seat of the neoplasm.

The hydro-myomata (incorrectly termed cysto-fibromata) are in the greater number of cases subserous, and sometimes attain a large size: I have myself removed one weighing thirty-two pounds. They are generally of rapid growth, and are characterized by containing a variable amount of fluid between their interstices, which usually coagulates on exposure to the atmosphere, or is in cavities formed within the tumor by the intervening solid stroma between such interstices having broken down: hence they resemble ovarian cystomata to such a degree that in the majority of instances they have been mistaken for them, the error not becoming apparent until the time of the operation. It is obvious that the ordinary fibro-myoma becomes œdematous, and then the cystic changes follow. The usual course is for the growths to decrease in size after the menopause, and in some instances to disappear entirely; in other instances they undergo calcareous degeneration, as previously stated, but this is not always the case; on the contrary, it may be that they begin to increase at this time. Subserous growths, if pedunculated, occasionally become entirely separated from the uterus, and if they are adherent to other parts their nourishment takes place through the adhesions; if no adhesions are present, they may remain in the peritoneal cavity without producing symptoms.

The submucous fibro-myomata not infrequently become pedunculated and are entirely expelled, but when partially extruded from the uterus that portion which is exterior to the os externum is liable to become gangrenous if the circulation is much impeded by the contracture of the cervix around the tumor. Enucleation may also take place in interstitial tumors by the mucosa covering the growth being in some way partially destroyed or injured. Again, either in submucous or in interstitial tumors the entire bed of the growth may become inflamed or suppurate, the tumor subsequently undergoing similar changes or becoming gangrenous. When gangrene and suppuration have ensued in the tumor, death, if this is the termination, is as often due to peritonitis as to pyæmia or septicæmia. It may, however, be possible for softening to take place in submucous tumors without any discernible cause, the whole tumor being expelled piecemeal without the production of any symptoms indicative of gangrene. Careful examination of such expelled particles shows them to be softened masses of the tumor in fatty disintegration. Should pregnancy occur, the tumors usually grow more rapidly, but after parturition they may completely disappear. I have also seen one instance of complete disappearance of an interstitial fibro-myoma larger than an infant's head, without the influence of the menopause or parturition. Pregnancy is not frequent: it is least of all liable to occur in connection with submucous tumors.

Diagnosis.—The symptomatology should always be considered in connection with the result of the physical exploration, which will be an aid, especially in complicated cases. The bladder and rectum should be emptied prior to examination. Ordinarily it is not difficult to determine the existence of a tumor if careful bimanual examination is made; but a marked difference will be found in most cases, according as such an examination is made during menstruation or in the interval, because at the former time the neoplasm has a greater blood-supply, and consequently is more succulent, especially if it abounds in connective tissue, when its size is more or less increased.

A small subserous tumor, if pedunculated, may be mistaken for an ovary. The former is usually firmer to the touch than is the ovary, has a smoother surface, and is not sensitive on bimanual compression. When the tumors attain the size of a uterus, especially if they have a broader base, they may be mistaken for that organ—if posteriorly situated, for retroflexion; but the difference to touch between uterine structure and fibro-myomatous tumor is usually sufficiently well marked, the consistency of the neoplasm being harder; by carefully tracing the direction of the cervix, one can generally determine the position of the uterus. With the aid of the probe or sound we can with certainty make out the direction of the uterine canal, if the other points are insufficient. Careful antisepsis is required if a sound is used. The larger the tumor and the broader its base, the more difficult is it to determine whether it belongs to the uterus or is only in close connection with the organ. If it is a solid tumor of the ovary, the uterine cavity will not be found elongated and there are not likely to be any menstrual disturbances; moving a solid ovarian tumor which is not adherent to the uterus will have no effect on the mobility of the womb; but any ovarian tumor with very tense and thick walls closely adherent to the uterus is practically impossible to distinguish unless fluctuation can be elicited. Exploratory puncture can be resorted to, but I shall not consider it as a means for differential diagnosis, on account of its danger, preferring to make an exploratory incision, which can, if necessary, be immediately followed by the proper operation.

Large interstitial fibro-myomata coexisting with ovarian tumors can be diagnosed by the recognition of two tumors, one uterine, the other independent of the first and giving evidence of fluctuation.

Interstitial tumors invariably cause elongation of the uterine cavity, a sound often entering its whole length; but if several interstitial growths are present, the canal may be so tortuous that a sound, or even a probe, cannot be introduced at all. From pregnancy the diagnosis is rarely difficult: the history and physical examination are usually sufficient. There may be cases of pregnancy with considerable bleeding, caused by threatened abortion: in such cases the direct exploration of the uterine cavity is necessary. When the tumor is complicated with pregnancy, greater difficulties arise, and the diagnosis will depend upon our ability to distinguish the tumor by its hardness and the degree of its protuberance from the uterus. There are, however, exceptional cases of fibro-myomata in which it is practically impossible to determine the coexistence of pregnancy in its early stages. Small interstitial growths are often exceedingly difficult to diagnose; they may give rise to the belief that the patient has a chronic metritis. On palpation, we can often distinguish the hard fibro-myomatous nodules in the wall of the uterus, which is softer to the touch: thus, if we feel a circumscribed induration somewhat protuberant on the surface of the uterus, we are justified in diagnosing a small interstitial fibro-myoma. Very small growths cannot be diagnosed with any degree of certainty. Small submucous tumors may resemble chronic metritis or endometritis, which also cause bleeding. The curette and direct exploration are the only means of deciding the question. When the submucous tumors are somewhat larger they resemble in some degree early pregnancy with threatened abortion, but the uterus containing them is harder and more globular.

The nearer the tumor approaches the cervix the shorter the vaginal portion will become. In addition, we have the direct examination of the interior of the uterus to aid us.

A partially extruded growth of this character may be mistaken for cancer of the portio vaginalis, especially when the former is gangrenous; in both conditions there is an offensive and profuse vaginal discharge and a somewhat similar sensation on palpation, but with care we shall be able to demonstrate the cervix surrounding the protruding mass: besides, a fibroid does not give rise to bleeding, as is the case with cancer which is breaking down.

Fibro-myomata of the pelvic variety may resemble pelvic exudations. If the tumors are not adherent, they can be displaced by the examining fingers, do not encroach so closely upon the pelvic wall, and are generally harder to the touch; but if the tumors are adherent and are surrounded by old exudation, it is occasionally impossible to distinguish between them. In such cases time must be the diagnostician; the exudate becomes smaller and often disappears entirely. Acute exudations should not cause much hesitation in diagnosis, because they are always accompanied by more or less febrile reaction, the onset is sudden, with acute pain and fluctuation, or elasticity is more or less distinct.

Intra-ligamentous fibroids are distinguished by their close connection with the uterus and their unyielding feel to the touch. Such growths developing from the supra-vaginal portion of the cervix frequently cause the vaginal portion to become retracted and to form practically a portion of the tumor, which we feel low down, hard, and nodular.

The symptoms of compression are extremely marked in this variety. Growths in the vaginal portion of the cervix are usually readily recognized by the protuberance in the lip affected, whereas the other lip is thinned out and hugs the part affected, the cervical opening resembling a laceration of the cervix. Intra-uterine polypi yield symptoms analogous to those of fungous endometritis or some of the malignant diseases of the corpus. Curetting and microscopical examination of the scrapings will determine the condition.

In the telangiectatic or cavernous tumors the very great increase in size and greater tensity at menstruation are important, and auscultation elicits a peculiar bruit, although the latter is found in ovarian tumors and also in soft myomata, as well as in pregnancy. It is often impossible to distinguish them from ovarian cystomata; but, in addition to the points mentioned, it is necessary to establish the relation between the uterus and the tumor.

The prognosis for the great majority of fibro-myomata is good so far as life is concerned, provided that the growth does not undergo one of the more serious degenerations, as malignant, gangrenous, cystic, etc. The cavernous variety may lead to a rapidly fatal issue by the rupture of a blood-sinus. The submucous and some interstitial tumors may eventually cause fatal anæmia.

Treatment.—This may be divided into palliative and radical, or surgical and medical. Our aim should be to free the patient of existing pain and to remove any condition which jeopardizes life. A serious operation should never be undertaken just because the woman has a fibro-myomatous tumor; the growth must in some manner menace life or health and not be amenable to other treatment before this is permissible. All medicinal treatment is absolutely useless in pedunculated subserous tumors. The hypodermic use of ergot, sometimes called the Hildebrandt treatment, has in some instances caused a cessation of growth in interstitial tumors, and even their extrusion, the latter especially in submucous growths; so we must conclude that the treatment is applicable only to interstitial and submucous tumors; the action of the ergot is to cause compression of the blood-vessels by producing more or less marked contraction of the muscle structure of the tumor. The drug should be used in the form of solution of ergotin, twelve centigrammes (two grains) being injected twice daily into a fleshy part, the thighs, the buttocks, or in some cases the abdominal parietes. The solution should be prepared fresh every few days, and the part where the injection is made must be thoroughly washed with soap and water and then with alcohol and finally with some bichloride of mercury solution (1 to 1000); the needle should also be passed through the flame of an alcohol lamp just prior to use. After the injection the part must be massaged for a few minutes, to insure rapid distribution. The addition of chloral hydrate to keep the ergotin solution has been abandoned by me on account of the burning sensation which the drug causes. A preparation called "ergotole," manufactured by an American firm, may be advantageously substituted for ergotin. The patient can be taught to make the injections herself, because it would be too expensive for ordinary patients to come to their physician every time for an injection, inasmuch as these must be continued for a long period. It may require two hundred injections before any marked benefit is noticed, and in all probably from one to two thousand will be needed. Abscesses are avoided only by strict attention to asepsis. The other remedy which may be used with benefit in similar cases is the fluid extract of gold seal (hydrastis Canadensis) in half-teaspoonful doses three times daily; in case of gastric disturbance the dose must be diminished. A number of favorable results have been reported as regards the hemorrhage, and a few instances of decrease in the size of the tumor. Among the other remedies employed are potassium bromide and iodide, arsenic, phosphorus, chloride of calcium, mercurials, etc.; none of these, however, possess any positive therapeutic value. Various mineral baths and mud baths are of more or less benefit.

Among recent remedies, galvanism plays the most important *rôle*, whether justly or not remains to be seen. Though formerly a strong advocate of this treatment, I have been forced by repeated failures to discard it. In only one variety of tumor does its application offer a prospect of the alleviation of symptoms,—viz., the intra-mural; in this class of cases it certainly does relieve many patients. Apostoli has brought this therapeutic measure into repute and has found many ardent advocates to follow him.

The method introduced by Cutter—puncturing the tumor through the abdominal walls with needles—has been almost universally discarded, so that I shall briefly describe Apostoli's method only. The implements necessary are: a galvanic battery with enough cells to generate a sufficiently strong current, a forty-cell battery being ordinarily required, or in cities having the Edison current the latter may be utilized, with the aid of an adapter and a proper rheostat to give sufficient resistance; a large clay electrode, several intra-uterine electrodes, and an electrode for electro-puncture (see Fig. 11) ; a rheostat and a galvanometer to measure the intensity of current used.

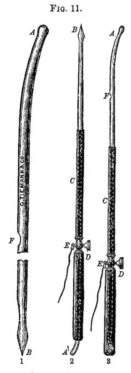

Fig. 11.

Apostoli's uterine electrodes.—1, natural size; *A*, ordinary hysterometer; *B*, trocar for puncture; *F*, notch marking average depth of uterus; 2 and 3, entire instrument reduced to one-third size; *C*, celluloid handle to protect the vagina; *E*, electrode; *D*, thumb-screw to regulate the length of the exposed sound.

The treatment by electricity is to a certain degree a surgical procedure : hence the utmost cleanliness is required. The vagina and vulva must be carefully cleansed with soap and water and douched with solution of bichloride of mercury; the intra-uterine electrode is sterilized in an alcohol flame and is kept in a carbolized solution. The hands of the operator are likewise scrubbed and disinfected after the application of the abdominal electrode, which must be large enough to cover the abdomen. The skin upon which the clay electrode is to be applied must be inspected, and any existing excoriations covered with a thin coating of collodion to prevent acute pain at such points. In place of clay electrodes, others have been proposed and used. The kind of electrode is immaterial, so long as it adapts itself evenly to the skin and covers a large area. The electrode is introduced into the uterus by means of touch alone, the patient being on her back ; if it is intended to check hemorrhage, the anode or positive pole is used within the cavity ; otherwise we employ the cathode.

The current is turned on very slowly, so as not to give any shock. The strength of the current must necessarily vary with different individuals. I have never been able to use more than one hundred milliampères, often not more than fifty, the patients complaining of intense pain when higher intensity is resorted to. Under an anæsthetic, I have used the strength advocated by Apostoli,—namely, two hundred and fifty to three hundred milliampères. If the anode is applied within the uterus, it must be of platinum or carbon; steel or copper will corrode. The active part of the electrode is insulated with a rubber cover over that portion which does not enter the uterine cavity. In cases where an intra-uterine electrode cannot be introduced, owing to the tortuous condition of the cavity, and where the tumor is accessible to the trocar-pointed electrode, which must always be made the negative pole, this is pushed directly into the growth from one-fourth to one-half inch, the precaution being used to have the non-active part of the electrode insulated. Care must be taken to turn the current on and off very gradually, so as to avoid the production of shocks; and the operator must always wait for any uneasiness or pain produced by the introduction of the electrode to subside. The action of the current should be continued from five to ten minutes. After the electrode is removed, a vaginal douche of some antiseptic solution must again be used.

The existence of suppurative salpingitis contra-indicates electrical treatment, death having occurred several times from an aggravation of the inflammation, with spontaneous rupture of the pyosalpinx, causing fatal septic peritonitis. Benefit should not be expected at once from this treatment, but it must be continued for several months, unless conditions arise which contra-indicate it,—namely, if instead of improvement the contrary takes place. It is a question as to what the mode of action is: however, that the positive pole possesses more than the cauterizing effect claimed for it by many seems certain to me. It is uncertain what the so-called "interpolar action" is.

Fig. 12.

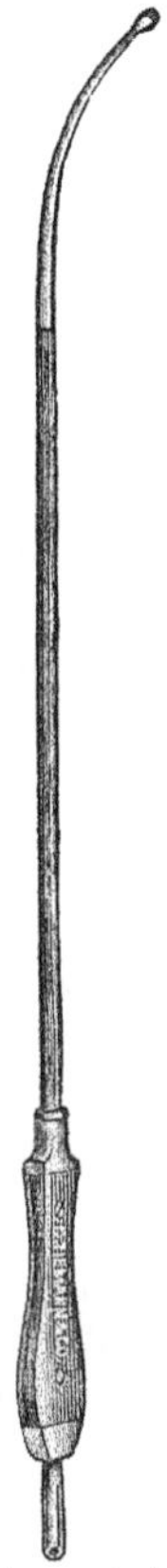

Subperitoneal tumors filling the pelvis and causing agonizing distress can at times be dislodged by placing the patient in the genu-pectoral position and pushing them above the promontory of the sacrum by pressure from the vagina or rectum. A Sims speculum should also be employed, to obtain the advantage of the air-pressure.

In case of hemorrhage, curetting, with subsequent local applications of tincture of iodine or pure carbolic acid, is often sufficient to afford relief for a long time. The patient, having been prepared with due care, is anæsthetized, and placed in the lithotomy position; the hypertrophied endometrium, upon the presence of which the bleeding is usually dependent, is removed with a Recamier's or a sharp curette; a dull instrument is useless. After the scraping an application is made to the interior by means of a Braun's syringe. The patient should be kept in bed for three or four days subsequently.

This treatment is applicable only to interstitial and to subperitoneal tumors with a broad base. I regard it as especially advantageous for anæmic patients, and repeat it

Platinum electrode.

in a few weeks, so as to gain time to build up the constitution for a possible radical operation. There are dangers connected with this treatment; for instance, in a tumor of medium size just beneath the mucosa the capsule may be injured and the bed of the tumor may become inflamed, with suppuration and gangrene as the result. A. Martin, however, purposely splits the endometrium covering the tumor, so as to permit the inflamed mucosa and blood-vessels to retract, which frequently causes a cessation of the bleeding.

Dilatation of the cervix occasionally affords benefit in this class of cases, relieving both the bleeding and the dysmenorrhœa, when the latter is due to narrowness of the cervical canal and the tumors are not large.

Ligation of the uterine arteries through the vagina has undoubtedly a very beneficial effect on many tumors, the pedunculated subperitoneal excepted. The operation is new. To Dorsett, of St. Louis, belongs the credit of proposing this treatment, although the scientific work of Sigmund Gottschalk in this direction should not be underestimated. Küstner did the operation in September, 1892, with good result. The stress laid upon the cutting off of the nerve-supply to produce additional change, as proposed by F. H. Martin, seems unnecessary. The main feature is the blood-supply. The operative technique employed by me begins with the disinfection of the patient; she is then placed in the position for vaginal hysterectomy; next the cul-de-sac of Douglas is opened, so that the needle can be guided by a finger introduced through the opening. A large full-curved needle armed with heavy catgut is now passed around the base of the broad ligament, including the uterine artery, and the ligature is tied.

The treatment of large tumors by this method should not be undertaken, and in tumors drawing the uterus high up it is not practicable.

Morcellation is applicable to submucous tumors of moderate size, and is sometimes practised in interstitial growths by some operators: we advise

FIG. 13.

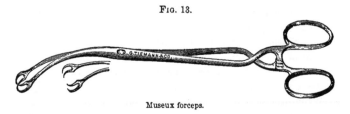

Museux forceps.

against the operation in this class. The cervix is first liberated at its lower segment by a circular incision and is then split bilaterally; the bleeding is checked by ligatures in preference to clamps. The fibro-myomatous uterus is drawn down as low as possible by Museux forceps placed in the anterior

FIG. 14.

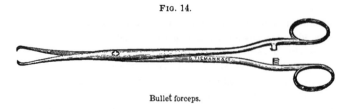

Bullet forceps.

and the posterior lip of the cervix. The tumor is examined with the finger to determine its relations with the uterus, and then an incision is made directly into the growth, which has been grasped by a strong volsella and drawn forcibly downward ; a piece is thus cut out with scissors or knife. In this manner the process is continued until the entire growth is removed, the Museux forceps being replaced at times by dentated cyst-forceps or by the serrated forceps of Péan. Large pieces of the tumor may

FIG 15.

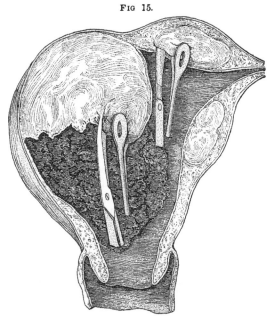

Removal of fibro-myomata by morcellation. (Péan.)

sometimes be enucleated by traction and rotation with the forceps. The last portions of the growth present a smooth, convex surface. Sometimes an additional growth is found, on examination, near the one enucleated ; this is also removed. To all bleeding points hæmostatic forceps are applied, the entire operation being done under constant irrigation. After completion of the work, strips of iodoform gauze are packed between the forceps and an occlusion pad is placed on the vulva. The forceps are removed in twenty-four hours, and the gauze packing is taken out in two or three days, after which douches may be used, if necessary. The main danger in morcellation lies in septicæmia, pyæmia, peritonitis, and thrombosis or embolism.

Pedunculated submucous tumors and small interstitial growths should always be removed per vaginam where it is apparent that they can be enucleated from their bed when the cervix is dilated, especially such as are already partly expelled by the efforts of nature. If the fibro-myomatous uterus is small enough to be removed by vaginal hysterectomy, that opera-

tion may be done. It is, however, rare for small tumors to produce such serious symptoms as to require this mutilating operation. The method will be discussed under the section on vaginal hysterectomy for cancer.

**Castration for Fibro-Myomata.**—We have stated that at the menopause it is usual for many of these tumors to undergo retrograde changes, and that the symptoms formerly produced by them gradually disappear when menstruation has ceased. With this end in view, castration is frequently performed to bring on a sudden climacteric, and if the case has been properly selected the operation will in nearly every instance produce the effect desired. The error committed by operators is not in the operation, but in the choice of the case in which it is applied.

Large tumors, those which are soft or œdematous, pure submucous growths, subserous ones with broad bases, such tumors as produce agonizing pressure-symptoms by filling the pelvis, hydro-myomata or fibrocystic growths, and the telangiectatic variety, should not be treated by castration; not only because the result is frequently unsatisfactory, but also because the operation often leads to a dangerous condition: in submucous and soft tumors, gangrene and suppuration are occasionally produced. In cavernous tumors the danger of thrombosis is to be borne in mind. There is but one class of tumors in which I advise the operation,—namely, interstitial fibro-myomata of medium size which produce hemorrhage but no marked pressure-symptoms. Some operators, however, advise castration for nearly all varieties of these neoplasms, even for fibro-cystic growths. There are cases in which it is impossible to remove the ovaries *in toto*, owing to adhesions. I have myself met with a case in which my intention had been to remove the adnexa only, but owing to hæmatosalpinx and distorted adherent ovaries, not previously diagnosed, it was impossible to do less than a hysterectomy.

The operation should never be undertaken unless the surgeon is ready to do any other which may become necessary; although we may open the abdomen with the expectation of removing the adnexa, conditions may be found which make this impracticable; further, we should never attempt to remove the adnexa except by the median abdominal section, and the incision should be made at the level at which, from the size of the tumor, we expect to find them. The length of the cut is not of great importance, although it is preferable to make it as short as possible; usually from two to three inches will suffice, care being taken not to wound the surface of the tumor, on account of the bleeding which might follow such injury. The adnexa are tied off with catgut, and the abdominal wound is closed with superimposed buried sutures of catgut,—peritoneum, fascia, and skin each separately.

**Myomectomy.**—Whenever it is possible to remove a tumor from the uterus without destroying the organ, it should be done, thus leaving the woman with functionating pelvic organs. The operation is called myomectomy, and was introduced by A. Martin, of Berlin, although it had previously been done by Spiegelberg and Spencer Wells. It is suitable for all subserous growths, and for such interstitial ones as can be enucleated without entering the uterine cavity, or by opening it to but a small extent.

After the abdominal incision has been made the fibro-myomatous uterus is brought outside of the abdominal cavity, and with a few provisional sutures as much of the wound is closed as is practicable. The uterus rests upon a sterilized towel; over the most prominent part of the tumor an incision is made and the growth or conglomeration of growths is enucleated. Sometimes the uterine cavity is opened in this procedure; hence it is well to curette and irrigate it with an antiseptic solution prior to the abdominal operation, because the mortality is far greater in cases in which the cavity is opened than in those in which this is avoided. The bed of the tumor is closed with successive tiers of catgut sutures. If the uterine cavity has been opened and previously disinfected, the danger is not aggravated, and the mucosa need not be closed separately. A rubber ligature around the cervix during enucleation should also be discarded, but care must be taken to stop all bleeding from the uterus before closing the abdominal walls. The ovaries should not be removed: in cases requiring removal of these glands, the indication is to do a hysterectomy.

Supra-vaginal hysterectomy with extra-peritoneal treatment of the pedicle is rapidly losing ground, yet under some circumstances it is advisable,—namely, when the patient is very anæmic, or when there is reason to believe (for we cannot always diagnose it with certainty) that there is a cardiac lesion or any condition which requires a rapid operation. After opening the abdomen by an incision as long as is necessary to allow of the dislodgement of the fibro-myomatous uterus, the adnexa are tied off at either side, and another ligature is placed on each side of the broad ligament, low down, so as subsequently to liberate the upper part of the cervix. A long clamp is placed on the uterine side, and the ligament cut between it and the ligature. Now a rubber ligature or a Koeberlé wire clamp is tightened around the cervix, care being taken that a fold of the bladder is not included, which danger is lessened by putting a sound into the viscus and letting an assistant outline the attachments, or by filling it partially with a mild solution of boric acid. The uterus with the tumor is amputated about half an inch above the constriction. Immediately above the ligature two long steel needles are passed crosswise through the cervix, the peritoneum being previously attached all around it below the constriction and closed through the entire wound, while the stump is held by an assistant with a volsella. The abdominal wound is closed in layers with continuous catgut sutures, or, if preferred, interrupted silkworm-gut sutures can be passed through the entire thickness of the abdominal parietes after the peritoneum has been attached to the stump: the latter method, however, though it saves time, is not so effective as the first in guarding against subsequent hernia. The pins rest upon the abdomen: to prevent their cutting into the skin, a small roll of gauze or rubber plaster is placed under them. The stump is carefully dried, then dusted with some powder, aristol, subnitrate of bismuth, or iodoform, and covered with gauze. The wire clamp is tightened as necessity demands immediately after the operation, and subsequently a little more each day. After the lapse of from ten days to two weeks or more the pedicle drops off entirely from the constrictor. The important point in the operation is to constrict only the cervix, and not a part of the body of the uterus or a part of the tumor. The growth, if extending below the constriction, must be enucleated; then there will be a thin pedicle, just as Hegar, who was the first strong advocate of the extra-peritoneal treatment by this method, demands.

FIG. 16.

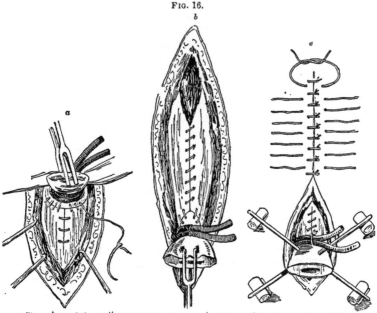

a. The suture of the peritoneum to the lower part of the pedicle is begun, the pedicle being drawn upward, so that its distance from the pubes is much increased.

b. Suture of abdominal walls above the pedicle, of the musculo-aponeurosis.

c. Peritoneum sutured in a ring about the lower part of the pedicle, the stump being depressed to show the suture. Deep sutures for integument in place, and superficial ones tied above the pedicle. The wound is shown with the cutaneous sutures below the pedicle not yet in place. (Pozzi.)

The advantages of this method are the rapidity with which the operation can be completed, if necessity requires, and the safety from hemorrhage. Its disadvantages are the protracted convalescence, the danger of hernia at the lower angle of the wound, and some risk of infection from the stump.

*Intra-Peritoneal Treatment of the Pedicle.*—The operation, in its first stages, is similar to that previously described; but after turning the tumor out and tying off the adnexa it differs, inasmuch as no elastic ligature or wire clamp is required around the cervix. The broad ligament should be tied low down, so as to secure the uterine artery. Anteriorly, a transverse incision is made a little above the attachment of the bladder and a corresponding incision posteriorly; a cup-shaped cavity is cut out, which should include the upper part of the cervical canal. This cavity is now closed with continuous buried catgut sutures. A separate row is used to unite the peritoneum over the stump. No bleeding should be present after completing the work.

Another method of supra-vaginal hysterectomy is lauded very highly by Dr. Baer and others who have adopted it. I give the description in Baer's own words:

"After the required abdominal incision is made, all existing adhesions of omentum, intestines, etc., are separated in the usual way, and the tumor lifted out of the abdominal cavity. If the incision has been an unusually lengthy one, several sutures are then placed at its upper end for the better protection of the intestines. The patient may now be elevated to the Trendelenburg posture, if deemed best, and the parts thoroughly studied, so that a clear idea as to the character and location of the tumors and pedicle may be obtained before the ligation and separation are begun. The

FIG. 17.

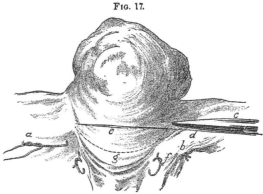

*a*, position of first ligature, transfixing broad ligament and including ovarian artery and veins; *b*, same tied: *c*, pedicle forceps grasping broad ligament under Fallopian tube and ovary to prevent reflux from uterus, when *d*, broad ligament, is severed just below forceps; *e*, incision of peritoneum above reflection of bladder, and peritoneum stripped down below *g*; *f*, ligature transfixing broad ligament at side of cervix, including uterine artery; *g*, dotted line, excision of tumor and amputation of cervix.

first step in the operation is the passing of a single silk ligature through the broad ligament near the cervix. This ligature is again made to transfix the broad ligament near the outer edge, to prevent slipping; it is then tied. A stout pedicle forceps is next placed under the Fallopian tube and ovary and made to grasp the broad ligament, for the purpose of preventing reflux from the uterus. The ligament is now severed just below the forceps, the incision being carried close to the tissues of the tumor. If deemed necessary, another ligature is now passed through the broad ligament farther down along the side of the cervix. This ligation and cutting are now repeated on the opposite side. The knife is then run lightly around the tumor an inch or two above the peritoneal reflection of the bladder in front, probably a little lower behind, and the severed edge of the peritoneum stripped down with the handle of the scalpel, for the purpose of making peritoneal flaps. The next step is a most important one: it is the ligation of the uterine arteries. This is done in the broad ligaments, outside of, but close to, the cervix. Care must be taken to avoid the ureter on the one hand and the cervical tissue on the other. The ligature may either be placed within the folds of the severed ligaments or, which is preferable, made to encircle the double fold of the ligament and artery in one sweep; action here will depend upon the size of the pedicle and the consequent separation of these folds. The constant traction which is made upon the pedicle by the assistant who is holding the tumor serves to draw out and elongate the cervix after the peritoneal covering has been incised, and thereby to permit deeper incision into the neck, which is next amputated with the knife by a wedge-shaped incision. The stump is now grasped with a small volsella forceps and further trimmed and reduced, if necessary, so that the entire supra-vaginal portion is removed before it is dropped back into the pelvis. The cervix being now released, it immediately recedes, and by the retractive and elastic properties of the vagina is drawn deeply into the pelvis, where it is buried out of sight by the peritoneal flaps covering it. These flaps have been rendered so taut by the ligatures which have

Fig. 18.

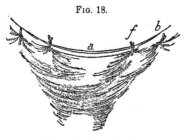

*a*, centre line, infolded edges of broad ligament lying closely in contact, having been rendered taut by ligatures *f* and *b*, which have included both layers of the broad ligaments and the ovarian and uterine arteries and veins.

been placed that usually as the cervix recedes into the pelvis they close over it like elastic bands. The cervix is now in its natural position, and without a ligature or suture in its tissues. The operation is finished by infolding the edges of the peritoneal flaps, which may be secured by Lembert sutures, if necessary. I have not found this necessary if the ligatures which secured the uterine arteries had also grasped the severed folds of the broad ligaments, for this so tightens them that the sides are brought forcibly together when the cervix is drawn under. The bladder and surrounding tissues aid also in closing the pelvic cavity. Nothing whatever is done to the cervical canal. The portion of the broad ligament embraced in the first ligature is the same structure that forms the ordinary ovarian pedicle, minus the Fallopian tube. The other ligatures close the opened broad ligament, as a rule. If any other vessels are found spurting, they are, of course, ligated. I have not found it necessary to employ the temporary elastic ligature. The steps of the operation vary somewhat to suit the complications which may be present in the individual case, but the general direction and conclusion are practically the same in all cases."

## Total Extirpation of the Fibro-Myomatous Uterus. *Technique of the Operation.*—The patient is prepared as for a vaginal hysterectomy, and then the operation is commenced from below, if the case is suitable for this, by ligating the broad ligaments as high up as possible, in the same manner as in vaginal hysterectomy for cancer, except that we do not ligate far away from the cervix. The vagina is likewise detached anteriorly and posteriorly from the cervix, and the bladder is dissected off as high as possible, the cul-de-sac of Douglas being opened first or last, whichever is the more convenient. No rule can be laid down : the operator must use his judgment as to which step should be taken first. The object to be attained is to free the lower segment of the cervix, when the operation from above is materially simplified : this becomes especially apparent in cases in which the pelvic floor is rigid. Now the vagina is packed with iodoform gauze, a strip of which protrudes into the peritoneal cavity by way of the posterior opening.

Next the abdominal section is made in the usual way, and the rest of the uterine attachments are tied off in sections and cut. To avoid injury of the bladder, the viscus, just prior to its detachment above, especially if it is spread over the tumor itself, should be partly distended with a weak boric acid solution to show its relation ; then about half an inch above its point of attachment to the uterus an incision is made and the remainder of the bladder is separated.

After excision of the fibro-myomatous uterus the vagina and floor of the pelvis are closed ; all that should be seen from above are the continuous catgut suture with which the pelvic peritoneum has been closed and a few small pedicles from the upper parts of the broad ligaments. The adnexa are tied off at the beginning, or as soon as practicable. The abdominal wound is then closed. In large tumors which do not crowd into the pelvis, but, on the contrary, pull the cervix and vagina towards the upper part of the pelvic cavity, so that the portio vaginalis can hardly be reached by the examining finger, this technique is out of the question, and the whole work must be done from above. But under these circumstances the operation from above offers no particular difficulty ; it is, in fact, decidedly easier than most operations for the removal of suppurating adnexa. The broad ligaments are secured in the same manner by successive ligation from above. The floor of the pelvis is closed in precisely the same way ; the only difference is, that the cul-de-sac of Douglas is opened from above, which, however, may also become expedient in the cases in which I advise the work to be done from below. Sometimes the opening cannot be readily made into the peritoneal cavity after the vaginal fornix has been opened ; we should then not endeavor to accomplish it, as the vagina has already been separated all around the cervix. The peritoneum is easily opened subsequently. It is obvious that in cases where the pelvic floor is rigid— especially in that class of tumors which crowd into the pelvis and produce pressure symptoms or develop between the broad ligament folds—not only

37

time, but much tedious and difficult work, will be saved if the operation is commenced as I have described. The only requisite for operating in this way is practical familiarity with vaginal hysterectomy. I should not employ clamps, unless time were an important element in the case. If the tumor is of small size (not larger than a new-born infant's head), and is impacted in the true pelvis, or if it is intra-ligamentous, and if the portio vaginalis in consequence is pressed down so low in the vagina that it can be easily palpated, we have reason to believe that the pelvic floor is rigid. Then, if the vagina is sufficiently voluminous, the operation can be done with greater advantage as above described.

During convalescence the patients operated upon according to this technique will have a vaginal discharge more or less profuse and usually more or less offensive, owing to the sloughing off of the parametric stumps constricted by sutures in the vagina. In addition, then, to the vaginal douches, if such are used, it is well to apply an occlusion pad.

Pan-hysterectomy is applicable to all tumors; its advantages are that there is nothing left in the peritoneal cavity which can give rise to sepsis, provided that the technique of the operation has been carried out surgically, as we now understand this term. Convalescence is more rapid than in extra-peritoneal treatment of the stump, and the danger from hemorrhage is almost *nil*. I am an advocate of pan-hysterectomy if an abdominal hysterectomy is required.

**Trendelenburg's Posture.**—Pelvic elevation is familiarly known under the term Trendelenburg's posture, because it was first extensively used and advocated by Trendelenburg in his clinic in Bonn. In medical literature it became known through the writings of Dr. Willy Meyer, who at the time was assistant in the Bonn clinic.

The object of the posture is to afford a clear view of the pelvic contents, so that the surgeon can work aided by sight. The intestines gravitate towards the diaphragm, unless adherent in the pelvis, and every step of the operation is conducted with the aid of the eye. There cannot be a bleeding point in the pelvis without its being detected.

Its application is called for chiefly in operations in which the surgeon works in the pelvis. Dr. H. C. Coe states in an article in the *New York Polyclinic* that the position is likely to lead to secondary hemorrhage, owing to the sudden change brought about in the pelvic circulation when the patient is lowered to a horizontal position. I have as yet not met with such a complication, and it can, I believe, be prevented by the employment of a table which can be lowered very gradually.

The table depicted on the following pages (Figs. 19, 20, and 21) meets this requirement: besides being readily portable, it prevents contortion of the vessels of the neck during elevation.

It is, however, not necessary to have a table or frame expressly made, as the posture can be readily obtained in any household. An ordinary wooden chair has been frequently made use of by me, and is admirably

FIG. 21.

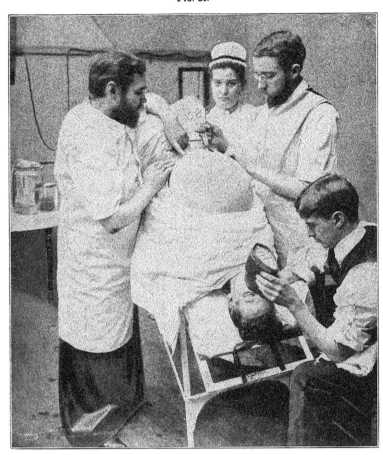

Table when in use, showing even plane between trunk, neck, and head.

adapted to the purpose. The two hind legs are cut off up to the cross-bar,

FIG. 19.

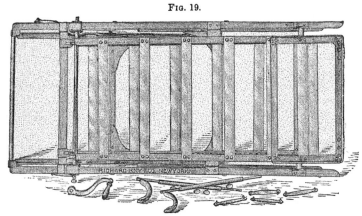

Table folded.

the chair is secured to the table, and the improvised structure is covered with blankets; or a sufficiently high box can be made use of; a board is fastened

FIG. 20.

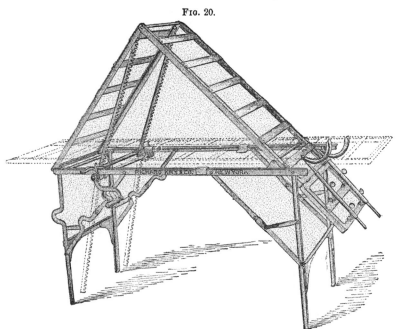

Table when elevated and when horizontal.

to it on the table, and all is covered. Such home-made contrivances have,

of course, great disadvantages, but still it is better to employ these than
to do without the benefit obtained from the position when a difficult pelvic
case is dealt with, such as a pan-hysterectomy.  If we cannot see, there is
more danger of injuring the bladder and ureters, and of insufficient security
in the ligation of vessels, than when pelvic elevation is used.  No complicated operation should be undertaken in the small pelvis without making
use of the aid derived from this posture.

*Intra-Ligamentous Tumors.*—When growths of this character are large
and broad-based, their removal is a formidable operation.  The anterior
surface near the upper border of the broad ligament is cut horizontally,
and the growth is enucleated with the fingers and scalpel handle, an assistant making traction on the tumor with Museux forceps, and applying
hæmostatic forceps wherever needed ; the vessels are subsequently tied and
bleeding surfaces are sewed over with continuous sutures ; the whole bed of
the growth should be closed in this manner.  In supra-vaginal cervical
tumors and those developed from the lower segment of the uterus there is
always danger of coming in contact with the ureters : hence their situation must be constantly borne in mind.  It is in the case of such tumors
especially that pan-hysterectomy is advisable.  Drainage is seldom necessary, but, if used, gauze drainage per vaginam is preferable.

Growths embedded in the infra-vaginal portion can usually be enucleated with ease.  The most dependent part of the tumor is grasped with
a volsella, and traction is made, so as to bring it as near as possible to the
vulvar orifice.  If the growth is not too large, an incision can be made at
or near its cervical junction and the neoplasm enucleated, or it may be
removed by an elliptical incision and any remaining remnant shelled out.
In large infra-vaginal cervical fibro-myomata this is sometimes not feasible ;
then the bulk of the growth is removed piecemeal (morcellation) until the
base of the tumor can be reached.  If the bed is smooth, the wound should
be closed at once with a buried suture ; but if it is otherwise, the edges of
the wound should be trimmed and packed lightly with iodoform gauze.

Small subserous or mixed (subsero-interstitial) fibro-myomata, not exceeding the size of an English walnut, on the anterior surface of the supra-
vaginal portion of the cervix, producing vesical disturbance, have been
removed by me several times by cutting the cervico-vaginal junction anteriorly to its full extent, stripping the bladder off the cervix sufficiently
to reach the tumor, then making an incision into the tumor through its
capsule, enucleating the growth, closing the bed with catgut, and again
uniting the first incision.

The after-treatment of the abdominal operation is very simple if the
pedicle has not been fastened in the abdominal wound.  The patients receive one hypodermic injection of morphine an hour or two after the operation if the pain is very intense.  Later no narcotics are permitted.  For
the thirst I have for the past ten years used hot water, in teaspoonful doses,
repeated every half-hour or hour.  The Koeberlé wire clamp, if used, is

tightened a little every day, and after the third day the stump is examined to see whether the process of mummification is progressing properly; if there is any moisture, it is carefully dried and the stump is touched with a fifty-per-cent. solution of chloride of zinc, and fresh powder, gauze, and cotton are applied. The transfixion pins are always guarded by a layer of gauze beneath them, to prevent pressure on the skin. The clamp usually comes off from the tenth to the fourteenth day, but sometimes it remains three weeks. Drainage, although still resorted to under exceptional circumstances, is practically a thing of the past. It is permissible, however, when complication with pyosalpinx exists and much pus has come in contact with the peritoneal cavity, and also when many adhesions are present: the latter are rare in connection with fibro myoma.

**Pregnancy.**—Pregnancy complicated with these tumors requires special consideration, and the responsibility resting upon the physician is an unusual one. In discussing the pathology we have learned that their growth is rapid during gestation, and hence due appreciation of their seat is of the utmost importance. A subserous tumor near the fundus should be treated on the expectant plan. Pelvic tumors, if subserous and more or less pedunculated, sometimes recede from the pelvis spontaneously; at other times they can be pushed up and out of the true pelvis during the progress of labor, and thus delivery can take place unaided or be terminated with forceps. Sometimes this cannot be accomplished, and we must be ready to deal with them by abdominal section, this being the only operative procedure admissible with comparative safety to the mother, and usually affording a good prognosis to the child. Cæsarean section, followed immediately by removal of the tumor, is the operation to be performed. In cases of pelvic fibro-myomata, such as were described as tumors of the supra-vaginal portion of the cervix, and growths in the lower segment of the uterus, it must be left to the judgment of the operator whether a Cæsarean section with or without removal of the ovaries, pan-hysterectomy, or a Porro operation should be done. The latter should be preferred whenever practicable.

Interstitial tumors, if gestation is permitted to go to term, are always best treated by the Porro operation,—supra-vaginal amputation of the pregnant uterus, with extra-peritoneal treatment of the pedicle. Whether a Porro operation or a Cæsarean section is contemplated at the time of the viability of the child, it is always best to make it elective,—that is, to choose a time which corresponds to a period a few days prior to the natural termination of the pregnancy. Sometimes it is advisable to do a myomectomy about the middle of gestation: the cases to be selected for this are those of broad-based, subserous tumors and such interstitial growths as we have reason to believe are nearer the peritoneal surface than the mucosa of the uterus, as manifested by the symptoms prior to pregnancy.

Another very important therapeutic procedure to be considered is the production of abortion. A positive rule cannot be laid down, but the following may serve as a guide. If the choice is given at an early period of gestation (up to the third month), abortion should be produced, this being then, with ordinary precautions, practically free from danger; but after the fourth or fifth month I prefer to wait for the termination of gestation and then to do whichever operation is indicated, because at the latter period of gestation abortion is not free from danger; besides, after its accomplishment the patient is not relieved of the tumor. Infra-vaginal tumors of the cervix, if discovered before the sixth or seventh month, should be at once removed, but during the first two and a half to three months they should not be interfered with, on account of the liability to abortion. If not discovered until near the termination of pregnancy, it is just as well to wait until labor has set in and remove the growths then.

Operations for fibro-myomata are ordinarily the cleanest of all abdominal operations, and drainage should be regarded as a complication. Our aim should be to stop bleeding at every point in the peritoneal cavity, so that there shall be no occasion for the draining off of secretions.

The mortality of the operation for the removal of fibro-myomatous tumors differs with individual operators, but depends chiefly upon the kind of tumor, and the circumstances (the physical condition of the patient) under which the operation is done. As to the method of operation, i.e., with intra-peritoneal or extra-peritoneal treatment of the stump, or pan-hysterectomy, statistics are in favor of the first-named; we must not forget, however, that the other operative procedures are as yet in a state of evolution, and that extra-peritoneal treatment of the stump has such obvious disadvantages that it is our duty to seek a method which will overcome them. The mortality in the case of broad-based intra-ligamentous tumors as well as those developing from the supra-vaginal portion of the cervix is large; we can count on twenty-five per cent.; whereas in interstitial tumors of the body of the uterus, for which hysterectomy is done, it is only from ten to fifteen per cent. The average mortality of all abdominal operations for these tumors may be put down as fifteen per cent. in the hands of operators of ordinary skill and experience, castration excepted, in which it should not exceed three per cent. Removal of tumors from the infra-vaginal portion of the cervix should cause no deaths referable to the operation. We have noted that the causes of death are as variable as the operations in vogue; yet the largest death-rate is yielded by sepsis and hemorrhage, or sequelæ due to the latter, complications which are avoidable in pan-hysterectomy, as first performed by Bardenheuer, but promulgated among the profession by August Martin, of Berlin.

### CAVERNOUS ANGIOMA OF THE UTERUS.

Angiomata in various portions of the body are quite common, and the theories as to their origin are numerous. In the uterus the existence of such neoplasms is exceedingly rare.

The patient from whom the specimen figured was obtained is thirty-seven years old and a nullipara.  For nearly a year she had bled more or less, the hemorrhages during the last four months being profuse and the intervals short.  A number of curettings with a sharp instrument, with short intermissions, had only a temporary effect on the metrorrhagia.  The endometrium showed nothing malignant; only a hyperplastic endometritis could be diagnosed with the microscope.  The bleeding finally became so profuse at the expected time of her menstruation that, in view of the previous failures to cure with the curette and local applications, it was resolved to do something radical, especially as the patient was becoming very anæmic and much discouraged.  Vaginal hysterectomy was decided upon rather than castration, first, because it seemed highly probable that she would be cured if she recovered from the operation; and, second, although no malignancy could be shown as yet, it seemed rather suspicious for the bleeding to recur so persistently shortly after curetting.

After removal of the uterus it was bisected anteriorly, when a tumor was found, of the size and shape of an English walnut, located in the anterior upper corner of the organ, and reaching to the fundus.  The tumor protruded into the uterine cavity, and appeared lobulated, of a dark mahogany-red color, and of a consistence somewhat firmer than that of the surrounding uterine walls; it extended, especially in its posterior portion, a little more than half the thickness of the uterine wall.  Its transverse section appeared mottled, exhibiting a large number of dark-purplish and whitish spots, both of which varied in diameter from the transverse section of a raven's quill down to a pin-head.  To the touch the purplish spots appeared soft, corresponding to the consistence of recently coagulated blood; whereas the consistence of the whitish spots was very firm, almost approaching that of cartilage.  Still more conspicuous was the difference in the color of the circular spots in their transverse section through the tumor, where the dark-purple or blood-colored circular fields were distinctly marked from the whitish spots alluded to.  With low powers of the microscope the most striking feature was an abundance of cavities, varying greatly in size and shape, filled with blood.  Obviously these were transverse sections of large veins separated from one another by intervening fibrous connective tissue, in which a considerable number of capillary blood-vessels could be seen.

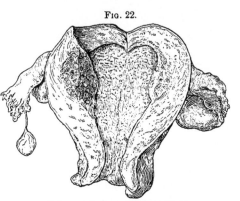

Fig. 22.

Cavernous angioma of uterus, half size.

The blood was not uniformly distributed throughout the veins, some of which showed clots consisting mainly of red blood-corpuscles and comparatively little fibrin; other cavities, on the contrary, held a good deal of fibrin and serum, but not many red blood corpuscles.  This peculiar fact may be accounted for by the circumstance that the blood did not enter all the veins of the tumor, a number of veins being partially or completely obliterated, and consequently presenting an obstacle to the circulation of the blood even within the permeable portions.  With high powers of the microscope the endothelial wall of the permeable cavities could be seen without difficulty : hence the tumor was regarded as a cavernous angioma.  The appearance of the tortuous arteries at the border of the tumor was that of the condition

FIG. 23.

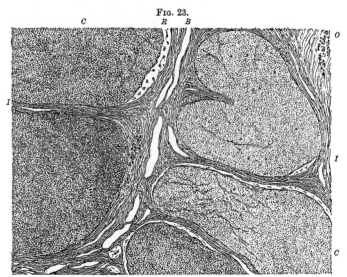

C, C, cavernous veins filled with blood and coagulated fibrin; I, I, interstitial fibrous connective tissue; B, capillary blood-vessels in the interstitial tissue; R, light highly refracting rims along the walls of the veins; O, obliterated blood-vessel marked by clusters of pigment.

described by pathologists as waxy degeneration.  The interstitial connective tissue contained at different points a dark yellow-brown pigment which was probably the outcome of previous extravasations of blood.  In other portions there were larger masses of pigment clusters, which, from the configuration of the fields holding such pigment, were considered as the residues of obliterated cavernous veins.  The large venous cavities penetrated into the muscle wall of the uterus, as already stated.  The tortuous arteries and the enlarged capillaries were most numerous at the periphery of the tumor. There was no distinct boundary-line between the peripheral cavernous veins and the adjacent muscle tissue, which latter bordered directly upon the venous cavities.  Small light patches in the interstitial connective tissue admitted of no other explanation than that they were completely obliterated arteries or capillaries. Considerable interest attaches to the obliteration of the cavernous veins throughout the tumor. Whether the involution of the veins was due to the repeated scraping and subsequent application of carbolic acid I am unable to say with positiveness, but presumably this was the case. A number of the obliterated veins appeared of such peculiar shape that I was forced to believe that the venous cavities were in a collapsed condition when obliteration began. Another possibility is that some parts of the tumor were deprived of blood by preceding obliteration of a certain number of venous cavities, which likewise may have resulted in the locking up of the blood-current and collapse of the veins thereupon.

FIG. 24.

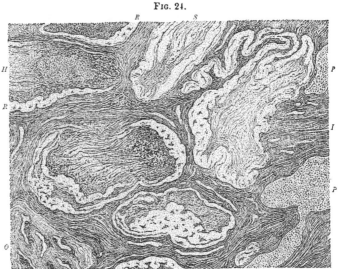

Cavernous angioma of uterus; obliteration of veins. × 50.—*P, P,* permeable cavernous veins filled with blood ; *H,* half-permeable vein ; *S,* solidified cavernous vein ; *R, R,* hyaline rim around both permeable and solidified veins ; *O,* completely obliterated vein ; *I,* interstitial fibrous connective tissue carrying capillary blood-vessels.

All veins either in the process of obliteration or thoroughly obliterated were marked by hyaline or waxy rims around the walls. Such rims were occasionally found doubled, or even trebled ; in the latter instance a narrow rim of medullary tissue could be traced between the waxy layers. The central portions were occupied by either myxomatous or fibrous connective tissue, and in the latter instance the fibrous tissue was often found in hyaline or waxy degeneration. Occasionally a portion of the calibre of the vein remained permeable to blood, whereas a large amount of the previous calibre had disappeared, the vein being transformed into one of the above-named tissues. Again, these tissues were often found intermixed with medullary tissue, which in my specimen was stained deeply with ammoniacal carmine, while the waxy portions took either no carmine or

very little. Another feature was the varying breadth of the waxy rim,
which at one periphery was broad, occupying almost the whole previous
calibre of the blood-vessel, while the opposite periphery was occupied
only by a narrow rim.

In my case the calibre of the previous vein was in a measure still
preserved and permeable to blood. The greater amount, however, was
solidified and transformed into a myxomatous and myxo-fibrous connective tissue. The latter was unquestionably the outcome of a proliferation
of the endothelial wall of the vein, much in the manner in which arteries

FIG. 25.

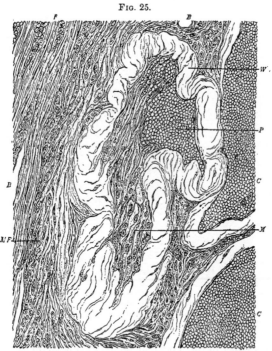

Cavernous angioma of uterus; obliteration of veins, × 200.—W, wall of vein in waxy infiltration;
P, permeable portion of calibre filled with blood; M, myxomatous tissue filling the interior of vein;
C, C, cavernous veins bordered by a rim in waxy infiltration; F, fibrous connective tissue; MF, myxo-
fibrous connective tissue; B, B, capillary blood-vessels.

are rendered solid in the process of endarteritis obliterans by an outgrowth
of the endothelium. Around the partially obliterated vein was seen myxo-
fibrous tissue, obviously the outcome of an inflammatory process accompanying or preceding the obliteration of the vessel. Then followed the smooth
muscle wall of the uterus, in which were clusters of medullary or inflammatory corpuscles in the interstitial connective tissue, either the outcome of
inflammation or the first step towards the new formation of cavernous angioma, an extension of the tumor from its periphery. There are good reasons

for upholding the latter view, especially because of the presence of hæmatoblasts or undeveloped red blood-corpuscles within the medullary nests. To-day it is fully admitted that Rokitansky's assertion, made fifty years ago, that the formation of red blood-corpuscles precedes the formation of cavernous angioma, is correct. How peculiar the outcome of obliteration of a cavernous vein may be is shown in Fig. 26. Here the convolutions of the waxy rim are so pronounced that one is almost compelled to believe that the vein was collapsed and empty before the process of obliteration began. The convoluted rim here is but faintly striated, and contains a limited number of branching protoplasmic or fibrous tracts. This means

Fig 26.

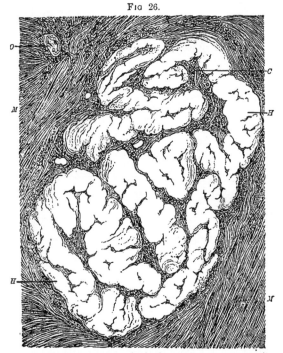

Obliterated vein, × 200.—*H, H,* hyaline convoluted tracts; *C,* medullary and fibrous tissue between the convolutions; *M, M,* smooth muscle-bundles of uterus; *O,* obliterated capillary or artery.

a high grade of waxy infiltration. Between the convolutions we notice tracts of medullary tissue intermixed with fibrous connective tissue. The supply of this tissue with capillary blood-vessels is small. The whole formation is surrounded by a zone of medullary tissue directly bordering upon unchanged smooth muscle tissue. In the left upper corner we notice a waxy patch, evidently an obliterated capillary or artery. What the waxy rim is can be determined only with higher powers of the microscope.

From a histological stand-point I would not hesitate to compare the

waxy rims of the cavernous veins with an anomalous formation of cartilaginous tissue in certain chondromata.    The basis substance is in both
instances not devoid of structure, being traversed by an exceedingly delicate reticulum of living matter, discernible with a power of six hundred
diameters, in the shape of branching tracts of minute granules.    Only one
other case of cavernous angioma of the uterus is as yet on record, that
described by Klob in his " Pathologische Anatomie der weiblichen Sexual-
organe," page 173.

FIG. 27.

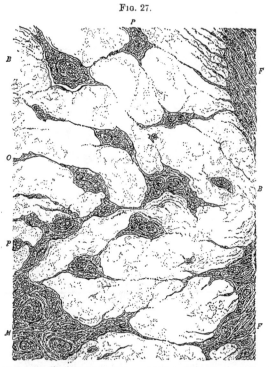

Cartilaginous rim of obliterated vein in cavernous angioma of uterus, × 600.—*M*, medullary tissue
in centre of obliterated vein; *F, F*, fibrous tissue on periphery of obliterated vein; *P, P.* coarsely
granular protoplasmic bodies; *O*, offshoot of protoplasmic body; *B, B*, cartilaginous basis substance.

From the facts described I have little doubt that the tumor was slowly
progressive, though partially, at least, healing by the obliteration of a
number of veins.    In consequence of the almost constant bleeding, extirpation of the organ was a perfectly legitimate procedure.    Another
deduction may be made from this case,—that it was not the curetting
which gave the temporary relief, so much as the local use of pure carbolic
acid.    On the contrary, the bleeding was always quite profuse when the
curette was used.

## ADENOMA.

Glandular tumors are of frequent occurrence in the cervix as well as in the body of the uterus. Allusion has been made on a preceding page to a combination of glandular new formation with myxomatous tissue. Since glandular tissue cannot exist without some adjacent myxomatous or fibrous connective tissue, the name adenoma will be applied only to glandular

Fig. 28.

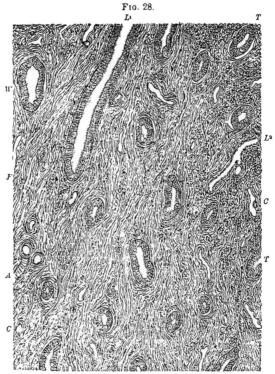

Chronic endometritis fungosa with acute recurrences, × 100.—$L^1$, utricular gland in longitudinal section; $T$, $T$, utricular glands in transverse section; $W$, slightly widened utricular gland; $F$, fibrous connective tissue between the glands; $L^2$, accumulation of lymph-corpuscles, denoting acute inflammation; $A$, artery, $C$, $C$, capillaries.

tumors in which the epithelial new formation is prevalent. In the cervix these lead to prominent raspberry-like formations protruding over the surface of the mucosa. They undergo cystic degeneration, and then produce what older gynæcologists have erroneously termed ovules of Naboth.

*Lympho-Adenoma.*—This name I propose for a morbid process in the mucosa of the uterus hitherto but little understood, and frequently mistaken for fungous or glandular endometritis. The so-called fungous endometritis, like any other inflammatory process, is confined to the interstitial lymph tissue, and at the utmost may lead to an enlargement of the utricular glands with a simultaneous widening of their calibres.

No pathologist will admit that an inflammatory process will cause a new formation of glandular structures; yet we frequently meet, in fungous endometritis, with a large number of utricular glands, freely bifurcating and exhibiting alternate widening and constriction of the tubules. Such a condition cannot be simply the result of inflammation, but must be considered as a neoplasm; and since both elements of the uterine mucosa, the

Fig. 29.

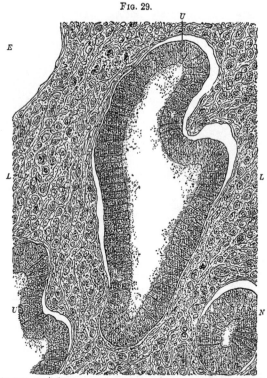

Lympho-adenoma of uterine mucosa, × 500.—*E*, empty space of utricular gland; *U, U*, newly-formed utricular glands with wide calibres; *L, L*, lymph-tissue; *N*, normal utricular gland in transverse section.

lymphatic as well as the glandular tissue, are noticeably augmented in bulk and increased in size, the term lympho-adenoma becomes applicable. Although other writers speak of a benign adenoma (Ruge, Veit, Pozzi, and others), no sufficient differentiation has as yet been attempted between a simple inflammatory process and a new formation of tissue.

The term fungous endometritis is, in my opinion, applicable only to a slight nodular thickening of the mucosa, in which the microscope reveals a considerable increase in lymph-corpuscles, but no augmentation of the utricular glands. At most some of the tubules may exhibit moderate widening of their calibres. Lympho-adenoma, on the contrary, will produce nodulated protrusions over the mucosa, frequently of considerable size, and the microscope shows not only an increase in the number of the lymph-corpuscles, but also a pronounced increase in the number of the utricular glands. In fungous endometritis an augmentation of the number of lymph-corpuscles occurs only in the acute stage: when the process be-

Fig. 30.

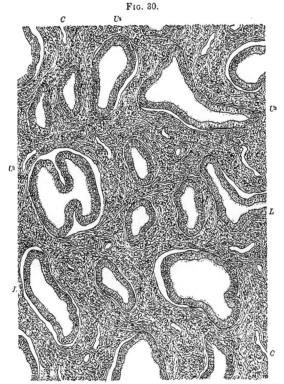

Lympho-adenoma of uterine mucosa, × 100 — $U^1$, utricular gland with folded epithelial lining; $U^2$, three successive transverse sections of a utricular gland; $U^3$, oblique section of a utricular gland, L, L, lymph-tissue; C, C, capillary blood-vessels.

comes chronic they will decrease in number and the original myxomatous net-work will be transformed into myxo-fibrous or even fibrous connective tissue, terminating in atrophy of the mucosa. In such a case the utricular glands are conspicuously diminished in number and some of them are found transformed into cysts. In lympho-adenoma the number of the lymph-corpuscles is not so considerably augmented as in acute hyperplastic endometritis, but, the disease being progressive, as in all tumors, atrophy of the lymphoid tissue will not take place. In both instances hemorrhages occur.    In fungous endometritis simple curetting and local applications

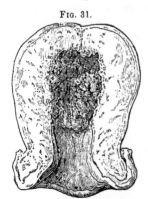

Fig. 31.

will effect a cure; in lympho-adenoma, on the contrary, such a procedure will result in a permanent cure only if the disease is not far advanced and is confined to a small area. In spite of repeated curetting, the hemorrhages may recur, so that vaginal hysterectomy is indicated.

The microscope furnishes the only means of deciding whether we have to deal with simple fungous endometritis or with progressive lympho-adenoma.   The microscopic examination of the scrapings becomes still more important when it is necessary to determine whether we have to deal with a benign lympho-adenoma or with an incipient myeloma (sarcoma).   L. Heitzmann in 1887

Lympho-adenoma of uterus (benign adenoma) —Uterus was extirpated on account of recurrences after curetting.

called attention to the fact that in the early stage of myeloma the epi-

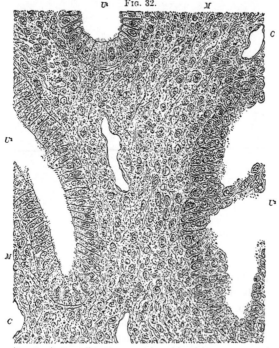

Fig. 32.

Transformation of epithelia of utricular glands into myeloma tissue.  From a specimen of Charles D. Jones's, × 500 —$U^1$, utricular gland with normal epithelia; $U^2$, utricular gland whose epithelia are coarsely granular and have augmented nuclei; $U^3$, utricular gland with epithelia partly transformed into myeloma tissue; $M$, $M$, lympho-myeloma; $C$, capillary blood-vessels.

thelia of the utricular glands will soon become transformed into myeloma elements. This will occur indifferently whether the sarcoma attacks a normal or an inflamed uterine mucosa. Heitzmann's assertion has attracted little attention ; but my own numerous microscopical researches in this line have convinced me that it is correct. So long as the epithelial layer of the utricular gland is perfect, we may have to deal with fungous endometritis or lympho-adenoma, but the process will invariably be a benign one. When, on the contrary, we find the epithelia of some utricular glands transformed into lymph-corpuscles, penetrating even into the calibre, the diagnosis of lympho-myeloma (small round-celled sarcoma of Virchow) is established. As soon as this diagnosis is reached, the removal of the uterus is the only means of saving the patient's life.

Quite recently Charles D. Jones has examined a number of scrapings and uteri extirpated on account of the diagnosis of lympho-myeloma made on microscopical examination of the scrapings. To this gentleman I am indebted for the accompanying drawing (Fig. 32).

The microscopical examination of scrapings in such cases is the more important since it enables us to recognize malignant disease at the earliest stages of its development, and by prompt removal of the uterus to save the patient's life.

38

# CHAPTER XII.

## MALIGNANT NEOPLASMS OF THE UTERUS.

BY HER MANN J. BOLDT, M.D.

### MYELOMA OR SARCOMA.

THESE malignant tumors were for a long time considered to be rare. To-day we know that they are not of exceptional occurrence. The clinical features I shall not dwell upon, since all that will be said of cancerous tumors holds good for sarcomatous. They are equally infectious, therefore equally malignant, and the symptoms are much the same in both.

Virchow has distinguished three varieties of sarcoma: (1) the round-celled, (2) the spindle-celled, and (3) myxo-sarcoma. A fourth variety has recently been added to this list by Sänger, sarcoma deciduo-cellulare.

The round-celled sarcoma of Virchow is the most common form. The small round-celled sarcoma, or, as I would prefer to term it, lympho-myeloma, is far more common than the large round-celled sarcoma of Virchow, or globo-myeloma. Whenever a diagnosis is necessary on account of frequent hemorrhages from the uterus, the cervix should be dilated and the mucosa curetted with a sharp instrument, both for diagnostic and for therapeutic purposes.

The diagnosis of lympho-adenoma, a benign form of tumor, is established when the utricular glands are found not only widened, but increased in number, and the epithelial lining unbroken, being composed of columnar ciliated cells. The adjacent myxomatous lymph-tissue may be increased in a varying degree and crowded with small non-nucleated bodies, the lymph-corpuscles. So long as the epithelial layer is unbroken, the diagnosis of benign lympho-adenoma is permissible, as is illustrated and explained more fully in the section on adenoma.

The condition is quite different when the original lympho-adenoma or the previously unchanged mucosa of the uterus becomes affected with lympho-myeloma. In this case we notice first an increase in the bulk of the nuclei of the columnar epithelia; next some of the neighboring epithelia lose their intervening cement-substance and fuse together, forming multinuclear protoplasmic bodies, which finally split up into a large number of small solid or vacuolated bodies, thus accomplishing the transformation into lympho-myeloma.

L. Heitzmann and recently Charles D. Jones have called attention to

594

this fact. The latter examined the mucosa of several uteri extirpated on account of the diagnosis "incipient myeloma," made after the microscopical examination of pieces removed with the curette, and found more or less advanced myeloma. There is a possibility of recognizing under the microscope the earliest stages of a myelomatous growth by means of the changes in the epithelia. We frequently notice an interruption in the epithelia of the utricular glands, through which the myelomatous tissue penetrates the calibre of the glands. In an advanced stage only vestiges of the previous epithelia are discernible, the whole tissue consisting of a more or less vacuolated lympho-myeloma.

FIG. 1.

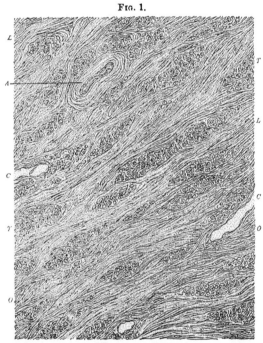

Small spindle-celled sarcoma of uterus, × 500.—L, L, longitudinal bundles of spindles; T, T, transverse sections of bundles; O, O, oblique sections of bundles; A, artery collapsed; C, C, capillaries.

Spindle myeloma is comparatively rare, and is composed of spindle-shaped protoplasmic bodies with irregular, coarsely granular nuclei, freely interlacing and somewhat resembling fibro-myoma. I observed a case of this variety of tumor which started from the body of the uterus and extended to the broad ligament, the tubes, and one of the ovaries. All the tissues of the organs named were transformed into spindle-shaped myeloma-corpuscles. The diagnosis of this tumor was made from scrapings, and extirpation of the uterus and adnexa was performed. The microscopical appearance of the tumor is represented in Fig. 1.

FIG. 2.

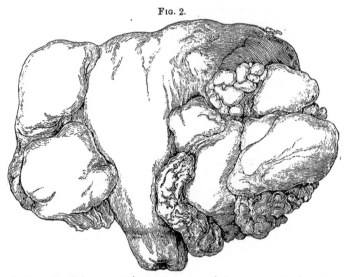

Small spindle-celled sarcoma of uterus and adnexa: posterior view, one-half natural size.

FIG. 3.

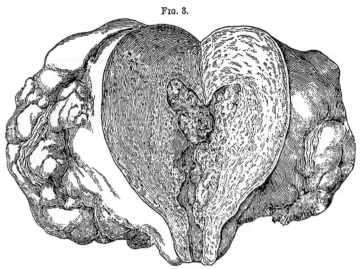

Small spindle-celled sarcoma, showing interior of uterus.

MALIGNANT DECIDUOMA (SARCOMA UTERI DECIDUO-CELLULARE).

Although many authorities dispute this variety of sarcoma as a particular form, deeming it simply a mixed sarcoma, Martin Sänger insists upon its origin from decidual elements, because the protoplasmic bodies constituting the tumor exhibit a close resemblance to decidual elements, and also because, thus far, the neoplasm has been found only in patients who shortly prior to its observation were pregnant.

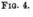

FIG. 4.

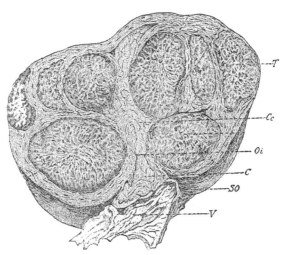

Uterus with tumors divided anteriorly in the median line.—*T*, neoplasm; *Cc*, cavity of uterine body; *Oi*, internal os, *C*, cervix; *SO*, peritoneal surface of the uterus; *V*, vagina. (Sanger.)

The symptoms are similar to those of some retained secundines after delivery or abortion. The prognosis is favorable only if the condition is recognized very early and the diseased uterus then immediately extirpated.

The recognition is based upon a microscopical examination by a competent pathologist of the débris obtained by the use of a *sharp* curette, which should be done in all cases of prolonged sanguineous discharge after premature or normal evacuation of the products of conception.

If the disease is allowed to run its natural course, death ensues in from seven to twelve months from complications similar to those in cancer.

One case was seen in consultation by me. A woman aged thirty-three years had aborted at about the fourth month. Shortly after abortion sanguineous discharges again occurred, and she was curetted by her family physician, under the impression that placental remnants were left *in utero*. When seen by me about four months subsequently, the uterus was greatly enlarged and the patient anæmic. An examination of the débris resulted in the diagnosis of a peculiar form of sarcoma. The patient died a few months subsequently of asthenia, pleurisy with effusion having previously taken place. Unfortunately, no post-mortem was permitted.

### CANCER OF THE UTERUS.

This disease occurs most frequently between the ages of forty-five and fifty years, although early periods of life are not exempt. I have seen several cases in patients between twenty and thirty which were too far advanced for radical operation.

It was formerly thought that it was limited to the cervix; later experience, however, especially since vaginal hysterectomy has been generally performed, has shown that cancer of the corpus uteri, although not nearly so frequent as cervical carcinoma, is not rare.

For clinical reasons cancer of the body will be considered separately from cancer of the cervix. Cancer of the portio vaginalis, the so-called "cauliflower growth," has no tendency to invade the uterine mucosa, though exceptions to this rule occur. The papillary growth begins on the surface, and the thickened epithelial covering extends into the depths of the portio, when, breaking down, new papillæ are formed, which subsequently undergo neerotic destruction; or it is of a fungous appearance, sometimes partly filling the vagina, and hiding the cervical opening beneath it. Although it remains limited for a considerable period to the part from which it originated, in the course of time the periuterine tissues and the vagina will be involved, or it may spread along the cervical canal.

It is conceded that there is always an inflammation of the endometrium accompanying cancer of the cervix, but the truth of the assertion of Abel and Landau, that the lesion is sarcoma, is greatly doubted and even denied by many; yet those authors have shown me specimens which were sarcomatous beyond a doubt. In other cases cancer of the cervix begins in the form of a nodule situated beneath the mucous membrane, and this is not transformed into an ulcerating surface until the disease has been present for a comparatively long time. When cancer begins in the cervical mucous membrane, it rapidly causes destruction of the cervix; and though the disease may not be noticeable on inspection, the introduction of the finger into the cervical canal will often show this to be extensively destroyed. The broad ligaments become affected early, and not seldom the lining membrane of the corporal endometrium. In all varieties of cancer the advanced stages resemble one another in consequence of induration of the broad ligaments and the presence of a greater or less amount of exudative material in the pelvis which is of either an inflammatory or a malignant character, and produces pressure upon the vessels and nerves and not rarely upon the ureters: hence in such advanced stages the patients have intense pains in the pelvis and lower extremities.

The uterus under such circumstances is firmly fixed and immobile to the touch; the bladder is also frequently involved by the extension of the disease. In consequence of the necrotic process a vesico-vaginal fistula is formed; the rectum is only exceptionally affected. Kidney lesions are very common in connection with cancer of the uterus: for example, hydronephrosis may be produced by compression of the ureters, especially near their insertion into the bladder.

**Pathology of Cancer of the Uterus.**—Cancer of the cervix is generally divided into several varieties with reference to its seat, such as cancer of the portio vaginalis, cancer of the supra-vaginal portion of the cervix or of the cervix proper, and cancer of the mucosa lining the cervix. I lay no stress upon the localization, since this is of comparatively small importance to the practitioner.

In the cervical portion of the uterus we meet mainly with four varieties of carcinoma: (1) dermoid, (2) scirrhus, (3) adenoid, and (4) medullary.

1. *Dermoid cancer* is of comparatively rare occurrence. Under the microscope it exhibits nests and pegs, composed of flat epithelia, containing lumps of colloid masses, the so-called cancer pearls. For illustration, I refer the reader to the chapter on neoplasms of the vulva (Fig. 9).

It is this form which produces pronounced papillary elevations on the surface of the mucosa, assuming later the aspect of a so-called cauliflower growth. The epithelial depressions between the papillary connective-tissue formations, as such, arouse the suspicion of an incipient cancer, especially when some of the epithelia are enlarged and show an increase in the size of their nuclei, or a splitting of the latter into several lumps,—so-called endogenous new formation.

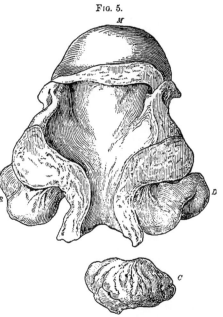

Fig. 5.

Villous cancer of the vaginal portion of the uterus (so-called cauliflower growth) combined with fibro-myoma of the fundus uteri, double hydrosalpinx, and cystic ovaries—*M*, fibro-myoma; *R*, right ovary and tube; *L*, left ovary and tube; *C*, amputated cancer of vaginal portion.

The fibrous connective tissue produces long and narrow papillary elevations, frequently with finger-like branches; their blood-vessels are rather numerous wide capillaries, and the connective tissue is more or less crowded with so-called inflammatory corpuscles, or, according to Virchow, is in a condition of small-celled infiltration which to-day we consider the incipient stage of cancer, since we know that the more pronounced is the infiltration of the connective tissue the more malignant is the type of cancer.

2. *Scirrhus.*—This is likewise a rare form, and always occurs in the depth of the tissue. (See Fig. 13.) It consists of nests, either isolated or in associated alveoli, filled with small, distinctly polyhedral epithelia. Between the nests there is a large amount of dense fibrous connective tissue,

FIG. 6.

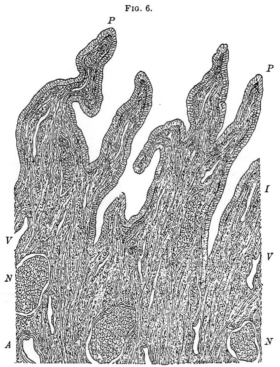

Papillary or villous cancer of the vaginal portion of the uterus (so-called cauliflower growth).—*P, P,* papillæ on surface of tumor, lined by columnar epithelia; *I,* fibrous connective tissue in inflammatory infiltration; *N, N,* cancer-nests in deeper portions; *V, V,* veins; *A,* artery.

lacking the small-celled infiltration seen in the initial stages. Obviously this form cannot be diagnosed under the microscope if clippings from the surface of the mucosa are examined. The surface, as a rule, shows only papillary excrescences, freely supplied with blood-vessels, and covered with a single row of ciliated columnar epithelia of a normal appearance.

3. *Adenoid cancer* is the most common form, and sooner or later changes into the medullary type. (See Fig. 8.) At first we notice under the microscope, aside from papillary elevations on the surface, numerous

FIG. 7.

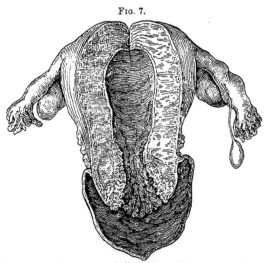

' Cancer of cervix, the disease starting in the cervical mucous membrane.

FIG. 8

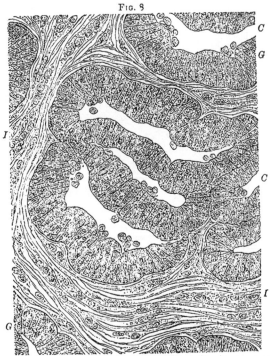

Adenoid cancer of mucosa of uterus, × 500 —*G, G,* hyperplastic utricular glands, lined with columnar epithelia; *C, C,* irregular calibres holding corpuscles; *I, I,* inflammatory infiltration of fibrous connective tissue.

tubular glands coursing irregularly in the fibrous connective tissue, an appearance which we may describe as adenoma.    As soon, however, as we notice clusters of protoplasmic bodies in the connective tissue in the neighborhood of the newly-formed glands, we are enabled to determine the presence of the preliminary stage of cancer.    Experience has taught us that every adenoma of the cervix uteri is prone to change into cancer, and this is indicated by incipient infiltration of the connective tissue with small

FIG. 9.

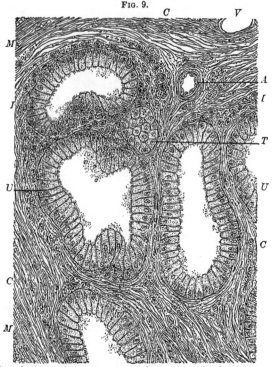

Adenomatous stage of carcinoma of the cervix uteri, × 250.—U, U, utricular glands, the columnar epithelia in small portions coarsely granular; T, segment of a utricular gland, the epithelia in top view; I, I, so-called small-celled infiltration of connective tissue on the borders of utricular glands; C, C, fibrous connective tissue; M, M, smooth muscle-bundles in longitudinal and transverse sections; A, artery; V, vein.

protoplasmic bodies.    The diagnosis "cancer" is thoroughly established when we observe the newly-formed tubular glands branching and with partly widened calibres.    Along the epithelial lining we see a varying number of epithelia, with nuclei augmented both in size and in number. Preceding this we note karyokinetic figures in the nuclei, indicating a more rapid outgrowth of the living matter within the protoplasm of the epithelia. In pronounced cases of adenoid cancer the tubules exhibit manifold convolutions, and frequently only one side of the wall of the contorted tubule is discernible, the rest having perished in a crowd of protoplasmic bodies varying in aspect from a small solid lump to a larger globular, nucleated, protoplasmic mass. Even at the height of this infiltration, which means a transition to the medullary type, we frequently notice single or clustered, somewhat angular, bodies, vestiges of previous epithelia.

4. *Medullary Cancer.*—This is the most malignant form, and usually arises from an adenoid cancer (see Fig. 8), though any variety of cancer, including dermoid and scirrhus, may in the course of time be transformed

FIG. 10.

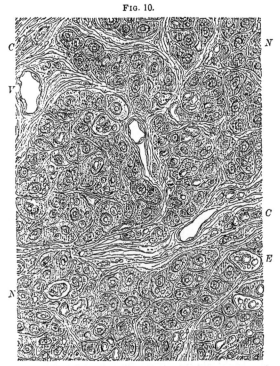

Medullary cancer of uterus, × 500—*C, C,* fibrous connective tissue crowded with protoplasmic bodies; *V,* vein in transverse section; *N, N,* epithelial nests; *E,* endogenous new formation of living matter.

into medullary. The diagnosis of this form is easy enough so long as we find vestiges of previous tubular glands, consisting of a single row of columnar epithelia or clusters of such epithelia. It is difficult, or may even be impossible, when such vestiges are absent. In the latter instance we meet with protoplasmic bodies of varying sizes and shapes closely packed together, holding, as a rule, only scanty, wide capillaries. These are the cases which were termed by former pathologists encephaloid tumors, owing to their resemblance to brain-tissue. Virchow first maintained that cancer may lose its histological characteristics and assume those of sarcoma, an assertion the correctness of which, originally much doubted, may to-day be considered established.

The cancerous origin of the tumor is indicated by the greatly varying sizes and shapes of the protoplasmic bodies, which in myeloma (sarcoma) are more uniform. Evidently, Abel and Landau examined cases in which a medullary cancer had attained its ultimate and most malignant stage, that of myeloma.

To the clinician this is of small importance, because medullary cancer and myeloma are equally dangerous to life. Some authors speak of a flat ulcer upon the mucosa of the cervix as a form of cancer. As mentioned previously, ulcers due to lacerations or to the corrosive properties of the endometrial discharge may become the seat of cancer. The latter diagnosis becomes admissible only if we are able to establish the presence of an outgrowth of the epithelial structure, which in simple ulcers is more or less destroyed, but is never augmented.

**Etiology.**—We may consider a long-continued cervical catarrh with erosions, and also cervical lacerations causing such pathological changes, as direct etiological factors. I myself have seen one case in which the primary seat of the cancer was in the angle of the laceration. Age, as has been noted, is a predisposing factor.

**Symptoms.**—Unfortunately for the patients, the beginning stage of cancer of the cervix causes no symptoms. It is not until the neoplasm begins to ulcerate that bleeding and leucorrhœal discharges are usually present, although occasionally an irregular "spotting of blood" may be noticed, which is not due to an ulcerating cancer, but to accompanying inflammation of the lining membrane of the uterus. Frequently the first evidence is a slight bloody discharge after coitus. If the disease makes its appearance during the period of sexual activity, the hemorrhage manifests itself only in a more prolonged and profuse menstruation. Very often the sanguineous discharge which occurs after the menopause assumes the appearance of expressed meat juice. This appearance is also found sometimes in the early stage of dermoid cancer.

A vaginal discharge having an offensive odor, whether mixed with blood or not, should always arouse suspicion, especially if profuse and occurring in a woman over thirty-five years old. Although the bleeding is not generally profuse, I have seen as the first symptom alarming to the patient a copious hemorrhage, which continued to a less extent for several days. This symptom can be explained only by a rupture of a large blood-vessel in the tissue necrosed by the process of ulceration. The continuous oozing of blood so often seen is caused by a rupture of the dilated capillaries in the ulcerating neoplasm. Among the earliest symptoms, then, we must class bleeding, in the form either of spotting or of prolonged or irregular menstruation, and offensive leucorrhœa.

Pain is not a characteristic symptom until the neoplasm has encroached upon tissues outside of the uterus, except in cases—by no means rare—

where a concomitant pelvic inflammation exists. When, however, the malignant infiltration has passed into the broad ligaments and the pelvic peritoneum, variable pains are present, which resemble those of pelvic peritonitis, and consist of backache, hypogastric pains, and inguinal pains frequently radiating down the thighs, caused by pressure upon the nerves. They are often described as lancinating in character. When vesical symptoms are present, it is a certain sign that the disease has encroached upon the cellular tissue between the bladder and the cervix. The presence of rectal symptoms may be ascribed to inflammation of the peritoneum forming Douglas's pouch. Œdema of the lower extremities may occur in consequence of thrombosis of the veins or of the marasmic state of the patient, which produces an hydræmic condition of the blood. The nutrition of the patient suffers very much, the digestion is greatly impaired, vomiting is not rare, and loss of appetite is a prominent symptom. The skin assumes a pale-yellow tint, usually described as the cancerous cachexia. The cystitis which so frequently is present is very painful. Eventually, in many cases, uræmia more or less pronounced develops; it is caused by pressure on the ureters, either by the malignant neoplasm or through distortion of the ducts by inflammatory changes in the pelvic cellular tissue. When a vesico-vaginal fistula has formed by the ulcerative process penetrating the bladder, the painful symptoms of cystitis are relieved; but the discomfort of being constantly wet and soiled is almost as distressing to such patients.

The cause of death is, in the majority of cases, exhaustion; next to this, peritonitis is the most frequent factor. Among other conditions leading to a fatal issue may be mentioned thrombosis of the large pelvic veins, as the common and internal iliac, etc., which sometimes gives rise to pyæmia. Pyelonephritis, embolism of the pulmonary artery, pneumonia, pleurisy, uræmia, the formation of secondary tumors in distant organs, such as the lungs, liver, kidneys, etc., may all be enumerated among the direct causes of a fatal termination of uterine cancer. Pregnancy occurs in many cases of cancer of the portio vaginalis, and it has seemed to me that the disease, under such conditions, progresses more rapidly. When conception does take place, abortion is apt to occur; yet not a few such patients carry to full term. Hanks says that abortion takes place about the third month; although this is correct, it is not due to the fact that the patient has cancer, but rather to the coexisting endometritis, which, as experience teaches, favors the occurrence of abortion at that period of gestation. The accompanying endometritis and the diseased condition of the cervix are, however, to a great extent hinderances to conception.

Diagnosis.—The early stage of cancer of the cervix can never be diagnosed with certainty without a microscopical examination of an excised piece of the suspected part, and even with this aid it is by no means always easy to decide the question; in fact, it is sometimes impossible, so that the clinical features must often settle our course of procedure, and in some cases we are justified in proceeding with a minor operation rather than in waiting long for the case to clear up. The malignant disease may resemble a follicular erosion, though it differs from it in having somewhat elevated and indurated edges. The raw surface in both conditions may bleed with equal readiness on manipulation, but if papillary projections are already present, in cancer these break down with much greater readiness on being scraped lightly with the finger-nail. There is a possibility of mistaking cancer for a submucous fibro-myoma protruding from the os externum, especially when this is becoming gangrenous; yet, if care be exercised, the healthy ring of cervical tissue will be found, on examination, encircling the benign neoplasm. Still more difficult will the diagnosis be if the disease begins in the cervical canal; it may have made considerable progress, and yet there may be nothing abnormal in appearance, the portio being seemingly normal; but when the tip of the finger or a sound is introduced into the canal, a considerable cavity may already be present. The chief clinical distinction between beginning cancer and cervical endometritis will be found in the fact that the discharge in the latter condition retains its mucous consistency, which is always lost in cancer. The sanguineous discoloration and offensive odor are sometimes present in endometritis. Great difficulty in making a diagnosis is experienced when cancer assumes the form of a nodule beneath the vagino-cervical mucosa, before it begins to break down. We may suspect such a nodule to be malignant if it is hard and protuberant, the exterior being of a bluish-red color, and the patient more than thirty-five years old. We should always, under such circumstances, excise a piece for microscopical examination. · Advanced stages of cancer of any part of the cervix are readily diagnosed, but in such instances it is usually impossible to recognize from what part of the cervix the malignant disease originated.

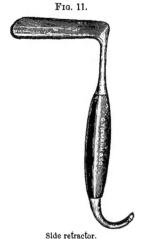

FIG. 11.

Side retractor.

### Treatment of Cancer of the Uterus.

—This may be divided into palliative and radical. The former is indicated in all cases where the disease has progressed to such an extent that the malignant structure apparently cannot be removed *in toto*. Among the various remedies and forms of treatment, that which has stood the test best is curettage, with subsequent cauterization with the Paquelin or the galvano-cautery. The course to be pursued is preparation of the patient as for vaginal hysterectomy, the instruments consisting of a speculum to depress the perineum, one for the anterior vaginal wall, with attachment for constant irrigation, and side retractors. (Fig. 11.) One or two volsellæ, two bullet-forceps, a needle-holder, two full-curved needles, and a large sharp curette or scoop make up the armamentarium, which requires sterilization.

Other needful accessories are a Paquelin cautery, a uterine dressing forceps, heavy catgut or silk (to tie the uterine arteries, if necessary), a sufficient number of pledgets of absorbent cotton, and five- to ten-per-cent. iodoform gauze in strips two inches wide. The patient is anæsthetized, and then placed in the dorsal position. All tissue readily removable is gouged out with the large sharp curette or scoop, under continuous irrigation ; then the bleeding is stopped as much as possible by packing strips of iodoform gauze tightly into the cavity, leaving it in contact a few minutes, and then removing it. Then the round ball point of a Paquelin cautery at a red heat is used to cauterize thoroughly the interior. Subsequently, douches of a solution of boric acid (1 to 20) may be used. Another very efficient treatment is to pack the crater, after curettage, with pledgets of absorbent cotton as large as an English walnut, which have been impregnated with a fifty-per-cent. solution of chloride of zinc. A non-absorbent cotton tampon is placed over these. Any chloride of zinc that may have come in contact with the vaginal mucous membrane is neutralized by a saturated solution of bicarbonate of sodium. The chloride of zinc produces a still further separation of cancerous tissue, and in about a week or ten days the slough will have loosened sufficiently to be removed. Iodoform gauze may be packed in the excavation in case of any bleeding after separation of the slough. Later, should the discharge become very offensive, and if a second curettage with subsequent cauterization is contra-indicated, subnitrate of bismuth mixed with aristol or iodoform may be dusted into the cavity. Antiseptic douches are of great value. Not infrequently the disease has progressed so far that it may happen that the uterus is pierced with the curette during the operation. If rigid antisepsis has been adhered to and the operation is stopped at once, this will not be apt to produce a serious result.

Dr. John Byrne, of Brooklyn, uses the galvano-cautery for his work, and in an address before the American Gynæcological Society he gave his results, which are unequalled, according to his analysis, by those of any other method of treatment,—viz., in nearly four hundred cases, not a single death due to the operation. In forty out of sixty-three cases of cancer of the portio vaginalis (twenty-three patients having been lost sight of) the periods of exemption ranged from two to twenty-two years, the average period being over nine years. Of eighty-one cases involving the entire cervix, thirty-one patients were lost sight of, ten relapsed within two years, five had no recurrence for two years, eleven for three years, six for four years, eight for five years, six for seven years, two for eleven years, one for thirteen years, and one for seventeen years. Thus in fifty of this class whose histories could be followed up the average period of exemption was nearly six years.

Narcotics will invariably become necessary at some time during the course of the malady, but we should wait as long as the patients can bear the pain without their use, and should then begin with the smallest possible dose which will alleviate suffering.

With Dr. Byrne's consent, I describe his operations both palliative and radical, because of the remarkable immediate and remote results obtained by him, concerning which his statements are absolutely reliable.

After having removed all broken-down tissue by the use of a sharp curette, the cavity is sponged repeatedly with a mixture of commercial acetic acid, 3i, glycerin, 3iii, and carbolic acid, 9i; then the cavity is packed with absorbent cotton, which is allowed to remain for a few minutes or longer, as the case may be. On removing this, if bleeding is found to have ceased and the cavity is fairly dry, the cautery is applied. If, however, oozing of blood to any extent should still continue, it will be best to pass into the cavity a tampon saturated with the above styptic, allowing it to remain for forty-eight hours before the application of the cautery. Cauterization in all such cases should be conducted in the following manner:

The diseased organ should be exposed to view and the vagina protected by a Sims speculum and an anterior and two lateral retractors; it may be necessary to seize the edges of the excavation with one or more volsellæ. Before introducing the cautery electrode, a wad of absorbent cotton is to be passed into the cavity, held there for a moment, and as soon as it is withdrawn a dome-shaped electrode, brought to a cherry-red heat, is to be rapidly and repeatedly passed over the bottom of the cavity mainly. The surface is then again dried by wads of absorbent cotton held in dressing forceps, and cauterization is resumed as before. This process is to be repeated until the deeper parts of the cavity have become dry and charred, when the sides are to be treated in precisely the same manner and roasted to the same crisp condition. The seat of operation will now present the appearance of a perfectly black and dry cavity. All ragged and overlapping edges are next trimmed off by the cautery knife; a firmly-rolled tampon of suitable size, with silk thread attached, and saturated with the styptic compound, is then placed in the cavity, and finally a supporting vaginal tampon is applied and the patient removed to bed. The vaginal tampon may be removed on the following day, but the one in contact with the charred surface should be allowed to remain for forty-eight hours or longer. The subsequent treatment will consist of antiseptic vaginal douches, twice daily.

*High Amputation.*—In conditions admitting of high amputation, the following is the method usually resorted to. The uterus is to be exposed and the vaginal walls protected in the manner already described. The diverging volsella (Fig. 12), being passed well into the cervical canal, should now be expanded to a proper degree and locked, so as to afford complete control of the uterus during the entire operation.

By alternate traction and upward pressure on the uterus, an accurate idea should be obtained as to the proper point at which to begin the circular incision, so as to avoid injuring the bladder or opening into the cul-de-sac of Douglas. As to the latter, however, should it be found that the disease has involved the retro-uterine tissues, and that its excision or destruction by the cautery cannot be effected without opening the peritoneal cavity, there need be no hesitation in doing this, as no harm is apt to result from it, whether done accidentally or by design. Should it be evident at the outset that the operation, in order to be thorough, must include a portion of the cul-de-sac, it will be better to make the line of incision anterior to this until the cervix has been removed, leaving the excision of the retrouterine parts by the cautery knife as the final proceeding. Under these circumstances all that will be needed will be an antiseptic tampon properly applied.

In making the circular incision, the *cold* cautery knife (Fig. 12), slightly curved, should be applied close up to the vaginal junction, and, from the moment that the current is turned on, should be kept in contact

Fig. 12.

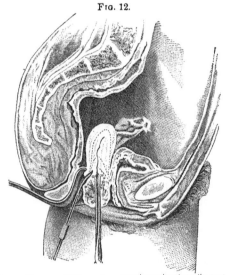

The carcinomatous cervix exposed by speculum, the uterus steadied with double diverging tenaculum, and the cautery knife applied. The lines show the course which the knife should take, according to the invasion of the neoplasm.

with the parts to be incised. Before removing the electrode for any purpose, such as change of position or altering the curve of the knife, the current should be stopped, and before continuing incision the instrument should be placed in position while cool. In other words, if the knife be heated before operation, even though to only a dull red, and applied to parts at all vascular, more or less hemorrhage will certainly follow; whereas if the cool platinum blade is already in contact with moisture as the current is being transformed into heat, vessels are shrunken or closed even before they are severed. This is a very important point, and should never be lost sight of in cautery operations.

The circular incision having been made to the depth of a quarter of an inch, it will now be observed that by increased traction the uterus may be drawn much farther downward, and by directing the knife upward and inward the amputation may be carried to any desired extent. In cases calling for amputation above the os internum it will be better to excise and remove the cervix first, then, after dilating the canal sufficiently to admit the diverging volsella, to proceed as in the first instance, taking care, however, to keep within bounds. It will be found that the cupped stump can now be drawn down and made to project as a more or less convex body.

In all cases the dome-shaped electrode should be repeatedly passed over the entire cavity, so as to render the cauterization complete.

In carrying the knife towards the sides of the cervix, circular and other arterial branches are apt to be encountered, and hence, in this locality particularly, a high degree of heat in the platinum blade is to be carefully avoided. As an additional security against hemorrhage, the convexity of the knife should be pressed against the external surface of each particular section cut, so as to close vessels more effectually. The metallic parts of the electrode for the distance of about two inches should be covered with a strip of thin flannel, so that the vagina may be protected against injury from the reflected heat.

Injections of pyoktanin blue in inoperable cancer of the uterus have been given a very careful and thorough trial; I am unable to note a single instance of cure from the use of the remedy. The advantage to be gained, in my experience, is the prolongation of life, with a temporary improvement of the symptoms in most cases.

The pyoktanin should be in the form of a freshly-prepared solution (1 to 300), to be injected with a hypodermic syringe at several points in the infiltrated tissue, a few drops being used at each place of puncture, and in all about thirty minims being consumed. The dry powder is used in the interior of the uterus, or the entire surface may be brushed with a cotton swab dipped in a one-per-cent. solution. The injections should be made at intervals of from twenty-four to forty-eight hours. Thorough curettage should always precede the pyoktanin treatment.

We now come to the consideration of the radical treatment by means of the knife.

High amputation of the cervix for cancer, although promising in its results if the disease is limited to the vaginal portion, is not upheld by me, and will not be further discussed, first, because unquestionable cases of independent cancerous nodules in the body of the uterus have been observed; and, second, the operation, if properly performed, is just as difficult and nearly as serious as complete extirpation of the uterus. I hold that the entire uterus should be removed, even if the cervix is only slightly diseased, if the patient gives her consent to such a procedure. We shall therefore consider that operation only. If the organ is too large to be removed per vaginam, it should be extirpated by cœliotomy, as was proposed by Freund, of Strasburg, before vaginal hysterectomy came again into vogue.

The technique is similar to that used in total extirpation of the uterus in fibro-myoma, except that the necrosed tissue is first removed per vaginam with a curette, and the raw surface is touched with the actual cautery in order to avoid infection. Other methods—the sacral and the sacrococcygeal—for removing the uterus for cancer are not acceptable to me, because a uterus in which the disease has progressed so far that it cannot be removed per vaginam, on account of malignant infiltration of the parametria, should not be removed at all.

FIG. 13.

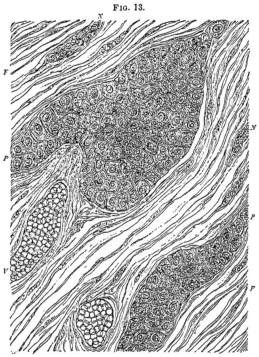

Scirrhus of body of uterus, × 500.—P, P, plugs composed of small epithelia; F, F, dense fibrous connective tissue between the plugs; N, N, nests of medullary corpuscles; V, blood-vessel filled with blood.

The frequent hemorrhages of greater or less degree, the fetid vaginal discharges, the pains of various character, the rectal and vesical tenesmus, the marasmic appearance of the patient, with impairment of the functions of the stomach, the indurated vagina, unyielding and hard to the touch, the ready breaking down of the cervix on manipulation, or of the already formed crater from the necrosed portion of the cervix, and the general induration of the pelvis around the immovable uterus,—all these are characteristics of cancer of the cervix too far advanced for a radical operation.

Cancer of the corpus uteri starts invariably from the mucous lining.

It appears principally in two forms, the adenoid and the medullary.  A great
rarity is scirrhus of the body, of which I have seen one case.  (Fig. 14.)
All that I have said of the adenoid and the medullary form of disease of
the cervix holds good for cancer of the body.

I may add that recent researches have established the fact that the
so-called small-celled infiltration of the fibrous connective tissue (Virchow),
termed inflammatory reaction by Waldeyer, must be considered as the
formative stage of cancer.  This fact is of great clinical importance.  If,
after removal of the uterus, the connective tissue at the cut surface, especially of the vagina, either in cervical or corporeal cancer, reveals under

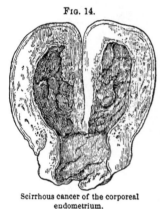

FIG. 14.

Scirrhous cancer of the corporeal
endometrium.

the microscope ever so little of such infiltration, we may be sure that the disease
will recur.  The same is true of the peritoneal cut surface in corporeal cancer.

The chief symptom in cancer of the
uterine body is hemorrhage.  I have
stated that in carcinoma of the cervix
bleeding is not apt to occur until the neoplasm begins to break down ; if the disease
is situated in the body, we shall have, on the
contrary, hemorrhage at a very early stage.

The amount of bleeding varies : in the
case of patients who have not reached the
menopause, it takes the form of menorrhagia in the beginning ; later, however,
the hemorrhages occur irregularly and con-

tinue for a varying period, from three or four days to as many weeks.  I
have seen several instances of acute anæmia due to continued bleeding in
cancer of the uterine body.

The diagnosis cannot be made until the interior of the uterus has been
explored and the suspected tissue has been examined microscopically.  It
is for this reason that in all cases of uterine hemorrhage in women more
than thirty years old, in which the uterus is but little increased in size,
curettage with a sharp instrument is indicated, after which the scrapings
should be examined by a competent pathologist.  If these show malignant
disease beyond a doubt, there is but one course left to pursue.  It is of
great advantage to dilate the cervical canal and to explore the uterine cavity
with the finger directly, to determine whether this is smooth, or whether a
tumor or numerous papillary projections are present in the interior.

The question which must necessarily be of importance to all physicians
is, What are the remote results of vaginal hysterectomy for cancer?  No
absolute percentage can be given ; it must necessarily depend upon two
important factors : first, the time at which the diagnosis is made, and,
second, the distance from the apparently diseased structures at which the
operator works.

The earlier the diagnosis of malignant disease the better are the prospects of radical cure by operation. If the disease is in its early stages, before infiltration of the adjacent structures has taken place, we can

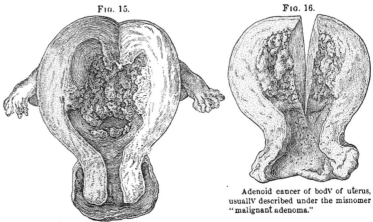

FIG. 15.

FIG. 16.

Medullary cancer of body of uterus.

Adenoid cancer of body of uterus, usually described under the misnomer "malignant adenoma."

probably count upon not less than fifty per cent. of permanent cures in the hands of expert operators,—*i.e.*, those who operate sufficiently far away from the diseased organ and take precautions not to produce infection during the operation.

*Technique of Vaginal Hysterectomy.* — The bowels are thoroughly emptied on the day prior to operation, and a warm bath is given. Before operation the mons and the external genitals are shaved, the abdomen, thighs, buttocks, external genitals, and vagina are vigorously scrubbed with ten-per-cent. creolin-mollin soap, then with a 1 to 1000 corrosive sublimate solution, after which the external genitals are washed with ether, subsequently with alcohol, and finally again with sublimate solution. The vagina is wiped out or thoroughly irrigated once more with a solution of corrosive sublimate (1 to 250), and then all is irrigated with plain water. The surroundings of the vulva are guarded with dry sterilized towels or with towels wrung out of a 1 to 1000 sublimate or a five-per-cent. carbolic acid solution, which are exchanged for clean ones when occasion demands it. The operator and assistants must disinfect themselves just as scrupulously.

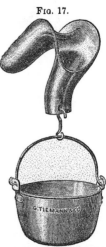

FIG. 17.

Edebohl's self-retaining speculum, used in vaginal hysterectomy, etc.

The instruments required are sterilized by boiling in a two-per-cent.

sal-soda solution for ten minutes, and are then rinsed off with plain water two or three times, after which they are placed in plain warm water for use. After the operation has begun, plain water only is used. In cancer of the portio and cervix, such portions as readily break down are removed by scissors and the sharp curette, then volsella-forceps are used to pull the uterus down; but when there is no structure left which can be grasped by the volsella, as is not infrequently the case, the vagina surrounding the cervix is grasped anteriorly with one or two bullet-forceps half an inch or farther from the margin, and an incision is made as far away from the

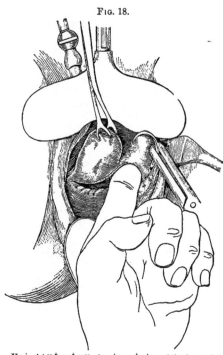

FIG. 18.

vagino-cervical border as is thought necessary; the mucosa is now stripped down and the bladder is peeled off for a short distance, when we can readily place a volsella. At this stage of the operation I prefer to open the cul-de-sac of Douglas, since with my index finger I can then better guide my needle in suturing the base of the broad ligaments. After opening the cul-de-sac the peritoneum is attached to the margin of the vagina by a continuous catgut suture. Sometimes I suture and ligate all around the cervix before cutting the vagina, but only when the uterus can be readily drawn down and is small, and a sufficiently large vagina is present. The operation then is practically bloodless, an impor-

Vaginal hysterectomy, showing suturing of the base of the broad ligaments, the cul-de-sac having already been opened and the peritoneum attached to the vaginal mucosa with a continuous catgut suture.

tant desideratum in a patient in poor physical condition. After placing a ligature, the tissues are cut; the uterus then gradually becomes more and more movable; if the parametria on one side are thickened, that is the side which ought to be liberated first. The base of the broad ligaments being ligated and cut, we shall have no trouble in stripping off the bladder entirely, upward and outward, and then the peritoneum is at once secured to the anterior edge of the vagina by a continuous suture of No. 2 or No. 3 catgut. We now have a clear field in which to work. We place a ligature first on one side and then on the other, and cut; the uterus can be drawn lower and lower as we proceed. The needle is introduced near the margin of the vagina, and, guided by the left or the right index finger, as the case may be, secures as much of the broad ligament as is deemed proper; on emerging, it is again brought out in the vaginal margin, thus securing the stumps so that they are subsequently readily placed completely outside of the peritoneum. This also aids in preventing the ligatures from slipping off. If possible, I bring out the tubes and ovaries without first detaching them from the uterus. In cancer of the body the adnexa should always be removed, on account of the danger of carcinoma either being already present or developing subsequently. After having removed the uterus, which is done under almost constant irrigation, by means of a speculum constructed especially for such work by Fritsch, the iodo-form gauze tampon or sponge, which I usually place within the peritoneal cavity after opening the cul-de-sac of Douglas, to prevent the intestines and omentum from prolapsing and hindering the work, is removed, and the pelvic cavity is irrigated with a stream of warm water. The stumps of the broad ligaments are now drawn down with bullet-forceps sufficiently to give a clear

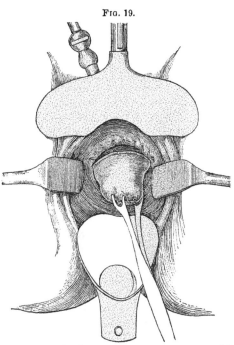

Fig. 19.

Vaginal hysterectomy. The bladder has been separated from the cervix and the peritoneum, and the vaginal mucous membrane united with a continuous catgut suture. The external cervical opening is closed with a continuous silk suture at the beginning of the operation.

view and to bring them completely into the vagina, and a full-curved needle is introduced through them on either side, entering anteriorly through the vagino-peritoneal margin and emerging posteriorly in the same manner, and the ligature is tied. The opening in the vagina still remaining is closed with two or three sutures. All remaining ends of sutures are cut off, the vagina is irrigated with Thiersch's solution, and a small strip of iodoform gauze is introduced.

This is the best method, and patients so treated have been dismissed within ten days. It must, however, be frequently modified according to the case, one of the most frequent variations being, if ligatures are used for the operation, to put a small strip of gauze in the vaginal slit still left, and to drain for twenty-four or forty-eight hours. This is done when peritoneal adhesions have been separated which give rise to oozing. Formerly I did not suture the peritoneum to the vaginal mucous membrane, neither was I particular about attaching my stumps in the vagina, yet my patients made good recoveries; but the convalescence was longer, and the procedure is obviously not so surgical, and necessarily, from a theoretical stand-point, is more dangerous. The gauze drainage in such cases was left from a week to ten days, and it was usual to see temperatures of 100° to 101° or 102° F. from the third to the eighth or even as late as the fourteenth day,—a resorption fever. When it is easier to retroflex the uterus or to anteflex it in order to secure the broad ligament, it should be done; this, however, is very seldom the case. Where the uterus is large and the vagina quite small, the latter may be dilated with a colpeurynter from two to three days before the intended operation, or a perineal incision may be made at the time of operation.

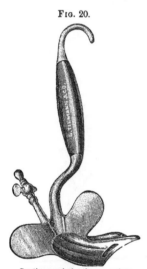

Fig. 20.

Continuous irrigation speculum.—
Thumb-screw to regulate the amount
of irrigating fluid, and attachment for
tube of irrigator.

Catgut is used for sutures and ligatures throughout the operation. The best quality of gut is selected in the numbers desirable for use, which for heavy ligatures vary from Nos. 4 to 6, for plastic work from Nos. 2 to 4. For two weeks or longer it is placed in sulphuric ether and the jar is shaken daily once or twice; then it is removed and for a few hours (two or three) is wrapped in a dry, sterilized towel to allow the ether to evaporate. It is then placed in a watery solution of corrosive sublimate (1 to 1000) for eighteen or twenty-four hours, from which it is removed to a jar of absolute alcohol, in which it is boiled in a waterbath for several hours; the paper tied over the jar is pierced at several points with a needle, to prevent an explosion. Finally it is removed and placed in another jar of absolute alcohol. For an operation only about as much gut as will presumably be used should be taken out, and put into another smaller jar or dish of alcohol, in order to avoid unnecessary opening of the large jar.

In patients who have had attacks of parametritis and perimetritis, and in whom the broad ligaments have been thickened by the former inflammatory processes, the operation will be exceedingly difficult, since it is almost impossible to draw down the uterus; in such cases the incision is made anteriorly, and then the cul-de-sac of Douglas is opened, the posterior cut is extended laterally, and the peritoneum, if it be convenient to do so at this stage of the operation, is attached to the margin of the vagina. Now the bladder is stripped from the cervix as far as can be conveniently done, and, guided by the finger, a clamp is placed on the base of the broad ligament the required distance from the cervix, and the parametria cut close to the inner border of the clamp; the same is done on the other side. It will now generally be found that the uterus can be drawn a little lower down, so that the bladder can be entirely separated from the cervix, when the remaining part of the broad ligament can be included in the next clamp applied, and then the rest of the broad ligament is cut. The same course is pursued on the other side, and any bleeding points which may still be found are secured by smaller hæmostatic forceps.

The handles of all forceps are securely tied with silk to prevent them from springing open subsequently, and the vagina is lightly packed with iodoform gauze, a strip of which is also wrapped around the forceps to prevent pressure on the soft parts. A heavy pad of absorbent cotton is secured

Fig 21.

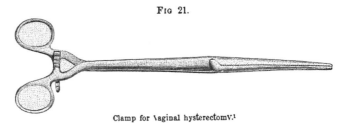

Clamp for vaginal hysterectomy.[1]

to the vulva by a T-bandage loosely applied. After the lapse of from twenty-four to thirty hours the clamps may all be removed without hesitation. To leave them longer would be injurious to the soft parts, and is entirely unnecessary. It has been argued against the use of hæmostatic forceps that when they are taken off the stumps of the broad ligament will retract and thus give rise to the danger of septic infection; also that along the handles of the instruments septic material may travel into the peritoneal cavity. However this may hold in theory, practice has disproved it. I have given this method a fair trial, and have not found a single instance to give cause for regret. It is positively a time-saving method; and not only so, but cases will be found operable when clamps are used in which ligatures cannot be employed. I refer to cases in which the parametria are very much thickened, because we can place clamps nearer the outer part of the broad ligament, if this is at all infiltrated, than it is possible to place a ligature. My only reasons for not using them always are, as previously

---

[1] The model of clamp here depicted has given me the best satisfaction of all varieties. Caution should be given to the maker that each instrument is first to be tried upon some material, such as a towel folded three or four times, to ascertain that the jaws grasp with equal firmness on both the distal and the proximal end.

stated, first, the convalescence is longer, and, secondly, I prefer from a surgical stand-point to leave a completely closed wound, because such patients after the operation are in as good condition as a woman after a normal confinement. It is the ideal operation, in my opinion. Unfortunately, however, we do not always have cases in which we are able to carry out this procedure. Another reason for preferring to close the peritoneal cavity entirely is that, in my opinion, there is less risk of ileus. Olshausen, of Berlin, treats the stumps of the broad ligaments intraperitoneally, and closes the peritoneum and vagina completely, but he admits, in his discussion before the Tenth International Medical Congress, that several patients so treated have had elevations of temperature and abscesses have formed and ruptured into the vagina.

One of the principal points in the technique of the operation, to prevent a recurrence of the disease, in cancer of the cervix, is to make the primary incision a considerable distance from the apparently diseased structures and to ligate the parametria as far from the uterus as possible. I have satisfied myself that in a certain number of cases of seeming recurrence it is not in reality a recurrence; the disease simply continues from some of the neoplasm left behind in the parametria, which may readily be overlooked. Other cases, of actual recurrence, take place through infection with carcinomatous material in healthy tissue. Examples of this are seen in the extensive parametric recurrences after operations for cancer of the portio, whether the operation has been supra-vaginal amputation or total extirpation. Such infection takes place during the operation. It is for this reason that, so far as my personal observation goes, the malignant disease of the uterine body and that developing in the cervical canal give a better prognosis in regard to recurrence than cancer of the vaginal portion, or that involving the cervix proper, because in the latter classes we come directly in contact with the disease during operation.

The difference between recurrence through infection and that due to diseased tissue left at the time of operation is, that in the former the manifestations are more general, the disease taking in a larger area in the parametria, whereas in the latter it is in the beginning more local and the general invasion takes place later. It is of great importance to understand the condition of the pelvic organs in a given case as thoroughly as possible before beginning the operation, and this can usually be learned only by examination under an anæsthetic.

We must determine the mobility of the uterus; if the parametria are infiltrated; if the disease has encroached upon the bladder or the rectum, and, if so, to what extent; if retro-uterine adhesions are present, and their nature: in short, we must decide whether the case is one still fit for operation, or, rather, whether we can make our incisions in non-malignant tissue. Up to within four years ago I held that we should always remove the carcinomatous uterus, if it was a surgical possibility, even should it prove necessary to operate in tissues already infiltrated by carcinoma, believing (1) that the life of the patient would be prolonged; (2) that her sufferings would be diminished; (3) that, no uterus being present, we should have little or no bleeding and no disagreeable and ichorous discharge, and that, on the whole, the patient would at least be far more comfortable as long as she survived. This view is still held by a number of operators; but I have changed my opinion, and during the past two years I have seen enough patients to justify me in having done so. The patients, in the first place, do not live so long; secondly, they suffer excruciating pain; thirdly, there is fetid discharge and some hemorrhage,—indeed, occasionally quite profuse; fourthly, they are in no way more comfortable than they would have been if a total extirpation had not been done and the case had been treated on sound surgical principles, if as comfortable. To the second and third objections there are exceptions; I have myself seen them: hence the support I gave to the operation, even when the indications seemed doubtful. Some patients suffer intense pain in the pelvis, rectum, and bladder after recurrence and "continuous disease" after hysterectomy. By "continuous disease" I mean a continuation of the neoplasm when the operation is done in already diseased structures.

We now come to consider points in the diagnosis which serve to limit the operation from a clinical stand-point, premising that the terms upper and lower line of limitation for total extirpation for cancer should be discarded. There is only one line. Either the uterus can be entirely removed with a presumably good result—by operating in healthy tissue, so that we have no continuous invasion of the neoplasm—or we cannot remove it. No matter how recent the disease and how limited it may appear, the invariable rule, if the choice of the operation is given, should be to remove the organ completely; consequently, the lower line of limitation must be rejected.

1. Does a movable uterus always indicate operation?

2. Is hysterectomy contra-indicated because the parametria or the folds of the peritoneum posteriorly are thickened?

3. Does a fixed or an adherent uterus contra-indicate total extirpation?

4. Is total extirpation of the uterus contra-indicated when the disease is apparently limited to the cervix?

1. In answer to the first question, I would say that we can generally operate if the uterus is freely movable; but there may be a movable uterus because the broad ligament and the utero-rectal ligaments are not infiltrated, yet the disease may have involved the bladder to such a degree that a radical operation is out of the question. In such cases we gain much knowledge from the use of the sharp curette just before operation. We gouge out all the readily removable structure from the cervix, and if the disease has passed through the cervix into the cellular tissue between the bladder and the cervix, and into the former viscus, it is now readily discernible. It behooves us to explore the bladder with the finger, and so to determine the mobility of the vesical mucosa and muscularis against the

diseased part, which can be readily done per urethram after dilatation, the patient being thoroughly anæsthetized. If we find that only a limited portion of its wall is involved, we can proceed, that being no contra-indication; we must simply be able to remove all of the diseased part without interfering with the ureters, and to close the defect completely at the time of operation, the same as in a vesico-vaginal fistula. The same indication would hold good for moderate involvement of the rectum; it would be necessary to resect in the same manner as in cancer of that structure. If, on the other hand, we find that the bladder or rectum is already involved to such an extent that we cannot entirely remove the disease, we are not justified in operating, no matter how movable the uterus may be: the sharp curette and the vesical and rectal examination have done their duty in clearing up the case. Usually, of course, such invasions are marked by other signs of advanced disease, yet exceptions may occur.

2. A woman may have passed through one or more attacks of parametritis or perimetritis, or both, due to traumatism or incident to a puerperium, and, as a consequence, the uterus may have become more or less immovable, the broad ligament may be infiltrated, and the folds of Douglas in a like condition, and yet the operation be not only justifiable, but necessary. Here the individual experience and judgment of the operator must decide whether such induration is inflammatory or carcinomatous. The examination is best made with one or two fingers of one hand in the rectum and with the other hand on the abdomen. We can thus feel and map out the pelvic contents, so as to determine the extent of the induration, and—a very important feature—whether it possesses elasticity; if it does, there exists an inflammatory infiltration. Carcinomatous infiltrations have a peculiar resistance and are generally more bulky than inflammatory infiltrations. Here the superiority of touch is on the side of the operator who has practised to any extent pelvic massage according to Brandt's method. All this, of course, necessitates narcosis for the purpose of precision.

3. It is obvious that, although a cancerous uterus may be firmly fixed in the pelvis, its removal by means of vaginal hysterectomy is not contra-indicated, provided the adhesions fixing it are not infiltrated by the malignant neoplasm.

4. Inasmuch as vaginal hysterectomy involves but little more danger than high amputation of the cervix, and is obviously a more radical operation, it is always to be preferred, although the cancer is apparently limited to the cervix.

# CHAPTER XIII.

## NEOPLASMS OF THE OVARIES, TUBES, AND BROAD LIGAMENTS.

BY HENRY C. COE, M.D.

## INTRODUCTORY.

THE importance which this subject has assumed during the past decade is due to the corresponding interest awakened in abdominal surgery, an interest which has steadily increased so as almost to overshadow minor surgical gynæcology. In this busy age it is impossible for the practitioner, when seeking information on a special subject, to review all that has been written: while it is important that he should possess a fair amount of theoretical knowledge, it is a well-recognized fact that the clinical side must always assume more importance to him than the pathological. For this reason the sections on pathology in this article are limited to the brief presentation of attested facts, mooted questions and discussions of theories being omitted.

While it is true that the successful abdominal surgeon, aside from his inherent qualifications, must have served a long and severe apprenticeship, it has been conclusively demonstrated that the occasional operator may obtain results which fully justify him in attempting operations which were once deemed unjustifiable for him. The writer does not believe that, in this country at least, abdominal work will, or should be, kept in the hands of a few men. Circumstances arise in which it is necessary for the general practitioner to perform ovariotomy: hence the importance of his possessing clear, well-defined ideas regarding indications and technique.

Every teacher of gynæcology must have arrived at the conclusion that the main thing which should be thoroughly mastered by the profession is the diagnosis of pelvic troubles. In most text-books this subject has been rendered too complicated by the introduction of many rules. Precision in diagnosis is the result of two factors,—the exercise of common sense and the cultivation of the *tactus eruditus*. The recognition of the presence of a pelvic or abdominal tumor, and of its probable nature and relations, at once implies the formation of a definite opinion as to the line of treatment advisable under the circumstances. The final decision concerning the performance of a radical operation may require counsel, but let the practitioner

621

at least learn to recognize that there *is* a tumor, at such a stage in its development as to be operable.

In order to gain a clear idea of the origin and mode of development of the neoplasms which will be considered in this chapter, the reader must refresh his memory in the anatomy of the broad ligament and the organs between its folds, especially the upper portion, known as the mesosalpinx. A study of Doran's diagram will suffice for pages of description indicating

FIG. 1.

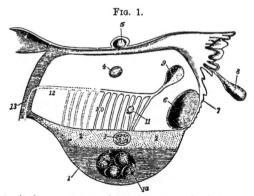

Diagram of the structures in and adjacent to the broad ligament, with tumors of the ovary, tube, and broad ligament.—1, Framework of parenchyma of ovary, the seat of (1a) simple or glandular multilocular cyst; 2, tissue of hilum, with (3) papillomatous cyst; 4, cyst of broad ligament, independent of parovarium and Fallopian tube; 5, similar cyst in broad ligament above the tube. but not connected with it; 6, similar cyst developed close to (7) ovarian fimbria of tube; 8, hydatid of Morgagni; 9, cyst developing from horizontal tube of parovarium (cysts 4, 5, 6, 8, and 9 always have a simple endothelial lining); 10, parovarium (the dotted lines represent the inner portion, always more or less obsolete in the adult); 11, small cyst developing from a vertical tube; cysts that have this origin, or that spring from the obsolete portion, have a lining of cubical or ciliated epithelium, and tend to develop papillomatous growths, as do cysts in (2) the tissue of the hilum; 12, duct of Gärtner, often persistent in the adult as a fibrous cord; 13, track of that duct in the uterine wall; unobliterated portions are, according to Coblenz, the origin of papillomatous cysts in the uterus.

the difference between ovarian and parovarian cysts, concerning which even some gynæcologists have vague notions. It is also necessary to review the minute anatomy of the ovary, and to recognize the fact that it consists of two distinct portions from which neoplasms may develop,—the *oöphoron*, or follicular zone, and the *paroöphoron*, otherwise known as the hilum. Bearing in mind, moreover, the fact that the ovary not only contains the tissues and cells found in both desmoid and epithelial growths, but is also the seat of many degenerative processes, some of which are not yet satisfactorily explained, it is not difficult to understand why it should be so frequently the point of origin of neoplasms, solid as well as cystic. The reader should study carefully every pelvic tumor removed by himself or others, and, if possible, submit it to a competent pathologist. Many operators of great experience fail to utilize their anatomical material, so that unique and valuable specimens are lost, or else are described so inaccurately that the reports possess no scientific value.

## NEOPLASMS OF THE OVARY.

Several different classifications of ovarian tumors may be adopted, according as they are studied from a developmental, an anatomical, or a clinical stand-point. Clinically, they are distinguished as solid or cystic, and again as benign or malignant. The latter terms are used somewhat loosely, for the fact of malignancy cannot always be determined until after careful microscopical examination, and even then a cyst which is anatomically benign may be viewed with grave suspicion by reason of the accompanying conditions found at the operating-table.

### OVARIAN CYSTS.

**Pathology.**—Cysts of the ovary are called *oöphoritic* or *paroöphoritic*, according to that portion of the gland in which they develop, and unilocular or multilocular, according as they contain one or many cavities. Dermoids, which clinically are included among cysts, form a peculiar class which it is customary to consider separately, at least as regards their pathology, though their close relation to ordinary cysts is shown by the not infrequent occurrence of a transition form,—so-called multilocular dermoids.

The subject of the origin of ovarian cystomata has long been the *bête noire* of students, who have been puzzled to reconcile the various theories that have been offered to account for the wide variations from simple follicular dropsy to the complex multilocular tumors containing various kinds of fluids and studded on their interior with numerous cystic and papillary outgrowths. So different do they appear that it seems impossible to refer them to a common origin. What the practitioner needs is a good working theory which will not only be clear in his own mind, but will have a direct relation to the questions of diagnosis and treatment. This will be obtained not by combining several theories, but by keeping steadily in mind the fact before mentioned of the division of the ovary into two distinct parts, one containing ovisacs, the other not. In one portion the cyst (whether simple or compound) has its origin in degenerative changes, occurring in the Graafian follicle, while in the hilum the mode of development is essentially different. When both portions take part in the process, the result is a neoplasm sharing the peculiarities of both seats of origin.

*Oöphoritic Cysts.*—(a) *Unilocular Cyst* (*Hydrops Folliculi; Follicular Cyst; Dropsy of the Graafian Follicle*).—These terms have been used so loosely that the reader often derives the impression that they are synonymous. The inference that every dropsical follicle may become a large cyst naturally carries with it the deduction that a cystic ovary is a source of positive danger and should be promptly extirpated,—one which is opposed to the principles of modern conservative surgery. The importance of the practical surgeon having a clear idea of this subject is at once apparent, since on his decision at the operating-table depends the preservation of an ovary after the removal of a neoplasm involving the opposite one. There is no time then for pathological refinements.

Dropsy of the Graafian follicle is sufficiently explained by its name,—a simple dilatation of the ovisac with an accumulation of serous fluid. These cysts, which are mostly peripheral, vary in size from that of a pea to that of an English walnut, and are often really unilocular, though even in such small cysts an examination of the wall will show traces of septa marking the presence of former loculi representing adjacent dilated ovisacs. This wall is thin and transparent, being composed of fibrous tissue. In a young cyst the lining may be the original membrana granulosa of the follicle, while the larger cysts have an inner layer of stratified epithelium, which may atrophy and disappear entirely in consequence of pressure. The contained fluid is a limpid serum, having a low specific gravity, and containing sodium chloride and a trace of albumin. Unchanged ova have been found in cysts as large as cherries.

FIG. 2.

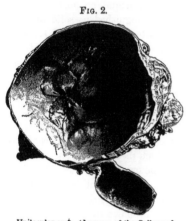

Unilocular cyst. (Museum of the College of Physicians and Surgeons.)

Dropsy of the follicle is essentially a retention cyst, due to a simple hyper-physiological process. The true cause of the non-rupture of the ripe follicle is not always clear, Rindfleisch's theory of a "deficient bursting force" being rather vague. A careful examination of the affected ovary usually justifies the inference that previous cirrhotic changes in the cortex or stroma have caused such thickening in the follicular wall as to prevent its rupture. Degenerative changes in these small cysts are rare. Spontaneous or traumatic rupture (during examination) probably occurs with considerable frequency and with harmless results; in fact, it may lead to a cure.

True unilocular cysts of a size sufficient to assume surgical importance rarely originate in the oöphoron, so that when an operator encounters a tumor which seems to be oligocystic he is usually safe in inferring that it is either parovarian or was originally multilocular.

(b) *Multilocular Cysts of the Oöphoron.*—Without desiring to involve the reader in a discussion of the various pathological theories which have been advanced to account for the protean forms observed in ovarian cysts, it is only proper to state that weighty authorities refuse to accept the explanation which commends itself by its simplicity and clearness,—*i.e.*, that multilocular cysts develop by the simultaneous distention and coalescence of contiguous dropsical follicles, as illustrated by Tait's familiar simile of the group of soap-bubbles. The transition from cystic degeneration of the ovary to the enormous neoplasm which fills the entire abdomen seems too great to be bridged over so easily. Yet it does not seem forced to refer all multilocular cysts to a common origin,—the non-developed or degenerated follicle,—assuming that in the simpler form the follicle alone shares in the process, while in the glandular and proliferating forms there is accompanying activity of the glandular and connective-tissue elements.

To begin with the simplest variety of multilocular cysts. Whether these are originally of inflammatory origin or the contrary does not especially concern us, though they probably do represent the result of a previous so-called general "cystic oöphoritis," and not a simple hydrops folliculi, the distinction between which has already been pointed out. In its incipiency such a tumor would be represented simply by an agglomeration of small grape-like cysts forming a mass the size of an orange. These grow, some rapidly and some more slowly, until they reach the size of the adult head (which they seldom exceed), and various internal changes occur which,

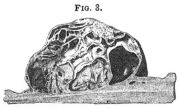

Multilocular cyst, incipient stage. (Museum of the College of Physicians and Surgeons.)

it should be remembered, are purely mechanical. There is no proliferation of epithelium or formation of new cysts, in which they differ from true cysto-adenomata. On section they present a characteristic honey-comb appearance, contiguous cysts being separated by their respective walls, which become thinned by increasing pressure and eventually give way, throwing two loculi into one. Localized thickenings, general hypertrophy of the cyst-wall, etc., occur, though rarely the degenerative changes seen in the larger neoplasms. The fluid preserves its original serous character, with the occasional admixture of blood, débris, etc. The simple epithelial lining previously described is preserved in the smaller cysts, but disappears in the older ones.

Passing to the more complex variety of multilocular cysts, we are given the choice of two theories,—either to regard them as identical in their mode of development with the simpler form already described, or as originating in a more complex manner, according to the various theories of Waldeyer, Pflüger, et al. The reader will find the former to be preferable from a clinical stand-point, and, indeed, it has the sanction of some of the best pathologists, notably of Sutton. The latter distinguishes multilocular oöphoritic cysts as simple and adenoid, with a third variety, multilocular dermoids, which will be described later. The adenoid feature, which many have found such difficulty in explaining, is referred by him to simple proliferation of the original lining epithelium of the cyst. In a similar manner, with the additional element of connective-tissue hypertrophy, may be explained the presence of the dendritic or papillomatous masses which spring from its inner wall.   The commonest form of cyst is the so-called "proliferous glandular," characterized, as its name implies, by the development of secondary glandular outgrowths from the walls of the larger cysts (which are simply retention-cysts), which may increase in size and coalesce so as to fill the cavity of the parent cyst; or the newly formed follicles may not dilate, and, being surrounded by a dense stroma, may present the appearance of solid growths.   On section of such a cyst, the relation of the primary and secondary loculi to the parent cysts will be at once apparent, as well as the mode of formation of larger cavities through the coalescence of adjacent loculi.   If the connective tissue of the cyst-wall undergoes proliferation, there result vegetations or cauliflower growths, which project into and may fill the cyst-cavity; when these predominate, the growth is characterized as a "proliferous papillary cyst."   Both glandular and papillary formations may coexist in the same cyst.

Fig. 4.

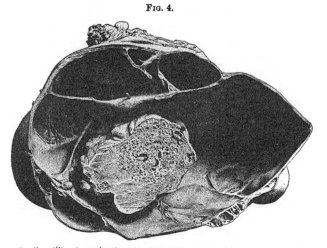

Small multilocular cyst.   (Museum of the College of Physicians and Surgeons)

The exterior of a multilocular cyst which has not undergone marked degenerative changes presents a characteristic smooth, glistening appearance, its color being uniformly whitish, except at spots where the wall is quite thin or has undergone inflammatory or necrotic changes, where it may show grayish-green or brown spots.   It varies in thickness according to the age of the cyst, the amount of distention, and the presence of localized hypertrophy, adhesions, etc.   Some hint as to the character of its contents may be obtained from its external appearance.   As Doran observes, "the smoother and shinier and the more silvery the cyst-wall appears when exposed by abdominal incision, the better the case will be both for the patient and for the operator."

The wall of the main cyst, especially in the vicinity of the pedicle, can usually be separated into three layers, though if it has become much thinned the middle coat may disappear entirely, the outer and the inner being then fused together. The outer surface is covered with a layer of endothelial cells. Cubical epithelium has been found on the surface of small growths. The middle coat is composed of white fibrous tissue, containing smooth muscular fibres which seem to be derived from the ovarian ligaments. The blood-vessels supplying the tissues are found in this layer, as well as large lymphatics, especially in the neighborhood of the pedicle. Nerves have been traced to the cyst-wall, but their ultimate terminations have not been made out. As before stated, ovarian tissue may sometimes be found even in cysts of considerable size, especially the remains of the hilum. The writer has seen a corpus luteum in the wall of a large cyst, showing that ovulation still persisted. This would explain those cases in which pregnancy has occurred with double ovarian tumors. The

FIG. 5.

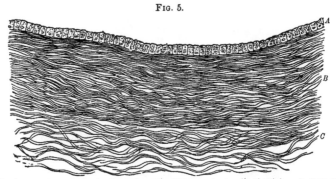

Section through the wall of a simple ovarian cyst. (Olshausen.)—*A*, epithelial lining; *B*, dense fibrous layer; *C*, loose fibrous layer.

smaller secondary cysts are lined with a single layer of columnar epithelium, which in the larger cysts becomes flattened by pressure, so as to assume an endothelial appearance; the cells eventually atrophy or undergo fatty degeneration, desquamate, and disappear entirely. Changes in the color, thickness, and consistency of the inner wall of the cyst represent various inflammatory and degenerative changes. Acute inflammation may terminate in actual suppuration, necrosis, or gangrene, with perforation of the wall, while chronic inflammation may result in localized thickening, deposits of lime salts, etc. Changes in the walls of blood-vessels lead to thrombosis, ecchymoses (either punctate or extensive), or actual rupture of vessels, with more or less profuse hemorrhage into the cyst. The cyst-fluids vary greatly in their physical characteristics, specimens of entirely different color and consistence being often obtained from the different loculi of the same cyst. The main cyst may contain a thick chocolate-colored fluid, one of the secondary cysts a transparent jelly, another a thin limpid secretion, while others may be greenish, milky, or (in the case of a dermoid) thick and pultaceous. These modifications in color are due to admixture of blood, pus, fat, epithelial cells, cholesterin, etc. The original fluid consists of two portions,—one a simple transudate from the blood, the other due to a change in the protoplasm of the epithelial cells. Its specific gravity varies from 1010 to 1050; it usually has a neutral or an alkaline reaction. Spontaneous coagulation does not occur unless it contains a considerable amount of blood, a peculiarity which distinguishes it from ascitic fluid. It contains albuminoids, fats, and salts; cholesterin is often present; mucin and albumin are very frequent; paralbumin is a constant component, being precipitated in fine flocculi on passing carbonic acid gas through the fluid. It was formerly considered pathognomonic of ovarian cyst-fluid, an error which was pointed out long ago.

FIG. 6.

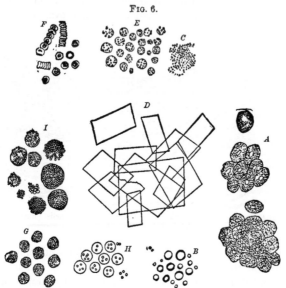

Microscopical appearance of ovarian fluid. (Drysdale.)—*A*, epithelial cells; *B*, oil-globules; *C*, free granular matter; *D*, crystals of cholesterin; *E*, granular cells; *F*, blood-corpuscles; *G, H*, pus-corpuscles; *I*, inflammatory globules of Gluge.

Much stress was once placed upon the importance of examining cyst-contents with the microscope. The formed elements observed are blood- and pus-corpuscles, fatty globules, cholesterin-plates, and epithelial cells in various stages of degeneration. The so-called "ovarian granular cell" which Drysdale regarded as peculiar to ovarian cyst-fluids is not pathognomonic, since it may be found wherever epithelial cells are undergoing fatty degeneration. As a matter of fact, however, the presence of numbers of these bodies in fluid withdrawn from an abdominal tumor would possess some diagnostic value, though their absence would not. Some hint as to the presence of degenerative changes in the cyst-wall might be derived from a careful examination of the fluid withdrawn through an aspirating needle. There is also room for considerable bacteriological work in this direction, in order to throw more light upon the septic character of fluids which macroscopically appear innocent, while others which present a suspicious appearance cause no irritation when they escape into the peritoneal cavity.

(c) *Cysts of the Paroöphoron; Papillomatous Cysts.*—Doran refers all papillomatous cysts to the hilum of the ovary, explaining the presence of papillary growths in oöphoritic glandular cysts by the presence of remnants of the epithelium of the Wolffian body in the stroma of the parenchyma. Sutton does not go quite so far as this, but believes that the majority of papillomatous cysts spring from the paroöphoron. Williams, on the contrary, thinks that they are derived either from the germinal epithelium or from the Graafian follicle,—a view which harmonizes with the

FIG. 7.

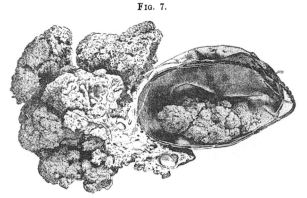

Papillomatous ovarian cyst. (Museum of the College of Physicians and Surgeons.)

theory already proposed, that all ovarian cysts are of follicular origin. The two former observers hold that papillary cysts developing from the hilum tend to invade the broad ligament, as distinguished from those originating in the parenchyma, which leave it intact. Without entering further into the discussion of their mode of origin, it is sufficient to say that these cysts seldom attain a large size as compared with the glandular variety, and present a similar appearance externally, except when the papillary growths have perforated the cyst-wall. On section they are seen to be filled with dendritic masses, varying in size from that of a millet-seed to that of the fist, and either sessile or having long, slender pedicles. According to their vascularity, they may present a whitish or a reddish color. They are soft and friable, sometimes having a gritty feel from the presence of psammomatous bodies. They proliferate rapidly, often causing rupture of the cyst, when they spread over its outer surface and to the adjacent peritoneum. The fluid, unlike that contained in glandular cysts, is usually clear and watery, but has about the same chemical and microscopical characteristics, though mucin is rarely found. Microscopically the cyst-wall is seen to consist of the usual fibro-muscular layers and an inner cylindrical epithelial lining, which is continued over the papillary outgrowths, sometimes being ciliated. The latter are formed by prolongations of the stroma, which has become looser and more myxomatous and is highly vascular. Many calcareous bodies (psammomata) are found throughout the stroma and on the surface of the papillary masses.

The tendency of these tumors to undergo cancerous degeneration is well known, though so sweeping a statement as that of Wells, that they are all malignant, is, of course, based on clinical rather than on anatomical observations. The cancerous change may be limited to small portions of the cyst, discoverable only on careful microscopical examination, or it may involve the entire growth and be accompanied by metastases in distant organs. The question of metastasis in connection with simple non-malignant papillomatous cysts is an interesting one, and is of great importance surgically. By metastasis we understand not the direct extension of the growths to adjacent organs (the bladder, rectum, or uterine cavity) after perforation of the cyst, but the development of independent secondary growths on the peritoneum, with accompanying ascites. These are produced by the implantation of fragments of the original growth which are detached, float about in the peritoneal fluid, and lodge at various points, where they become fixed and undergo an independent growth. Cases of true metastasis in the lungs have been reported, emboli being carried by the vessels in the usual manner.

FIG. 8.

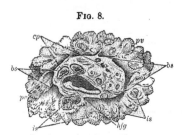

Section of papillomatous ovary. (Coblenz) —*hfg*, dropsical Graafian follicle; *cp*, cysts filled with papillary vegetations; *bs*, pedicle; *is*, interpapillary spaces; *pv*, superficial papillary vegetations.

As regards their frequency of occurrence, papillomatous cysts are now known to be more common than was usually supposed, their proportion to· the glandular being about one to ten.

Closely related to these cysts is the interesting condition known as superficial papilloma of the ovary, or clinically "warty" ovary. This is quite rare, many gynæcologists with a large experience in abdominal surgery never having encountered a case. In a typical specimen the ovary is enlarged to the size of a walnut or a goose-egg, its exterior being studded with cauliflower growths identical in appearance with those found in papillomatous cysts, which may appear as minute sessile warts or large, friable, pedunculated masses. Although the ovary itself may be little changed, it is sometimes so covered with the neoplasm as to be apparently transformed into the same. Section of a warty ovary shows that the growth is entirely superficial, the stroma being often unchanged or presenting merely the ordinary appearances of fibrous hyperplasia. Microscopically the papillary masses are identical with those already described; they are vascular connective - tissue outgrowths, covered with a single layer of cylindrical epithelium, often ciliated, which, as Williams has shown, is continuous with the germinal epithelium of the ovary, processes of which can be traced down into the stroma. This simple and satisfactory explanation serves to clear up a good deal of the mystery which has been attached to these peculiar neoplasms. From their position on the surface of the ovary it will naturally be inferred that they tend, even more than do papillomatous cysts, to form secondary deposits in adjacent organs and on the peritoneum, and are equally prone to malignant degeneration.

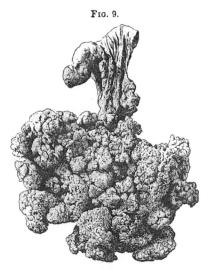

FIG. 9.

Papilloma of ovary. (Cleveland.)

The occurrence of ascites in connection with the cystic and solid growths

FIG. 10.

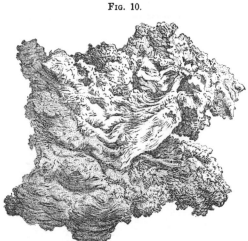

Papilloma of ovary. (Williams.)

above described is so common as to deserve mention in connection with their pathology. Its clinical significance will be considered in another

FIG. 11.

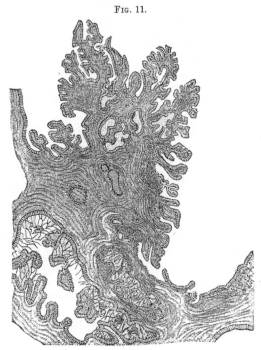

Interior of papillomatous cyst. (Williams.)

FIG. 12.

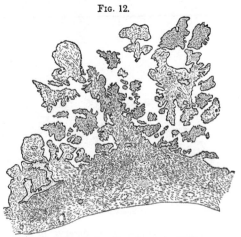

Section through wall of papillomatous cyst. (Williams.)

place.   Although ascites may develop without rupture of the cyst, it is usually to be regarded as an evidence of general peritoneal irritation, due to metastatic deposits, rather than as a transudation from the growths themselves.   Viewed in this light, it of course offers no reliable clinical evidence of the malignancy of a neoplasm.   Hydrothorax has been noted in some cases, though not due to metastasis in the pleura.   As Freund remarks, this is not necessarily a contra-indication to operative interference.

### TUBO-OVARIAN CYSTS.

The term "ovarian hydrocele" was formerly used as synonymous with tubo-ovarian cysts.   Sutton has pointed out that there is an essential anatomical difference.   A tubo-ovarian cyst consists of a simultaneous dilatation of the ovary and of the Fallopian tube, which have become adherent; whereas ovarian hydrocele is formed by a collection of fluid within the fold of peritoneum which sometimes surrounds the ovary.   The latter is distinguished anatomically from tubo-ovarian cyst by the fact that the tube opens into a sac on the posterior fold of the broad ligament, that there is no evidence of inflammation, and that the ovary is found projecting through the wall of the sac.   The contents of a hydrocele may occasionally escape through the tube into the uterus,—the so-called "intermitting ovarian hydrocele."

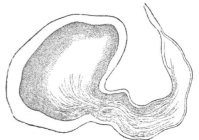

FIG. 13.

Tubo-ovarian cyst.   (Olshausen.)

Various theories have been advanced to account for the development of tubo-ovarian cysts, the most plausible of which seems to be that it begins as a catarrh of the tube, the fimbriated extremity becoming attached to the ovary at the site of a Graafian follicle, that the tube and the ovary enlarge simultaneously, and that the septum between the two cavities subsequently gives way.   But, since this combination may occur in connection with large multilocular cysts (and even with those of the broad ligament), it seems fair to infer that there may be previous formation of the cyst before the diseased tube becomes adherent to it.   Such cysts present a characteristic shape, there being a gradual dilatation of the tube from its proximal extremity outward, the elongated cyst ending in a large bulbous extremity.   They are generally of small size, but may contain two or three pints of fluid.   The disease is usually unilateral.   According to the length of time during which it has existed, the line of demarcation between the tube and the cyst becomes less and less distinct, until the fimbriae disappear entirely.   The outer surface of the cyst is covered by peritoneum, and its wall consists largely of smooth muscular fibres which become much thinned through distention. It is lined with a layer of columnar ciliated epithelium, but the cilia soon disappear. It contains serous fluid with few cellular elements, which, in consequence of hemorrhage, may assume a chocolate color. It is not possible to recognize positively such a growth before operation; it is most apt to be confounded with hydrosalpinx, nor is the diagnosis always clear till the specimen has been carefully examined by a pathologist.

### EXTRA-PERITONEAL CYSTS.

A peculiar form of cyst described by Tait,[1] which develops from the patent urachus, is clinically indistinguishable from an ovarian or a parovarian cyst. Although cysts of this form are rare, the surgeon should bear in mind their existence, in order that he may not be confused by the peculiar relations of the tumor noted on opening the abdominal cavity. They develop outside of the peritoneum, and, lifting up the peritoneum first over the anterior abdominal wall, may then dip down into the pelvis and make their way upward along the spine. These growths are usually small, but Tait mentions one which contained a gallon of fluid. They sometimes communicate with the bladder, and they have been known to rupture at the umbilicus. They grow rapidly, and may often undergo suppuration, leading to hectic fever and other symptoms of sepsis.

The diagnosis is difficult, and the surgical treatment far from easy. Since they have no pedicle, it is necessary to enucleate them, and, as the peritoneum must be stripped off over a wide surface, there is great danger of subsequent necrosis of this membrane.

### DERMOID CYSTS.

It is hardly necessary to call the reader's attention to the various theories which have been presented to explain their origin, notably that of inclusion of the epiblast. The theory of Johnstone is not only the simplest, but is in perfect harmony with that already suggested to account for the origin of ordinary cystomata,—i.e., that they originate from the Graafian follicle, through a faulty development of the ovum itself, which contains the germ of all varieties of tissue; hence tissues and organs are found in dermoid cysts which spring not from the epiblast alone, but from the mesoblast and the hypoblast as well. This suggestive theory seems to explain satisfactorily the occurrence of dermoid elements in ordinary multilocular cysts.

Dermoids may be classified for convenience as pure dermoids and unilocular or multilocular cysts with dermoid loculi. Dermoids constitute about five per cent. of all ovarian tumors, and may be found in patients of every age, from the new-born child to the woman of eighty, though they are most common during the period of functional activity. The majority of ovarian cysts in children are of the dermoid variety. Both ovaries are

---

[1] British Medical Journal, November, 1886.

affected in about one-fourth of the cases. They seldom exceed in size a man's head, differing from ordinary cystomata not only in their slow

FIG. 14.

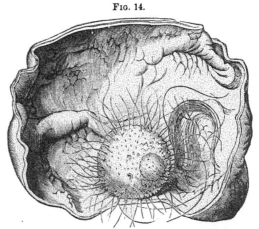

Ovarian dermoid, containing pseudo-mamma. (Sutton.)

growth, but also in the fact that after reaching a certain size they may remain stationary for years, although prone to undergo degenerative changes and to contract adhesions to adjacent organs.

FIG. 15.

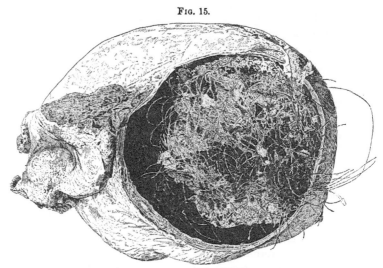

Dermoid cyst. (Museum of the College of Physicians and Surgeons.)

Macroscopically a dermoid presents a decided contrast to an ordinary multilocular cyst, having a dull appearance and a darker color (instead of being white and glistening), with yellowish patches where the caseous contents are seen through the thinned wall. The wall is usually thicker than in an ordinary cyst, and is lined with a layer of tissue, either smooth or thrown into folds or projections, presenting the appearance of skin. Dermoids nearly always contain hair, which may spring from the inner surface singly or in tufts, or may be rolled into balls. This hair is usually of a coarse texture, and either light or dark, its color bearing no relation to that of the patient's hair. Sections through elevated patches on the cyst-wall show that they contain several layers, the inner consisting of several strata of epithelial cells, the superficial being flattened and non-nucleated,

FIG. 16.

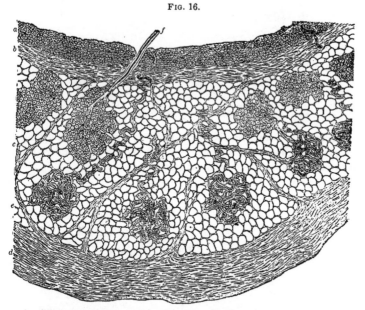

Section through the wall of a dermoid cyst, showing—*a*, flattened epithelial cells; *b*, deep layer of connective tissue; *c*, loose adipose tissue; *d*, superficial connective-tissue layer; *e*, sweat-gland; *f*, hair follicle and sebaceous gland. (Wyder.)

the deeper layers polyhedral. Below these is a layer of connective tissue corresponding to the corium, and more externally the panniculus adiposus. In addition to hairs, which show the same microscopical structure as in true skin, normal sweat and sebaceous glands are seen, though these, as well as the hair, may atrophy and disappear.

Various other structures are frequently found in dermoids, bone and teeth being most common, though cartilage and nervous and muscular tissue may be present, and even well-formed organs, especially mammæ. Bone occurs either in the form of thin laminæ embedded in the connective tissue of the cyst-wall or in various bizarre shapes, resembling rudimentary cranial bones, alveolar processes, etc. Microscopically, these present the ordinary structure of bone. Teeth are of quite common occurrence, and may vary in number from two or three to several hundred, the usual number being ten or twelve.

The contents of dermoid cysts vary in consistence from an oily liquid to a thick caseous mass (after exposure to the air), its peculiar appearance being due to the substances of which it is composed,—*i.e.*, the secretion of the sebaceous glands mixed with epithelial débris and cholesterin in which are mingled masses of hair. In a few instances the caseous material has been found arranged in the form of spheres, which on section showed fat deposited in concentric layers. This phenomenon has been ascribed to axial rotation of the cyst. The contents of a dermoid seldom exceed three or four pints. The presence of blood may change the color from the ordinary white or dirty gray to brown or chocolate.

Tumors of this variety, though anatomically benign, are to be viewed with suspicion, since cases have been reported in which they have undergone sarcomatous degeneration. Moreover, the development of malignant disease within the pelvis has been observed after the removal of dermoids. Peritoneal metastases have several times been noticed, developing in the same manner as in connection with papillomatous cysts. It is not certain whether these are due to bursting of the cyst or are examples of true metastasis. The secondary masses present a structure similar to that of the parent cyst, containing the same caseous material, but hair has been found in them in only a single instance.

It should be noted that true dermoid cysts are invariably unilocular, the formation of secondary cysts by proliferation never occurring. If, as rarely happens, separate loculi are found, their presence is to be explained rather by the coalescence of separate adjacent cysts (three or four of which may develop independently in the same ovary) than by the actual growth of septa within a unilocular cyst, as Tait suggests. So-called multilocular dermoids (Fig. 17) are not, as the name would seem to imply, pure dermoids

FIG. 17.

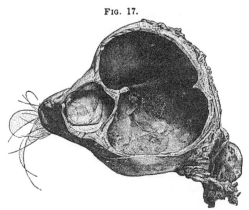

Small multilocular dermoid cyst. (Museum of the College of Physicians and Surgeons.)

containing several compartments, but are ordinary proliferating cysts, one or more loculi of which present the ordinary structure of a dermoid, as regards the presence of skin, hair, bone, etc. These growths, which are not uncommon, possess considerable interest for the surgeon as well as for the pathologist, since the presence of the dermoid element may modify the prognosis of an otherwise simple neoplasm by introducing certain complications (peritonitis, suppuration, perforation, etc.) peculiar to the latter class of tumors.

*The Pedicle.*—In order to understand the formation of this structure the reader must familiarize himself with the normal relations of the ovary to the Fallopian tube and mesovarium. According as a tumor arises from the parenchyma or from the hilum, it will tend to grow upward into the abdominal cavity or between the folds of the broad ligament; in other words, its development will be respectively intra-peritoneal or extra-peritoneal. Under the former conditions the cyst will be pedunculated, under the latter sessile or non-pedunculated. In the case of certain small tumors which are not intra-ligamentous there may be no true pedicle, the growth being sessile and attached by the mesovarium alone. The typical pedicle contains the mesovarium with the ovarian and the tubo-ovarian ligaments and the Fallopian tube. The round ligament is not properly included, and is not usually ligated at the time of operation.

Pedicles vary greatly in size, some being long and slender, others broad, thick, and fleshy, the difference being due to atrophy or to hypertrophy of the existing structures, not to any change in their number, since they are quite constant. There is no constant relation between the size of the cyst and the character of the pedicle, except that in the case of small movable tumors (especially the solid variety) it is apt to be long and slender. As the cyst continues to enlarge and the mesosalpinx is stretched, the outer end of the tube approaches it until it lies in direct contact with the growth. There is no feature in the anatomy of the pedicle so important from a surgical stand-point as the distribution of the vessels. The arteries are branches from the uterine as well as from the ovarian. Those from the latter enter the pedicle from the outer side, the uterine branches from the inner extremity. The veins which are derived from the pampiniform plexus are sometimes enormously dilated, so that the central portion of the pedicle may have an appearance resembling that of varicocele. Both arteries and veins may present a formidable appearance by reason of their size, it being not uncommon to see an artery as large as the radial in the stump. Connective tissue and smooth muscular fibres are naturally found in the pedicle, and nerves and lymphatics may be traced along it to the cyst, though their ultimate distribution in the latter has not been positively made out.

## SOLID TUMORS OF THE OVARY.

These are of infrequent occurrence as compared with cystomata, forming about five per cent. of the whole number of ovarian neoplasms. The benig-

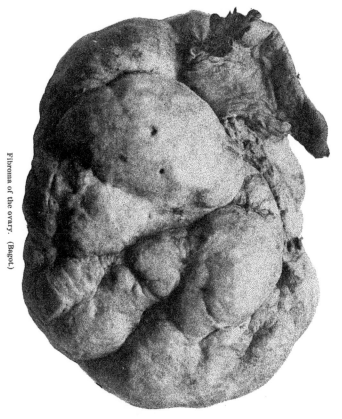

Fig. 20.

Fibroma of the ovary. (Bagot.)

nant class are represented by fibro-myomata, the malignant by sarcomata and carcinomata.   They are especially interesting from a clinical stand-point.

*Fibromata and Cysto-Fibromata.*—Considering the amount of fibrous tissue in the stroma of the ovary, the rare occurrence of fibrous growths,

FIG. 18.

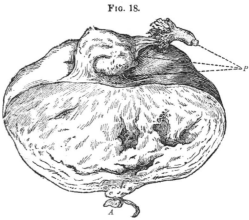

Fibroma of the ovary, with beginning cystic degeneration.  (Mundé.)—*P*, pedicle; *A*, adhesion.

especially as compared with their frequency in the uterus, is worthy of note. Several writers have practically denied their existence, while others have stated that they are often observed.   This discrepancy is doubtless due to the fact that sufficient care has not been exercised in distinguishing between fibro-myoma and spindle-celled sarcoma, which often present the same appearance macroscopically.   A true fibrous neoplasm is to be distinguished from fibroid hypertrophy of the ovary, which may cause an enlargement of the gland to the size of a hen's egg. Careful microscopical examination of the specimen is necessary in order to determine its true character.

FIG. 19.

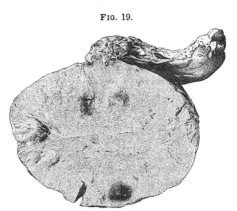

Fibroma of the ovary.  (Museum of the College of Physicians and Surgeons.)

Pure fibromata of the ovary are more rare than fibro-myomata,—a curious fact, when we remember that the smooth muscle-fibres in the ovary are comparatively few in number and are confined to the paroöphoron.   The entire ovary may be transformed into a fibrous growth, or only part of the gland may be involved, the remaining portion being the seat of ordinary fibroid degeneration. The tumor is smooth, hard, and lobulated, being identical in appearance with a subperitoneal uterine fibroma; in fact, those who have denied the existence of these ovarian neoplasms have described them as subserous pedunculated fibroids that have become detached from the uterus. But the anatomical relations of the tumor and its pedicle, similar to that of a cystoma, at once show its true origin. On section they present the gross and microscopical appearances of an ordinary fibroma. They vary in weight from a few ounces to seven or eight pounds. Fibro-myomata attain a larger size than fibromata, since specimens have been described ranging from fifteen to sixty pounds in weight. Tumors consisting almost entirely of unstriped muscular tissue have been described, but it is probable that most of these were of a sarcomatous character. On section they present a reddish appearance, are softer than fibromata, and often show evidences of myxomatous and other degenerative changes. Microscopically they have a fibrous structure, with longitudinal bands of unstriped muscular fibres extending into it from the paroöphoron. The scarcity of blood-vessels in ovarian fibromata is noticeable, and has been offered as an explanation of the fact that they rarely attain a large size.

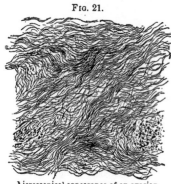

FIG. 21.

Microscopical appearance of an ovarian fibroma. (Howell.)

The secondary changes observed in these growths are similar to those seen in uterine fibroids, such as cystic, myxomatous, fatty, and calcareous degeneration. Interstitial hemorrhages occur in the larger growths, and suppuration as the result of torsion of the pedicle. Of these, cystic degeneration is the most interesting. In the smaller growths it may be limited to simple local softening, dropsy of a central follicle, or the result of interstitial hemorrhage. True fibro-cysts originate, as in uterine fibroids, from the dilatation of adjacent lymph-spaces ("geodes"), which finally coalesce and form large cavities filled with a clear serous fluid; through fatty degeneration, hemorrhage, etc., the fluid may become thick and turbid. True fibro-cysts of the ovary (*fibroma lymphangiectodes*) are exceedingly rare.[1]

It is a curious fact that ascites is a common accompaniment of ovarian fibromata, though a satisfactory explanation of the phenomenon has never been offered, since it occurs in connection with small neoplasms, when neither pressure on neighboring vessels, torsion of the pedicle, nor peritoneal irritation can be urged as a cause of the effusion. The practical importance

---

[1] For additional information on the pathology of these tumors, consult the author's paper in the American Journal of Obstetrics, vol. xv. p. 561.

of this fact is this,—that the surgeon usually associates ascites with malignant disease, and thus might be deterred from operating upon a solid tumor of the ovary which was really of a benign character.

*Sarcoma.*—A study of the normal ovarian tissue, especially in fœtal life, would lead to the inference that this variety of neoplasms should be the most common met with in this locality. While this is not the case, ovarian sarcoma is certainly more frequent than is stated by Schroeder (one in sixty). The relative frequency of sarcomata in children holds true in the ovary, where they form (according to Sutton) a considerable percentage of the entire number. The round-celled variety occurs, but is very rare as compared with the spindle-celled. It is probable that the majority of solid ovarian growths are fibro-sarcomata. Sarcoma is essentially a disease associated with sexual activity, and hence occurs in younger women. Both ovaries are usually primarily affected, an exception to other solid tumors, benign and malignant. They do not ordinarily reach a large size, their bulk seldom exceeding that of a man's head. Tumors weighing twenty or thirty pounds are generally sarcomata. Macroscopically, they may be

FIG. 22.

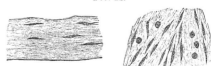

Spindle-celled sarcoma of the ovary. (Doran.)

FIG. 23.

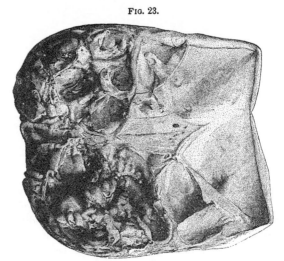

Myxo sarcoma of the ovary. (Boldt)

identical in appearance with pure fibromata, though sometimes they are softer and of a more reddish hue. They also present a similar appearance on section, though in the majority of cases more vascular.

Medullary sarcoma of the ovary cannot be distinguished from cancer, except by microscopical examination.

Mixed forms have been described, such as the mixed round and spindle-celled, myxo-sarcoma, alveolar sarcoma (Billroth), and sarcoma carcinomatodes (Virchow), which are sufficiently described by their names. Fatty degeneration, hemorrhages, thrombosis, calcification, etc., are among the occasional degenerative changes. The statement made regarding the frequency of ascites and the consequent rarity of adhesions applies to the malignant as well as to the benign solid tumors of the ovary.

Sutton insists upon a separate classification for malignant ovarian tumors in children, describing them under the term *oöphoromata*. He calls attention to the following peculiarities: histologically they are identical in structure with the connective tissue of the fœtal ovary, they are bilateral, are rarely seen after puberty, may be associated with dermoids, tend to recur, and towards puberty assume an alveolar arrangement.

Reference has already been made to the possible sarcomatous degeneration of dermoids.

FIG. 24.

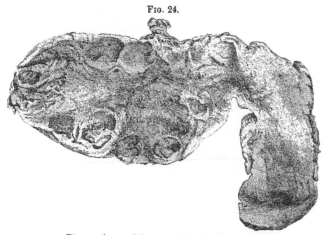

Fibro-carcinoma of the ovary (primary). (Chambers.)

*Carcinoma.*—In referring to "primary" and "secondary" cancer of the ovary we must bear in mind cancerous degeneration of a pre-existing tumor, especially of a cystoma. The reader will readily understand that a cysto-carcinoma may be a primary neoplasm, but a carcinomatous cyst never. Again, a distinction should be made between cancer of the ovary secondary to disease in an adjacent organ, as the uterus, and the same disease accompanying malignant growth in some distant locality, as the breast.

Primary cancer is now held to be much less frequent than secondary. The medullary form is most often met with, and presents the ordinary histological peculiarities. The disease occurs quite frequently in women under thirty, like sarcoma, but, unlike the latter, affects both ovaries in only one-half of the cases. They rarely attain a large size, and appear as whitish, lobulated masses, having usually a doughy feel. In the initial stage there is simply a general symmetrical enlargement of the ovary. A section of the tumor at this stage may show either a diffuse homogeneous development of the disease, or the presence of small foci marking the sites of degeneration of the epithelium of separate follicles. In the latter case the gland might retain its functional activity for some time, as shown by the persistence of ovulation, and even by the occurrence of conception. These growths are the most vascular of the solid ovarian neoplasms, and are especially prone to undergo fatty degeneration. Necrotic changes lead to the formation of pseudo-cysts filled with bloody or colloid fluid. Myxomatous and colloid degeneration also occur. Extension to the

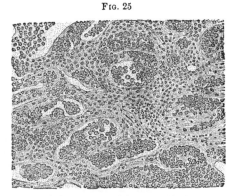

FIG. 25

Medullary cancer of the ovary. (Tait.)

tubes, peritoneum, and uterus takes place early in the form of multiple nodules. Adhesions ultimately occur, but less early than would be expected, on account of the development of ascites, which in this connection is generally due to irritation of the peritoneum by the development of secondary nodules.

Metastatic deposits may develop in distant organs, especially in the liver and intestines. The retro-peritoneal glands are apt to be affected in the later stages of the disease.

Secondary cancer of the ovary is most often met with in connection with cancer of the body of the uterus, though rarely before the disease is considerably advanced. Its comparative infrequency in connection with epithelioma of the cervix—a fact which has been noted by those who have had much experience with total extirpation—is doubtless due to the peculiar distribution of the lymphatics at the bases of the broad ligaments, their connection with the ovary being less intimate than those in the upper borders. Lymphatic infection is also observed in ovarian abscess following puerperal septic endometritis.

Metastatic deposits have been observed in the ovary in cancer of the breast, and less often in primary disease of other viscera, especially the melanotic form. We must distinguish true metastasis from direct extension of the disease from the uterus, where there is also general involvement of the pelvic viscera and peritoneum. Here the organs are often so fused together and united to coils of intestine that it is impossible to distinguish the ovarian growths until they have been dissected out, and even then their

FIG. 26.

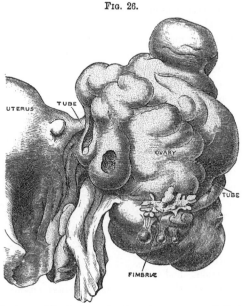

Carcinoma of the ovary secondary to carcinoma mammæ. (Sutton.)

original relations cannot be determined. Such cases interest the pathologist rather than the surgeon, since they are the ones in which the latter must confine himself to an explorative incision.

### MODE OF GROWTH.

As regards the etiology of ovarian tumors, it cannot be said that the various attempts to explain their origin have been very successful. Traumatism, sexual excess, and oöphoritis have been mentioned as exciting causes. The latter might be properly urged in the case of some fibrous and cystic growths in which there is well-marked evidence of fibrous hyperplasia due to former inflammation. The frequent occurrence of dermoids and sarcomata before puberty would seem to indicate that they bear a close relation to the period of formative activity. It may be stated in a general way that ovarian tumors develop most frequently during the period of sexual activity, and their frequent appearance in unmarried and sterile women suggests that constant ovulation, without the periods of rest enjoyed during pregnancy, is to some extent an etiological factor. On the other hand, it is fair to infer that the increased congestion of the pelvic organs incident to pregnancy will accelerate the growth of a pre-existing tumor, as in the case of uterine neoplasms, though to a minor degree.

Clinically, two stages may be recognized in the growth of an ovarian tumor,—the intra-pelvic and the abdominal. Formerly the latter was alone supposed to interest the surgeon, since the fact was not considered that the surgical importance of the neoplasm is not dependent upon its size alone. A tumor the size of an orange, impacted within the pelvis, may give rise to more serious disturbances than one which distends the abdomen.

In its initial stage an ovarian cyst tends to sink downward behind the broad ligament as in ordinary prolapsed ovary. This presupposes a somewhat elongated pedicle; with a short, fleshy pedicle it may be sessile from the outset. To this rule there are, of course, numerous exceptions, since tumors of small size are found above the brim of the pelvis and even in the abdominal cavity, about which they can be moved freely, while they gravitate to the dependent side as the patient changes her position in bed. Rarely the growth may be situated in front of the broad ligament and uterus instead of behind them: this has been noted in the case of dermoids. It is, of course, the rule when the uterus is already retroverted. The degree of prolapse of the incipient cyst varies. It may reach the bottom of Douglas's pouch and cause bulging of the posterior vaginal fornix. Its unilateral situation with regard to the uterus is an important diagnostic point.

The disturbances caused by a small movable tumor the size of an orange are usually slight, being limited to moderate anterior or antero-lateral displacement of the uterus, with resulting vesical irritation, and mechanical pressure on the rectum. The resulting pelvic congestion naturally leads to a certain amount of uterine enlargement and increase in the menstrual flow, though it is not uncommon to meet with a small uterus in connection with a large abdominal tumor of long standing.

As the cyst enlarges, it begins to slip out of the pelvis and to encroach upon the abdomen, still retaining its unilateral position. The intestines are pushed upward and backward, while the uterus is either drawn upward (if the pedicle is short) or is pressed downward and to the opposite side of the pelvis, being usually retroverted, sometimes anteverted. As the tumor continues to grow, it approaches the median line of the abdomen, which, instead of presenting an asymmetrical distention, becomes uniformly enlarged. The intestines are displaced upward, and their normal peristaltic movements are interfered with. Later the entire abdomen is filled by the growth, which compresses the stomach, rests against the under surface of the liver, and leaves a minimum of space for the viscera. Pressure upon the large vessels leads to œdema of the lower limbs, while the renal circulation is interfered with. The thoracic viscera share in the general disturbance, the breathing-space being encroached upon and the heart displaced.

The variations in growth shown in the case of the different forms of ovarian neoplasms are numerous. The description above given applies to a simple multilocular cyst. Dermoids are notorious for their slow growth and intra-pelvic development. They are apt to become impacted in the cul-de-sac of Douglas, so as to cause marked pressure-symptoms. Of the solid tumors, fibromata, unless quite small, are distinguished by their slow growth, free mobility, and situation at the side of and above the uterus. Sarcomata may at first grow quite as slowly, but eventually they increase rapidly, remaining unilateral until they attain a large size. Secondary nodules and metastases are apt to occur during the later stage of the disease.

In primary cancer of the ovary the gland is often uniformly enlarged, and is apt to have nodular masses on its exterior. The tumor is not usually prolapsed, but remains high up in the pelvis, being often fixed by adhesions. The disease is frequently bilateral. Not only does the tumor grow rapidly, but it early extends to the adjacent tissues, and is attended by peritonitis which causes general matting together of the pelvic contents. When the neoplasm encroaches upon the abdomen, the latter often presents an irregular, nodular form, due not only to the peculiar shape of the original tumor, but also to the presence of secondary disease of the omentum and peritoneum.

Papillomatous cysts which develop between the folds of the broad ligament are of relatively slow growth, and at first simply distend the ligament, displacing the uterus laterally and pressing upon the bladder. They may enlarge principally in one direction, or in several, extending downward to the floor of the pelvis, where they may compress the ureter, inward to become adherent to the uterus, and outward until they reach the pelvic wall. They may force their way upward into the abdomen, distending the lower part of it. When the papillary masses have perforated the wall of the cyst and extended to the peritoneum, the original contour of the tumor may be lost, so that it resembles a solid malignant growth. Double cysts of this character are more likely to become fused together than are those of the glandular variety. Union of opposite cysts usually occurs while they are in the intra-pelvic stage, and may be so intimate that their separate character is not recognized until after they have been enucleated and two distinct pedicles have been identified.

The size which an ovarian cyst may attain without being noticed either by the patient or by the physician is remarkable. The writer recalls a case in which he assisted in the removal of a cystoma weighing upward of forty pounds, six weeks after a normal delivery. No suspicion of its presence had been aroused until after the puerperal week, when the patient herself called attention to the fact that her abdomen had not diminished as much as usual. It is not uncommon for a gynæcologist to discover tumors of considerable size of which the patient had no knowledge whatever.

As regards the duration of the disease, we have no positive data. Fortunately, in these days no attempt is made to see how long a patient will survive. Lee has stated that the usual duration is from one to two years. While writing this article, the author has removed a tumor the weight of which was nearly one hundred pounds, and which had existed for twelve years without reducing the patient's strength beyond the possibility of an easy convalescence.

There is no regularity with regard to the growth of benignant neoplasms of the ovary, whether solid or cystic. Small cysts may apparently remain unchanged for a long period, and large ones, especially if oligocystic, may reach a certain size and remain stationary for years. Rapid growth after a long period of quiescence, sudden enlargement or change in contour, and the development of new, especially *acute*, symptoms mean the occurrence of certain changes within the tumor itself, or in its environment, which will now be described.

*Changes within the Tumor.*—Reference has already been made to certain degenerative processes which may take place within the tumor. These involve principally the cystic variety. The changes in solid tumors present no especial differences from those observed in the same growths elsewhere in the body. Fibromata and spindle-celled sarcomata may undergo softening and cystic degeneration, either through general œdema, or in consequence of hemorrhages, necrosis, etc. The tendency of certain sarcomatous and cancerous neoplasms to undergo softening is well known.

The degenerative changes which occur in the wall of an ovarian cyst are usually, though not always, most marked in the main cyst. Areas of local degeneration may represent simple fatty changes or actual inflammatory processes which end in suppuration and necrosis, or may terminate by fibrous thickening or the deposit of lime salts. The blood-vessels over the degenerated patch may rupture spontaneously, causing a moderate amount of hemorrhage into the sac, which, as it takes place slowly, possesses no clinical importance. Of more serious import is the rupture of large vessels in consequence of overstretching during the growth of the cyst, traumatism (especially from puncture), or interruption of the venous return, either gradually from pressure or suddenly from torsion of the pedicle. Proliferous cystomata seem to be particularly prone to hemorrhages, by reason of the vascularity of the papillary outgrowths. The accident may occur several times in succession, or a single profuse hemorrhage into the main cyst may distend it to its utmost capacity. The contents of the cyst will be changed to a thick, chocolate-colored fluid, a tarry coagulum, or a mass of solid fibrin, according to the age of the effused blood. Through complete interruption of the circulation, or infection, the clot may break down and exhibit the appearance seen in infected surgical cavities.

Reference to the localized degenerative processes in the cyst-wall leads naturally to the subject of general inflammation and suppuration, although it should be clearly understood that there is no direct causal relation between the two. Simple inflammation of the sac is most often due to traumatism, or to twisting of the pedicle. Dermoids, from their frequent impaction within the pelvis, are most liable to direct injury, especially during parturition, as will be noted subsequently. Doubtless the peculiar character of the cyst-wall, as well as the nature of the contents, predisposes them to acute degeneration, but it is more in accordance with modern pathology to attribute the majority of cases of acute suppuration to external infection.

Undoubtedly when tapping was frequently performed, in pre-aseptic days, many innocent cysts were transformed into suppurating sacs by direct infection, but this cause is now rare. In a certain proportion of the cases the infection may be transmitted through a diseased adherent Fallopian tube, but the most frequent channel is unquestionably the intestine ; indeed, the common occurrence of degenerative changes in dermoids may be attributed quite as much to their intimate relation with the rectum as to the fact that they are the most subject to traumatism. Intestinal adhesions are quite common, suppuration is comparatively rare. Why infection should occur in one case and not in another is not always clear. Doubtless extreme thinness of the cyst-wall at the point of adhesion favors the osmosis of gas, even when there is no fistulous communication. Every abdominal surgeon must have noted the frequency with which the diseased appendix vermiformis is found adherent to ovarian cysts, and is prepared to subscribe to the view that infection is readily transmitted to the latter through this channel. The subsequent course of the suppurative process may be similar to that of a true pelvic abscess, with this difference, that in the latter the purulent focus is extra-peritoneal, and the pus tends to burrow along certain well-defined planes, pointing either externally or towards the most dependent point. A suppurating cyst may perforate into the peritoneal cavity, though this is rare, on account of the surrounding adhesions. Cases have been reported in which perforation of the abdominal wall occurred, but most frequently the cyst (especially a suppurating dermoid) discharges its contents into one of the adjacent hollow viscera, such as the small intestine, rectum, bladder, or vagina, when a permanent fistula is usually established. Rarely the sinus closes spontaneously and the sac collapses and eventually remains as a mass of indurated tissue. The cystitis occasioned by the communication of a dermoid with the bladder is of a peculiarly severe and obstinate type, and is apt to result in serious renal disease.

Gradual perforation of the cyst-wall may occur independent of previous inflammation. As before stated, this is of common occurrence in connection with papillomatous cysts. There is under these circumstances a gradual leakage of fluid into the abdominal cavity, but, as this is usually of an innocent character, it seldom causes more than a localized peritonitis, the fluid being absorbed or mingled with the accompanying ascitic fluid. Perforation may also occur from simple localized thinning of the cyst-wall in consequence of degenerative processes. This may occur on several occasions in the same case, as may be inferred from the finding of old cicatrices at the time of operation. Cases of spontaneous cure of ovarian cysts were doubtless of this nature when the fluid was bland and non-irritating. Small secondary cysts may rupture into the peritoneal cavity, just as adjacent loculi communicate by perforation of their septa, without any ill results. There is, of course, a certain amount of leakage in every case in which a cyst is tapped through the abdominal wall, the consequences of which depend entirely upon the character of the growth and the contained fluid. It is the rule for a localized inflammation to occur at the site of the puncture, as shown by the development of parietal adhesions. In the case of a papillomatous cyst, tapping may be followed by the same results as spontaneous perforation,—*i.e.*, extension of the papillary growths to the peritoneum. Cysts may discharge their contents into adherent viscera through simple thinning of their walls, without previous suppuration, though this is the exception; if the sac communicates with the gut it is apt to become infected, when the condition will be the same as that already described.

Rupture is an accident of far greater clinical significance than perforation, since it means not the gradual leakage of fluid, but the sudden discharge of nearly all the cyst-contents into the abdominal cavity, with results more or less serious, according to the character of the same. The accident may be spontaneous, being due to gradual thinning of the wall and over-distention, or may be due to traumatism, as a fall or blow, or to extreme pressure from the pregnant or parturient uterus. Excessive venous congestion, due to acute torsion of the pedicle, is another well-recognized cause. The rupture of secondary cysts may be unattended by serious consequences; so, too, the watery contents of a unilocular cyst may escape into the peritoneal cavity, where it is readily absorbed and is carried off by the kidneys. If the rent is not large, it may close and the sac may refill, perhaps to rupture again at the same or at another point. If a fistula remains, there is an intermittent discharge of fluid, which accumulates as a pseudo-dropsy, or occasions a low grade of peritonitis which results in a true ascites that may entirely mask the original condition. There is apt to be more or less hemorrhage from the over-distention of the vessels following the sudden diminution of pressure; this may reach serious proportions, especially when rupture follows axial rotation.

The contact of fluid from a suppurating dermoid cyst causes great irritation of the peritoneum, setting up a general inflammation of that membrane that may be rapidly fatal. Colloid material is not only quite irritating, though not infectious, but is not absorbed. It is often distributed through the entire cavity, covering the viscera with a thick viscid layer and causing a more or less acute peritonitis which may soon be fatal (especially if there is an admixture of septic matter), or may assume a low grade with resulting ascites. Sometimes the colloid matter may become organized, or may apparently develop secondary growths on the peritoneum,—the so-called *pseudo-myxoma peritonei* of Werth. When papillomatous cysts rupture there is a general diffusion of the outgrowths, which become engrafted upon the parietal and visceral peritoneum, the formation of secondary growths and the development of ascites being much more rapid than in cases of gradual perforation. The same phenomena in the case of a cyst that has undergone cancerous or sarcomatous degeneration are, of course, of more serious import. On the whole, the accident is a serious one, since it has been estimated that before the days of prompt surgical interference the mortality was at least forty per cent. In some instances the patient has actually succumbed to shock, while in others the resulting peritonitis was so virulent that it terminated fatally in three or four days. The character of the fluid, the amount which escapes, as well as the suddenness of the accident and the occurrence of profuse hemorrhage, modify the result.

Torsion of the pedicle, as the most common cause of the complications just described, deserves our careful study. Sutton states that it occurs in about ten per cent. of all cases of ovarian and parovarian tumors. Axial rotation of an ovarian tumor implies perfect mobility, a comparatively long pedicle, and the application of one or more forces (either sudden or continuous) acting in such a way as to cause the rotary movement. Small movable tumors are much more liable to rotate; non-adherent dermoids seem to be peculiarly liable to the accident. Fibromata and sarcomata with long, slender pedicles offer favorable conditions, the reverse being the case with solid tumors which have such short pedicles as to be practically sessile. Rotation may be partial, so that there is only a half-turn of the pedicle, the cyst returning to its former position after the initial pressure is removed. Many of these cases are doubtless overlooked at the operating-table. There may be one or three or four complete turns; Croom reports a case in which the pedicle was twisted twelve times. (!)

Torsion may be "acute" or "chronic;" i.e., it may take place suddenly or gradually. The acute cases are far more serious than the chronic. Rotation may occur in either direction,—from left to right, or the reverse, —though rotation towards the median line seems to be the rule. Cases of double torsion have been reported where tumors of both ovaries were present.

Various ingenious explanations have been suggested to account for the phenomenon, but it must be evident to any one who has studied the subject that no single etiological factor can be made to apply to all cases. That there is a direct relation between pregnancy and parturition and axial rotation is well known. It was noted in twenty-five per cent. of the cases reported by Thornton. Torsion during pregnancy is more apt to be gradual, while after abortion or delivery at full term it takes place suddenly, in consequence of the rapid lessening in the size of the uterus and the consequent sinking of the tumor towards the pelvis.

The primary result of torsion is interruption of the circulation in the vessels of the pedicle, the consequences of which are more or less serious, according to the suddenness and completeness of the arrest; this depends upon the length and thickness of the pedicle and the tightness of the torsion. As the thicker-walled arteries resist compression longer than the veins, blood is carried to the tumor, but is unable to return, so that extreme venous congestion results. The veins become enormously dilated and may rupture, thus increasing the tension of the cyst-wall, which may also rupture, fatal hemorrhage occurring. This is, fortunately, rare, the more common result being moderate hemorrhage or extravasation.

The appearance of a rotated cyst at the operating-table is characteristic. Instead of the usual white, glistening hue, it presents a deep-red, sometimes almost black, color, the veins near the pedicle being prominent. Section of the cyst-wall shows that its color is due not to gangrene, but to the uterine congestion and extravasation. The fluid may present the ordinary chocolate color, or may be black and tarry from the presence of coagulum, as in a case in which the writer had an opportunity to make a post-mortem examination. While necrosis may result, actual moist gangrene of the cyst must be rare if there has been no infection from without. What does occur in these acute cases is the rapid development of peritonitis, which is naturally of a virulent type. Simultaneous twisting of a coil of intestine, leading to complete obstruction, has been noted in a few cases, a fatal termination being inevitable if there is not prompt surgical interference.

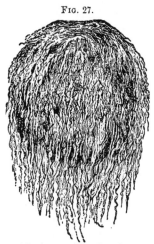

FIG. 27.

Adhesions on the surface of an ovarian cyst which had been separated from its pedicle by torsion. (Doran.)

The phenomena seen in cases of acute rotation where the pedicle is so thick that the circulation is not completely arrested, as well as those in which it takes place gradually, simply differ in degree from those already described. The pedicle becomes thickened and œdematous, its vessels are thrombosed, and it may undergo such degeneration through fatty changes as to be entirely separated from the uterus. Meantime a circumscribed peritonitis surrounds the tumor, rendering it immovable. These adhesions may develop new vessels sufficient to nourish the growth, even when the pedicle has been completely separated, though it ceases to grow and may undergo partial atrophy.

*Changes outside of the Tumor.*—The most important changes in the environment of an ovarian neoplasm directly due to its presence are peritonitis with the formation of adhesions, ascites from irritation of the peritoneum, and pressure-effects on neighboring or distant viscera. Since these have a direct bearing upon prognosis, they deserve some attention. Allusion has already been made to several causes of peritonitis referable to the presence of cysts, torsion of the pedicle, suppuration, and rupture being followed by the most acute and virulent type; whereas perforation of the wall of a papillomatous cyst, with extension of the growths to the peritoneum, leads to a subacute form of inflammation which is not of a threatening character.

Localized peritonitis is apt to be present in connection with large multilocular cysts of long standing, probably due purely to mechanical irritation of the apposed serous surfaces.  Yet immense tumors which have existed for years have been found entirely free, while small intra-pelvic cysts are often firmly adherent.  In fact, it is impossible, in most cases where there has been no history of traumatism or external infection, to assign a cause for the complication.  There may be one or several attacks, which may be strictly localized or general.  It must have been noted by every operator that the condition of the accompanying tube (especially if it contains pus) has much to do with the initial attack.  There is nothing peculiar about the progress of the inflammation, as it usually results either in general thickening of the peritoneum or in the development of adhesions, which differ in size, firmness, etc., according to the more or less intimate relation of the affected serous membrane to the outer surface of the tumor.  Surgically, adhesions are recognized as parietal, visceral, and intra-pelvic.  The first are slight or firm, according to their age and the close apposition of the tumor and abdominal wall during the process of organization.  Mobility of the neoplasm implies the development of thin bands, or even long, slender filaments.  The cyst-wall and parietal peritoneum may be so intimately united that it is almost impossible to separate them at the operating-table. Adhesions to the abdominal viscera are more or less serious, according to their extent, firmness, and vascularity.  If recent, they are often friable and easily separated ; but if of long standing, there is apt to be a rich development of new blood-vessels, sufficient to give rise to serious hemorrhage if they are torn.  This applies most of all to omental adhesions.  Strange to say, the presence of general intestinal adhesions does not seem to interfere with the peristaltic movements to any great extent, so that obstruction is a rare complication.  When this occurs (excluding cases of axial rotation), it is more apt to be due to a single band of adhesion than to the agglutination of several coils.  The worst forms of adhesions are found in connection with cancer, especially in secondary deposits.  The appendix vermiformis, as before stated, is not infrequently adherent to an ovarian cyst ; the danger of infection through this source, as well as through a firmly adherent loop of intestine, has been alluded to.  Adhesions to the stomach and liver are met with only in cases of long-standing tumors of sufficient size to fill the entire abdomen, and are not usually very firm or especially vascular. Such tumors are, fortunately, rarely met with at the present day.

Intra-pelvic adhesions constitute one of the worst complications with which the surgeon has to deal, not only from the difficulty of separating them, but from the danger to important structures during the process. Dermoids become adherent to the uterus, rectum, and Douglas's pouch, while small tumors situated laterally are fixed in such a position as to press upon the uterus, iliac vessels, and sacral nerves.  Repeated attacks of peritonitis lead to fusion of the pelvic organs, which may be completely shut off from the abdominal cavity by overlying coils of adherent intestine.  As before stated, the causes of such repeated attacks of pelvic inflammation are often unknown.  Infection of a retro-uterine cyst in close proximity to the rectum is doubtless a common cause, while traumatism (especially in the case of dermoids) is another. Simple unilocular cysts, with watery contents, are often found to be buried in firm adhesions, possibly the result of recurrent attacks of inflammation referable to the presence of a diseased tube. Intra-ligamentous cysts, either simple or papillomatous, are subject to the same complication, being adherent to the bases of the broad ligaments, in dangerous proximity to the ureter and uterine artery. Large abdominal tumors may also contract adhesions to the pelvic viscera and the peritoneum. The bladder may be drawn up in front of the tumor and become so firmly attached to it that its recognition and separation at the time of operation are no easy matter.

By the term "pressure-effects" we understand the results of mechanical pressure of the tumor at any stage of its development. The visceral changes thus occasioned are to be distinguished from coexisting disease of the abdominal or thoracic viscera which is independent of the neoplasm, though it may be aggravated by it.

One of the first results of the presence of an intra-pelvic tumor is displacement of the uterus, often a flexion sufficient to cause more or less dysmenorrhœa, especially if the organ becomes adherent in an abnormal position. Intra-ligamentous cysts simply displace it to the opposite side of the pelvis. If the tumor becomes impacted in Douglas's pouch, the pressure on the rectum causes not only obstruction of its lumen, but venous obstruction, resulting in hemorrhoids, proctitis, etc. At the same time, pressure on the neck of the bladder leads to vesical irritability, though rarely to actual cystitis, with its secondary complications, ureteritis and pyelitis. Perforation of a suppurating cyst into the bladder results in the development of a peculiarly obstinate cystitis. Calculi are often formed around hair, teeth, etc., discharged from a dermoid cyst. The writer has noted a fatal suppurative nephritis in two or three cases. Pressure on the ureter by a small impacted tumor may lead to the most serious consequences, varying with the partial or complete occlusion of the duct, hydronephrosis being the result of the latter condition. Venous obstruction may be confined to the intra-pelvic vessels, causing œdema of the lower limbs, or rarely the vena cava itself may be compressed, leading to the development of ascites. Large abdominal tumors press directly upon the viscera, causing more or less serious disturbances, which are not to be explained by simple displacement. Intestinal obstruction does not occur from mere pressure independent of adhesions, as the intestines are able to accommodate themselves to the smaller space allowed to them, just as in pregnancy; but cases of ileus have been reported from the strangulation of a loop of gut by the pedicle. Minor degrees of obstruction are indicated by the presence of tympanitic distention and obstinate constipation.

That the kidneys, although not subject to direct pressure, are seriously affected by a tumor of long standing is evident from the condition of the urine, which is often diminished in amount and loaded with urates. Renal congestion is caused not only by pressure on the urine, but by venous obstruction. "Reflex irritation" has also been mentioned as an element in the renal disturbance. This condition of affairs, if allowed to continue, must lead to structural changes, even to chronic interstitial nephritis. Deaths from acute suppression and uræmia following ovariotomy, where no evidence of organic kidney-trouble had been discovered before operation, must be attributed to this cause. The stomach may be displaced by a large cyst and its functions seriously impaired. If the pressure is long continued, chronic gastritis is the result. As regards the thoracic viscera, the heart seems to escape, except in cases of long standing, when dilatation of the right auricle and ventricle and fatty degeneration have been noted. Fenwick believes that this is a direct result of the presence of the neoplasm, and constitutes a formidable complication of ovariotomy.

Not only is the diaphragm pushed upward and the thoracic cavity diminished by the growing tumor, but the sternum and lower ribs are pushed outward, so as to constitute a permanent deformity. Collapse of the air-cells in the lower lobe, pulmonary œdema, bronchitis, and pleural effusion are resulting complications which seriously affect the prognosis of an operation. It should be noted that pleural effusion in these cases is due rather to obstruction of the circulation than to actual inflammation of the pleura, as shown by its rapid disappearance after removal of the pressure.

These are, briefly stated, the principal results of mechanical pressure, such as have been noted in cases of long standing. It is hardly necessary to add that the majority of them are avoidable by an early operation, for which they furnish a forcible argument, rendering further comment unnecessary. Among the purely mechanical effects may be mentioned extreme distention of the abdomen, with thinning of the wall, distention of the superficial veins and anasarca, umbilical (rarely inguinal) hernia, varicose veins of the labia and lower limbs, general œdema of both lower extremities, and neuralgiæ, attributable to pressure on the sacral plexus, all of which speedily disappear when the cause is removed. These are not important in themselves, except so far as they add to the discomfort of the patient by wearing out her general health and thus hastening the fatal termination of the case, unless she is relieved by surgical art.

### COMPLICATIONS OF OVARIAN TUMORS.

These may exist in connection with either the pelvic, the abdominal, or the thoracic viscera, and will be considered in this order.

(a) *Pelvic Organs.*—Complications in connection with the uterus may be either physiological or pathological, the former being both more common and more important.

The subject of pregnancy as a complication of ovarian tumors is one which possesses unusual interest for the obstetrician as well as for the abdominal surgeon. It is impossible, in view of the limitations imposed in this article, to discuss it exhaustively. For further information the reader is referred to monographs and works on obstetrics.

The occurrence of pregnancy in connection with neoplasms of the ovary has been observed so frequently that it is no longer regarded as a pathological curiosity. There is no reason why conception should not occur when one ovary is in a normal condition, as ovulation and menstruation proceed as usual; but why it should occur when the unaffected adnexa are buried in adhesions is not clear; still less so when both ovaries are the seat of neoplasms. So long as any of the normal stroma remains, even though it is represented by a localized thickening in the wall of a large cyst, it is fair to infer that, provided that the tube remains pervious, conception is still possible. More difficult of explanation are those curious cases in which this has occurred in connection with double malignant tumors, the most careful examination failing to reveal any traces of the normal parenchyma. The only plausible explanation is that the disease made such rapid progress after impregnation had taken place as to destroy such slight remains of the stroma as sufficed for the maintenance of the function of ovulation.

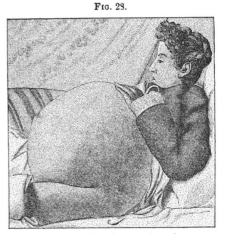

Fig. 29.

Pregnancy complicated with an ovarian cyst.   (May.)

It is important to consider, in turn, the effect of pregnancy and parturition on the tumor and the manner in which the pregnant uterus is affected by the latter. The treatment of the complication will be discussed in another section. There is little doubt that the increased pelvic congestion incident to the physiological state furnishes an additional stimulus to the growth of an incipient cyst. Any one will be prepared to admit this who has had an opportunity to examine the normal or diseased ovary during Cæsarean section. Provided that the growth is movable and has a sufficiently long pedicle, it is first crowded over to one side of the pelvis, then slips above the brim into the abdominal cavity, where it may attain an immense size before its expansion is interfered with by the growing uterus. Such small, freely movable tumors are especially liable to undergo axial rotation, as already stated. But the tumor may become imprisoned below the sacral promontory, even though it is non-adherent, when it cannot develop upward, but must expand laterally and towards the posterior vaginal fornix. Prolapse of the uterus from mechanical pressure may result during the early months. Impaction of a retro-uterine dermoid cyst is a serious complication, since the resulting pressure may lead to rupture, inflammation, and suppuration. The pressure-symptoms due to the tumor itself are increased by the presence of the large uterus. An attack of peritonitis may cause the fusion of the two, with a necessary interruption of the

Fig. 29.

Fig. 30.

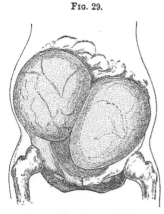 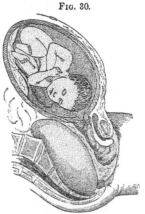

Pregnancy with an ovarian cyst. (Barnes.)

Labor complicated with an ovarian cyst.
(Barnes.)

pregnancy. In the case of movable abdominal tumors, as the uterus rises out of the pelvis it pushes the neoplasm to the opposite side of the abdomen, which may accommodate both tumors, with no serious results except a natural augmentation of the usual pressure-effects, which may become so extreme, especially dyspnœa and disturbance of heart-action, as to threaten the life of the patient. Axial rotation and rupture are still possible dangers, the latter especially in the case of thin-walled adherent cysts. It is remarkable how much compression a cyst will stand. Fortunately, large abdominal tumors do not seem to share in the impetus of pregnancy to the same degree as the intra-pelvic variety, their growth being probably somewhat retarded by the pressure to which they are subjected.

The question of labor complicated with ovarian tumors is one that concerns us here principally from a pathological stand-point. Although any tumor, no matter what its size or position, is liable to serious injury during evacuation of the contents of the uterus, either prematurely or at full term, it is astonishing how little influence it may have on the growth. Small retro-uterine tumors, if movable, may slip out of the pelvis before the head engages, or, if caught between the head and the sacral excavation, may be so compressible as to suffer no harm. Rupture of the cysts under these circumstances would be attended by the results already mentioned, varying in severity according to the character of their contents. Even though labor may terminate normally, the cyst may be so bruised from prolonged pressure that suppuration occurs. The risk of axial rotation from sudden emptying of the uterus applies principally to cysts with long pedicles which have slipped out of the pelvis.

As regards the influence of the tumor itself on the course of pregnancy and parturition, the statistics of former writers are clearly at fault. Modern observers agree that the risks have been much exaggerated. Doubtless abortion is a not uncommon result of the impaction of small tumors within the pelvis, simply from interference with the progressive enlargement of the uterus, and this is in itself a useful and conservative process. Premature delivery also occurs from the presence of large abdominal growths. Adhesion of the neoplasm to the uterus might be a cause of dystocia, as well as of post-partum hemorrhage. There is no reason to infer any injury to the organ itself from the presence of the tumor, except so far as absolute obstruction of the parturient canal would lead to the danger of rupture during labor. The situation, in a word, is this. The uterus during the early months is displaced forward or laterally by a small tumor; rarely it is prolapsed. As it rises out of the pelvis it develops in the direction of least resistance, moving to the opposite side of the abdomen from the growth, and gradually encroaches upon the median line at the expense of the more compressible cyst. After the organ is emptied, the tumor, if large, expands and occupies its usual position, descending towards the pelvic cavity if of moderate size and freely movable, otherwise remaining in the abdomen. The intestines, hitherto pushed upward, now descend and resume the position which they occupied before pregnancy. The statements made with regard to the complication of ovarian tumors with pregnancy apply largely to cysts, solid tumors being comparatively rare. The risks in connection with solid growths (especially the softer malignant ones) would be most from degenerative changes incident to pressure. Twisting of the pedicle is also liable to occur in the smaller fibrous and sarcomatous tumors. Impaction of a solid tumor within the pelvis would naturally cause marked dystocia, in view of its unyielding character.

Neoplasms of the uterus may coexist with ovarian tumors without giving rise to any special disturbances. Uterine fibroids, if small, may have no effect on the ovarian growth; the conditions in the case of large fibroids are much the same as in pregnancy, except that the uterine tumor is now relatively of much slower growth. Axial rotation of a cyst may be produced as in pregnancy. Adhesion of the cyst and fibroid may occur and lead to serious pressure-symptoms. The writer recalls a case in which a subperitoneal fibroid which had become fused with an ovarian cyst was detached from the uterus and received its nourishment entirely through the latter. In general, the pressure-effects resulting from the presence of both ovarian and uterine tumors partake of the peculiar characteristics of both, those from the latter being more intra-pelvic. The tendency of the opposite ovary to become cystic in connection with fibro-myoma of the uterus is a familiar fact and has a direct bearing on the question of its removal during ovariotomy.

42

Since extirpation of the uterus for malignant disease has become so common, the frequency of coexisting cystic degeneration of the ovaries and small ovarian cysts, both single and double, has been remarked. The writer has seen only one instance in which carcinoma of the cervix was associated with a large ovarian cyst, but there is no reason to regard the coincidence as especially rare. The increased congestion due to the presence of the tumor may readily accelerate the progress of the malignant disease, and, on the other hand, a simple cyst has been known to undergo cancerous or sarcomatous degeneration secondary to a similar condition in the corpus uteri. The indication to remove an ovarian cyst, if possible, during vaginal extirpation (it would naturally be done at the time of an abdominal hysterectomy) is therefore a clear one; but, on the other hand, there would be no object in performing ovariotomy upon a patient with inoperable cancer of the uterus.

The presence of accompanying disease of the adnexa deserves some mention. The condition of the opposite ovary is a point of much practical interest, since the surgeon must be able to recognize it promptly at the operating-table. We should naturally expect to find it in every case the seat of chronic congestion and well-marked organic changes, in view of the extra work thrown upon it, so to speak. On the contrary, it is not infrequently perfectly healthy, as shown by the perfect performance of all its functions for years after ovariotomy; yet the writer believes that it is the rule to find macroscopical evidence of pathological changes in the gland in the shape of enlargement, thickening of the cortex, and follicular dropsy (both central and peripheral). Not infrequently a small unilocular cyst, either simple or dermoid, exists in connection with a large tumor on the opposite side. Any marked enlargement of the opposite ovary in connection with a solid tumor is to be viewed with suspicion as an evidence of incipient malignant disease. Hæmatoma has been noted in some instances, —an evidence of extreme venous congestion with hemorrhage into a pre-existing cyst. Abscess is rare, and is either secondary to tubal disease or the result of infection through adhesion of the ovary to the gut. Allusion has already been made to the simultaneous development of two tumors, so that it need only be said that there is no rule regarding the relative rapidity of their growth. One may remain intra-pelvic, while the other fills the abdomen. The earlier fixation of one by peritonitic adhesions may explain their different behavior. Fused cysts are those which have literally grown together and have a common cavity, through absorption of the septum, but separate pedicles. An ordinary ovarian cyst may be associated with a parovarian or an intra-ligamentous cyst on the opposite side.

The changes in the tubes are recognized by the modern surgeon as extremely significant; more so, in fact, than those in the opposite ovary. Salpingitis is a common accompaniment of small ovarian cysts, and, as before stated, is doubtless responsible for the attacks of pelvic peritonitis which result in parietal and visceral adhesions. Although the Fallopian tube undergoes marked changes during the growth of a large tumor, it is less apt to be the channel for infection than in the former case, probably because it is less pervious. Pyosalpinx is a serious complication of intra-pelvic tumors which are otherwise innocent. Hydrosalpinx is met with not infrequently, the distended tube being often as large as the accompanying cyst. The mode of development of tubo-ovarian cysts has already been mentioned. Cystitis with resulting pyelitis, not due to the presence of the tumor, is a serious complication.

(b) *Abdominal Viscera.*—Acute or chronic disease may develop independently of the neoplasm. Renal affections are especially serious from a surgical stand-point. In the writer's experience, contracted kidneys are by no means rare, their presence being unsuspected until the post-mortem. Chronic diffuse nephritis is less common. Hydronephrosis has been noted from pressure on the ureter by inflammatory nodules within the pelvis, and pyelitis (with or without the formation of calculi) secondary to cystitis of independent origin. The increased congestion due to the presence of the tumor would naturally tend to aggravate pre-existing troubles.

The writer has found at autopsies on patients dying after ovariotomy, nutmeg and fatty livers, distention of the gall-bladder, and numerous gall-stones, none of which seemed to have given rise to any symptoms during life. Cirrhosis is a much more serious matter. Chronic catarrh of the stomach, ulceration, and dilatation may exist, conditions which would be aggravated only by the mechanical pressure exerted by an unusually large tumor. Complications on the part of the intestines may seriously affect the prognosis. Old adhesions and stenoses from the cicatrices following ulceration have given rise to complete obstruction independently of the tumor, as in a fatal case reported by the writer. Enteritis, both simple and tuberculous, has been noted, and at one post-mortem he found a diphtheritic colitis, evidently of long standing, which had led to perforation.

Inflammatory thickening of the omentum and peritoneum may antedate the development of a simple cyst. The possibility of miliary tuberculosis is to be borne in mind, since it may be of extra-pelvic origin and coexist with an ovarian tumor.

Reference has already been made to ascites as the direct result of ovarian tumor, due sometimes to the mere irritation of the peritoneum caused by the presence of the neoplasm, sometimes to the development of secondary papillomatous or malignant growths, less often to mechanical pressure on the great vessels. Attention was also called to the pseudo-ascites which has its origin in rupture or perforation of the cyst, with leakage. But, aside from these local causes, it should be borne in mind that ascites, with or without anasarca, may result from the usual visceral causes,—chronic disease of the heart, liver, or kidneys. It is important to distinguish between the two forms of hydroperitoneum in connection with the question of operative interference. Chronic peritonitis (and especially the tuberculous variety) may also be mentioned. So-called encysted ascites may complicate ovarian cyst, as in the case of a patient recently operated upon by the writer, when a collection of fluid within the pelvis was mistaken for a second cyst.

(c) *Thoracic Viscera.*—It is important to distinguish between functional and organic cardiac troubles in deciding as to the propriety of operative interference. The ordinary rules of physical examination will guide us in this respect. Valvular disease is not as serious a complication as might be supposed, provided that compensatory hypertrophy exists. Fatty degeneration and dilatation render the prognosis far more grave. This will be referred to in connection with the contra-indications to ovariotomy. Pericarditis and permanent displacement of the heart by old adhesions are regarded by some authorities as constituting a condition which may be seriously, if not fatally, affected by the pressure of a large tumor. The writer performed an autopsy upon a patient with an immense tumor, who died from cardiac paralysis without operation; the right cavities of the heart were only moderately dilated, no other visceral lesions being found.

Acute pulmonary affections, such as bronchitis, pleurisy, and pneumonia, are peculiarly obstinate when occurring in connection with large cysts, the symptoms being aggravated by the diminution of the breathing-space. Chronic bronchitis, especially in old subjects, is a bad complication, in view of anæsthesia and confinement in the recumbent posture after operation. Old pleuritic effusions are equally unpleasant: the writer witnessed a sudden death from this cause during anæsthesia. Pleuritic adhesions, atelectasis, and emphysema are of frequent occurrence and are comparatively unimportant.

It has been stated by some authorities that pulmonary phthisis is a rare complication of ovarian tumors. This agrees with the writer's experience. Should it develop in a subject with a large abdominal growth, the disease would be affected unfavorably, for the reasons already mentioned. In addition to the affections above mentioned there are many other local and general diseases which may coexist with ovarian tumors and render the patient's condition more serious, as well as complicate the operation. Of these, it is only necessary to mention syphilis, marked anæmia and leukæmia, malaria, and other similar disorders. Diseases of the nervous system are most important. The question of ovariotomy in the insane has been settled satisfactorily. The necessity of brevity forbids our dwelling any longer upon this interesting subject. To summarize: any acute or chronic disease may coexist with an ovarian tumor, and may either pursue its usual course or be subject to aggravation directly due to the presence of the neoplasm, thus impairing the patient's health more rapidly than would otherwise be the case, and increasing the risks of delay in operative interference. That, in spite of all these complications, the statistics of ovariotomy are so favorable furnishes a strong commentary on the state of modern abdominal surgery.

## CLINICAL HISTORY.

As has been stated, the presence of the tumor may be unknown to the patient until her attention is attracted to it by enlargement of the abdomen and a vague sense of discomfort due to its increasing size. The graphic clinical picture presented by the older writers of women who have suffered for years with immense abdominal growths is not often witnessed at the present day, thanks to the general intelligence of both the profession and the laity. Since every case presents features peculiar to itself, the reader will naturally infer that the lists of symptoms detailed in text-books do not represent a single typical case, but such as have been noted in many different ones. Thus, one cyst may occasion marked disturbances during the initial stage of its development, few or none of the ordinary pressure-effects being noted after it rises out of the pelvis, while another attains a considerable size before it gives rise to any symptoms, either from mechanical pressure or from the development of inflammatory complications.

One would expect to observe well-marked local symptoms during the early development of ovarian tumors, in view of those commonly noted in connection with chronic hyperplasia and cystic degeneration of the ovary. Why localized pain should be present in one case and not in another is not always clear, even after the abdominal cavity has been opened. Doubtless the position of the organ (in Douglas's pouch), the presence of inflammatory thickening of the unaffected portion of the stroma, and, above all, the coexistence of tubal disease with perioöphoritic adhesions, explain the stormy inception of some cystic tumors.

, Menstruation may be perfectly regular as to its recurrence and the amount of the flow, but dysmenorrhœa of the usual type will of course result from the condition of the ovary and tube described. Menorrhagia is the rule, due to chronic congestion and resulting endometritis fungosa. The gynæcologist's attention is sometimes attracted to the presence of a small cyst while seeking for an explanation of this symptom. Amenorrhœa in the early stage usually means the simultaneous development of two tumors, especially if they are malignant. If associated with enlargement of the breasts, nausea, etc., pregnancy may readily be suspected. As a later symptom, scanty menstruation or amenorrhœa is simply an expression of the general depreciation of the system. There may be irregular discharges of blood; such metrorrhagia in women at or near the climacteric might awaken suspicions of the development of malignant disease of the uterus. Sterility, when present, may be due to causes outside of the ovaries, such as stenosis, endometritis, etc. Pregnancy would be less likely to occur in connection with a bilateral tumor. As a growing tumor encroaches upon the pelvic organs, there are bearing-down pains in the back, sacral (less often sciatic) neuralgia, with pressure on the rectum leading to obstinate constipation, proctitis, hemorrhoids, etc. Defecation is rendered difficult, and is followed by distressing tenesmus. Pressure on the neck of the bladder leads to frequent micturition, vesical tenesmus, or dysuria. Cystitis may develop from the retention of urine. Since compression of the ureter is nearly always unilateral (except rarely with double malignant tumors), hydronephrosis may develop without being suspected, as in a case observed by the writer. Diminution in the amount of urine, lumbar pain, or (in case of disease of the opposite kidney) uræmic symptoms may show the serious effects of such compression. The reader should bear in mind that such marked disturbances are most common in the case of tumors that have become impacted within the pelvis in consequence of one or more attacks of peritonitis. This is peculiarly true of dermoids, which are generally attended with more pain than any other class of tumors, even malignant. Reference has been made to the results of pressure on the intra-pelvic veins,—œdema of the vulva and lower limbs, distress in walking, etc. In general, it may be said that the presence of the pressure-symptoms mentioned should at once arouse the suspicion that an intra-pelvic tumor exists, though this may be a fibroid or a retroverted pregnant uterus instead of an ovarian neoplasm.

The element of pain in connection with ovarian tumors is a variable one, being dependent less on the growth itself than on the accompanying peritonitis. This is noted in cases of cancer, where the pelvic organs have become matted together from repeated inflammatory attacks. The pain is then more of a dull ache than the spasmodic, lancinating pains which are popularly supposed to be pathognomonic of malignant disease. Severe abdominal pain in this connection may be regarded as evidence that the peritoneum is extensively involved. On the other hand, the early development of ascites in connection with cancerous and papillary deposits seems to retard (though it does not prevent, as some writers affirm) the formation of adhesions, and thus there may be a notable absence of pain, even towards the end of life. Extensive intestinal adhesions may exist without causing either severe pain or any evidence of interference with normal peristalsis, but the writer has noted most agonizing colicky pains in connection with circumscribed adhesions of the small intestine; in fact, these are apt to occur more often than when a considerable length of the gut is anchored to the cyst or abdominal wall. Fibro-myomata and spindle-celled sarcomata with long pedicles, which move freely with changes in the patient's position, may cause severe pain by rolling from one side of the abdomen to the other as she turns in bed. Unless these are sessile and cause pressure-symptoms, they, however, rarely cause much discomfort, except from the accompanying ascites.

The principal discomfort caused during the abdominal stage of an uncomplicated multilocular cyst is the feeling of weight and distention, associated with gastric irritability and interference with breathing. As time goes on, even though the tumor is apparently stationary, the patient's nutrition becomes seriously impaired, as shown by progressive emaciation and feeble heart-action. The urine becomes scanty and concentrated, and may contain albumin and casts; food is no longer retained; dyspnœa becomes extreme, so that the patient is unable to lie down, and can obtain only occasional snatches of sleep. Even when sitting, the weight of the tumor, as it rests on her swollen limbs, renders this position unbearable. Icterus may result from disturbance of the portal circulation and pressure on the biliary duct. The skin, especially over the abdomen, is dry, and is often the seat of eruptions which add to the sufferer's distress. The "ovarian facies," which has been so graphically described by Sir Spencer Wells, is simply an evidence of the general emaciation plus the expression of anxiety and suffering seen in other wasting diseases. A patient with malignant disease may present a somewhat similar appearance, though it appears earlier. It is impossible to describe either satisfactorily, or to define the delicate shades of difference between them; their recognition is entirely a matter of experience. Towards the end of life the patient develops hectic, the pulse becomes more rapid and feeble, and, if not relieved, she sinks into a typhoid condition and dies from exhaustion, provided that some intercurrent complication does not hasten the fatal termination. This picture (though, happily, the original is rarely seen now) is not an exaggerated one, since the writer has recently observed a case of many years' standing which presented almost an exact counterpart. That the symptoms were entirely due to the presence of the tumor, and that even under these conditions such patients are not beyond the reach of surgery, was shown by the complete transformation of this patient within a month after ovariotomy had been performed.

It is important for the reader to be able to recognize promptly the symptoms of these accidental changes in ovarian tumors, which have been described at length. Acute inflammation and suppuration of the sac are denoted by the sudden development of localized pain and tenderness, with a rapid pulse and elevation of temperature (with or without an initial chill) ranging from 100° to 101° F. in the morning to 103° or 105° F. in the evening, sweating,—in short, the ordinary symptoms of septic infection. General peritonitis may develop, when the case soon terminates fatally; or, if the tumor is intra-pelvic, adhesions may shut off the inflammatory focus from the general cavity, when the symptoms are those of ordinary pelvic peritonitis. Provided that the pus does not find an outlet, the symptoms of septicæmia may persist for weeks, the patient has the usual diarrhœa, and eventually dies of exhaustion. Fortunately, rupture into the peritoneal cavity is usually prevented by dense adhesions, so that the sac empties into the bowel (especially the rectum, in the case of dermoids), less often into the vagina or bladder, this accident being recognized by the sudden discharge of pus, bones, hair, etc. Cases have been reported in which the pus has made its way through the abdominal wall either at the umbilicus or in the groin. The subsequent history of these patients is a miserable one. Rarely the sac may be entirely emptied and may be obliterated by granulation, but, as a rule, irregular discharges of pus or dermoid contents occur, sometimes during defecation, the sac alternately filling and collapsing, until after the lapse of months the patient succumbs from exhaustion or dies during an acute attack of septicæmia. The case is different when the sac communicates with the bladder, when a virulent form of cystitis is occasioned, which eventually leads to fatal pyelitis. If a dermoid cyst communicates with the bladder, calculi are apt to form around the hair, teeth, or bones which find their way into the viscus.

The symptoms of perforation of the cyst-wall, with gradual escape of its contents into the abdominal cavity, vary according to the nature of the fluid. If the latter is non-irritating there may be no clinical evidence of the accident. In the case of papillomatous cysts there may be a low grade of peritonitis, with the gradual development of ascites and increase of pain, but the symptoms are so little characteristic that unless the patient had been under constant observation for a considerable interval, and a marked change in the size and shape of the tumor had been noted, no suspicion of the extension of the papillary growths would be entertained. The only circumstance under which this condition might be reasonably inferred would be the appearance of these phenomena soon after tapping, especially if the cyst was intra-ligamentous or parovarian.

The symptoms of rupture differ according to the amount of fluid discharged, as well as its character. A sudden attack of severe abdominal pain in a patient with an ovarian cyst, following a blow, fall, or unusual effort, is succeeded by a distinct change in the shape and tension of the tumor. If the fluid is non-irritating, the amount of shock may be insignificant, and there may be little, if any, subsequent elevation of temperature. There is increased diuresis, and the cyst gradually enlarges again. Rupture of a colloid or dermoid cyst, as Sutton has stated, is rarely followed by the escape of a large amount of material, as it is too thick to make its way readily through the opening; consequently there is less noticeable diminution in the size of the tumor, though its shape is usually changed. The amount of shock depends upon the accompanying hemorrhage, which is sometimes quite profuse, and upon the virulence of the fluid. Colloid material is often, though not always, quite irritating, and may promptly set up acute diffuse peritonitis, as evidenced by pain, distention, and the characteristic rapid pulse and elevation of temperature. That the symptoms may be slight was shown in the case of a patient upon whom the writer operated successfully, removing a large multilocular dermoid which must have ruptured several days before. There was intense congestion of the parietal and visceral peritoneum, but only a slight evening rise of temperature, without pain, increased tenderness, or any apparent change in the tumor, though over a pint of pultaceous material was found among the intestines. The patient made an uneventful recovery, though drainage was not employed. The peritonitis following rupture may be localized and of a subacute type, resulting in the formation of adhesions which give rise to more or less constant pain. Reference has been made to the development of ascites in consequence of the irritation of the peritoneum, also to the engrafting of colloid material. Any one who has seen a case of acute torsion of the pedicle will seldom fail to recognize the accident on another occasion. In a typical case the patient is suddenly seized with a violent pain in the abdomen (more severe than in rupture), with symptoms of shock, and it may be also of internal hemorrhage. Vomiting follows, the tumor becomes larger and more tense, and the patient may feel as if she were going to burst. The writer has been struck with the resemblance of the symptoms to those of accidental hemorrhage into the gravid uterus, there being in both cases a sudden overdistention of a sac from the rapid accumulation of blood. The shock and actual loss of blood may be fatal. In some cases the characteristic symptoms of acute intestinal obstruction soon appear. Peritonitis rapidly develops, and, if it does not soon terminate fatally, destruction of the vitality of the cyst is indicated by the septic symptoms already described. Should the cyst rupture under the increased tension, the patient might die at once from internal hemorrhage.

Gradual torsion of the pedicle is not attended with any marked symptoms by which it could be recognized before operation, unless we accept Doran's suggestion that it may be inferred from the presence of " dull, constant abdominal pains in a patient who keeps in good health and bears a cystic tumor that increases but little, or not at all, in the course of many months or years." It is obvious that at the present day no intelligent observer would deliberately watch the growth of a tumor for any length of time without settling the diagnosis by an explorative incision. It should be added that the symptoms of axial rotation in the case of solid tumors are less severe than in the cystic variety. There may be sudden pain, more or less shock, and intestinal obstruction, but the dangers of intra-cystic hemorrhage and rupture are absent. Œdema and extravasations of blood may cause a sudden increase in its size, and cystic degeneration is a frequent result of torsion of the pedicle. Localized peritonitis may result, but suppuration would occur only in semi-solid neoplasms of low vitality, such as cysto-sarcomata or cysto-carcinomata. Ascites may develop in consequence of the interruption of the circulation, or from peritoneal irritation.

### DIAGNOSIS.

In considering the question of diagnosis it will be found most convenient to adopt Olshausen's division of all tumors into three classes,—viz., (a) those which are strictly intra-pelvic, (b) those which occupy the lower part of the abdomen, and (c) those which extend to the epigastric region. This is the division which is practically recognized by every gynæcologist, who instinctively, as soon as he notes the size of a tumor, runs over in his mind the possible conditions which might cause a corresponding enlargement.

Small pelvic tumors are not infrequently detected during an ordinary routine gynæcological examination; in fact, it sometimes happens that one finds them in patients who have been examined and treated by former physicians. It is always a good plan to make a careful search for a neoplasm in patients who complain of marked pressure-symptoms, such as have been detailed, as well as in cases of prolapse of the uterus without much enlargement of the organ or injury of the pelvic floor. The writer makes it a rule to examine thoroughly every patient under anæsthesia previous to the performance of a minor operation, having on several occasions discovered neoplasms of the ovary which he had before failed to detect. The recognition of a simple cyst the size of a hen's egg in the usual situation behind the broad ligament or at the bottom of Douglas's pouch demands but an elementary knowledge of gynæcological examination. Its lateral position, globular form, peculiar elastic feel, and mobility independent of the uterus are quite characteristic. It is readily pushed upward, and under favorable conditions (in a thin patient, with relaxed abdominal wall) can be mapped out bimanually and its connection with the uterine cornu established. Palpation through the rectum serves to confirm the diagnosis already made. A rectal examination alone may be advisable in the case of young girls. Should the disease be bilateral, the two tumors can be felt on either side, or one may be behind the broad ligament and the other in the cul-de-sac. If it is intra-ligamentous, its position with regard to the uterus will be more strictly lateral, and it cannot be dislodged in either direction. Rarely the tumor will be found anterior to the uterus, though still a little to one side. Küstner has affirmed that dermoid cysts are found in this location more commonly than the simpler variety, and are recognized by the fact that when displaced upward they tend to return to their original position.

When the cyst reaches the size of the fœtal head at term it usually displaces the uterus antero-laterally, so that, if still movable, its separation from the organ can be readily defined. Its size can now be readily appreciated bimanually, and fluctuation is more or less distinct if the fluid is thin. The most exquisite sense of fluctuation is obtained in a thin-walled monolocular cyst. It may be possible at this stage to distinguish either the semi-solid, gelatinous feel of a multilocular colloid cyst, with its irregular outline, or the peculiar doughy sensation communicated to the finger on palpating a thick-walled dermoid. A small fibroma or fibro-sarcoma with a long pedicle is distinguished by its hard, nodular feel, its mobility, and its isolation from the uterus; but such growths, especially if sessile, are usually mistaken for subperitoneal fibroids. The slow growth, the absence of pain, and the good general condition of the patient would be points in favor of a benignant neoplasm. Fibrous tumors are rarely bilateral like cancer, do not form secondary deposits, and ascites is less frequently present. There are, however, cases in which the mere recognition of a solid tumor is alone possible, no hint being obtained as to its character.

When a small cyst is fixed by inflammatory exudate the diagnosis becomes much more difficult, not only because the sensitiveness of the patient does not permit so thorough an examination, but also because the inflammation leads to thickening of the cyst-wall, obscuring the former fluctuation. The smooth, globular outline of the tumor can no longer be mapped out bimanually, while its adhesion to the uterus or walls of the pelvis may be so firm that its origin from the ovary becomes problematical. If the existence of the tumor was not previously known, the history of an attack of pelvic inflammation might readily lead to the inference that the ill-defined enlargement was an abscess. Should suppuration occur in the cyst, an inference as to its original character would be well-nigh impossible. Under these circumstances an examination under anæsthesia is indispensable to the making of even a probable diagnosis. Although such an examination should be as thorough as possible, it must not be forgotten that the cyst may be ruptured by too rough manipulation when the patient is not in a condition to give the danger-signal. When the muscles are completely relaxed by ether it will often be found that a cyst which was supposed to be adherent is simply impacted in the pelvis and can be pushed up readily, or one which was thought to be absolutely fixed will have a certain range of motion, so that its separation from the uterus can be made out. The examiner should seek to insinuate his index finger or index and middle fingers into the sulcus between the uterus and the tumor. Provided that the patient is sufficiently thin, he may with the aid of the external hand grasp the entire organ and draw it forward, away from the tumor. Drawing down the uterus with the volsella, in order to decide whether the tumor moves with the uterus or not, is not practised so much now as formerly. It would not give much information in the case of a small cyst firmly adherent to the posterior surface of the uterus. The sound gives little information in such a case; reference will be made to its use in connection with the differential diagnosis.

The importance of fluctuation as an evidence of the presence of a cyst has been overestimated. Even with the patient anæsthetized, the examiner is liable to be deceived, mistaking the doughy feel of a soft fibroid for that of a thick-walled dermoid; conversely, it is a common occurrence to find at the operating-table a simple ovarian cyst (even a thin-walled unilocular one) so buried in exudate as to simulate a fibroma. Explorative puncture is now regarded as a legitimate procedure only in the case of intra-pelvic cysts which the surgeon has good reason to suppose contain fluid. The cautious gynæcologist will not only feel comparatively sure that he has to do with a collection of fluid, but will not thrust his needle into the sac unless it is either adherent in Douglas's pouch or causes a bulging of the posterior vaginal fornix, so that there is no fear of irritating material escaping into the pelvic cavity. A needle of moderate calibre should be used, at least two inches long, the ordinary aspirating-syringe being sufficient, though some prefer a regular aspirator. It is hardly necessary to add that the strictest aseptic precautions should be observed with regard to cleansing the vagina and the instrument. The fluid obtained may be watery, bloody, or purulent. The contents of a dermoid or colloid cyst can, of course, not be withdrawn through an ordinary needle. The resistance experienced during its passage may furnish a hint as to the solid or semi-solid consistence of the tumor. If pus is withdrawn, it is an easy matter to make an incision into the sac at the time and to irrigate and drain it.

When a tumor has risen out of the pelvis and has attained such proportions as either to cause a visible enlargement of the abdomen, or to be palpated readily through the abdominal wall, the diagnosis no longer depends upon the result of the vaginal examination. When consulted with regard to the nature of such a tumor, the first thing to determine is whether one really exists. In deciding this important question the physician must endeavor to be entirely independent, not allowing himself to be biassed either by the positive statements of the patient or by the opinions of former examiners. By reviewing the history carefully, he may elicit facts which will render him suspicious of the existence of a neoplasm, such as the presence of a strong hysterical element, especially in connection with the climacteric, a marked tendency to adipose or tympanites, symptoms of pregnancy, obstinate constipation, etc. His knowledge of human nature and a previous experience with similar cases will stand him in good stead.

In making a physical examination the patient is placed upon her back on a table or sofa, with her abdomen entirely exposed and her limbs slightly flexed, in order to relax the muscles as much as possible. The skirts should be loosened and the corsets unfastened or, better, removed. As these preparations are sure to make a timid patient nervous, the examiner should avoid a brusque, business-like air, and should endeavor to gain her confidence and allay her fears by a few words of encouragement. Gentleness, either natural or acquired, contributes not a little to the success of the gynæcologist, and is of decided advantage in the class of cases under consideration.

Before touching the abdomen one should inspect it carefully, noting especially whether it is symmetrical or not, the prominence of the navel, the presence of equal bulging in the flanks, of prominence of the superficial veins, œdema of the skin, etc. In order to estimate the amount of sagging of the abdomen it may be well to have the patient sit on the edge of the table, or even to stand erect, when a practised eye will often detect the contour presented by excess of adipose, ascites, or pregnancy. At the same time the general aspect of the patient, especially as to the development of fat, should be noted. (Compare Figs. 34–37, ante, pp. 61 and 62.)

In the case of a stout woman, whose symptoms indicate the presence of the climacteric, it is well to begin our manipulations by picking up the abdominal wall and rolling it between the thumb and fingers in order to estimate its thickness. If the wall is sufficiently relaxed, we may draw the fold strongly forward and palpate deeply *beneath* it over the site of the supposed tumor. Additional information may be gained by having the patient sit up, when the fatty folds are brought out more distinctly. The examiner then touches the entire abdomen with one hand, noting the general doughy feel, instead of the peculiar resistance offered by a tumor.  He then palpates with both hands, first together and then on opposite sides of the abdomen, observing the ordinary surgical rule *not* to palpate in the long axes of muscles.  The pseudo-fluctuation in a fat subject may be easily mistaken by the experienced for the sensation given by cyst-fluid.  In case of doubt, compare it with the thigh, where the same phenomenon will be noted.  Note that the wave is not transmitted from one side of the abdomen to the other, especially if, as Goodell suggests, an assistant " muffles this fat-thrill" by pressing upon the abdomen between the hands of the examiner.  Finally, percuss strongly, sinking the hand deeply into the wall, when uniform resonance will be noted instead of the flatness which marks the presence of a neoplasm.  The vaginal examination will be negative as regards

Fig. 31.

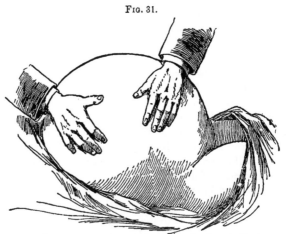

Palpating the abdomen in a case of ovarian cyst.  (More Madden.)

the detection of any intra-pelvic tumor, though in a very stout patient the bimanual will, of course, be unsatisfactory.

Under these circumstances, and in the absence of pressure-symptoms and other signs of an ovarian cyst, the practitioner can be reasonably certain that the patient has been deceived.  However, if, from the thickness or resistance of the abdominal wall and the nervousness of the subject, he has been unable to obtain positive evidence as to the absence of a tumor, it will be wiser for him not to hazard an opinion until he has made an examination under anæsthesia, especially if a former examiner has not only asserted that a tumor is present, but has even proposed an operation.  A small growth *may* exist, though it does not cause the uniform enlargement which the patient has mistaken for one.  The confidence with which the physician expresses his opinion must be determined by his experience.

The same class of patients (women at the climacteric) are commonly troubled with tympanitic distention of the intestines, which leads them to believe that they have a tumor. Their attention is first attracted to it by the fact that their clothing is uncomfortably tight. Careful questioning elicits the fact that the swelling is not permanent, but "comes and goes," being usually most marked a little while after eating. They are much troubled with rumbling of the bowels, eructations of gas, and flatulence, often with colicky pains. The "tumor," when first noticed, was not unilateral, but appeared in the hypogastrium. The examination of these patients is usually rendered difficult by the fact that they have a thick deposit of adipose as well as tympanitic distention. Inspection is often misleading, since the abdomen may present a globular swelling such as we are accustomed to associate with a tumor. Palpation furnishes contrary evidence, as before, while percussion gives a uniform resonant note. On auscultation, the gurgling produced by gas in the intestines will be heard. These patients are usually hyperæsthetic, but deep percussion will furnish conclusive evidence in spite of their resistance. So-called "phantom tumors" in young hysterical women may be exceedingly puzzling, whether due to tympanites or to tonic spasm of the abdominal muscles, especially as the attendant may be thrown off his guard by the patient's plausible history. The necessity for a thorough examination under ether is evident, especially as the condition has been observed in women with ovarian or uterine tumors, as well as in pregnancy. Œdema of the abdominal wall has been mistaken by the patient for a neoplasm, but no physician should fall into this error, since he will not only recognize the ordinary pitting on pressure, but will find a cause for the phenomenon. It has been noted as a late accompaniment of abdominal tumors.

Having reviewed briefly the common sources of error in deciding as to the existence of an abdominal tumor, we shall next consider the ordinary physical signs presented by an ovarian cyst, first, when it occupies the lower part of the abdomen, and, second, when it extends to the epigastric region. The diagnosis may be quite easy,—as Sutton remarks, "more certain than most things in clinical medicine,"—or it may be simply impossible unless the abdomen is opened. The principal difficulties in the way are a doubtful history, thick or resistant abdominal walls, and the presence of the various complications before mentioned, especially adhesions, ascites, and other tumors.

An uncomplicated ovarian cyst of moderate dimensions (the size of a man's head) usually causes, especially in a thin subject, a distinct bulging in one flank, which the patient has herself noticed. On palpation, its globular outline is readily made out, its borders being defined with the fingers, except below, where it is lost in the pelvis. It has a firm, elastic feel which to the expert is quite characteristic, though, in the words of Tait, this sense of resistance "it is quite impossible to teach." Fluctuation may or may not be present. In a unilocular cyst, or in the large cavity of a multilocular one with thin walls, especially if the abdominal wall is not too thick, an exquisite wave may be felt by tapping with the finger on the inner side of the cyst while the hand is placed over its outer side. Its surface is either smooth or nodular. It will be found to extend over to the median line of the abdomen, or past it. On manipulating the tumor, it will be found to have a certain range of mobility, sometimes enough to be appreciated by the patient, who feels it roll over to the opposite side as she turns in bed.

On percussion, there is dulness over the tumor, with tympanitic resonance above and laterally, there being no change in the area of dulness as the patient is turned alternately on one side and the other, unless the tumor is so movable as to gravitate to the dependent side. Auscultation furnishes no additional evidence, an occasional bruit being the only adventitious sound heard over the tumor.

On making a vaginal examination it may be impossible to feel the cyst; if a portion is still intra-pelvic, the presence of a short pedicle or adhesions may be inferred. The uterus, of normal size or only moderately enlarged, will be felt, either ante- or retroverted, more often in the latter position. Not infrequently the entire organ is drawn upward with the vagina, when the fundus can be felt above the symphysis in contact with the abdominal wall: it will usually be pushed over to the opposite side of the pelvis by the growth. It is unnecessary to use the sound in these cases. The examiner should note how much, if any, motion is communicated to the organ while manipulating the tumor, as he can thus gain some idea as to the length of the pedicle. Palpation of the other ovary should always be attempted, since a second incipient cyst may be discovered. A rectal examination will settle the position of the uterus in case of doubt.

A large abdominal tumor of ovarian origin presents certain physical peculiarities which should be carefully noted, as they will be referred to again in connection with the subject of differential diagnosis. The abdomen is uniformly enlarged, but is most protuberant in the region of the umbilicus; the latter may be flattened as in pregnancy, or protrudes if hernia is present. It may present an irregular outline, the bulging being more marked in one flank than in the other. On deep inspiration a downward movement may be observed in the tumor. Dilatation of the superficial veins is not pathognomonic; the *lineæ albicantes*, commonly observed in pregnancy, may be well marked. The difference in symmetry between the physiological and the pathological condition will be shown by measuring the distance from the umbilicus to each anterior superior iliac spine. The upper limit of the growth can be made out by palpation, while below it is not to be separated from the pelvis. Its lateral borders are now not clearly defined. The peculiar elastic feel of the tumor is readily appreciated, while deep fluctuation is felt with more or less distinctness. It is often possible in the case of a colloid cyst to make out not only the location of the large sac, but the presence of secondary cysts of different consistence. Percussion furnishes the same results as before, the transverse colon, which now lies just above the tumor, giving tympanitic resonance in this region. As the tumor continues to grow it may be no longer possible to define its upper border, which lies beneath the ribs, so that a certain amount of tympanitic resonance is obtained only at the sides, and may be lost even there as the neoplasm, unable to grow any farther in an upward direction, spreads out laterally, the shape of the abdomen being changed accordingly.  The ribs and sternum are bent outward, and the belly becomes more pendulous. Percussion over the stomach, liver, and spleen shows that these organs are displaced upward, while examination of the thoracic viscera indicates the pressure to which they are subjected from below.  The facies and general condition of the patient present the appearance already described at this advanced stage.

While modern surgeons attach less importance to the refinements of diagnosis than did those of a former generation, not only because experience has shown that few, if any, of the clinical signs which have been described are absolutely reliable, but also because the question of prognosis has been essentially modified by improvements in operative technique, it is not well for the practitioner to be content with the mere recognition of a large ovarian tumor.  He should at least try to find out all that can be learned about its character and environment before opening the abdomen.  He may, with more or less success, gain by a physical examination some information as to whether it is solid or cystic, benign or malignant, single or double, slightly or firmly adherent.  At the same time a careful examination will show if the patient has visceral complications which may affect her chances of recovery from an operation.  Solid tumors rarely reach so large a size as to fill the entire abdomen.  Such a growth of moderate size may be recognized by its greater firmness and the absence of elasticity and fluctuation.  With a thin, relaxed abdominal wall it may be possible to make an accurate diagnosis, but experts are frequently deceived, since a thick-walled colloid cyst may readily be mistaken for a solid tumor.  Rapid growth, the early development of ascites, and progressive depreciation of the general health, point to its probable malignant character, the suspicion being strengthened by the detection of secondary nodules in the omentum and peritoneum and by the condition found by vaginal examination.  Cysto-sarcoma and cysto-carcinoma may present the same physical conditions as an ordinary multilocular cyst, but the accompanying conditions denote a more malignant process.  The same symptoms may be produced by an ordinary cyst that has undergone malignant degeneration, but ascites is apt to develop later under the latter conditions.  If a cyst which has existed for some time without causing serious symptoms begins to grow rapidly, or if the patient's health declines more quickly than would be explicable by the mere presence of the tumor, a malignant change may be reasonably inferred.

Double cysts may be recognized while they are still of moderate size, but when they fill the abdomen, and especially when they are fused together, it is impossible; nor is the diagnosis a matter of any practical importance.

The side from which the cyst sprang is often inferred from the history, the displacement of the uterus, the position of the intestines, the greater prominence of the affected side, and the position of the pedicle. These signs are manifestly wanting in the case of a tumor that fills the abdomen. Surgeons pay little or no attention to this point.

The determination whether a cyst is unilocular or multilocular, papillary, dermoid, or multilocular dermoid, is sometimes possible. Thus, a smooth, uniform tumor in which fluctuation is the same at every point, the wave being easily transmitted from one side to the other on slight tapping with the fingers, is either a unilocular cyst containing a thin fluid, or an oligocystic tumor with a large cavity. The slow growth of the latter is a point in favor of the diagnosis. The difference between thin and gelatinous contents is better appreciated when the cyst-wall is relaxed than when it is tense.

A multilocular cyst may be recognized by its size (since it attains the largest dimensions of any ovarian tumors), irregularity, semi-solid consistence, and the fact that fluctuation, if present, is limited to a certain area. Under favorable conditions a peculiar vibration may be felt, such as would be given by the agitation of a quantity of jelly. Secondary cysts are sometimes felt as detached masses, or give the impression of being pedunculated like a group of subperitoneal uterine fibroids. Under these circumstances they may be mistaken for cancerous nodules in a collection of ascitic fluid, especially if symptoms are present which seem to suggest malignant disease.

The positive recognition of true papillomatous cysts is seldom possible. Certain anatomical peculiarities should be borne in mind, such as their moderate size, the frequency with which they are bilateral, their relatively rapid growth, without other evidences of malignancy, and the development of ascites, not early, but after they have existed for some time. On palpation they give the sensation of being semi-solid, in spite of their thin fluid. On the other hand, a cyst has often been diagnosed as unilocular the principal cavity of which contained numerous secondary cysts and papillary outgrowths too small to affect the wave of fluctuation. The prediction that a multilocular cyst contains such masses is always unsafe, since its semi-solid feel may be due to secondary cysts with thick colloid contents. The inference that the sac contains pus or blood is usually impossible, even when the history points to probable axial rotation or acute inflammation. This doubt, as well as the impossibility of determining that an apparently simple cyst is not papillomatous, furnishes a forcible argument against explorative puncture.

Reference has already been made to the diagnosis of intra-pelvic dermoid cysts. Pure dermoids seldom exceed the "second stage" of development. Their slow growth, especially in a young subject, frequent complication with peritonitis, and the unusual amount of pain accompanying them are by some writers regarded as characteristic. As a rule, their true character is recognized only at the operating-table, or when they perforate into and discharge their contents through one of the mucous canals. On palpation they give an obscure doughy sensation different from that of a colloid tumor, and exceptionally it is possible to feel a tooth or a bony nodule in the cyst-wall. That the latter is by no means a positive sign is shown by reports of cases in which calcareous plates on the exterior of simple cysts, or the bones in ectopic sacs, have been mistaken for dermoid contents. Multilocular dermoids are seldom recognized as such before opening the abdomen, since the dermoid loculi are relatively small and are masked by the general colloid character of the tumor. Under exceptionally favorable conditions, as in a thin patient, where the dermoid portion is in contact with the abdominal wall, its doughy feel and the presence of bones might furnish a sufficient contrast to the other portions of the tumor to suggest the complex nature of the growth. Its rapid growth and large size would render it certain that it was at least not a pure dermoid. A good deal of attention was formerly bestowed upon the diagnosis of adhesions, which were an object of peculiar dread to the ovariotomist. Many now go to the opposite extreme, and affirm a profound scepticism with regard to the possibility of recognizing them before operation. There is no doubt that increased experience renders one distrustful of his ability to predict either their presence or their absence. The reader's time will not be taken up with refinements of diagnosis, but it is important that he should learn to apply certain rules for the detection of the more obvious adhesions on account of their bearing on the question of prognosis, always being prepared to find at the operating-table that he has been entirely mistaken in his inferences.

The method of recognizing the fact of the fixation of intra-pelvic neoplasms has already been outlined. In the case of a medium-sized abdominal tumor the history of a former attack of peritonitis, with tenderness on moderate pressure and limited mobility (or entire absence of the same) on manipulation, indicates the probable existence of adhesions. The suspicion is strengthened if the growth remains unilateral, not developing in the usual way towards the median line. Firm attachments to the abdominal wall can be made out when the latter is quite thin and relaxed and there is not too much local sensitiveness to prevent free manipulation of the tumor. A history of previous tapping would help to support the diagnosis. The presence of crepitation on rolling the tissues over the surface of the tumor is not pathognomonic of recent adhesions, since the same sensation may be caused by nodules or calcareous plates on its exterior. The supposed independent movement of the parietal and visceral serous membranes may be deceptive. Moreover, apparent fixation of the dependent portion of the tumor within the pelvis may be due to a short pedicle.

In the case of a large tumor of long standing it may usually be assumed that parietal adhesions are present, though subjective symptoms are absent. The exceptions are few, but the pseudo-membranes may be limited and filamentary. Clinically, the presence of free peritoneal fluid is no evidence that general adhesions do not exist. Occasionally a layer of ascitic fluid is detected between the tumor (especially if it is solid) and the abdominal wall by practising gentle palpation with the finger-tips. Olshausen has called attention to the fact that when the fluctuation is no longer transmitted freely across the abdomen, but is confined to isolated spots over the tumor, it is an indication that the fluid is confined in interstices of the pseudo-membranes. Fixation of the neoplasm may be inferred when by inspection or percussion it shows no downward movement on deep inspiration; but thickness of the abdominal wall may easily obscure this sign.

The presence of visceral (especially intestinal) adhesions may be suspected from a history of obstinate constipation and severe colicky pains, from the intimate relation of a coil of intestine to the cyst, and especially from the discharge of cyst-contents per rectum. Exceptionally a loop of gut may lie in front of the tumor, where, in a favorable subject, its presence might be recognized by the localized tympanitic note on percussion. It may be safely assumed that a tumor fixed within the pelvis is covered by a layer of adherent gut, though we question if many examiners possess Winckel's ability to palpate the coils per rectum. It is doubtful if adhesion of the omentum to the anterior surface of a cyst can be recognized before operation, unless under the exceptional circumstances referred to by some writers when there exists at the same time a large umbilical hernia. Vaginal palpation enables one to demonstrate the relations of the intra-pelvic portion of an abdominal tumor, though the question of its fixation is generally doubtful, as it is so impacted by reason of the superincumbent weight that it may not share in the movement imparted to the main tumor. Upward dislocation of the uterus is not a positive sign of its close attachment to the growth, and, on the other hand, the retroverted organ may be rendered immovable purely by the pressure of the neoplasm. The length of the pedicle makes considerable difference in this respect. It is well to remember that the bladder is occasionally drawn upward and attached to the anterior surface of the tumor so as to be in danger when the abdominal incision is made. The passage of a catheter will readily establish this point and put the surgeon on his guard, though the experienced operator never loses sight of this possible complication. The coexistence of uterine with ovarian tumors may render the diagnosis quite difficult, especially if these are fused together by inflammatory exudate, or if free peritoneal fluid is also present. The differential diagnosis will be discussed in the following section. In arriving at a conclusion the physician should pay particular attention to the menstrual history, and note the size of the uterus and its relations to the suspected fibroids. The difference in density between a hard uterine fibroid and an ovarian cyst is readily appreciable to the practised touch, but the coexistence of solid growths of both organs cannot be made out with any degree of probability. These are cases in which an explorative incision is clearly indicated.

The diagnosis of early pregnancy in a patient with an ovarian tumor

presents no especial difficulties, provided that the history is clear and that the previous existence of the growth is known. But when she consults the physician for the first time his attention is apt to be so concentrated on the neoplasm that he forgets the possibility of an accompanying physiological condition. If, from her age, her irregular menstrual history, and the absence of the ordinary subjective symptoms, the possibility of pregnancy seems doubtful, the most experienced may err, especially if the uterus is so displaced or masked by the tumor that it cannot be clearly mapped out bimanually. Retroversion of the pregnant uterus plus an impacted cyst constitutes a puzzling combination. When both the uterine and the ovarian tumor have slipped out of the pelvis, not only do they cause a peculiar broadening of the lower part of the abdomen different from that due to either enlargement alone, but the limits of the two tumors can be defined, with a well-marked depression between them. The latter sign, as well as independent mobility of the cyst, is wanting when the latter is adherent to the uterus. However, it will be noted that one tumor is continuous with the portio, while the other is not. If the uterus is dislocated upward, the results of the vaginal examination (internal ballottement, etc.) may be negative. As pregnancy advances, external ballottement and fœtal movements and heart-sounds will serve to establish the diagnosis, aside from the difference in the rate of growth in the two tumors, the symmetrical contour of the one and the irregular form of the other. It need hardly be added that in a case of this kind, in which an exact diagnosis is so important, the practitioner should keep the patient under careful observation, noting carefully any change in the condition of affairs, and should share the responsibility with a more experienced *confrère*. Delay of a few weeks during the early period of pregnancy is advisable in order to make sure of the progressive enlargement of the uterus, but during the latter half it may subject the patient to too great a risk. It should not be forgotten that tubal gestation may occur in a woman with an ovarian tumor, as will be discussed later. In short, it is possible for cysts to coexist with neoplasms of abdominal as well as of pelvic origin, as shown by the complicated conditions daily encountered in the operating-room.

The duty of the surgeon is by no means fulfilled when he has exhausted all the means of arriving at a conclusion regarding the character of an abdominal tumor and the presence of local complications. A general survey of the patient should be made in order to determine if she is suffering from any organic visceral trouble. It is not necessary to describe the ordinary routine practice of the careful diagnostician, except to add that the examination should be *thorough*, in view of its direct bearing on surgical treatment. The question of indications and contra-indications will be discussed elsewhere. Suffice it to say that there is ample room for the exercise of the highest skill and acumen in deciding how far an ominous sign is to be interpreted as due to an independent lesion of an organ, and how far to the presence of the neoplasm, or to what extent a pre-existing trouble is aggravated by the growing tumor.  The condition of the heart and kidneys should receive the keenest scrutiny, as it is to complications in these organs that the majority of the non preventable deaths after ovariotomy are due.  Other things being equal, the most successful surgeon is he who is most thorough in this respect.  In a doubtful case a single examination is not sufficient to determine these points.  The patient must be kept under careful observation for several days, preferably in a hospital, where she can be under constant surveillance.  Serious cardiac and renal complications have been entirely overlooked by a too prompt operator impelled by one of the strongest motives to haste in this age of competition,—the fear of losing a good case.

### DIFFERENTIAL DIAGNOSIS.

Sutton remarks emphatically that "there is no organ in the belly, except the supra-renal capsule, which has not at some time or other given rise to signs resembling those presented by an ovarian cyst."  When we add to this the fact that the exact origin of a tumor can sometimes not be determined even after the abdomen is opened, the reader will infer that the subject is a somewhat broad one.  But it will be evident as we proceed that the same process of elimination is followed as in any other branch of medicine, and that, however great may be the number of conditions which we may assume to be present, they can be rapidly narrowed down to two or three by dismissing such as are, from the history and results of the physical examination, manifestly improbable.  Instead of trying to recall indiscriminately the score of different causes of abdominal enlargement enumerated in the text-books, the beginner should accustom himself to a certain routine, when he will be surprised to find how much simpler the matter is than he had at first supposed.  The writer's practice is to divide all tumors into two classes,—those which originate in the pelvis, or, more broadly, below the umbilicus, and grow upward, and those which spring from the upper half of the abdomen and grow downward.  A second subdivision into lateral and median tumors then suggests itself, when the mind at once reverts to the tissues or organs in the given locality from which it might develop.  It will be found that this rule is practicable even in the case of neoplasms that are apparently quite symmetrical and fill the entire abdomen, so that at first sight it appears impossible to assign them to either class.  Before entering upon this subject it is important to consider at some length a condition which may be mistaken for the presence of an ovarian cyst.

There ought to be no difficulty in distinguishing between ovarian cyst and a dropsical effusion due to general causes, such as chronic disease of the heart, lungs, or kidneys, or even to a depraved state of the blood, since the history of the case and the fact that the patient has been for some time under observation should prevent error.  The history of a large cyst may extend over many years.  That it is possible to overlook so obvious a cause has been impressed upon the writer by his seeing abdominal section performed by prominent gynæcologists, who found, to their dismay, not the supposed ovarian cyst, but (as shown by autopsy) in one instance cirrhosis of the liver and in another contracted kidneys, while in a third the true cause of the effusion could not be determined. The simultaneous occurrence of œdema of the lower limbs (a rare and late complication of ovarian tumor) should lead the practitioner to make a thorough search for some visceral lesion. More puzzling are those cases in which hydroperitoneum is due to local causes, such as subacute or chronic peritonitis (especially tuberculous), obstruction of the portal circulation, or malignant disease, especially the latter, when the effusion occurs so rapidly as to obscure the original condition. It may be said that there is nothing which tests a man's general medical knowledge so thoroughly as an investigation of the causes of ascites. He who has not enjoyed the advantages of a careful training in physical examination will find that the proper study of a single case furnishes invaluable mental discipline.

Assuming that the history gives no positive clue to the true condition in a patient seen for the first time, the practitioner must enter upon the examination with his mind as unbiassed as possible. For obvious reasons, the greatest difficulty will be experienced in deciding between extensive ascites and a cyst which fills the abdomen, since with a smaller tumor or a moderate amount of effusion the peculiar characteristics of each are more apparent.

In a patient with ascites it will be noted on inspection of the abdomen that it is enlarged symmetrically, but is somewhat flattened, not showing the prominent swelling seen in ovarian cyst, while there is a marked bulging laterally. The lower ribs are not bent outward as in the case of a large tumor. The motion imparted to the latter on deep inspiration is wanting. Turning the patient upon her side, the free fluid will gravitate accordingly, causing a change of form which is not seen in the case of a cyst. With the patient in the sitting posture, the difference in the shape of the abdomen will also be apparent. To the initiated, simple palpation will at once reveal the absence of that resistance peculiar to a multilocular cyst, though a large, thin-walled oligocystic tumor may present precisely the same sensations to the fingers. In a favorable case a visible superficial wave of fluctuation may be observed following a light tap, and will be clearly appreciated by the hand placed on the opposite side of the abdomen. In a cyst, even when its borders cannot be clearly defined, fluctuation is limited to the cyst-area, may be more distinct in the upper portion of the tumor than in the lower, and is absent in the semi-solid portions. Comparing the results of percussion, the fluctuation in ascites is not confined to the dull area.

The distinguishing characteristic of ascites is a tympanitic percussion-note in the region of the umbilicus, with dulness in the flanks, the reverse being true in the case of a cyst, except in rare cases in which the latter contains gas by reason of its communication with the intestine.  In some cases in which the tympanitic note is not appreciated, Wells has suggested placing a pillow under the patient's hips, in order to cause the fluid to gravitate towards the diaphragm, when the intestines will float upward. Change in position brings out a change in resonance varying with the level of the fluid.  This is best appreciated when it is not present in excess. Thus, its upper level can be mapped out when the patient is sitting, and when she is turned alternately on one side and the other a tympanitic note will be heard over the upper flank.  Deep pressure and strong percussion may be required in the case of a patient with a thick abdominal wall, or where the latter is so distended with fluid that the intestines lie some dis-

Fig. 32.

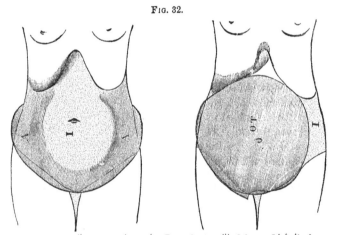

Area of dulness in ascites and ovarian cysts. (Barnes.)—*A*, ascitic dulness; *I*, intestinal resonance; *OT*, dull area of ovarian tumor; *I*, intestinal resonance.

tance behind it.  The characteristic signs may be absent when the omentum is greatly thickened by cancerous or tuberculous deposits, fat, etc., or where the intestines are generally adherent.  Here the examiner must rely upon the sensation of fluctuation and the variations noted on change of position. A vaginal examination often throws considerable light upon the diagnosis, for while in ascites the pelvic organs are often normal, the uterus being in its proper position and freely movable, with an ovarian cyst it is apt to be either retroverted or drawn upward.  The bulging of the posterior vaginal fornix by free fluid in the pelvis gives an entirely different sensation from a cystic tumor, while the wave of fluctuation transmitted from above is much more distinct.  When the pelvic organs are entirely shut off from the abdominal cavity by inflammatory exudate, this evidence is, of course, wanting.

Sometimes a collection of ascitic fluid is confined by adhesions, causing a circumscribed enlargement which may readily be mistaken for an ovarian cyst. There is a history of an acute or a subacute peritonitis (which is nearly always tuberculous), with corresponding impairment of the health and often persistent localized pain. The abdomen is not prominent. The tumor, the boundaries of which are ill defined, is fixed among the intestines, so that fluctuation is limited and the percussion-note is dull in front, as in the case of an ovarian cyst, there being also no variation with change in position. It is most often found in the middle of the abdomen rather than at one side. Vaginal examination is negative as regards the detection of a tumor or a fluctuation. It is evident that a diagnosis is often impossible without the aid of an explorative incision. The writer was once completely deceived in a case of tuberculous peritonitis which gave all the physical signs of a typical multilocular cyst, the semi-solid portion being a mass of thickened omentum, while the supposed main cyst was a collection of ascitic fluid among the adherent coils of intestine.

The association of ascites with an abdominal neoplasm at once raises the question whether the latter is of ovarian origin. If the tumor is large and there is only a moderate amount of ascitic fluid, an application of the usual method of palpation and percussion will enable the examiner to map out the tumor, and to distinguish the deep elastic feel, or fluctuation, in the latter from the superficial wave obtained by tapping on the opposite side of the abdomen. Should the tumor be deep-seated, alternate light and firm pressure will bring out the delicate shades of difference. With double cysts the diagnosis will be more difficult. In the case of solid growths of medium size, especially if these are bilateral, the suspicion of malignancy will be aroused by the history of rapid growth and serous exudation, cachexia, and especially the detection of secondary nodules in the omentum and peritoneum.

It will be remembered that ascites may accompany small fibrous tumors. Its association with a small cyst in a patient in good health usually suggests the papillary variety, while its gradual development in connection with a multilocular tumor may follow perforation. It would rarely be possible to distinguish cyst-fluid in the peritoneal cavity from the ordinary exudation, unless a sufficient quantity had escaped to allow of comparison with the cyst. Olshausen has described a peculiar crepitus imparted to the palpating finger by colloid material in the peritoneal cavity.

When the tumor is small and the abdomen is much distended with ascitic fluid, the neoplasm may be completely masked. Under these circumstances, when the general causes of hydroperitoneum have been eliminated, the vaginal examination is negative and the practitioner suspects a local cause, and, if his leanings are surgical, he begins to think of the propriety of making an explorative incision. Before proceeding so far he should ask himself whether it may not be better first to withdraw some of the fluid. The value of explorative puncture as a means of diagnosis has doubtless been greatly overrated, but that does not prove that the careful observations of our more cautious predecessors should be dismissed as entirely valueless. It is true that few abdominal surgeons would hesitate before making an explorative incision in a doubtful case because of the result of the chemical and microscopical examination of a drachm of fluid withdrawn by the hypodermic syringe. On the other hand, the withdrawal of a few pints of free fluid may clear up the diagnosis most satisfactorily, especially where malignant disease is suspected. The writer, though opposed to the practice of tapping ovarian cysts, has frequently resorted to the aspirator under the above circumstances, and never with any bad results, though he has always been prepared to operate promptly if it seemed necessary. Although in several instances the fluid was found to be ovarian instead of dropsical, the patient was none the worse for the puncture. At the same time the possible dangers of puncture, even when a small needle is inserted to a slight depth, should not be lost sight of. An adherent loop

of gut or superficial vessel may be punctured, septic fluid may escape from a cyst, a vascular solid tumor may be wounded: all of these accidents have occurred. Yet these can nearly always be avoided by proper care in the selection of the point of puncture, and by remembering that, since the object is merely to remove the excess of free fluid, the needle need not be introduced so deeply as to reach the neoplasm. The purpose of the operation may be defeated through blocking of the needle by lymph or a thick fluid. Ascitic fluid is of a yellowish or greenish color, frequently bloody, has a specific gravity seldom above 1015, and contains a considerable amount of albumin, but no paralbu-

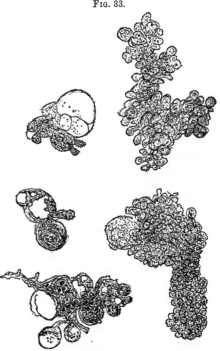

Fig. 33.

Sprouting cell-groups in ascitic fluid: malignant disease of ovary and peritoneum.

min. The viscidity noted even in thin cyst-fluids is absent. It coagulates spontaneously, and, when examined microscopically, contains few, if any, of the cell-elements so common in the contents of ovarian cysts. It is evident that the fluid from a paroarian cyst, when mixed with blood, might present the same peculiarities. Of more diagnostic value are the " sprouting cell-groups" described by Foulis, the presence of which in free peritoneal fluid the writer still believes (in spite of the positive contrary assertions of some observers) to render highly probable the existence of malignant or papillomatous growths in the peritoneum. Figure 33 represents the actual appearances observed under the microscope in a drop of ascitic fluid removed from a doubtful case of the writer's, in which the diagnosis of cancer was confirmed by an explorative incision. A similar diagnosis, based on the same grounds, was made in several other instances, each time correctly. While the absence of these cells is by no means an argument against the presence of malignant disease, the writer's personal experience has led him to believe that they possess considerable diagnostic value,—an opinion recently expressed by so accurate an observer as Osler.

Echinococcus hooklets and scolices are sometimes found in ascitic fluid where the existence of the parasites had not been suspected.

Any inference as to the rupture of an ovarian cyst from the examination of free fluid would be open to grave doubt, though the finding of numerous "ovarian cells," cholesterin plates, etc., might serve to confirm a diagnosis of ruptured cyst based on other more probable signs.

But, as before stated, the most useful application of explorative puncture lies in the removal of a sufficient amount of fluid to enable the observer to unmask tumors and secondary nodules, to the differentiation of which he can then proceed according to the usual rules, being governed in his decision as to the performance of explorative cœliotomy by the presence or absence of advanced malignant disease and the condition of the patient.

The differential diagnosis of intra-pelvic ovarian tumors presents greater difficulties than does that of abdominal growths, since it involves a high degree of cultivation of the *tactus eruditus*. Several experts examining the same patient not only may receive different impressions with regard to what they feel, but, if they agree as to facts, may interpret them differently, even after they make a thorough examination under anæsthesia, while explorative cœliotomy may prove them all to have been in error. The pelvic tumors to be distinguished from ovarian are encysted collections of serum, pus, or blood, enlargements of the tube, fibroid tumors of the uterus and broad ligament, retroflexion of the gravid uterus, and last, but not least, ectopic gestation.

Reference has already been made to the difficulty of recognizing the nature of an encysted collection of serum in the abdominal cavity where the symptoms of peritoneal tuberculosis are not clear. Such a collection in the pelvis it is practically impossible to distinguish from an ovarian or parovarian cyst. The history of former attacks of peritonitis is not conclusive, since inflammation of the adnexa almost invariably exists, and the tissues and organs are so matted together that the bimanual examination conveys no definite information. Explorative puncture per vaginam, in case the tumor is accessible, throws little light on the diagnosis, since the fluid obtained bears a close resemblance to that of a hydrosalpinx or a parovarian cyst, though cylindrical epithelia (especially the ciliated variety) are, of course, absent. It has been the writer's experience that the diagnosis is made only by cœliotomy, which is clearly indicated in these cases.

The recognition of an intra-pelvic collection of pus does not present great difficulty when there is noted the characteristic history of a traumatic (*i.e.*, *septic*) or puerperal origin,—continued elevation of temperature, pain, and the usual septic symptoms. An abscess in the folds of the broad ligament is distinguished from a cyst in the same locality by its sensitiveness on pressure, immobility, irregular shape (often by its prolongation upward towards the iliac fossa), and firmer consistence. Should the extra-peritoneal abscess point towards the vagina, its intimate relation with the posterior fornix and the distinctness with which fluctuation can be obtained would be noted only in the case of a broad-ligament cyst : the history of the case and the aid of the exploring-needle would then be necessary. It should be remembered that appendicitis is by no means rare in the female, and that the pus in a retro-peritoneal abscess thus resulting may gravitate into the pelvis : its origin would hardly be overlooked if proper attention were paid to the ordinary symptoms of appendiceal trouble. Localized extra-peritoneal purulent foci around the rectum and beneath the vesico-uterine fold may be exceedingly puzzling. Intra-peritoneal abscesses secondary to disease of the tubes seldom attain a considerable size, and, in addition to the history of tubal trouble, they are so surrounded by inflammatory exudate that fluctuation cannot be obtained, while the difficulty of exactly locating them renders puncture a somewhat hazardous procedure. Ovarian abscesses seldom reach a sufficient size to be mistaken for cysts, and the symptoms are much more acute. It is evident that it must frequently be impossible to distinguish a small suppurating cyst from a pelvic abscess, especially when the history is indefinite and when perforation occurred some time before. A clue to the true condition would be obtained when the examiner is able to distinguish the globular outline of the cyst, to detect a certain degree of mobility, however slight, and the usual absence of the extensive exudate which surrounds an old abscess-sac. The cyst is more nearly retro-uterine, and may be felt to refill and empty itself more distinctly than an abscess-cavity. If by reason of exudate the evidence afforded by the bimanual examination is negative, any chance of an exact diagnosis being made is out of the question.

Enlargements of the tube from hydro- or pyosalpinx have been mistaken for small ovarian cysts. This is likely to occur in the case of pyosalpinx, since, aside from the history of pelvic inflammation, if it reaches a sufficient size to form a considerable tumor, its elongated shape, the tenderness on pressure, and the obscure boggy sensation imparted to the finger, instead of distinct fluctuation, would point to the probable condition. Bilateral hydrosalpinx uncomplicated by inflammatory exudate ought to be recognized without much difficulty. Such an enlargement confined to one tube is marked by its peculiar, elongated, tortuous shape. When the tube terminates in a globular cystic tumor the diagnosis of tubo-ovarian cyst may be made with more or less probability. A hydrosalpinx of unusual size, the distal end of which is adherent in Douglas's pouch, may present all the physical signs of ovarian cyst, nor would positive information be gained by the withdrawal of a specimen of fluid for examination. The same comments apply to pseudo-hæmatosalpinx resulting from hemorrhage into a previously dilated tube.

Fibro-myomata of the uterus, tube, or broad ligament, of the ordinary consistence, would hardly be mistaken for an ovarian cyst. A subperitoneal pedunculated fibroid may occupy a similar position to a cyst, and if it springs from the uterine cornu may present the same physical signs. Unless the abdominal wall is too thick, however, its greater density is at once apparent to the practised touch. A diagnosis between such uterine fibroids and fibromata and fibro-sarcomata of the ovary is possible only when the uterus can be clearly mapped out and the fact established that the tumor is connected with it by too long and slender a pedicle to be of uterine origin. Multiple fibroids surrounded by exudate, especially if ascitic fluid is present, may be mistaken for cancerous nodules, if the patient is in poor general condition. Time, or an explorative incision, will clear up all doubts. The sensation imparted by a small thick-walled cyst (especially a dermoid) intimately adherent to the posterior surface of the uterus may be almost exactly like that of a soft fibroid in a similar locality. Menorrhagia and enlargement of the uterine cavity may be common to both, as well as simultaneous movement of the uterus and tumor. When examined under ether the difference in consistence may be made out, as well as the more intimate relation of the fibroid to the organs. The pressure-symptoms due to an impacted fibroid are usually more marked than are those resulting from a cyst similarly situated. The writer has mistaken a semi-solid ovarian cyst adherent to the fundus uteri for a fibroid, the error being demonstrated at the operating-room. In another instance a semi-solid intra-ligamentous cyst which had become fused with the uterus was supposed by several experts to be a fibro-myoma, the history and physical signs being quite characteristic of the latter.

Retroversion of the gravid uterus at the third or fourth month would hardly be overlooked if the history of pregnancy was clear, but if the symptoms were masked by those due to pressure of the incarcerated organ, an incautious examiner, who did not bear in mind this possibility, might think that the globular, elastic (or even fluctuating) swelling in Douglas's pouch was a cystic tumor. A careful bimanual examination, under ether, if necessary, will demonstrate the absence of the fundus uteri in its usual position and the continuity of the cervix with the tumor, as well as the presence of Hegar's sign and other evidences of early pregnancy.

Other pathological conditions of the uterus, such as pyo- and hæmatometra, and congenital anomalies and atresiæ resulting in the retention of menstrual blood in one horn of a uterus bicornatus, pregnancy in a double uterus, etc., though rare, should be considered. Errors are often unavoidable, though a careful review of the history and close observation of the patient will do much to clear up the diagnosis.

Ectopic gestation, with the resulting conditions hæmatosalpinx and hæmatocele, has become so familiar to us of late years that we naturally think of its possibility whenever we discover an intra-pelvic tumor. The symptoms and diagnosis of this condition have been so thoroughly discussed in a special chapter that it is unnecessary to call the reader's attention to any but the cardinal points,—a history of suppression or irregularity of menstruation, symptoms of pregnancy, colicky pains, and, in case of rupture, a sudden tearing pain in the lower part of the abdomen with more or less characteristic signs of internal hemorrhage. Before rupture a distinct boggy (often pulsating) tumor is felt behind and at one side of the uterus, while after rupture there is a diffuse fluctuating or boggy mass in the broad ligament, or filling Douglas's pouch. With this evidence a positive diagnosis can often be made; but with an uncertain history, or with an almost entire absence of the usual symptoms, there might be considerable room for doubt whether the retro-uterine tumor was not a dermoid, especially as the pressure-effects with the two enlargements may be identical. Normal pregnancy with a small ovarian cyst may lead to an error, as in a case of the writer's in which he opened the abdomen under the mistaken impression that he was dealing with an ectopic sac. It is quite possible, also, that axial rotation and rupture of a cyst in a woman who presented symptoms of pregnancy should be regarded as rupture of such a sac. In a patient seen for the first time great care is necessary in order to avoid error, and even then the surgeon frequently opens the abdomen with the expectation of finding something quite different from what he had diagnosed.

As regards the difference between pelvic hæmatocele and a small ovarian cyst, aside from the acute history and rapid formation of the former, it presents a less regular, circumscribed outline and fluctuation is indistinct. If situated between the folds of the broad ligament, the tumor is somewhat elongated laterally and does not present the same globular swelling as a cyst. Its relation to the mass of the ectopic sac is also apparent. An intra-peritoneal hæmatocele the extension of which is limited by previously formed adhesions may cause a bulging in the posterior fornix similar to that of a retro-uterine cyst, but the distinct fluctuation obtained on palpating the latter is wanting, and there is absolute immobility. On puncturing, either pure blood is obtained, or no fluid at all. An old encysted ectopic sac may be unrecognized until suppuration and the discharge of fœtal bones reveal its true character. The writer has recorded a case in which the fœtal bones felt through the wall of the sac were supposed to be bony nodules within a dermoid cyst, especially as the patient had the severe pain and pressure-symptoms so often noted in connection with the latter. The history in these cases, as well as in those of old hæmatocele, is often entirely misleading, so that the practitioner is most excusable for overlooking the condition. When the pelvic organs have been fused together as the result of one or more attacks of peritonitis, an autopsy alone may enable one to determine the nature of the tumor which was felt during life. It should be noted that ectopic gestation may coexist with an ovarian cyst on the opposite side; in fact, any of the conditions above mentioned may exist as complications. This only serves to show how difficult may be the differential diagnosis, so that the most experienced gynæcologist often refuses to commit himself before he has opened the abdomen,—a procedure which is clearly justifiable in case of doubt, especially in the presence of urgent symptoms.

Among other pelvic enlargements which may be encountered are hydatids, especially in the broad ligament,—an exceedingly rare affection in this country,—retro-peritoneal tumors, and malignant growths springing from the muscles or the pelvic bones. A kidney may be so far displaced as to occupy the hollow of the sacrum behind Douglas's pouch (as in a case reported by Mundé), and the sac of a spina bifida may be found in nearly the same locality. Post-rectal dermoids have been described. Retroperitoneal malignant disease, as well as sarcomatous and osteoid growths, could hardly be taken for tumors of ovarian origin. The writer has known of a fæcal mass in the sigmoid flexure being mistaken for a pelvic tumor,—an inexcusable error.

Adhering to the division of abdominal enlargements which has been proposed, we note the following which grow from *below* upward. In the median zone are enlargements of the uterus, due to pregnancy, hæmatometra and fibroids or fibro-cysts, distended bladder, also large hæmatoceles, encysted collections of serum and pus, while in the inguinal and iliac regions are found pedunculated subperitoneal fibroids, pelvic and appendiceal abscesses, malignant disease of the cæcum and colon, herniæ, and various tumors of the abdominal wall. The distinguishing characteristics of all those tumors which lie between the brim of the pelvis and the umbilicus is that their origin is indicated by a zone of tympanitic resonance between their superior border and the lower ribs, which is preserved even when they rise into the epigastrium, and the fact that they cannot be moved into the upper part of the abdomen. Under this category may be included displaced viscera (kidney and spleen) which have become adherent in the lower half of the abdomen, so that it is impossible to return them to their original site.

It would seem as if advanced pregnancy ought never to be mistaken for ovarian cyst, yet the practitioner cannot afford to forget the possibility of error, in view of the recorded (and unrecorded) mistakes of prominent abdominal surgeons. The writer long since arrived at the conclusion that in the absence of the characteristic symptoms the diagnosis of normal pregnancy at any stage may be one of the most difficult in the whole range of medicine. He who has never made a mistake certainly has that experience before him. Having watched a patient for three or four months before he

arrived at the positive conclusion that she had a cyst of the broad ligament instead of being pregnant, and having recently seen in consultation
a patient supposed to be *in labor* who had an ovarian cyst with ascites,
he is inclined to urge the need of caution in every doubtful case; for it
is the doubtful cases—those of young girls and those of women who are
supposed to have reached the climacteric, both of whom deny or conceal
symptoms of pregnancy—that errors are most likely to be made. It is
unsafe to base a diagnosis upon a single point; it must be supported by
other evidence. In an ordinary case the history and physical signs at once
establish the existence of pregnancy; but the history may be negative,
menstruation being persistent, while the enlargement of the uterus does not
correspond to the supposed period of pregnancy, or else it is enormously
distended in hydramnios, fœtal movements cannot be appreciated either by
the patient or by the physician, and there are no heart-sounds; even the
characteristic rhythmical contractions cannot be felt. Under these circumstances it may be necessary to suspend judgment for several weeks, making
several examinations, if necessary, since fresh evidence may be obtained
at subsequent interviews. The recognition of a median, symmetrical enlargement which has been progressive, the lower part of which is continuous with the cervix, should at once awaken suspicion. Bimanual palpation
may cause contractions of the organ. External ballottement—the sensation
of a small body bobbing about in fluid within a closed sac—is a valuable
sign, which can be simulated only by a small solid tumor or a colloid cyst
floating in free ascitic fluid. The general condition of the patient and the
physical signs of ascites should indicate the pathological condition.

Rectal palpation may enable one to exclude pregnancy by the detection
of the small, unimpregnated uterus. There are cases, however, in which,
as the symptoms are not urgent, we are justified in counselling delay. The
complication of ovarian cyst with pregnancy has already been discussed.
It should be remembered that it may occur even in cases of bilateral
malignant disease of the ovaries.

Hydatidiform degeneration of the chorion may, on palpation, simulate
colloid cyst, especially if the enlargement of the uterus is irregular and continues beyond the ordinary period of pregnancy. After this time one would
be justified in exploring the interior of the uterus, although the peculiar
watery discharge, mingled with hydatids, would usually give a clue to the
true condition beforehand. Enlargement of the uterine body from a polypus,
malignant disease, hæmato-, pyo-, and physometra, have all been mentioned
as conditions which sometimes resemble ovarian tumors. Hydrometra would
seldom present a sufficient enlargement. Wells calls attention to the fact
that in many reported cases of hydrometra the discharge of fluid was probably really due to the escape of the contents of an ovarian cyst through
the tube into the uterus.

The writer has reported a case in which he performed cœliotomy for
abdominal pregnancy a month after full term in a case originally supposed

to be hydramnios with a dead fœtus, where it was impossible to decide positively, even under ether, whether the patient had a cancerous ovarian cyst or ascites from cancer of the omentum, so rapidly had her general health declined and fluid accumulated in the abdomen. The history in this instance was most misleading, and the vaginal examination showed the general bulging of the posterior vaginal fornix, with the fluctuation, seen in ascites.

An interstitial fibro-myoma of the uterus causes a symmetrical enlargement in the median line of the abdomen, the history showing a slow growth and an increase in the normal menstrual flow, while the patient is either in good health or is simply anæmic from loss of blood. The uterus is enlarged, as shown by palpation and the introduction of the sound, and is continuous with the tumor, moving with it. The cervix often disappears or is much shortened. The tumor has a hard or elastic feel which is quite characteristic, and is more likely to be mistaken for pregnancy than for a large ovarian cyst. Pregnancy may occur in a fibroid uterus, a point to be remembered before sounding its cavity. In the case of multiple fibroids, their firmer consistence, and the facts that they cluster around a median tumor and often move with it, and that there is considerable elongation of the uterine cavity (to four inches or more), would be arguments against the presence of a multilocular cyst. The detection of separate nodules in the uterine wall, or a hard retro-uterine tumor, would be additional evidence in favor of a fibroid growth. The diagnosis may be very difficult in the case of a subperitoneal tumor of softer consistence, attached to the uterus by a long pedicle and situated in the flank, especially since the uterus may be of nearly normal size and menstruation is not affected. While an examination under ether may enable one to distinguish such a growth from a semi-solid ovarian tumor, there is no certain means of distinguishing it from a fibroma or fibro-sarcoma of the ovary. Percussion usually furnishes negative results, but on auscultation a venous murmur corresponding to the pulse-beat will be heard in a considerable proportion of large uterine fibroids; this is rarely heard in ovarian cysts. The association of an ovarian cyst and a pedunculated fibroid does not give so favorable an opportunity for comparison as might be supposed, since it is frequently impossible to decide which tumor is the cyst and which the fibroid.

The difficulty of distinguishing between cysto-fibromata of the uterus and semi-solid ovarian cysts has been emphasized by all writers. Less stress is now laid on the importance of an exact differential diagnosis, since the surgeon is no longer appalled at the prospect of being obliged to perform hystero-myomectomy instead of a proposed ovariotomy. It may be stated in general that fibro-cysts are not only relatively infrequent, but are rarely found in women under thirty. They grow more slowly than ovarian cysts, but after attaining a certain size may enlarge rapidly, the general health, as a rule, not being seriously affected. Menorrhagia is not a constant sign, neither is elongation of the uterine cavity, especially if the tumor is subperitoneal. The presence of distinct hard nodules would be significant, though semi-solid colloid cysts might give the same sensation. On palpation, fluctuation, when present, is seldom distinct, the tumor having rather an elastic feel. The cervix is often felt continuous with the tumor, and motion imparted to it is shared by the uterus. The advice formerly given to puncture the tumor in case of doubt is to be rejected in view of the great vascularity of fibro-cysts; moreover, the fluid removed is seldom characteristic. An explorative incision is the natural resort in case of doubt, when the dark vascular appearance and firm fasciculated structure of the fibro-cyst distinguish it from the pearly, glistening look of an ovarian cyst. A thorough exploration with the whole hand in the abdominal cavity may be the only means of settling the question of the origin of the tumor.

Hæmatocele seldom attains such a size as to form a large abdominal swelling. When it does, the history of the case, its irregular, indistinct outline as felt bimanually, its immobility, and its softness when recent, will indicate its character. An old encysted collection of blood may present the form of a smooth, round, dense tumor which crowds the uterus forward but does not move with it. In the absence of a clear history, it is practically impossible to distinguish an old hæmatocele that has undergone softening or suppuration from a suppurating cyst. Explorative puncture per vaginam gives little or no information, except in a recent case.

Reference has already been made to encysted ascites. A similar circumscribed collection of pus in the lower part of the abdomen presents the same physical signs, with an additional history of suppuration. The zone of indurated tissue and adherent gut around such an abscess is quite different from the environment of a suppurating cyst.

Tumors situated in the flanks which are most apt to be mistaken for ovarian cysts are subperitoneal fibroids and abscesses. The situation, elongated shape, and fixation of an extra-peritoneal pelvic abscess, as well as the history, are sufficiently characteristic. Intra-pelvic abscesses rarely form an abdominal enlargement, and their relation to inflammatory trouble of the adnexa can ordinarily be made out. They may complicate ovarian cyst, when the true condition can be made out only by direct examination through an abdominal incision. The collection of pus in appendicitis is too distinctly localized to be mistaken, while the pain and other symptoms should prevent error, except possibly in a case of adhesion of the diseased appendix to a small suppurating cyst.

Cancer of the intestine gives rise to a lateral tumor, which is recognized according to the ordinary rules of surgical diagnosis. The writer made an autopsy upon a patient with colloid cancer of the descending colon, which had been pronounced by experts to be a fibroma of either the uterus or the ovary. Hernia and desmoid tumors of the abdominal wall should be recognized with proper care. When the patient is very stout, however, or the tumor grows into the peritoneal cavity, it may be taken for an intra-peritoneal growth.

44

Reference has been made to tuberculous and cancerous nodules of the omentum and peritoneum, and the necessity which the practitioner is often under of being obliged to remove some of the ascitic fluid before these can be recognized.  With tubercle there is seldom an excess of fluid, and fluctuation is limited.  If encysted, the diagnosis may be exceedingly obscure, as already stated.  It is not safe to depend too much on the history in cancer, since absence of pain and cachexia are frequently noted even in somewhat advanced cases.  In an unusually stout patient with a limited amount of ascites the diagnosis may long remain uncertain.  The characteristic feel of the thickened omentum is a valuable guide, though the same peculiar cake-like mass may be present when the omentum is loaded with fat or is thickened in consequence of ordinary inflammation.  A small benign solid tumor of the ovary, accompanied by ascites, may be mistaken for a malignant growth.  The slow accumulation of fluid and the absence of symptoms will convince the examiner, especially if the patient is kept under careful observation, that cancer is not present, especially if the tumor is unilateral.  The slow growth and apparent benignancy of fibrosarcomata should, however, not be forgotten.  It has not infrequently happened that one surgeon has refused to operate, thinking that the tumor was malignant, when another has removed it and cured the patient,—a strong argument in favor of explorative cœliotomy in every case in which the condition of the patient is not evidently hopeless.  Hydatid cysts of the omentum, as Sutton points out, being multiple, are more likely to be mistaken for cancerous nodules than for a multilocular ovarian tumor, especially when the characteristic fremitus cannot be detected.  A simple cyst of the omentum may give all the physical signs of an ovarian cyst; indeed, the writer has found in fluid removed from such a cyst numerous cells identical in appearance with the so-called "Drysdale's corpuscles."

Ordinary care would prevent even an inexperienced examiner from mistaking a mass of impacted fæces in the descending colon for a neoplasm, but in the case of a circumscribed tumor as large as a man's head, situated in the transverse colon, there is a chance for error, especially when the length of the mesocolon is such that the tumor sags downward below the umbilicus.  The history of constipation cannot always be obtained.  In a case in the Woman's Hospital the patient had several diarrhœal movements daily, and presented a cachectic appearance which might have suggested the possibility of malignant disease.  The tumor was dull on percussion, and could be moved freely in all directions, but on deep pressure could be compressed like dough, the pitting being persistent after the pressure was removed.  Vigorous purgation and the use of high enemata of ox-gall soon caused its disappearance.  There should be no doubt as to the condition when the history and symptoms indicate organic stricture of the gut.

Ordinary distention of the bladder from atony would be mistaken for an ovarian cyst only by a careless examiner, though cases have been reported in which the bladder has been tapped.  One's obstetrical experience should lead him to recognize at once the characteristic median pyriform swelling and distinct wave of fluctuation, as well as the relation of the swelling to the uterus. Mistakes are most liable to occur in cases where the retention of urine is due to the pressure of a pelvic tumor,—a retroverted uterus, fibroid or small ovarian tumor, benign or malignant; the practitioner, on detecting the smaller tumor, jumps to the conclusion that it has a direct connection with the fluctuating swelling in front. The caution to insert a catheter in every doubtful case is by no means superfluous.

The rare extra-peritoneal cysts which develop from the patent urachus have been mentioned, and should be considered in this connection, as they sometimes communicate with the bladder as well as rupture at the umbilicus. They are of rapid growth, and usually contain a clear fluid, though they are liable to suppurate, especially if urine enters them from the bladder. It is doubtful if they can ever be distinguished from ovarian or parovarian cysts before the abdomen is opened, and even then such a cyst would be extremely puzzling to one who encountered it for the first time. The tumor lies in front of the uterus and bladder. A peculiarity noted by Tait is the presence of dulness over the lower part of the cyst, with increased resonance towards and above the umbilicus, "yet the physical signs above the umbilicus are clearly those of encysted fluid."

A displaced kidney or spleen, situated in the lower part of the abdomen, may easily be mistaken for a small ovarian tumor, especially if the organ has undergone cystic degeneration. Careful questioning of the patient may elicit the fact that the tumor gradually descended from the original site of the viscus, to which it can be returned by manipulation. In a thin subject the peculiar shape of the kidney or spleen can often be detected. The writer once felt in the region of the umbilicus a secondary cyst in a multi-locular tumor which presented the same shape, mobility, etc., as an enlarged and displaced spleen. A sufficient number of cases have been reported in which the true condition was discovered only at the operating-table to cause the practitioner to bear in mind this rare form of abdominal enlargement.

Retro-peritoneal malignant disease is accompanied by severe localized pain, with or without rapid depreciation of the general health. In a case under the writer's observation there was an almost immovable globular tumor, the size of a man's head, situated in the hypogastrium a little to one side of the median line, and inaccessible from the pelvic side. There was tympanitic resonance over it, except when the intestines were displaced by deep pressure. It was supposed to be intra-peritoneal before its true location was determined by making an explorative incision.

Want of space forbids our considering other enlargements in the lower abdomen which have been mistaken for ovarian tumors, or *vice versa*. The enumeration of too many would only puzzle the reader, who will find it the safest rule in every case of doubt to consider first the most probable conditions, rather than to run over in his mind the long list of rare ones. It is possible for one to be hampered by too many facts at the bedside. A few, well digested, are of more practical use than a confused mass of them which have not been properly arranged.

Tumors originating in the upper part of the abdomen are distinguished, at any rate in their earlier stages, by the existence of a distinct zone of tympanitic resonance between their lower borders and the pelvis. This distinction is important, especially when there are *two* tumors, one of pelvic and the other of abdominal origin. A neoplasm seldom attains such a size that this peculiarity is not to be noted. An obscure history, particularly if the patient is unintelligent, with especial difficulties in the way of an exact physical examination (thickness of the abdominal wall, matting together of the intestines, adhesion of the tumor to the pelvic brim, etc.), may render the diagnosis uncertain.

Enlargement or displacement of the kidney, liver, or spleen is the most frequent condition to be looked for. Less frequently dilatation of the stomach, cyst of the pancreas, enlargement of the gall-bladder, and hydatid cyst may require to be considered.

Renal tumors, either solid or cystic, might be mistaken for ovarian, though, as Sir Spencer Wells observes, there are few exceptions to the rule that the former press the intestines forward, while the latter displace them backward. On the other hand, a loop of intestine might slip between a small ovarian cyst and the abdominal wall, or might be adherent to its anterior surface in consequence of a former inflammatory process. Another contingency is the presence of a renal tumor so large that its usual relations are obscured. The history generally gives a clue to its origin. The frequency with which malignant growths of the kidney develop in young subjects is well known. It will nearly always be ascertained that the enlargement was first noted below the false ribs, and gradually extended inward towards the umbilicus, then downward to the lower part of the abdomen, the reverse being true in the case of an ovarian cyst. The history of hæmaturia, pyuria, or nephritic colic is an important point, as well as variations in the size of the tumor accompanied by a sudden increase in the amount of urine. The latter sign may be present in connection with rupture of a simple cyst, as before stated; but this accident is so rare that stress need not be placed upon it.

Pyonephrosis is accompanied by other symptoms which should indicate its presence to the surgeon. Hydronephrosis may complicate ovarian cyst. Catheterization of the ureters may then afford valuable information. Cystic degeneration and semi-solid tumors of the kidney are most likely to be mistaken for multilocular cysts and cysto-sarcoma. In the case of a renal tumor percussion will show dulness over its outer side, with tympanitic resonance anterior, due to the presence of the ascending or the descending colon, according as the right or the left kidney is affected.

A movable kidney would not be mistaken for an ovarian tumor with a long pedicle, unless it was displaced into the lower part of the abdomen; it is not necessary to repeat the rules for recognizing the displaced organ.

Examination of the urine may be entirely negative, as well as the examination of a specimen of cyst-fluid obtained by explorative puncture,—a procedure not to be recommended for diagnostic purposes alone.

Ordinary enlargements of the liver are generally made out without much difficulty, especially when the lower edge of the organ can be felt and an area of tympanitic resonance intervenes between this point and the brim of the pelvis. An excessive amount of ascitic fluid may obscure the true condition, in which case it becomes necessary to remove enough of the fluid to permit a more thorough examination. By this means the writer was once enabled to detect cancerous nodules in the liver and omentum of a patient whose youth and the absence of the usual history had led her physician to believe that she had a large ovarian cyst. Cystic disease of the liver, either simple or hydatid, is less easy to differentiate; but the history of the case, the origin of the tumor from the upper part of the abdomen, and the presence of intestine below it should place the examiner on his guard.

Enlargement of the spleen from malaria or leucocythæmia would hardly puzzle the general practitioner, though specialists have been caught napping, especially when the tumor extended as low down as the pelvis. Its origin from the left hypochondrium, its relation to the stomach, its mode of growth downward and inward, and its peculiar shape, as well as its downward movement on deep inspiration (a test which should be applied to all abdominal tumors), mark its true character. A history of malaria and the examination of the blood furnish additional corroborative evidence. Displacement of the normal spleen (unless as low as the pelvis) is not so likely to give rise to error as is extreme mobility of the enlarged organ. The writer has seen two explorative cœliotomies performed for the latter condition,—both fatal. When the organ is both displaced and cystic a mistake is pardonable, especially if it cannot be pushed upward to, or near, its original site.

Pancreatic cysts are not so rare as was once supposed, between thirty and forty having been operated upon, though the diagnosis has rarely been made beforehand. The cyst is usually first noted in the epigastrium below the left lobe of the liver, the stomach being displaced forward and the transverse colon downward, and generally moves on inspiration and expiration. Fluctuation is not always distinct. On making explorative puncture an alkaline fluid has been obtained of low specific gravity, containing a large amount of albumin and fat-globules, but no epithelial cells. The fæces may contain free fat and the urine sugar in these cases.

Dilatation and displacement of the stomach have been mentioned as possible causes of error, but a careful review of the history and the practice of the ordinary methods of percussing and palpating that viscus should enable the physician to guard against them. Unusual distention of the gall-bladder has deceived even so skilful a diagnostician as Tait, while other rare conditions, such as chylous cyst of the mesentery, have been mistaken for ovarian cysts.

Hydatid disease of the kidney, liver, and spleen, though so rare in this country, should be borne in mind.  They give a history of rapid and irregular growth, and of beginning in the hypochondriac region and extending downward.  Their thin, irregular outline, peculiar jelly-like feel, and characteristic fremitus distinguish them from an ovarian cyst.  When they surround coils of intestine, the latter give areas of resonance in the midst of the general dulness which are never heard over a cyst.  On puncturing a hydatid, the hooklets and scolices of the parasites will be found in the fluid.

Even from this hasty review of the question of differential diagnosis the reader will infer that it is a large subject, not to be fully mastered except after many years of experience and observation.  It will be admitted that the general practitioner who has been accustomed to take a broad view of each case is, on the whole, less likely to make serious errors of diagnosis than the specialist, who relies too much on his intuition and is accustomed to resort promptly to an explorative incision in order to discover without delay the nature of a doubtful tumor.  It is perhaps fortunate that the practitioner is seldom so situated that he can advise such an operation at the first interview,—fortunate for himself as well as for his patient.  It cannot be denied that explorative cœliotomy, on account of its ease and comparative safety, has often been abused, being employed in many cases where not only is the tumor clearly of extra-pelvic origin, but all the clinical evidence is against the possibility of its removal.  It is now constantly performed for every possible enlargement, actual or supposed, under circumstances which a few years since would have caused it to be regarded as little short of criminal.  Surgeons have encroached on medical cases so much that it seems as if there would soon be no organic visceral lesion (except cardiac) which might not be studied by direct inspection or palpation.  Whatever may be the advance in surgical skill and boldness in this tentative direction, we advise the occasional operator to confine his explorative incision to those cases in which he has to do probably with an *operable* tumor, the nature of which he has been unable to determine by the exercise of the ordinary methods of physical examination, conducted deliberately on several occasions, if necessary, and with the aid of anæsthesia.  Moreover, humanity as well as a proper regard for his art should deter the surgeon from making such an incision in a patient who is so evidently weakened that she may not survive it.

It is only necessary to caution the beginner that by an explorative incision is meant the simple opening of the abdominal cavity and the introduction of one or more fingers, seldom the whole hand, in order to palpate the tumor, which may also be inspected as far as possible through the incision.  The breaking down of adhesions or any injury to the growth by rough manipulation at once introduces another element into the case, from the risk of hemorrhage or inflammation, so that the patient is worse off than before.  Many an explorative cœliotomy has ended in a serious, it may be fatal, operation which the surgeon had no intention of performing. Moreover, an incomplete operation is very different from a simple exploration. The aim of the latter is to settle a doubtful diagnosis without serious risk to the patient. Whether a radical procedure is attempted at the time or not will depend upon the urgency of the case, the judgment of the surgeon, and the previous understanding which he has had with the patient and her friends. In private practice this matter is naturally viewed in a somewhat different light from that in which it is regarded in hospitals, where so much more is left to the decision of the surgeon.

### TREATMENT OF OVARIAN TUMORS.

It is not necessary at the present day to reiterate the statement made by all writers that there is only one form of treatment for ovarian cysts, and that is extirpation. Medicinal treatment, electrolytic puncture, the injection of iodine and other astringents into the cyst, would now be regarded as malpractice. It is only a few years since that it was a frequent practice to tap a cyst several times before its removal, a procedure which has been abandoned by all who recognize its dangers. There are, of course, circumstances under

Fig. 34.

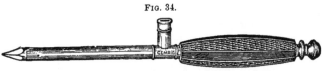

Trocar for puncturing cyst through abdominal wall.  (Goodell.)

which it may be impossible to perform ovariotomy on account of the objections of the patient or the friends (though it is seldom that these cannot be overruled), or the presence of cancer, extreme weakness, or grave visceral complications, which would render an operation inevitably fatal. In acute, sometimes in chronic, pulmonary affections it may be necessary to tap in order to relieve dyspnœa; but in any case, unless, as Greig Smith puts it, tapping is resorted to "simply to promote euthanasia," it should be regarded merely as a step in the improvement of the patient's condition preliminary to a radical operation. In a recent case in which the writer withdrew eighty pints of fluid in order to relieve acute pulmonary œdema which promised a speedy fatal termination, the improvement was so rapid that he was able to perform ovariotomy successfully three weeks later, removing a cyst then weighing thirty or forty pounds. It will be evident from what has been said that he disapproves of diagnostic puncture through the abdominal wall, except in cases in which a suspected tumor is obscured by ascites.

The dangers from tapping are the wounding of large vessels in the walls of the cyst, the puncture of adherent intestine, the direct introduction of sepsis, or the escape of septic or irritating fluid from the cyst, following the withdrawal of the needle. That these dangers are not exaggerated is shown by cases in which the abdomen has been opened a few days or weeks after puncture and an innocent fluid has been found to be transformed into an irritating one, or where the tapping has resulted in a localized peritonitis, causing parietal adhesions in a cyst which was previously movable. The tendency to a rapid dissemination of secondary growths after the tapping of an intra-ligamentous papillary cyst has been emphasized.

The aspirator is safer than the trocar, although the emptying of a large cyst by this instrument is slow and tedious. Strict aseptic precautions should be observed, the needle being boiled and kept in antiseptic fluid. If an ordinary canula is used, a rubber tube should be attached to it, the end being placed in a basin of carbolic solution to prevent air from entering the cavity. A point is usually selected midway between the umbilicus and the pubes where careful percussion has demonstrated the fact that no coil of intestine is in the way, though if fluctuation is more distinct on one side of the median line the needle can be introduced there. The skin should be prepared by thorough scrubbing and the application of ether, alcohol, and bichloride, as in an ordinary abdominal section. The operation is practically painless, or it may be rendered so by freezing the site of puncture with ether or rhigolene spray. The patient may lie on her side at the edge of the bed, or, if the cyst is unusually large, she may be supported in a sitting posture.

A few cautions to the inexperienced are pertinent. Having selected the point at which it is proposed to puncture, avoiding large superficial veins, the surgeon plunges his needle into the cyst to the depth of two or three inches, withdraws it quickly, and then holds it steadily. If no fluid escapes, the probability is that it is too thick to run. Instead of pushing the needle in deeper, an attempt may be made to clear its end with a blunt stylet; the same manœuvre is adopted when it becomes clogged with a mass of lymph. As the cyst collapses, so that the fluid escapes more slowly or not at all, the end of the canula may be raised or turned to one side, while steady pressure is made on the sides and upper portion of the sac. The advice sometimes given to empty secondary cysts by re-introducing the sharp stylet and puncturing them is hardly safe for the beginner. Empty the main cyst entirely, if possible, in order to prevent subsequent leakage into the peritoneal cavity. As the canula is removed, the opening is at once covered with sterilized gauze, which may be secured by means of collodion or rubber plaster. The hollow left in the abdomen is then filled with cotton and a firm binder is applied, as much to relieve the patient's feeling of relaxation as to keep the dressings in place. She should remain in bed from four days to a week, until all danger of inflammation is over, the diet being light and the bowels being moved regularly.

Tapping per vaginam has been referred to as a means of establishing a doubtful diagnosis, though as the surgeon acquires increased experience and boldness he will be less apt to resort to it, except where he suspects the presence of pus. At the present day no one would think of emptying an abdominal cyst in this way. Tapping through this route should be confined to impacted or adherent intra-pelvic cysts, where the pressure-symptoms are extreme and the patient refuses to undergo a radical operation.   The sac must lie in contact with the vaginal fornix, so as to cause a distinct bulging behind the uterus.   The median line is the point of safety.   None but an expert should introduce a needle close to the posterior surface of the broad ligament, since there is danger of wounding the uterine artery or even the misplaced bladder,—accidents which the writer has seen happen to a justly celebrated gynæcologist.   On the other hand, puncture per vaginam may reveal pus and enable the operator to incise and drain an adherent suppurating cyst with far less risk to the patient than if he attempted its removal, and with the same ultimate benefit.

It is hardly necessary to remind the reader that the aspirator is the only proper instrument to be used here, or that the vagina must be just as thoroughly scrubbed and disinfected as if one intended to perform a vaginal hysterectomy.   The needle is best introduced by the sense of touch, the patient being in the dorsal position.   If the operator desires to see the point of puncture, he can easily do so with the aid of a Sims speculum. Select a place just behind the uterus, where fluctuation is most distinct and no pulsating vessels are felt, and plunge the needle in boldly, directing the point upward in the axis of the pelvis.   If pus escapes, introduce a narrow-bladed bistoury or sharp-pointed scissors alongside of the needle and make an opening sufficiently large to allow proper drainage.   The subsequent treatment is that of an ordinary pelvic abscess,—curettage, irrigation (especially with peroxide of hydrogen), and drainage with iodoform gauze or a tube.   It is better to give an anæsthetic, so that a thorough examination of the pelvis can be made.

It is a question if this method of treatment is not to be recommended to the practitioner in the case of firmly adherent cysts which are readily accessible through the vaginal fornix, in preference to cœliotomy, especially when the patient is weak and an evening rise of temperature points to pusformation.   Under these circumstances ovariotomy is certain to be attended with special difficulties, which, though they may not deter the experienced surgeon, may well cause the occasional operator to hesitate before confronting them.

## OVARIOTOMY.

By this term is now understood the removal of tumors of the ovary and broad ligament through an abdominal incision.   Vaginal ovariotomy may be dismissed as an operation which has fallen into disrepute, though its revival under proper indications may be expected.   The reader is referred to special monographs for information regarding the history and statistics of the operation ; suffice it to say that it is now established on so firm a basis that the average mortality, including all cases, varies from five to ten per cent., the latter being considered as too high in the present age of abdominal surgery.   As regards operations for cystoma, it has been said that the number of contra-indications has been so lessened that practically the presence of a tumor is a sufficient indication for its removal. The long list of contra-indications formerly mentioned in text-books has now been shortened so as really to include only disease of the thoracic and abdominal viscera so advanced as to interfere with the performance of any other major operation. The risk of immediate death from shock from lesser degrees of cardiac and renal disease is now regarded as no bar to the successful performance of ovariotomy.

As Greig Smith justly remarks, "No writer is justified in doing abdominal surgery unless he is prepared to cope with every emergency which may arise, to do so promptly, and according to the well-recognized rules." The occasional operator may meet with a series of uncomplicated cases, the favorable result of which renders him over-confident. The successful ovariotomist must have a practical acquaintance with general surgery. The idea that no preliminary training is required is a most erroneous one. Ovariotomy may be one of the simplest or it may be one of the most difficult operations in surgery, and it is impossible to predict which it will be before the abdomen is opened. Any intelligent physician who has witnessed a few operations may remove a simple non-adherent cyst; whereas the enucleation of an intra-ligamentous tumor, or of one which has many intestinal adhesions, may call for the exercise of the highest surgical skill and experience. The beginner had better abandon the operation and close the abdomen than blindly to attempt such a procedure. The necessary experience can be gained only by a careful study of the anatomy of the pelvis, prolonged observation of the work of the best operators, and, above all, an apprenticeship as an assistant. Even then one learns only through his own errors. Reading and a theoretical familiarity with the details of an operation can never take the place of practical experience. This is said not to discourage the reader, but to convince him that boldness and self-confidence cannot be substituted for surgical knowledge. The factors of success in ovariotomy are rapid, careful work, the instant recognition of complications, and the power of dealing with them. These may convert an apparently hopeless case into a brilliant success. The word "luck" should be banished from the surgical dictionary : care and good judgment, not good fortune, insure success.

Every surgeon has a certain number of inevitable deaths from shock, hemorrhage, or visceral complications, but even these will become less frequent as his diagnostic skill and surgical experience increase. Sepsis is now rightly regarded as a direct reproach to the surgeon. Asepsis cannot be learned by intuition ; it must become a second nature with the surgeon, the result of long routine practice. A single flaw may vitiate the most carefully planned and skilfully executed operation. Unless a man firmly believes in the vital importance of cleanliness, there will always be an element of doubt as to his results. Operators differ in many minor details, as to the use of antiseptic fluids, etc., but the cardinal principle of cleanliness underlies the practice of all modern surgeons. While it is wise to imitate the methods of the best operators, every ovariotomist finds that he must work out a certain technique which is best for *him*. The time has passed when numerous complicated instruments and a multiplicity of assistants are deemed necessary for the proper performance of abdominal surgery; the more experienced the operator, the simpler are his preparations and the smaller is the number of his assistants. In this respect the inexperienced observer may gain a false impression from witnessing operations in hospitals. In private practice, a single assistant, the anæsthetizer, and a nurse to wash the sponges, are all that are required, while the necessary instruments may be carried in a hand-bag. The elementary details which will be given are deemed necessary, since it is assumed that the reader has not enjoyed the advantages furnished by hospital training.

To the surgeon of wide experience the question of assistants may not assume such importance, but even with him it involves one of the most vital elements of success. The writer has often observed that distinguished cœliotomists have been apparently so much annoyed and hampered by the absence of their usual assistants that the operation has been anything but a success. After working for a long time with a man who is intimately acquainted with the surgeon's peculiar methods, the latter is often greatly embarrassed by the presence of a strange assistant. To the beginner, then, we would offer this important advice: unless in a case of emergency, never attempt ovariotomy unless the gentleman who stands opposite to you has had the same practical experience as yourself, or even greater. Few men can do a complicated operation without feeling the necessity of advice or suggestion. This is not a confession of ignorance nor an evidence of want of decision, but is a proof of the difficult nature of the task and of the importance of securing every element of success.

Before considering the operation itself, certain preliminary statements are *à propos*. We cannot insist too strongly on the importance of keeping the patient under observation for several days prior to the operation. It is of course assumed that there is no emergency to render immediate interference necessary. The surgeon must become thoroughly acquainted with the patient, for a superficial examination on the day of the operation is not sufficient. Obscure visceral complications may exist which can be recognized only by prolonged observation. If possible, a week should intervene before the operation; though the nervous condition of the patient may be such as to render it necessary to shorten the period of suspense. Aside from disturbances incident to the presence of the tumor, she may have some affection of the thoracic or abdominal viscera, such as would lead to a fatal result. These should be recognized and a careful history of the case obtained and repeated physical examinations made. Routine examination of the urine is not sufficient to reveal the presence of obscure renal trouble. A diminution in the amount of urine is a more significant symptom than the mere presence of an occasional trace of albumin or a few casts. In private practice the surgeon cannot leave these matters to others, but must attend to them himself. The presence of chronic disease of the heart, lungs, or kidneys is not necessarily a contra-indication with the present rapid methods of operating. Under these conditions the patient may be greatly benefited and her life prolonged by the removal of the tumor; but, since these always constitute an element of doubt, the beginner may well hesitate before touching a case of this nature. Each must be judged on its individual merits alone. The patient should be clearly informed of the risks incurred. At the present day statistics are more apt to be impaired by the disregard of such complications than by sepsis.

*Season of the Year.*—The writer had occasion some years ago to inquire into the truth of the opinion held by some writers that the mortality after operation during certain months was greater than during others. This is entirely erroneous.

*Time of Day.*—Other things being equal, the morning is the most favorable time for operation; the patient is then refreshed after a night's rest and is spared the anxiety of a day's waiting, the surgeon and his assistants feel fresher, and the light is good. In this country operations are usually done in the afternoon.

*Preparatory Treatment.*—As soon as the day of the operation has been fixed, the general health of the patient should be carefully attended to; the bowels should be thoroughly regulated by daily laxatives; frequent baths should be given, in order to increase the action of the skin. During the last three or four days the diet should be regulated, being confined to broths and easily digested food, milk being withheld in view of its constipating effect. Special attention should be paid to the stomach. If it is very irritable, suitable diet and medication should be employed.

It was formerly the custom to operate as nearly as possible midway between the two menstrual periods; it is now well known that the presence of menstruation has no deleterious effect: nevertheless, in view of the increased pelvic congestion which occurs at this time, many still believe it wiser for the surgeon not to select this time, unless some special emergency calls for an immediate operation.

*Preparation of the Room.*—It is not necessary to describe the preparations usually made in hospital. In private practice the room should be prepared by removing the carpets, curtains, portières, pictures, and movable furniture. The walls, floor, and wood-work should be thoroughly scrubbed, then mopped off with 1 to 2000 bichloride solution. Many surgeons hold that these precautions are unnecessary. Perfectly aseptic operations have been performed in tenement-houses with the most unfavorable environment. Recent investigations have demonstrated the presence of septic germs in the air, the injurious effect of which is lessened by keeping the room moist with steam.

*Instruments and Dressings.*[1]—The following instruments are all that

---

[1] For further details the reader will consult Chapter II.

are absolutely necessary for the performance of ovariotomy : a scalpel, one pair of curved blunt-pointed scissors, one pair of angular scissors, two pairs of mouse-tooth forceps, half a dozen small and two or three long bæmostatic forceps, two pairs of cyst-forceps, an aneurism-needle or ligature-passer, a trocar, a needle-holder, curved needles, large and small, braided or twisted pedicle-silk, catgut, silkworm-gut, silver wire (No. 26 or 27), a dozen small sponges, and three or four large flat ones. A Paquelin cautery, aspirators, retractors, volsella, écraseur, rubber tubing, and extra clamps should be at hand in case of need. In view of the possible necessity of repairing injuries of the intestine, the proper needles threaded with fine silk should not be omitted.

On account of the difficulty of preparing and keeping sponges, many surgeons now use pads of sterilized gauze, four by six inches, consisting of four or five layers sewed together. These can be used both for sponging the wound and for introduction into the abdominal cavity. Three or four dozen of these should be prepared ; they should be thrown away at the end of the operation. The writer now uses them in preference to sponges, especially in septic cases.

The dressings consist of powdered boracic acid, iodoform, aristol, or dermatol, and sterilized gauze, to be held in place by broad strips of rubber adhesive plaster. The surgeon should also be provided with a number of bandages of ten-per-cent. iodoform gauze, two inches in width and two or three yards long, for packing the pelvic cavity. These should be prepared with the greatest care, and should be kept in an aseptic glass or rubber box. Half a dozen drainage-tubes of small calibre and various lengths should be provided. The writer prefers a tube from one-eighth to one-fourth of an inch in diameter, closed at the bottom, with lateral openings in its lower third. The reader is referred to the chapter on general technique for information regarding the preparation of sponges and dressings and the care of the instruments. Instruments may be wrapped in a towel or piece of gauze and dropped into a kettle of boiling water containing a teaspoonful of soda, as soon as the surgeon reaches the house. The boiler described in Chapter II. (Fig. 13) meets all the requirements, and is simple and portable. Successful operators now agree that the field of operation and everything which comes in contact with the wound should be rendered aseptic previous to the operation, and that nothing but simple boiled water should be used at the time. It is not necessary, as it was formerly supposed to be, to place the instruments in strong carbolic-acid solution, or to wash the hands in 1 to 2000 bichloride at frequent intervals during the operation, unless they come in contact with pus, when, of course, they should be at once thoroughly disinfected.

It is not sufficient that the surgeon and his assistants should be scrupulously clean ; the operator must see to it that his nurses are just as careful as the doctors, and to this end no nurse should be employed in an ovariotomy case who has not had a thorough aseptic training. It is impossible for the operator to watch every one during the operation, but his principal assistant should keep an eye on the nurses and see that they do not omit to disinfect the hands thoroughly after touching any unclean object. This caution is by no means superfluous, since during the excitement of an operation the most careful nurse may momentarily forget herself and pick up an instrument or a sponge which has dropped on the floor.

*The Table.*—An ordinary kitchen table that has been thoroughly washed, first with soap and water and then with bichloride solution, will answer perfectly well. It need only be sufficiently long to sustain the trunk of the patient, the feet being placed upon a chair. Ingenious tables have been devised for operations in the Trendelenburg posture, which are described elsewhere in this work. Some of these are portable, and may be carried to a private house. In a case of emergency the patient may easily be placed in an inclined posture by flexing the knees over the back of an inverted kitchen chair. The reader must not forget that Trendelenburg's posture is not secured by simply elevating the foot of the table.

The table should be prepared by the nurse with a clean blanket, over which are spread a rubber cloth and a sheet. Two small blankets should be in readiness, one to cover the legs and the other the chest of the patient, with two pieces of rubber cloth to be placed over these. There should be likewise a small stand for the instruments, two bowls and pitchers, a slop-pail or foot-tub, and plenty of boiled water, both hot and cold.

The night before the operation the patient receives a warm bath and a thorough scrubbing, especially the abdomen; the pubic hair is shaved by the nurse, and a gauze compress wrung out of bichloride solution (1 to 2000) is placed on the abdomen and held in position with a bandage, which is not removed until the patient is placed on the operating-table. Some use a dressing of soft soap. If the operation is to be at nine o'clock in the morning, the patient is given a laxative the night before, a light supper, and, if she is restless or sleepless, a little bromide at bedtime. At seven o'clock the next morning the lower bowel is thoroughly emptied with an enema, even if the medicine has acted freely. She is kept quiet in bed, receiving nothing by the mouth until an hour before the operation, when she is given half an ounce of whiskey.

In the mean time the nurse sees that the room and necessary appliances are in readiness. She has provided two dozen sterilized towels, an abdominal binder, safety-pins, stimulants, etc. A wash-boiler is filled with water, and a clean kettle is provided for boiling the instruments, unless the surgeon uses his own sterilizer.

At the proper time the administration of the anæsthetic is begun in an adjoining room. As regards the choice of anæsthetics, it may be regarded as the general practice in this country to use ether, cases being excepted in which there is marked albuminuria or some bronchial affection in which œdema of the lungs is feared. The administration of ether during ovariotomy should be intrusted only to one thoroughly familiar with this duty, who will give his entire attention to it. A stimulant should not be given within half an hour of etherization, as the patient will be likely to vomit it before the operation begins. If she is very weak, if her stomach is irritable, or if the surgeon fears that the operation will be a long and difficult one, attended with considerable shock, it is good practice, as soon as she is sufficiently under the influence of the ether, to give a high rectal enema of a half-pint or a pint of hot salt solution, containing one or two ounces of whiskey or brandy. It has always seemed to the writer better to do this at the beginning of the operation than to wait until the patient is exhausted by shock or loss of blood and to interrupt the operation in order to give the enema.

While the anæsthetic is being administered, the surgeon and his assistant, who have previously sterilized their hands according to the rules familiar to all,—that is, by scrubbing for five minutes with soap and hot water, immersing for two or three minutes in alcohol, then in a solution of bichloride (1 to 1000) for the same time, and lastly in boiled water,—remove the instruments from the sterilizer and place them in warm boiled water.

In an operation conducted in the ordinary posture[1] the surgeon stands

Fig. 35.

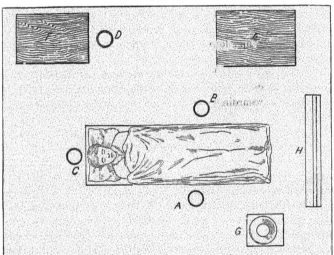

Positions of patient, operator, and assistants in ovariotomy. (Modified from Thomas-Munde.)— A, operator; B, assistant; C, anæsthetizer; D, nurse; E, table for instruments; F, table for sponges; G, basin for boiled water or bichloride solution; H, window.

on the right of the table, his assistant opposite. Behind the assistant is the nurse with the sponges. If the surgeon prefers to handle the instru-

---

[1] For the full description of cœliotomy in the inclined or Trendelenburg posture the reader is referred to the section on hystero-myomectomy.

ments himself, which is the better plan if he has a strange assistant, a small stand at his right will contain the instruments arranged in one tray and the needles and sutures in another. The necessary dressings and extra instruments, rolled in a sterilized towel, should be at the left of the assistant. The foot of the operating-table is placed as close to a large window as practicable.

The patient, having been anæsthetized and her bladder emptied by catheter, is brought in and placed on the table, wearing a night-gown, thick drawers, and an undershirt and woollen stockings. The night-gown and undershirt are drawn up over her chest and the drawers down over her knees; her feet are placed upon a chair at the foot of the table, the thighs being slightly flexed by a pillow or a rolled blanket placed under the knees. Her chest and lower limbs are protected with blankets, over which are placed pieces of rubber sheeting.

The assistant now removes the bandage which was applied the night before, and thoroughly disinfects the abdomen as follows: it is scrubbed first with soap and water, using a sterilized brush (a soft plate brush); it is then washed with ether, special attention being paid to the umbilicus, then with alcohol, and finally with bichloride solution (1 to 1000). As it may be necessary to perform hysterectomy, the vagina should also be thoroughly cleansed according to the rules laid down elsewhere. The assistant again disinfects his hands, and pins warm bichloride (or sterilized) towels over the abdomen, chest, and lower limbs, the median line of the lower part of the abdomen alone being left exposed.

It is good practice for both the operator and his assistant to palpate the abdomen carefully before beginning the operation, in order to satisfy themselves again regarding the presence of a tumor and of its probable character.

Having satisfied himself that the patient is thoroughly anæsthetized, the surgeon is ready to begin. The operation has been divided into four stages: 1, the abdominal incision; 2, separation of adhesions; 3, emptying and extraction of the cyst and ligation of the pedicle; and, 4, toilet of the peritoneum and closure of the abdomen.

1. **The Abdominal Incision.**—A few years ago the length of the incision was supposed to have an important bearing upon the prognosis of the operation. This idea has been abandoned. It makes no difference to the patient in an aseptic operation whether it is two or four inches in length, whereas it makes an essential difference whether the surgeon wastes ten minutes in trying to deliver a large tumor through a small opening, or at once makes a free incision through which he can remove it without difficulty. The experienced operator will be able to judge beforehand, to some extent, whether he will be able to operate through a three-inch incision or one twice as long. It should not be less than three inches in length, and should be made with a bold, free cut, and not with a series of irresolute nicks. If the abdominal wall is quite thin, care must be exercised not to

open the peritoneum and perhaps to wound underlying intestine at the first cut; this is an accident which has happened to good surgeons. On the other hand, in the case of a patient with three inches of adipose tissue between the skin and the fascia, it is manifest that a long, deep incision must be made at the outset. It is a cardinal rule that the peritoneum should be exposed and incised as quickly as is consistent with safety, the surgeon always bearing in mind that a loop of intestine may be adherent directly in the line. It was formerly supposed to be necessary that it should be made directly in the median line; but this is comparatively unimportant. Some hold that a firmer cicatrix will be secured by dividing the muscles. A director is not needed: its use shows that the operator is either timid or inexperienced. Having cut down upon the fascia, it is divided and the properitoneal fat exposed. This is often so thick as to lead the operator to

Fig. 36.

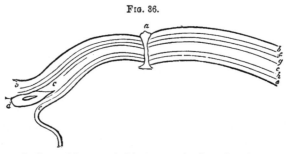

Diagram showing tissues divided by an incision in the median line of the abdomen.—*a*, umbilicus; *b*, skin; *c*, linea alba; *d*, symphysis pubis; *e*, peritoneum; *f*, superficial layer of areolar tissue; *g*, deep layer of areolar tissue; *h*, properitoneal fat. (Wells.)

believe that he has already entered the peritoneal cavity and has the omentum before him; but the color of the fat and the absence of vessels constitute an important difference. Spouting vessels are caught with pressure-forceps, so that all the hemorrhage may be stopped before the peritoneum is opened. The peritoneum, which may be recognized by its smooth, glistening appearance, is caught up with two mouse-tooth forceps and lifted well out of the wound, and a small nick is made between them. The operator now introduces his forefinger and satisfies himself as to the absence of parietal intestinal adhesions. If these are present, another opening should be made higher up, in order to reach a spot which is free from them. Sometimes the cyst is firmly adherent along the line of incision, so that careful inspection is necessary in order to distinguish cyst-wall from peritoneum. Good operators have stripped off the peritoneum over a considerable area before they discovered that they were not peeling off an adherent sac. The surgeon then introduces his forefinger as a guide, and enlarges the peritoneal incision with angular scissors to a length corresponding with that of the external wound, being careful to cut upon the finger, in order to avoid wounding omentum or gut. Two fingers are now introduced, or

45

the whole hand, and the abdomen is thoroughly explored, in order to make out the nature of the tumor, its relations, the presence of adhesions, and possible secondary growths on the peritoneum.

The operation is thus far simply explorative, and, provided that no damage has been done to the tumor and adhesions have not been generally broken up, it may be terminated at this point, if the surgeon deems that it is wiser not to proceed. His decision will be based in each instance on his own experience and judgment, the advice of his colleagues, and the previously expressed wishes of the patient. Happy is the cœliotomist who is not haunted by memories of fatal cases in which, against his better judgment, he did not rest content with a simple exploration.

If he finds that he has to do with a simple ovarian cyst, with few or small semi-solid portions, the original incision may be sufficiently long, and he may proceed at once with the second step; but if he encounters a large solid or semi-solid tumor which can be only partially emptied with a trocar, if at all, it is wiser to extend the incision to the necessary length (five to eight inches), which is done with the scissors as before. The incision may be carried around or straight through the umbilicus. In the mean time, the assistant seizes the bleeding points with pressure-forceps, and with a flat sponge or gauze compress protects the lower portion of the wound, preventing the escape of intestine. Hot towels should be frequently applied to the abdomen during the course of the operation. The intestine and bladder, especially where the latter is drawn up in front of the tumor, have been wounded by premature opening of the peritoneum. This accident should not discourage the operator, but he should at once close the viscus with a Lembert suture of fine silk and then proceed with the operation. Sometimes the peritoneum is so thickened from previous inflamma-

FIG. 37.

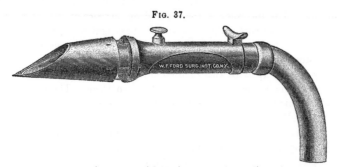

Trocar to prevent escape of cyst fluid into the abdominal cavity.   (Bissell.)

tion, or is so fused with the cyst-wall, that the surgeon may strip off the peritoneum under the mistaken impression that he is separating the cyst. In order to avoid this error, if there is any doubt whatever, he should extend his incision upward till he reaches a point above that at which the cyst is adherent, when he can easily proceed to effect a separation from above downward. Under some circumstances, however, it is better to tap the cyst before making this separation, especially if the contents are purulent or infectious.

2. **Separation of Adhesions.**—(*a*) *Adhesions to the Abdominal Wall.* —These are separated by introducing the flat hand between the cyst and the wall and sweeping it around over the whole surface of the tumor until all the bands are broken up.

(*b*) *Omental Adhesions.*—Slight adhesions may be broken up in a similar way, but if these are somewhat firm it is best to draw them into the wound and ligate them between two catgut sutures. If time is an important element, they may be temporarily secured with forceps, ligatures being applied subsequently.

(*c*) *Intra-Pelvic Adhesions.*—These adhesions, especially in the case of small, impacted tumors, must be broken down by the finger with great care. It is in these cases that Trendelenburg's posture is especially valuable, because the surgeon can *see* exactly what he is doing, and will not make the mistake of taking an intra-ligamentous cyst for a tumor lying behind the broad ligament and shut in by old adhesions.

(*d*) *Intestinal Adhesions.*—The management of intestinal adhesions requires much care and delicacy of manipulation. It is better to separate them when they are in plain view than to trust entirely to the touch. Slightly adherent loops of gut may be separated by light sponging; in any case, the pulp of the forefinger is to be used, the surgeon working against the wall of the cyst rather than against the intestinal wall. Oozing is controlled by pressure. If a considerable extent of the serous surface of the gut is stripped off, a few Lembert sutures of fine silk should be at once introduced. Under some circumstances it is better not to attempt the separation of the gut at all, but to detach a portion of the cyst-wall, leaving it adherent to the intestine. The presence of firm, general intestinal adhesions may determine the surgeon either to abandon the operation or to be content with simple drainage of the cyst. Each case is to be treated according to its merits and according to the experience of the surgeon. There is sometimes considerable shock from such prolonged manipulations. One man will be able to finish successfully an operation that would be hazardous in the hands of another of less skill and experience. It sometimes happens that during the attempts at separation either a hole is torn in the gut or it is torn completely across. According to the extent of the injury, the surgeon will be called upon to perform at once either linear suture of the gut or enterorrhaphy. He should not be appalled at this accident, since it by no means implies a serious result. The operator must determine for himself whether it is best to separate all the adhesions before tapping the cyst, or to reduce its size and draw it out of the wound, separating adherent loops of intestine as they appear. In the case of a large tumor the latter is sometimes the better course to pursue: at any rate, only the principal cyst should be evacuated previous to the separation of the adhesions.

3. **Emptying and Extraction of the Cyst and Ligation of the Pedicle.**—(*a*) *Tapping the Cyst.*—The cyst having been exposed, the edges of the abdominal wound are protected with flat sponges or gauze pads and a trocar is plunged into the sac. Most surgeons do this with the patient on the back; a few prefer to turn her upon the side, in order to avoid the possibility of any fluid escaping into the peritoneal cavity. The care which the surgeon exercises in this respect will depend upon the importance which he attaches to the contact of the cyst-fluid with the peritoneum. The writer was convinced by an unfortunate experience that it is impossible to predict from its macroscopical appearance whether a fluid is infectious or not. A quantity of thick caseous matter and hair from a dermoid cyst may escape into the cavity and give rise to no irritation; whereas a thin, apparently innocent, fluid from a simple cyst may possess the most virulent properties, as noted in a recent case. It is certainly better, if it can possibly be avoided, to allow no fluid to trickle down into the cavity, whether the patient is on the side or on the back. It is easier to prevent this when she is in the former position.

Immediately after plunging the trocar into the cyst, the surgeon should seize it with a hook, draw it up into the wound, and grasp it with cyst-forceps. As the sac collapses it should be drawn still farther out of the wound, the assistant in the mean time so thoroughly surrounding it with sponges and towels as to prevent any escape of the fluid. If the fluid is too thick to flow through the trocar, or if a sufficient quantity has been evacuated to allow the cyst to be dragged partly out of the wound, the surgeon should at once remove the trocar, enlarge the opening in the sac with scissors, and rapidly evacuate its contents. The whole hand is now introduced into the principal cyst-cavity, the colloid material is rapidly turned out of it, and secondary cysts are broken through so as to discharge their contents into the central cavity. Traction is in the mean time kept up on the cyst until it is sufficiently reduced in size to be dragged out of the wound. As it is drawn out, the assistant is ready with flat sponges to prevent the escape of the intestines.

Unsuspected omental or intestinal adhesions may still remain to be separated with sponge or fingers, bleeding vessels being ligated, if necessary.

(*b*) *Ligation of the Pedicle.*—If it is found that the fluid is colloid or is distinctly purulent, it is the practice of some operators to irrigate the cyst freely with boiled water or an antiseptic solution. This takes extra time, and is unnecessary if the adhesions have been thoroughly separated so that the surgeon will complete the operation.

Having drawn the cyst out of the abdominal wall so as to expose the pedicle, the surgeon now proceeds to ligate it. An ordinary aneurism-needle is generally used for passing the ligature: the instrument devised by Dr. Clement Cleveland will be found especially convenient. (Fig. 38.)

Some surgeons prefer stout catgut, which has the advantage of being absorbable material, but the majority are still rather afraid of it, on account of the danger of slipping. Twisted Chinese silk, thoroughly sterilized, is the most reliable material for the ligature, and is practically non-irritating.

FIG. 38.

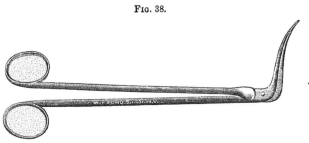

Cleveland's ligature-passer.

The aneurism-needle is threaded with a double ligature at least two feet long, and is passed through the pedicle just above the round ligament, within from half an inch to an inch of the uterine cornu. The loop is now divided, the aneurism-needle is withdrawn, the ligatures are crossed by one or two turns, and are tied with a surgeon's knot. While the surgeon is tying the ligature the assistant should lessen his traction on the cyst a little. It is unnecessary to add that the knot should be tied slowly and deliberately, not so tightly as to cut into the tissue, yet so firmly that slipping will be impossible. After cutting one ligature short, the two ends of the other should be passed around the entire pedicle, and again tied in the same manner. The cyst is now cut away at a distance of about a quarter of an inch from the ligature, two pairs of compression-forceps having been placed on the pedicle just below the point of section. The stump is touched with the Paquelin cautery, is sponged dry, and carefully inspected. If the vessels are of unusually large size, it is good practice to ligate the principal ones separately with fine silk. Although it is desirable to avoid a multiplicity of ligatures, if there is the least doubt with regard to the security of the stump it is better to transfix and to tie below the original ligature, or to place a single piece of silk around the whole. In the case of a broad, fleshy pedicle it is necessary to ligate it in sections, using the so-called cobbler's stitch.

The ligation of the pedicle, although a simple procedure, is one of the most important steps of the operation, which fact is thoroughly appreciated by those who have been so unfortunate as to lose patients from hemorrhage due to slipping of the ligature. The stump should not be dropped back until the surgeon is sure not only that the ligature is firm, but also that there has been no undue retraction of the included tissues. Nearly all the fatal cases of so-called " secondary hemorrhage" after ovariotomy have been due clearly to careless or improper application of the ligature, or to the fact that the surgeon did not leave a sufficient amount of tissue beyond it.   The application of the cautery furnishes an additional safeguard against hemorrhage, as well as against infection from a septic surface.

FIG. 39.

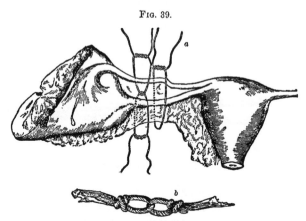

Ligation of the pedicle.—*a*, ligation with a single and a double ligature; *b*, double ligature after it has been tied.   (Modified from Spencer Wells.)

If a large fleshy stump is left, it is well to cover the raw surface with peritoneum, without cauterizing, provided that such traction is not made as to imperil the firmness of the ligature.   Doubtless this little procedure will often prevent subsequent adhesion of the stump to a contiguous loop of intestine.

After the stump has been dropped back, the opposite ovary is brought up into the wound and is carefully examined.   Surgeons will often differ as to the indications for its removal.   The wishes of the patient, especially with regard to a future pregnancy, must always have considerable weight.   In a general way it may be stated that when the ovary is enlarged to three or four times its normal size, and is clearly the seat of general cystic degeneration or fibroid hypertrophy, there can be little doubt as to the propriety of sacrificing it.   Even if it is not notably enlarged, but is buried in adhesions (especially if there be accompanying disease of the tube necessitating its removal) and has given the patient considerable trouble, most surgeons would not hesitate to extirpate it.   On the other hand, if the patient earnestly desires to preserve the function of menstruation and the capacity for conception, the superficial cysts may be punctured, or diseased portions of the ovary may be excised and the tube rendered pervious, as described in Chapter XII.   It is proper to caution the reader not to carry his conservatism so far as to attempt to save an ovary which is practically an incipient cyst, since cases are sufficiently common in which it has been necessary to remove a second tumor as large as the first within a year or two after the former operation.

**4. Toilet of the Peritoneum and Closure of the Abdomen.—** The last stage of the operation consists in cleansing the peritoneal cavity, securing any bleeding vessels, and closing the wound. This is an exceedingly important step, and should not be slurred over, even though the operation may have been so long and bloody that the patient is in a serious condition from shock or loss of blood. To leave several bleeding vessels, or a quantity of cyst-fluid, within the cavity in order to finish the operation hurriedly, is often to vitiate the most rapid and brilliantly executed ovariotomy.

The first point is to thoroughly sponge out the abdomen. Most of the blood or other fluid will have gravitated into the pelvic cavity, from which it can easily be removed. If the blood rapidly accumulates, it is a sign that bleeding is going on somewhere. It is the practice of many surgeons to attempt to arrest this bleeding by the use of hot-water irrigation. The writer holds that it is better to search for and to secure the bleeding points first, then to irrigate, if desired. This bleeding will be either arterial or venous. If arterial, it probably comes from a spouting vessel in the omentum or raw surface of the intestine, or there is possibly a point deep in the pelvis. The omentum should be carefully inspected, being spread out on a hot towel, if necessary. Bleeding points are to be tied with silk or catgut as quickly as possible and the viscera replaced. Oozing from fine parietal or intra-pelvic adhesions may be disregarded, since it can usually be stopped by sponge pressure. The surgeon should actually *see* where the hemorrhage comes from, and for this end the Trendelenburg posture possesses obvious advantages. If blood alone escapes into the cavity, and the patient has no severe shock, irrigation will be unnecessary. The hæmostatic and stimulating effects of hot water within the peritoneal cavity are well known. No special apparatus is necessary. Boiled water or saline solution at a temperature of 110° F. may be poured freely into the abdomen from a pitcher and allowed to circulate among the intestines. From one to several gallons may be used. This is quickly removed with hand sponges, the pelvic cavity is wiped dry, and, if there is much oozing, the cavity is temporarily packed with sponges or gauze.

We have thus far referred to the escape of blood alone into the cavity. Many surgeons employ irrigation for the removal of pus, colloid material, and other ovarian fluids. This may be good practice when such fluids have been disseminated throughout the abdominal cavity, but the writer is convinced that when they have been confined to the pelvis it is better surgery to remove them thoroughly with pads or sponges, rather than to disseminate them among the intestines. It is a question whether the practice of attempting to arrest free oozing with hot water is not equally unscientific.

If there is troublesome oozing from the depths of the pelvis, it is the surgeon's duty to satisfy himself that there are not still some bleeding vessels which can be secured. Haste or carelessness in this respect has cost the lives of not a few patients. Provided that the oozing is general, from a large raw surface deep down in the pelvis, it is best controlled by packing with strips of iodoform gauze which are brought out through the lower angle of the wound.

*Drainage.*—This leads us to a consideration of the question of drainage, one which has been widely discussed, but which may be regarded as still unsettled. All experienced abdominal surgeons hold decided opinions on this subject, yet such opinions differ widely. Some drain in nearly every case in which they have had extensive adhesions, oozing, or the escape of a suspicious fluid; others adopt the general principle of draining in every case in which they irrigate. Some do not irrigate at all, and yet drain; others irrigate frequently, and rarely drain. It is difficult to lay down a fixed rule for the guidance of the inexperienced. The general application of the advice "when in doubt, drain" would be a mischievous one. Probably the reverse would be the better working rule: "when in doubt, do *not* drain." It should be remembered that the drainage-tube is a necessary evil. Its proper care requires a thorough knowledge of the rules of aseptic surgery and entails much extra care and responsibility on the part of the surgeon: he cannot delegate this work to any but an experienced nurse or assistant. Probably few cases of ovariotomy really require drainage. The writer would limit it to those in which a quantity of pus or suspicious fluid has escaped during the operation and has been disseminated among the intestines, and in which a large raw or sloughing surface remains which it has been necessary to pack with gauze. One of the most valuable applications of the drainage-tube is its indication of hemorrhage during the first twelve hours following the operation. The writer has little confidence in gauze alone as a drain for the pelvic cavity, and has been accustomed to use a tube—at least for a few hours—in a case in which gauze packing has been employed.

Personal experience and an observation of the work of successful operators have convinced him that the use of the drainage-tube is becoming more and more limited as the rules of aseptic surgery are more generally applied, and that the ideal method of drainage is per vaginam. In hospital practice, abdominal drainage may be followed by the most satisfactory results, but in private operations, especially where the patient must be left in the care of a general practitioner, the surgeon must feel the greatest anxiety if he has left in a drainage-tube, to be attended to and removed according to the judgment of the inexperienced physician.

Provided that there has been persistent oozing, with a large raw surface within the pelvis, we first introduce the necessary amount of gauze, which may vary from five to ten yards; then we carry a drainage-tube down to the bottom of Douglas's pouch, choosing one of sufficient length to project an inch above the level of the abdominal wound. The tube is now filled with a strip of gauze, and the surgeon is ready to close the wound, which may be done with silver wire, silk, or silkworm-gut.

*Closure of the Wound.*—Silkworm-gut is probably the cleanest and least irritating form of suture, since it can be rendered absolutely aseptic, and can be left *in situ* for three or four weeks, if desired. The surgeon must bear in mind not only the desirability of immediate coaptation of the edges of the wound, but the avoidance of complications, such as mural abscesses and the subsequent development of ventral hernia. The former are eliminated by absolute asepsis during the operation, and by avoiding, as far as possible, bruising of the edges of the wound by forceps or rough manipulation.

It is desirable to cleanse the edges of the wound thoroughly before and after inserting the sutures. These are introduced in the following way. After drawing down the omentum to its proper position, a small flat sponge or pad is placed in the cavity beneath the wound. Beginning at the upper angle, the surgeon inserts a curved needle at a distance of an eighth or a quarter of an inch from the edge, according to the thickness of the wall, and passes it through all the layers of the wound, being careful to include the fascia. In order to insure this, the assistant seizes it with forceps and draws it forward. The needle is reintroduced at a corresponding point at the opposite edge, and is carried through the peritoneum, fascia, and skin as before. Some surgeons prefer to suture the peritoneum and fascia separately with a continuous catgut suture. This takes a little more time, and is a refinement which should not be practised at the end of a long operation, where the patient's strength is much reduced. However, if the wound is a long one—over four inches—it is a good plan to suture at least the fascial edges separately. As the sutures are introduced, the ends are secured with compression-forceps. They are usually half an inch apart; the mistake is often made of placing them too close together. If there is a thick layer of adipose tissue, it is occasionally desirable either to allow the skin wound to close by granulation, or to drain the adipose layer by a small rubber tube or strip of gauze introduced at the upper and lower angles of the wound. A suture is introduced in the track of the drainage-tube, but it is not tied until after the tube has been removed.

FIG. 40.

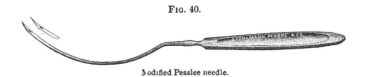

Modified Peaslee needle.

For rapid work a modified Peaslee needle (Fig. 40) will be found convenient.

Previous to suturing the fascia the flat sponge is removed, and the surgeon satisfies himself, by inserting a sponge to the bottom of the pelvis, that hemorrhage has ceased. The presence of a small amount of blood or water need cause no apprehension, since it is readily absorbed by the peritoneum.

The assistant now lifts up the abdominal wall by the sutures while they are tied, in order to prevent the omentum from becoming entangled in them. The sutures are tied from above downward, with an ordinary surgeon's knot, sufficiently tight to secure exact coaptation of the edges, but not to strangulate the tissue,—a common cause of suppuration. A few superficial sutures are usually necessary to secure exact union.

*The Dressing.*—The wound and its neighborhood are now sponged off with bichloride or boiled water, powdered with aristol, boracic acid, or dermatol, iodoform or sterilized gauze is applied, and one or two layers of borated absorbent cotton, the whole being held in position by broad strips of rubber plaster carried over the hips and abdomen. If a drainage-tube has been used, a collar of gauze is placed under it to prevent its being forced down into the pelvis. The strip of gauze is now removed from the tube, in order to note the amount of fluid which it contains. Additional strips are inserted and removed until the tube is dry; it is then plugged with gauze, and its opening is thoroughly covered with gauze dressing secured with plaster. The patient is then dried with warm towels, a many-tailed bandage is applied to the abdomen, and she is removed at once to her bed, hot bottles having been placed in readiness. If she is weak from loss of blood, or collapse threatens, an enema of hot salt solution may be given at once.

The nurse now gives her undivided attention to the patient, and the room is at once cleared, so that there may be no traces of the operation when she recovers consciousness.

**Accidents and Complications during Ovariotomy.**—1. *Escape of Fluid into the Cavity.*—This was formerly regarded as of serious significance, especially in the case of cysts with thick colloid contents. Most surgeons now consider that it does not add to the danger of the operation. Personally, the writer thinks that it is best to use caution, lest even a small quantity of the most innocent looking fluid enter the cavity, since it is not possible to judge from its macroscopical appearance whether or not it is of an infectious character. In a recent case, in which a cyst of moderate size, absolutely without adhesions, was removed through a two-inch incision, the entire operation occupying less than twenty minutes, two or three drachms of fluid oozed out at the side of the trocar and entered the peritoneal cavity, from which it was promptly removed. The operation was conducted with the strictest aseptic precautions, yet within thirty-six hours the patient developed virulent septic peritonitis, to which she succumbed on the third day. The post-mortem showed that the stumps were healthy; the pelvis contained a quantity of stinking fluid, and there was general adhesion of the intestines, which were covered with flakes of organized lymph. The only explanation which could be given to account for the infection was that a careful examination of the cyst-wall showed that it had undergone necrosis at one point. The fluid was not examined bacteriologically, but was evidently not so innocent as it appeared to the naked eye.

Fluid can be prevented from entering the cavity, even when the patient is not turned upon her side, by seizing the cyst with a hook or forceps as soon as the trocar has been plunged into it, and drawing it out of the wound, the edges of which are compressed by an assistant, who protects the latter thoroughly with hot towels or pads. If fluid escapes into the cavity, unless there is general diffusion of colloid material among the intestines, it is better to sponge than to wash it out, although the writer has had good results by the latter method, even when a large quantity of dermoid material had escaped into the cavity twenty-four hours before the operation.

The question of drainage after irrigation has already been mentioned; it is now practised not so much because of the fact that irrigation has been performed on account of the escape of fluid into the cavity, as because the latter is of a purulent nature, and also because a large raw surface or "dead space" has been left within the pelvis.

2. *Hemorrhage.*— General oozing from the separation of slight adhesions seldom assumes serious proportions, since it may usually be stopped by pressure. Firm adhesions, especially to the intestine, should not be separated by touch alone, but should be divided between ligatures, or by forceps if haste is necessary. Large spouting vessels should be caught with clamps as soon as they are seen. The greatest loss of blood occurs during the removal of malignant tumors. The surgeon should not be appalled by the extreme vascularity of the tissues, but should work rapidly, securing adhesions *en masse* with forceps, first removing the tumor, then quickly sponging out the blood, and, as soon as bleeding points are seen, seizing them with clamps, ligating them at his leisure. In these cases it is desirable to lose as little blood as possible, and haste is an important factor in the success of the operation, to avoid shock. Hemorrhage deep within the pelvis is apt to be most annoying to the inexperienced operator, who sees the blood welling up as fast as it is sponged away, without being able to locate the source of the bleeding. Under such circumstances, elevation of the patient in Trendelenburg's posture gives a most favorable view of the bleeding points. No time should be lost in working through a small incision; the original wound should be rapidly enlarged to six or eight inches, if necessary. The intestines should be held back with towels and flat sponges, and the operator should actually *see* the points from which the oozing occurs. Extensive raw surfaces may often be covered in with a continuous catgut suture passed with a curved needle. This is a procedure which sometimes takes considerable time and patience, but it should not be neglected, since the patient's life may depend upon its proper performance. Persistent venous oozing can usually be checked either by hot-water irrigation or, better, by pressure, the pelvis being packed full of sponges, which are not removed till after the sutures have been inserted. The writer would again caution his readers against relying upon the use of hot water alone for checking hemorrhage: he has frequently seen operators lose valuable time by pouring gallons of water into the abdominal cavity in the attempt to arrest arterial

bleeding, which could be stopped only by finding and ligating the bleeding points.

3. *Injury to Viscera.*—In wounds of the liver the bleeding can be nearly always controlled by pressure or by the use of the actual cautery at a dull heat. Applications of subsulphate of iron have fallen into merited disfavor.

Injuries to the intestine may involve the serous surface alone, or the muscular layer, or may result in complete tearing across of the gut. Extensive losses of tissue are readily repaired by a Lembert suture of fine silk, as are also complete perforations which do not involve more than one-third of its calibre. More extensive injuries of the muscular coat and complete tearing require enterorrhaphy. These are accidents which try the nerve of the operator, who is obliged to prolong the operation often when the patient is already exhausted; but he should not therefore neglect the smallest detail which is necessary to secure safety. The rectum is often wounded during the enucleation of deep intra-pelvic tumors. The opening should be at once closed and a drainage-tube inserted. As a further precaution, the wounded area should be isolated from the rest of the cavity by gauze.

Wounds of the bladder are comparatively rare during ovariotomy, though cases have been reported in which it has been opened. They are closed in the usual manner with a Lembert suture. The wound heals rapidly, and there is little danger of the escape of urine into the peritoneal cavity if a catheter is kept in for a few days.

In peeling off cysts which are adherent to the posterior surface of the uterus, its serous covering is often extensively lacerated, leading to free oozing. The raw surface sometimes requires to be closed with a suture, though the oozing can often be readily controlled with the cautery. The tumor is sometimes so fused with the uterus that it is necessary to remove a portion or the whole of the organ. When supra-vaginal amputation has been performed, the stump is fixed in the lower angle of the wound, and is treated in the ordinary manner. Total hysterectomy is preferable.

By operating in the inclined posture it is often possible to recognize and to avoid the ureter during the enucleation of intra-ligamentous cysts, but the duct is sometimes either torn or cut across, is ligated, or is temporarily grasped with forceps in such a way as to occlude its lumen. If the ureter is actually divided, and the accident is recognized at the time, several courses are open to the surgeon,—either to make an opening into the bladder and to suture the distal end of the ureter to it, to suture the ureter in the lower angle of the wound, or, if this is impossible, to remove the corresponding kidney at once, which has been done in several instances with success. The condition of the patient might contra-indicate the latter heroic measure. Kelly has performed uretero-ureterostomy under these circumstances with the most satisfactory result.

4. *Shock.*—As before stated, in the case of a patient whose strength is much reduced, or when it is likely that the operation will be a long and

severe one, precautions should be adopted to avoid shock by the administration of stimulating enemata and the application of hot-water bags to the
chest and extremities; at the same time the patient should receive only
sufficient ether to prevent her from struggling. Shock during operation is
combated by hypodermic injections of camphorated oil and strychnine and
by rectal enemata of hot salt solution and whiskey. Irrigation of the
abdominal cavity with hot water has been mentioned. Infusion of salt
solution should be resorted to in desperate cases as soon as the abdominal
cavity has been closed.

5. *Complications on the Side of the Tumor.*—(*a*) *Intra-Ligamentous Cysts.*
—In these cases the operator is obliged to enucleate or to peel out the cyst
from between the folds of the broad ligament, a procedure the proper performance of which requires a thorough knowledge of the anatomy of the
parts, great delicacy of manipulation, and promptness in dealing with emergencies. It is often impossible to form a pedicle, so that after the tumor
has been removed there remains only a large bleeding cavity between the
folds of the broad ligament. Under these circumstances the latter must be
ligated in sections, its upper portion cut away, and the peritoneal edges
turned in and sutured. It is sometimes good practice to ligate the tube
and upper portion of the broad ligament close to the uterus, to divide
this portion between two ligatures, and then to begin the enucleation from
within outward, tying bleeding vessels as they are divided. The caution
has already been given to avoid injury to the ureter when working deep
within the pelvis.

(*b*) *Incomplete Operations.*—These will become more rare as the surgeon's experience increases. Many cysts were once regarded as impossible
of removal which are now easily extirpated. The presence of firm, general
adhesions, of an intra-ligamentous cyst which cannot be enucleated without
extreme shock and loss of blood, or the sudden collapse of the patient in
the middle of the operation, may lead the surgeon to conclude it as rapidly
as possible. In this case the cyst is emptied, is drawn up into the wound,
as much of the sac as possible is excised, and it is then sutured in the lower
angle of the wound, and is drained with gauze or an ordinary glass tube.
Convalescence is protracted on account of the necessary suppurative process
and consequent granulation, but most patients make a satisfactory recovery,
only they cannot always be regarded as cured. The writer has succeeded
at a second operation in removing a cyst which he had previously drained
in this way on the supposition that it was impossible to extirpate it. After
enucleating an intra-ligamentous cyst, the cavity within the broad ligament
is sometimes so extensive that it cannot be closed with sutures. In this
case it is treated in the same manner as above described,—that is, the peritoneal sac is stitched into the lower angle of the wound and is drained
as before. The method of vaginal drainage presents many advantages,
especially in the case of suppurating cysts firmly adherent to the floor
of the pelvis.

Instead of adopting the combined abdomino-vaginal drainage, practised by Sims, the method suggested by Hanks in the case of suppurating cysts offers many advantages,—that is, to empty and irrigate the sac from above, thoroughly disinfecting it with peroxide of hydrogen, then to carry a rubber or gauze drain through into the vagina. The upper opening in the cyst is then carefully sutured and the abdominal wound is closed. Drainage is perfect, and the treatment of the case resolves itself into that of a simple pelvic abscess.

Special complications in operations on malignant tumors have been mentioned. There is considerable room for the exercise of judgment. The surgeon will be more apt to err on the side of rashness than on that of caution. He should study well the nature, vascularity, and environment of the growth, and note the presence or absence of secondary deposits, before he converts an explorative incision into a radical operation. Having once begun to separate adhesions, there is no retreat; the operation must be finished, frequently at the expense of the patient. It is impossible to lay down any fixed rule, since each case presents individual peculiarities which can be recognized and dealt with only at the time. It may be stated, in general, that the size of the tumor is no criterion of the difficulty of its removal or of the amount of shock that will be experienced by the patient. Small intra-ligamentous cysts, in which at first sight the operation appears simple and uncomplicated, may require more time for their removal and occasion more profound shock to the patient than the extirpation of immense abdominal tumors.

In some cases the cyst may be so firmly adherent to the parietal peritoneum that the line of demarcation cannot be made out. The inexperienced operator may peel off the thickened peritoneum over a wide area under the mistaken impression that he is separating the cyst-wall. In such a case it is better to cut away the flap of peritoneum, since it may become gangrenous.

Numerous cases are on record in which instruments or sponges were left within the peritoneal cavity, the result having been either fatal peritonitis or the escape of the foreign body through the wound or into one of the hollow viscera after a long suppurative process. Theoretically, this accident ought never to occur, as it is a cardinal rule that all the instruments and sponges should be accounted for before the wound is closed. It is usually due to the fact that the responsibility of counting these is shared by several, instead of being left to a single nurse. The writer's plan is never to introduce a sponge into the cavity without calling the attention of both his nurse and his assistant to the fact, and to have each sponge verified as it is removed; but even with these precautions he once left a pad in the cavity. There is no excuse for losing forceps, since only long clamps should be applied. The writer once reopened a wound twice in order to remove a flat sponge which a nurse insisted was still in the cavity: it was subsequently found in a slop-pail. It has been his painful experience to find no fewer than three sponges in the peritoneal cavity at the post-mortem table, which had been left there by experienced operators.  If there is any doubt as to the fact of a foreign body being left behind, the wound should be at once reopened and a thorough search instituted for it.  The same advice is applicable whenever the mistake is discovered, even though it be twelve hours or twenty-four hours after the operation.  The writer assisted a colleague in removing a small sponge which was found among the intestines eighteen hours after operation, the patient having had no bad symptoms.  She made a good recovery.

**After-Treatment.**—The cardinal principle to be observed in the after-treatment of an ordinary case of ovariotomy is to leave the patient alone as far as possible.  Nothing should be given during the first twenty-four hours except an occasional sip of hot water.  The rectum may be used for the administration of nourishment or stimulants in the case of patients who are very much exhausted, or when the stomach remains irritable for several days.  During the second twenty-four hours a little hot tea, gruel, clam-broth, or beef-extract may be given by the mouth, not more than half an ounce every two hours.  Most patients will be able to take milk, either with lime water, sterilized, or peptonized.  The objection to milk on account of its tendency to constipate is outweighed by the fact that it is usually retained by the most delicate stomach.  If rectal enemata are given, they should not be repeated more frequently than once in five or six hours, the amount being limited to three or four ounces.  Beef-extract or sarco-peptones with whiskey and such drugs as may be needed may be given in this way with advantage.  The patient may be very much troubled with nausea and vomiting, persisting even for forty-eight hours after operation.  The latter is to be carefully distinguished from the vomiting of acute peritonitis, which is not only more violent in character, but consists in the ejection of a quantity of dark-brown or greenish fluid and is accompanied by the other well-known symptoms of this complication.  The inexperienced physician as well as the nurse should be cautioned against yielding to the patient's entreaty for cracked ice, since she may continually take it for several hours and then eject the entire quantity of water at once.

No internal medication should be employed, if it is possible to avoid it.  The writer believes that the wide-spread objection to opium is not entirely rational.  It is, of course, not desirable to administer it freely for the relief of pain, but there is no objection to giving a small hypodermic two or three times after an abdominal section if the patient is unusually restless and sleepless.  It also acts well in cases of obstinate vomiting.  One-eighth of a grain of morphine with one-hundred and-fiftieth or two-hundredth of a grain of atropine is usually sufficient.  Nor has he observed at any time that this checks normal peristaltic movements.  The injection should be given only by the direction of the surgeon, not as a routine measure, but exceptionally, when he regards it as especially indicated.

The bowels may be moved on the third or fourth day in a simple case, though it may happen that there will be no movement before the fifth or sixth. Symptoms of peritonitis indicate an early resort to purgation, as will be stated subsequently. Moderate tympanites alone is no indication, since this can be relieved by the passage of a rectal tube, with the injection of a little turpentine and water, if necessary. It is a good plan to give on the third or fourth day a tablet triturate of calomel, one-half or one-fourth of a grain every hour until six doses have been given, to be followed by teaspoonful doses of a saturated solution of Rochelle salt, continued until the patient feels as if the bowels would move. A similar effect may be produced by administering a rectal enema containing two ounces of a saturated solution of salts, half an ounce of glycerin, and a pint of warm water. This should be given through a soft-rubber rectal tube, introduced high up into the bowel and allowed to enter slowly. The discharge of flatus per anum within a few hours after the operation is regarded as a favorable symptom, showing that the bowel has recovered its normal function and that there is no obstruction.

If the patient can pass her urine she should be allowed to do so from the first; otherwise it may be drawn every six or eight hours for the first day or two. Great care should be used in keeping the catheter absolutely aseptic, in order to avoid the development of cystitis, which is a most annoying complication. The attendant need not be alarmed if the amount of urine secreted during the first twenty-four hours does not exceed twenty ounces; it may be several days before the normal amount is passed.

The former objection to moving a patient during the first few days has been dismissed. She should lie on her back during the first twelve to twenty-four hours, after which she may be turned upon her side and supported in this position by pillows placed behind the back. It is desirable to pass a rectal tube in this position. A small roll of blankets or a pillow is placed under the knees, so as to flex them slightly.

The wound is not disturbed until the eighth day, when the dressing should be changed, with aseptic precautions, and the wound cleansed and carefully examined. Many surgeons remove the sutures at this time; it is probably better to leave some of them for two or even three weeks, especially if silkworm-gut is used. Induration at the site of the sutures, or the development of a mural abscess, would, of course, require the prompt removal of the offending ones.

The patient should be kept in bed at least two weeks, and longer if complications have arisen, such as mural abscesses, pelvic exudates, etc. She should be provided with a properly fitting abdominal bandage, to be worn as soon as she leaves her bed; the plaster and the light dressing over the wound may be employed for two weeks longer. If she can be persuaded to remain in bed for three weeks, so much the better. The bandage is to be worn for six months or a year after the operation, especially if there is a weak spot at the lower angle of the cicatrix, due to the use of a drainage-tube.

**Complications after Ovariotomy.**—*Shock.*—This is the first danger to be overcome. It usually follows a severe operation in a weak patient in whom a cyst has been enucleated or many adhesions separated. It is common after the removal of malignant tumors The immediate treatment of shock consists in the application of heat by hot-water bottles (especial care being taken that they are carefully covered, so as not to burn the patient), stimulating enemata, and hypodermic injections. The writer cannot forbear repeating the caution which he has frequently given against the too frequent and indiscriminate resort to hypodermic stimulation. Great care should be used in the administration of such powerful alkaloids as strophanthin, digitalin, nitroglycerin, strychnine, etc. Of these, strychnine is probably the safest. It may be given in doses of one-sixtieth to one-fortieth of a grain, repeated every two or three hours until one twentieth or one-fifteenth of a grain has been given. The hypodermic injection of alcohol in any form, or of ether, is not to be commended. It frequently gives rise to painful indurations or abscesses which annoy the patient more than the operation itself. The desire to obtain an immediate effect in these cases may lead an inexperienced surgeon to over-stimulate the already exhausted heart. Hot beef-tea and whiskey, or hot saline solution given per rectum, are both safe and efficient means of combating collapse. Sterilized camphorated oil, one part in four or five, injected deep into the muscles of the thighs, is a powerful stimulant, and, if given through a *clean* needle, causes no irritation. In every case time should be given the patient to recover from the shock, which may last for twenty-four or thirty-six hours.

*Hemorrhage.*—So-called "secondary hemorrhage" after abdominal section is really primary, being due either to the slipping of a ligature or to persistent oozing. The writer has called attention to the increased danger from the latter cause when the operation has been performed in Trendelenburg's posture. It is now his practice to lower the patient to the dorsal position before inserting the sutures, and to satisfy himself before closing the abdomen that the venous return consequent on the change of posture has not given rise to fresh bleeding.

The diagnosis of hemorrhage is not difficult when a drainage-tube has been used, because bright-red blood then wells up through the tube in such quantity as to leave little doubt as to the existence of the accident; but when no tube has been used, and the operation has been long and difficult, it is sometimes extremely difficult to distinguish between prolonged shock and progressive hemorrhage. The experienced surgeon will judge of the presence of hemorrhage in these cases by the general appearance of the patient, the increasing pallor, the cold extremities, the rapid respiration, and the fact that her pulse, instead of responding to stimulation, continues to grow more feeble. The writer has had occasion to reopen the cavity in several instances,—twice in his own practice,—and was only once led into error in the diagnosis by depending on these signs.

46

It is manifest that if anything is done it must be done promptly,—that is, within an hour or two after the operation. In the only instance in which the writer succeeded in saving the patient the wound was reopened within less than an hour. If there is any doubt, one or two stitches at the lower angle of the wound should be cut and its edges pulled apart, when the fresh blood wells up into the opening. Almost every abdominal surgeon has had deaths from this cause, but they should become more and more rare as greater care is exercised in the ligation of the pedicle and in the checking of hemorrhage before the abdomen is closed. It is sometimes difficult to distinguish between serious hemorrhage and the moderate oozing which not infrequently follows complicated operations: the latter, however, does not produce that profound effect upon the patient's pulse and general condition which is invariably observed in the case of active hemorrhage.

The secondary operation, although done hastily, should be performed, so far as possible, with strict aseptic precautions, since it is always to be hoped that the patient may recover, and that sepsis will not be introduced in consequence of reopening the abdomen. There are few emergencies which call for more promptness and coolness on the part of the operator. In this respect it is comparable to operations for ruptured ectopic gestation, although it is really of a more serious nature, since the patient is subjected to a second abdominal section immediately after the first. No time should be lost after opening the abdomen in seizing the pedicle, drawing it up into the wound, and seeing if the ligature has slipped: if it has, the stump should again be transfixed and tied in the usual way, after which the cavity is irrigated with hot salt solution, is quickly sponged dry, and is closed again. If it is impossible to locate the source of bleeding, a firm gauze tampon should be introduced.

The ordinary treatment followed after post-partum hemorrhage is then indicated,—stimulating rectal enemata and the infusion of saline solution. The subcutaneous injection of the same solution has been employed with good results. It is better to give the patient a few whiffs of chloroform in order to husband her strength, but it may be necessary to operate without an anæsthetic.

*Peritonitis.*—This was once the great dread of the abdominal surgeon, who distinguished a traumatic as well as a septic variety. A localized, non-septic peritonitis probably accompanies many severe operations in which numerous adhesions have been separated, but this possesses little significance as compared with the peritonitis which is a result of sepsis. It may be an acute form, developing within thirty-six or forty-eight hours, possibly after an operation which may have been aseptic, but in which a small quantity of irritating fluid has been left in the cavity. Great stress was formerly laid upon high temperature; this is now regarded as the least important sign. It may not rise above 101° F. until just before death. The heroic measures formerly taken to reduce fever after ovariotomy have all been abandoned. We now aim at treating the cause, *not* the effect.

Cold sponging and the ice-cap are usually sufficient to keep the patient comfortable. The cold pack has been employed with good results. The pulse is a much more reliable evidence of trouble, added to a peculiar facies which to the experienced surgeon is an unfavorable indication even in the absence of other symptoms. Persistent vomiting after entire recovery from the anæsthetic, with distention of the abdomen, and a small, wiry, rapid pulse (120 to 140), point to a very grave condition, in which the prognosis is most unfavorable. However, the surgeon should by no means abandon hope, since cases which are apparently rapidly progressing to a fatal termination may suddenly take a favorable turn under prompt and efficient treatment. The cardinal rule is to suspend the administration of everything by the mouth, nutrient enemata being given every five or six hours. Immediate attempts should be made to move the bowels by laxatives, if possible; if not, by a high enema of turpentine and saturated solution of salts. As regards the administration of morphine under these circumstances, the pendulum has swung somewhat in the other direction. It is still regarded by many as absolutely contra-indicated, yet this is doubtless an extreme view, since a full dose of morphine may relieve the shock to the splanchnic plexus, which is a possible cause of the paralysis of the bowel, and thus actually assist the action of the purgative. In cases of obstinate vomiting of a large quantity of fluid, lavage of the stomach has been employed with benefit. It is probable that some cases of intestinal obstruction are really due to toxæmia. These are cases in which prompt relief follows the free movement of the bowels. It is doubtful if septic peritonitis is ever arrested in this way.

After attempts at moving the bowels have been continued for thirty-six or forty-eight hours without success, and it is evident that the patient is growing rapidly worse and the tympanites increasing, with persistent vomiting, whether fæcal or not, the surgeon should not hesitate to reopen the lower angle of the wound, and to wash out the abdominal cavity with boiled water, breaking up such adhesions as exist and evacuating all collections of pus or serum, and inserting a drainage-tube. Recovery has followed this treatment, though the chances are desperate.

*Intestinal Obstruction.*—This may be immediate or secondary. Acute obstruction may be due to the simple adhesion of a loop of gut to a raw surface on the abdominal wall or within the pelvic cavity. Under these conditions, reopening the abdomen and separating the loop may be successful; but the adhesive inflammation is more often of septic origin, and the prognosis is doubtful. The element of shock in secondary cœliotomy is one which seriously affects its success. Chronic obstruction may occur several weeks or months after ovariotomy, following adhesion of the gut to the wound or abdominal parietes, or imprisonment by bands of organized lymph. The obstruction is recognized not merely by the presence of obstinate tympanites, but by the non-passage of flatus or intestinal contents, by localized pain, violent and limited peristalsis, and obstinate vomiting, which may or may not be fæcal. The surgeon who waits for fæcal vomiting in these cases before operating usually waits too long.

*Renal Complications.*—Renal complications following ovariotomy are among the most severe with which the surgeon has to deal. These may vary from simple insufficiency, which yields to treatment within forty-eight hours, to actual suppression and uræmia, which may terminate fatally on the second or third day. The use of chloroform instead of ether may prevent these to some extent, but not absolutely. Where the surgeon has recognized before operation, as he should have done, the presence of kidney-trouble, he will be on the lookout for the first manifestation afterward. The amount of urine secreted must be carefully noted, and it should be daily examined by a competent observer for albumin and casts. In cases in which it has been necessary to enucleate intra-ligamentous cysts, ligation of the ureter may be suspected. It is difficult to recognize this, especially if the patient has had no symptoms referable to the affected kidney. Simple diminution of the amount of urine without change in its character may awaken anxiety, but if the patient's general condition is good and her pulse not rapid or of high tension, we should not be in haste to adopt heroic treatment. Suppression, partial or complete, a rapid, high-tension pulse, a rise of temperature, dry tongue, and great restlessness, with or without delirium, are serious indications, which must be met by prompt treatment,—that is, by the use of hot poultices, local stimulation and dry cupping, a calomel purge, diaphoresis with hot packs, the free administration of fluids, the withholding of stimulants, and the giving of small doses of nitroglycerin, and especially of the fresh infusion of digitalis in half-ounce doses, every six hours, either by the mouth or by the rectum.

It is important to distinguish cases of uræmia from those of acute sepsis, since many of the symptoms are similar, especially the rapid elevation of temperature and increase in pulse-rate, with or without distention of the abdomen. The previous history of the patient and a careful examination of the urine will generally give a clue to the true condition.

*Cardiac Complications.*—Some patients in whom no organic cardiac lesion can be detected may have a rapid, feeble heart-action, continuing for several days after the operation, even if the latter has not been specially severe. The writer has known a case in which the pulse remained at 150 to 160 for a week or ten days without any other unfavorable symptoms, the patient eventually making a good recovery. There was a strong hysterical element in this case. The possibility of the latter factor should always be borne in mind, since it may save the surgeon much anxiety. In the writer's experience, patients with valvular disease of the heart usually do well after ovariotomy, though the possibility of complications from this source should always be borne in mind.

*Pulmonary Complications.*—Acute bronchitis and pneumonia may follow the administration of ether. In most of the cases which have come under the writer's observation the patient was allowed to take cold from being imperfectly covered either during the operation or immediately afterward. Special attention should be directed to protecting the chest with a flannel sack when she is on the table and after she has been placed in bed.

Other less frequent complications are parotiditis, tetanus (which is extremely rare in this country), acute mania, and various vascular disturbances, such as thrombosis and embolism, a fatal case of the latter having been reported by Thornton. Among the later complications are ulceration and perforation of the intestine, which may be due either to the pressure of the drainage-tube or to sloughing of a loop of gut the serous covering of which has been stripped off while separating adhesions. Fortunately, perforation generally occurs in the track of the tube, and thus leads to a temporary, more rarely a permanent, fæcal fistula at the lower angle of the wound.

Among the annoying sequelæ of ovariotomy are indurations and abscesses around the pedicle, which not only retard convalescence, but may lead to subsequent adhesions and persistent pelvic pain. Absolute asepsis of the ligature and careful disinfection of the pedicle, especially by means of the cautery, will minimize the risk from this source, but it is impossible to prevent it entirely.

It has been asserted that the use of catgut ligatures avoids the complications which may result from the employment of silk ; but most surgeons still prefer to take the risks of subsequent irritation of silk rather than those of hemorrhage from slipping of the pedicle. In an aseptic operation the ligature is encysted, and may remain *in situ* for several years. The writer found one perfectly preserved two years after a former operation. Trouble is less apt to follow from this source in ovariotomy where the pedicle is aseptic than in suppurative disease of the ovaries and tubes, when it may be necessary to leave diseased tissue in the stump.

*Mural Abscesses.*—This complication is usually more annoying than dangerous, although cases are on record in which such abscesses have ruptured into the peritoneal cavity with fatal result. They may be due to several causes,—primarily sepsis. Theoretically they should not occur, but practically every surgeon meets with them under circumstances in which they appear unaccountable. They are due not only to imperfect cleansing of the skin at the site of the incision and to the use of unclean needles and sutures, but to tying the sutures too tightly, to undue handling or bruising of the edges of the wound, to prolonged compression of masses of tissue with forceps, and, above all, to the contact of septic material. The latter cannot always be prevented, neither can the infectious material be entirely removed by careful sponging with a weak antiseptic solution.

The formation of a mural abscess is usually manifested within from five to eight days after the operation. It may give rise to so much systemic disturbance that the operator will believe that he has to do with general sepsis ; the temperature may be elevated to 103° or 104° F., the pulse being rapid and wiry ; the patient has local pain, and yet her facies, the absence of tympanites, vomiting, etc., prove that general infection is absent. Examination of the wound may show a normal appearance, but careful palpation of its edges reveals one or more indurations at the site of the sutures. The offending suture should be promptly removed and the pus evacuated either through the needle-puncture or by separating the edges of the wound over it. It is not necessary to remove all the sutures unless there is general induration. Threatening abscess may be averted by the use of an ice-bag, or, better, warm carbolized compresses. The abscess, after evacuation, should be syringed out with a solution of peroxide of hydrogen, full strength, packed with iodoform gauze, and later treated with balsam of Peru to promote granulation. If there is general induration of the wound, it is good practice to lay it open down to the fascia, which will have united firmly by the seventh or eighth day, and to break up all the purulent foci, so as to allow it to granulate from the bottom. Convalescence may be protracted two or three weeks on this account, but the resulting cicatrix is often firm and unyielding, so that under proper treatment there is even less danger of ventral hernia than when the healing has been by first intention. A fistulous track at the site of the drainage-tube is apt to occur if the latter is allowed to remain too long, or if proper care is not exercised in keeping it absolutely aseptic. The fistula may persist for weeks or months. Under these circumstances the surgeon should suspect that there is a foreign body at the bottom of the wound, such as an infected ligature, and should keep the fistula open until the latter either has come away or can be reached and removed. This is a rare complication after simple ovariotomy. If the upper portion of this track is allowed to close over, pus may accumulate at its bottom, constituting a true pelvic abscess and requiring a second operation. Sometimes it is necessary to establish a counter-opening in the vagina before the abdominal fistula will close.

*Ventral Hernia.*—Every abdominal surgeon who follows up his cases must acknowledge that this accident occurs in the practice of even the most experienced. Those who deny the imputation are apt to be corrected by their surgical *confrères* who have occasion to operate upon patients reported as permanently cured. Ventral hernia is in effect a separation of the wound, more or less extensive. This separation occurs in the fascia, and may be due to several causes,—either to imperfect closure of the wound at the time of the operation, or to imprudence on the part of the patient, who has neglected the caution to avoid undue exertion for a sufficient period after operation and to wear an abdominal bandage for at least a year. The use of a drainage-tube, especially if the edges of the wound are not brought together immediately after its removal, leaves a weak spot which is very apt to become the seat of a small hernia. More extensive hernia results in wounds six or eight inches in length, in which the surgeon has not taken the precaution to bring the fascial edges into exact apposition, or to suture peritoneum, fascia, and skin separately.

The treatment of this complication need not be described here; it is sufficient to say that there is only one radical cure,—that is, to reopen the abdomen, to excise the old cicatrix, separating all omental and intestinal adhesions, and to close the wound with four layers of sutures, one including the entire thickness of the wall, and a separate set each for the peritoneum, the fascia, and the skin. Any treatment less radical than this is almost certain to result in failure. This secondary operation is not always an easy one, especially if there are firm parietal adhesions.

Among the later complications of ovariotomy may be the development of a cyst on the opposite side, where an apparently healthy ovary has been left. The possibility of this occurrence should lead the surgeon to remove the second ovary if there is reasonable doubt as to the presence of cystic degeneration; provided, of course, the patient so desires. In the hands of the experienced surgeon, a second or even a third abdominal section offers no special difficulties; but the beginner should remember that it is very common to find the omentum or intestine adherent to the old cicatrix, which is also quite thin, so that an incautious use of the knife might result in injury to the gut. Some surgeons make their incisions a little to one side of the original cicatrix. A better practice is to begin the incision above, and to open the cavity at this point, so that adherent gut or omentum lower down may be detected at the outset.

Some mention should be made of the phenomena observed after the removal of both ovaries, especially in young women. Among these are:

(1) *Persistent Metrostaxis or Pseudo-Menstruation.*—The writer has two cases now under observation in which a flow has recurred at regular intervals for upward of a year, unaccompanied by pain. In both instances an induration exists around one of the stumps. The attempt to refer the hemorrhage in these or any other cases to the presence of a third ovary is unscientific. The writer is fully in accord with Sutton in his statement that there is no authenticated instance on record of a third ovary. He has been able to explain persistent hemorrhage in all the cases which have come under his observation on the theory that a portion of ovarian tissue was left in the pedicle, that pelvic congestion was induced by the presence of adhesions or indurations, or that the uterus remained enlarged and congested in consequence of displacement, endometritis, or the presence of a fibroid.

(2) *Vaso-motor disturbances* are exceedingly distressing in a certain proportion of cases. They are the phenomena commonly observed in connection with the normal menopause, and may last from a few months to two or three years. There is no medicinal treatment which is capable of general application.

It is hardly necessary now to call attention to the exploded idea that double ovariotomy necessarily causes any change in the sexual condition, such as atrophy of the breasts, loss of sexual appetite, etc. The latter is either unaffected or increased; in a few instances it may be diminished or lost. Obesity is often observed, though usually in women who have a tendency in this direction. In general, it may be stated that the opinion of Sir Spencer Wells agrees with the observation of other ovariotomists, that those patients who recover from ovariotomy are permanently cured.

## NEOPLASMS OF THE TUBES.

These possess more pathological than clinical interest, not only because of their rarity, but by reason of the fact that they seldom attain such a size as to be recognized as distinct tumors. When we reflect that the tubes are simply prolongations of the uterus, their walls being identical in structure, it would appear strange that they are not more frequently the seat of similar morbid growths, especially as they are so subject to inflammatory conditions which in other organs have been regarded as an etiological factor in the production of neoplasms. As in all fibro-muscular tissues, simple hypertrophy of the tubal wall must be carefully distinguished from a true neoplasm. Primary malignant growths are especially rare, while secondary involvement is less common than would be supposed, considering the relative frequency of malignant disease of the uterus and ovaries.

Tubal neoplasms fall naturally into the two subdivisions benign and malignant. The former are, in the order of their frequency, adenomata, fibro-myomata, cysts, and lipomata.

### BENIGN NEOPLASMS.

**Adenoma.**—Since Sutton has settled the much-disputed question of the presence of glands in the mucous membrane of the Fallopian tube by proving from his studies in comparative anatomy that the depressions

FIG. 41.

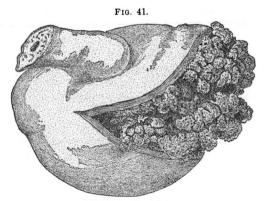

Papilloma of the tube. (Doléris.)

between its folds in the oviduct of the human female are to be regarded as true glands, it is a natural inference that adenomata can develop from them just as in the endometrium. Doran was the first to describe a true papillary adenoma of the tube, and two or three other similar specimens have since been examined. The tube was considerably enlarged, and was filled with a cauliflower-like mass, which in one instance protruded from the distal end in the form of a number of vesicular bodies. These papillomatous and

Fig. 42.

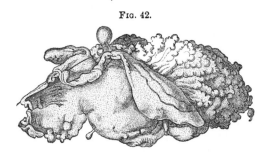

Papillary adenoma of Fallopian tube. (Doran.)

vesicular masses sprang directly from the mucous membrane. Under the microscope the growths presented the ordinary anatomical structure of adenoma. A peculiar clinical feature of these cases is the fact that hydro-peritoneum was present, the fluid having been derived from the tube; there was no reaccumulation after removal of the latter. The similarity between the condition and the ascites accompanying papilloma of the ovaries and peritoneum will be at once apparent. It is evident that this affection must be distinguished from hypertrophy of the tubal mucous membrane, which is sometimes seen as the result of a chronic catarrhal salpingitis.

**Fibro-Myoma.**—As before stated, the infrequency of fibroid growths as compared with those of the uterus is quite remarkable. Sutton calls attention to the fact that hyper-trophy of the muscular wall of the tube often accompanies general fibroid degeneration of the uterus; but this is, of course, entirely differ-ent from a true neoplasm. Fibro-mata or fibro-myomata of the tube are usually not larger than a marble, so that they rarely possess a clinical interest. Simpson's reported case, in which the tumor was said to have been as large as a child's head, is viewed with considerable suspicion.

Fig. 43.

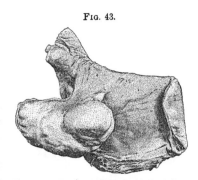

Fibro-myoma of tube. (Museum of the College of Physicians and Surgeons.)

Spaeth reports a more reliable case in which the enlargement was about two inches in diameter. These little growths are usually subserous, some-times pedunculated, but interstitial nodules have been described. Microscopically, they show a predominance of the muscular over the fibrous tissue.

Cysts.—These are insignificant in size, never larger than a walnut, and usually much smaller. They may readily be mistaken for cysts in the mesosalpinx, to which reference will be made subsequently. They may exist either beneath the serous covering of the tube or within the muscular wall. The little vesicular bodies not infrequently seen in the tubal mucous membrane of the ampulla suggest either an inflammatory origin or possibly a retention of the secretion of the simple tubules, as seen in the familiar *ovula Nabothi*. The subperitoneal cysts, which are sometimes pedunculated, have a lining of epithelium (rarely ciliated) and contain a clear mucous fluid. They may rupture spontaneously like hydatid cysts. Sutton refers to a cyst the size of a walnut within the muscular wall of the tube, the description of which corresponds with the "atheromatous cyst" found by Faye in a similar situation. A form of cyst found by Kiwisch in the submucosa was probably of inflammatory origin; in fact, it would seem as if this were the explanation of all the cysts situated in the muscular layer of the tube.

Lipoma.—Fatty tumors are so rare as to deserve only a passing mention. Such a growth the size of a walnut has been described by Rokitansky.

### MALIGNANT NEOPLASMS.

Cancer.—The fact that the tubes often remain unaffected in cases of advanced malignant disease of the uterus and ovaries is one that has been commented upon by pelvic pathologists. True metastasis through the lymphatics has rarely been observed. When the tubes are secondarily affected, it is nearly always by direct extension from the corporeal endometrium, but even this occurs less often than one would suppose,—according to Kiwisch, in one-fourth of the cases of diseases of the uterine body. Orthmann has collected only four cases in which it extended from the ovary to the tube. Until a few years ago the possibility of the development of primary epithelioma of the tubal mucosa was denied, but now at least five authentic cases have been reported. The development of the disease and the consequent enlargement of the tube result in an appearance similar to that observed in adenoma.

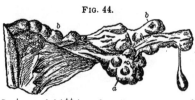

FIG. 44.

Carcinoma of right tube and ovary.—*a*, cancerous nodules in ovary; *b, b*, nodules in tube. (Winckel)

The histological appearances are identical with those of epithelioma of the corporeal endometrium. According to Henning, medullary cancer may develop in the submucosa or beneath the peritoneum and may extend to the muscular tissue. He doubtless refers to secondary nodules, such as those figured by Winckel. (Fig. 44.)

**Sarcoma.**—Primary sarcoma of the tube is still more rare than cancer, not over three or four authentic cases having been thus far recorded. A specimen presented by Dr. J. E. Janvrin to the New York Obstetrical Society was thus described by the pathologist: "The general histological construction of this newly-developed tissue would argue against its being classified as an inflammatory growth, but would place it among the mixed connective-tissue growths. Owing to the large variety of histological elements found, it is impossible to give it any single name which will in any adequate manner express the condition. It may well be classed under one of two headings,—either as a composite fibro-sarcoma or a composite myxosarcoma, the latter being the more accurate of the two."

*Symptoms and Diagnosis.*—It may be stated that in all the cases of neoplasms of the tube above described the true condition was unsuspected, having been found either at the time of operation or post mortem. Even in cases of secondary involvement in connection with general malignant disease of the pelvic organs a diagnosis must be made rather by inference than from any positive evidence, since there is always such a formation of adhesions as to obscure the outlines of the affected tubes. In cases in which fibromata were situated in the tube it would be practically impossible to decide that this was their primary seat. No characteristic symptoms have been noted, except in Doran's case of primary cancer, which gave rise to a peculiar sanious discharge, while curettage demonstrated the fact that the endometrium was healthy. Malignant disease of the tube usually develops after the primary affection in the uterus has made considerable progress, and pursues a slow course. Enlargement of the tube would be evident on examination, yet, from the accompanying inflammation of the mucosa, it would be difficult to distinguish it from ordinary salpingitis. The phenomenon of ascites before referred to might serve as an indication of more serious trouble.

*Prognosis.*—The benign neoplasms are of insignificant importance, if we except adenoma, in the few cases of which the accompanying ascites indicated a condition of irritation which might lead to serious consequences, aside from the resulting perisalpingitis. In primary malignant disease of the tubes the prognosis is absolutely unfavorable, since its fatal termination is merely a question of time. Secondary involvement of the tube in cancer of the uterus and ovaries presupposes a stage of advancement of the disease at which operative interference is hopeless. Primary tuberculosis of the tubes is a serious affection, since it tends to extend to the peritoneum. When they remain localized, the tuberculous masses may break down to form abscesses, which either rupture with a rapidly fatal result from peritonitis, or, if the pus remains encapsulated, eventually exhaust the patient. If secondary to pulmonary or general tuberculosis, they simply increase the hopelessness of this condition. (See Chapter VII.)

*Treatment.*—The indication to extirpate the diseased tubes is clear, except in advanced malignant disease, when the general affection of the pelvic tissues contra-indicates it. That the adnexa should be removed, if possible, in all cases in which the uterus is extirpated for malignant disease of the corporeal endometrium, whether primary or secondary to cancer of the cervix, is self-evident.

## NEOPLASMS OF THE BROAD LIGAMENTS.

The following neoplasms may develop primarily within the folds of the broad ligament, especially in that portion between the ovary and the tube known as the mesosalpinx : cysts, fibro-myomata, lipomata, and sarcomata. It has been stated that dermoid cysts have been found within the broad ligament which had no connection with the ovary, but their independent origin in this region seems extremely doubtful.

### PAROVARIAN CYSTS.

The parovarium consists of a row of parallel blind tubules radiating from the paroöphoron to join another tubule which extends at right angles to them.

Three distinct parts have been distinguished in the parovarium: Kobelt's tubes, the vertical tubes, varying from five to fifteen in number, and the one at right angles to the latter, which represents the remains of Gärtner's duct. Kobelt's tubes, which usually number four or five, are free at one end, while at the other they spring from the outer extremity of Gärtner's duct. From these develop certain small pedunculated cysts, to be distinguished from the hydatid of Morgagni (*q. v.*), which are of no importance clinically. Parovarian cysts proper originate in the vertical tubules, are nearly always non-pedunculated, and present certain peculiarities which clearly distinguish them from intra-ligamentous ovarian cysts. (Fig. 1.)

It is a peculiar fact in regard to these cysts that they do not seem to develop until puberty, due possibly, as Sutton suggests, to the stimulation which the parovarium receives at this time. The writer is inclined to accept this theory, since it agrees with the fact which he has noted in several instances, that these cysts often develop after the removal of an ovarian tumor, in cases in which the presence of continued pelvic congestion is indicated by persistent menorrhagia.

Parovarian cysts are more common than was formerly supposed, though the writer does not agree with Sutton in estimating their relative frequency at ten per cent. The opinion expressed by earlier writers that they seldom exceed the size of the fœtal head at term is erroneous, since all operators agree that they may attain considerable dimensions, so as to contain several quarts of fluid. There is no doubt that before these growths were carefully studied the " unilocular" cysts of the ovary which were mentioned in former monographs were really of parovarian origin. Polycysts of the parovarium have been described by Bantock and Tait, but, if they occur at all, they must be exceedingly rare, and must be due to the simultaneous enlargement of adjacent tubules. They are in no way comparable with multilocular ovarian cystomata. The reader is safe in inferring that a true unilocular cyst is parovarian.

Papillary parovarian cysts sometimes occur histologically similar to those which spring from the paroöphoron, and invest these neoplasms with

FIG. 45.

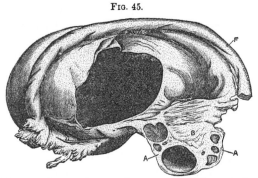

Cyst of the parovarium, showing its relation to the ovary and tube.—*A*, oöphoron; *B*, paroöphoron; *F*, Fallopian tube. (Sutton.)

a clinical importance far greater than was once assigned to them, as will be explained subsequently. Parovarian cysts, whether small or large, present certain distinct anatomical characteristics with which every operator should familiarize himself. Since they grow between the folds of the broad ligaments, they are entirely enveloped in a delicate layer of peritoneum, which is freely movable over them and can be easily stripped off, as peritoneal adhesions are rare in connection with these formations. The relations

FIG. 46.

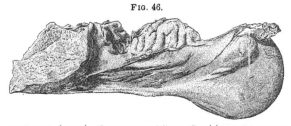

Small parovarian cyst. (Museum of the College of Physicians and Surgeons.)

of the tube and ovary to the cyst are important. They are at first entirely distinct, but as the cyst enlarges, separating the layers of the mesosalpinx, the tube stretches over its anterior surface and becomes closely united with it, the fimbriæ remaining distinct, while the ovarian fimbria may be greatly enlarged. The tube is necessarily elongated with the growth of the tumor, and has been found as long as sixteen inches and quite slender. The peculiar relation of the tube is explained by the fact that the outer and inner edges being fixed by the uterus and tubo-ovarian fold respectively, it cannot unfold laterally, but only in the middle; hence the stretching of the portion which lies between these points.

The ovary is often found unchanged below the cyst, though it, too, may be so stretched and compressed by the growing tumor as to be almost indistinguishable except as a localized thickening on the cyst-wall. When the atrophied gland is incised, however, its identity will be disclosed by the presence of the characteristic cortex and Graafian follicles.

The walls of these simple cysts are very thin, and are composed of connective tissue with some smooth muscular fibres. They are lined with a layer of columnar epithelium which is sometimes ciliated in the smaller cysts; but it may be cubical, or stratified, or may atrophy and disappear entirely in the larger cysts, as the result of long-continued pressure. Small warty prominences or papillæ not infrequently spring from the inner surface; these must be distinguished from the papillary masses to be described.

A typical parovarian cyst-fluid is limpid, often opalescent, with an average specific gravity of 1005; it has a neutral or a slightly alkaline reaction, and contains less albumin than the fluid from an ovarian cystoma. The statement that albumin and paralbumin are entirely absent is not susceptible of general application, and should not be relied upon for differential diagnosis. We often find merely a trace, however. Admixture of blood, degenerative changes within the cyst, etc., may so modify the appearance and chemical composition of the fluid that it is no longer characteristic. Few formed elements are discovered under the microscope, save an occasional epithelial cell or red blood-corpuscle. Ciliated epithelia are not confined to parovarian cysts, hence their presence has no great diagnostic value. Suppuration is extremely rare. Briefly, a parovarian cyst would be distinguished from an ovarian cyst at the operating-table by the following peculiarities: the peritoneal coat is easily detached, the ovary is distinct and not involved, even though greatly atrophied, the cyst is unilocular and contains a limpid fluid with low specific gravity and only slightly albuminous. The Fallopian tube crosses the anterior surface of the cyst and is closely attached to it; in short, there is no distinct mesosalpinx, as in the case of an ovarian cyst.

The various accidents and degenerative changes described in connection with ovarian cysts rarely affect those now under consideration. Adhesions are particularly rare, and suppuration occurs only in consequence of septic infection from tapping. Spontaneous rupture is probably of not infrequent occurrence, but as the fluid is non-irritating and escapes between the layers of the broad ligament, it is readily absorbed without bad consequences. Spontaneous cure after rupture should be regarded as the exception rather than the rule, and does not furnish a valid argument in favor of tapping *versus* a radical operation. In spite of the absence of a distinct pedicle, a parovarian cyst may suffer axial rotation, and may even become entirely detached. Its vascular supply, being derived largely from its peritoneal covering, is sufficient to prevent any danger of gangrene. Papillary cysts of the parovarium may be readily mistaken for similar growths developing from the paroöphoron, which they resemble histologically. When the ovary is entirely distinct and unaffected, the origin of the cyst is clear; but if the papillary growths are closely associated with the hilum, only a careful microscopical study of the specimen will enable the pathologist to decide. The papillary masses grow from the inner wall of the cyst; if the latter ruptures, they readily invade the peritoneum, both visceral and parietal, as previously described. The question of the possible malignancy of these secondary growths has already been discussed.

Clinical History and Diagnosis.—It will be inferred from what has been said concerning the comparative innocuousness of these growths that they seldom give rise to serious symptoms, except as they furnish a starting-point for the development of general papillomatous outgrowths on the peritoneum. There is no rule as to rapidity of growth. Cases have been reported in which such cysts attained a noticeable size within six weeks, others in which they had existed for as many years without growing any larger. While still small and intra-pelvic, they simply displace the uterus to the opposite side of the pelvis, causing dysmenorrhœa and menorrhagia. The patient has no sense of discomfort, and is unaware of the existence of the tumor. As it rises into and fills the abdomen, it may cause the disturbances noted in connection with uncomplicated ovarian cysts, due to mechanical pressure on the viscera,—dyspnœa, palpitation, disturbance of the alimentary tract, etc. Emaciation is rare; in fact, the general health is usually perfect so far as the effect of the tumor is concerned.

The diagnosis of cyst of the broad ligament offers few difficulties during the early stage. Its position on one side of the uterus, in the median plane of the pelvis, distinguishes it from cysts of the tube and ovary, which lie behind the broad ligament or in Douglas's pouch. From collections of pus or blood within the folds of the broad ligament it is distinguished not only by the absence of febrile symptoms, but by its symmetrical outline and distinct fluctuation. The introduction of an exploring needle per vaginam, under strict aseptic precautions, would give a clue to the character of the cyst. After it has attained the size of a man's head, it is not easy to distinguish it from an ovarian tumor. The fact that it is a symmetrical monocyst of slow growth, with a thin wall, and with a distinct wave of fluctuation transmitted freely in every direction, especially through the vaginal vault, the uniformity of the cyst, and the absence of semi-solid portions, are, of course, important negative evidences. Non-impairment of the general health in a patient who has had a tumor for several years argues in favor of a parovarian rather than of an ovarian cyst, since the latter generally leads to complications which occasion pain and various disturbances of a more or less serious nature.

A thin-walled monocyst which fills the abdomen is commonly mistaken for ascites. A careful review of the history of the case and the application of the rules already laid down for distinguishing this condition from ovarian cystoma should prevent error. It should be noted that hydro-peritoneum may coexist with a papillary cyst and thus mask the true condition, which is recognized only after the ascitic fluid has been withdrawn. It is, of course, impossible to distinguish clinically (even at the operating-table) the origin of such a cyst.

**Treatment.**—*Palliative.*—Arguing from the well-known fact that broad-ligament cysts often rupture spontaneously and do not refill, tapping was formerly recommended as the proper treatment. Such a course is now regarded as opposed to the spirit of modern surgery. A small cyst of this character, not larger than an orange, may be safely aspirated per vaginam, and it may not refill; the same may be true of a large one which can be reached in the same way. But a small cyst may just as well be let alone, and a large one should be removed. In short, it is better not to tap any cyst, unless for purely diagnostic purposes, for the following reasons. We can never be absolutely certain of the character of a neoplasm until the abdomen is opened. The probabilities are that it will refill, and the tapping may convert a simple into a complicated case by setting up a localized peritonitis. Again, the cyst may be papillomatous, when tapping would simply hasten the dissemination of the outgrowths previously confined to the cavity of the cyst.

*Radical.*—The removal of a parovarian cyst is simple or difficult according as there is a pedicle developed or not. Under the former condition, the technique is precisely the same as in an ordinary ovariotomy; but if the cyst is intra-pelvic and sessile, and especially if it has burrowed downward between the peritoneal folds to the base of the broad ligament, the indication is to split the broad ligament and to enucleate the cyst in the manner which has already been described. This is often an exceedingly delicate and difficult manœuvre, so that if the operator is inexperienced he would be wiser not to attempt it, since he exposes the patient to the risks of shock and hemorrhage for the removal of an innocuous neoplasm. After enucleating the cyst, the base of which often dips down to the floor of the pelvis, and ligating bleeding vessels, the best way is doubtless to excise the redundant portions of its peritoneal covering and to turn in and unite the opposite folds with a running catgut suture. Two-thirds of the broad ligament may be safely removed in this way. This, to my mind, is preferable to the plan, once more common than now, of stitching the peritoneal sac in the lower angle of the wound and draining it as in an ordinary incomplete operation. Of course, if the surgeon cannot enucleate the sac, it must be treated in this way, which is safe enough, though the subsequent process of granulation may be long and tedious. The writer cannot insist too strongly on the importance of the reader's recognizing clearly the relations of a parovarian cyst before he attempts its removal.

On the one hand, it may be the easiest operation in abdominal surgery, with a mortality which is practically *nil*, while, on the other, it may be one of the most difficult. In either case the mortality may be sufficiently low in the hands of an experienced operator to justify the rule that parovarian cysts the size of a fœtal head at term should be extirpated, but for the occasional operator the rule should be rather as follows : Make an explorative incision, puncture, and remove the cyst if a pedicle can be found; otherwise let it alone, or you may get into a dilemma from which it will be difficult to extricate yourself with credit, and, above all, with safety to the patient.

SIMPLE CYSTS OF THE BROAD LIGAMENT.

Various other cysts, of minor importance, may develop in the broad ligament, such as the hydatid of Morgagni, a little pear-shaped body springing from one of the lower fimbriæ of the Fallopian tube. This is to be distinguished from the sessile cysts which often grow behind the ovarian fimbriæ. Cysts may develop at the outer extremity of the horizontal tube of the parovarium ; these are also pedunculated, and are lined with a layer of non-ciliated epithelium. They may spring from the vertical tubes of the parovarium and also from the interior layer of the broad ligament. A sort of local dropsy of the broad ligament, due to congestion or œdema, is often seen in connection with uterine fibroids.

These little bodies have been distinguished as simple cysts of the broad ligament, and are to be clearly distinguished from parovarian cysts, already described ; in fact, the unchanged parovarium may be found on their outer surface. They are unilocular, are lined with endothelium, and are covered by the two layers of the broad ligament until they come in contact with the ovarian fimbriæ of the tube ; then, if they become larger, they may often present an appearance identical with that of parovarian cysts. They possess no particular clinical importance, and are the variety most likely to be cured after tapping or rupture.

SOLID TUMORS.

There are probably many fibromata which are supposed to originate in the broad ligament, but which are really subperitoneal uterine fibroids that have developed between its folds. True myomata may grow in this region at points where unstriped muscular tissue is normally found,— namely, in the round ligament, in the ovarian ligament, and in the connective tissue between the folds of the broad ligament. They are usually of small size, but Doran describes a specimen weighing sixteen pounds. Clinically, it would be practically impossible to distinguish these from uterine fibroids. If pedunculated, they may be easily removed ; but if, as sometimes happens, they are situated between the folds of the ligament, it is necessary to enucleate them in the same manner as intra-ligamentous cysts.

Lipomata have been occasionally observed in this locality ; sarcomata

47

and carcinomata are secondary to disease in the uterus or ovaries. Warty growths found in the folds of the broad ligament are usually secondary

FIG. 47.

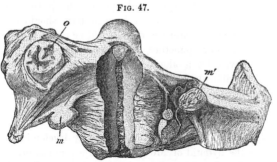

Myomata of broad ligament (*m, m'*).—*o*, small ovarian cyst. (Winckel.)

to papilloma developing in the parovarium, or in a parovarian cyst. Such a neoplasm may originate in the Wolffian remains within the folds of the ligament and involve the ovaries subsequently. Only careful examination of the specimen would reveal its true origin.

FIG. 48.

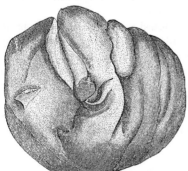

Fibroma of the ovarian ligament. (Doran.)

Echinococcus cysts, though extremely rare in this country, may develop within the pelvis in the subperitoneal connective tissue, whence they may grow upward between the folds of the broad ligaments, and, lifting up the peritoneum, extend into the iliac fossa. They are round, elastic, and not connected with the uterus or the ovaries, and on explorative puncture the characteristic hooklets are found in the fluid.

### PAROVARIAN VARICOCELE.

Winckel has called particular attention to this condition, which was originally described by Richet. The latter recognized two varieties, one lying between the tube and the ovary and the other beneath the ovary. True varicocele is to be distinguished from simple varicose dilatation of the veins of the pampiniform plexus, such as is frequently found in connection with neoplasms both of the uterus and of the ovaries. In the former there is permanent dilatation of the vessels, the walls of which are thickened, and the veins themselves often contain thrombi or pheboliths. It is doubtful if a close comparison can be drawn between varicocele in the

male and in the female, since venous congestion is so much more common
in the latter under physiological conditions, the anastomosis between the
vessels being so free that extreme hyperæmia and dilatation are possible
without leading to actual changes in the structure of their walls.   The
attempt has been made to endue this condition with considerable clinical
and surgical importance, on the ground that it may lead to serious secondary

FIG. 49.

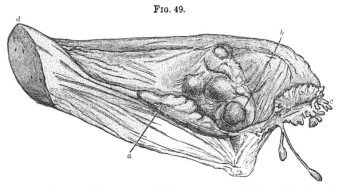

Parovarian varicocele with thrombosis.—a, right ovary; b, enlarged veins containing thrombi;
c, fimbriated end of tube; d, right horn of uterus.   (Winckel.)

changes in the ovary.   The symptom described in connection with varicocele, which has been frequently noted as a complication of retro-displacement of the uterus, is dull, aching pain extending upward to the region of
the kidney, disappearing after the patient has occupied the recumbent position for some time, and reappearing as she stands erect, as in the male.
Winckel calls attention to the fact that these dilated veins may rupture,
leading to retro-uterine hæmatocele; but no cases have been reported in
which this accident has been verified at autopsy.   It has been asserted
that the diagnosis of this condition could be made bimanually, one finger
being in the rectum.   Under favorable circumstances, a peculiar knotted
condition of the vessels is felt at the upper portion of the broad ligament.
This would be more apparent if the veins contained phleboliths.   The
alternate filling and emptying of the vessels according to the change
of posture might give some clue to the true condition, but it would be
extremely difficult to distinguish the enlarged and thickened veins from
ordinary indurations in the broad ligament due to former perisalpingitis
and ovaritis.   There is usually accompanying disease of the uterus or of
the adnexa sufficient to give rise to the symptoms.

While the writer does not deny the existence of the condition, he is disposed to regard it as of secondary importance, and is still sceptical as to
the possibility of clearly detecting it at the examining-table.[1]

_____

[1] See American Journal of Obstetrics, vol. xxii. p. 504.

The operative treatment of this condition is practically associated with that of the coexisting affection in the uterus or adnexa. For example, in supra-vaginal amputation and complete extirpation of the fibroid uterus the broad ligaments are so thoroughly ligated as to remove the affected veins. In removing the adnexa, if the veins cannot be entirely included within the ligature, additional ligatures may be passed through the broad ligament at a lower point, so as to enable the operator to excise the varicocele. Kelly has practised an ingenious procedure of ligating the veins *in situ*, but this is not calculated to be of permanent benefit, because of the free intercommunication of the vessels within the broad ligament.

### TUMORS OF THE ROUND LIGAMENT.

Physiological enlargement of these ligaments during pregnancy is well known. It may become extreme, so that they may be readily seen and felt through the abdominal wall to be as large as the forefinger. The enlargements found in this region are cysts, fibro-myomata, and fibro-sarcomata.

*Cyst or Hydrocele.*—This is supposed to be developed within the canal which represents the original round ligament. It is at first hollow instead of solid. It may appear in the form of several cysts, or of a collection of fluid either within the inguinal canal or at the external ring. Schroeder reports a case in which there seemed to be a communication between the cyst and the peritoneal cavity, since the fluid could be reduced within the abdomen.

*Fibroma and Fibro-Myoma.*—These are the most common, especially fibro-myoma. Myxo-fibroma and fibro-sarcoma have also been described. They are rarely situated within the intra-peritoneal portion of the ligament, though they are most often found within the inguinal canal or at the external ring; also at the insertion of the ligament. They usually begin at the external ring and grow downward towards the labia. They are found most often upon the right side, being rarely bilateral. In some cases pregnancy has seemed to be an exciting factor, though they have been thought to result from trauma.

The differential diagnosis from hernia, either inguinal or ovarian, is made from their hardness, their slow growth, the absence of pain, especially during menstruation, and the absence of dysmenorrhœa. They are distinguished from the inguinal glands by their hardness and by the fact that, when small, they may be often reduced within the canal. A pedunculated tumor in this region may grow from the round ligament or may be a fatty hernia. The latter is soft, painful, and ill defined. Hernia of the ovary has an oval shape, is very tender, and increases in size during menstruation. If the tumor develop towards the labium, it may be mistaken for a cyst of Bartholin's glands. In this case the history of its original location and its insertion at the external ring will show its origin from the round ligament. Of course, if the tumor is intra-peritoneal, it will be almost impossible to distinguish it from a subperitoneal uterine fibroid or a solid ovarian tumor.  Abscesses are to be distinguished by their history and location ; malignant disease by the absence of pain and by the rapid depreciation of the general health.  It may be impossible to distinguish a neoplasm of the round ligament from sarcoma growing from the adjacent muscles or pelvic bones.  Malignant degeneration is to be feared because of the location of the tumor and its rich blood-supply from the epigastric artery.  In a doubtful case an explorative incision furnishes a positive means of diagnosis.  The only treatment is extirpation, which is easy when the tumor develops from the external ring.  When situated within the internal ring and projecting into the peritoneal cavity, its removal involves the performance of cœliotomy, which may be a difficult and bloody operation.

# CHAPTER XIV.

## ECTOPIC PREGNANCY.

### BY WILLIAM T. LUSK, M.D.

AFTER coitus the spermatozoa may make their way through the Fallopian tubes to the pelvic cavity.[1] It is therefore possible for the ovum to be fecundated in any portion of the route from the ovary to the uterus. In exceptional cases the ovum may, after fecundation, be arrested in its travels and develop at a point external to the uterine cavity. To these cases the term ectopic pregnancy is now applied.

Until the publication of Mr. Tait's " Lectures on Ectopic Pregnancy," in 1888, it was the common belief that the ovum might, after fecundation, develop primarily in the tube, within a Graafian follicle, or in the peritoneal cavity; but in the work referred to, Mr. Tait expressed the belief, based upon the examination of a large number of specimens, that all cases of ectopic pregnancy are *ab initio* of tubal origin. The possibility of a primary abdominal pregnancy he denied. The ovarian form he regarded as possible, but not proved. Subsequent research has tended to sustain Mr. Tait's position. In any event, the ovarian and abdominal forms are extremely rare. Nearly all the cases once quoted in support of their primary occurrence have been found to lack the requirements of serious scientific evidence, and even the few which cannot be summarily laid aside are not free from critical objection.

Tubal pregnancies, once regarded as rare events, and usually discovered only at post-mortem examinations, are now known to be frequent mishaps, and the possible cause of a large number of ordinary pelvic disturbances.

**Tubal Pregnancy.**—The ovum may find lodgement in any part of the tube. The cause is most frequently to be found in the various forms of chronic salpingitis. Owing to the associated loss of epithelium, to dilatation, and to other changes in the tubal wall, the two active forces which propel the ovum through the tube—ciliary movements and peristalsis—are

---

[1] Mr. Tait has long advocated the doctrine that, under normal conditions, the ovum first encounters the spermatozoa after its entrance into the uterine cavity. This view has been maintained still more recently by Wyder and Martin. *Vide* discussion on Martin's paper, Aetiologie der ektopischen Schwangerschaft, Zeitschr. f. Geb. und Gyn., Bd. xxvii. S. 205 *et seq.*

742

weakened and destroyed, while unimpeded ingress is afforded to the spermatozoa.

Again, the passage of the ovum may be interfered with by the secondary results of catarrhal inflammation, such as mucous polypi and sac-like dilatations, or constrictions, flexions, and dislocations of the tube, due to adhesions and bands, the products of associated peritoneal inflammations.

Abel,[1] in a case in which tubal pregnancy occurred a second time in the same patient, found a spiral rotation of the tube on the uterine side, a condition which had previously been shown by Freund to be a sign of arrested development. He ascribes the presence of diverticula to a similar origin. He suggests that these spiral turns and diverticula resulting from an infantile state of the tube are accountable in many instances for recurrent ectopic gestation where adhesions, polypi, and catarrhal inflammations can be excluded as etiological factors.

Because of its frequent connection with inflammatory processes, the occurrence of tubal pregnancy is often preceded by a long period of sterility. When due to constriction, the closure of the tube may be only partial, permitting the spermatozoa to reach the ovum, while the latter, owing to increase in size attendant upon fecundation, finds its onward progress arrested; when complete, on the contrary, the spermatozoa can gain access to the ovum only by first passing through the patulous tube, and then migrating across the rear of the uterus to the ovary, or to the open abdominal end of the tube upon the opposite side. In a considerable number of cases the corpus luteum has been found upon the side opposite the tube containing the fecundated ovum. With the present prevailing views[2] this phenomenon is to be accounted for only by the hypothesis of the migration of the ovum across the peritoneal surface of the pelvis, or across the uterine cavity from one tube to the other. That the external migration of the ovum is possible has been shown experimentally by Leopold,[3] who found that, after tying the right tube and removing the entire left ovary in a couple of rabbits, uterine pregnancy took place. The doctrine of the internal migration of the ovum is more a matter of dispute. The normal mechanism by which the ovum is conveyed into the uterus is presumably peristalsis of the tubes and the current produced by the lining ciliated epithelium,—both forces which would naturally offer resistance to the passage of the ovum from the uterine cavity into a tubal canal.[4]

---

[1] Abel, Wiederholte Tuben-Gravidität bei derselben Frau, Arch. f. Gyn., Bd. xliv. S. 72.

[2] Mayshofer, Ueber die gelben Körper und die Ueberwanderung der Eies, denies the whole doctrine of a distinct corpus luteum of pregnancy, and holds that corpora lutea are found at stated intervals—perhaps monthly—through the entire period of pregnancy.

[3] Leopold, Die Ueberwanderung der Eier, Arch. f. Gynaek., Bd. xvi. S. 24.

[4] Wyder (Beitrage zur extrauterin Schwangerschaft, Arch. f. Gynaek., Bd. xli. S 188 et seq.) believes that a specimen examined by him furnished the anatomical evidence of the occurrence of the phenomenon in question. He argues that it is rendered possible by the loss of the ciliated epithelium and by pressure exerted directly upon the ovum by the

Of late a number of observations have been placed on record showing that a recurrence of ectopic pregnancy in the same patient occasionally takes place. Abel, whose paper has already been referred to, furnishes ten cases reported as belonging in this category, eight of which he regards as indisputable. More recently, Dr. Henry C. Coe[1] has published a novel instance in which pregnancy occurred a second time in the same tube. (Fig. 1.)

FIG. 1.

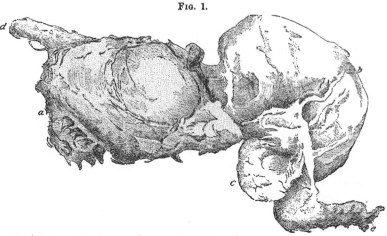

Repeated pregnancy in the same tube.—*a*, old sac; *b*, recent sac; *c*, atrophied ovary; *d*, divided proximal end of right tube; *e*, fimbriated extremity of tube. (Coe.)

Tubal pregnancy is associated with the formation of a uterine decidua which differs in no wise from that of pregnancy, except that the distinction into three layers is less marked.

A complete decidua within the tubal sac enclosing the ovum is, at least during the early stages of growth, exceptional. Thus, Zedel[2] found the cells

---

uterus, a pressure resulting from antiperistaltic movements supposed to occur during coitus, or from uterine contractions at the menstrual period. D. Veit (Die Frage der inneren Ueberwanderung der Eier, Zeitschr. f. Geb. und Gyn., Bd. xxiv. S. 327) discredits the anatomical value of Wyder's specimen.

[1] Coe, Internal Migration of the Ovum, etc., Am. Jour. Obstetrics, June, 1893, p. 855. Hayden's case, referred to in Coe's report, is regarded by Abel as pregnancy in the rudimentary cornu of a uterus bicornis. The list of recurrent ectopic pregnancies includes the cases of Schwarz, Tait, Winckel, I. Veit, Hermann, Leopold, Meyer, Olshausen, and Frommel. The case of Henkelom of Leyden, and a second case of Hermann, are reported as doubtful.

[2] Zedel, Zeitschr. f. Geb. und Gyn., Bd. xxvi. S. 78. It should be mentioned that the opinions regarding the anatomical changes which take place during the development of the ovum in ectopic pregnancies have undergone considerable modification during the past few years. Those given are derived especially from the recent studies of Abel, Klein (Zur Anatomie der schwangeren Tube, Zeitschr. f. Geb. und Gyn., Bd. xx. S. 288), and Zedel. The net outcome would seem to indicate an ever-diminishing difference between the conditions existing in normal and those existing in ectopic gestations.

of the mucous lining for the most part flattened and atrophied by pressure, while the decidual changes were limited to the vicinity of the insertion of the ovum.

In the decidua serotina the cells have the same shape and character as those of the uterine mucous membrane. They consist chiefly of large spindle-shaped and polyhedral cells with vesicular nuclei, between which are scattered round cells like leucocytes and narrow cells of connective tissue. Giant cells are found here and there, especially in the median layer. Next to the muscular coat there is a transitional zone in which decidual cells are intermingled with muscular and connective-tissue fibres. The inner surface is covered with the so-called canaliculated fibrin, due, according to Zedel, to an increase of the intercellular substance with separation of the cells, loss of cell-contours, and disappearance of the nuclei. A homogeneous mass is thus produced with occasional striæ, to which the name is due.

Concerning the decidua reflexa opinions are conflicting. Frommel, Winckel, Werth, Veit, Orthmann, and Zedel maintain its existence. None was discovered by Langhans, Leopold, and Klein. Zedel thinks Klein's failure to find the reflexa was due to his not examining an intact ovum.

The placental circulation does not differ from that of ordinary pregnancy. The veins traverse the walls of the tube in an oblique direction. No important changes occur before they penetrate the decidua; they then widen (eight to ten times) and are speedily lost in the serotina. The arteries, after reaching the decidua, make increased spiral turns, and pass obliquely to the decidual elevations, where the muscular walls are gradually lost, and the vessels consist of endothelium and the connective tissue of the adventitia only. Zedel believes that it is the pressure of the blood-stream, and not the growth of the villi, which opens up the thinned walls of the vessels and leads to the formation of the intervillous communications.

The development of the chorion is like that in uterine gestation. The lumen of the tube, both at the central and at the distal extremity of the ovum, remains normally patent.

In the early months the development of the ovum leads to a spindle-shaped dilatation of the tube, associated with hypertrophy of the muscular walls, due to increase in the length and thickness of the individual fibres. As regards the degree of hypertrophy, very great individual variations have been observed. Indeed, in the same sac a thickening at one point may be accompanied by an excessive degree of tenuity, due to eccentric growth of the ovum, at another. Now, the ultimate fate of a tubal pregnancy is in large measure dependent upon these anatomical differences. Unquestionably, early rupture is the rule. Mr. Tait says, "Out of an enormous number of specimens which I have examined, I have entirely failed to satisfy myself that rupture has been delayed later than the twelfth week." It seems to me, however, carrying scepticism too far to refuse credence to the positive observations of others, made apparently with the utmost care and with full knowledge of possible sources of error, which seem to show that a tubal pregnancy may exceptionally reach an advanced stage or even full term. At present it seems fair to assume that when the sac which surrounds the ovum is composed of muscular and connective-tissue fibres with an external peritoneal envelope, and directly communicates with the Fallopian tube, the sac-walls are of tubal origin. Of course it is not possible to assert that no rupture has taken place in the course of development. It is only known positively that rupture occurring at the site of placental attachment gives rise to hemorrhage fatal to the fœtus ; and the same is true, with rare exceptions, when rupture occurs at any point of the peritoneal surface. That rupture into the cavity of the broad ligament has first occurred in all the cases which go on to the period of viability does not seem so absolutely certain. The anatomical appearances, in some instances at least, indicate that the exposure of the fœtal membranes here and there through the maternal sac results not so much from laceration as from the gradual separation of the muscular fibres due to excessive stretching.[1] In most of the cases in which the pregnancy reaches an advanced stage the development of the tube takes place principally between the folds of the broad ligament. The support furnished the tubal sac by the gradual unfolding of the layers of the ligament hinders rupture. More rarely pregnancy may reach the period of viability without encroaching upon the intra-ligamentous space. The tumor then rises above the pelvic brim, and is furnished with a sort of pedicle consisting of the uterine end of the tube and of the broad ligament.

The first, or intra-ligamentous, form lies close to the uterus, which it not infrequently crowds upward and forward. The uterine end of the tube varies greatly in length. The fimbriated extremity is unrecognizable. Usually no traces of the ovary are found. In the so-called pedunculated form the uterus is crowded to one side or is retroverted. The uterine end of the tube is usually long and thickened. The corresponding ovary has generally been discovered. In both cases the relations of the sac are often obscured by adhesions to adjacent viscera. In the second half of pregnancy rupture of the sac and the escape of the fœtus into the peritoneal cavity may occur without noticeable hemorrhage, or without interruption of pregnancy. As the pressure is removed by the escape of the amniotic fluid, the placental borders curl inward so as to furnish a cup-like space, while the membranes sink downward and cover the upper placental surface. The fœtus in these cases may occupy the abdominal cavity, or a sac may be formed by the agglutination of the adjacent viscera.

Werth was the first to report a case in which the death of the embryo, occurring in the second month, was followed by hemorrhage, which poured through the abdominal end of the tube into the pelvic cavity and gave rise to intra-peritoneal hæmatocele. This form he termed tubal abortion. In a

---

[1] *Vide* tables of Werth, Beiträge zur Anatomie und zur operativen Behandlung der Extrauterinschwangerschaft.

case described by Wyder the fimbriated extremity of the tube was oblit-erated, and, as a consequence, the hemorrhage following the separation of the ovum converted the ampulla of the tube into a blood-cyst the size of the fist. Many similar observations have since been made by others.

**Pregnancy in the Rudimentary Cornu of a One-Horned Uterus.**—This anomaly so closely resembles the tubal form of pregnancy that the diagnostic distinction can rarely be established during life. When the muscular structures of the cornu are sufficiently developed the preg-nancy may advance to term.[1] Indeed, cases have been reported by Grinew, Schultze, Litschkus, and Handfield, where labor-pains at the end of gesta-tion were followed by the expulsion of the child; but, according to the estimates of Stoll,[2] based on statistics gathered by himself, by Sänger, and by Himmelfarb, eighty per cent. terminate in rupture. To this a special predisposition is created by the obliteration, after conception, of the lower portion of the rudimentary cornu, which thus becomes an impervious cord. Stoll therefore advises, in cases where the diagnosis has been made at an early period, to pass the finger into the cervix to ascertain whether a communication with the pregnant cornu exists. Should such be the case, abortion would be indicated; whereas if the cornu was impervious the proper procedure would be cœliotomy and amputation.

**Interstitial Pregnancy.**—The term "interstitial pregnancy" is ap-plied to cases in which the ovum is developed in the uterine portion of the tube. The latter measures about seven lines in length by one line in diam-eter. At first the muscular walls hypertrophy and form around the ovum a sac which projects from the upper angle of the uterus. Since, ordinarily, the growth of the muscular tissue does not keep pace with that of the ovum, rupture occurs at an early period. In twenty-six such cases collected by Hecker, all ruptured before the sixth month. Tait says that, "so far as known, interstitial pregnancy is uniformly fatal by primary intra-perito-neal rupture before the fifth month." Schwarz,[3] however, reports a case belonging to this category in which the fœtus was expelled into the uterine cavity.

The patient was known to be pregnant. Repeated hemorrhages indi-cated a threatened abortion. To avoid further dangers, the cervix was dilated with the view of emptying the uterus. On examination with the finger the uterine cavity was found to be empty, but there was a piece of membrane at the uterine opening of the left tube, which was removed.

---

[1] Turner, Edinburgh Medical Journal, May, 1886, p. 974; Werth, Arch f. Gynaek., Bd. xvi. S. 281; Salin, Centralblatt f. Gynaek., 1881, S. 221.

[2] Stoll. Beitrag zur Graviditat des Uterus bicornis, Zeitschr. f. Geb. und Gynaek., Bd. xxiv. S. 275.

[3] Schwarz, Wiener Med. Blätter, 1886. In the abstract furnished by Grandin in the American Journal of Obstetrics (January, 1887, p. 101) the date of pregnancy is not given. Similar cases have been reported by Dr. Charles McBurney (New York Med. Jour., March, 1878, p. 273) and by Dr. Cornelius Williams (Ibid., December, 1878, p. 595), both of which were followed by the recovery of the mother.

The next day the finger detected membrane at the same site, and, beyond, a hard body. The uterus began to contract energetically. On the fifth day a fœtus was passed by the vagina, the pains ceased, the tumor became much smaller, and the patient made a good convalescence.

FIG. 4.

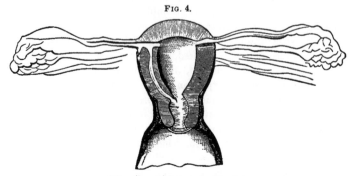

Bifurcation of tubal canal. (Hennig.)

Martin removed a male fœtus thirty-three centimetres long (six months) from the left uterine cornu. The patient recovered. Duvelius, who examined the specimen, concluded that the ovum had partly grown into the tube and between the folds of the broad ligament. He thought that rupture had been prevented by the number of the muscular elements in the sac-wall.[1]

A possible form of interstitial pregnancy is furnished by the occasional existence of a canal, open at its two extremities, and apparently a continuation or a bifurcation of the Fallopian tube. A case reported by Dr. Gilbert in the *Boston Medical and Surgical Journal* (March 3, 1877), in which the head of the child could be felt just above the os internum, covered by a thin mucous membrane, and in which delivery was successfully accomplished by an incision through the partition, probably belonged to this variety. A similar case, in the practice of Dr. H. Lenox Hodge, is reported by Parry.

In the post-mortem examinations the distinction between an interstitial pregnancy and one in a rudimentary cornu is not easy to make out. The chief point of difference consists in the fact that in interstitial pregnancy the sac communicates by an orifice with the uterine cavity, or is separated from the uterus by a partition, while in pregnancy in a rudimentary cornu the two halves of the uterus are united by a muscular band, which is situated not at the upper angle, but near the os internum.

**Ovarian Pregnancy.**—In spite of modern scepticism, there is little question as to the occasional occurrence of ovarian pregnancy. The specimen discovered by Patenko[2] in the Pathologico-Anatomical Museum of St.

---

[1] Martin, Zeitschr. f. Geb. und Gynaek., Bd. xi. S 416.
[2] Patenko, Casuistische Mitteilungen, Arch. f. Gynaek., Bd. xiv. S. 156.

Petersburg seems to answer all the requirements of a demonstration. The right ovary was of the size of a hen's egg, and contained a cyst with smooth walls filled with serum. In this he found a body of a yellow color, of the size of a hazel-nut, which contained cylindrical and flat bones. The most careful microscopical examination established the fact that the bones were those of a fœtus, and not merely the chance products of a dermoid cyst. The presence of corpora lutea and follicles in the walls of the envelope proved that the body was an ovary. The tube on the corresponding side was nowhere adherent to the sac. The abdominal extremity was closed, and there were no traces of fimbriæ.[1]

Paltauf[2] relates a case of extra-uterine pregnancy in which there was a sacculated condition of both tubes which communicated with a cyst of ovarian origin. The ovaries were closely united. By means of the ovarian cyst a complete communication was established between the two tubes. In the large central ovarian cyst a clot was found which contained an embryo corresponding in size to one of from forty-five to forty-eight days' development. The origin of the condition here met with is naturally a matter of speculation.

**Abdominal Pregnancy.**—In most cases of abdominal pregnancy a connective-tissue proliferation is set up about the ovum, which surrounds it with a vascular sac. The latter often attains a degree of thickness which renders it comparable to the gravid uterus. (Klob.) The walls keep pace, as a rule, with the growth of the ovum, and, as they extend into the abdominal cavity, form adhesions to the intestines, the mesentery, and the omentum. It is stated that organic muscular fibres have been found in the sac, especially near the uterine attachment. In this form the fœtus most frequently reaches maturity.

In rare cases the ovum develops free in the abdominal cavity, without the formation of pseudo-membranes, the fœtus being surrounded solely by the amnion and chorion.

The greater number of so-called abdominal pregnancies are unquestionably of tubal origin. In reality, they are for the most part extra-peritoneal, and result from a rupture in the tube-walls occurring between the folds of the broad ligament. In these cases the conditions are not incompatible with continued fœtal development, and gestation may reach an advanced stage.

The question as to the occurrence of primary abdominal pregnancy must be regarded as unsettled. The discovery of an ovum growing in the peritoneal cavity, with the tubes and ovaries demonstrably intact, would

---

[1] Mr. Tait, in his work on Ectopic Pregnancy, refers to a specimen described by Dr. Walter as one of primary ovarian pregnancy (the sac had ruptured at the fifth month and the fœtus had escaped into the peritoneal cavity), which is now in the Dorpat Museum, and suggests a careful investigation as to its real character. At Werth's request, this has since been made by Runge, with a complete confirmation of the significance given to it by Walter in his original publication. Werth, *loc. cit.*, p. 64.

[2] Paltauf, Arch. f. Gynaek., Bd. xxx. S. 456.

suffice to establish the abdominal variety.  In the early months, before the
anatomical conditions are obscured by secondary changes, there is no pre-
tence that such proof has been obtained.  In more advanced stages a good

FIG. 5.

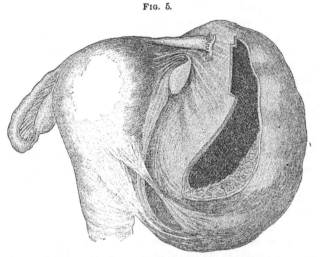

Case of supposed abdominal pregnancy.  At first it was reported as such bV Zweifel, but later, after
careful microscopic examination, it proVed to haVe beeu primarilV tubal.

many cases of assumed abdominal pregnancy have been placed in evidence.
These, so far as my investigations permit me to judge, are divisible into two
classes :

1. Cases in which the tubes are reported as intact, but in which there
exists a direct communication between the tube upon the affected side and
the sac-cavity.

2. Cases in which the tubes are reported as intact and not in communication with the sac.

Few of these merit criticism.  In many, without doubt, the ovum was
primarily implanted in the fimbriated extremity of the tube, from which
later it grew either outward into the abdominal cavity or downward between the folds of the broad ligament.

In certain cases rupture of the sac and the fœtal membranes may occur,
and the fœtus pass into the abdominal cavity ; these are termed secondary
abdominal pregnancies.  Most often the child dies at or soon after rupture,
but instances have been reported in which it continued to develop within the
abdomen.  The presence of the child usually excites an active proliferation
of connective tissue, by means of which a secondary sac is formed, though
in Jessup's case the child was absolutely free in the abdominal cavity, and
in one of my own, eleven years after rupture, the child was found attached
to the omentum, but without any special investment.

A few histories are on record of the coexistence of extra uterine and intra-uterine pregnancies; the latter occur at the same period as the former, or subsequent to the death of the extra-uterine fœtus.

**Tubo-Abdominal and Tubo-Ovarian Pregnancy.**—When the ovum becomes lodged near the trumpet-shaped extremity of the Fallopian tube it may grow outward into the abdominal cavity. Local peritonitis is then set up, and plastic exudation is thrown out, forming an envelope around the ovum, which is likewise bounded by the contiguous organs. In this way the ligamenta lata, the ovaries, the mesentery, the intestines, the bladder, and the uterus may all contribute to the investment of the fœtal membranes. In case of rupture in the tubal portion, inflammatory products may form and limit the extent of the injury. At first, owing to its weight, the distended tube drops into the cul-de-sac of Douglas. In advanced pregnancy, the spleen, kidneys, and liver may become involved and form part of the sac-walls around the ovum. Usually the placenta is developed in the pelvic cavity.

When the investment of the ovum is furnished by the tube and the ovary the term tubo-ovarian pregnancy is employed. The course in either case does not differ materially from that of an abdominal pregnancy.

**Symptoms.**—The earlier symptoms of extra-uterine pregnancy do not materially differ from those of the intra-uterine form. Menstruation usually ceases, though not with the same regularity as in normal pregnancy. The recurrence of the monthly flow for one or two periods is not an uncommon incident. In some cases, too, a nearly continuous sero-sanguinolent discharge of moderate extent has been observed. Up to a certain point the hypertrophic changes of the uterus take place in the usual manner. The mucous membrane is converted into a decidua, and a mucous plug fills the cervix. In general terms, the length of the uterus is greater the closer the contiguity of the ovum to the uterus. In a few cases of tubal pregnancy there has been no increase in the size of the uterus. The extra-uterine ovum may, in the course of its growth, drag the uterus upward, or push it downward, forward, or to the side, according to the site of its development.

Characteristic symptoms of extra-uterine pregnancy do not occur until the ovum has reached a certain degree of growth, and in some cases not until after rupture has taken place. Often preceding rupture, or, in abdominal pregnancies, before the death of the fœtus, the patient suffers from paroxysmal pains in the sac and uterine pains like those of labor. The latter are associated with a sero-sanguinolent discharge, and are followed by the expulsion of portions of the decidua.

The symptoms of rupture are the usual ones of internal hemorrhage,—viz., yawning, languor, fainting, clammy perspiration, rapid pulse, intermittent vomiting, collapse, and acute anæmia. After the death of the ovum these symptoms may cease and not return again; whereas if the ovum continues to grow there may be repeated attacks of hemorrhage and local peritonitis.

When the death of the ovum does not occur within the first three or four months, the pressure of the tumor usually gives rise to dysuria and constipation.

**Terminations.**—The investigations resulting from the recent widespread interest in diseases of the uterine appendages have shown that tubal pregnancy is by no means of rare occurrence. Whereas in tubal and interstitial pregnancies it was formerly believed that the usual terminations were rupture of the sac, hemorrhage, peritonitis, and death, it is now known that in a pretty large percentage of cases the ovum perishes at an early period of development, and, though the sequelæ of these so-called tubal abortions may cause discomfort or lay the foundation of chronic invalidism, they do not necessarily lead to a fatal result. As in cases of uterine abortion, the death of the ovum is for the most part followed by hemorrhage, which may be confined to the tube (hæmatosalpinx), or the blood may escape by the fimbriated extremity into the peritoneal cavity, or, if circumscribed by adhesions, it may give rise to the intra-peritoneal form of pelvic hæmatocele. Even when rupture takes place the hemorrhage is not necessarily fatal. Mr. Tait insists on the relative harmlessness of most cases of hæmatoma due to rupture occurring between the folds of the broad ligament; while the records of cœliotomy show that, even with intra-peritoneal rupture, the hemorrhage has often been found moderate in amount, and did not in itself furnish the occasion for surgical interference.[1]

In abdominal pregnancies, which it has been seen are usually, if not always, secondary to the tubal form, the ovum or fœtus, as a rule, excites a local peritonitis, attended with pain and fever, and followed by the formation of pseudo-membranes, which exercise a conservative influence by shutting off the ovum from the peritoneal cavity. Indeed, in the exceptional instances in which these inflammatory conditions do not develop, the movements of the fœtus within its own membranes may give rise to such intense suffering as to cause the woman to die from exhaustion. (Schroeder.)

In abortions at an early stage it often happens that no trace of the embryo is found, and the diagnosis must be made from the presence of the chorionic villi. Even when abortion does not occur in the first few weeks the child is apt to die prematurely. Sometimes, however, gestation may advance to full term; in this case labor-pains set in, the decidua is expelled, and the child dies during the expulsive efforts. In the majority of cases the dead fœtus excites a suppurative inflammation in the sac by which it is enclosed, and the patient dies either from general peritonitis or from profuse suppuration. In cases in which the peritonitis remains local and the suppuration is tolerated, fistulous communications may form with one of the hollow viscera or the abdominal walls, through which the contents of the sac may be eliminated. Most frequently the opening takes place into the large intestine, quite often through the abdominal walls, more rarely

---

[1] For example, the cases reported by Orthmann from Martin's clinic.

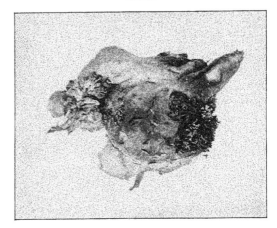

Tubal pregnancy.—Development of ovum between folds of broad ligament; secondary rupture into peritoneal cavity.

FIG. 3.

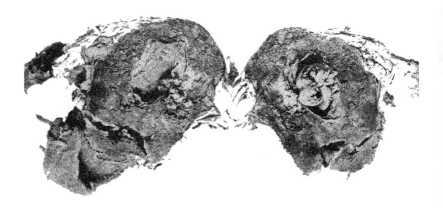

Rupture of tube.—Ovum surrounded by coagulated blood between folds of broad ligament

into the vagina and bladder. In any case, the process of elimination is slow, often lasting months and even years. When the bones and the soft tissues have all been discharged, complete recovery may take place. In the larger proportion of cases, however, if nature is not assisted, the patient perishes from exhaustion and blood-poisoning before the process is ended.

Sometimes the foregoing inflammatory changes do not occur as the result of the death of the fœtus, in which case the fluid contents of the sac are reabsorbed and the walls collapse and come in contact with the fœtal cadaver. The skin of the latter, and at a later period the deep-seated soft tissues, undergo fatty degeneration, and form a greasy substance consisting of fat, lime salts, cholesterin-crystals, and blood-pigment. Afterwards the fluid portions are absorbed, and the fœtus may shrink up like a mummy, preserving its shape and organs to the minutest detail; or partial calcification of the fœtus and membranes may ensue. A fœtus thus altered is called a lithopædion. A lithopædion in the sense of a complete petrifaction does not exist.

Küchenmeister distinguishes three conditions to which the term is applicable:[1]

1. When, after absorption of the fluid, the membranes alone calcify and the fœtus undergoes mummification.

2. When, after absorption or escape of the fluid, the membranes calcify and calcification of the fœtus occurs at points where the membranes adhere to the fœtal surface.

3. When the fœtus escapes into the abdominal cavity and cretaceous matter is deposited in the smegma covering the fœtal surface. In this way calcified strata form around the fœtus and exert compression upon the contained tissues. Beneath the chalky layers the tissues are mummified.

A lithopædion may remain embedded in connective tissue for years without injury to the mother. In a case reported by me the child was found attached to the omentum eleven years after the rupture of the tubal sac. The lithopædion of Leinzell was removed in 1720 from a woman ninety-four years of age, who had carried it for forty-six years. The presence of the lithopædion does not prevent pregnancy from taking place. In some cases it may, after years, excite suppuration, a result which is fostered, according to Spiegelberg, by pregnancy and labor. Recovery may follow the artificial extraction of the foreign body, or death may result from inflammation and the discharge of pus.

**Diagnosis.**—The diagnosis of extra-uterine fœtation is based upon the existence of the signs of pregnancy, the exclusion of an ovum within the uterine cavity, and the presence of a tumor external to the uterus.

There is a wide difference of opinion as to the practicability of early diagnosis. The problem seems simple enough. Given pregnancy, and

---

[1] Ueber Lithopädien, Arch. f. Gynæk., Bd. xvii. S 153.

having ascertained that the ovum is not in the uterus, the diagnosis is effected. But we all know that the subjective symptoms of pregnancy are deceptive, and that the pigmentation and the mammary and utero-vaginal changes are not always so clearly defined in the first three months as to make it safe in every case positively to diagnosticate pregnancy in even the intra-uterine form. The advice to use the sound to demonstrate the vacuity of the uterus in suspected cases has been the cause of many needless abortions. Fortunately, the sound often does no other harm than to add to our sources of error.

In the main, we must depend upon local changes and local symptoms. Thus, a tubal swelling and enlargement of the uterus, associated with suppression of the menses, often followed after a brief period by sero-sanguinolent discharges and increased flow at the menstrual period, with paroxysmal pains radiating from the side of the pelvis upon which the affected tube is situated, and with the expulsion of the uterine decidua at the end of the second or in the course of the third month, are to be regarded with suspicion. But a tubal sac is the product of a variety of pathological conditions.[1] The uterine changes in the early months are inconstant. These sometimes correspond to those of ordinary uterine gestation, but often there is neither perceptible enlargement nor cervical softening to indicate pregnancy. Paroxysmal pains are frequent in other forms of tubal disease, and menstrual disturbances are common phenomena in uterine derangements. The expulsion of the decidua, though a valuable sign, is not of constant occurrence. In many tubal abortions the only symptoms are those of pelvic hæmatocele. In many instances of early rupture of the tube with hemorrhage into the peritoneal cavity there are no antecedent symptoms, or only those of ordinary pregnancy. In reading the reported cases of the operative removal of pregnant tubes, it is surprising to note in how many of them the diagnosis was established only by the subsequent detection in the removed tubes of decidual cells and chorionic villi. Undoubtedly a probable diagnosis prior to rupture might be made in many instances if the patients could be subjected to frequent examinations from the beginning of the pregnant state, but this, in the nature of things, is rarely practicable.

In the intra-ligamentous form the conditions for diagnosis are more favorable. Here gestation is apt to be prolonged, and if rupture occurs between the folds of the broad ligament the hemorrhage is limited in amount. In this class the patients are apt to seek early professional advice, owing to the discomforts from which they suffer. The swelling at the side of the uterus is easily reached through the vagina, and we have as distinc-

---

[1] Veit regards as an important distinction in the early stage, that whereas in other forms of tubal enlargement the swelling may be hard, or tense, or fluctuating, when due to an intact ovum it possesses a characteristic soft feel. Verhandlungen der Deutschen Gesellsch f. Gynaek., Third Congress, Leipsic, 1890, S. 162.

tive signs a rapidly growing tumor, early fluctuation, and the presence of pulsating vessels over the site of the tumor. Bimanual examination under an anæsthetic, especially if the thumb be introduced into the vagina and two fingers into the rectum, makes it possible to determine that the tumor is independent of the uterus.[1]

After the third month it is not ordinarily difficult to determine the existence of the pregnant state. Ballottement is usually perceptible at an early date, the fœtal movements are apt to be very painful, and the fœtal heart makes the diagnosis certain ; but the greatest care needs to be exercised in the examination of the patient and in the formation of an opinion concerning the extra-uterine situation of the ovum. In a suspected case, violence in the attempt to separate the tumor from the uterus may cause rupture of the sac. Mr. Tait cites as a misleading condition an abnormal thinness of the uterine walls. In my own experience, lateral flexion of the uterus often simulates ectopic gestation to a surprising degree. In these cases the fundus containing the ovum lies upon one side of the pelvis. The cervix is crowded to the opposite side. Between the two a deep sulcus is felt. If the patient is hysterical, these deranged relations are exaggerated by contraction of the abdominal muscles. No difficulty in detecting the error is experienced when the patient is anæsthetized, except in cases where the fundus is fixed to the side by adhesions. In two cases seen by me the intra-uterine nature of the pregnancy was determined only by the forcible introduction of the finger through the cervix. Cases of retroflexion of the gravid uterus, with incarceration, are likewise often difficult to distinguish from extra-uterine pregnancy.

The distinction by physical signs between the tubal, the ovarian, and the secondary abdominal form is scarcely practicable so long as trained anatomists fail to agree concerning them when the abdomen has been opened and the organs are exposed to view.

A review of the subject of diagnosis makes it apparent that many cases of ectopic pregnancy present no symptoms previous to rupture. In another class the existence of a suspicious tumor with few or none of the corroborative signs should lead to a waiting policy, or, when the symptoms are of a threatening character, to an explorative cœliotomy. It is well, however, to remember that, with reference to this latter procedure, recent popular interest in abdominal surgery has a tendency to invest trifling anomalies occurring in gestation with a sinister importance ; but there still remains a considerable class in which an early diagnosis can be reached with reasonable certainty.

---

[1] According to Smolsky's observations, the tube in the first two months is the size of a pigeon's egg ; at the end of the second month, of an English walnut; at two and a half months, of a hen's egg ; at three months it reaches the size of the fist ; and at four months the size of two fists. Variations may result from hydramnios, hæmatosalpinx, malformation, etc. Smolsky, Diagnostie et traitement de la grossesse tubaire, Nouvelles archives d'obstétrique et de gynécologie, December, 1890, p. 649.

**Treatment.**—The treatment of extra-uterine fœtation varies in accordance with the stage of pregnancy and the condition of the fœtus. For the sake of convenience, we distinguish: 1. Cases of early gestation; 2. Cases of advanced gestation (with a living fœtus); 3. Cases of gestation prolonged after the death of the fœtus.

1. *Cases of Early Gestation.*—The indication for treatment in the early months varies with the conditions. If rupture has occurred, care should be employed to ascertain, if possible, whether the resulting hemorrhage has taken place between the folds of the broad ligament, or, if intra-peritoneal, whether the blood is free in the abdominal cavity or is restricted to the pelvis by old adhesions. Circumscribed effusions of blood due to ruptured tubes do not, as a rule, threaten life, and disappear with time and with little other treatment than rest in the recumbent posture.

If the outpouring of blood has taken place primarily into the abdominal cavity, or as a secondary occurrence after the giving way of the first barriers, cœliotomy is unquestionably demanded. While it is not denied that even in these extreme cases the effused blood may be circumscribed by an adhesive inflammatory process, and that a few patients may recover under expectant treatment, the waiting policy is a gamble with life. On the other hand, the opening of the abdomen for the purpose of removing blood and clots and for the extirpation of the tube-sac has been the means, since Mr. Tait demonstrated the practicability of the operation, of saving multitudes of women from impending death. The operation is not, as a rule, difficult. It involves the separation of adhesions, where these exist, the tying of the pedicle, and the removal of the ruptured sac. In the intra-ligamentous form it may be necessary to ligate the attached portion in sections. Where a pedicle cannot be readily formed, Veit recommends the tying of the broad ligaments at the two extremities of the sac before proceeding to ligate the base. Previous to closing the abdominal incision great care should be taken to insure the arrest of hemorrhage not only from the stump, but from the separated adhesions.

When the diagnosis is made previous to rupture the choice lies between cœliotomy and the employment of measures to destroy the life of the embryo. In practice, the decision is pretty certain to be governed by other than theoretical considerations. Thus, an experienced operator, who possesses trained assistants and can command for his patient the surroundings which are needful for success, will be apt to select cœliotomy. The risks have been proved to be small, and the patient is relieved from possible future troubles due to retention of the products of conception. But all men are not experts in pelvic surgery. The danger which threatens the life of the patient is often imminent, and assistance from afar is not always easy to obtain. Under these conditions the question arises, how far reliance is to be placed upon measures designed to destroy the life of the fœtus, and thus, by arresting the growth of the ovum, to diminish the chances of immediate rupture and hemorrhage. Of the various methods heretofore proposed to accomplish this object, only two merit discussion,—viz., the injection of morphine solution and the faradic and galvanic currents.

*Injections into the Sac of Solutions designed to destroy the Fœtus.*—This method was first suggested by Joulin.[1] He proposed injections of sulphate of atropine (one-fifth of a grain dissolved in a few drops of water) into the sac by means of a long hypodermic syringe. His suggestion was successfully carried into effect in two cases by Friedreich,[2] of Heidelberg. The needle of the syringe, he advised, should be introduced into the sac through the abdominal or vaginal walls, a few drops of fluid should then be withdrawn, and its place supplied by the solution containing the poison selected. Friedreich employed by preference one-fifth of a grain of morphine. The operation was repeated every second day, until the diminished size of the ovum afforded evidence that the result sought for had been accomplished. The operation seemed to produce but slight inflammatory disturbance, and the maternal system did not feel the influence of the narcotic. Rennert[3] has since succeeded in destroying the life of the fœtus in the fifth month of extra-uterine gestation by means of a single injection containing about half a grain of morphine. The patient recovered after a protracted illness. Koeberlé reported to the Gynæcological Section of the Eighth International Medical Congress at Copenhagen a case of advanced abdominal pregnancy where the child was destroyed by morphine injections. The fœtus and placenta were absorbed. The recovery was complete. Ten cases have been observed by Winckel and one by Fournier. Of the sixteen cases, three have ended fatally.

Winckel,[4] who is the chief modern advocate of this method, makes an injection of the strength of half a grain of morphine through the abdominal wall, above Poupart's ligament, and repeats the same after six to eight days. Two to three injections usually suffice. As a result of the death of the fœtus, the pains subside, the abdomen becomes soft, the swelling rapidly diminishes in size, the appetite returns, and convalescence follows. The method is applicable up to the end of the fourth month.

*The Faradic Current.*—The transmission of the faradic current is accomplished by passing one pole into the rectum or vagina to the site of the ovum and pressing the other upon a point in the abdominal wall situated two to three inches above Poupart's ligament. The full force of the current of an ordinary one-cell battery should be employed for a period varying from five to ten minutes. The treatment should be continued daily

---

[1] Traité complet des accouchements, p. 968.

[2] Cohnstein, Beitrag zur Schwangerschaft ausserhalb der Gebärmutter, Arch. f. Gynaek., Bd. xiv. S. 355. Hennig likewise reports a case operated on by Koeberlé, where profuse hemorrhage occurred. It is not stated whether the patient recovered. (Die Krankheiten der Eileiter und die Tubenschwangerschaft, S. 138.)

[3] Extrauterinschwangerschaft im funften Monate, Arch. f. Gynaek., Bd. xxiv. S. 266.

[4] Lehrbuch der Geburtshülfe, zweite Auflage, S. 269.

for one or two weeks, until the shrinkage of the tumor leaves no doubt as to the death of the fœtus.

The successful employment of the faradic current in extra-uterine pregnancy we owe to Dr. J. G. Allen, who reported two cases of recovery through its instrumentality in 1872. His first case occurred in 1869 and the second in 1871. So little pains did he take regarding his discovery that the subject was nearly forgotten, until a new success was reported by Drs. Lovering and Landis, of the Starling Medical College, in 1877. Since then, Brothers [1] has collected fifty cases in which electricity was employed. In twenty-five cases, to which I can add a twenty-sixth from my own practice and not included in Brothers's list, the health of the patients was ascertained to be good at the end of periods varying from one to eight years.

There were no evil results in any of the cases traceable to the electricity. Of the four fatal ones, in that of Janvrin rupture of the tube had undoubtedly taken place before the galvanism was employed, in that of Wylie the eight months' fœtus was killed by injections of morphine into the sac after electricity had been discarded, and in the cases of Duncan and Steavensen and Boulton and Steavensen electro-puncture was employed.

The treatment by means of faradism is available only during the first three months, and in the intra-ligamentous form of ectopic gestation.

The arguments against faradism are the usual ones urged against all conservative measures,—viz., that reported successful cases were simply examples of diagnostic errors, and that hesitation to resort in every case to abdominal section is *prima facie* evidence of surgical incompetence. The difficulties of diagnosis, however, are small in the case of a growing intra-ligamentous fœtal sac, and it is not necessary to abandon a tenable position simply because of slurring comments. In conclusion, I am willing to admit theoretically that the ovum, after its vitality has been destroyed, may be a source of discomfort and may require removal; but it must be borne in mind that a small dead ovum between the folds of the broad ligament is usually innocuous and gives rise to few of the symptoms resulting from tubal distention.

2. *Cases of Advanced Gestation.*—After the third month it has now come to be regarded as a settled rule that the removal of the fœtus, the placenta, and the investing membranes should be attempted as soon as the diagnosis has been made. If complete extirpation of the sac proves impracticable, it should be removed to the fullest extent possible, as its presence when left *in situ* is capable of leading to intractable sinuses and persistent suppuration. The older method of stitching the sac to the abdominal wall and leaving the placenta to come away spontaneously furnished a certain number of favorable results after the death of the child and the arrest of the cir-

---

[1] Subsequent Behavior of Cases of Extra-Uterine Pregnancy treated by Electricity, American Journal of Obstetrics, vol. xxiii., No. 2, 1890.

culation had taken place. During the life of the child, death from hemorrhage was the usual result.[1] The conclusion drawn from this experience was to await the death of the fœtus before operating; but the statistics of Schauta confirm the apprehension that, what with rupture of the sac, intestinal and visceral perforations, and sepsis, there is but slender hope of a happy issue when a waiting policy is adopted.

With clearer anatomical views of extra-uterine pregnancy, it is more and more recognized that the treatment of that condition is subject to the ordinary rules of abdominal surgery.

The difficulties encountered in the removal of the fœtal sac are the result of excessive vascularity and extensive adhesions, but these obstacles to success have of late been found in many cases not to be insurmountable. The first operator to move in the right direction to lessen the risks of hemorrhage and sepsis was Martin, who detached the placenta after tying the supplying vessels in the broad ligament beneath the placenta and at the side of the uterus. This he did in 1881, in the days of imperfect Listerism. The patient was in the seventh month of pregnancy. The sac was afterwards closed on the peritoneal side, and drainage was accomplished through an opening made into the vagina.

Breisky,[2] however, was the first to place the operation on a solid surgical basis by showing that it is practicable to remove the entire ovum. His patient was at the end of the eighth month of pregnancy. He first stitched

---

[1] John Williams has reported a successful case belonging to this category (thirty-five weeks' gestation). The placenta continued to discharge for about five weeks. The patient returned home at the end of two months. (Obstetrical Transactions, London, vol. xxix. p. 482.)

Jessup (London Obstetrical Transactions, 1876, p. 261) and John W. Taylor (Ibid., 1891, p. 115) removed at term children that were free among the intestines. In both cases the cord was drawn out of the lower corner of the wound, and through the opening thus left the putrescent placenta was gradually discharged. Jessup's patient left the hospital after two and one-half months; Taylor's, after three and one-half months.

Dr. Jordecai Price, of Philadelphia, delivered a living child by section in the tenth month of pregnancy, October 23, 1892. The sac was adherent to the transverse colon and to the small intestine to a small extent. The placenta was attached to the left tube, to the entire pelvic viscera on the left side, and to the descending colon. Owing to the certainty of fatal hemorrhage in case of detachment of the placenta, the sac was stitched to the abdominal wall. At the end of the third week the patient's condition seemed desperate, but she ultimately recovered, and the child was living at the end of fifteen months. (Philadelphia Medical and Surgical Reporter, May 20, 1893.)

Bruhl (Arch f. Gyn., Bd. xxxi. S. 404), in a patient presumably six months pregnant, stitched the sac to the abdominal walls and packed with iodoform gauze. The child breathed a few times. The patient was discharged at the end of seven weeks.

Treub (Zeitschr. f. Geb. und Gyn., 1888, Bd. xv. S. 384) operated successfully three weeks before the end of gestation. The placenta was removed and the sac was partially resected. The latter was then stitched to the abdominal wall and tamponed with iodoform gauze.

Lihotzky (Wien. Klin. Wochenschr., 1891, S. 184) operated after the same method at the seventh month, with good recovery of the patient.

[2] Wiener Med. Presse, No. 48, 1887.

the sac to the abdominal wound, opened it, and removed the fœtus. He then removed the stitches, ligated the broad ligament on the side of the uterus, and separated the tumor, tying at the same time any large vessels found bleeding in the cut surface. By progressive ligation of the base from within outward towards the pelvic wall, the sac with the contained placenta was detached with slight loss of blood. Packing the cavity with iodoform gauze was subsequently resorted to.[1]

A year later our own Eastman[2] removed the entire sac in an ectopic pregnancy of the tubal variety at the eighth month. He was able to clamp the uterine end of the tube and the broad ligament and to cut away the portion which contained the ovum. He afterwards quilted the stump with iron-dyed silk. The patient made an excellent recovery. The operation of Eastman stands as one of the finest achievements of American surgery.

Olshausen[3] found the placenta attached to the right broad ligament. By tying the ligament beneath the placenta, the latter was removed without loss of blood. Again, in a like case, Braun Fernwald[4] tied the broad ligament to which the placenta was attached, and thus removed the upper portion without difficulty, but on the posterior surface of the uterus and in the cul-de-sac the separation was not practicable. He therefore amputated the fundus of the uterus, after applying an elastic ligature, and stitched the funnel-shaped cavity of the cul de-sac of Douglas to the abdominal wound and filled it with iodoform gauze. The operation was performed on the 11th of February, and the patient was discharged cured on the 13th of April.

Now, while these successes favored the belief that a large number of cases of ectopic pregnancy in the second half of gestation were amenable to surgical treatment even when the child was living, it has been maintained that in cases in which the sac occupies the entire extent of the ligamentous folds it is the part of wisdom to refrain from interference until the death of the child takes place and the placental circulation is arrested. But on the 10th of January, 1891, Schauta[5] successfully applied to a case of the kind the principles which govern the removal of intra-ligamentous ovarian cysts. After tying the ovarian artery at the peritoneal fold, which constituted the residue of the ligamentum infundibulo-pelvicum, he incised the peritoneal covering in a circular line corresponding nearly to the largest circumference of the sac. The enucleation of the latter was readily accomplished without rupture of the sac-walls. Considerable hemorrhage resulted from the detachment of the ovum from the uterus. This was temporarily

---

[1] Lazarewitsch, of Kharkoff, reported in 1886 a case in which he extirpated the entire sac with a favorable result. The particulars I have not been able to obtain.

[2] American Journal of Obstetrics, vol. xxi., September, 1888.

[3] Deutsch. Med. Wochenschr , 1890, S. 174.

[4] Arch. f. Gynaek, Bd. xxxvii. S. 286.

[5] Beiträge zur Casuistik, Prognose und Therapie der extrauterin Schwangerschaft, Prag, 1891.

controlled by pressure and later by sutures. The peritoneal borders of the cavity were then sutured to the parietal peritoneum, and the cavity itself was drained by a Mikulicz tampon.

On the 4th of February, 1890,—*i.e.*, nearly a year previous to the case of Schauta,—Professor Rein,[1] of Kiew, reported a successful operation in the thirty-seventh week of pregnancy. He stated that the fœtus, the placenta, and all the membranes were removed by enucleation from the peritoneum in precisely the way resorted to in intra-ligamentous ovarian cysts. The mother made a good recovery. The child was alive two years later. The particulars of this interesting case are not given.

After a careful study of Schauta's case, I decided to operate on the 19th of April, 1893, upon a patient presumably six months pregnant. As the case is one which illustrates most of the difficulties of removing an intra-ligamentous sac, I shall take the liberty of relating it *in extenso*. The abdominal incision extended from about two inches above the navel to the symphysis. The exposed tumor had the reddish-blue aspect of the pregnant uterus. The small intestines were everywhere adherent to its upper portion. The descending colon was displaced inward and pursued an oblique course from the iliac fossa towards the ensiform cartilage. The uterus was attached to the tumor by its lower posterior surface and was deflected to the right of the median line; its fundus and lateral surfaces were well defined. On the right side a portion of the tube about half an inch in length extended from the right cornu to the sac. The left tube was of normal dimensions, and was apparently attached to the sac by a short fold.

The sac was subperitoneal. Its lower segment occupied the entire pelvic space. It was attached to the posterior surface of the uterus beneath the peritoneal covering. There was no pedicle indicated. It was clear that the pregnancy had started in the right tube and had subsequently developed to a great extent between the folds of the broad ligament. The abdominal portion of the tumor contained, as shown by the contractions, and subsequently by microscopical examination, muscular fibres, presumably derived from the tubal walls.

I at first attempted to separate adherent intestines; this, however, was somewhat difficult and was associated with profuse bleeding from the sac-surface. I was therefore obliged to desist and to proceed first to tie the ovarian arteries. Access to the vessel at the right ligamentum infundibulo-pelvicum was difficult, as the sac was everywhere in close contact with the pelvic wall. Two ligatures were easily applied at the uterine insertion. For further security I tied the left ovarian artery, which apparently distributed vessels to the covering of the ovum. These ligatures controlled the bleeding to a marked degree. I then cautiously cut down through the walls of the enveloping sac to the ovum, about two inches above the fundus

---

[1] Zur Laparotomie bei extrauterin Schwangerschaft, Centralblatt für Gynaek., No. 60, December 17, 1892.

of the uterus, and rapidly enlarged the opening in a transverse direction with blunt-pointed scissors. The separation of the ovum was easily effected by the fingers. I had intended to follow the example of Schauta and remove the ovum entire, but before the work was completed the sac ruptured and a living fœtus escaped. As rupture was followed by increased hemorrhage, I directed my assistant to compress the aorta while the enucleation was completed. Fortunately, this was accomplished in a few seconds. The hemorrhage which followed from the placental site was promptly controlled by packing the cavity with iodoform gauze. My assistant next transferred his fingers from the aorta and pressed the gauze firmly downward into the bleeding space.

Afterwards I was able to detach leisurely the remnants of membrane which were adherent to the intestines and to tie off the residue of the sac-walls which extended from the uterus along the site of the affected tube. When the work was finished, there remained of the original cavity only the space between the ligamental folds and the denuded posterior uterine wall.

After the trimming had been completed, the packing was withdrawn and was quickly replaced by a Mikulicz pouch, into which were crowded two strips of gauze, each a yard and a half in length by a half-yard in width. The abdominal incision, so far as the pouch permitted, was then closed. The operation lasted about fifty minutes, and was performed in the presence of upward of one hundred and fifty spectators.

The child moved its limbs after its birth, and, though nothing was done for its preservation, it lived for twenty-six minutes. It measured between eleven and twelve inches in length, and weighed about twenty-four ounces. It had fine hair upon its head. There was some fat in the cellular tissue, but no lanugo and no vernix caseosa. The eyelids were separate, and the pupillary membrane was still distinct. The nails did not reach to the tips of its fingers. It was evidently well advanced in the sixth month.

The patient suffered a good deal from shock following the operation. The temperature sank to 95.6° F., but in the evening she rallied. At nine P.M. the dressings were found soaked with serum tinged with blood. Afterwards the amount of discharge was moderate.

The pulse was rapid (112 to 140) during the first two days. The temperature remained normal until the fifth day. It then rose to 101.8° F., and the patient suffered a good deal from tympanites. She was given three grains of calomel, and an enema of chamomile infusion was administered. A portion of the gauze dressing was removed. On the following day (the sixth) the patient had many watery stools; the pulse and temperature were thereafter normal, but she had much discomfort, and the face had a pinched aspect until the 28th of April (the ninth day), when the stitches and the remainder of the gauze were removed. Convalescence has since then been uninterrupted. The patient has regained her flesh and color, and the sinus has nearly closed.

So far as I have been able to obtain records, there have now (1894) been reported sixteen successful cases of cœliotomy performed with the fœtus living in the second half of ectopic pregnancy,—viz., those of Breisky, Braun, Eastman, Jessup, Rein, Lazarewitsch, Lusk, Martin, Olshausen, Schauta, Taylor, Treuh, John Williams, Brühl, Lihotzky, and Mordecai Price.

While it is evident that much remains in the way of perfecting the technique of the primary operation in advanced extra-uterine gestation, the evidence herewith presented is sufficient to show that under the most difficult circumstances it is not necessary to fold the hands and await the occurrence of a miracle.

As an example of modern surgical resources, Mackenrodt relates that, in the case of a woman who was insensible and pulseless from internal hemorrhage due to a ruptured tube, he inserted at the time of operation a tranfusion-tube into each mamma, and thus introduced into the system an abundance of a saline solution. No chloroform was given. The operation was short. During the application of the binder the pulse returned to the wrist. The patient became conscious and recovered. Dührsen reports a similar success.

3. *Cases of Gestation after the Death of the Fœtus.* After the death of the fœtus the same principles hold good so long as the sac-contents have not been infected. After putrefaction or pus-formation has set in, the older method of stitching the sac to the abdominal incision previous to opening it is still the best.

The question as to whether the placenta should be detached and the sac filled with a Mikulicz bag, or whether it should be left in place to separate spontaneously, is unsettled. In the latter case it has been found useful to strew the inner surface of the sac with a mixture of tannin and salicylic acid, to act as a styptic and disinfectant. In many instances the walls are too friable to admit of gauze packing.

### THE INTRA- AND EXTRA-PERITONEAL FORMS OF PELVIC HÆMATOCELE.

The term pelvic hæmatocele is applied to encysted collections of blood in the pelvic cavity. It is customary to distinguish the intra-peritoneal form, situated, as a rule, behind the uterus, and the extra-peritoneal variety, or, as it has been better termed, "hæmatoma," between the folds of the broad ligaments.

**Intra-Peritoneal Pelvic Hæmatocele.**—In intra-peritoneal hæmatocele the encysted blood is usually situated behind the uterus, which it pushes upward and forward against the pubis, while below it forms a tumor between the rectum and the vagina. The effusion itself is shut off from the abdominal cavity by adhesions between the small intestines, the sigmoid flexure, the cæcum, the genital organs, and the abdominal walls. In extreme cases it may reach as high as the navel. The sac is subject to movements communicated to it by the diaphragm. When the hemorrhage is considerable, the blood may rise above the ligamenta lata and the uterus and occupy space to the front as well as to the rear of these organs. In very rare cases the encysted blood occupies an anterior situation between the vagina and the bladder.

According to Nélaton, Bernutz, and all the earlier French writers, the visceral adhesions which serve to complete the capsule in which the blood is contained form after the outpouring of the blood. Virchow and his followers, on the other hand, have maintained that antecedent adhesions rendered hæmatocele formation a possibility.

While it may be true that, in moderate hemorrhages, the blood-escape may be circumscribed by secondary adhesions, it is to be borne in mind that ordinarily normal blood is rapidly absorbed by the normal peritoneum. A hæmatocele requires either a hemorrhage of an irritating character which excites a local peritonitis, or a peritoneum thickened by previous inflammation. Modern cœliotomies have shown that the way is, in many instances, prepared by the peritonitis and the matting together of the pelvic viscera incident to a variety of tubal disorders.

The outpoured blood rapidly undergoes coagulation. Membranes, at first soft and glutinous, but speedily becoming of a cartilaginous consistency, form around the clots. Subsequently the peritoneum thickens and fills with vessels of new formation. These membranes, when of long duration, frequently leave behind a permanent thickening between the vagina and the rectum.

The blood in hæmatocele is largely of tubal origin, and is effused most frequently at the menstrual period. A considerable number of cases of hæmatocele is doubtless the result of ruptured tubal pregnancy and of tubal abortion, where favoring conditions—viz., peritoneal thickening and matted viscera—often exist at the time of the hemorrhage. The theory of ectopic pregnancy as the exclusive source of the affection has been rightly disputed. In the non-pregnant state autopsies have shown that blood may be poured from the tubes as a consequence of menstrual disturbances or of rupture of varicose veins. In rare cases, too, hemorrhages may proceed from Graafian follicles, or from hemorrhagic peritonitis, or may be due to a reflex from the uterine cavity in excessive menorrhagia or metrorrhagia.

The symptoms vary according to the severity of the attack. There is no initial chill. The attack is sudden, the patient often complaining at the outset of a feeling as though something had given way; at the same time a sharp pain is experienced, of a peritoneal character, which compels the sufferer to go to bed. The pains are confined to the pelvis, or radiate over the entire abdomen, or down the thighs along the course of the crural or sciatic nerves.

The hemorrhage which forms the basis of a hæmatocele occurs usually at a menstrual period. Menstruation is often temporarily suppressed, returning later, however, as an irregular hemorrhage. For the first week the latter is often profuse; afterwards it has a dark, grumous character, and may continue for weeks. Fehling believes the bleeding to result from an associated interstitial endometritis. If the hemorrhage is very profuse, the patient may become pallid, and suffer from palpitation, yawning, and vomiting, due to acute anæmia. Owing to peritonitis and anæmia, the pulse becomes more rapid (100 to 140), the appetite is lessened, thirst is experienced, and the tongue is dry and coated. Fever is usually absent, or, if present, the temperature rarely exceeds 101° to 102° F. Constipation is the rule. Urination is frequent, difficult, and painful.

So long as the blood is fluid it cannot be well made out by percussion. After coagulation the tumor can be readily determined by bimanual palpation. At first it has an elastic softness; later it becomes dense, nodular, or preserves a partly fluctuating character. By it the rectum is flattened antero-posteriorly, the bladder is dragged upward, and, as has been already mentioned, the uterus is pushed upward and forward against the pubic wall. With the dislocation of the pelvic organs the patient experiences a constant desire to empty the bladder and the rectum.

The prognosis is generally favorable, though, as a result of exertion, of digital examinations, of purgative medicines, or of a return of the menses, a renewal of the hemorrhage is possible.

The usual outcome is absorption. The tumor becomes smaller, harder, and less painful, the uterus returns to its normal position, and the visceral and rectal tenesmus cease. Very rarely, in consequence of the invasion of pathogenic germs, fever is set up, the pains return, suppuration occurs, and perforation takes place usually into the rectum, or more rarely into the bladder or vagina or through the abdominal walls. When the discharge takes place externally, relief is afforded to the patient; when into the peritoneal cavity, death speedily ensues.

The diagnosis is usually easy. The sudden attack, its occurrence at the time of menstruation, the signs of internal hemorrhage, the absence of fever, the rapid formation of the pelvic tumor, and the displacement of the pelvic viscera are sufficiently characteristic. By careful palpation, if necessary under an anæsthetic, it is possible to outline through the rectum the posterior surface of the hæmatocele, and to determine through the vagina the independence of the uterus.

The treatment is mainly expectant. At the outset, cold to the lower abdomen to restrain hemorrhage, prolonged rest in bed, the use of the catheter, if required to empty the bladder, and time (four to six weeks) usually suffice for a cure. I do not personally remember a single instance where surgery was needed to secure a happy issue. In a case of excessive distention of not too recent origin, or suppuration, there is no valid objection to a vaginal incision made with the intent to empty the sac-cavity. Gusserow [1] employed this method in a number of instances to shorten the period of convalescence or to relieve serious symptoms resulting from local press-

---

[1] Arch. f. Gynaek., Bd. xxix. S. 389.

ure. His plan consisted in washing out the vagina with corrosive sublimate solution (1 to 2000), in vaginal incision, and in irrigation of the
sac with a solution of salicylic acid. If the cavity had distinct walls, these
were attached by sutures to the vaginal wound; afterwards a drainage-
tube was introduced into the sac and the vagina was packed with iodoform
gauze. Gusserow deprecates the use of the curette, and warns against
making an opening per vaginam before time enough has elapsed to insure
against a renewal of the hemorrhage. Indeed, should circumstances arise
calling for interference at an early stage of the malady, an opening from
above, after cœliotomy, would possess the advantage of enabling the operator to secure bleeding points under the guidance of the eye.

**Extra-Peritoneal Pelvic Hæmatocele (Hæmatoma).** — This
term is applied to effusions of blood which take place beneath that portion
of the peritoneum which covers the pelvic space. Usually it results from
the rupture of vessels during menstruation, or it may be secondary to tubal
pregnancy, or to rupture of the lower segment during childbirth. As a
rule, the hæmatoma develops between the folds of the broad ligament, sometimes occupying the entire space, or, again, forming circumscribed tumors
in the upper portions of the ligament. Less frequently the peritoneum
may be lifted from the cervix and the bladder. As a rule, the swelling
occupies one ligament only. Sometimes the effusions are bilateral. They
may even dissect up the entire pelvic peritoneum so that the pelvic viscera
are bathed in blood. The sac thus formed is of irregular shape, with
pocket-like recesses, and is here and there traversed by filaments of connective tissue. The effused blood undergoes the usual changes. Coagulation takes place, followed by absorption of the fluid portion; the clot
then adheres to the ragged surface of the sac and is slowly absorbed, or may
remain in part unchanged for months.

Rupture of the peritoneal walls may take place either at the beginning
of the attack as a consequence of pressure, or at a later date as the result
of a disintegration of the sac-contents. Disturbances of circulation are
produced by the presence of the tumor, as evidenced by œdema and thrombi
in more remote tissues, by apoplectic effusions into the ovaries, and by the
development of a hemorrhagic endometritis in the uterus.

The disease is characterized by the suddenness of the onset, by the
colic-like pains, by the intense anæmia ensuing from the loss of blood, and
by the absence of fever. The menstruation is often, at first, arrested for a
short time. The patient experiences a constant inclination to empty the
bladder and the rectum. The tumor is usually at the side of the uterus;
only in exceptional cases it has a bilateral seat, or is found in front of the
uterus. On the side not affected the uterus can be outlined by the finger.
Through the rectum the cul-de-sac of Douglas is found to be empty. In
contradistinction, inflammatory exudations are characterized by a long
preceding illness and are attended by chills, high temperature, and acute
pain.

Gusserow[1] lays stress upon the convexity of the tumor at the pelvic brim in hæmatoma, while the effusion is reached with difficulty through the vagina. In hæmatocele, on the other hand, the blood poured into the cul-de-sac pushes down between the vagina and the rectum, and is definable above only when the space is filled to a marked degree. The prognosis is favorable. Fatal results from internal rupture are exceedingly rare. The treatment is for the most part expectant. In the rare cases where either the local disturbance or the non-absorption of the clots renders interference advisable, an incision can be made as in hæmatocele per vaginam, with due regard to asepsis and drainage; but the irregular, sacculated character of the tumor-walls and the uncertainty attending work done from below lead one to ask whether greater safety is not obtained by abdominal section, as has been especially advocated by Martin.[2] By this method the entire contents can be removed, bleeding points can be secured, and, after drainage has been established by the vagina, the peritoneal incision can be closed by sutures.

---

[1] Arch. f. Gynaek., Ueber Hæmatocele periuterina, Bd. xli. S. 400.

[2] Pathologie und Therapie der Frauenkrankheiten, dritte Auflage, S. 396.

# CHAPTER XV.

## FUNCTIONAL DISEASES.

BY CHAUNCEY D. PALMER, M.D.

### MENSTRUATION.

MENSTRUATION is a periodic function of the uterus, the rhythmic performance and physical changes of which, local and general, occur in the human female for about thirty years.

*Synonymes.*—Menses, courses, periods, turns, catamenia, and "unwell." Of all these terms the most appropriate are "the menses" and "menstruation."

What is it? The menstrual flow consists of blood associated with broken-down epithelium, squamous and ciliated, mucous secretion of the uterus and vagina, and at times débris of the uterine mucous membrane with tubular glands. The latter is very properly called *decidua menstrualis*.

At first slimy, because of the accompanying mucus, thin and pale, it soon becomes dark, of the color of venous blood, growing pale towards the close of the function. Its odor is peculiar and characteristic, and is due to fatty acids and the secretion of the genital glands.

The average quantity is from four to five ounces. There are great variations within the bounds of health. Every woman is a law to herself.

The blood discharged is alkaline in reaction, like ordinary blood, and free from clots, because of its admixture with mucus. There is a hypersecretion from the uterus and the vagina prior to, during, and after the flow, which if slight and temporary is purely physiological, but if excessive and long continued is morbid. A uterine leucorrhœa always begins in this manner.

The duration of the flow varies greatly: the average is from four to five days.

The appearance, odor, quantity, and quality of the menstrual flow are subject to many variations within the bounds of health and disease. Thus they are modified by age, social condition, diet, climate, the degree of physical exercise to which the female is accustomed, and her amount of physical vigor. How the flow is altered by disease will be mentioned hereafter.

768

The menstrual flux comes from the corporeal cavity of the uterus above the internal os. In some cases it may come partly from the Fallopian tubes ; but this is exceptional.

The age at which menstruation first appears is influenced by race, climate, mode of life, and other conditions. Tilt's observations were that Hindoo women in Calcutta menstruate before they are twelve years old, while negroes in Jamaica begin at the average age of fifteen. The usual time of inception of menstruation in temperate climates is at the age of fourteen. In tropical climates it begins earlier, as at twelve ; in extremely cold climates, as in Northern Russia or in Greenland, later, between sixteen and twenty-three. It is estimated that for every ten degrees of latitude farther north or south the menstrual commencement is one year later or earlier. Brunettes generally menstruate earlier than blondes. The earliness of its inception is likewise influenced by city life. City girls commence earlier than their rural sisters, owing to the stimulating influence of social life and more frequent communication with males in recreation and play. Its early appearance in Turkey and India is partly due to premature and improper association of the sexes. It is also earlier in higher life, where there are luxurious habits and indiscreet reading and society. Premature sexual excitement does not necessarily coexist.

Severe labor, hardships, and privations retard it. Its late appearance is sometimes the *result* of constitutional ill health, and not its cause, as is so often supposed. Aside from this, it may be due to tardy or imperfect development of the internal genitalia.

Normal menstruation, when the function has been well established, recurs about once in twenty-eight days, or a lunar month. More rarely it appears at or near the same day of each calendar month.

When menstruation is about to occur, the whole aspect of the female changes : she becomes more modest and shy, the face easily flushes, and the entire demeanor changes. Coincidently with this performance of the uterine function, from a renewal of the growth of the uterus, there is a noticeable mammary growth, and widening of the form, from a development of the pelvis. There is also a growth of hair on the pubes and in the axillæ. The whole contour of the body becomes more rounded and attractive. The uterus, the mammæ, and the pelvis continue developing until the age of twenty, when they are matured—the time of nubility.

**Precocious Menstruation.**—Numerous cases are on record in which menstruation has occurred at a very early age, as from a few days after birth to within the first, second, third, fourth, or fifth year of life, soon followed by the other evidences of puberty above enumerated. In these cases there is a premature, but well-formed, miniature woman, physically speaking, but the mental development is not correspondingly precocious, and the bodily appearance oftentimes leads to uncalled-for expectations and unnecessary exactions from her instructors. The ability for procreation, though rarely tested, no doubt exists. In one case pregnancy and parturition at term occurred at nine years and seven months. This girl commenced to menstruate at twelve months, became pregnant about six weeks before she was nine years old, and after a labor of six hours was delivered of a child weighing seven pounds. The youngest American mother on record was ten years and thirteen days old. She weighed one hundred pounds and was four feet seven inches high; she commenced to menstruate at one year.

Hemorrhage from the genitals of new-born girls must in general be owing to the same causes as hæmatemesis, melæna neonatorum, umbilical hemorrhage, or the epistaxis of infants. These conditions are involved in more or less obscurity. The blood then is always faulty in its composition, with a feeble coagulability, and with a marked fluidity; or there is some abnormal state of the walls of the minute vessels, and a diathesis of hæmophilia, inherited, or dependent on obscure causes, if there is a good family history. A hemorrhagic diathesis may pass from one generation, to reappear in another, in cases of this kind. Congenital syphilis is a recognized cause, creating marked blood dyscrasia in an infant. There may also be a disturbance of circulation, leading to a congestion of the finer capillaries.

Menstruation commonly ceases at about forty-five; earlier, if it has begun very early in life. Morbific influences may cause either its much earlier cessation or its undue continuance. Thus, chronic metritis, in its third stage of sclerosis or cirrhosis, may cause a premature cessation at thirty, thirty-five, or forty; so, also, may superinvolution of the uterus. More often it is continued until later than forty-five, as to fifty or even fifty-five or sixty. Abnormally prolonged menstruation has a satisfactory explanation in many morbid causes, as granular endometritis, or uterine fibroids, polypoids, or cancer.

Menstrual cessation indicates ovarian atrophy. The ovaries shrink, shrivel, and become harder, whiter, and less vascular. Corresponding changes take place in the uterus, vagina, and mammæ. Thus, most of the sexual organs shrink and undergo a physiological atrophy. We are not to infer that the ovaries have ceased their function because menstruation has stopped. As ovulation is in many instances carried on before the menses appear, so it may be continued many years after their cessation.

The interval between the beginning and the end of menstruation constitutes a period of about thirty years, subject to many variations, physiological and pathological, mental, moral, and physical. As stated, many years may be consumed in the total suppression of this function. If the woman is perfectly healthy, her menses appear less and less frequently, the intervals becoming gradually longer, the duration of each time of flow shorter, and the quantity less. In this way the system becomes accommodated to the local and general menstrual changes, with the least physical and mental disturbance.

Menstruation is attended by certain phenomena, local or pelvic, general or constitutional, which are to be considered. The mucous membrane of the uterus thickens, becomes softer and of a deeper color, and is folded and mammillated. The uterine glands enlarge, and their secretion becomes excessive in amount. The decidua menstrualis is formed from the uterine mucous structure. Its maximum growth immediately precedes a menstrual flow, a few days prior to which it undergoes a fatty granular degeneration, and during which it is exfoliated more or less, leaving bare many bleeding blood-vessels. Just how much of the membrane is cast off at each menstruation, and whether the mucous glands are destroyed or not, is a debatable question.

The views of Williams, who has studied this matter much, are as follows. The uterine mucous membrane undergoes fatty degeneration, its vessels rupture, and an extravasation of blood ensues, especially near the surface, for it is there that fatty degeneration is most advanced. The glandular portion of the mucous membrane is shed. This theory presupposes an entire removal of the mucous membrane, down to the muscular fibres, and a regeneration from groups of round cells of the mucous coat.

It is more generally believed that the deeper layers and glands of the mucous tissue remain intact, and that the exfoliated layers are replenished with rapidity after a menstrual period has passed, ten days being sufficient. Ercolani thinks that the decidua menstrualis is formed by a rapid growth of cells derived from and replacing the ciliated epithelium. Kundrat and Engleman maintain, what is probably true, that only the superficial layer of the mucous membrane is shed at each menstrual period. Möricke asserts that during menstruation the mucous membrane disappears entirely. These expressed views show how widely microscopists differ.

Menstruation probably marks a destructive process, following a constructive process of growth of the decidua and the development of the Graafian follicles. The decidua is formed in preparation for the reception of the ovum. Should impregnation result, the decidua menstrualis is converted into the decidua vera, the same tissue in kind, but larger and thicker.

The uterus is always larger and heavier (volume one-third more) and somewhat softer during menstruation than at the middle of the inter-menstrual periods. The pampiniform plexus becomes engorged and enlarged. The cervix is larger, softer, and of a violet color. The os externum and os internum are more open. The physiological hyperæmia and the results do not pass away altogether until one week after the cessation of the flow.

Menstruation is a neurosis, indicating anatomical changes, a hyperplastic action, a degeneration of tissues, and a reparative process. This periodical discharge of blood is the result of a physical conformation, inherent and peculiarly dependent upon ultimate cell changes in the cerebrospinal centres, transmitted to the generative ganglionic system, producing a pelvic fluxion, a uterine and ovarian hyperæmia. A menstrual hypertrophy ensues. The fatty degeneration and the disintegration of the uterine lining are not the causes, but the results, of the menstrual molimen. They corroborate the theory that menstruation is the result, and not the cause, of uterine action.

The trophic nerves govern and equalize the movements of fluxion and the erectility of the female pelvic organs. Emotional and psychical causes give rise to molecular changes, evidenced by a sudden menstrual suppression.

Ovarian erectility and motility are not unlike erection in the male. The corpora cavernosa and corpus spongiosum of the male organ are made up of venous sinuses; so the uterine and peri-uterine spaces are furnished with cavernous sinuses and plexuses, possessed of the same wonderful capacity of rapid unloading and filling. The female generative tract is capable of enormous venous engorgement.

The general phenomena attending menstruation are a somewhat diminished appetite, impaired digestion, and not infrequently diarrhœa and increased micturition. Pigmentation under the eyes and on the face is sometimes noticed. Meteorism is at times present. The glandular system is stimulated. The sudoriferous and sebaceous glands are more active. There is general malaise, with frequent yawning. Both physical and mental vigor are diminished, and there is some mental depression. The face is usually wan and pale. There is a small decrease in weight and a slight fall in temperature. Vascular and nervous tension are somewhat on the decline. Following the cessation of the menstrual flow there is, coincident with a repair of the corporeal mucous membrane, a gradual reconstructive process going on in the body at large. The blood-supply generally increases, the body gains in weight, vigor heightens, vascular and nervous tension augment, and the temperature of the body rises about one-half a degree Fahrenheit (Kiwisch), all of which phenomena, local and general, conclusively prove that menstruation is not a local process, but a general physiological action, a menstrual cycle, finding its local expression in the generative organs. Corroborative evidence of this accepted theory of the menstrual cycle is afforded in the changes which occur at times in some of the morbid processes of the body. Nævi enlarge and assume a deeper color prior to the menses; so do varicose veins of the lower extremities. Menstrual headaches are quite often due to the vascular and nervous changes incident to this function.

To a certain degree the menstrual flux has a depurative influence on the blood: it is a process of purification, in the Mosaic sense. To this periodical discharge of blood the body at large becomes habituated. Its sudden arrest induces abnormal symptoms, from vascular and nervous disturbances. Nature, from conditions of the nervous system back of and beyond the internal genitalia, at times attempts to give vent to this vascular tension by establishing a vicarious discharge of blood from other parts of the body, as the nose, the bronchi, or the rectum. Finally, menstruation is a miniature gestation and parturition,—a gestation, so to speak, of from twenty-three to twenty-five days, and a parturition of four or five days.

As menstruation, conception, gestation, and parturition are the various functions of the uterus, and as these are intimately connected with the function of the ovaries, or ovulation, it becomes necessary to consider their mutual relationship.

When does the Graafian follicle discharge its ovule? The older view is that the ovule is discharged following menstruation. The newer view, advanced by Raciborski, is that when the menses have commenced the ovule has already escaped. Both views are doubtless correct, for there is no invariable rule for all cases. Most impregnations occur within a week following the end of the menses. Many, without doubt, occur before, as proved by the duration of gestation and the conduct of the last menstruation. Some women are at times cognizant of the escape of the ovum, and may prevent an impregnation by avoiding coitus for a week after the end of the menses.

How many ova are discharged at each time? There is no rule as to this. One ovum or many may be expelled, from one or more Graafian follicles, in one or both ovaries, at a certain period of ovulation.

It was formerly held that menstruation was dependent upon ovulation. The newer view, which is well supported, is that menstruation and ovulation are more or less independent of each other.

What reasons are there for believing that women have ovulation without menstruation, not considering cases where there is no uterus?

(a) Ovules have been found in the ovaries of young girls; (b) ovarian tumors, presumably developed from Graafian follicles, have also been found in young girls; (c) pregnancy has occurred prior to menstruation and puberty; (d) pregnancy has occurred during lactation; (e) pregnancy has occurred after the menopause; (f) post-mortems have shown the evidences of previous ovulation, by the existence of a corpus luteum, when there has been no previous menstruation.

All these facts are rather negative evidence and proof of that regarding which we all agree, the occurrence of ovulation without menstruation. But what proof have we that menstruation may, or does, occur without ovulation? This fact is of course more difficult to prove. The evidence is:

(a) The occurrence of menstruation when no Graafian vesicles have ruptured, as shown post mortem; (b) the occurrence of menstruation after single, and especially after double, oöphorectomy or ovariotomy.

Many cases—at least several hundred—are now reported in which menstruation has continued after both ovaries have been removed. The majority of these patients had regular monthly fluxes, and the minority had irregular fluxes. The majority of double ovariotomies or oöphorectomies have been followed by a total and permanent menstrual cessation. So that, as a law, we are justified in saying that menstrual continuance, regular or irregular, after these operations, is exceptional. These exceptions are doubtless explained by:

(a) The law of habit or periodicity; (b) the presence of some ovarian stroma unintentionally allowed to remain; (c) the exceptional presence of a third ovary, or an anomalous distribution of ovarian stroma within the folds of the broad ligaments (Beigel found accessory ovaries eight times in three hundred and fifty autopsies); (d) metrostaxis from chronic uterine disease, fungoid endometrium, polypi, etc.

The cases of pregnancy (Emmet, Garrigues) after double oöphorectomy prove either that a third ovary must have been present, or that ovarian stroma was left behind. Thomas has well remarked that the reason why menstrual cessation is more apt to follow a Tait's than a Battey's operation is that the ovaries are more deeply excised in the former.

All these facts warrant the following statements: Menstruation has never occurred in any female who had no ovaries. A complete extirpation of the ovaries prior to the beginning of menstruation would doubtless have prevented its original occurrence. The prime moving factor of menstruation is a preliminary ovulation. The latter function is established for months, sometimes for years, prior to menstruation. Menstruation being once established, and its law of periodicity having become fixed, it may continue for an uncertain period in the future, without any ovarian stimulus.

Most of the exceptions to the rule of menstrual cessation after oöphorectomy are explainable by the facts above mentioned. A sanguineous discharge from the uterus one or more times following oöphorectomy is usually not menstrual, but the result of some morbid uterine condition. The local irritation of an ovarian ligature applied in the operation of oöphorectomy or ovariotomy not uncommonly creates a sanguineous discharge a few days following these operations.

" Propter uterum est mulier," we used to say. We should rather say now, " propter ovarium est mulier."

## THE MENOPAUSE.

" The menopause" is a term expressive of the conditions existing at the time of the menstrual cessation. This period is also called the climacteric, and the critical period of life. It really comprises all that time of life beginning with the gradual physiological menstrual irregularity, and ending with its entire cessation, after which there is a complete restoration to health. Menstruation may cease abruptly, but more often it is irregular as to time, quantity, and duration during an indefinite number of years. Usually the menopause is attended by a perfectly normal condition, general and local. Manifestations of certain nervous phenomena, mild and evanescent, are by no means uncommon, and if there should be some organic uterine disease, the general and local symptoms at this time become much more serious. Hence, very properly, it is called the critical period of life. Physiologically speaking, it is to the system at large of the elderly woman what the period of puberty is to that of the girl, or what the period of dentition is to that of the infant. It is not fraught with danger, unless there has been some serious local disease in former years.

**Symptoms.**—Sometimes, previous to the menstrual cessation, certain vague nervous symptoms are felt. The most common is what is called " hot flashes," a purely nervous phenomenon, implying a congestion of the nerve-centres, from an arrest of the flow, and relieved by a vicarious hemorrhage, as epistaxis, diarrhœa, or leucorrhœa. The temper at times becomes irritable, and headaches, hysterical attacks, an unnatural fear, or melancholia may be noticed.

There are changes in the physique: the woman grows more fat and develops a growth of hair on the chin or face. Fat in the abdominal walls, simulating pregnancy, is not uncommonly observed. Symptoms of pseudocyesis are at times well pronounced. Pruritus vulvæ and eruptions on the skin are also noticed. Sexual activity where there was previous sexual frigidity is not uncommon.

## DISORDERS OF THE UTERINE FUNCTION.

Menstruation, one of the special functions of the uterus, may be deranged in several ways: as, more or less absent in amenorrhœa; more or less excessive in menorrhagia; or painful in dysmenorrhœa. These are not distinct diseases of the uterus, but derangements of its functions, which are expressive of many conditions, both general and local. Pathological conditions quite different, and even dissimilar, may enter into their causation; hence, like cough and dropsy, they are but symptoms. Medical inquiry must at once be directed to the special underlying morbid conditions giving rise to them. There are great difficulties in the way of a thorough investigation in many of these cases. Fortunately, very correct inferences can be drawn as to their underlying causative factors, by the symptoms of the case and by the age and the social condition of the patient. On the other hand, at times a direct and thorough examination of the concerned organs is absolutely essential for a rational treatment. A successful and scientific treatment of these functional disorders in all their manifestations implies a thorough knowledge of gynæcology.

### AMENORRHŒA.

Amenorrhœa signifies the absence of menstruation. This technical term has an absolute and a relative application. Absolute amenorrhœa means a complete absence of menstruation, and of course implies a duration of at least several months; relative amenorrhœa denotes menstruation which is delayed, scant, and comes on at prolonged intervals. Again, the term applies to those who have never menstruated, a condition called *emansio mensium*. Cessation of the function after it has once been established is called *suppressio mensium*.

Amenorrhœa is a normal condition during pregnancy and lactation; but when, from the age of fifteen to that of forty-five, there is menstrual suppression not from pregnancy or lactation but from disease, it is a true amenorrhœa. As it is based upon general and local conditions, a study of these is most satisfactory.

**Etiology.**—The general causes are:

(*a*) *Acute Diseases.*—The menstrual flow usually ceases during couvalescence from acute diseases, on account of the general debility and anæmia; hence its return is always an indication of a restoration to health.

(*b*) *Chronic diseases*, depressing and exhausting in their nature, cause menstrual suppression. Among these may be noticed chronic diseases of the liver, the stomach, the intestines, the kidneys, and especially the lungs. No better illustration could be afforded than the ordinary manifestation of amenorrhœa in the tubercular diseases, almost always a lung disease. In most of these chronic constitutional diseases the menstrual flow becomes more and more scant and irregular, the intervals being lengthened. Women who suffer from chronic albuminuria or general cancer become amenorrhœic. Anæmia, chlorosis, malaria, syphilis, and general struma, in which diseases the general organs lack sufficient nourishment to carry on this function, are followed by amenorrhœa. Defective hygiene causes it. In some of these conditions there may be no sanguineous menstrual discharge, but instead a profuse muco-purulent leucorrhœa. All cachexiæ are constitutional causes of amenorrhœa.

(c) *Psychical causes* are not uncommon. Sudden and unexpected news, fright, grief, and great anxiety are causes of this kind of menstrual disorder.

An abrupt change in the place of living, association, and climate frequently so acts. Young ladies who go from home to a boarding-school are apt to have amenorrhœa; so are immigrants to this country. There must be some change in the nervous system through the emotions. Again, we are often consulted by the newly married, who, of course, have suspected the possibility of pregnancy. The fear of pregnancy following an illicit coitus not infrequently leads to temporary amenorrhœa. All these are conditions which very properly can be called psychical amenorrhœa. Insanity is almost always associated with amenorrhœa.

The local causes are:

(*a*) An absence or a very imperfect development of the uterus. The uterus is oftener imperfectly developed than any of the other genital organs, certainly much more frequently than the ovaries. Such a condition is found when the whole female physique is otherwise well matured. Then there is also, of course, sterility. The uterus may be fairly well developed, but it is delayed in its growth. The ovaries may be absent or ill developed, so that the sexual changes of puberty have not taken place. Such a condition is usually associated with the absence or imperfect anatomical and physiological changes of the uterus, tubes, and vagina. Cases of the presence of the ovaries, with ovulation, and an absence of the uterus, are often attended by the most aggravating nervous symptoms.

(*b*) Atresiæ, congenital or acquired, are generally causes of menstrual retention, not of menstrual suppression. There is far greater intolerance from the acquired than from the congenital causes. An imperforate hymen is the most frequent and least dangerous of these malformations.

(c) Diseases of the ovaries do not rank first in frequency and importance as local causative conditions creating amenorrhœa. Acute or chronic ovaritis comparatively rarely causes this symptom, and cystic degeneration, passing on to the tumor formations, very seldom does so. Women with large ovarian tumors become amenorrhœic towards the last, from a serious drain on the general health.

(d) Chronic metritis, in its third stage of cirrhosis or uterine atrophy, has for a prominent symptom the amenorrhœic condition. Superinvolution of the uterus, a rare condition, first described by Simpson, is at times a cause.

Acute, followed by chronic, pelvic peritonitis leads to amenorrhœa, from local structural changes induced in the ovaries and tubes.

The diagnosis of amenorrhœa is very easy, but the differentiation of the varied conditions creating this symptom may require the most skilful perception and extended experience.

The prognosis depends upon the cause. Most cases are amenable to treatment; some are utterly incurable.

**Treatment.**—No better example of the importance of a correct diagnosis in determining the line of treatment could be offered than a case of amenorrhœa. We must survey the body at large, to ascertain if the cause is there, and finally explore, if necessary, the pelvic organs. In this diagnostic investigation we first come to a satisfactory conclusion as to whether the amenorrhœa is physiological or pathological. If the former, no treatment is needed. If the latter, the treatment will vary according to the special cause. It must aim at the correction of the underlying morbid conditions.

Amenorrhœa from acute diseases is overcome by such means, dietetic, hygienic, and medicinal, as will restore the general health. A nutritious and well-regulated diet, fresh air, and fair exercise, with general medicinal tonics, are called for. When the special diseases are cured menstruation will in due time return. As progressive decline of the general health from chronic tubercular disease is evidenced by menstrual cessation, so reappearance of menstruation may be regarded as a favorable prognostic symptom. No special attention is to be given this pelvic symptom, but the whole treatment is directed to the pulmonary lesion. Anæmic patients need iron; always, however, after the stomach, if deranged, has been regulated, the appetite improved, and constipation overcome. Iron will fail to increase the quantity and improve the quality of the blood unless the stomach is in a fair condition to receive and assimilate it. Chlorosis calls for iron and arsenic; malaria, for quinine, quinidine, cinchonine, cinchonidine, and chinoidine, and a dry climate. A condition of syphilis needs the mercurials and the iodides.

Amenorrhœa from plethora is an indication for the use of belladonna; from obesity, a dietetic management, especially a skim-milk diet, and an abundance of physical exercise.

Rheumatic amenorrhœa calls for the salicylates. Physiological experimentation with the salicylates shows that they stimulate the menstrual as well as the hepatic secretion. Cimicifuga is a well-selected remedy for rheumatic amenorrhœa, and especially for delayed and painful menstruation. Guaiacum is also a good remedy under similar circumstances.

Strychnine is a good muscle and nerve tonic, and will assist the action of iron. Pulsatilla is indicated when the menses have been stopped by mental shock or fright.

Apiol or apiolene is one of the most safe and efficient emmenagogues. It is not contra-indicated if there is a beginning pregnancy. It may be given in capsules of five to six drops for a dose, two or three times a day, for a few days preceding the expected flow.

Aloes has been regarded as an emmenagogue. It stimulates the functions of the lower intestines and indirectly stimulates the internal genitalia. Therefore, if there is a coexisting constipation, a pill consisting of aloes, or its active principle, aloin, is a good remedy.

A great many American drugs have of late been loudly recommended for the amenorrhœic states, as caulophyllum, aletris farinosa, and polygonum hydropiperoides. At times they are useful.

The hygiene of all amenorrhœic patients needs most careful looking after. A good diet, an abundance of fresh air, out-door exercise, and cold shower-baths are never to be neglected. Sea-bathing is always useful. A change of place is often highly beneficial, particularly from inland to the sea-side. Marriage, too, is at times to be considered.

The use of the so-called direct emmenagogues, as rue, savin, and cantharides, is objectionable. The uterine function should never be forced, when the general system is struggling for existence. Very few remedies have any direct stimulating effect on the lining membrane of the uterus. Some of them, when given in large doses, cause the expulsion of the uterine contents by stimulating its muscular fibres to contract.

Hot hip- and foot-baths are generally useless, unless the function is about to appear.

Acute suppression is best treated by rest in bed, local warmth, hot pediluvia, and hot drinks.

Massage is a therapeutic means which is usually beneficial in the cure of retarded and suspended menstruation. Strong movements involving the pelvic muscles and the adductors of the thigh are useful. The uterus and the ovaries may be manipulated, as it were, through the abdominal walls. Reference is not here made to the methods of Thure Brandt.

As it is not uncommon for the menstrual function to be more or less irregular—seemingly suspended—for the first few years after its beginning, no special medicinal treatment is needed. The delay of the oncoming menstruation from fourteen to twenty years of age also calls for no treatment other than attention to hygiene in diet, dress, exercise, and baths. The uterus in these cases being imperfectly developed, time must be allowed for its normal growth. Look less to the intellectual training of such girls, and more to their physical development.

Iron is the hæmatic tonic, and of course stands first. It has an emmenagogue action, increasing the blood-supply of the pelvic organs of either sex. When the stomach is ready to receive tonic doses of iron, the dried sulphate, the carbonate, the muriated tincture, or the syrup of the iodide may be chosen ; these are the best. The virtues of iron may be increased by quinine and nux vomica. The following is a favorite pill with the author :

> R Ferri sulphatis exsiccati, Ʒii ;
> Quininæ sulphatis, Ʒii ;
> Strychniæ sulphatis, gr. i ;
> Extracti gentianæ, q s.
> Misce et fiat in pil. xl.
> S.—One pill after each meal.

Or the pill of the carbonate of iron—Blaud's pill—may be given. Wyeth's glycerole of the chloride of iron is an excellent preparation. Iron is not contra-indicated if there is obesity. Obese women may be anæmic and hydræmic.

The potassium permanganate and the binoxide of manganese are new additions to our list of emmenagogues. Experience has shown that they are very efficacious. Administered for a few days or weeks preceding menstruation, in doses of from one to two grains three times a day, they have been found to be quite serviceable. The union of the elements of these medicines is so feeble that they readily undergo decomposition. A gelatin-coated pill or a compressed tablet is the best form for their administration.

If there is atresia of the vagina or the uterus, the treatment is surgical. When the occlusion is low down, from an imperforate hymen, or in the vagina above the hymen, a free crucial incision, with thorough antiseptic drainage, is needed. When higher up, an opening in the vaginal tract should be obtained, if practicable ; if not, and there is accumulated menstrual secretion, the distended tract may be perforated through the rectum, and a free opening thence maintained.

Electricity is the most reliable of all the emmenagogues, being the most direct uterine stimulant that we possess. The current may be utilized in either the faradic or the galvanic forms, the former always being tried first. Of the faradic, only the primary or the direct form should be used. The pelvic sympathetic may be stimulated by general faradization or central galvanization. The primary faradic current is best applied as follows : the negative pole is placed within the uterus, by an appropriate intra-uterine electrode, while the positive pole is applied externally to the abdomen or the sacrum. A séance of about fifteen minutes may be held every third day. Simpson's intra-uterine galvanic pessary, as modified by Thomas, need not be used, being purely a local uterine irritant. The galvanic current, in the strength of from five to ten milliampères, may be used if the faradic fails.

The local use of electricity is especially adapted for stubborn, long-continued cases which have resisted the hygienic and medicinal treatment, —for instance, those cases in which the uterus is quite small and ill developed or has been atrophied from superinvolution or chronic metritis, or in which the internal genitalia are markedly dormant and atonic. The good results at times attained have been very surprising. Personally, I have seen fertility follow this intra-uterine treatment when given for amenorrhœa and sterility.

### VICARIOUS MENSTRUATION.

Vicarious menstruation is a condition closely allied to amenorrhœa. It means a condition of the female system in which there is a regularly recurring discharge of blood from other parts of the body besides the uterus. This vicarious sanguineous flow comes from the nose, the bronchial tubes, the stomach, the intestines, or the rectum, generally from a mucous surface; but it may take place from the skin or at the site of a wound or a scar, when the structures are favorable for its exit. In most cases there is also absolute amenorrhœa. Its explanation is easy when we consider the physiological phenomena in the nervous and vascular systems which attend menstruation. As already stated, menstruation is not by any means a purely local pelvic matter, but is always general in its *modus operandi*.

The treatment applicable for vicarious menstruation is that which is adapted for amenorrhœa. Few, if any, means should be made use of to stop the vicarious flow, unless possibly its continuance might be hurtful. Measures calculated to restore the normal direction of the sanguineous discharge have been dwelt upon in discussing the management of amenorrhœa.

### MENORRHAGIA.

Menorrhagia is an excessive menstrual flow, being expressive of a condition the opposite of amenorrhœa. There are menorrhagic conditions as to time, quantity, and duration, as well as an absolute menorrhagia. Thus, if menstruation appears too often, is excessive in quantity, or continues too long, the condition is menorrhagic.

"Menorrhagia" is a term often confounded with "metrorrhagia," which means non-menstrual uterine hemorrhage.

As the amount, the duration, and even the frequency of menstruation vary greatly within physiological limits, it becomes difficult at times to say when normal menstruation ceases and menorrhagia begins.

Etiology.—Both menorrhagia and metrorrhagia are generally dependent upon a common cause, and both usually exist at the same time. They depend upon many and widely different causes, both constitutional and local.

The constitutional or general causes are plethora, anæmia and chlorosis, debility from excessive lactation, hæmophilia, purpura, scorbutus, chronic valvular diseases of the heart, chronic pulmonary diseases, as pneumonia and emphysema, hepatic disease, as chronic cirrhosis, chronic splenic and renal diseases, chronic constipation and abdominal tumors, and psychical influences.

The local pelvic causes are ovarian and peri-uterine congestions and inflammations, tubal inflammatory diseases, hæmatosalpinx, uterine congestion, chronic metritis (first and second stages), subinvolution of the uterus, chronic endometritis, with fungoid granulations, cervical lacerations, uterine displacements, especially retroversion and retroflexion, uterine fibroids and polypi, cancer of the uterus, and retention of the products of conception. Uterine and ovarian congestion followed by menorrhagia may be provoked by excessive coitus. Menorrhagia occasionally accompanies plethora. Stout, obese women generally have scant menstruation.

Thus it will be seen that any cause which essentially alters the quantity or deranges the quality of the blood—plethora, anæmia, chlorosis, or hæmophilia—may lead to excessive menstruation. Women who have had an excessive drain of milk during lactation are apt to have menorrhagia.

Any causes which impede the normal return of the venous blood, as valvular diseases of the heart, chronic pneumonia or emphysema, hepatic, splenic, and renal diseases, abdominal tumors, or loaded bowels, are almost always attended by prolonged and profuse menstruation. Psychical causes also act in the same way. Fright, fear, and excessive mental or emotional disturbances act as potently as do morbid physical conditions.

One of the most common causes is the presence of fungosities within the uterine cavity, either from chronic endometritis or from a retention of some of the products of conception. The profuseness of a menorrhagic attack is by no means in proportion to the size of an intra-uterine growth ; a small polypus and fungosities may act as potently as large tumors.

Malignant disease of the uterus is almost invariably followed by menorrhagia and metrorrhagia. These are among its first symptoms, and they diminish only late in its progress. Many, if not most, women become so accustomed to lose blood per vaginam that any beginning hemorrhage may be neglected. Many women labor under the impression that the change of life must be attended by an excessive menstrual flow. The cause of any excessive menstruation should always be sought, as this is invariably indicative of some disease.

Laceration of the cervix uteri is a very common cause of cervical erosion, eversion, and a general endometritis, with fungoid granulations, hence menorrhagia. Parametritis and perimetritis have metrorrhagia as a common symptom. In all uterine displacements and flexions the uterus is the seat of more or less hyperæmia, from an impeded venous circulation. Of the various displacements retroversion is most commonly so attended.

Subinvolution of the uterus, in which the organ is enlarged, softened, imperfectly contracted, and congested, has menorrhagia for a symptom. Subinvolution is often the first stage of chronic metritis. The second

stage of chronic metritis, or chronic hyperplasia, is also attended by excessive menstruation, and the menorrhagia does not cease until the third stage,
or cirrhosis of the uterus, has commenced.

Treatment.—The treatment of menorrhagia is that appropriate for
the attack proper and for the menstrual interval.

For the attack the first consideration is rest in the recumbent posture.
By this position of the body the pelvic organs, whether the seat of active
or of passive hyperæmia, are, through the influence of gravity, relieved to
no inconsiderable extent of an increased blood-supply. All tight clothing
should be removed. The bed should be hard and cool.

The food should be light and non-stimulating. It is always prudent to
keep the bowels open and the rectum and colon unloaded, and to favor
the return of the portal venous circulation, which is intimately connected
with the pelvic. An occasional so-called cholagogue, followed by a saline,
not too active, may be advantageously employed. Chronic constipation is
always to be overcome by mild doses of salines, and by such agents as small
doses of podophyllin with nux vomica.

Which are the best medicinal hæmostatics will depend entirely upon the
provoking causes. Should the fault lie in the heart's action or in a retarded
venous circulation, one of the best medicines is digitalis. A good tincture
made from the English leaves or a pure infusion is the best form. Digitalis has not a wide range of application, but in certain conditions is a
fairly reliable hæmostatic agent. Temporarily beneficial in uterine hemorrhages resultant on cardiac disease (mitral insufficiency), it may prove curative in other cases. An atonic condition of the circulation, a weak heart,
with slow or rapid action, and low arterial tension—conditions which aggravate, if they do not produce, excessive hyperæmia of the uterus, and hemorrhage—may be combated by digitalis.

Morbid psychical conditions are best relieved by the bromides. Menorrhagia from excessive coitus also calls for bromides.

Faulty conditions of the blood, from anæmia, chlorosis, excessive lactation, hæmophilia, or defective hygiene, are best improved by a good hygiene
and weaning of the child, and by the internal administration of iron and
other tonics. As a rule, iron is contra-indicated during menstruation, especially if the flow is excessive; but to this rule, as to all others, there are
exceptions. Iron, in the form of the muriated tincture, proves to be an
excellent means for checking excessive menstruation dependent on marked
anæmia, hydræmia, and hæmophilia. In most cases iron is to be utilized
only during the menstrual interval.

Menorrhagia from plethora calls for a restricted diet and the use of the
salines and the bromides.

Arsenic is a most valuable hæmostatic in the menorrhagic conditions of
young girls, as well as of women nearing the menopause. Menstruation
which at either time of life comes on too frequently, continues too long, or
is too profuse, being purely functional, is best met by Fowler's solution in

doses of from three to five drops every few hours to two or three times a day. It seems to be indicated when iron is contra-indicated, and may be given during the time of the flow as well as during the interval.

We have seen good results follow the use of gallic acid internally, but do not place much dependence upon it.

Ergot stands at the head of the list of all medicines as a uterine hæmostatic, because of its well-proved physiological effect in stimulating contractions of the involuntary unstriped muscular fibres, wherever found. It is singularly well adapted to conditions of the uterus in which there are well-developed but relaxed muscular fibres with dilated and engorged blood-vessels. Hence such pathological states of the uterus as chronic hyperæmia of the active or passive kind, chronic metritis in its first stage, and sub-involution are controlled best by ergot. These conditions, for manifest reasons, are less marked in the nullipara than in the multipara. The more soft, flabby, relaxed, and engorged with blood the uterus is, the more pronounced will be the good effects of ergot.

Quinine is, of course, the remedy when the disease is of malarial origin. The efficacy of ergot is at times enhanced by combining it with quinine and nux vomica.

One of the most useful of all remedies given internally is hamamelis, in the form of the fluid extract. It is an American remedy, and has been utilized for hemorrhages from all parts of the body and for varicose veins. Hamamelis does not seem to be equally efficient for all kinds of uterine hemorrhage. For the sudden outburst or for active and profuse hemorrhage it is inferior to ergot, but for a slow, long-continued flux, when the blood is dark and venous and the hemorrhage is passive in character, it is the remedy *par excellence*. These are conditions always present in flabby, enlarged, subinvoluted uteri after delivery at term and after abortions, also in some forms of chronic endometritis, before or following the removal of fungosities, and in chronic retroversion, some fibroids, etc. I have also found hamamelis to exert a favorable influence upon urinary hemorrhages in several cases of papilloma of the female bladder. The fluid extracts of secale cornutum and of hamamelis make an efficacious combination.

Viburnum prunifolium has been successfully used, especially when the menorrhagia has been coupled with dysmenorrhœa. Cannabis indica is highly recommended by Churchill and Thomas.

Hydrastis canadensis has been favorably reported upon by various European authorities. By them it is regarded as a vaso-constrictor in congested states of relaxed mucous membranes. For uterine hemorrhages due to metritis, endometritis, myomata, or incomplete involution it has been found to be invaluable. It combines well with the fluid extract of ergot. Hydrastinin appears to be the best form for the administration of hydrastis. A ten-per-cent. solution of hydrastinin may be given hypodermically, but an excellent form for its use is a preparation made by Lloyd Brothers, of Cincinnati, called " Lloyd's Specific Medication." This possesses all the active ingredients of the drug, without any of the extraneous materials found in fluid extracts.

The action of all medicinal agents should be supplemented in bad cases by local applications. Cloths wrung out of cold water, or a rubber bag filled with ice-water, may be applied to the hypogastric region. Quite cold water may be injected into the rectum. Heat is also a good remedy, better than cold. This is admirably illustrated in the treatment of post-partum puerperal hemorrhage. A large quantity of very hot water, from 125° to 135° F., may be injected into the vagina in bad cases. Should the patient become profoundly anæmic and swoon from loss of blood, an excellent way to revive her is to inject a pint or more of hot salt water into the rectum, thereby directly stopping the flow, and sustaining her by the absorption of the saline fluid.

The best non-surgical local means is the use of the vaginal tampon. When the hemorrhage is severe, and when on account of distance it is not practicable to visit the patient often, the whole vagina and the cervical canal may be tamponed with dry absorbent cotton, after the use of hot-water vaginal irrigation. To add to the efficiency of these tampons, those in contact with the cervix may be medicated with glycerite of alum. These tampons are allowed to remain from twelve to twenty-four hours and are then removed; the vagina is then again irrigated with hot water, and is again tamponed, if necessary. Internal medication suited to the case is continued. If the flow is excessive and life is endangered, any oozing should be detected by frequent inspections. Should the vaginal packing fail, the uterine cavity is to be packed with tampons of appropriate size, after dilatation with the metallic forceps. Dilatation, curettage, and uterine packing with iodoform gauze, applied with a suitable intra-uterine forceps, are not to be neglected in many of these cases of chronic hemorrhagic endometritis.

The following principles are ever to be borne in mind in the treatment of menorrhagia and metrorrhagia. In all cases, if any local interference is needed, see that the uterine canal is kept open ; obtain and maintain a patulous uterine canal. This of itself tends to arrest the bleeding. Then remove all foreign bodies, products of conception, fungoid granulations, intra-uterine polypoids, and fibroid tumors. During the intervals, the judicious and thorough use of the intra-uterine curette is one of the best means of promptly and safely curing many of these cases. Its use should precede any intra-uterine medication. The best local uterine medicaments are Churchill's tincture of iodine, iodized phenol, and iodo-tannin. These medicaments may be applied with a cotton-wrapped probe or with the intra-uterine syringe.

Intra-uterine injections are safe if the cervical canal is patulous, if the fluid is warm, if no air is injected, and if no force is employed.

Puncture of the cervix to abstract blood, followed by applications of tampons of boro-glyceride, does good in some cases of chronic congestion of the uterus.

Removal of the uterine appendages should be adopted only as a last resort in any case. Cancer of the uterus calls for hysterectomy, partial or complete.

Malpositions of the uterus which give rise to menorrhagia are treated by rectification of the position of the organ, by tampons, by electricity, and by pessaries. Any coexisting chronic endometritis is to be combated by dilatation, curettage, and packing. Lacerations of the cervix, and their sequelæ, call for curettage and trachelorrhaphy.

Local galvanization of the uterus is a therapeutic agent worthy of the highest consideration in bad cases of uterine hemorrhage dependent upon uterine fibroids and chronic affections of the endometrium. It is often best to use the curette a week before commencing the use of the galvanization. The positive pole, a suitable sterilized electrode of iridium or platinum, should always be applied within the uterus. The effect of the positive pole is to coagulate the albuminous particles in its immediate vicinity, and thereby to produce a hardness of these tissues. This characteristic action varies with the strength of the current, from slight congealing and hardening of the tissues, to general coagulation and solidification for a considerable space around. Positive galvanization is, then, a most potent uterine hæmostatic.

Chronic endometritis with hemorrhagic vegetations is more amenable to positive galvanization than are uterine fibroids. Chronic metritis, associated as it usually is with chronic endometritis, is also greatly benefited by local galvanization of the uterus, the positive pole being utilized in the first and second stages, and the negative pole in the third stage. The absorption of the hypertrophied tissue is stimulated by the inter-polar effect, while the polar effect is localized on the diseased endometrium and its immediate surroundings. The séances may be for fifteen minutes once in three days, the strength of the current being from ten to fifty milliampères.

### DYSMENORRHŒA.

" Dysmenorrhœa" means difficult or obstructed menstruation, and refers to pain preceding, accompanying, or following the menstrual discharge.

A certain sense of pelvic fulness and discomfort doubtless almost always attends the menstrual function, but, as normal menstruation is not attended with any special pain, any menstrual period which is painful is called one with dysmenorrhœa. All chronic inflammatory pelvic diseases attended with pain at the menstrual interval have more pain at the time of the flow, but this is not dysmenorrhœa; nor are those cases in which inter-menstrual pain comes on with marked regularity about the middle of the inter-menstrual period instances of dysmenorrhœa.

Dysmenorrhœa is one of the most common of the various menstrual derangements, and manifests itself by pain, which varies greatly as to frequency, duration, time, and severity. As it simulates other pelvic affections, they are sometimes taken for it, and *vice versa*.

Dysmenorrhœa may properly be divided into the following varieties:

the neuralgic, the congestive or inflammatory, the obstructive, and the membranous. All these forms have symptoms more or less in common, but, as they are different in their essential morbid conditions, it becomes necessary for the purpose of treatment to determine each variety presenting itself. The dividing line between the varieties is not always well marked. Normal menstruation depends almost as much on a good condition of the constitution at large as on a healthy state of the intra-pelvic organs. Hence dysmenorrhœa may be constitutional or local in its origin. The variety known as ovarian differs from the others more in location than in kind. Spasmodic dysmenorrhœa is a term applied to the neuralgic form in which there is a spasm of the circular fibres about the os internum.

### Neuralgic Dysmenorrhœa.

Neuralgic dysmenorrhœa is a variety in which no special disease of the uterus or the appendages may be detected. Ordinarily, on the most careful physical exploration, no alteration in size, shape, position, consistency, or vascularity of the pelvic organs or structures will be noticed ; or, if any is observed in any case, the morbid condition is quite uncertain as to location, quantity, or variety, no two cases being alike. Again, a seeming causative local disease may be cured, but the dysmenorrhœa continues, showing us that the pathological entity, as appreciated by our senses, is not pathognomonic. The most severe types of the malady are seen in nulliparæ in whom there is no structural lesion of the uterus. There is a neuralgic or hyperæsthetic, it may be at times a congested, condition of the corporeal uterine membrane. The insertion of the uterine sound or an electrode to the os internum uteri and along the mucosa elicits pain identical in kind and degree with the dysmenorrhœic pain. A slight discharge of blood sometimes follows this method of exploration, even when carefully done. Then there must be a congestion of the endometrium ; but the pain produced cannot be the result of this condition alone, being out of all proportion to it. The sentient nerves of the endometrium are in a state of hyperæsthesia —a neuralgia. This hyperæsthesia is mostly at the os internum. It is not improbable that a fissured state of the neighboring endometrium, inducing a spasm, may at times excite a contraction such as we see in anal fissures. In such a state menstrual pain will be excited by the influx of blood into the tissues. The greater the tension and the rigidity of these tissues, other things being equal, the greater the pain ; and this is probably one explanation of the greater relative frequency of dysmenorrhœa in the unmarried and the nulliparous. A similar unyielding character of tissue is present in some cases of chronic metritis. With it there are undue vascular tension and a compression of the end nerves, which are always irritable. When the flow is well established, the swelling subsides, and tension is relieved.

Causes.—In no variety of dysmenorrhœa is it more important to determine the constitutional condition. There is present a local neurotic state provoked to the excitation of pain by the stimulus of the physiological pelvic congestion incident to the oncoming menstruation. This pain is increased by the presence of the hemorrhagic flow within the uterine cavity. The local neurosis, an expression of the nervous system in which there is an exalted sensibility to pain, shows itself by general hysterical phenomena, spinal irritation, neurasthenia, and local and general neuralgiæ. Pain, like age, is relative. The causes may be the same, but no two patients suffer alike. Anæmic and chlorotic states of the blood always predispose to neuralgic dysmenorrhœa.

Rheumatism and gout are direct exciting causes. The rheumatic dysmenorrhœa much resembles the neuralgic. All habits of body conducive to indolence, want of proper physical exercise, and faulty methods of dress, by enervating the nervous system, indirectly lead to dysmenorrhœa. Hence the disease is relatively more common in the upper classes. Excessive venery and masturbation favor its development. General ill health retards any easy and physiological disintegration of the intra-uterine membrane.

These diseases are too often the penalty of a poor inheritance, a defective hygiene, a forced education, and the false stimulus of our modern and artificial life.

Symptoms.—Every possible kind of pain may be experienced as to time, duration, severity, and location. Some cases are so pronounced that the pain is felt at the very inception of the menstrual function, and continues with an increasing force for years after, until it becomes very severe, most dreaded, spasmodic, and agonizing. In this neurotic variety the pain is intermittent, remittent, or continuous. Again, it may start after years of painless menstrual life, for instance, commencing after marriage. Severe types of the disease are often associated with reflex headaches, sympathetic nausea and vomiting, or neuralgic pains elsewhere, at the menstrual times, seemingly supplementing or superseding the localized uterine pain. Other organs of the pelvis, as the bladder and rectum, become affected by sympathy. The breasts become tumid and tender. Sometimes there are periods of uncertain length during which there is little or no pain, after which there may be a relapse. Such periods are noticeable after physical or mental recreation, a change of habits, and during and after a time of travelling, with its manifold divertisements.

Severe dysmenorrhœal attacks are always attended with and followed by much prostration, so that weeks may be needed for a full recuperation.

The pain is located in the uterine or ovarian regions, but oftentimes is felt also in other parts of the body. It comes on soon after the commencement of the flow, is most severe during the first day, becomes less during the second day, and least towards the last. The discharge may be scanty or profuse, or consist of clots. The severity of the pain seems to be in inverse proportion to the quantity of the flow. The diminution of pain following the flow is not so manifest in the neuralgic as in the congestive variety.

The diagnosis is made by an exclusion of the other varieties, after a physical exploration and after a careful analysis of the local and general symptoms. Neuralgic dysmenorrhœa is by far the most frequent variety. Commencing early in life, at or soon after puberty, or in early married life, it is found oftenest in those who are subject to the various neurotic diseases.

As stated, although physical exploration quite generally fails to find any morbid conditions of the uterus and its surroundings, one of the most common pathological lesions in this variety is anteflexion or some congenital defect of the uterus. That the flexion itself does not cause the painful menstruation must be apparent. Probably the dysmenorrhœa exists when there is anteflexion because the uterus is ill developed and neurotic.

### Congestive or Inflammatory Dysmenorrhœa.

**Pathology.**—This variety of the disease has a more distinct pathology. Any cause, constitutional or local, which promotes or perpetuates active or passive hyperæmia of the uterus may lead to it. The inflammatory types of the affection are usually of a chronic form, and may not only implicate the uterine tissues proper, but likewise involve the parametric structures,— tubal, ovarian, and peritoneal.

**Symptomatology.**—Pain is usually present for days prior to menstruation, increasing each day as that function approaches, and mitigating more or less after its appearance. The woman feels more at ease after the flow is established, contrary to the clinical phenomenon of the neurotic variety.

The diagnosis is based on the symptomatology and on the signs which are elicited by a physical exploration.

Ovarian dysmenorrhœa implies ovarian congestion or inflammation. Some developmental defect of these organs predisposing to neuralgia, or a varicocele of the pampiniform plexus of the organ, is present. Scanzoni suggested that the ovarian pain in dysmenorrhœa might be due to the maturing of a Graafian vesicle lying deep in the ovarian stroma.

### Obstructive Dysmenorrhœa.

The essential condition of this variety of dysmenorrhœa is a retention of the menstrual secretion. The inference that painful menstruation is mechanical in its origin has seemed most natural because of its directness, simplicity, and plausibility. This theory, popularized by Macintosh, of England, in 1832, and subsequently by Simpson and Marion Sims, has too often swayed professional opinion. In the light of modern gynæcology, and with the present thoroughness of physical pelvic exploration, it cannot be doubted that in a certain proportion of cases obstructions of the uterine canal do exist, and that these may serve to create pain in menstruation.

Abnormities of the uterine cervix, congenital and acquired, with stenosis, are by no means uncommon. Of the congenital form, there is especially the elongated and conoid infra-vaginal cervix, with the pin-hole os; of the acquired, that arising from chronic inflammation of any of the tissues, and especially that resulting from the vicious use of certain caustics. This stenosis is sometimes very great, and there may be.almost complete occlusion. Flexions of the uterus can create obstruction only when they are sharp and the curvature is present to the second degree. Dysmenorrhœa associated with anteflexion does not come from any obstruction of the canal.

Some standard as to the average size of the cervical canal is usually accepted. Tilt has ventured to say, " When the cervical canal will not allow an ordinary sound to pass through it easily, the cervix should be dilated or divided." Sims denied that the easy passage of a medium-sized sound into the cavity is proof that there is no need of surgical interference.

But the size of the canal, like the quantity of the menstrual flux, is relative and not absolute. A much better evidence of obstruction is obtained when immediately following the withdrawal of a small-sized sound pent-up secretion or menstrual blood escapes.

Besides, there are narrowings and tortuosities of the uterine canal from the presence of intra-uterine and interstitial fibroids. Membranous dysmenorrhœa is clearly due to impeded menstrual flux, for as soon as the false membrane is expelled pain is relieved and the uterus is at rest. Under all these circumstances the seat and kind of pain, intermittent, expulsive, and resembling the throes of labor, and the duration and the intermission of the flow, may be more or less characteristic. Such pains are called expulsive, for the uterus is struggling to overcome a resistance and to expel its contents.

It is not difficult to understand how, in a certain sense, all the varieties of dysmenorrhœa (but not all cases) may at times be attended with a certain narrowing of the uterine canal: the neuralgic, by a spasm of the circular fibres, especially at the internal sphincter of the cervix ; the congestive, by a swollen endometrium, clots of blood, and broken-down mucous membrane; and the membranous, by its false membrane. It is clearly understood how long and oft-repeated attacks of pain may lead to structural changes. The neuralgic may become congestive, and conversely. To regard all dysmenorrhœa as practically obstructive seems not only erroneous in theory, but pernicious in practice, and for the following reasons.

There is want of conformity between the seeming causative lesion or abnormity and the symptoms. Not only, as stated, may there be dysmenorrhœa when no abnormal conditions of the uterus as to size, shape, position, or condition can be detected, but, on the other hand, well-defined abnormities of the uterus, as the pin-hole os, the elongated cervix, the contracted canal, the flattened and ill-developed uterine body, and flexions, may be present and there may be no dysmenorrhœa.

Stenosis of the os externum, marked in kind and degree, resulting from chronic inflammation or the unwise use of caustics, and well-defined acquired flexion, are not always attended by menstrual pains. Instances are not wanting of uteri with patulous canals and much attending dysmenorrhœa.

Allowing four days for the menstrual period, and two ounces of fluid for each day,—an amount in excess of most cases,—some forty drops are emitted each hour, or about two-thirds of a drop each minute, a quantity which would easily pass through almost any cervical canal. Therefore we are forced to believe not only that dysmenorrhœa is in most cases not obstructive, but also that any obstruction rarely exists.

Associated with organic diseases or not, sometimes developed but more often aggravated by them, clinical evidence points to the conclusion that the neurotic feature is the only one in many cases, and that it is manifested to a greater or less extent in all.

### Membranous Dysmenorrhœa.

**Pathology.**—This variety, the least common, consists in a casting off, in shreds or in complete sections, of the superficial layer of the uterine mucous membranes. The cast-off film resembles a product of conception, and its expulsion has been mistaken for an early abortion. When complete,

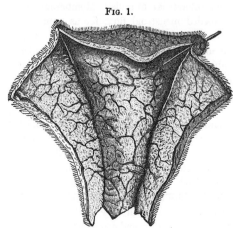

FIG. 1.

Dysmenorrhœal membrane (Coste).

it represents the triangular cavity of the corpus uteri. It is soft, comparatively thick, with many perforations, the sites of the utricular follicles. It is the uterine lining membrane, hypertrophied in all its structures, as in pregnancy, hence called the "menstrual decidua." But the absence of the chorionic villi and the decidual cells proves that it is not a product of pregnancy.

Two views, in the main, are held: that its production is the result of some ovarian disease (Olshausen and Tilt), and that it is a desquamation or exfoliation of the uterine mucous membrane (Raciborski and Simpson). Klob, whose opinions are widely accepted, says that it is an exudation from endometritis. Braun also accepts this view.

**Symptoms.**—The dysmenorrhœic pain begins at the inception of the flow, and increases in severity until the sac is completely expelled. The pains resemble those of early abortion or the first stage of parturition. The menstrual flux increases in quantity until the expulsion occurs. The pain and the flow cease together.

**Diagnosis.**—As it may be mistaken for the products of an early abortion or a mass of blood-clots, polyps, or diphtheritic exudations spontaneously expelled, a careful physical and microscopical examination may be required: this once made, no doubt will remain.

**Prognosis for all Varieties.**—The prognosis of dysmenorrhœa is for the most part favorable. The longer the duration, however, other things being equal, the more difficult it is to effect a cure. The difference in the curability depends largely on the fact that the impressionability of patients to pain becomes more and more marked. Nothing so much increases the susceptibility of the nervous system to pain as the almost constant use of opiates in some form by many of these patients. The abuse of opium and of the whole list of narcotics and stimulants under these circumstances is very great. They induce a condition of the nervous system—a subjective state of pain, exaggerating the patient's sufferings and demanding relief at any cost—more difficult to overcome than the original disease. The neuralgic variety of the malady is more amenable to treatment than formerly, and the great majority of cases are entirely curable. The congestive form is easily relieved, the obstructive is controllable, but the membranous is the most stubborn to combat.

**Treatment of Dysmenorrhœa.**—In this disease there is a practical exemplification of the fact that the underlying essential of all treatment is diagnosis. Having determined the variety of the painful menstruation, and especially the local pelvic condition of the uterus, the ovaries, the tubes, and the parametric tissues, in all cases in which any local examination is justifiable, we are prepared to form a rational plan of management. The treatment may be divided into that which is appropriate for the time of the flow, to relieve pain, and that which is suitable for the menstrual interval, to prevent pain. The latter, then, in a curative sense is more important than the former. Almost all cases of dysmenorrhœa, irrespective of kind, call for some constitutional treatment. A bad constitutional condition favors the disease, and in all long-continued cases the general health is undermined.

Let us now consider first the constitutional treatment appropriate for the menstrual times, in general.

For the attack of pain, of course no local treatment is needed except what the patient employs herself. A great many remedies have been employed to mitigate the menstrual pain, but reference is here made only to such as the author's experience has found useful.

The tincture of pulsatilla is an excellent remedy in a few cases. Unfortunately, it fails more often than it succeeds. It is indicated only in the neurotic types of the disease, especially in young women, but is not contraindicated in any form. It is best given in ten-drop doses three times a day for at least three days preceding the inception of any painful period, and should be continued in similar doses, given more frequently at the time for pain, if pain is then present.

The tincture of cimicifuga may be administered in a similar manner. It is indicated for the neuralgic form of the disease. Unlike pulsatilla, it is generally efficacious. Experience has taught us its usefulness in chronic rheumatism, and it is admirably adapted for the rheumatic types of this disease. In many cases it may be given three times a day during the whole interval, and more frequently at the menstrual time. The salicylates influence the menstrual flow, making it more free and less painful, especially if it is of a rheumatic type. In cases distinctly rheumatic the salicylates may be given three times a day during the menstrual interval, and every two or three hours at the time of the flow. Guaiacum in the ammoniated tincture seems especially adapted for the rheumatic forms. Many years since, a preparation called Fenner's tincture—gum guaiacum and mercuric bichloride—was in common use for dysmenorrhœa, but, like many other remedies in medical practice, had then an uncalled-for application.

A combination of mercuric bichloride and potassium iodide, administered for a long season, is at times very efficacious. Its benefits have not been due to the relief of any syphilitic complications, or to the melting down of any parametric inflammatory infiltrations, the only lesion being a chronic endometritis, with spasmodic dysmenorrhœa.

Viburnum prunifolium is another remedy now much prescribed, and for some cases has a well-deserved reputation. The following is the author's formula for its use:

> ℞ Ext. viburni prunifolii fluidi, ℨj;
>     Tinc. cardamomi comp , ℨss;
>     Syrupi simplicis, ℥ss.—M.
> Sig.—One teaspoonful every two or three hours.

Caulophyllum and viburnum opulus have a similar use. All these last-mentioned remedies act best when the flow is not scanty. The bromides of potassium and sodium seem best indicated in the ovarian types of dysmenorrhœa. Gelsemium is the remedy for cases with rigidity of the cervix and for the spasmodic forms of the disease. Five drops in water may be given each hour.

Cannabis indica is a nerve-stimulant, an anodyne, and an antispasmodic. It acts somewhat like ergot, but more promptly and energetically. It would seem to be indicated in cases where the ovarian neuralgic condition is present. It is certainly to be preferred to opium.

Nitroglycerin, in doses of one drop of a one-per-cent. solution, may be prescribed in cases accompanied with vaso-motor spasm and characterized by pallor and coldness of the skin. Antipyrin would appear to be indicated in a class of cases the opposite of those calling for nitroglycerin, when there is vaso-motor dilatation and flushing of the skin, with an increased temperature.

Apiol or apioline, in capsules of three minims each, every two to three hours, when severe pains precede the appearance of the flow, and in the amenorrhœic forms of dysmenorrhœa, is useful.

The medicine most frequently given is opium, in some of its forms. No remedy is more abused; none should be prescribed less frequently. More harm than good has been done by its administration. It is the easiest matter to create a fondness for its use and favor a physical dependence upon its continuance. Only an extreme necessity would justify its use by the mouth or hypodermically. All its good effects may be obtained and some of its ill effects obviated by giving it in the form of a suppository composed of the aqueous extract of opium combined with the extract of belladonna, only as needed.

All cases of dysmenorrhœa are relieved by rest in a recumbent posture, by hot applications to the lower abdomen, and by the use of the hot vaginal douche. The extremities should be kept warm.

**Treatment during the Interval.**—This is subdivided into the constitutional and the local.

The constitutional treatment implies first the correction of all defective hygienic conditions. Every dysmenorrhœic patient should observe the greatest care in diet, bathing, dress, exercise, and mental exertion. The bowels should be evacuated daily, while systematic cholagogue and saline purgation is called for in the congestive and inflammatory varieties.

Marriage is at times to be considered favorably. Many women with dysmenorrhœa are sterile; but if fertility follows marriage, parturition and lactation may cure the disease. Marriage is often beneficial in the neurotic types of the disease, but is contra-indicated in the congestive, obstructive, and membranous varieties.

Many, if not most, patients with dysmenorrhœa are more or less anæmic, and a scanty menstrual flow is more common than one which is profuse. Hence iron in some form is a very good remedy to begin with. The best preparations are the dried sulphate, the pill of the carbonate, and the muriated tincture. The system at large may be fortified by other tonic remedies, as quinine, strychnine, arsenic, phosphorus, and cod-liver oil, given alone or in combination with iron. Arsenic is called for if the flow is profuse, and mercuric bichloride, with tincture of cinchona, if there is chronic endometritis. The general nutrition may be improved by cod-liver oil, the malt extracts, and a full diet. Arsenic and mercuric bichloride, in minute doses long continued, are the best remedies for the membranous form of the disease.

All excitements, both general and local, as well as undue sexual intercourse, dancing, and the prolonged use of the sewing-machine, are to be avoided.

All morbid conditions of the uterus and the parts surrounding it are to be remedied as far as possible during the interval by proper medical and surgical treatment. One of the most common of these morbid conditions is chronic endometritis. When this is present, thorough uterine curettage, after cervical dilatation, is the first thing needed. Dilatation by expanding forceps after the Ellinger pattern or some of its modifications (as Goodell's or Palmer's) has been practised to a considerable extent, and no doubt many cures have resulted. The method is not employed so frequently as formerly. On theoretical grounds, it would seem to be indicated in cases where there is a highly sensitive, if not a fissured, state of the endometrium about the os internum.    It benefits these cases in the same way that a thorough stretching of the sphincter ani relieves cases of fissures of the anus.

A forcible dilatation repeatedly made with the metal instrument is to be regarded as a surgical operation to be conducted with thorough antiseptic precautions, always followed by a few days' rest in bed.    Curettage may be done at the same time.    Performed with care and special precautions, it is not a dangerous procedure, and almost always does good, at least for some months.    Many relapses occur, however.

Theoretically, electricity appears to be strongly indicated in most cases of dysmenorrhœa, and experience has substantiated this view.    It is especially indicated in the neuralgic form of the disease, but is not contra-indicated in any variety.    General and possibly local faradization (extra-pelvic and intra-pelvic) often do good.    The secondary faradic current (that of tension) is to be preferred to the primary, and might properly be utilized first.    But the galvanic current is far more potent for good.    It should always be given with an intra-uterine metallic electrode, a method which implies that the best antiseptic precautions are to be called into requisition. The vagina should be washed out with an injection of hot mercuric bichloride solution (one to two-thousand), and the intra-uterine electrode, first cleansed and then dipped in a stronger solution of the bichloride, is applied to the fundus uteri, while the other electrode is placed over the abdominal wall.    The polar effect should always be considered.    The positive pole is used if the uterine canal is patulous and the menstrual flow· is too free or too long continued.    It is more useful in controlling pain, diminishing congestion, and lessening irritation than is the faradic.    Hence, as a rule, it is to be chosen.    When, however, the menstrual flow is very scanty, the uterus small, and its canal contracted, the negative pole applied topically will do more good.    The séance should continue for fifteen minutes at least once a week during the menstrual interval, and the strength of the current should be from twenty to forty milliampères.    Very few cases will resist this treatment.    If it is given with antiseptic precautions and followed by necessary rest, bad results need never be expected.

The congestive form may be treated in the same manner, after purgation, rest, and local depletion, if the neurotic element also enters as a factor into the local condition.

Believing that stenosis exists much oftener at the external than at the internal os uteri, it can readily be understood why sterility is far more frequent and persistent than dysmenorrhœa.    It is easier for the menstrual discharge to escape than it is for the spermatic fluid to effect an entrance. It is well-nigh impossible for sterility to continue over a period of five years of married life without causing local disease,—catarrh, parenchymatous congestion, displacements of the uterus, and, finally, sympathetic disorders of the ovaries.    So vascular are these organs that they cannot be subjected for years to the hurtful influences of oft-repeated, as well as the periodical, influxes of blood, without a rest, and yet suffer no disturbances in circulation. From this cause, and perhaps others less active, the quantity of the glandular secretion, as well as that of the menstrual discharge, is increased, and any existing stenosis is made relatively greater. The only rational treatment is to strike at the original cause, and to remove the first link in the chain of the disease. Open up the stenosed canal. Painful menstruation is thereby mitigated, and the chances for fertility are increased. Galvanization is an admirable remedy under these circumstances, the negative pole, for its local dilating effect, being chosen.

**Treatment of Membranous Dysmenorrhœa.**—This variety is the most intractable of all, dependent, as it generally is, on some morbid condition of the corporeal endometrium. It is best treated by a certain amount of cervical dilatation, followed by a thorough curettage of the endometrium with a sharp instrument and packing with iodoform gauze. This operation is done about one week preceding the expected menstrual period, and may be repeated about one week after its close. Intra-uterine galvanization may follow in another week. The intra-uterine electrode should be the negative pole, because of its dilating effect. I am disposed to attribute greater therapeutic power in these cases to careful, thorough galvanization (from ten to twenty-five milliampères) than to very frequent curettage and intra-uterine medication.

### STERILITY.

This is another functional disorder of the uterus, and implies an inability for impregnation during normal reproductive life.

Sterility is either relative or absolute. In the former condition there is diminished procreative power, in the latter procreation is impossible.

Sterility is sometimes congenital, resulting from faulty development. It is said to be acquired when it arises from disease after an uncertain period of fertility.

Matthews Duncan says that one marriage in ten in Great Britain is sterile. Probably the percentage is larger in the United States. Many women are childless in early married life from intentional causes.

A marriage may be unfruitful from causes pertaining either to the male or to the female. More women than men are sterile, in the ratio probably of six to one, though de Sinéty makes it four to one. Sterility exists, however, in men much oftener than is commonly supposed. Its greater frequency in women is easily understood when it is remembered that the function of the male in reproduction ends with the discharge of the semen, but that the function of the female only begins then, and continues for a long time afterwards. If impregnation or fecundation occurs, some morbid action may interfere with gestation at any time in its course. Sterility then, of course, follows. Fertility implies, therefore, normal fecundation and gestation.

Let us first see how these processes may be thwarted in the female, and then consider in general the causes of sterility in the male.

1. Sterility may arise from an inability to perform coitus. Semen must be deposited by the male within the genital canal of the female. But impregnation becomes impossible from absence or very incomplete development of the vagina, atresia of the vagina, vaginismus, and imperforate hymen.

Most of the faulty developments of the external genital organs of the female may prevent coitus. Not infrequently the meatus urinarius is situated in a mere depression between the labia majora, and sexual intercourse has repeatedly taken place within the urethra.

The vagina may be partitioned (double vagina) so that there is stenosis. Intromission is then impossible. The labia minora may be adherent through their whole length. Great hypertrophy of the labia or clitoris may result from elephantiasis or tumors of some kind.

The hymen may be not only tough and imperforate, but also greatly distensible. If it is perforate, although it impedes coitus, pregnancy may ensue, for a drop of semen may be sufficient to give rise to fecundation, if it enters any minute orifice of the vaginal tube.

Vaginismus is a condition of the vulvar orifice in which all attempts to introduce the penis within the vagina cause extreme suffering. The sphincter vaginæ or the muscles of the pelvic floor may also be thrown into a spasmodic state. A digital examination or the insertion of a vaginal tube is attended by a similar spasm. A vulvar or vaginal inflammation, an erosion, or a fissure about the carunculæ myrtiformes is usually at the bottom of this trouble. A vulvar or vaginal hyperæsthesia explains some cases. Vaginismus also, but more rarely, exists in the upper vagina, from which the semen is then immediately expelled.

Sterility may ensue when there is pain in coitus, a condition called by Barnes dyspareunia. The causes of dyspareunia are manifold. These are vulvitis, vaginitis, milder forms of vaginismus, rough attempts of the male at coitus, excessive sexual intercourse, lacerations of the cervix uteri, uterine inflammations and displacements, ovarian inflammation and prolapse, peri-uterine inflammations, urethral caruncles, fissures of the rectum, painful hemorrhoids, etc. As, however, none of these prevent intromission or the deposit of the semen within the vagina, they need not prevent impregnation. If sterility results from any of them, it is not because of the symptomatic dyspareunia, but from the disorders themselves preventing impregnation or thwarting gestation.

2. Sterility may result from inability of the semen to enter the uterine cavity. Under these circumstances coitus may be painless and complete, but fecundation becomes impossible from atresia or stenosis of the os externum uteri or the cervical canal, flexions and displacements of the uterus, tumors of the uterus, and alterations in the quality and the quantity of the uterine discharge.

Rarely indeed do we see a completely imperforate os uteri. Much more frequently there is observed a partial occlusion or stenosis, which is congenital or acquired. The congenital form shows itself in what is called the pinhole os, with an elongated conoid cervix, a very common but not a certain cause of sterility. Quite generally this condition is associated with dysmenorrhœa. Acquired stenosis of the canal may be the result of a pernicious use of caustics, especially the nitrate of silver, so commonly employed years ago. Again, it may arise from a cicatricial contraction of the parts, from injuries during parturition, or after certain surgical operations, as trachelorrhaphy. This stenosis may be present in any part of the cervical canal, but most commonly it is at the os externum. No doubt in many of these cases of sterility other conditions enter into the causation. A very small os may allow the entrance of spermatozoids, as they very often pass through a smaller opening into the Fallopian tubes. Then fecundation may occur, although there may have been an obstructive dysmenorrhœa, and with it some mucous as well as menstrual retention. A secondary endometritis in time follows, and this adds to the causes of sterility. A coexisting dysmenorrhœa is always more easy to relieve than a sterility. A pinhole os externum, with a conoid cervix, is the most common of the congenital conditions creating sterility.

Various theories have been propounded to explain the entrance of the spermatozoids within the uterus. The uterus after a sexual orgasm has a certain suction power, but the chief agent is the inherent activity of the spermatozoids.

Uterine flexions and displacements lessen the chances of fertility. Both of these conditions are extremely apt to coexist with endometrial catarrh, which oftener causes the sterility than the obstruction. Malpositions are always associated with disorders of circulation, and the latter become the chief etiological factors of sterility.

Uterine tumors cause obstructions, but are followed sooner or later by uterine catarrh, and this clinical factor is always to be considered.

Anteflexion is a frequent cause of congenital sterility. Chronic endometritis, cervical, corporeal, or general, invariably increases the quantity and alters the quality of the uterine discharge. The spermatozoids are washed away and thus prevented from entering the uterine canal; their vitality also is impaired. There is no more common cause of sterility than this; certainly it is the most common of the acquired causes.

The vitality of the sperm may be destroyed by excessive acidity of the vaginal mucus. This condition exists, for the most part, in married women after one or more deliveries, and constitutes a variety of acquired sterility. Any cause which prevents the entrance of healthy sperm within the uterine canal may prevent fecundation; nevertheless, fertility may exist when seeming obstructions are found. Women vary greatly in their procreative powers. I have known conception to occur when the cervix uteri was seriously diseased from cancer, and when there was a vesico-vaginal fistula, although the urine is considered poisonous to the spermatozoids.

3. Sterility may result from an incapacity for proper ovulation. This is a cause of impairment of fecundation or insemination which is not so easily recognized as are the morbid conditions of the uterus that may be detected by touch and by sight. Under this head may be included any condition of the ovary which impairs the ovule, as chronic ovaritis in some of its forms, peri-oöphoritis, and cystic degeneration. These conditions of the ovary explain many obscure cases of sterility. Imperfect development of the ovule may also result from any general debilitating disease, as anæmia, scrofula, tuberculosis, or syphilis. Obese women are often sterile, no doubt from imperfect ovulation. A rich diet and a life of luxury diminish fertility; a spare diet and poverty seem to favor it.

Gonorrhœa, it matters not how contracted, is a very common cause of sterility in women. Gonorrhœa in women not only causes vulvitis, vaginitis, and an inflammation of the vulvo-vaginal glands, with urethritis and cystitis, but, as a rule, it also causes endometritis, salpingitis, pelvic peritonitis, and oöphoritis. To Dr. Noeggerath we are indebted for a thorough elucidation of this subject. While experience has established much which he enunciated in 1872, it has been clearly demonstrated that some of his statements, as to the frequency of the continuance of gonorrhœa in men and women after its seeming disappearance, are exaggerations. Gonorrhœa in either sex is a stubborn and long-continued disease. It has many complications in both sexes, but especially in women. In some cases, no doubt, it has an indefinite continuance; but cures are by no means impossible.

Ovulation may be perfect in the development of the ovule, but, owing to organic changes in the ovary or in the Fallopian tubes (hydro-, pyo-, or hæmato-salpinx), or to pelvic peritonitis, mechanically preventing an instinctive application of the fimbriæ to the ovaries, sterility results. To Bernutz and Goupil we are indebted for much of our knowledge concerning pelvic peritonitis. In many of these cases the ovule escapes from the ovary, but fails to reach the uterine cavity.

4. Sterility may arise from inability to continue and complete gestation. Although the sperm has entered the uterine canal and the fecundated product is within the uterine cavity, conception and gestation having taken place, still, this last physiological process of fertility is, for various reasons, not completed. Abortions occur early in gestation, and with great frequency. Ninety per cent. of all child-bearing women abort once or oftener during their lives. One out of twelve pregnancies ends in an abortion.

Abortions may also take place from traumatic causes, emotional violence, and pelvic and general diseases. The fecundated ovule, having entered the uterine cavity, may fail to find a suitable soil for its attachment and development. The causes of abortion are paternal, maternal, and fœtal. Syphilis is a very common cause. The development of the embryo depends very much on a normal condition of the decidua, and the healthy decidua depends greatly on a healthy endometrium. Catarrhal and syphilitic inflammations prevent and arrest gestation.

5. Sterility may result from a want of physical adaptation of the parties,—sexual incompatibility. A married life may be sterile for years, yet when either party obtains a new companion fertility may follow. Napoleon Bonaparte, for instance, had no child by Josephine, which led to his unlucky and inhuman divorce; he married again and had a child. Josephine was fertile by her first husband. There must be some physiological difference in the spermatozoids or the ovules of different persons. The sperm of some may be more active; the germs of others may be more susceptible of impregnation.

Contrary to what has been commonly believed, phthisical subjects do not show diminished fertility. The progress of phthisis seems to be retarded during pregnancy, but is always hastened after delivery.

Women very young in years have conceived long before puberty, while others advanced in years have been delivered long after the menopause.

Sexual enjoyment is not necessary for impregnation. Conception has occurred after a rape, or when the female has been under the influence of an anæsthetic or stupefied by alcohol or narcotics, and not unfrequently when she is perfectly passive or is disgusted with sexual intercourse.

Sterility is temporarily physiological after delivery, and usually, but not always, during the whole period of lactation. Not a few women avoid another pregnancy by prolonging the time of suckling, though conception during lactation is by no means uncommon.

The causes of sterility in the male are impotency, and also azoöspermia, when the seminal fluid contains no spermatozoids or only such as have a feeble vitality. The microscope alone detects this condition, which is found at times in men otherwise in good health and of normal sexual vigor. When normal spermatic fluid is deposited in the healthy vagina or cervical canal, the vitality of the spermatozoids ought to be maintained from five to ten hours or more.

**Diagnosis.**—The diagnosis of the morbid condition producing sterility is of the utmost importance. A judicious appreciation of the actual pathological state impairing or destroying the normal fertility is by no means an easy matter. Success in the management of sterility depends largely upon a correct diagnosis. At times all the means of diagnosis may be required. Touch, bimanual exploration, the speculum, the sound, the dilator, and the volsellum, together with inspection, palpation, percussion, and auscultation of the genital organs, are to be called into play, as needed.

**Prognosis.**—The prognosis is certain and favorable in some cases, uncertain and unfavorable in others, according to the conditions present. There is often great disappointment in the treatment of sterility.

**Treatment.**—The special treatment of all varieties is the removal of the cause, if practicable. This, of course, presupposes a correct diagnosis, and a determination as to whether the sterility is the fault of the wife or of the husband. In all cases of long-continued sterility, after having thoroughly examined the female without finding a satisfactory cause for the same, the investigation should be commenced with the male. Obtain some semen from the vagina of the wife, within a short time after a coitus, for a microscopical examination. In case the cause is found with the husband, treatment of the wife is useless.

It is not in place here to speak of the management of sterility in the male. For barrenness of the female we remove and correct, as best we can, all causes which impede coitus. An atresia of the vagina, an imperforate hymen, or a bad vaginismus is to be overcome by appropriate, mostly surgical, means. Conditions, congenital or acquired, may be detected which render the treatment not only unsatisfactory but useless. If there is dyspareunia from vulvitis, vaginitis, vulvar hyperæsthesia, chronic endometritis, chronic metritis, chronic pelvic peritonitis, chronic salpingitis, chronic ovaritis, ovarian prolapse, displacements of the uterus, or a diseased urethra, bladder, or rectum, these need special care and attention. Removal of these diseases may prolong life, make it more comfortable, and increase the chances of impregnation.

If semen fails to enter the uterine cavity because of displacements or flexions of the uterus, this organ is to be replaced and maintained in a normal position. Most displacements of the uterus are secondary to, and associated with, endometritis or metritis, the correction of which is of the first importance.

Stenosis of the os uteri may be remedied by a crucial incision, dilatation, and galvanism with the negative pole within the cervical canal. Mild cases of stenosis are best treated by negative galvanization, which tends also to correct any coexisting cervical catarrh. If, however, there is a decidedly elongated conoid cervix, with a pinhole os externum, the best procedure is to curette the uterine cavity, for the resulting uterine catarrh, and then to excise a wedge-shaped piece from the infra-vaginal conoid cervix and to stitch the opposing cervical lips together. If thorough antiseptic precautions are taken, and if no peri-metric inflammation is lurking behind, this operation is simple and unattended with danger; otherwise it may be followed by an acute peritonitis and death, as simple discission of the cervix not unfrequently was in times past. Symmetry of the parts is best obtained by good incisions and a careful suturing.

Under no circumstances ought the woman's life to be endangered by any surgical measures. No operation should be undertaken unless it is absolutely certain that the fault is hers. Results are too uncertain and the risks too great to allow of unnecessary manipulations.

Chronic endometritis in its many forms is best combated by dilatation, curetting, and packing with gauze, followed by intra-uterine medication or intra-uterine galvanization.

"No grass grows on a well-trodden path." Prostitutes rarely conceive, partly, at least, because of their frequent coition. Rare indulgence favors fertility. If children are desired, great moderation is advisable.

Abstinence from sexual intercourse for months at a time is in some cases beneficial, not only by curing the disease which causes the sterility, but also by increasing the chances of impregnation. A separation of husband and wife for considerable periods is under many circumstances advisable.

If the uterus is absent or very small, less than an inch and a half in length, all efforts to insure fertility would seem to be hopeless. An ill-developed uterus, not less than two inches long, may be stimulated to grow if the patient is young and otherwise healthy.

In correcting by trachelorrhaphy the eversion, erosion, and hypertrophy of the cervix uteri following bad lacerations, it is important that the cervical lips be not so closely sutured together as to impair fertility, a not unfrequent result. A stenosis caused by the improper use of nitrate of silver needs correction by incisions or dilatations. A laceration of the cervix may cause sterility by impairing the retentive power of the uterus. Trachelorrhaphy is then indicated.

When is impregnation most likely to occur? Fecundation may in some cases result from coition at any time during the month. Nevertheless, it is true that it is most apt to occur within a week after the cessation of the menstrual flow. Doubtless a prolonged dorsal decubitus, with elevated hips, favors the retention of the seminal fluid within the vagina and aids impregnation, especially if there be a vaginismus of the upper part of the vagina.

Impregnation may occur and an early unsuspected abortion may take place. Most of these abortions result from undue frequency in coitus, from violence in the act, or from some impairment of gestation by endometritis.

Excessive acidity of the vagina is to be overcome by the internal use of alkaline Vichy water, and by vaginal injections of potassium carbonate in solution just prior to coition.

All the best-known tonics, iron, quinine, strychnine, arsenic, phosphorus, cod-liver oil, and faradic electricity, by improving the general health, favor fertility.

*Artificial Impregnation.*—Can anything be done artificially to promote impregnation? In those cases in which there is a serious obstacle to the passage of the sperm into the uterus this fluid may be introduced within the uterine canal by mechanical means. Being first assured by a microscopical examination that the husband's semen is capable of causing fecundation, and that there is otherwise no serious obstacle to gestation, the consent of both parties having been obtained, the following method may be resorted to. Normal coitus is practised. The woman maintains the recumbent posture, and within an hour afterwards a small quantity of the semen from the vagina is sucked into a properly constructed syringe warmed to the body temperature, and a few drops of the same are injected into the uterus beyond the internal os. The woman remains in bed for a few hours following this procedure.

Marion Sims has had the greatest experience with this operation, and it has been successful in the hands of Gérault, de Sinéty, and others. There is no reason why it should not be tried, in otherwise unsuccessful cases, when legitimate reasons make offspring desirable.

### CHLOROSIS.

Chlorosis, one of the most common disorders of nutrition, is a form of anæmia characterized by certain blood peculiarities. It is rare in the male, but quite common in the female. In most instances it is associated with disturbances of menstruation, and it is usually present at the time of puberty, when the reproductive organs are especially developing. That it is a special disorder of nutrition is evidenced by its frequency among ill-fed, over-worked girls. Defective hygiene, in the way of poor food, lack of sufficient exercise, and impure air, and undue strain in mental exertion, are causes. It is, however, met with also in the upper classes of society and in girls of a good physical inheritance. There is always an anæmic state of the blood, the red corpuscles being deficient in number and lacking richness in hæmoglobin. There is weakness in the blood-forming and blood-propelling apparatus, the cause of which is to be sought for in some faulty condition of the mesoblast. In this disease the heart and the blood-vessels are usually small, but a compensatory hypertrophy of the heart may at times be present. The absolute number of the corpuscles may be diminished one-half, although the relative number may remain normal, while in the corpuscles themselves the hæmoglobin is greatly diminished. The percentage of hæmoglobin may be reduced from the normal one hundred to sixty or even fifty, making the red corpuscles noticeably pale. The serum may be normal in quantity, but the solids are reduced in amount.

There may be a defective growth of the ovaries and the uterus in chlorosis.

These changes and those of the circulation are not constant features. The disease in many instances undergoes rapid relapses. The symptoms are those of anæmia, as shortness of breath, palpitation of the heart, and swooning phenomena. The pulse is accelerated and easily excited. The complexion is peculiar,—not the blanched color of hæmoglobin loss, but the curious yellowish-green color which gives the disease its name of "the green sickness." The appetite is disordered, and there are indigestion and constipation. Cardiac murmurs are heard, simulating organic diseases of the heart. Menstruation is almost always deranged, and hysterical manifestations are frequent. Menorrhagia is very rare, amenorrhœa very common.

In diagnosis we must bear in mind the possibility of the symptoms being due to constitutional syphilis or to some organic disease of the stomach or the kidneys.

**Treatment.**—Iron is almost a specific. It should be given in fair doses and continued for a long time. Blaud's pill of carbonate of iron is one of the most efficacious preparations. The other preparations of iron are the dried sulphate, tincture of iron, and glycerole of chloride of iron. The red corpuscles will often greatly increase in number and improve in quality under the use of iron. The progressive development and the increase in number of the red corpuscles can be estimated with the bæmo-cytometer.

In rare cases the beneficial results of iron cease after its administration is discontinued. It is well then to give arsenic for a period, or iron and arsenic may be combined, as follows:

R Pulv. ferri redacti, ℈ii;
Quiniæ sulphatis, ℈ii;
Acidi arsenosi, gr. i;
Ext. gentianæ, q. s.
M. et ft. massa in pil. xl div.
Sig.—One pill after each meal.

Chalybeate waters are always beneficial. The tincture of nux vomica with hydrochloric acid is an efficient remedy for chlorosis. While medicines are given, a strict attention is to be paid to hygiene in food, air, and exercise. The diet should be rich in albumen and easy of digestion. Lean and spare patients need fats and the carbohydrates. Malt and cod-liver oil are useful in certain cases. Exercise in the open air, taken as freely as can be borne with comfort, is needed.

Iron is sometimes very disappointing in its therapeutic effects. Unfortunately, its medicinal administration as commonly practised has little or no scientific foundation. The etiological factors entering into the production of anæmia and chlorosis in consequence of digestive disorders and faulty assimilation are not so clearly understood as might be wished. Anæmia and chlorosis have a multiplicity of causes, some of which are quickly amenable to iron, while many others persist uninfluenced by this remedy. All the salts of iron seem to be most efficacious if first acted upon by the hydrochloric acid of the gastric juice and thus converted into chlorides: hence the tincture of the chloride acts better than any other chalybeate, when it is tolerated by the stomach.

Hæmogallol and hæmal are new préparations, which Professor Kobert has highly recommended for these and other conditions indicating the use of iron. They are said to be more easily transformed into blood-coloring matter by the organisms of debilitated persons than any other ferruginous preparations.

## DISEASES OF THE NERVOUS SYSTEM DEPENDENT UPON DISORDERS OF THE PELVIC ORGANS.

The various systems of the female economy are in intimate relations with the pelvic organs in health and in disease. We call these hysteroneuroses when the symptoms resulting are from disease. Hystero-neuroses are phenomena simulating morbid conditions in an organ anatomically healthy, but due to morbid changes in the uterus and ovaries. Of these two the uterus is generally the offending organ. There is a sympathetic hyperæsthesia, due to reflex action, from the uterine derangement. This is proved by the fact that these phenomena are intractable to treatment addressed to the symptoms, but are amenable to treatment directed to the causative pelvic disorder.

It is a matter of daily occurrence to witness the disorders of pregnancy. Almost as frequently we see the physiological changes in the system at large which result from menstruation, particularly at puberty and at the menopause. They are varied in character, as determined by ramifications of the ganglionic and spinal nerves and centres. When the organ receiving the impulse is in a state of lowered vitality and lessened resistance or of hyperæsthesia, or when the nerve-tracts are in a condition of morbid irritability, these reflexes are stimulated and heightened. Hence disorders of many parts of the body, the nervous system in particular, arise from functional or organic changes of the pelvic organs. Excitability is a common property of all living parts, and is an essential condition of life. A great variety in the alterations, as regards seat, character, and intensity, renders it impossible to connect them at all times with the symptoms of any definite kind.

Menstruation in its systemic phenomena modifies and aggravates goitre, the diseases of the skin, varicose veins, fibroid tumors, and the circulatory changes of the brain, in health and in disease. The influence of disordered menstruation manifests itself in the brain (sleeplessness, melancholia, dementia, and mania); in other parts of the nervous system (local paralyses, epilepsy, and catalepsy); in the larynx (aphonia); in the heart (palpitation); in the lungs (cough, asthma, and dyspnœa); in the stomach (nausea, vomiting, and indigestion); in the intestines (tympanites, diarrhœa); in the kidneys (hypersecretion of urine); in the skin (eczema, acne); in the breasts (disturbances of the lacteal secretion, pain, localized enlargements); in the joints (pain, false ankyloses), etc. But for all practical purposes we may say that the resulting disorders of the nervous system partake of the nature of chorea, hysteria, epilepsy, hystero-epilepsy, migraine, and neurasthenia. These, together with nymphomania and other varieties of a perverted sexual appetite, onanism, and insanity, will be especially referred to.

An irritation starts from the site of an organic lesion, and proceeds to the nerve-cells at the base of the brain and the upper part of the spinal cord. Reflex action of the sympathetic explains many of the diseases of women. Any irritation will travel on the lines of the least bodily resistance, and the degree of transmission depends also on the subject affected. Through this irritation the nerve-cells undergo alteration of their nutrition, and after a time acquire a morbid excitability which is the essence of the disease. We may never know what cells are altered. The changes in them may be more dynamical than physical: the microscope may be unable to detect any differences. No special lesion is constantly present.

Recent pathology has taught us how serious distant diseases may be started through reflex action. All the hystero-neuroses may persist after molecular changes have continued for an undue length of time.

Let us now consider each of these diseases in a more definite manner.

## CHOREA.

This nervous disease has a very obscure pathology. It is beyond the scope of this chapter to give the theories which have been advanced or to refer to the morbid conditions which have been found in connection with it.

Chorea consists in an exaggeration of those muscular movements which are constantly taking place, especially in children, who have not as yet acquired the power of governing the actions of their muscles. The movements are incoherent and devoid of character or rhythm. Chorea is most probably a functional disorder, beyond the reach of an anatomical demonstration. Among the causes, predisposing and exciting, we must not neglect to recognize those of a reflex nature, as intestinal worms, rectal fissure, and disorders of the genital functions. Pregnancy is a very common cause,—the disease commencing early in the third month, in those who have had it in childhood and who are otherwise predisposed to it, and subsiding after parturition. The disease is three times as frequent in girls as in boys, especially at the time of its most common occurrence, puberty. It can at times be distinctly traced to retroversion of the uterus, laceration of the cervix uteri, or dysmenorrhœa.

The best treatment consists in removing any tangible cause. The administration of a highly nutritious and easily digested diet is essential. Fats are a necessary element of the diet. Quiet and rest combined with nutritious food do more good than medicines. Sea-air and sea-bathing are to be highly recommended.

A moderate labile galvanic current applied daily to the spine, and arsenic, given internally, at first in small and then in gradually increasing doses, followed by cimicifuga, strychnine, iron, and quinine, are the best remedies.

Moral treatment is indispensable. Remove mental strain, control study, correct improper habits, and strengthen the will-power. These are potent means to regulate the life of a choreic patient, and are always conspicuous for good.

## HYSTERIA.

In this disease there is a functional disturbance of the nervous system, with much mental perversion. Although confined almost entirely to the female sex, it is not always so limited. Herein lies the proof that hysteria is not dependent alone on uterine or ovarian diseases. When the malady is present in a female, there may be no tangible evidence of any pelvic disorder. But there is no doubt that local affections of the genital organs have much to do with the causation of hysteria. It is more common during pregnancy, and its symptoms are most apt to appear at the catamenial periods. Erosions or lacerations of the cervix, chronic endometritis, malpositions of the uterus, and dysmenorrhœa produce and perpetuate hysterical phenomena in subjects predisposed to it by inheritance, sedentary habits, idleness, vicious practices, or any excessive development of the emotional nature. Hysterical symptoms subside when the local disease is cured. Ovarian diseases also, as oöphoralgia, ovaritis, and ovarian prolapse, are causative.

Hystero-epilepsy, for the elucidation of which we owe much to Charcot and his pupils, is a disease in which certain convulsions like epilepsy occur in hysterical patients, especially at or near the menstrual times. It is unlike epilepsy in its typical form, although cases with both disorders in one person may present difficulties in diagnosis. Hysteria alone is generally present, but it takes on a semblance to epilepsy. The attacks may be very frequently repeated, but are less severe and much less grave than those of epilepsy.

Firm pressure over the ovaries during an attack modifies or causes a complete relaxation of the spasm, and a return to consciousness, followed by a relapse on removal of this pressure. Hystero-genetic zones exist in various parts of the body, as over the breasts and ovaries, especially the latter.

Treatment.—In the treatment of these disorders, ascertain the cause or causes, and deal with them, if practicable. If there are symptoms of any uterine or ovarian disease, a pelvic examination should be made, but never unless there are strong reasons to anticipate that such diseases may thus be detected and that some benefit will result. While unnecessary examinations are to be avoided, an hysterical patient should not be allowed to continue in her sufferings without an examination being suggested, if indicated by the symptoms.

Always improve the appetite, if it is poor; correct the digestion, if it is impaired. Direct a regular and nutritious diet. Secure daily normal alvine evacuations. Open-air exercise, to the extent of fatigue, should be insisted on. The reading of sound, wholesome literature, avoiding cheap and sensational novels, supplies good food for the mind. Cold baths —better, cool sea-baths—are valuable adjuncts. Anæmia and debility are to be combated by iron and vegetable tonics. Strychnine generally aggravates the disease. Cimicifuga is a valuable remedy if there are menstrual derangements. The use of alcohol and narcotics is always to be avoided.

For the convulsions, when there is no doubt that they are due to hysteria, a sudden shock may be given to the nervous system, as by the pouring of cold water over the head and face, which is often followed by a return to consciousness, and a suggestion of its repetition may prevent another hysterical attack.

Amyl nitrite will arrest the paroxysm of hysteria or hystero-epilepsy. The bromides and arsenic are the best remedies during the intervals between the attacks. Local paralyses are best managed by massage, passive motion, and electricity. Aphonia generally yields to electricity.

Diseases of the uterus and its appendages, when present, should be rectified. Always avoid unnecessary manipulations of the genital organs.

Change the surroundings, if the family and friends are deleterious in their influence. Excessive sympathy is as injurious as are ridicule and abuse. Over-solicitude during attacks aggravates them and renders them more frequent. Gain the confidence of the patient, and arouse her to a systematic exercise of her will-power and self-control. Electricity is very beneficial, in the form of general faradism.

In obstinate cases, uncontrolled by other means, the Weir Mitchell treatment, by seclusion, rest, forced feeding, massage, and electricity, is highly advisable.

Although cures may be effected by hypnotism, its practice involves the risk of aggravating the patient's condition. Oöphorectomy for hysteria and hystero-epilepsy has been much abused.

Graily Hewitt contends that hystero-epilepsy is largely due to reflex irritation having its seat within the uterus, and that this irritation is caused by flexion of the uterus. This is no doubt true of some cases, but their number is relatively small. A more common cause is a diseased condition of the Fallopian tubes and ovaries.

In all cases which are clearly due to some reflected pelvic irritation, medicinal and hygienic measures should be tried first. After these have had a fair and continued trial, surgical operations may justly be considered. Unrelieved local pelvic disease, causing much pain, impairing usefulness, and exciting hystero-epileptic attacks, may be combated by surgical means. The gynæcological records of the last few years point unmistakably to the direct relationship, as cause and effect, of the two diseases, and prove that cœliotomy performed as a *dernier ressort* is not only justifiable, but necessary. But not every case so operated on has been bettered. Again and again have the attacks continued as bad as before. Past experiences warrant the following directions. Do not perform cœliotomy for hystero-epilepsy unless unmistakable evidence of some structural or organic change can be detected within the pelvis. Be assured that this is the source of irritation, and that the nervous phenomena cannot be relieved by general medicinal and hygienic measures.

### MIGRAINE.

Migraine, or hemicrania, is a very common form of headache, and an extremely distressing complaint. Because so frequent and so intractable, it deserves most earnest consideration. Generally accompanied by certain vaso-motor changes, it indicates circulatory disturbances.

We recognize two forms of this nervous disease, the spastic and the paralytic. In the first the painful side of the head, generally the left, becomes pale and shrunken, the pupils are dilated, the ear is cold and pale,

the temporal artery is tense and hard.    The pain in the temple is increased
by pressure on the carotid.

In the paralytic form of the disease the face and ear are hot, red, and
swollen, the eye is injected, and the pupil is contracted.    The pain in this
variety is diminished by carotid pressure.            .

The vaso-motor symptoms are at times very imperfectly defined.    In
the spastic form the vessels of the affected half are more or less contracted,
due to an irritation of the cervical sympathetic ; in the paralytic form there
is a vascular dilatation, from paralysis of the sympathetic nerves.    The
cervical sympathetic is the site of this pathological lesion.    Fluctuations
in the arterial supply set up irritation of the sensory nerves in the skin,
the pericranium, the cerebral membranes, and the sensory portion of the
cerebral cortex.

That two such opposite conditions, anæmia and hyperæmia, can cause
such a nerve-storm seems rational when we know that epileptiform convulsions may be so caused.    Some cases show a marked regularity, attacks
recurring at intervals of varying length.

Migraine is very often an inheritance, direct or indirect, being directly
inherited from the disease itself in one or the other parent, or indirectly
transmitted from some other neurosis, as epilepsy, insanity, etc.    Prolonged
wear, mental strain, loss of sleep, and sexual excesses are causes, especially
in the anæmic or debilitated.    Gout is sometimes a cause.

Females have this disease more often than males, particularly at the
period of puberty and towards the climacteric change of life.    Many women
have it only just before, during, or immediately after menstruation.    Of
course, genital diseases, functional or organic, may aggravate it, but we do
not believe that the disease originates exclusively from this source.    Recognizing the systemic changes incident to menstruation, and that the menstrual
phenomena are followed by intermenstrual phenomena in the nervous and
circulatory systems, we can understand how this disorder is more apt to be
aggravated by this pelvic function, and how it may show itself only at the
menstrual periods.    All women are more susceptible to neurotic manifestations at such times, and all the sympathetic disorders are then most apt
to show themselves.    Vascular tension, like nerve-tension, is diminished
after the menstrual epochs.

Treatment.—In order that any permanent relief may be obtained,
the state of the general health must receive special attention.    We must
do what we can to elevate the standard and increase the stability of the
health of the whole system.    All tangible diseases must be removed and
all recognized functional disorders corrected.    During the interval iron
and quinine are called for if there are anæmia and debility.    The last of
these remedies may be given before, and the former after, meals.    Constipation must be relieved.    Cod-liver oil is highly useful when given during
the cooler months.

If there is a gouty diathesis, give the iodides.    If visual refraction be at fault, this error should be corrected by appropriate glasses. The diet should be regulated. A change of air, scenery, and association almost always does good, and sometimes effects a cure. Menstrual disorders may call for attention.

The best medicines to prevent attacks or mitigate their frequency and severity, besides those previously mentioned, are arsenic, cannabis indica, and zinc phosphide. Fowler's solution may be given, in doses of from three to five drops, after meals, for weeks or months. Its use lessens the frequency of the attacks of migraine. A good plan of treatment is to give two grains of quinine before meals and three drops of the arsenical solution after meals. To do good, they must be continued steadily for a long time.

Cannabis indica, in the form of the extract, is also very useful when administered for a considerable period. Arsenous acid and extract of cannabis indica may be combined, or the extract of cannabis indica may be given with zinc phosphide. A very efficacious combination of remedies is:

> ℞ Zinci phosphidi, gr. ii ;
> Strychniæ, gr. ss ;
> Ext. cannabis indicæ, gr. x.
> M. et ft. massa in pil. xx div.
> Sig —One pill three times a day during the intervals.

For the attack itself the following remedies are very beneficial. Tincture of nux vomica in doses of one drop every fifteen minutes is useful in cases attended with stomach disturbances. Cases of the spastic form of the disease call for nitro-glycerin or nitrite of amyl, while those of the paralytic type call for ergot or antipyrin.

These medicines are too often prescribed indiscriminately, without regard to the variety of the migraine. Those remedies are most effective which counteract the existing abnormal vaso-motor condition. Thus, in migraine accompanied with vaso-motor spasm, glonoin, amyl nitrite, alcohol, or quinine will relieve pain and abort or arrest the attack. They dilate the cerebral blood-vessels. Such remedies as the bromides and antipyrin, which contract the capillaries, act best if given when there is vaso-motor dilatation. Antipyrin may be given in doses of five grains every two hours during the attack, from its commencement, or smaller doses may be given oftener. Antipyrin and bromide of sodium unite well in an effervescing mixture. Antipyrin and phenacetin owe their analgesic properties to their effects on the sensory cells of the central nervous system, diminishing their irritability. Antipyrin and ammonium bromide form an excellent combination.

Sodium salicylate, in doses of three grains every half-hour, is sometimes quite efficacious in similar cases ; so also is salipyrin.

The bromides are admirably adapted for headaches attended with cerebral irritability and excitability. They arrest functional activity of the brain, secure sleep, and diminish pelvic congestion.

Brain-weariness and exhaustion are most favorably influenced by caffein and guarana. The effervescing salts bromo-caffein and phospho-caffein are very good. Caffein is a powerful cerebral stimulant; it is also a heart-tonic, increasing the arterial blood-pressure. It is one of the best reme-dies that we have to increase absolutely the activity and the capacity of the human brain for work. Headaches due to brain-exhaustion and anæmia indicate its use.

One of the most trustworthy remedies for the attacks of sick-headache is cannabis indica. This remedy is not only reliable when given for a long time during the intervals between the attacks, to prevent another attack, but is also very valuable during the attack itself, given in doses of ten drops every three hours. Its use is clearly called for in cases asso-ciated with or dependent on such menstrual disorders as menorrhagia and dysmenorrhœa.

All cases are benefited by maintaining the horizontal posture and by perfect quiet in a darkened room. Cold to the head will do good in the paralytic form of the disease, and hot water in the spastic form.

The hypodermic use of morphine has been greatly abused in the treat-ment of this disease. Of course pain is relieved thereby and sleep is secured, but if continued for any length of time its future use is depended upon, and the morphine habit is created. Antipyrin and phenacetin are antipyretic, analgesic, and hypnotic.

Galvanism persistently used has produced good results. It is both prophylactic and curative. Almost every attack is relieved by it, but its successful employment must be based on scientific principles. The polar effect is always to be sought. While it has been applied over the mastoid process, in the spastic form of the disease it will often be found better to place the anode over the sympathetic nerve, at the site of the pain, or in the auriculo-maxillary fossa, while the cathode is placed over the upper cer-vical region. In the paralytic form of the disease the cathode should be substituted for the anode. A good way is to apply the anode over the frontal region and the cathode to the lower cervical region. In the spastic form the positive pole is applied to the forehead and the negative pole is held in the hand, while in the paralytic form the negative pole is applied to the forehead and the positive pole is held in the hand. The polar effects are thereby best secured.

### NEURASTHENIA AND SPINAL IRRITATION.

Neurasthenia is a constitutional neurosis which is due to deficiency or exhaustion of nerve-force. Spinal irritation, a local spinal neurosis, is a symptom of spinal exhaustion. Both of these conditions, especially the latter, are much more common in women than in men. Spinal irritation to some degree is most frequent in the higher classes of society, in women between fifteen and forty-five.

Coccygodynia is at times a distressing form of spinal irritation, affecting the tip of the spine in the region of the coccyx. It often accompanies irritation of other portions of the spine.

In neurasthenia there is a weakness of the nervous apparatus, associated with undue irritability, mental and physical. These manifestations of weakness and irritability show themselves after the least provocation, by undue excitement and fatigue. There is also a lack of vigor, efficiency, and endurance, a want of mutual support and control in the different parts of the nervous organization. The patient is unequal to the ordinary tasks of life. Everything is done with undue exertion. Even talking and thinking are exhausting. She becomes a subject of many morbid fears.

These symptoms may coexist with some functional disorder of the brain, with an incapacity for mental exertion, and with much mental irritability, some disturbance of the special senses, and insomnia; or they may show themselves in other parts of the nervous apparatus, as the spinal and the sympathetic system, by disorders of the sensory or of the motor functions, and by vaso-motor changes. All such patients are easily agitated, very sensitive and timid. They are often, though not always, spare in body, anæmic, broken down in health, and at times bedridden. There is a predisposition to chorea, hysteria, or hystero-epilepsy. These functional nervous disorders may be associated with neurasthenia.

There is no known distinct anatomical change underlying the manifold symptoms of neurasthenia. Affecting all parts of the body, the symptoms are too often referred to the generative organs, especially in women.

Doubtless this disease is much more frequent in this than in any previous century. Clearly our modern American life favors it, for nowhere is it more common than in our larger cities. Here the wear and tear of life are in excess. Our climate may have something to do in producing the disease, but, at any rate, the social exactions of our modern society are very great, and housekeeping is much more complex than formerly.

Neurasthenia can be ascribed to a great variety of causes. A bad inheritance in the way of temperament, lack of judicious physical exercise in youth, undue strain of the brain in study or occupation, social disappointments, sexual excesses, business and domestic excitements and anxieties, and pelvic diseases, enter into the causation of this trouble. The latter conditions particularly concern us here. Female sexual diseases may be direct causes. More often they are but associated or, it may be, resultant conditions.

Any female pelvic disease which gives rise to pain, frequent and excessive menstruation, or profuse leucorrhœa may directly bring about neurasthenia. There is a difference in the effects of chronic uterine and ovarian diseases in these respects, as there is a difference in the inherent and acquired vital resistances of constitutions. In some cases grave disease causes little or no disturbance, while in others a slight local disorder is followed by a multiplicity of symptoms. The most potent local pelvic affections creating reflex disorders are chronic oöphoritis, ovarian prolapse, and especially lacerations of the cervix uteri. Cervical tears almost always heal by second intention, and by the formation of some cicatricial tissue. They bring about eversion, erosion, granular degeneration, cystic degeneration, and chronic uterine catarrh. Pain is created, and reflex disturbances are set up. Not all lacerations of the cervix need trachelorrhaphy, but in some cases nothing else will be efficacious for good. Few, if any, morbid conditions of the cervix demonstrate in a greater degree these results of the varying susceptibility of the nervous system to pain and reflex irritation.

Treatment.—The cause of the disease is to be removed, if recognized. Unfortunately, the causes are at times not satisfactorily made out, and we are forced to address ourselves to the general condition. The next indication is to improve nutrition as well as we can. The nervous system should be fortified by food to do its work at the best possible advantage. The wear and tear of life are thus diminished, by calling into service a fuller reserve, and thus we conserve the vital expenditures.

Since many neurasthenics are such only in certain surroundings of climate, business, home and friends, and enjoy good health when leading a simpler life, involving less care and responsibility, we do such patients the best service by changing their places and methods of living.

Sufficient sleep is always to be secured, not by means of medicines, but by systematic muscular exercise in the open air, by a quiet life, and by an early retiring to rest, aided, it may be, by the administration of some food at this time. An hour of rest each afternoon is always desirable. Mellin's food, with hot milk, or malted milk, is often very good for this purpose. The partaking of a glass of pure rich milk some two hours after the breakfast, at luncheon, and at bedtime, is to be favorably considered. Alcohol needs to be very cautiously prescribed for neurasthenics. Wyeth's liquid malt is one of the best forms.

The best medicines are arsenic, cod-liver oil, iron, and phosphorus. Arsenic acts best on persons of the lymphatic or nervous temperament. Coexisting menorrhagic disorders are also best controlled by its use. Cod-liver oil, pure, or emulsified with the syrup of lacto-phosphate of lime, is to be prescribed during the colder months, after a proper regulation of the stomach. Phosphorus, in the form of zinc phosphide, or free (in Fairchild's elixir of calisaya bark), is an excellent remedy.

Cases of pronounced invalidism from neurasthenia require a special treatment. The rest-cure, elaborated by Weir Mitchell, is pre-eminently useful. The more chronic and more pronounced the case, especially when hysterical phenomena are present, the greater the prospect of a speedy and complete cure. Seclusion, forced feeding, rest, massage, and electricity, all are of signal benefit. No one of these can be safely omitted.

Abundant rest is thus secured; a tired brain is put at ease, for the mind is diverted and not excited; and, with massage administered once or twice daily, exercise is given to all parts of the body, without exertion. Sleep, also, is thus secured. Pelvic congestion is diminished by the recumbent posture of the body. The circulation of the blood is equalized by massage. Nutrition is favored by forced feeding. Excretion is not neglected. The tonic effects of electricity are obtained by a well-regulated administration of this agent. By all, life is started anew; a complete transformation is inaugurated.

Patients with spinal irritation are likewise benefited in this way. But in the treatment of these cases galvanism should not be neglected. Hammond has contended that spinal irritation is the result of spinal anæmia, because the spinal pain is almost always ameliorated by the recumbent posture and is aggravated by the erect position.

Such cases are most improved by a labile upward galvanic current, the positive pole being applied to and below the regions of the spinal tenderness, while the negative pole is placed at the sixth or seventh cervical vertebra. The experience of the author convinces him of the efficacy of this method of applying the constant current. Whether the improvement caused by it is the result of increasing the spinal circulation is not so conclusively proved.

General faradization, and especially local pelvic faradization, with a very long thin wire for the secondary current of tension, one pole being within the vagina or rectum, is an admirable remedy in cases associated with, or dependent upon, intra-pelvic disease. Not only is there mitigation of any existing pelvic pain by an improvement of the pelvic circulation and an increased tonicity of any relaxed muscular fibres, but the common attendant symptom of constipation is relieved without laxative medication.

In no class of diseases within the domain of the gynæcologist and the neurologist is it more obvious than in this that success in the management of the various neurasthenic conditions is largely in proportion to the degree in which we win the confidence and stimulate the faith of our patient. All intelligent co-operation will surely be rewarded.

### INSANITY.

A great many theories about this disease have in times past governed the medical mind. The importance of clearly distinguishing what may cause and maintain insanity, and of determining which of two diseases present exists independently, cannot be overestimated.

Insanity is either of central or of reflex origin. For our present purposes all cases may be classified as follows: first, those which are purely central, from cerebral causes; second, those which are the result of female sexual diseases, from reflex causes.

It is the province of this chapter to speak only of cases which are purely reflex from pelvic causes. These cases are noticed about the age of puberty, after marriage, during and following parturition, and at the climacteric period. These times appear to be periods of special susceptibility in women.   At the same time we must remember that purely central conditions produce or arrest pelvic symptoms and modify female pelvic functions. A few cases of female sexual disease are bettered by the cerebral disturbance; most are made worse.   Again, the two conditions, cerebral and pelvic, may coexist, or they may be purely independent.   Mental derangements frequently disturb the functions of several organs of the body, or modify action, healthy or diseased, in them.   Why not the pelvic viscera?   Menstrual disturbances are to be regarded as both cause and effect.   The vast majority of all cases of insanity arise from conditions and circumstances which depress and exhaust the nervous system.   Extraordinary functional activity of the sexual organs involves a great demand upon the whole organization.   Frequent child-bearing, with lactation, causes an excessive drain on the whole body.   The most frequent occurrence of insanity in women is under such circumstances.   In most women mental depression, to a greater or less degree, is experienced at the menstrual times, from causes entirely physiological.   Many cases of insanity, even those not reflex in their origin, are worse at the catamenial periods.

Insanity at the menopause we all recognize, and it is very properly called climacteric.

The most common cause of amenorrhœa is impaired general nutrition. Most of the anæmic conditions favor menstrual suppression.   Mental shock and prolonged anxiety so act.   Insanity always impairs the general nutrition of the body and disorders innervation.   Hence the insane are very often amenorrhœic.   The uterine function is restored only after an improvement of the general health.

Any disease of the uterus or ovaries in a highly sensitive organization may cause mental derangement, which subsides only when the causative disease is overcome.   The irritation and exhaustion from the pelvic disease may be the exciting cause of insanity, while the predisposing cause resides either in an altered or deranged nervous system or in some lesion of the brain, inherited or acquired.   Horatio R. Storer, in his excellent work on insanity in women, contends that this disease when developed during the existence of uterine or ovarian affections is the result of reflex irritation. Unquestionably his statements are in the main true, but they are too positive.   While the reproductive organs exert a potent influence on the mind in health and in disease, not all cases of insanity in women are caused by pelvic diseases.   These affections do not occupy so important a position in the etiology of insanity as one would be disposed to think from Storer's statements.   Insanity in women proceeds from the same general causes as insanity in men, though possibly oftener, on account of the general impressibility of their nervous system and their higher emotional nature.   Not only are women subject to a host of diseases peculiar to their sex, but these diseases greatly modify their natural disposition and character.   Their lives are subject to perpetual changes.   Sex is in reality the predisposing, the exciting, and the continuing cause of much of the insanity in women.   The relative frequency of insanity in the two sexes is a subject of much observation. Mental disorders are probably more common in women than in men. The vast amount of statistical information on this point is not altogether reliable. More females than males are found in the asylums of our country, though more females than males recover from their first attack of mental aberration.

Fifteen per cent. of all cases of insanity in women arise during the discharge of the maternal functions. Depressing emotions, as shame and mental distress in the unmarried, and other accessory causes, vary greatly in different cases, but the inherited or acquired neuropathic condition is fundamental.

Puerperal insanity is brought about by the exhaustion of nerve-force and the anæmia in the puerperal state. Septic causes also doubtless favor its occurrence. Lactation causes insanity by producing exhaustion and anæmia. In these cases an hereditary tendency can often be traced. Insanity following pregnancy is brought about, in part at least, by impairment in the quantity and quality of the blood. When it manifests itself early in pregnancy, it is, no doubt, in many cases reflex.

The menopause is to woman, in her physical relations, a most critical period of life.

We must not misapprehend the sexual manifestations of insanity. Symptoms should not be taken for causes. The perversion of the appetites is one of the premonitory symptoms of this disease, and is the essence of all mental aberrations, the sexual instinct being no exception to the rule.

Some inherited weakness of the nervous centres must be assumed, in order that any uterine or ovarian disease may produce such functional mental changes.

From seventy to eighty per cent. of all cases of insanity are curable, if judicious treatment is instituted in the first month of the disorder. A longer duration than six months of the disease is attended by a rapid decline in the rate of recoveries. In the first manifestations of the mental derangement the brain is affected only functionally, but destructive molecular changes are likely in time to occur insidiously. Puerperal insanity furnishes a large percentage of recoveries,—probably eighty per cent. at the least.

Treatment.—To deal even in the briefest way with the treatment of the various forms of insanity is beyond the scope of this article. A great variety of pathological conditions—mania, melancholia, dementia, monomania, etc —the alienist will be called on to treat. As insanity is a disease of the whole nervous system, and as the entire physical organization, with every function of the body, becomes involved, the system at large must be treated. We are to recognize causes and circumstances depressing and exhausting the nervous system in all cases. There is no specific treatment. We are to treat patients irrespective of the form of the malady. Thus the broadest principles of treatment should guide us. Urgent symptoms,

as constipation and insomnia, may first need attention. To secure sleep
the bromides and chloral are called for. The bromides are especially useful
because of their quieting influence upon the brain, and because they tend
to diminish pelvic congestion. Hyoscin is particularly serviceable when
there is excessive motor irritability. When it secures sleep, this change
indicates the first improvement in the disease. Dangerous exhaustion is
always to be guarded against.

In all cases of insanity referred to in this chapter, those dependent
upon pelvic causes, and, in fact, in all cases in women, a careful inquiry
is to be made in reference to existent pelvic symptoms and to signs of intra-
pelvic affection. If there is the least indication, from the history obtained,
of uterine or ovarian disease, a thorough gynæcological examination is to
be made, always in the presence of one or more witnesses.—The questions
now come up, Which disease started first? Which disease is the seeming
cause? Is the case post-puerperal or climacteric? Does the mental aberration exist independently, or do the two diseases, the pelvic and the cerebral,
hold any relationship? This examination involves inquiry as to the age,
the social relation, the menstrual functions, and the existence of any organic
sexual disease. Obscene talk on the part of the patient does not indicate
the presence of such disease.

The intra-pelvic examination may demand the employment of an anæsthetic. Ether or chloroform may be used for this purpose, but experience
teaches us their inferiority to nitrous oxide gas, which may be administered
in the method employed by dentists. Anæsthesia is induced by it, and the
effect on the disturbed cerebral functions is generally very beneficial. Dr.
Shaw, medical director of Kings County Insane Asylum, Flatbush, has
observed no unpleasant effects from its use. On the contrary, it has proved
to be a valuable tonic in cases of extreme debility of the nervous system,
and experience has shown its use in the treatment of insane women with
pelvic disease to be a valuable contribution to gynæcology.

Nothing will be said here as to the general management of cases, with
regard to diet, baths, stimulation, medication, how and when to divert and
to amuse, or how and when to restrain, if necessary. Any pelvic disease
which may be the immediate or seeming cause of the insanity, as endometritis, erosions of the cervix, chronic pelvic peritonitis, ovaritis, ovarian
prolapse, and cervical cicatrices, with uterine displacements and neoplasms,
should have special treatment. Whether the cause or not, they certainly
exert an unfavorable influence on the mental derangement, and should be
corrected as soon as practicable. I firmly believe that the staff of every
large insane asylum for women should have for one of its members a competent gynæcologist, with broad and comprehensive views of pathology and
treatment. The greatest tact and experience will be needed to determine
when to resort to local medication, and how often to repeat it, or when
to interfere surgically. A judicious local treatment will at times be rewarded by the disappearance of the cerebral irritation and insomnia, as

if by magic. The promptness of the relief will depend largely upon the duration of the insane phenomena. Secondary disease does not always disappear when the primary cause has been removed. Chronic mania will at times remain unchanged. Not only should gynæcological examinations be made in the presence of a witness, as already stated, but care should be taken to avoid undue frequency of local inspections and applications.

When the disease is far advanced, the details of treatment can be carried on only in institutions designed for the purpose and furnished with all needed appliances for isolating, watching, exercising, amusing, and instructing patients. Confirmed cases certainly should be placed in an asylum, but very mild cases, at least at the beginning, may be better managed in certain homes and surroundings.

In the management of insanity no fixed, machine-like treatment is adapted for all cases. Treatment must be adapted to cases and conditions, and will be efficient and satisfactory in proportion to the degree of individual care and attention bestowed.

## NYMPHOMANIA.

"Sexual feeling," says Maudsley, "is the foundation for the development of the social feeling." When the sexual feeling in the female is excessive or perverted, it is called nymphomania. This form of erotomania is a disease in the female like satyriasis in the male. There is mental perversion always attended by uncontrollable sexual passion. To gratify the sexual appetite, in advanced and confirmed cases, all the decencies and proprieties of life are sacrificed. It is a delirium of lust, a psychical desire engrafted on a markedly neurotic temperament, or a disease excited by impure reading or association. The imagination calls up sexual images, which may lead to hallucinations and illusions. Nymphomania in its most severe forms is associated with or dependent on certain varieties of insanity, with or without gross brain-disease. Although this disease is observed in children and in octogenarians, it occurs most frequently at the beginning or at the end of menstrual life. The genital organs are constantly in a state of turgescence. There is the greatest perversion of the sexual act, gratification being sought not only in masturbation, but also with others of the same sex, the patient playing the active or the passive rôle. In many instances this disorder is a reflex manifestation, from an irritation of the genital organs. Thus, certain diseases of the uterus and of the appendages give rise to nymphomania. The local exciting causes are intestinal, especially rectal, the presence of worms, hemorrhoids, inflammations of the vulva, vagina, or rectum, various eruptions on the external genitalia, inflammations of the urethra and bladder, and diabetic urine. Medicines, even cantharides, have very little, if any, such effect. Nymphomania may result from masturbation and sexual causes, as well as cause them. Some cases of nymphomania assume a periodic form. Vangrado speaks of a woman who, although chaste, was seized with excessive sexual passion in the intervals between pregnan-

cies, and became lascivious beyond expression, but when pregnant there was a total suspension of her erotic desires.  Sometimes nymphomania is developed from a sudden cessation of normal coitus, in women of a highly erotic temperament.   The gynæcologist at times comes in contact with women who show a fondness for gynæcological examinations.  Various subterfuges are resorted to by them to induce a handling of their sexual organs.   Cases calling for a frequent and unnecessary use of the catheter are instances in point.

In most cases where accusations of rape while under the influence of an anæsthetic have been brought against physicians, no doubt the women believed that they had been so violated.   Not only, however, should the former life of the accusing party be considered, but also the well-known medico-legal fact should be recognized that such erotic symptoms may be developed by the anæsthetic itself.

**Treatment.**—The best results are obtained by moral suasion, by good and thorough occupation, by diversion, and by free physical exercise in the open air, to the point of fatigue.   Early rising, cold bathing, regulation of the bowels, the use of a plain but nutritious diet, and the internal administration of the bromides are the best remedies.   When local diseases are suspected, search for them, and remedy them by appropriate treatment. Marriage is contra-indicated until a cure has been effected.   Clitoridectomy, though seemingly justified, is only exceptionally beneficial.   Oöphorectomy, having almost invariably failed to give relief, is unwarranted.   Experience teaches that the removal of the ovaries does not always impair sexual desire, but that the female is permanently sterilized.   Dependent as this disease almost always is upon some faulty mental or cerebral conditions, inherited or acquired, treatment should be addressed chiefly to their relief.

### PERVERTED SEXUAL APPETITE.

Most women are passive, not active, in sexual intercourse.  Women, sexually speaking, may be divided into three classes.   With most women coitus is at first not pleasurable, but if the sexual organs remain healthy during married life the performance of the act gradually becomes less distasteful, and is enjoyed, at least at times, if not too frequently indulged in, by virtue of a love for, or a sense of duty to, the husband.   A large number of women never experience a sexual impulse impelling them to the act; to them the sexual orgasm is unknown.   Another class of women are, like men, active and aggressive for sexual gratification, and they suffer if there is sexual continence.   Such an active sexual passion may be acquired by a perfectly virtuous woman.

The relative proportion of these three classes stands very much in the order mentioned.   Colored women enjoy sexual intercourse more fervently than do their Caucasian sisters, and there are doubtless differences in this respect in women of different nationalities.   The great majority of women who take to a life of prostitution do so not for sexual enjoyment, but from mercenary motives, love of idleness, fondness for ease, and a desire for display in dress. Sexual passion is not so great in females as in males. Many women fall into perverted sexual habits for the purpose of pandering to a patron. Sexual feeling, unknown to most women until marriage, may be unduly exercised and stimulated. It is then an acquired faculty, which is greatly perverted. Sexual continence, enforced by the death of a husband, after the free exercise of the sexual function during married life, is at times followed by unpleasant results. Sexual excesses are borne better by most women than by men, because of their inherent passivity.

Dyspareunia, painful or unpleasant coition, generally denotes some disease of the vulva, vagina, uterus, ovaries, or parametric tissues. While diseases of these parts generally cause dyspareunia, the opposite state, that of an abnormally strong sexual appetite, may result from them. Sexual perversion may be either congenital or acquired. It is congenital when it arises from defects in the sexual structure—hermaphrodism—or from some defect in the cerebral structure, as idiocy. It is acquired from pregnancy, the menopause, hysteria, ovarian disease, or through a stimulation of the nerves of sexual sensibility from sexual excesses or masturbation. It may be acquired from some cerebral disease. Heredity also constitutes an element in causation. Few bodily attributes are more readily transmitted to posterity than certain peculiarities of the sexual system.

Insanity, as has been stated, is very frequently attended by perverted sexual impulses. These sensations may be the symptoms of some local disease; more frequently they are cerebral in origin, existing when the former life has been pure and when there is no local disease.

Masturbation from erotic desires is practised much less frequently by girls and women than by boys and men. When it is indulged in by the female, it is, as a rule, the result of some local reflex irritation of the sexual or genito-urinary organs. Pruritus is a very frequent underlying pathological condition favoring masturbation.

## VAGINISMUS.

We owe much to Marion Sims for our first knowledge of this disease. Vaginismus is an abnormal contraction of the muscles of the pelvic floor. It is not a disease *per se*, but a symptom of various morbid conditions of the vulva, the vagina, and the surrounding parts.

Formerly it was supposed to involve the sphincter vaginæ only, but now it is understood to concern also the levator ani, the transversus perinæi, and the bulbo-cavernosus muscles. These muscles are abnormally irritable, and the reflex contraction occurs in them as a result of the following diseases: urethral caruncle; vulvar inflammation, erosion, and fissures; vaginal inflammation and erosion; inflammation and fissures of the hymen, with irritable caruncles; rectal fissures; cervical lacerations; uterine displacements, as retroversion and retroflexion; ovarian prolapsus; periuterine inflammation and exudations.

The diseased area is irritated by coitus, by digital touch, or by the use of the probe, and a reflex muscular spasm is evoked. Patients are always nervous, irritable, hysterical, subject to neuralgia, and easily depressed mentally. Sexual intercourse is always painful, generally very much so, and it may be impracticable. There is usually a neurotic dysmenorrhœa. Vesical and rectal irritability are very commonly present.

Generally only the lower portion of the vagina is involved, but its upper part may be solely affected, not only making coitus painful, but also causing a speedy and forcible expulsion of the seminal fluid from the vagina thereafter. In this form of vaginismus, which is not very uncommon, the levator ani is mostly involved.

Although not severe at the start, quite often, from motives of modesty, vaginismus is allowed to continue unrelieved until it causes severe suffering and much mental anxiety. Nevertheless it can be speedily controlled.

**Treatment.**—All attempts at sexual intercourse should be absolutely prohibited until the local painful areas are removed or healed and the parts have lost their unnatural hyperæsthesia.

The cause of the local irritation is to be removed, to effect a cure. An irritable urethral caruncle or any inflamed and irritable carunculæ myrtiformes are to be excised. An inflamed, hyperæsthetic hymen should be exsected after being ruptured. An irritable fissure of the anus must either be divided by the knife or gradually stretched. Vulvitis and vaginitis should be relieved by appropriate local applications, as boric acid, bismuth subnitrate, and hot-water vaginal injections. Keep the bowels open. Heal any erosions of the vulva or the vagina by the topical use of solutions of silver nitrate, iodoform, or aristol.

When the hymen and carunculæ myrtiformes are dissected away, the borders of the incisions should be stitched together and the parts dressed with iodoform or aristol, so that healing may take place by primary intention. Healing by secondary intention and by the formation of cicatricial tissue leads to local pain and reflex disorders.

Owing to its anæsthetic properties, the topical application of the secondary faradic current of tension with the long fine wire will at a proper time do great good.

Topical applications of solutions of cocaine (from two to five per cent.) are useful for hyperæsthetic conditions of the vulva and vagina, after the local inflammations have been subdued.

The general health should be improved by tonics. Gradual or forcible dilatation of the contracting muscles, or incision, if needed, should be practised. Gradual dilatation is effected by a series of dilators of hard rubber, a larger dilator being used and allowed to remain longer each succeeding day. Forcible dilatation, with the patient under the influence of an anæsthetic, similar to that which is practised for anal fissures, may be done, after which a good-sized hard-rubber dilator should be inserted and allowed to remain for several hours.

The fibres encircling the vaginal orifice may be divided with scissors, on each side, just within the fourchette. The mucous membrane should be united with sutures before a hard-rubber dilator is inserted.

## REMOTE EFFECTS OF OÖPHORECTOMY.

As a rule, extirpation of the ovaries stops menstruation. A slight hemorrhagic discharge per vaginam often follows this operation in a few days, due no doubt to the pressure-effects of the ligatures around the ovarian arteries. It ceases spontaneously in a short time. But, while there is generally no return of the menstrual flow, in exceptional cases it recurs at regular or irregular intervals, for the following reasons. Because a third ovary, unsuspected and untouched, remains. Beigel found a third ovary present in eight out of some five hundred post-mortem examinations. Because of failure to remove the whole of both ovaries. Tait's operation —salpingo-oöphorectomy—is more certain to be followed by menstrual cessation than Battey's or Hegar's operation, because in the removal of the uterine appendages by Tait's method the ligature is placed deeper, and a third ovary, if present, or any irregularly situated Graafian follicles, are more apt to be removed. Menstruation may continue irregularly or regularly for a while from force of habit or the law of periodicity. It in time ceases if all the follicles have been extirpated.

Many cases of irregular menstruation after oöphorectomy may be explained by the presence of some diseased condition of the cervix uteri or of the endometrium, or by the presence of some foreign body within the uterine canal.

There could be no more conclusive proof of the presence of remaining Graafian follicles than the fact that pregnancy sometimes occurs after double oöphorectomy.

So generally does complete removal of both ovaries cause complete cessation of menstruation that we confidently look for it. Hence we may with perfect propriety and justifiability perform this operation for the removal of certain organic diseases of the ovaries, with their resulting symptoms, and for the arrest of uncontrollable hemorrhages from fibroid tumors of the uterus not too large in size.

This operation has been performed also for many other pelvic diseases, and for nervous and mental disorders seemingly dependent upon, or aggravated by, a functional activity of the ovaries. Thus, it has been done for hysteria, menstrual epilepsy, hystero-epilepsy, nymphomania, chorea, the various forms of insanity, dysmenorrhœa, and pelvic pain indescribable and ill defined in character and position. The actual condition of the ovary, unfortunately, has not always been accurately determined. Just here oöphorectomy has been greatly abused. Battey's operation may be needed to bring about a premature change of life. Hegar's or Tait's operation may be justifiable in cases of organic disease of the ovary or ovaries and tubes which cannot be otherwise controlled. But the author contends that oöphorectomy has been more abused than any other operation in the domain of gynæcological surgery, because resorted to for ill-defined symptoms which were not altogether dependent upon ovarian functional activity or disease. When there is no organic change in the ovaries and has never been any, oöphorectomy is almost always contra-indicated. Cystic changes in these organs are very common; for the most part they are purely physiological. We should not be deceived by their appearance. That a recovery follows oöphorectomy proves only that the patient has survived the operation; it does not prove that she has recovered from the disease for which the operation was performed. Even if good results follow an operation, we should bear in mind the curative effects of surgical procedures *per se*,—the psychical influence produced on the body by a strong mental impression. Reflex action, through revulsion and counter-irritation, sometimes does good. The *post hoc* is not always the *propter hoc*. Hundreds, if not thousands, of women have had their ovaries needlessly sacrificed. Doléris several years ago said that in four out of every five cases of oöphorectomy done in Paris the operation was unnecessary. More careful consideration and a well-rounded treatment for women would save numbers of ovaries and tubes. Some women, chiefly prostitutes, have asked for the extirpation of their ovaries, to prevent the possibility of impregnation. Pain and dysmenorrhœa are not sufficient indications for female castration. With Hegar and Winckel, I believe that the gynæcologist should not venture on so radical a step unless the case demonstrates to his complete satisfaction the existence of some organic ovarian disease. Many symptoms supposed to be due to organic changes in the ovary are due to obscure peri-oöphoritis or to ovarian neuralgia. In a few of the cases in which the operation has been done the patients have been made worse, rather than better. Oöphorectomy is a comparatively safe surgical procedure. When properly done in selected cases relief is sometimes very speedy, but in other cases this may not be experienced for a year or more.

*Necessity is the only justification for ovarian extirpation.*

# CHAPTER XVI.

## DISEASES OF THE URETHRA, BLADDER, AND URETERS.

BY CHARLES JEWETT, M.D., Sc.D., AND JOHN O. POLAK, M.D.

## THE URETHRA.

*Anatomy.*—The inferior three-fourths of the urethra is embedded in the anterior vaginal wall, the upper fourth is separated from the vagina by an intermediate layer of cellular tissue. In its average normal position it courses backward and upward in a general direction nearly parallel with the pelvic brim. Its shape, however, is slightly curved, with its concavity toward the symphysis. Its inferior or anterior portion lies immediately beneath the pubic arch, suspended by the pubo-vesical ligament. Its relation to the superior and inferior triangular ligaments is similar to that in the male. The inferior opening of the urethra, the meatus urinarius, is situated in the median line at the lower margin of the vestibule, its posterior or superior orifice at the neck of the bladder. The average length of the urethra is one inch and three-eighths, and when not overstretched its diameter is about one-fourth inch, but it admits of considerable distention. The urethra when at rest is a closed tube. According to Henle, its cross-section at a point near the meatus presents an antero-posterior slit, near its vesical end a transverse slit, and in the intermediate portion is stellate, owing to the arrangement of the mucous membrane in longitudinal folds. These mucous folds, however, frequently extend to the meatus, giving it a puckered or star-like appearance. Sometimes this orifice is round.

The urethra has a mucous and two muscular coats. The mucosa, as already stated, is disposed in longitudinal folds. The epithelium of the lower portion of the urethra is of the squamous variety, that of the upper portion is partly of the cylindrical and partly of the pavement form. The mucous surface is studded with papillæ, and near the external orifice are numerous lacunæ. The urethral glands are most abundant near the meatus. The basement membrane is composed of fibrillar connective tissue richly supplied with elastic fibres. The submucous coat, not distinctly separated from the mucosa, contains a dense net-work of veins, giving it the character of cavernous tissue. The muscular coat is arranged in an inner longitudinal and an outer circular layer. The innermost fibres are smooth, the outer, in part, of the voluntary striated variety. The latter act as a

823

sphincter for the bladder; a similar function is performed by the compressor urethræ muscle between the layers of the triangular ligament. The muscular coat of the canal is enclosed by a fascia.

Just within the external orifice of the urethra are two glandular tubules. Skene, who first discovered them, describes them as follows: " Upon each side, near the floor of the female urethra, there are two tubules large enough to admit a No. 1 probe of the French scale. They extend from the meatus urinarius upward from three-eighths to three-fourths of an inch, running parallel with the long axis of the canal. They are located beneath the mucous membrane in the muscular walls of the urethra." The mouths of these tubules are found upon the free surface of the mucosa, within the labia of the meatus urinarius. The location of the openings is subject to slight variations according to the condition and form of the meatus. In some subjects, especially the young and the very old, and in those in whom the meatus is small and does not project above the plane of the vestibule, the orifices are found about one-eighth of an inch within the outer border of the meatus. When the mucous membrane of the meatus is thickened and relaxed, so as to become slightly prolapsed, or when the meatus is inverted, the openings are exposed to view upon each side of the entrance to the urethra. The upper ends of the tubules terminate in a number of divisions, which branch off into the muscular walls of the urethra.

### MALFORMATIONS OF THE URETHRA.

Atresia urethræ is a rare congenital defect. Most frequently it is due to a transverse membranous septum. Sometimes the urethra is reduced to a tendinous cord in a portion of its course or through its whole extent. The urine may be evacuated at the umbilicus through a pervious urachus, or it may escape by some other abnormal channel. When no exit exists, the bladder becomes distended during intra-uterine life by accumulation of urine. This condition usually renders the fœtus non-viable, and is liable seriously to complicate delivery.

In hypospadias, the lower or anterior portion of the urethra is either wholly absent or in its place there is a groove representing the upper urethral wall. The urethra thus opens at some point upon the anterior vaginal wall.

A case of bifurcation of the urethra is described by Fürst. From a point one-tenth inch below its vesical end the urethra was double. The two canals opened into the vagina at points about one-tenth inch apart.

*Treatment of Atresia.*—Urethral atresia with imperforate bladder is seldom amenable to treatment; the malformed fœtus generally dies during delivery or soon after. In a few instances the life of the child has been saved by the establishment of an artificial canal by puncture in the direction of the absent urethra or in the suprapubic region. Cases of atresia urethræ with urachal fistula have been successfully treated by ligating the umbilical excrescence and constructing a canal to supply the missing portion of the urethra.  A mere membranous septum should be perforated.

When only the inferior portion of the urethra is absent, the defect may be remedied by a plastic operation.  Flaps are formed by longitudinal incisions one on either side of the median line.  Their edges are dissected up and turned in towards each other in such a manner that the epithelial surface of the flaps shall form the lining of the canal.  The channel thus constructed is made continuous with the existing portion of the urethra above.  The flaps should be somewhat larger than are apparently needed, to allow for subsequent contraction.  A sound should be occasionally passed for a time, to counteract the tendency to narrowing.

### DISEASES OF THE URETHRA.

**Urethritis.**—Urethritis is in the great majority of cases of gonorrhœal origin.  Simple urethritis, while comparatively infrequent, may occur from a variety of causes.  Among these may be mentioned prolonged and unsatisfied sexual excitement, the irritating effects of concentrated urine or septic vaginal discharges, chemical irritants, and mechanical injuries.  Exceptionally urethral catarrh may occur as a complication of one of the exanthematous diseases.

Recent writers agree almost unanimously concerning the frequency of gonorrhœal urethritis, and that it is never absent in cases of recent infection of the vulvo-vaginal tract.  Zeissl, however, maintains that there are only five cases of urethral blennorrhœa to a hundred of gonorrhœal vaginitis.  This difference of opinion is probably to be attributed to the fact that in many instances the acute stage is mild and of short duration, and that chronic urethritis in the female may easily be overlooked.  The period of incubation in the specific form is from two to five days.

*Symptoms.*—Urethritis begins in sensitive patients with slight chilliness, malaise, and moderate burning and tickling upon urination, for several days.  These symptoms are frequently ignored or overlooked.  The prominent symptom in the acute stage is painful urination.  Scalding and burning are caused by the passage of the urine over the inflamed mucous membrane.  There is also frequent desire to urinate.  In occasional cases a few drops of blood escape during or immediately after micturition.  In hemorrhage proceeding from the urethra the blood is not intimately mixed with the urinary secretions, as is usually the case in hemorrhage from other portions of the urinary tract.  In non-specific urethritis the manifestations are of a milder character, and it usually runs its course in a few days.  The gonorrhœal form lasts about six weeks, the acute symptoms subsiding in from ten to fourteen days.  Disease in Skene's follicles runs a slow course, persisting long after all other manifestations have ceased.

*Diagnosis.*—In acute urethritis the meatus is swollen, reddened, and the urethral mucous membrane somewhat prolapsed, exposing the inflamed orifices of the urethral glands.  Per vaginam the urethra is felt as a firm ·

cord, tender to the touch. In any stage, by pressure through the vagina upon the urethra from above downward, except when the patient has voided urine immediately before, a purulent fluid can be pressed from the meatus. In the specific form the microscope will generally reveal the presence of the gonococcus.

Neisser contends that the microscopical examination for the coccus is at present the best and only strictly reliable diagnostic method. The cocci are to be looked for in urethral or vaginal mucus, in the urine, or upon threads which have been left for a short time in the vagina. The non-specific character of the inflammation can be established only after repeated and skilled examinations have failed to demonstrate the presence of the gonococcus.

If the patient voids a portion of the urine into one vessel and the remainder into another, during the acute stage, cloudy urine will be found in the first vessel, clear urine in the second; cloudiness of the second urine indicates cystitis.

In the female, gonorrhœal urethritis frequently passes into the chronic stage. In chronic urethritis there are no subjective symptoms, the diagnosis depending wholly upon physical examination. The patient not having urinated for several hours, a drop of thin, milky muco-pus may be obtained by pressure upon the urethra from behind forward. Urine passed after observing the precaution to cleanse the vulva will be found cloudy and containing shreds of mucus. The endoscope reveals the usual appearances of inflammation.

*Treatment.*—The treatment in acute urethritis, whether of specific origin or not, is conducted on the same general plan. It consists essentially in rest, a non-stimulating diet, the use of alkaline drinks, hot vaginal douches, warm sitz baths, and saline laxatives. In the subacute and chronic stages the oil of sandal-wood (ten minims every four hours) will be of service. The drug should be pure, and is best given in capsules. Salol, in doses of five grains every three hours, is useful, and is sometimes better borne than the sandal-wood oil.

Authorities differ as to the proper time to begin urethral injections. Most writers advise waiting till pain and smarting have nearly ceased. Neisser, on the other hand, begins in acute cases at the outset. He employs injections of nitrate of silver (1 to 4000), repeated four to six times daily. During convalescence the frequency is reduced to once a day. For the first few days after beginning this treatment the discharge is increased; it then becomes watery and contains more epithelium, the gonococci rapidly disappearing. This plan of treatment is also endorsed by Guyon. The injections are made when the bladder is moderately full, with an ordinary urethral syringe, a pipette, or Skene's reflux catheter, which is adapted for urethral irrigation. The bladder should always contain urine, in order to prevent direct action of the injection-fluid upon the walls of that organ. Great benefit is derived from douching the urethra two or three times a day with water as hot as the patient can bear, using the reflux fluted catheter (Skene) with a fountain syringe attached.   In subacute or chronic cases this may be followed by an injection of sulphate of zinc (gr. ½ to gr. ii ad ʒi), or by the use of a urethral suppository of iodoform (gr. x) in cacao butter.

FIG. 1.

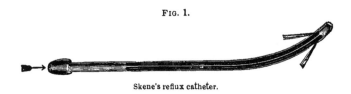

Skene's reflux catheter.

Ichthyol diluted with an equal volume of water is warmly praised as a local application.

J. William White recommends reflux urethral irrigation with gradually increasing strengths of nitrate of silver, beginning with one-half grain to the drachm, followed by gradually strengthened solutions of sulpho-carbolate of zinc.   Weisse passes an elastic or metallic catheter into the bladder, and, after withdrawing the contents, injects into it, by means of the irrigator, zinc sulphate, two to three parts, tannin, five-tenths part, in five hundred parts of water, at a temperature of 26° R. (90° F.)   The catheter is then withdrawn and the patient directed to empty the bladder.   Granular erosions yield to local applications of nitrate of silver.   Particularly good results are obtained by daily applications of a two- to five-per-cent. solution of nitrate of silver through a short endoscope, by means of applicators, which are easily made of smooth, narrow strips of wood wrapped with cotton.

Gradual dilatation with bougies is applicable to certain cases where hyperplasia of the walls has caused contraction of the canal to a greater or less degree.

In chronic cases with persistent suppuration in Skene's glands, these tubules must be laid open by slitting them up on the urethral surface and touching them with strong tincture of iodine or a solution of perchloride of iron.

**Stricture of the Urethra.**—Urethral coarctations are far less frequent in the female than in the male; they are for the most part acquired, congenital narrowing being extremely rare.   Strictures of a high grade are of very exceptional occurrence.   The causes of cicatricial contraction are chronic urethritis, most frequently gonorrhœal, injuries during child-birth and other forms of traumatism, caustic applications, and ulcers of syphilitic or tuberculous origin.   Atresia may arise from atrophy of the muscular coats.

*Symptoms.*—A history of injury during labor or of urethritis is sometimes obtainable.   Irritability of the bladder and dysuria are usually the most prominent symptoms.   Rarely there is incontinence or partial retention, which may give rise to cystitis.

*Diagnosis.*—Digital examination per vaginam will reveal more or less thickening and induration of the urethra at the strictured point. Cicatrices may be felt in the urethro-vaginal septum. The existence of stricture, too, is easily demonstrated and its location determined, as in the male, by a bulbous sound. Obstruction from pressure upon the urethra by pelvic neoplasms or from urethral dislocations may be confounded with stricture, but these conditions are readily distinguished from cicatricial contraction.

*Prognosis.*—In general, under proper treatment, the prognosis is good. In long-standing cases in which dilatation of the urethra or chronic cystitis has been established, while much may be done for the amelioration of the condition, complete recovery is seldom possible.

*Treatment.*—As a rule, the most satisfactory method of treatment is gradual dilatation as practised in stricture of the male urethra. A series of graduated dilators similar to those used by Kelly in dilating the urethra for diagnostic purposes may be used. Instruments should be sterile, and the urethral canal carefully cleansed before they are passed. Care must be taken to prevent laceration of the urethral mucosa, and the dilatation ought not to be carried far enough to cause permanent incontinence. The largest sound should never exceed sixty millimetres in circumference. Dense cicatricial bands which do not yield to the foregoing treatment may be incised with a dilating urethrotome after the method of Otis, as practised in stricture of the male urethra. The normal calibre of the urethra is then maintained by passing a full-sized sound at intervals of several days till the incision has healed. When the urethral obstruction depends on a constricting band of scar-tissue in the anterior vaginal wall, the cicatrix should be divided by multiple transverse incisions on the vaginal surface and subsequent contraction prevented by the use of the sound.

**Prolapse of the Urethral Mucous Membrane.**—Prolapse of the urethral mucous membrane sufficient to cause a marked protrusion at the meatus is rare. Slight ectropion is by no means uncommon. The process of eversion is usually a gradual one; acute prolapse is, however, possible. The prolapse generally involves the entire margin of the meatus; exceptionally it is limited to a portion of it. In recent prolapse the surface of the tumor differs little in appearance from the normal mucous membrane. In long-standing cases the protruding mass may become dark, œdematous, fissured, eroded.

Hofmeier observes that this affection is most frequently met with in young debilitated women. He mentions, however, two cases which occurred in children seven and nine years of age respectively. Portions of the prolapsed tumors microscopically examined by Ruge revealed a very vascular structure, consisting of widely dilated vessels set closely together, rather than a true primary prolapse of the urethral mucous membrane. Södermark has reported three cases, two of which occurred in old women, aged fifty-eight and seventy years respectively, while the third was found in a child of nine years.

The following cases recently published by Bagot, of Denver, Colorado, are of interest:

CASE I.[1]—A woman, aged thirty-three years, came to the Rotunda Hospital, April, 1889, stating that there was a swelling at the orifice of her vagina, from which a discharge was running, and that for the past week she suffered from intense pain on walking and during micturition. She had been delivered of her second child about four weeks and five days previous to this, and there had been nothing abnormal about her labor, but during the puerperium she had suffered from a slight attack of endometritis. On examination, a small dark-red tumor about the size of a walnut was found projecting from the vestibule. The central and most prominent portion of the tumor was sloughing, and in the middle of the sloughing mass the external orifice of the urethra was found, through which a sound was easily passed into the bladder. The tumor was simply dusted over with iodoform and the patient kept in bed. She was discharged in four weeks, the tumor having sloughed off in a day or two after admission, a spontaneous cure thus being brought about.

CASE II.—A child, five years of age. She had been suffering from pain during micturition for the past five weeks; her under-linen was constantly stained by a sanious discharge. Examination revealed a tumor of bright-red color, about the size of a large cherry; it was found projecting from the vestibule and filling up the vulvar orifice. The external meatus of the urethra, situated in the centre of the tumor, was dilated and funnel-shaped, resembling very much the ostium of a Fallopian tube greatly hypertrophied and swollen. The tumor bled easily when touched. The growth was removed with the scalpel, and the urethral mucous membrane stitched to the external mucosa with interrupted silk sutures. Recovery.

CASE III.—A child, seven years of age, had been suffering from hæmaturia for some days. Examination demonstrated a dark-red or purple tumor, about the size of a cherry,

FIG. 2.

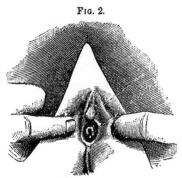

Prolapse of urethral mucous membrane in a child. (Bagot.)

projecting from the vestibule, the meatus being situated a little below the centre of it. It bled easily when touched, and on inquiry it was found that the child had from time to time suffered from hemorrhages, but had at no time complained of pain. The same procedure was adopted as in Case II., with entire success. (Fig. 2.)

*Etiology.*—A relaxed condition of the urethra, together with a loose

[1] Dublin Journal of the Medical Sciences, September, 1891.

attachment of its mucous membrane to the submucous structures, is generally assumed as a predisposing cause of the prolapse. Age and debility undoubtedly favor its development.

Vesical or rectal tenesmus of whatever origin, and, in children, violent and prolonged paroxysms of coughing, are regarded as exciting causes.

Bagot observes that in the cases reported by him the results of microscopical examination went to confirm the opinion that cases which are commonly described as complete prolapse of the urethral mucous membrane are rarely, if ever, instances of true primary prolapse, but that the prolapse of the mucous membrane is secondary to some neoplastic change in it, the most usual being, according to the investigations of Ruge and Martin, angioma.

*Symptoms.*—Vesical tenesmus and dysuria are marked in proportion to the degree of obstruction and the sensitiveness and irritability of the urethra and the displaced structures. Soreness and pain are increased on walking, and coitus is frequently painful. Pain, however, is not always present, especially in children.

*Diagnosis.*—When the displaced mucous membrane is not too much strangulated and swollen, mere prolapse may usually be distinguished from new growths by the fact that it may be replaced. The reduction of the tumor should be attempted with the patient in the lithotomy position. Again, urethral prolapse generally appears as a circular protrusion with a central opening. The tumor is of a less vivid color, is less prone to bleed, and is less sensitive to the touch, than caruncle.

*Treatment.*—In recent cases, and in others in which the prolapsed structures are in a comparatively healthy condition, simple measures may be tried. The protruding mass should be replaced, after reducing the swelling by applications of hot water or ice. After repositing the redundant mucous membrane, retraction of the urethral canal is to be promoted by the use of suitable applications, such as touching daily with a two-per-cent. carbolic acid solution or dilute tincture of iodine. Tannic acid bougies, weak solutions of persulphate of iron, or other astringent remedies may be tried. Meantime the patient must be kept in the recumbent posture and care used to guard against recurrence of the prolapse during micturition. Vesical or rectal tenesmus must, so far as possible, be relieved. The bladder should be examined for the possible presence of stone or vesical tumors.

These means failing, or being obviously inadequate, recourse must be had to more active measures. The writers have succeeded with linear cauterization of the prolapsed membrane. The fine point of a Paquelin cautery is used at a dull-red heat, three or four applications being made in a line with the axis of the canal and at equal distances about the circumference.

Excision of the redundant tissue is frequently necessary. After removal with the knife or scissors, the urethral mucous membrane is stitched to the margin of the orifice with fine sutures. Subsequent dilatation of the meatus may be necessary to counteract cicatricial contraction.

Vesico-Urethral Fissure.—Skene says that this lesion is by no means infrequently met with in the female. Reginald Harrison and Spiegelberg have recognized and described a similar condition in the posterior urethra and neck of the bladder in the male. In 1882, Harrison called attention to the condition sometimes found at the neck of the bladder after death, consisting in a crack or fissure of the mucous membrane, produced by ulceration commencing in the posterior urethra and involving the neck of the bladder. About two-thirds of the fissure is located in the urethra, while only the upper portion extends into the vesical neck, yet the entire lesion is within the grasp of the sphincter vesicæ in the majority of cases, and is thus a potent cause of irritable bladder which may often pass unrecognized by the physician. The cause of the fissure probably lies in a previous urethritis. Injuries during confinement favor the development of this affection, since repair of lesions within the grasp of the sphincter is seldom possible.

*Symptoms.*—The symptomatic importance of this lesion depends upon its site. Occurring, as it does, at the union of the bladder and the urethra, and because of the constant slight pressure by sphincteric contraction, the pain is continuous and severe. The upper portion of the fissure, which extends into the bladder, is exposed to the irritation of the urine, and excites a constant burning pain at the neck of the bladder. Pain is most severe during and after urination, and the patient strains to empty the bladder. Occasionally a few drops of blood escape at the end of micturition. The pain varies in degree, in some cases being intense when the urine is highly acid and less severe when it is neutral or alkaline.

*Diagnosis.*—Pressure with the finger upon the neck of the bladder and posterior urethra produces a sensation as though a knife were piercing the part. The symptoms of cystitis and urethritis very closely simulate those of urethro-vesical fissure. In fissure, however, the pain is acute and circumscribed, while in cystitis it is diffuse and frequently extends over the body of the bladder. In fissure, urination is followed by the maximum degree of pain, while in cystitis a sense of relief soon follows micturition. In urethritis the greatest pain occurs during micturition, and subsides shortly after the bladder is emptied. Examination of the urine will exclude cystitis, while the presence of fissure can be detected and urethritis excluded by careful endoscopic examination.

In a majority of the cases observed by him, Skene has found the fissure on the right side of the neck anteriorly. Through the endoscope, with the parts on the stretch, it appears as freshly torn and bleeding, from one-fourth to one-half inch in length, and from one-twelfth to one-sixth inch in width, tapering towards the ends. The deepest part has a gray color, like an indolent ulcer, while the edges appear actively inflamed.

*Treatment.*—This is one of the most troublesome affections of the urinary tract which the surgeon is called upon to treat. Injections of various remedial agents in different strengths are not only useless, but even seem

to increase the tenesmus and other distressing symptoms.  Direct applications of strong caustics, the actual cautery, or free linear incision with

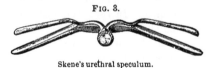

FIG. 3.

Skene's urethral speculum.

the knife, the fissure being exposed by the endoscope, yield
reasonably good results.  Dilatation of the urethra with
sounds gradually increasing in
size gives great relief.  Before
treatment by incising or dilating, salol, in doses of a drachm daily,
should be administered for a few days for its antiseptic effect upon the
urine.

Skene, in a recent paper,[1] recommends touching the fissure with the
galvano-cautery.  The method, however, is difficult of execution.  When
the fissure is on the vaginal side of the urethra, he uses a fenestrated endoscope, bringing the fissure into the field of vision.  (Fig. 4.)  He makes
pressure upon the endoscope from
the vagina with the finger, which
forces the diseased portion of the
mucous membrane into the fenestra and prevents the overflow of
urine.  He then dries it with a

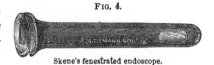

FIG. 4.

Skene's fenestrated endoscope.

small piece of bibulous paper and applies the cautery by simply drawing the
point slowly through the ulcer, so as completely to destroy its surface.  To
a certain extent, lateral fissures can be managed in the same way, but when
the fissure occurs above, which, fortunately, seldom happens, it is almost
impossible to employ this treatment.  The knife and argentic nitrate in
the mitigated stick are applied in a similar manner through the fenestra
of the endoscope.

When the foregoing methods fail, the establishment of a vesico vaginal
fistula, placing the fissure at rest, offers the only chance of recovery.

**Urethrocele.**—Urethrocele is a sacculation of the middle portion of
the urethra.  It consists most frequently in a bagging of the inferior wall,
the upper wall deviating little, if at all, from its normal position.  Less
often it is a diverticulum with a more or less constricted orifice.  The
tumor may attain a diameter of five or six centimetres.

*Etiology.*—The etiology of urethrocele is not settled.  That injuries
inflicted during childbirth have much to do with the etiology of simple dilatation is rendered probable by the fact that this lesion is most commonly
met with in women who have borne children.

Obstruction by organic stricture, and consequent dilatation of the
urethra immediately behind the stricture by reason of the impeded flow
of urine, have been assumed as causes.  As a fact, however, stricture and
urethral dilatation seldom coexist.  According to Englisch, the diver-

---

[1] Transactions of the New York Obstetrical Society, 1892.

ticular form results from the rupture of a congenital cyst of the urethral wall into the urethral canal.

*Symptoms.*—The symptoms of urethrocele are for the most part due directly or indirectly to the retention of a certain amount of urine in the sac. The residual urine becomes ammoniacal by decomposition and finally purulent. The sac-wall becomes inflamed and eroded. The ammoniacal urine causes urethritis; cystitis sometimes results from extension into the bladder. In many cases decomposed urine is expelled from the sac on sneezing, coughing, laughing, or other sudden muscular effort, giving rise to severe and troublesome excoriations of the surrounding external surfaces. There is frequent desire to urinate, and urination is painful. In case of the diverticular form of urethrocele with a very small orifice, so little residual urine may escape from the sac on micturition as to cause but little urethritis and little or no inconvenience.

*Diagnosis.*—Sacculation of the urethra is perceptible to the touch per vaginam and to ocular inspection of the anterior vaginal wall. When the pouch is of large size, it protrudes from the vulva. The retention of urine in the sac may be demonstrated by drawing it off with a catheter. Under pressure with the finger the sac collapses and the contents ooze from the meatus. On examination with the endoscope, the walls of the urethrocele are found inflamed and frequently eroded and covered with granulations. The existence of the pouch is also established by passing a curved sound into the pocket per urethram. The difficulty with which the sound enters the mouth of the sac and the globular expansion beyond serves to distinguish a diverticulum from simple dilatation. A periurethral abscess which has ruptured into the canal is differentiated by the history, and by the induration of the surrounding structures.

*Treatment.*—The plan of treatment will depend upon the form of the urethrocele and the degree of attending inflammation in the urethra and bladder. If the sac be of the diverticular variety, with little attending urethritis, it may be wholly excised and the resulting fistula closed by suture.

Fig. 5.

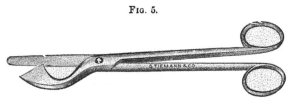

Skene's button-hole scissors.

In the presence of much urethritis, the opening remaining after excision of the sac should be left unclosed, to facilitate drainage and the use of remedial applications. The diffuse form is best treated by Bozeman's method of incision of the most dependent portion of the sac. A convenient instrument for the purpose is Skene's button-hole scissors (Fig. 5), or the Paquelin cautery knife may be used, cutting down upon a sound previously passed into the urethra. The urethritis is to be treated by the usual methods. After the parts have been restored to a comparatively healthy condition the fistula may be closed, with care to remove first any remaining redundant tissue. Cystitis, if present, is to be treated as in other cases. In moderate diffuse sacculation of the urethra with but little accompanying urethrocele, Skene advises dilating the lower part of the urethra and supporting the sacculated portion either with a pessary or with a tampon, together with the use of the usual topical applications.

**Urethral Dislocations.**—The only urethral dislocations of special clinical importance are downward displacements. Upward dislocation, as a rule, gives rise to no symptoms, save difficulty in passing the catheter. In downward displacement, on the contrary, varying degrees of suffering are experienced by the patient. The displacement may be partial or complete. In partial dislocation downward the "upper two-thirds of the urethra is prolapsed, that portion of the canal having a backward instead of an upward direction." When the prolapse is complete the bladder presents at the vulva, with the urethra protruding between the labia minora. A case is reported in which the bladder and the urethra lay between the thighs.

*Etiology.*—Downward dislocation of the urethra is invariably associated with prolapse of the anterior wall of the vagina. These conditions are almost uniformly the result of injuries during childbirth, sagging of the anterior vaginal wall occurring in perineal lacerations involving the levator ani muscle. The bladder or the upper portion of the urethra is thus permitted to fall below its normal position. The severer grades of urethral prolapse are possible only when the urethra has been partly torn from its supports.

*Symptoms.*—In minor degrees of displacement there are vesical irritability and partial loss of control of the bladder; urine escapes on coughing, sneezing, or laughing. In extreme displacement this unpleasant symptom is absent; the sharp bend in the urethra prevents incontinence, and difficult urination is the rule. The severity of the symptoms is much relieved by the recumbent position.

*Diagnosis.*—The diagnosis is readily made by a digital examination per vaginam or by inspection with the aid of a Sims speculum. Downward projection of at least a part of the urethra into the vagina will be observed.

*Prognosis.*—Under proper treatment, the prognosis is favorable in recent cases. After long-standing prolapse, restoration is difficult or impossible, owing to the development of structural changes.

*Treatment.*—As suggested by Skene, from whose work the foregoing facts have been largely drawn, the curative treatment must be addressed to the cause. Perineal injuries should be repaired, with a view to restoring the natural supports of the anterior vaginal wall. Temporary relief, with some degree of permanent benefit, may be gained by the use of vaginal tampons or the employment of a pessary so constructed as to support the entire prolapsed portion of the urethra.

**Fistulæ.**—Urethral fistulæ may be complete or incomplete; both forms, and especially the latter, are of rare occurrence. Complete fistulæ of the urethra open into the vagina; they result usually from injuries during childbirth. They give rise to comparatively little incontinence, as the urine is discharged through the fistula only during micturition. The method of procedure for the closure of complete urethral fistulæ differs in no respect from that employed in vesico-vaginal fistulæ, which will be found described under the treatment of the latter affection.

Incomplete urethral fistula is an opening leading from the urethra into the urethro-vaginal septum and ending in a blind extremity. A periurethral abscess rupturing into the urethra may leave such a fistulous tract. Rarely, cysts of the urethro-vaginal septum rupture into the urethra and cause this incomplete variety of fistula.

*Diagnosis.*—Pain during urination and a sense of heat in the urethra are common symptoms. A blind fistula in the posterior portion of the canal in the vicinity of the vesical neck gives rise to frequent urination and tenesmus. Pus may at times ooze from the urethra. Smarting during and for some time after urination is almost invariably present.

A history of periurethral inflammation materially aids the diagnosis. Examining by the vagina, the finger will detect thickening and induration of the urethral walls and in the urethro-vaginal septum at the seat of the fistula. Pus can be made to escape from the meatus by pressure from above downward upon the urethra with the finger in the vagina. When the lesion is situated in the floor of the urethra, as it most frequently is, it may be detected by a probe with the point slightly bent. This condition must be distinguished from the diverticular form of urethrocele.

*Treatment.*—The fistula should be made complete and the edges of the wound carefully denuded. The urethra and the fistulous tract are then to be kept clean by injections into the urethra of a solution of boric acid or some equally bland antiseptic. The urine is drawn with the catheter, to prevent irritating the wound; then the urethro-vaginal fistula may close of its own accord, or it can readily be closed by the usual operative procedure.

### TUMORS.

**Caruncle.**—Caruncle is a small raspberry-like growth at the external orifice of the urethra. Usually it is situated at the inferior portion of the meatus, though it may spring from any part of the circumference. In exceptional cases its location is above the orifice within the canal. These growths vary in size from that of a pin-head to that of a pea, and are usually single, occasionally multiple. They consist of hypertrophied papillæ, and are extremely vascular and abundantly supplied with nerve-filaments. To these growths Winckel has given the name papillary angiomata.

*Symptoms.*—The most prominent symptoms of urethral caruncle are exquisite sensitiveness to the touch and extreme pain during micturition; the severity of these symptoms is out of all proportion to the apparent importance of the lesion. Sexual intercourse is painful, frequently impossible, owing to the reflex spasm of the levator ani muscle. There is irritability of the bladder, giving rise to frequent urination and vesical spasm. In extreme cases cystitis may result: There is usually more or less hemorrhage from the tumor, sometimes to the point of exsanguination. Few affections of the urinary tract are capable of causing more serious injury to the general health. In neglected cases the nervous system is shattered by pain and loss of sleep and the patient is reduced to a condition of chronic invalidism.

*Diagnosis.*—Caruncle must be distinguished from urethral polypi and from prolapse of the urethral mucous membrane. A polypus is usually attached by a slender pedicle, while in papillary angioma the growth is sessile. Moreover, the former lacks the sensitiveness of the latter. In prolapse the protrusion is circular, with the urethral orifice at its centre, while caruncle springs from a portion only of the circumference. The vascular tumor, too, cannot be reduced. Angiomata in the deeper portion of the urethra may be differentiated from other urethral tumors by their sensitiveness to touch with the probe or to the pressure of the finger through the urethro-vaginal septum.

**Varices.**—These appear as bundles of irregularly distended, dark-blue or bluish-red vessels, most frequently occupying the urethral floor. Erectility has been observed in some of these vascular neoplasms. Occasionally a varix may rupture beneath the mucous membrane, forming a hæmatoma.

**Glandular Neoplasms.**—Urethral cysts may be located at any point in the canal. In early life they occur in the meatal portion, later near the vesical neck. Their origin is due for the most part to occlusion of the orifices of urethral glands. These small cysts are transformed into polypi by the absorption of their contents. The rarest form of neoplasm under this head is myxo-adenoma. This is small, vascular, and of a bright scarlet color, consisting of degenerated glandular tissue richly supplied with blood-vessels, the meshes being filled with myxomatous débris, supported by loose connective tissue.

**Fibroma and Sarcoma.**—The former, as a rule, lies embedded in the muscular wall of the urethra; it is frequently peduncular and protrudes from the meatus. In size fibromata vary from the bulk of a pea to that of a goose-egg. On section they are found to consist of densely packed fibrous tissue covered by stratified epithelium. As a class they are of infrequent occurrence.

Sarcoma of the urethra is so seldom met with that its mere mention in this connection will suffice.

**Carcinoma and Epithelioma.**—The existence of primary cancer of the urethra is very rare. Reginald Harrison and Mr. Beck each report a case in the male. In the female it is less frequent than in the other sex.

Goodell mentions a case in which the woman suffered severely from urinary obstruction due to cancerous growths in the urethra. The diagnosis is possibly open to doubt, as the patient was soon lost sight of and no microscopical examination was made. Lewers cites a case in a woman forty-nine years of age. She had had three children, the youngest being then fifteen years old. On examination in the situation of the urethral orifice, he found an irregularly-shaped ulcerated cavity admitting the tip of the finger. The walls of the cavity were formed of hard tissue, and the induration extended up the anterior vaginal wall for nearly two inches. The surface of the cavity bled easily on touch. The glands in both groins were involved. This may properly be regarded as a case of extension from the outer genitals. Even secondary malignant diseases by extension from uterus, bladder, or vagina rarely, if ever, reach the urethra before the patient dies.

Several cases have been recorded of periurethral carcinoma at the introitus vulvæ, near the meatus, and in the connective tissue surrounding the urethra.

*Symptoms.*—Pain is not necessarily present. The most frequent symptom is difficulty of micturition, owing to partial obstruction of the canal.

**Polypus.**—True polypus of the urethra is of rare occurrence. When present, it springs from a point high up in the canal, usually at the junction of the urethra with the neck of the bladder, and thus may readily escape detection. It is not painful, and gives rise to little trouble, except that sometimes it may cause obstruction to micturition. Goodell advises exploration of the urethra with the finger to confirm the diagnosis. The endoscope will reveal the condition with as much certainty and with less danger.

*Treatment of Caruncle.*—The use of chemical caustics, such as nitric, chromic, and carbolic acids, is unsatisfactory: the growth, as a rule, soon returns. Even when successful, unnecessary injury is done to the adjacent healthy structures. Total extirpation offers the only hope of permanent relief. This may be effected by excising the diseased structures and stitching together the edges of the healthy mucous membrane of the urethra. The most satisfactory method of extirpating the growth is by actual cautery. Skene recommends the use of the galvano-cautery as follows: "The neoplasm to be removed is seized by a narrow-bladed forceps at the junction of the normal and abnormal tissues, the forceps is closed and locked, and the neoplasm cut off. The cautery is applied to the forceps sufficiently to heat enough to desiccate, not char, the tissues held in its grasp. This being accomplished, the forceps is carefully removed by first unlocking it, then rocking it gently, so as not to pull the pedicle or stump apart and start bleeding. If the work is well done, the thin stump of desiccated tissue will project on the surface of the mucous membrane. The bladder should be emptied before operation, so that there will be no necessity to urinate for five or six hours after. This lessens the danger of reopening the stump, and usually but a small linear surface is left to heal by granulation after the eschar sloughs.  Applications of sterilized vaseline help to protect the stump while healing.  When the neoplasm arises from a chronic inflammation of Skene's glands, as is sometimes the case, the best method is to pass a fine probe up into the canal and cut down upon it with the fine cautery point from the vaginal surface.  In other words, lay the ducts of the glands open ; this divides the neoplasm on one side, and an incision should be made with the cautery on the opposite side, which divides the growth into two equal parts.  Then each part is grasped with forceps and removed in the manner already described."

*Treatment of other Urethral Tumors.*—Tumors of a vascular character with a broad base are readily removed by the ligature.  The growth being exposed and drawn into reach with a forceps, the base is transfixed with a needle from without inward in a direction parallel to the axis of the canal ; a ligature is then thrown around the base beneath the transfixing-needle, traction being made upon the tumor with forceps to bring the sides of the base into the grasp of the ligature, which is then tied tightly, care being taken to prevent cutting the tissues in the ligature.

Torsion is applicable in pedunculated neoplasms.  The base of the pedicle is seized with small thin-pointed forceps and the growth is twisted off with an ordinary pair of nasal forceps.  In employing this method it is well to touch the stump of the pedicle with the galvano-cautery, as a safeguard against hemorrhage, before letting go the grasp with the small forceps.

The curette has been utilized, notably by the Germans, for the removal of growths high up in the urethra.  After curettage the site of the tumor is to be dried and seared with the cautery.  Gouley and Skene employ a polypus snare for the removal of growths high up in the canal.  The technique is as follows : " The tumor being exposed with a urethral speculum, if the growth is pedunculated the loop of wire is passed over it and removal effected by constriction ; when there is a broad base the mass is raised with a pair of polypus forceps and the snare is then passed over and tightened."  Care should be taken to avoid breaking the wire.  The use of

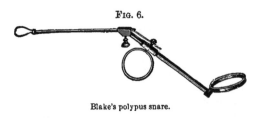

FIG. 6.

Blake's polypus snare.

the galvano-cautery for the destruction of urethral neoplasms has already been described : its value cannot be too highly estimated.

When the tumors are in the upper part of the canal and the meatus is constricted, gradual dilatation by sounds, or the employment of Simon's method of incisions into the external orifice of the urethra, is necessary before the removal of the neoplasm.  In the latter method one incision is made anteriorly, one-fourth centimetre in depth, the other one-half centimetre in depth, posteriorly. If the dilatation is confined to the lower portion of the canal, the growth can be exposed with little or no danger of subsequent incontinence.

The treatment of malignant growths is immediate and complete extirpation with the knife. The excised mass should include a wide margin of the adjoining healthy tissue.

### FOREIGN BODIES IN THE URETHRA.

Foreign bodies of various descriptions may find lodgement in the urethra.

*Diagnosis.*—The symptoms produced depend largely upon the size and character of the foreign body. Partial retention of urine is the chief symptom, accompanied with pain and a spasmodic contraction of both urethra and bladder. If the body be of irregular shape and its surface studded with sharp points, hemorrhage, ulceration, and even periurethral abscess may result. When the obstruction is total, retention, if persistent, may cause serious injury to the ureters and kidneys. The diagnosis is readily established by examining the urethra with the finger in the vagina.

*Treatment.*—The extraction of a foreign body may be accomplished by seizing it with a pair of long, thin-bladed forceps. The body is held in place by the finger passed per vaginam and pressed against the urethra at a point immediately behind the body during the attempt to engage it in the forceps. Sometimes the body can be removed by means of a wire loop or a smooth spoon curette. Dilatation up to the seat of obstruction and extraction with forceps, loop, or curette has been employed. When the object cannot be readily dislodged by these measures, it may, if friable, after being pushed backward into the bladder, be removed through a Kelly speculum with or without lithotripsy. If this be impracticable, incision of the urethra at the point of obstruction is permissible.

## THE BLADDER.

*Anatomy.*—The urinary bladder is a hollow muscular organ. When empty or moderately filled, it lies entirely below the plane of the pelvic brim, between the pubic bones in front and the uterus and vagina behind. In the infant it is an abdominal organ and is somewhat pear-shaped, the urachus corresponding to the stalk. In old age there is a partial return to the infantile condition. When over-distended, the bladder rises above the line of the pubic bones and is seen as a mesial projection above the symphysis. In extreme cases it may reach to the umbilicus, the female being more distensible than the male organ. In the mature female the transverse diameter is the greater, and the shape of the bladder when partially filled is ovoid, with its long axis directed transversely. The empty bladder is generally described as a collapsed sac, whose cavity, together with the canal of the urethra, appears in sagittal section either as a Y-shaped or an L-shaped fissure. This opinion is based on the study of frozen sections and the appearances found on the post-mortem table. Morris (Human Anatomy) says, " It is possible that this diastolic form of the empty bladder, as it has been termed, is the normal result of a relaxation preliminary to re-filling, but it appears more probable that it is due to the loss of the vital

FIG. 7.

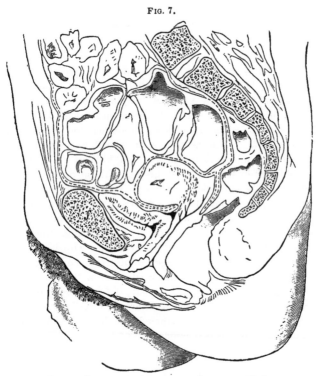

Frozen section of the pelvis, showing empty bladder.   (Fürst)

elasticity of the muscular walls, and that the healthy living bladder always maintains a rounded or ovoid form."

The bladder has three openings,—the ostium urethræ internum and the two ureteric orifices.  The former is described below; the latter are situated one on each side of the median line on the floor of the bladder, about three centimetres behind the vesical opening of the urethra and the same distance apart.  A transverse band stretching from one to the other is known as the inter-ureteric ligament.

The appearance of the ureteral orifice differs in different cases.  As stated by Kelly, " It sometimes appears as a dimple or as a fine slit in the mucous membrane; at others as a $\wedge$ with the point directed outward. Again, it may present the form of a truncated cone with gently sloping sides, the ureteral mons. The latter appearance is most apt to be developed in the knee-chest position." These appearances are of interest in connection with ureteral catheterization through the speculum.

The regional divisions of the bladder are: the apex or summit or superior fundus, the body, the base or inferior fundus, and the so-called neck. (Fig. 8.) The summit of the bladder is directed upward and forward and is attached to the urachus. The base is the part which looks downward and backward. The anatomical limits of these regional divisions, however, are not distinctly defined. The trigone is a triangular space at the base of the bladder whose apex is at the ureteral orifice and whose base is the inter-ureteric line. Over this area the mucous membrane is thinner and more closely adherent, having no submucous layer. The nerve-supply to this space is very abundant, and it is accordingly the most sensitive area of the bladder. The apex of the trigone where it merges into the urethra is the so-called vesical neck. The opening of the urethra into the bladder is, however, abrupt, not funnel-shaped, as the term neck might imply. In that part of the base which lies just behind the inter-ureteric line is a slight depression, the bas-fond, which in old age becomes a deep pouch holding residual urine.

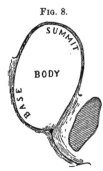

FIG. 8.

Regional divisions of the bladder.

The more important anatomical relations of the bladder are of clinical interest. In the erect posture the anterior inferior surface looks towards the symphysis. It is separated from the pubic bones by a space known as the cavum Retzii. This space contains a variable quantity of loose fat. Each lateral surface is partially covered with peritoneum. The posterior surface is intimately connected below to the cervix uteri and to the upper part of the anterior wall of the vagina, but is separated above from the body of the uterus by the shallow fold of peritoneum, the utero-vesical pouch. The superior surface lies in contact with the small intestines, sometimes also with a portion of the sigmoid flexure and with the appendix vermiformis.

The ligaments of the bladder are five false and five true ligaments. The false ligaments are formed of folds of peritoneum. This is reflected from the inner face of the anterior abdominal wall, at a point just above the symphysis, to the bladder, investing that organ, as has been already shown, superiorly, laterally, and in part posteriorly. It joins the bladder in front, dipping down over the superior vesical surface, and passes as far backward as the point of contact between the vesical base and the uterus at the junction of the uterine body and cervix. The superior peritoneal fold in front, which extends from the summit of the bladder to the umbilicus, covering the urachus, two utero-vesical folds, and the two lateral folds of peritoneum, constitutes the false ligaments. The true ligaments of the bladder are the superior (the urachus), two lateral, and two vesico-pubic, the last four being formed of the recto-vesical fascia.

The bladder has three coats,—a mucous, a muscular, and over a part of its surface a serous or peritoneal coat,—the relation of which to the viscus has already been described. The muscular coat consists of three layers, but the innermost is incomplete. The fibres run for the most part in longitudinal and in circular directions; at the neck the circular fibres are collected into a layer of some thickness, which immediately surrounds the upper end of the urethra, forming the so-called sphincter vesicæ of some writers. The mucous membrane is lined by transitional stratified epithelium and is arranged in irregular folds. Throughout the mucous membrane are minute glands and follicles.

The vascular supply of the bladder is derived from the superior, middle, and inferior vesical arteries, and from branches of the uterine, internal, pudic, hemorrhoidal, and sciatic. The veins form tortuous plexuses about the base, sides, and neck, and finally empty into the internal iliac veins. The lymphatic distribution in the submucous cellular tissues of the bladder is quite extensive, the lymph-vessels emptying into the hypogastric glands.

The nerves of the bladder are derived from the third, fourth, and, in rare cases, the second sacral nerves of the spinal system, and from the hypogastric plexus of the sympathetic. The latter plexus is situated in front of the last lumbar and the first sacral vertebra. The branches of the spinal nerves go mainly to the base and neck of the bladder.

### MALFORMATIONS OF THE BLADDER.

Congenital defects of the bladder, though of great variety, are of rare occurrence. Two only—exstrophy and double bladder—are of clinical interest.

**Exstrophy.**—Fissure of the bladder is the most common congenital defect of that organ. It is far more frequent in the male than in the female subject, eighty to ninety per cent. of cases occurring in the former sex. It is associated with partial failure in the closure of the ventral laminæ. It consists in a cleft, often an entire absence, of the anterior wall of the bladder and a median fissure of the anterior abdominal wall. Like other anomalies of development, it is rarely single. Frequently the urethra and the vagina are absent. Malformation of the vagina or uterus and developmental defects of other pelvic organs, and even hare-lip and spina bifida, are not uncommonly found associated with this anomaly. The ventral cleft may be limited to the region of the umbilicus, to the symphysis, or may involve the entire inferior half of the anterior abdominal parietes. When the ventral fissure is situated near the umbilicus, the pubic symphysis is closed, and the urethra, the inferior portion of the bladder, and the external sexual organs are normally developed. Fissure limited to the lower part of the bladder and the corresponding portion of the pelvis is very seldom found. When the malformation involves the lower portion of the abdominal parietes, there is usually separation of the pubic bones, the clitoris is cleft or undeveloped, the urethra and possibly the vagina are absent. The posterior bladder-wall is pushed forward by the intra-abdominal pressure and protrudes into the opening in the abdominal wall. The latter condition is known as exstrophy of the bladder. The exposed mucous membrane is inflamed and swollen. The ureteral orifices are usually exposed to view. The ureters are generally enlarged, sometimes having a diameter of two, or even eight or ten, centimetres, and their pelvic course and relations are altered. The exposed vesical mucosa of the posterior wall may take on to some extent the appearance of epidermis. The urethra either is impervious or, more frequently, is entirely absent.

*Treatment of Exstrophy of the Bladder.*—All devices thus far proposed for collecting the urine are useless. No plan offers any relief except a plastic operation, and this is only palliative. Even with the best result possible, the surgeon can do no more than diminish the annoyance which comes from the flow of urine over the surrounding external surfaces. Preparatory to operation the general health of the patient must be reinforced by the use of tonics and a suitable, hygienic regimen. As far as possible, morbid conditions of the urine should be corrected and the parts about the field of operation placed in a healthy condition. Whatever operative procedure is adopted, the urethra should first be restored. Of the numerous plastic operations that have been proposed for extroversion of the bladder, Wood's operation is a good example of the best general method of procedure. This consists first in dissecting a flap from the central portion of the abdominal wall immediately above the fissure and large enough to close the bladder completely; this should have a large pedicle. A lateral flap is taken from each groin, the superficial epigastric and the external pudic artery being included in the flap. The umbilical flap is turned down over the abdominal opening, with its skin surface towards the mucous membrane of the bladder. The margin of the abdominal fissure is vivified and the edges of the flap are stitched thereto. The groin flaps are then brought together with their raw surfaces in contact with the raw surface of the central flap and fixed in position by sutures. The parts may be protected after operation with a coating of iodoform and collodion. This plan, if successful, concentrates the flow of urine at a single point, but does not restore the function of the bladder. A urinal will still be required, and can then be used to advantage.

Berg (*Nord. Med. Ark.*, Bd. iii. Heft 3) recommends the following procedure, which he has employed with satisfaction. At a preliminary operation he takes from one inguinal region a single flap large enough to cover the abdominal opening and form the anterior bladder-wall. The raw surface of the flap he covers with epidermis according to Thiersch's method. At a second operation the flap, which now has two skin surfaces, is stitched to the edges of the abdominal fissure in the usual manner. When the capacity of the bladder permits and the mucous membrane is sufficiently healthy, he advises uniting the vesical edges in the median line without any preliminary operation. The abdominal opening is then to be closed with a skin flap.

**Double Bladder.**—Cases of supposed duplicity of the bladder have been described by several writers. Many of the recorded examples of double bladder, however, are susceptible of some other explanation. Sacculation of this viscus may simulate multiple bladder. Mollenetti's case, in which there were five bladders with a common urethra, was probably of this character. A distended urachal pouch or a congenital cyst may be mistaken for a supernumerary bladder. A complete division of the bladder into two halves by a septum is rare. Incomplete division is not so infrequently observed.

### CYSTOSCOPY.

Bruck, of Breslau, first proposed to effect the illumination of various parts and cavities by taking advantage of the diaphanous property of the tissues. For the examination of the bladder he suggested the introduction into the rectum of a properly protected platinum wire at a white heat. The interior surface of the bladder thus illuminated was then to be examined through a urethral speculum. This suggested to Nitze the principle upon which the present electrical cystoscope is based. In 1877 he conceived the plan of introducing a light into the cavity to be examined, with an optic apparatus which magnifies the part to be brought into view.

Leiter's cystoscope (Fig. 9) consists of a metal tube of calibre No. 22 French, with a single fixed angle near its distal end,—a *cathéter coudé*.

FIG. 9.

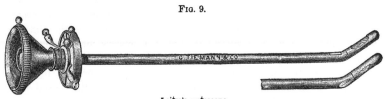

Leiter's cystoscope.

On the upper or concave surface of the beak is a window of rock-crystal. A miniature electric lamp is located within the instrument, behind this window, and is controlled by a switch at the ocular end. Its rays are projected through the window, illuminating the field to be examined. Another window is placed at the distal end of the straight portion of the tube, close to the angle and on the same side of the tube as the first; within the instrument at this window is a totally reflecting prism, which receives the rays from the illuminated field and reflects them along the shank of the cystoscope to the operator's eye. The image of the vesical surface thus brought to view is magnified by means of a telescope placed in the shank of the instrument.

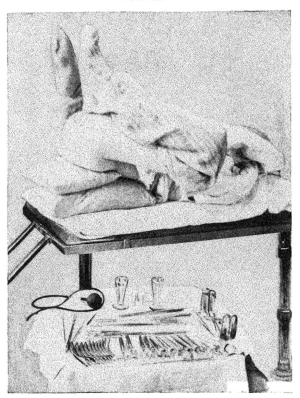

Hips in moderate elevation for cystoscopic examination and direct catheterization of ureters
Cystoscopic and ureteral instruments on the tray in the foreground.

FIG. 12

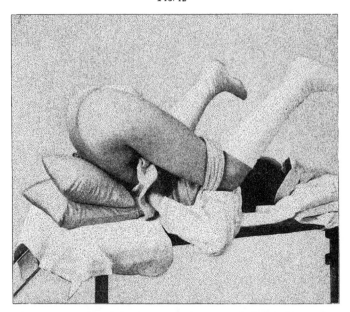

Hips in *extreme* elevation for cystoscopic examination and direct catheterization of ureters

FIG 16.

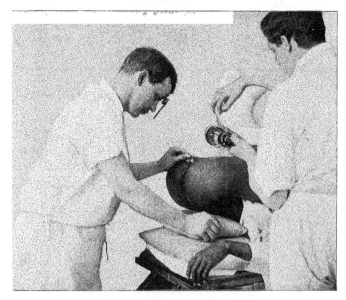

Direct inspection of bladder by reflected light.—Electric bulb with reflector held above symphysis pubis; hips in moderate elevation.

Two different instruments are desirable for exploration of the entire vesical surface: one with the window on the concave side, as above described; and, for the inspection of the base, one with the window on the convex side.

The conditions necessary for the employment of the cystoscope are as follows: first, the meatus and urethra must be of such calibre as to permit the passage of a No. 22 French sound; secondly, the bladder capacity must be from two to four ounces; thirdly, the fluid in the bladder must be transparent. One hundred and fifty cubic centimetres of fluid ($\zeta$v) expand the folds of the intra-vesical surface; more than this quantity places the anterior wall of the bladder so far away that it cannot be properly inspected. The minimum amount of fluid employed for the purpose is sixty cubic centimetres ($\zeta$ii): a bladder which holds less cannot be illuminated.

The filling of a diseased bladder to the proper extent is sometimes impossible because of irritability. This can be overcome by cocaine. Cases of poisoning from adopting Nitze's plan in its employment are, however, reported; Albarran has observed a fatal case. Morphine by suppository or by subcutaneous injection usually answers the purpose. Narcosis by ether or by chloroform is rarely necessary. If the urine be cloudy, the bladder must be previously emptied and washed out. Nitze recommends distention of the bladder with a half-per-cent. carbolic or normal salt solution. Before using the cystoscope the beak should be immersed in water and the light tested to see that it is in working order. Sterilized glycerin is used as a lubricant. The examination is conducted with the patient in the lithotomy position.

The dangers of cystoscopy, all of which are easily preventable with care, are burning of the mucous membrane, breakage of the lamp, and infection of the bladder.

*Direct Examination of the Bladder with the Pelvis Elevated.*—Dr. Robert T. Morris, of New York, has utilized straight endoscopic tubes for vesical examination. Kelly has recently demonstrated the advantage gained by extreme elevation of the pelvis for examining the bladder through the urethral speculum. By this method the interior of the bladder, including the ureteral orifices, can be brought under visual examination, and direct application of remedial agents can be made. For an account of Kelly's method we quote from his original paper:[1] "The following instruments and accessories are required for the examination: a female catheter, a series of urethral dilators, a series of specula with obturators, a common head-mirror and lamp (argand burner or electric light), long, delicate, mouse-toothed forceps, suction apparatus for completely emptying the bladder, ureteral searcher, ureteral catheter without a handle, several bran bags or an inclined plane for elevating the pelvis. The bladder is first emptied as completely as possible by the catheter; a residuum of from one to several

---

[1] American Journal of Obstetrics, January, 1894.

teaspoonfuls of urine always remains, even though the bladder is evacuated with the patient in the standing posture.    In order to determine the proper dilator to begin with, I calibrate the meatus urinarius externus by means of a slender metal cone ten centimetres long, marked in a graduated scale from its point (two millimetres) to its upper end (twenty millimetres in diameter).  (Fig. 10.)  The calibrator is pushed into the urethra as far as it will readily go, and the marking at the meatus externus is noted.  A dilator of the diameter indicated by the calibrator is then passed through the urethra by holding the handle at first well above the level of the external meatus, upon which the point rests, and carrying the dilator on through the urethra and into the bladder by a gentle sweeping curve of the hand downward and inward towards the urethra.  By introducing the dilators as

FIG. 10.

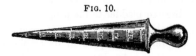

Urethral calibrator: the short lines indicate the diameter in millimetres.  (Kelly.)

they occur in the series, the average female urethra can easily be dilated up to twelve millimetres in diameter, with only a slight external rupture.  I have never seen a tear more than two or three millimetres in length and from one to one and a half in depth.  I have as yet had no occasion to incise the meatus to avoid extensive rupture.

"The metal dilators which I use for this purpose are double-ended and of a flattened S-shape, each end representing a single dilator in the series.  (Figs. 13 and 14.)  The points are conical; a flattened area in the middle, upon which the diameters are marked, affords a convenient grasp.  The series begins with No. 5 and runs in pairs up to No. 20: thus, Nos. 5 and 6 are made of one piece of metal, 7 and 8 of one piece of metal, and so on through the series.  The calibre of both dilators and specula is marked in millimetres.

"As soon as a dilatation of from twelve to fifteen millimetres is reached, a speculum (Fig. 15) of the same diameter as the last dilator is introduced and its obturator removed.  *The hips of the patient are now elevated* on the cushion or on a short inclined plane, twenty to thirty, or even forty centimetres, eight to twelve or sixteen inches above the level of the table.  (Fig. 12.)  There are sixteen specula, varying from five to twenty millimetres in diameter, the successive sizes increasing by one millimetre.  The specula are cylindrical, nine and one-half centimetres long, and each is provided with a conical trumpet-shaped mouth to assist in reflecting the light into the bladder.  Each speculum is fitted with an obturator.  The calibre is marked in millimetres on a little handle at the side of the speculum.

"The examiner now puts on the head-mirror and prepares to inspect the bladder.  An electric drop-light, an argand burner, a lamp, or a candle, in a dark room, is held close to the patient's symphysis pubis (Fig. 16), so that the light can be easily caught by the head-mirror and reflected into the bladder. A good direct light from a window will also suffice. Upon withdrawing the obturator, the pelvis being elevated, the bladder becomes distended with air, and, by properly directing the reflected light, all parts of the interior are accessible to direct inspection. If a pool of urine remains in the bladder, it should be withdrawn by means of a simple suction apparatus. (Fig. 17.) If there is a residuum of not more than two or three cubic centimetres, it can be easily removed by little

Fig. 13.  Fig. 14.

Fig 15.

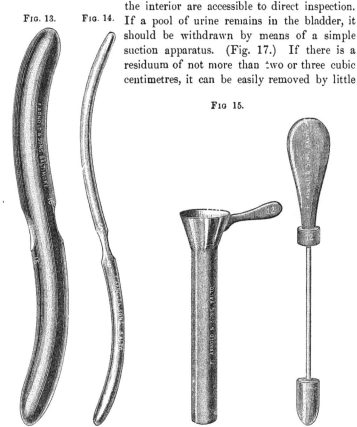

Double urethral dilators.—The smaller sizes, Nos. 5 and 6, are used only when the calibre of the urethra is very small or is narrowed by stricture.

Kelly's speculum and obturator.

balls of absorbent cotton grasped with long, delicate, mouse-toothed forceps, the teeth of which are slightly recurved. The facility with which foreign bodies are removed from the bladder by this method can be demonstrated by dropping a pledget of cotton into the bladder. It can be seen with the utmost ease, picked up, and removed without difficulty.

"The posterior wall of the air-distended bladder lies two to five centimetres distant from the anterior wall, and over this white background which presents itself to the eye of the observer is visible a beautiful net-work of branching and anastomosing vessels. The veins accompanying the arteries are easily distinguished by their dark color. The larger vessels evidently come to the surface from the deeper layers of the bladder, and they branch stellately, divide, and anastomose. By elevating the handle of the speculum, the field of vision sweeps over the base of the bladder until in some cases the region of the inter-ureteric ligament comes into view, often marked by a slightly elevated transverse fold or a distinct difference in color.

FIG. 17.

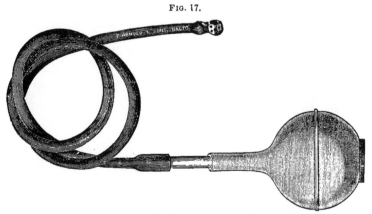

Kelly's suction apparatus (three-fourths natural size), used for withdrawing residual urine.

"By turning the speculum 30° to one side or the other and looking sharply, a ureteral orifice is discovered. The ureteral orifices and their surroundings are not constant in appearance; sometimes the orifice appears as a dimple or a little pit, or, in inflammatory cases, as a round hole in a cushioned eminence; again, it may be scarcely visible even to a trained eye, appearing as a fine crack in the mucosa; and occasionally it is so obscure as to be recognized only by the jet of urine as it escapes, or by a slight difference in the color of the mucous membrane at that point." The mucosa about the ureteral orifice is, as a rule, of a deeper rose color than the remainder of the mucous membrane of the bladder.

"A valuable aid for a beginner searching for the ureteral orifice is the following. A point is marked on the cystoscope five and one-half centimetres from the vesical end, and from this point two diverging lines are drawn towards the handle, with an angle of 60° between them. The speculum is introduced up the point of the V, and turned to the right or left until one side of the V is in line with the axis of the body. Then, by elevating the endoscope until it touches the floor of the bladder, the ureteral orifice will usually be found within the area covered by the orifice of the speculum. In order to ascertain whether it is the ureter which lies within the field, I use as a searcher a long, delicate sound with a handle bent at an angle of 120°, which is introduced through the speculum into the suspected

FIG. 18.

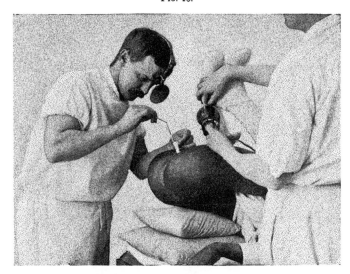

Left ureteral orifice exposed and searcher engaged.

FIG. 19.

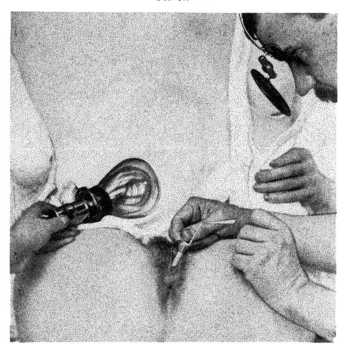

Speculum inclined thirty degrees to left, exposing right ureter; searcher being introduced.

Fig. 22.

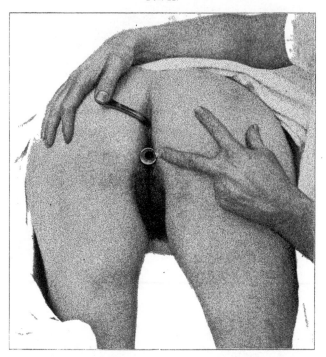

Cystoscopy in genu-facial posture —Speculum introduced into bladder; dilator under
right thumb indicates position of anus.

ureteral orifice which is under inspection. (Fig. 21.) The searcher passes easily from two to six centimetres up the ureter, and the lateral walls of the orifice are slightly raised, appearing as distinct folds with a dark pit between them. The searcher may be withdrawn and the ureteral catheter at once introduced if it is desired to collect urine direct from the kidney.

FIG. 20.

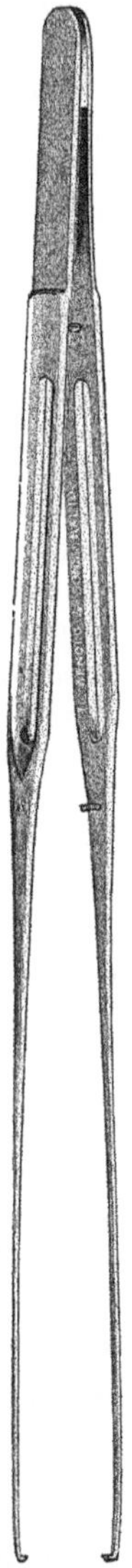

"The ureteral catheters which I use for direct catheterization are quite different from those heretofore employed. They are straighter, and either have no handle or only a small one which will readily pass through the No. 10 speculum. The catheter may be left in place some minutes or an hour or more. The urine which accumulates in the mean time in the bladder necessarily represents the discharge of the opposite kidney. In this way the urine of both kidneys may be isolated by simply introducing one catheter.

FIG. 21.

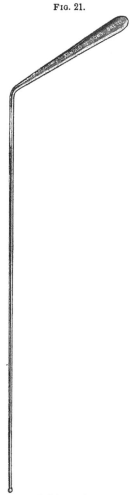

"By placing the patient in the genu-facial posture an extreme distention of the bladder is obtained, in the form of a flattened ovoid. In this posture the inter-ureteric ligament also comes sharply into view, but the ureters are not so readily seen." This posture, according to Kelly, is indispensable in some inflammatory conditions of the bladder resulting in thickening of its walls, thus preventing its ballooning in ordinary positions. Sims's position, modified by elevating the pelvis upon pillows, can be utilized in this method of examination, but with less success than the dorsal posture.

Kelly's delicate mouse-toothed forceps (three-fourths natural size).

Kelly's searcher.

"*Simple, Direct Catheterization without Pelvic Elevation.*—It is possible to catheterize the ureters with the patient simply in the dorsal position, without elevation of the pelvis. The success of such an attempt depends upon the examiner's familiarity with the position and appearance of the ureteral orifice on the posterior wall of the bladder. The manipulation necessary to expose the ureteral orifice becomes with practice almost instinctive. The bladder is emptied by the catheter, the ureter is dilated, and the speculum No. 10 or 12 introduced from five and one-half to six centimetres, and its outer end elevated until the base of the bladder appears, when it is turned 30° to the right or the left, and with a little patience in searching the ureteral orifice is found."

When dilating the urethra with specula smaller than No. 14, an anæsthetic is unnecessary, except in nervous women. When, in such cases, it is necessary to make a thorough examination, an anæsthetic is generally advisable. Local anæsthesia by means of cocaine may be used to facilitate dilatation, and is often the best form of anæsthesia. .

By this method of examination many apparently functional affections of the bladder will be found to belong to the domain of demonstrable diseases. To generalize from the cases lately under my care, I am able to say that cystitis is often a localized disease limited to a special area of the bladder. Tubercular and ulcerative cystitis can be detected at once. Tumors, calculi, and fistulæ are readily found, particularly with the patient in the genu-facial posture. Cicatrices stand out in sharp relief. Cases usually called irritable bladder show definite areas of hyperæmia surrounding and between the ureteral orifices. In a case of incontinence recently under my care I found an extreme injection of the mucosa over the inter-ureteric ligament.

In certain cases the knee-chest position may be used to advantage. In this posture the bladder is easily ballooned and the location of the ureteral orifices more readily detected.

### FUNCTIONAL DERANGEMENTS.

Cases relegated to this class were formerly more numerous than at present. Under improved methods of diagnosis many vesical disorders apparently functional are found to have an organic basis. The term irritable bladder, under which the functional derangements of the bladder are usually classed, is open to the objection that it implies a distinct pathological entity, while in fact the vesical disturbances in question are merely the symptoms of disease in other organs. The causes are various.

The local disorder may be one of the manifestations of a general neurosis. It is frequently observed in nervous and hysterical women. Frequent urination, incontinence, and spasmodic retention are often seen in this class of patients, from no other cause than disordered innervation. Any influence which acts to depress or excite the nervous system may be a contributing factor.

Vesical irritability is not an infrequent result of abuse of the sexual functions. Violent emotional disturbances are sometimes attended with loss of control over the vesical sphincter. This is illustrated in the occasional effect of severe fright. Examples of the extent to which mental influences may affect the bladder are the refusal of the sphincter to relax in the presence of another person, and the opposite effect of the sound of running water.

In many instances the vesical disorder is of reflex origin. Urethral caruncle, stricture, tumors, and other diseases of the urethra may furnish the source of the vesical irritation. Ureteral disease and painful affections of the vagina may act in like manner. Anal fissure, hemorrhoids, stricture at the lower portion of the rectum, ascarides, and other causes of rectal irritation are commonly recognized sources of retention and other vesical disturbances. Inflammatory disease of the uterus, tubes, ovaries, or pelvic peritoneum frequently gives rise to irritable bladder. Painful irritability is often observed after abdominal operations in which the adjacent pelvic viscera have been concerned. Greatly increased or diminished density of the urine makes it irritating to the bladder; so, too, do hyperacidity and other marked alterations in the composition of the urine.

Mechanical disturbances play a prominent part in the etiology. Cystocele, the traction of a misplaced uterus upon the vesical neck or of a tumor to which the bladder has become adherent, pressure of a gravid uterus or of a pelvic neoplasm, are potent causes of vesical disturbance.

*Symptoms.*—Functional derangements of the bladder often closely simulate organic disease. The symptoms resemble those of cystitis. There are dull pain and a sense of weight in the region of the pubes, often increased on standing or walking. The pain is felt most at the vesical base and neck, the nerve-supply being most abundant in this region.

Urination is frequently difficult, painful, or sometimes, owing to persistent urethral spasm, impossible. When the cause resides in some morbid property of the urine, the altered character of the secretion is apparent on inspection or with the aid of simple chemical tests.

*Diagnosis.*—Generally the diagnosis is made by a chemical and microscopical examination of the urine. A healthy condition of the urine excludes organic disease of the bladder; so, too, does the absence of albumin, pus, blood, and excess of vesical epithelium. Simple hyperacidity or alkalinity, extreme concentration or dilution, of the urine, are significant. Exploration of the bladder by abdomino-vaginal palpation, especially of the inferior portion of the organ, helps to exclude cystitis and foreign bodies. The uterus, ovaries, tubes, broad ligaments, the urethra, the pudendum, and the rectum must be examined for the recognized cause of reflex vesical irritation. The presence or absence of neurotic tendencies in the patient should also be taken into account. When in doubt, a careful cystoscopic examination is conclusive, best by the direct method.

*Treatment.*—The treatment must be ordered with reference to the cause. A suitable hygienic and tonic regimen will do much to improve the condition of the nervous system. Open air, sunlight, and a well-regulated system of physical culture are valuable remedial agents in the treatment of nervous women. To this must be added the correction of injurious habits. Tonics, including iron, and especially strychnine, are often potent aids in establishing a better nervous tone. Hot vaginal or rectal douches, hot sitz baths, and the application of moist or dry heat to the suprapubic region are valuable sedatives. Bromides in doses of twenty to thirty grains by the mouth, extract of belladonna, one-half grain, in suppository, or chloral, twenty to thirty grains, in solution by the rectum, and very rarely the use of opiates in the same manner, may be required to subdue the vesical irri_tability; the chloral may be injected in warm milk or in starch water. The food should be such as the patient can easily digest. Constipation must be prevented. Departures from the normal density or reaction of the urine should be corrected. Too concentrated urine calls for a more liberal ingestion of liquids and the use of mild diuretics. In excessive acidity the alkaline waters, such as Vichy or Apollinaris, are indicated. Alkaline conditions of the urine are corrected by the administration of the benzo-ates. When the vesical trouble is a reflex from disease of other pelvic viscera or is due to mechanical irritation, the provoking cause must, if possible, be removed.

In enuresis, belladonna pushed nearly to the point of intolerance is an agent of great value. The smooth galvanic current to the strength of five to twenty milliampères is frequently useful; one pole should be placed over the suprapubic region, and the other over the upper part of the sacrum or in the vagina against the vesical neck. The sittings may be repeated once or twice daily. Cold baths to the lumbo-sacral region at night are sometimes useful. The hypodermic injection of strychnine may be tried.

In this affection Sänger practises massage of the urethra as follows. He introduces a metal catheter five to seven centimetres deep into the bladder. While the index finger of the right hand closes the end of the catheter, the left index finger is placed on that part of the catheter which is just outside the meatus urinarius, and firm but elastic pressure is exer-cised by this finger, first downward and then to either side. In this manner the sphincter vesicæ and the muscles of the urethra are forcibly stretched.[1]

### CYSTITIS.

Cystitis in the female is of frequent occurrence. The process may be acute or chronic, local or general. It varies greatly in intensity and duration, lasting from a few days to several weeks. In the beginning stage the pathological changes consist mainly in congestion and swelling of the affected mucous membrane. In fully developed cystitis there is more or less inflammatory thickening of the bladder-walls, and the mucous sur-face is bathed with muco-pus and frequently eroded in patches. Slight hemorrhage may occur from the denuded areas. In the chronic stage the

---

[1] Weekly Medical Review, June 20, 1892.

structural changes are more pronounced; the thickening of the vesical walls is much increased and the capacity of the bladder diminished. The mucosa is studded with recent ecchymotic patches or with pigmentary stains left by former ones. It is ulcerated in patches, and is frequently the seat of polypoid growths. The ulcerated areas secrete pus freely, and sometimes bleed. The ulcerating process is aggravated by the irritant effect of the decomposing urine; sometimes it invades the muscular coat, and it may even perforate the bladder-walls. Hypertrophic thickening of the vesical walls may give rise to partial occlusion of the ureteral orifice, damming back the urine and resulting in dilatation of the ureters, hydronephrosis, and in some cases serious injury to the kidneys. Uretero-pyelitis and extensive organic disease of the kidney occasionally result from extension of the vesical inflammation.

In cystitis produced by over-distention the walls of the bladder are extremely thin. In these cases the inflammation is generally diphtheritic in character and the necrotic mucous membrane is partially or wholly exfoliated; the latter may come away entire or piecemeal. Rarely the phagedænic process involves the muscular and even the peritoneal coat. In the severest forms of diphtheritic cystitis the entire bladder may be destroyed by the sloughing process. A form of vesical ulcer analogous to round ulcer of the stomach has been described by Rokitansky.

*Etiology.*—The most frequent cause of cystitis is the introduction of infectious material upon the catheter or other instruments passed into the bladder. Any condition which lowers the resisting power of the bladder-epithelium favors the development of the septic process: cystitis is accordingly a frequent complication of the puerperal state. The mucous membrane of the inferior portion of the bladder is doubtless in all cases more or less contused and fissured after labor. The vestibule and vulva are bathed in germ-laden discharges. The passage of the catheter at this time is a fruitful cause of infection. Even with all the care that can be used, it is difficult to make the operation wholly aseptic; all else being clean, the urethra may be the source from which the offending bacteria are carried upon instruments into the bladder.

Cystitis by extension of the inflammatory process is a frequent result of urethritis, particularly of the gonorrhœal type. In occasional instances cystitis may result from extension of the septic process in vaginitis, ureteritis, salpingitis, pelvic peritonitis, carcinoma of adjacent viscera, or pelvic abscess contiguous to the bladder. Mechanical injuries, whether from external violence or from instrumentation within the bladder, are potent causes of vesical inflammation. The mucosa may be wounded in the unskilled use of the catheter. Retention and decomposition of urine induce cystitis. Extreme departures from the normal density of the urine it is believed may excite a mild vesical catarrh. Local chemical irritants, calculi, foreign bodies, entozoa, neoplasms, and tuberculosis are included among the causes of inflammation of the bladder. Vesical congestion may result from disturbances of the cutaneous circulation; exposure to cold is, therefore, a recognized cause of cystitis. Dupuytren, Nélaton, De Quest, Gouley, and others have observed that extensive burns of the skin bear an indirect causative relation to inflammation of the bladder.

In extreme over-distention the blood-supply to the mucosa and the sub-mucous structure is cut off by the urinary pressure. If the distention be relieved early, a simple cystitis follows; but if long continued, partial or total death of the mucous membrane takes place and it is exfoliated. In a case which came under the writer's observation the mucosa was thrown off in fragments per urethram after urinary retention for ninety-six hours with accumulation of over nine pints of urine.

*Symptoms.*—The symptoms vary according to the cause, extent, severity, and stage of the inflammatory affection. In all cases increased frequency of urination is the rule. Retention occurs rarely and incontinence never in acute cystitis. In the acute stage the desire to pass urine is almost constant, and is not relieved by the evacuation of the bladder. Micturition is attended with sharp, lancinating pains in the urethra and vesical neck, and is frequently accompanied with rectal tenesmus. Sometimes the urine is passed in short, interrupted spurts, even in drops, and often as many as a hundred times in twenty-four hours.

There is a feeling of fulness and heaviness in the bladder, with frequent violent paroxysms of pain, in the intervals of micturition. Sacral pain is persistent in most cases. In severe cystitis the affected organ is exquisitely sensitive, and the patient's sufferings are aggravated by the least jar or by the slightest pressure over the bladder. Finger lays stress upon increased pain on standing as evidence of trachelo-cystitis.

In septic and in diphtheritic forms the attack is usually ushered in with a chill and there are frequently repeated rigors. The temperature may reach 103° F. Grave constitutional symptoms soon follow. The patient falls into a typhoid condition, with dry tongue, cephalalgia, vomiting, sub-sultus, and delirium. Urination is sometimes obstructed by fragments of membrane, causing over-distention of the bladder. Total suppression and death by uræmia may result.

In acute cystitis the quantity of urine passed in twenty-four hours may be normal or slightly increased; the color may not be changed. The specific gravity varies from 1005 to 1020, and, if accompanied with fever, may rise to 1030. The reaction is feebly acid. After standing a few hours it becomes alkaline, and precipitates a diffuse sediment containing mucus, pus, and blood in greater or less amount, bladder-epithelium, and triple phosphates. Albumin is found owing to the presence of pus. Sometimes the urine becomes ammoniacal and exceedingly offensive.

In cystitis due to retention there is an abundant precipitate of ammonio-magnesium phosphate, the urine is alkaline, slimy, highly purulent, and contains mucus and much exfoliated vesical epithelium.

In chronic cystitis the symptoms referable to the organ itself and its contents are similar to those above described, but of a milder type. The urine contains pus, mucus, and exfoliated epithelium in large amounts. On standing, it precipitates an extremely tenacious sediment; it is of a neutral or alkaline reaction and is sometimes fetid. The endoscope reveals the evidences of inflammation. The mucous membrane is congested, ulcerated, and studded with ecchymotic patches.

*Diagnosis.*—In acute cystitis the bladder is found extremely sensitive on palpation through the bladder or rectum. In chronic inflammation the thickening of the vesical walls is generally appreciable to the touch on bimanual examination. Mere irritability is distinguished from inflammation mainly by the character of the urine. In the former condition the urine is not cloudy when recently passed, does not yield the characteristic precipitate on standing, and the microscopic examination reveals no pus. A careful examination of the urethra, the uterus, the rectum, and other pelvic structures will frequently disclose the source of the reflex disorder.

Cystitis is differentiated from pyelonephritis by carefully washing out the bladder and then observing the appearance of the first few drachms of urine withdrawn by catheter shortly after the irrigation. In cystitis it will be found clear, while in pyelonephritis it will be turbid.

The diagnosis should include the determination, if possible, of the cause of the cystitis.

*Prognosis.*—The duration of the disease will naturally vary with the cause and intensity of the inflammation. Mild catarrhal inflammation generally subsides within one or two weeks. Chronic cystitis is in most cases an exceedingly intractable disease, even under skilful treatment. In diphtheritic forms the prognosis is grave.

*Treatment.*—Especially important is the prophylaxis of vesical inflammation. Among the most fertile sources of cystitis are over-distention of the bladder after labor and the consequent use of the catheter. Distention of the bladder in the first few days of the puerperium may always be detected by palpation over the lower abdomen. The obstetrician, therefore, should not trust to the statement of the patient or the nurse that the urine has been frequently and freely voided; he should learn by palpating the abdomen at his daily visits after labor whether the bladder is full or empty. Even the nurse may be taught to recognize over-distention. The tumor can be felt by palpation over the lower abdomen, and pressure upon it causes a desire to urinate. The use of the catheter should be avoided, if possible. When the patient is unable to pass water in the reclining position, the attempt usually succeeds if she be allowed to assume the half-sitting or sitting posture. In all ordinary cases this liberty is justifiable as early as six or eight hours after labor, and it exposes the patient to less danger than does the passing of a catheter.

When the instrument must be used, the whole procedure should be managed with scrupulous care to make it aseptic. The soft-rubber instrument is least likely to do mechanical injury, especially in the hands of the nurse. It should be boiled for ten minutes immediately before and must be carefully washed after using. After sterilizing it must be handled only with hands that have been rendered aseptic. The meatus urethræ and its immediate surroundings are to be cleansed and washed with an antiseptic and the instrument passed under direct inspection of the parts. If this degree of care were always observed, infection of the bladder, even in repeated use of the catheter, would seldom occur.

In all instrumentation within the bladder similar precautions should be employed. As a preparation for the use of the lithotrite and for similar operations within the bladder, the exhibition of salol by the mouth for several days should be mentioned as a useful antiseptic measure.

In the treatment of acute cystitis, the first essential is rest in bed till the acute symptoms have subsided. Patients yield to this requirement the more willingly inasmuch as their sufferings are materially relieved thereby. The diet should be unstimulating. Fluid and semi-fluid foods, such as milk, eggs, and light broths, are most suitable ; a diet consisting largely of milk is particularly useful. Stimulants and stimulating condiments must be avoided. The free use of saline laxatives relieves vesical congestion. The skin should be kept active by warm bathing, friction, and suitable clothing. It is especially important that the extremities be warmly clad.

If the urine be acid, it should be rendered neutral and unirritating by the free use of alkaline drinks. Vichy water "with extra soda" may be given, or citrate of potassium, fifteen grains three to six times daily in dilute solution. When the urine is alkaline it may be rendered acid by benzoate of ammonium given in doses of ten grains every two hours. The liberal ingestion of a citric acid lemonade has a like effect. Salol is particularly useful in ammoniacal decomposition ; the dose should be five to ten grains every two hours, gradually increased till the urine is acid. Boric acid, in doses of ten to twenty grains every four hours per os, is a useful corrective when the urine is offensive. The ingestion of liberal quantities of pure water acts to dilute the urine and to render it more bland. To relieve the pain and tenesmus hot sitz baths or hot compresses to the hypogastrium may be of service. Ice-water injections per rectum may be used for the same purpose. More effectual for the control of pain is opium, belladonna, hyoscyamus, or chloral. These drugs are best given by the rectum. Opium must be used with caution, if used at all, owing to its tendency to produce constipation and vesical congestion as well as the danger of establishing the opium habit. Perhaps the most suitable preparation of opium for the purpose is Dover's powder. Chloral is one of the least objectionable of the foregoing narcotics ; it may be given by the bowel in twenty-grain doses, dissolved in two or three ounces of starch water or milk. In case of insomnia, one-half to one drachm of chloral may be given in this manner with most satisfactory effect. Bromide of sodium in twenty-grain doses by the stomach, and repeated once in four hours, often acts more kindly than opium for the relief of pain and tenesmus, especially in highly nervous women. Cannabis indica subdues the pain quite as effectually as opium, and with less injurious after-effect.

Irrigation of the bladder may be resorted to after the acute symptoms have subsided. Most useful for this purpose are boric acid in three-percent. solution, nitrate of silver in strength of one-tenth to one-half per cent., permanganate of potassium in one-tenth- to one-third-per-cent. solution, creolin one-half-per-cent. solution, gradually increased to two-per-cent., or carbolic acid (1 to 500).

In chronic cystitis special attention must be paid to the general health. A good diet and hygienic and tonic measures are essential. Opium is to be avoided if possible. Cannabis indica or the bromides may be used to relieve tenesmus. Alkaline reaction of the urine should be corrected as in the acute stage. If the urine be purulent, benzoic acid will be found of service. The following formula is recommended :

R   Acid. benzoic., ʒi ;
Aq. aurant. flor., ℥iss ;
Syrup., ℥iii ;
Aq., ℥xxvii.  M.
Sig.—A glass to be drunk between meals.

Of the balsamic preparations there is none better than a pure sandal-wood oil ; from three to eight capsules of ten minims each may be given daily. Eucalyptol, in doses of five to thirty minims three times a day, in emulsion or in capsule, is a useful remedy.

Here the treatment consists mainly in local measures. Much depends on the technique of vesical irrigation. A suitable instrument for this purpose may be improvised as follows. A soft velvet-eyed rubber catheter is joined to a piece of rubber tubing by a short piece of glass tube. A small glass or agate iron-ware funnel is connected with the other end of the rubber tube. The whole apparatus may be about sixty centimetres in length. (Fig. 23.) It is to be sterilized by boiling for twenty minutes immediately before using. After carefully cleansing the meatus urethræ and its immediate sur-

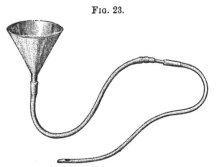

FIG. 23.

Apparatus for irrigating the bladder.  (Skene.)

roundings, the catheter, well lubricated with sterilized vaseline, is introduced and the urine withdrawn through the catheter tube and funnel. Great care is to be used to complete the evacuation very gradually, otherwise the bladder-walls may contract violently upon the catheter and be injured thereby. While the instrument is still *in situ* and its lumen filled with the column of urine, thus preventing the entrance of air, the funnel is filled with the solution for injection and gradually raised. In this manner the bladder is slowly distended. The quantity to be injected must depend upon the character of the solution and the degree of vesical irritability : in some cases an ounce is all that will be retained without causing pain. The maximum volume of fluid injected should rarely exceed two to four ounces. The funnel is then lowered and the bladder evacuated in the same careful manner as before. This process is repeated till the washings are perfectly clear. The patient lies in the dorsal position, with the knees drawn up and well apart. The bladder should be thoroughly washed out before throwing in the remedial injection. For this purpose the normal salt solution or a borax solution, one-half to one drachm to the pint, is less irritant than plain water. The temperature of the irrigating fluid should be 100° to 105° F. The remedial injections may be repeated once or twice daily. Suitable antiseptic solutions for irrigating the bladder are the mercuric chloride (1 to 10,000), the permanganate of potassium, the nitrate of silver, or the creolin solution already mentioned. Tyson praises as an irrigant a solution of salicylate of sodium (3i ad Oi). Methylene blue (gr. i to gr. ii ad 3i), and hydrogen dioxide, diluted with one to three volumes of boiled water, are useful injections, especially in purulent cases. Injections of ichthyol in water (one-half to one per cent.) have been highly recommended. Ichthyol is especially useful in gonorrhœal cystitis. In rebellious cases a two-per-cent. solution of resorcin may be used, or twenty drops of a strong nitrate of silver solution, ten grains to the ounce, may be employed. Iodoform injections have been used with excellent effect. The following formula is employed : iodoform fifty parts, glycerin forty parts, mucilage of acacia ten parts. An ounce of this mixture may be injected once daily; if well borne, the injection may be repeated two or three times daily.

In cases of much pain after the use of stimulating injections the bladder may be washed out with a solution of sulphate of morphine, one or two grains to the ounce. A still better calmative is hydrochlorate of cocaine; a few drops of a two- to four-per-cent. solution may be used. Care must be taken that a toxic dose of these agents be not left in the bladder. Recent observations have shown that most drugs are actively absorbed by the vesical mucous membrane, especially in the presence of erosions.

When other measures fail, the bladder must be drained. For this purpose the self-retaining catheter has been employed, but it is not to be advised, except where operative procedures are refused. When resort must be had to this method of drainage, the urethra is to be first dilated to the point of paralyzing the vesical sphincter. The dilatation is accomplished slowly by the use of a series of graduated dilators. The bladder is washed out daily with the normal salt or boric acid solution. When the vesical sphincter regains its tone the catheter should be removed, the dilatation repeated, and the catheter replaced.

More satisfactory for draining the bladder is the formation of a vesico-vaginal fistula. Emmet operates as follows. The patient is placed in the Sims position, under ether, and the perineum well retracted. A sound is passed into the bladder and its point made to press heavily against the septum at a point in the median line one centimetre above the vesical orifice of the urethra. The parts are steadied with a tenaculum and are incised upon the top of the sound. The blunt blade of the scissors is carried through the incision into the bladder, and the opening lengthened in the direction of the cervix uteri to the distance of three or four centimetres. To prevent the fistula from closing, the vesical and vaginal mucous membranes should be stitched together, or the patient may maintain the opening by passing the finger through it night and morning. Instead of the knife or scissors, the Paquelin cautery at a dull red heat may be used.

Byrne, of Brooklyn, has modified the operation, making it easy and expeditious, by the use of a specially constructed forceps, one blade of which is passed into the bladder, the other into the vagina, thus grasping the vesico-vaginal septum; the vaginal blade is fenestrated and the vesical blade grooved. (Fig. 24.) The thermo-cautery knife is introduced through

FIG. 24.

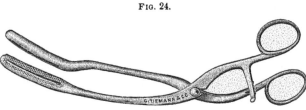

Byrne's cystotomy forceps.

the fenestra at a dull red heat and the septum divided, the knife being completely controlled and guarded by the fenestra and groove in the forceps. The operation must, of course, be done under an anæsthetic, best with the patient in the dorsal position. By the use of the cautery not only are hemorrhage and sepsis prevented, but the operation is accomplished with greater rapidity and the fistula is readily kept open. Suprapubic cystotomy has been done in obstinate cases of cystitis, but it offers no advantage over the vaginal operation.

**Tuberculosis.**—Tuberculosis of the bladder is regarded as a very rare disease. It is possible, however, that cystitis may yet prove to be more frequently of tuberculous origin than has hitherto been assumed. Rovsing found tuberculous bacilli in the bladder-discharges of three out of thirty cases of cystitis. In the great majority of instances it is dependent upon general tuberculosis, or is associated with tuberculous disease of the ureters and kidneys. It seldom occurs as a primary affection. As in tuberculosis of other organs, while no age is exempt, it is most commonly met with in the young.

*Pathology.*—The favorite seat of vesical tuberculosis is the neck of the bladder. In the earlier stages of the disease the mucosa is studded with miliary tubercles. These coalesce into caseous nodules, and later the tuberculous patches break down into ulcers.

*Symptoms.*—The symptoms are those of cystitis. Micturition is frequent and painful; the base of the bladder is extremely sensitive to pressure, and pain is increased by walking or riding. The urine may contain blood. Hæmaturia, however, is a more conspicuous symptom in the earlier than in the later stages of the affection; it is frequently the first to attract attention. In advanced tuberculous cystitis the urine contains pus.

*Diagnosis.*—If we look only to the symptoms, tuberculosis is very difficult of distinction from cystitis due to other causes. Absence of the usual causes of the cystitis is significant. Tubercular disease of the bladder is at once suggested by the presence of tuberculosis in other organs. Electrical cystoscopy is available for diagnosis when the urine is not bloody. Most conclusive are the direct examination of the bladder through the open speculum and the detection of the Koch's bacillus in the urine. The bacillus, however, is not always to be found.

*Prognosis.*—The prognosis is bad. In exceptional cases the patient may live eight or ten years; generally the duration of the disease does not exceed two. Death usually results from general tuberculosis.

*Treatment.*—The systemic treatment does not differ from that adopted in tubercular disease of other organs. Locally, injections of the glycerin-iodoform mixture have been found useful. Pain is to be controlled as in other forms of cystitis. In obstinate cases cystotomy may be advisable for the purpose of curetting away the tuberculous growths and also for drainage, the fistula being left open. The sufferings of the patient are thereby materially lessened, and in many instances a symptomatic cure is ultimately possible, so far as the local disease is concerned. Burrage, of Boston, has recently reported a case in which a tuberculous patch was satisfactorily curetted and cauterized with a nitrate of silver solution through a No. 14 Kelly endoscope.

### INVERSION OF THE BLADDER.

Inversion of the bladder or extroversion through the urethra is very seldom met with. It consists, generally at least, in a prolapse of all the coats, not, as some writers have assumed, of the mucous membrane alone. It may occur at any age, but is most frequently observed in children. It is sometimes brought on abruptly by violent straining efforts during defecation or micturition. McKay (*Canada Lancet*, February, 1892) reports a case caused by the straining and tenesmus attendant upon a prolapsus recti. More frequently the prolapse is gradually developed.

*Symptoms.*—In partial prolapse of the vesical wall, before the tumor makes its appearance at the meatus the symptoms do not differ essentially from those of a foreign body in the bladder. In adults there are abdominal pain and vesical tenesmus when the prolapse is complete; in children these symptoms are seldom noted. The tumor may reach the size of an orange, but is usually easily reducible. In chronic cases the vulva and thighs are eroded from the constant dribbling of urine. Continued traction upon the ureters sometimes results in ureteritis; extension to the kidneys and uræmia may then supervene. The prolapsed portion of the bladder-wall may become strangulated, with grave constitutional disturbance.

*Diagnosis.*—Inversion of the bladder must be distinguished from urethral or vesical polypi and from annular urethral prolapse. When reduction is possible, differentiation is readily made between vesical polypi and inversion by exploring the cavity of the bladder after replacing the protruding mass. Urethral polypi cannot be reduced within the bladder. The tumor in urethral prolapse springs from the margin of the meatus, while in vesical prolapse it is encircled by it. In the former, the urethral opening appears in the centre of the tumor; in the latter, it is annular, and surrounds the neck of the tumor. When the mouths of the ureters are exposed to view the diagnosis presents no difficulty.

*Treatment.*—The vesical protrusion should be carefully cleansed, and, if possible, replaced. This is to be attempted by first oiling the tumor and using gentle taxis. The use of a large sound helps to secure complete reduction, but should be omitted, if possible, owing to the danger of mechanical injury to the bladder. In partial inversion, slight forcible distention of the organ by means of a suitable injection may assist in repositing the prolapsed portion; in difficult cases the manipulation should be undertaken with the aid of anæsthesia. After reduction of the prolapse the patient must be kept for several days in the recumbent posture. A compress and T-binder may be used for retention. Straining at stool must be prevented by the use of laxatives or rectal injections, and vesical tenesmus controlled by suppositories of opium or of hyoscyamus, or by other suitable measures. More or less incontinence generally remains for a time or permanently. It is to be treated as in other cases of urethral dilatation.

### VESICO-VAGINAL FISTULA.

Vesico-vaginal fistula is a direct communication between the bladder and the vagina. It may involve either the trigone or the bas-fond, most frequently the latter. The size of the opening may be no larger than a pinpoint, or the whole vesico-vaginal septum may be destroyed. The aperture may be round, elliptical, angular, or a mere slit. The tissues about the edges of the fistula vary greatly in thickness, density, unevenness of surface, and color. Usually there is but one orifice; occasionally there are several.

A good example of the extent to which the vesico-vaginal wall may be injured in extreme instances is afforded in a case reported by H. M. Sims.[1] The base of the bladder and the corresponding portion of the anterior

---

[1] Transactions of the New York Obstetrical Society, 1893.

vaginal wall were entirely destroyed; the upper bladder-walls prolapsed through the opening, and the ureteral orifices were exposed to view. Dr. Malcolm McLean, in a personal communication to the writer, describes a case in which half the bladder was found prolapsed through a large vesico-vaginal fistula and protruding at the vulva. The fistulous opening extended from the cervical junction to within three-eighths of an inch of the pubic arch. The width of the fistula transversely was two and one-fourth inches. The urethra was also destroyed.

*Etiology.*—Vesico-vaginal fistulæ occur most frequently from difficult labors, in which the fœtal head is arrested in the lower portion of the birth-canal. Necrosis takes place from long-continued compression of the vesico-vaginal wall between the head and the pubic bones, and the injured structures subsequently slough, leaving a fistulous opening. Lacerations occurring during forceps or other instrumental deliveries seldom invade the bladder. In more than ninety per cent. of cases fistula results from neglected labors, not from measures adopted for delivery. Very rarely calculi or other foreign bodies in the bladder may perforate the vesico-vaginal septum.

*Symptoms.*—The most conspicuous symptom is the discharge of urine by the vagina between the acts of micturition. In case of a large fistula the flow will be constant. If the opening be small, the escape may be temporarily prevented by the pressure of the anterior vesical wall against the orifice. Sometimes a portion of the urine may be voided per urethram. The vagina usually becomes coated with urinary salts. In all cases the vulva and the inner surfaces of the thighs are excoriated by the irritating discharge, and the odor of decomposing urine is given off from the person and the clothing of the patient.

*Diagnosis.*—Large fistulæ may be detected by the vaginal touch; small ones can generally be located by ocular inspection with the aid of a small sound or probe. For this purpose the patient should be placed in the Sims position, and the anterior vaginal wall exposed by the use of the Sims speculum. In difficult cases the existence and location of a fistula are most readily demonstrated by injecting the bladder with milk and water or with a solution of methyl-blue, a grain to the ounce. When still in doubt as to the location of the fistula, Pozzi suggests that the anterior wall of the vagina be carefully dried and covered with a piece of dry absorbent paper; a moist spot developed on the paper betrays the seat of the fistula. The orifice once located, the direction and extent of the fistulous tract may be determined by the probe. Sometimes the examination is rendered difficult by cicatricial contraction of the vagina; preliminary dilatation may then be necessary to expose to view the seat of the fistulous opening.

*Preparatory Treatment.*—Before operating it is generally advisable to place the patient for a time under a course of tonic and hygienic treatment for the improvement of the general health. Time must be allowed after labor for the completion of the process of involution and for full convalescence; this will usually require not less than three or four months. The diseased structures about the fistula should be placed in the best possible condition for repair. Vaginal incrustations from urinary deposits are to be removed by the use of hot boric acid douches (two drachms to the quart), repeated two or three times a day for some weeks before operating. Erosions of the vagina may be pencilled with a two-per-cent. solution of nitrate of silver once or twice weekly for the same length of time.

Vaginal cicatrices which prevent easy access to the fistula, or may hinder the proper coaptation of the wound surfaces after denudation, must be divided by multiple incisions and stretched. The best time for operating is about a week after menstruation, as the healing process is thus least likely to be disturbed by the premature recurrence of the menstrual flow.

*Method of Operating for Closure of Vesico-Vaginal Fistulæ.*— The patient is placed in the Sims position, under an anæsthetic, the perineum being retracted with a Sims speculum. The lower end of the fistula is then seized with the tenaculum or a pair of long tissue-forceps. With a fistula knife, or scissors slightly curved on the flat, a strip of tissue is removed all around the margin of the fistula. (Fig. 25.) This strip should, if possible, be removed in one piece; there is thus less danger of leaving undenuded islets. The denudation is to be carried close to the mucous membrane of the bladder, but the latter must not be included, otherwise hemorrhage into the bladder may occur after the wound is closed. On the other hand, the strip of tissue removed should include at least a half-centimetre (one-fourth inch) of the mucous membrane of the vagina entirely around the fistula. The fistulous opening is thus funnel-shaped after the paring is completed, and the edges of the vesico-vaginal septum are evenly bevelled from the vesical to the vaginal side. This gives a broad surface for union, and is especially important when the edges are thin. The shape of the denuded opening should be such that the suture line will be straight or nearly so. Except in case of large fistulæ, it is desirable that the long axis of the opening should conform to that of the vagina, as there is thus the least strain upon the sutures. This is not always possible, the direction in which the wound is to be brought together depending largely upon the primary shape of the fistula. It is usually advisable to convert a round fistula into an elliptical one by exsecting two V-shaped pieces at opposite points on the margin.

Hemorrhage can generally be controlled by pressure with sponges or by a stream of hot water. Rarely a suture ligature of catgut may be required. The sutures are now introduced, beginning at the upper angle of the wound. The suture material used differs according to the fancy of the operator. For deep suture, silkworm-gut or plain sterilized braided silk No. 3 or No. 5 is recommended. The needles may be straight or moderately curved, and from one-half to three-quarters of an inch in length. The tissue being fixed with a tenaculum, the first suture is placed at the angle farthest from the operator. The needle is entered on the vaginal surface at a point from one-fourth to one-half inch from the line of incision, and swept in a curve, including all the tissues down to the vesical mucosa (Fig. 26). It is then passed symmetrically through the opposite lip of the wound. Care must be taken not to include the vesical mucous membrane. The applica-

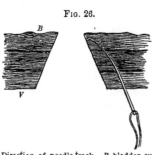

FIG. 26.

Direction of needle-track.—*B*, bladder surface; *V*, vaginal surface.

tion of each succeeding suture is greatly facilitated by steadying the edges of the wound by traction upon the suture last placed. The sutures should be one-fourth of an inch apart. All the stitches being in place, the bladder is washed out with care, to free it from blood-clots. The sutures are then tied, carefully approximating the wound surfaces. (Fig. 27.) Superficial sutures of fine silk are to be inserted as required to complete the coaptation of the wound edges. The ends of the sutures should be left about a half-inch in length, to facilitate removal. A light tampon of iodoform gauze is placed in the vagina.

Simon uses the dorsal position in this operation, with the hips elevated, exposing the fistula with his perineal retractors. This position gives easy access to the field of operation.

Edebohls points out that in extensive fistula the suprapubic method offers the great advantage that even if one could not draw together the vaginal wall sufficiently to close the entire aperture, he can at least close the opening by liberating the mucous membrane of the bladder itself from its vaginal and somewhat also from its bladder connections, and bringing its edges together. This will often succeed when no vaginal operation is practicable.

Cases are reported by Hirst, Armstrong, and Allen, in which the cervix was utilized to close the aperture. In a case of extensive complicated fistula, Pawlik removed the entire bladder, the vesical ends of the ureters being isolated, brought down, and attached in the vagina.

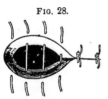

FIG. 28.

Two sutures tied.

After operation the patient is kept in the dorsal position for thirty-six hours; after that she is allowed to change her position when desirable for comfort. Opiates should be withheld if possible. The patient is catheterized every four hours for the first thirty-six hours, or oftener if there be desire to urinate; after that she may be permitted to void her urine. In case of small fistulæ the catheter may usually be wholly dispensed with, the patient being permitted to evacuate the bladder *per vias naturales* from the first. Permanent drainage by means of a catheter left in the bladder is seldom permissible.

FIG. 25.

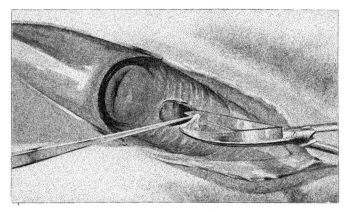

Paring the edges of the fistula

FIG. 27.

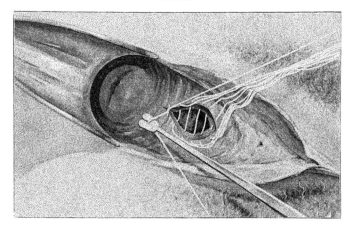

TVing the sutures.

The vaginal tampon is removed on the second day; sooner if offensive or soiled with urine. An enema is given to move the bowels on the third day, and the sutures are removed on the eighth day. The patient should remain in the recumbent position for at least two or three weeks.

## VESICAL CALCULI.

Stone in the bladder is a far less common affection of the female than of the opposite sex. This is accounted for mainly by the greater facility with which small stones are expelled through the female urethra.

They are oftener of the phosphatic variety than in the male. Foreign bodies from without frequently form the nucleus for urinary deposits. Roughened areas of the bladder-wall are liable to become incrusted, and such incrustations may serve as the starting-point of calculous formations. The formation of calculi is thus frequently observed after operation for vesico-vaginal fistula. The stone usually lies free in the cavity of the bladder, changing its position with the changing postures of the patient. Rarely it is incapsulated.

*Symptoms.*—The patient suffers from frequent urination, dysuria, tenesmus, and occasionally enuresis. The flow of urine may be abruptly cut off at micturition, owing to the occlusion of the vesical neck by the stone. A more or less severe cystitis always coexists. Hæmaturia may occur if the shape of the calculus be such as to cause abrasions. The urine contains pus, epithelium, and mucus, with amorphous crystals of triple phosphates.

The *diagnosis* is made with the sound, by a cystoscopic examination, by digital exploration through the urethra, previously dilated, or by conjoined abdominal and vaginal palpation.

As rigid an asepsis should be observed in the use of the exploring finger, the sound, or the cystoscope as is practised in major operative procedures. The bladder should be evacuated and thoroughly irrigated with Thiersch's solution. When the sound is to be used, the bladder should be moderately distended with a two-per-cent. boric acid, a half-strength Thiersch's, or a normal salt solution. The movements of the sound are thus unobstructed, and vesical folds which might envelop the stone are obliterated. The search is to be systematically conducted, first over the most dependent portion of the cavity, then over the rest of the bladder-walls, one or two fingers of the free hand guiding and assisting the manipulation through the vagina.

Cystoscopy or digital exploration may serve to discover an encysted stone which has escaped detection by the sound. Dilatation of the urethra sufficient to admit an index finger of not more than average size is rarely followed by persistent incontinence. The digital exploration is to be assisted with the fingers of the other hand through the vagina. Frequently a vesical calculus may be felt by the bimanual manipulation as employed in ordinary pelvic examinations.

The *prognosis* is good in the absence of renal and severe vesical lesions.

*Treatment.*—Calculi may be removed by way of the urethra or by vaginal or suprapubic cystotomy. Small calculi can be extracted through the urethra after dilatation with graduated dilators, or removed with slender forceps through a Kelly speculum. Moderately large and friable stones may be crushed by the usual method, or under direct inspection with the aid of the open speculum, and the débris washed out. If there be much cystitis, and the stone be of large size and too hard to be crushed, vaginal or suprapubic cystotomy is to be preferred, for not only may the stone thus be removed with less resulting injury to the bladder, but drainage for the diseased organ is secured.

Removal by the urethra without lithotrity is practicable only for calculi whose diameter does not exceed twenty millimetres. Greater dilatation is likely to result in permanent incontinence. The operation is conducted as follows:

The patient is placed, under an anæsthetic, in the lithotomy position, and the urethra dilated by the gradual method to twenty millimetres or less, as may be required. Small stones may frequently be best extracted by conjoined manipulation, the stone being pushed into the urethra and through it by the use of two fingers in the vagina. When this method fails, the stone is to be grasped and removed with forceps. Manipulation through the vagina will help to secure a proper seizure.

Friable stones which are too large for removal by the foregoing methods are to be crushed with a lithotrite and the débris washed out through a urethral speculum. The crushing is repeated till all fragments are small enough to pass. Care must be taken that no particle remains behind to act as a nucleus for a new concretion. When the lithotrite is introduced, the bladder should contain three or four ounces of a half-strength Thiersch's solution or some equally bland fluid. Lifting the handle of the instrument strongly upward, the beak is made to depress the posterior vesical wall. The stone, if free, rolls into the pocket thus formed, and with the aid of the finger in the vagina is easily engaged in the jaws of the lithotrite.

When cystotomy is required, the vaginal operation is generally preferred as the simplest and safest. In the suprapubic operation the preliminary distention of the bladder is best accomplished with air instead of water, as suggested by Dr. A. T. Bristow, of Brooklyn. The peritoneal fold is lifted farther above the symphysis than is possible with water, the danger of rupture is diminished, and the operator is saved the annoyance which comes from flooding the wound with water when the bladder is opened. If the distended bladder does not rise above the symphysis it may be pushed up on the tip of a large sound passed through the urethra.

### FOREIGN BODIES IN THE BLADDER.

Foreign bodies may be introduced into the bladder through the urethra either by accident or by intention. Lead-pencils, pipe-stems, ligatures, hair-pins, a crochet-needle, a rubber womb-protector, are among the articles that have been found in the bladder. Stumpff relates a case of hæmaturia due to the presence in the bladder of a pigeon's feather covered with ointment.

*Symptoms.*—The symptoms are substantially the same as in stone. Hemorrhage is more common than in the latter affection. The degree of disturbance depends upon the size of the foreign body and the character of its surface.

The *diagnosis* is made by the vaginal touch, by the use of the sound, or by direct inspection through the open speculum with the aid of the Kelly posture.

*Treatment.*—The treatment is substantially the same as for stone. The foreign body may generally be removed through the urethra, best with the aid of the open speculum.

### VESICAL TUMORS.

Neoplasms of the female bladder are of infrequent occurrence. They include papilloma, myxoma, fibroma, myoma, sarcoma, epithelioma, and carcinoma. The malignant forms are more frequently met with than the benign. Most commonly their site is the base of the bladder.

*Symptoms.*—The most constant symptom of vesical neoplasm is hæmaturia. Growths at the vesical neck give rise to frequent and painful urination. By falling over the urethral orifice they may interrupt the flow of urine at micturition, or may cause retention. Exceptionally, when the hemorrhage is free, retention may occur from obstruction of the vesical orifice by clots. Tenesmus is usually out of proportion to the size of the tumor. As a rule, cystitis sooner or later results. Ureteritis and pyelonephritis commonly supervene. Occasionally fragments of the tumor are expelled per urethram. Tenesmus aggravates the morbid condition of the mucous membrane; with the growing hypertrophy the hemorrhage increases. The urine contains pus, blood, mucus, epithelial scales, neoplastic shreds, and phosphates. The general health is in time impaired, the patient becoming thin, anæmic, and cachectic.

The *diagnosis* is made by conjoined abdominal and vaginal manipulation, by the electric cystoscope, by direct examination with the finger through the urethra, or by ocular inspection through the open speculum. An imperfect ballottement may be obtained in case of pedunculated growths, if the examination is made while the bladder is distended with fluid. Portions of the growth may be removed and examined under the microscope.

*Treatment.*—The tumor may be removed through the urethra, by a vesico-vaginal incision, or by epicystotomy.

Very small growths which are pedunculated may be twisted off and removed through the urethra. Troublesome hemorrhage is to be controlled by irrigation with warm water, or by gauze packing with counter-pressure over the abdomen. For several days after operation within the bladder the cavity should be washed out daily with a two-per-cent. solution of boric acid.   The urine meantime is to be kept bland by the use of alkaline drinks.

Byrne and Skene have employed the cautery in the treatment of vesical neoplasms.   The latter makes a vesico-vaginal fistula, brings the growth or sections of it into the opening and, when possible, through into the vagina, clamps the base (most of which should be normal mucous membrane) with forceps, cuts it off with the galvano-cautery, and desiccates the portion within the grasp of the forceps.   The bladder is carefully washed out with a half-strength Thiersch's solution and closed.   The catheter is passed every two hours for twenty-four hours after the operation, then every four hours.

Kümmel recommends the suprapubic operation for large benign or malignant growths.   The bladder wound is united by three rows of sutures,—the first through the mucosa, the second through the muscular coats, the third through the immediately overlying structures.   The skin wound is but partially closed, and the lower end tamponed with iodoform gauze.

In neglected cases in which the tumor is so large that total extirpation is impossible, thorough curettage of the growth, removing as much as possible, followed with cauterization of the whole diseased surfaces, may be employed.   The bladder is drained with iodoform wicking.   In rare instances partial resection or total extirpation of the bladder may be advisable, with implantation of the ureters in the vagina.


## THE URETERS.

*Anatomy.*—The ureters are two flattened white tubes which conduct the urine from each renal pelvis to the bladder.   Their diameter is about five millimetres (one-sixth of an inch) when distended.   They are of nearly uniform size throughout their length, save for a slight constriction usually found about two inches below the kidney. (Clark.)   The length has been variously stated at from thirty to forty-five centimetres.   According to Kelly and Morris, their length is about thirty centimetres (twelve inches).

The abdominal portion is from twelve to fifteen centimetres in length (five to six inches).   The ureter at its point of origin from the pelvis of the kidney lies concealed by the ribs at a distance of four to four and six-tenths centimetres from the median line.   They immediately underlie the peritoneum, coursing from the pelvis of each kidney obliquely downward and inward through the lumbar region until they reach the pelvic brim, where they are about five centimetres apart.

*The Pelvic Portion of the Ureter.*—The left ureter, after having crossed the left common iliac artery one and a half centimetres above its bifurcation, passes in front of the left hypogastric artery above its point of division, and reaches the left pelvic wall at the level of the angle of the larger sciatic notch.

The right ureter, at the distance of one and a half centimetres below the bifurcation of the right common iliac artery and vein, crosses over the external iliac artery and vein.   Thence it descends with the internal iliac

FIG. 29.

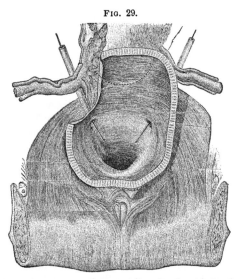

Base of the female bladder.  Anatomical relations of ureters at their entrance into the bladder.  (Sa\age.)

FIG. 30.

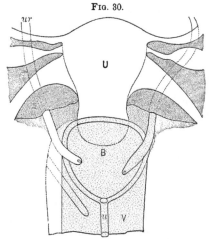

Uterus, ureters, and upper part of \agina of a woman forty years old.—U, uterus; B, bladder; u, urethra; V, \agina; ur, ureter.  (Garrigues.)

artery into the lesser pelvis.   For the rest of their course the ureters on both sides are alike.   Covering the point of origin of the obturator nerve, they cross, in their downward course along the lateral pelvic wall and floor, the points of origin of the obturator, umbilical, and uterine arteries, describe an arch the convexity of which is directed backward and outward, and then terminate in the bladder.

"The distance of the lower end of the ureter from the external os uteri is nearly constant at three to three and a half centimetres. The pelvic part of the ureter in the first portion of its course hugs the pelvic wall, later it reaches the pelvic floor (levator ani). It lies below the peritoneum, with which it is joined by cellular tissue, but not between the layers of the broad ligament. On entering the lesser pelvis, the ureters first diverge, then gradually converge downward; at the distance of four centimetres from the bladder the convergence increases rapidly." [1]

After passing from three-fourths of an inch to an inch obliquely downward and inward between the muscular and mucous coats, they open upon the mucous surface of the bladder by constricted orifices. These orifices are from two to three centimetres apart, and are connected by a band known as the inter-ureteric ligament.

### METHODS OF EXAMINING THE URETERS.

*Palpation.*—In most cases the ureters can be palpated in the usual bimanual method of pelvic examination; they can be rolled between the vaginal and abdominal fingers from their vesical termini to the point where they pass under the broad ligaments. The ureter is best found by first carrying the internal finger to the vesical neck, the cord-like urethra serving as a guide; hence the tip of the finger is carried for two or three centimetres obliquely upward and outward; here it rests over one posterior angle of the trigone. From this point the ureter sweeps outward and upward around the cervix. In favorable cases it may be readily detected by repeatedly rolling the intervening structures between the fingers of the outer and the inner hand. The normal ureter presents the feel of a narrow tape or flattened cord, without hardness. If the ureter be enlarged, palpation can be carried still farther by examining through the rectum, thus reaching that portion of the ureter behind the broad ligament and following it up over the posterior pelvic wall. It must not be mistaken in this position for the obturator artery or nerve, or the upper border of the levator ani, or the fibres of the obturator muscle, or the rim of the foramen. The diseased ureter becomes thickened and nodular, and is peculiarly prone to be mistaken for a cellulitis or an adherent ovary. (Kelly.) The ureter, when diseased, is identified by its knotty and cord-like feel, together with the fact that pressure upon it excites the desire to urinate, especially when applied to the lower portion of the tube. Kelly has shown that the normal ureter can be traced and minutely examined in the upper part of the pelvic course by introducing a ureteral bougie through the urethra and bladder

---

[1] Holl, Wiener Med. Wochenschr., Nos. 45 and 46, 1882.

into the ureter, carrying it to the brim of the pelvis, and palpating the tube through the rectum on the bougie. The internal iliac artery, which can readily be felt per rectum, affords a convenient landmark for locating the ureter in the posterior portion of its pelvic course. Here it lies generally along the inner aspect of the artery; exceptionally it is found on the outer side of the vessel.

*Catheterization of the Ureters.*—Ureteral catheterization as a means of diagnosis was employed by Simon in 1875. He catheterized the ureters under the guidance of the finger, after dilating the urethra with his graduated dilators. Pawlik, in 1880, introduced the method of catheterizing by the aid of external anatomical landmarks,—folds of the mucous membrane in the anterior vaginal wall. In 1886, Sänger defined the indications for ureteral catheterization. It remained for Kelly, in this country, to perfect the operation, catheterizing the ureters under direct inspection through the open speculum, as already described in connection with the methods of cystoscopic examination.

The ureters may be catheterized free-handed as follows. Pawlik, the pioneer in this method of exploration, places the patient in the genu-pectoral position. The operation, however, may be as readily done with the patient on the back, the legs strongly flexed upon the abdomen, and the pelvis well elevated. A careful antisepsis must be observed. The posterior vaginal wall is retracted by a large Simon or Sims speculum. With the bladder moderately distended, certain folds appear upon the anterior vaginal wall which serve as landmarks or guides to the location of the ureters. The degree of distention required is most accurately accomplished by first emptying the bladder with the catheter, removing residual urine with some form of suction apparatus, and then injecting one hundred and fifty to two hundred cubic centimetres (nearly six ounces) of a three-percent. solution of boric acid, or a methyl-blue solution (gr. i ad ℥i). On close inspection, two oblique folds may be seen on the anterior wall of the vagina which start from points a little way behind the level of the vesical neck. These folds diverge from before backward, and correspond very nearly in direction to the course of the ureters.

FIG. 31.

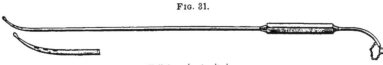

Kelly's ureteral catheter.

The Kelly catheter, which is a modification of that of Pawlik, is shown in Fig. 31. It is about thirty centimetres in length and two millimetres in diameter. The tip is slightly curved, and terminates in an olive-shaped point one and a half millimetres in diameter. The catheter is passed into the bladder and its point turned toward the vagina. By raising the handle the tip is made to press gently against the posterior vesical wall, and the course of the instrument is thus marked by the slight protrusion of the septum. The ureteral orifices are situated about three centimetres behind the vesical opening of the urethra and about the same distance apart, yet their location is not constant. Beginning near the median line, the catheter is made to glide up and down over the floor of the bladder above and below the level of the ureteral openings; it is then carried a little farther out and swept up and down in a similar manner, and this is continued till the ureteral eminence is found. A sensation of tripping is felt as it passes over this point. The tip of the catheter is then brought back to the site of the ureteral orifice, and the effort made to engage it in the ureter. Once entered, the instrument is felt to be in the grasp of the tube, and may be passed with little or no resistance for some length. On removing the stopper from the catheter the urine soon begins to flow; it trickles from the instrument in a broken stream, a few drops at a time. The operation is more difficult in the nulliparous than in the parous woman.

### MALFORMATION OF THE URETERS.

Ureteral duplicity is not extremely rare, some sixty cases having been reported. It may occur on one or both sides. Exceptionally duplicity persists throughout the course of the ureter. In a large proportion of cases of double ureter the kidney has two pelves, one tube arising from each and uniting with its companion before reaching the bladder. Beach[1] reports a case in which one division of the double ureter entered the bladder in the normal plane, the other terminating below as a cul-de-sac, which, post mortem, was found filled with pus. A case in which both kidney and ureter on the left side were absent is mentioned by Cutler; there was no left renal artery, nor was there any rudimentary indication in the bladder of the left ureteral orifice.

A supposed instance of congenital atresia of the ureter is reported by Colley.[2]

Occasionally one or both of the ureters, instead of emptying into the bladder, have an abnormal insertion into the vagina or rectum, or, as in congenital absence of the bladder, into the cul-de-sac which forms the inner termination of the urethra.

In a case of congenital absence of the bladder reported by Phillips,[3] the openings of the ureters appeared in the abdominal parietes as two small pouches on each side of the suprapubic region. Schatz[4] has in two instances observed a ureter communicating with the vagina, the bladder being normal in each case. Emmet, Von Massar, and Baker have reported ab-

---

[1] British Medical Journal, 1874, vol. i. p. 629.
[2] London Lancet, 1879, vol. i. p. 372.
[3] Lancet, 1879, vol. ii. p. 829.
[4] Medical Press and Circular, London, August 5, 1891.

normal ureteral insertions without any coexisting malformation of the bladder. A similar case is noted in the records of the Boston City Hospital.

*Treatment.*—Baker and Emmet have operated for this condition. Emmet attempted a plastic operation, making a uretero-vesical channel from the abnormal vaginal orifice to the point where the ureter should normally have entered the bladder, hoping by a subsequent operation to perforate the bladder-wall, lead the artificial canal into the vesical cavity, and close in the whole by a vaginal flap. The first part of the operation was successful, but the patient died of intercurrent pneumonia before the final step could be undertaken. In Baker's case the urine was found to escape drop by drop from a small orifice in the immediate neighborhood of the meatus urinarius. The external orifice was very small, and for a time escaped observation, yet behind the opening the canal appeared to be of considerable calibre. When a probe was introduced the ureter could easily be traced along the anterior vaginal wall to the left of the cul de-sac, passing directly over the site usually occupied by the vesical orifice of the left ureter, and separated from the vagina by a thin septum only. A probe was introduced into the ureter and cut down upon at a point about four centimetres from the meatus urinarius; the canal was found to be lined with mucous membrane. The ureter was then dissected up from the incision to a point in the vesico-vaginal septum corresponding to the normal situation of the left ureteral orifice; here an opening was made into the bladder, through which the ureter was turned in after the redundant portion was excised. Its extremity was united to the edge of the vesical mucosa at the inner border of the perforation by cotton sutures, and the vaginal edges of the mucosa were then drawn together around the ureter by silver wire; for eight days the bladder and vagina were washed out two or three times a day and the catheter used every four hours. The result was entirely satisfactory.

### DISEASES AND INJURIES OF THE URETERS.

**Stone in the Ureter.**—A calculus may pass through the canal and do but slight injury to its mucous membrane, or it may cause deep abrasions or become lodged in the tube. When a stone is arrested in its descent, it lodges most commonly either about two inches below the kidney, at the constriction of Bruce Clark, or at the vesical orifice of the ureter. Ureteritis follows, and, if the obstruction be not relieved, hydronephrosis and destruction of the kidney result.

*Symptoms and Signs.*—Renal colic ensues when a stone enters the ureter. The attack sets in abruptly, without apparent cause, or may be initiated by sudden muscular effort. It is characterized by agonizing pain, which starts in the flank of the affected side and passes down the ureter. Vomiting occurs during the painful paroxysms. Micturition is frequent, occasionally painful, and the urine is sometimes bloody. There is usually tenderness on the affected side. In very thin persons it may be possible on abdominal palpation along the course of the ureter to feel the stone *in situ.* When arrested in the pelvic portion, the stone may be located by palpation through the rectum.

*Treatment.*—When the obstruction is complete, as shown by negative catheterization of the affected ureter, the removal of the obstruction is indicated. A calculus in the intra-pelvic portion of the ureter may be reached by incision through the vagina, through the abdominal wall, or by Kraske's method of sacral resection. When the stone lodges in the extra-pelvic portion of the ureter, the extra-peritoneal method of removal is advised by Van Hook and by Fenger as the easiest and safest procedure. In exceptional instances it may be necessary to open the peritoneal cavity for the purpose of locating the stone. Its seat once determined, its removal is to be accomplished by the retro-peritoneal route. Intra-peritoneal ureterotomy is to be done only when the foregoing method is impracticable. The ureteral incision is closed by immediate suture. In case the parts have sustained serious injury from pressure of the calculus and consequent inflammatory changes, limited resection of the tube and restoration of its continuity by Van Hook's method of anastomosis are justifiable. Cabot believes that, by a properly selected operation, a stone can be removed from any part of the ureter by an extra-peritoneal incision. The management of the ureteritis after passage of the stone consists in flushing the urinary tract with diluents. Boro-citrate of magnesium, in doses of one drachm in a glass of warm water three times a day on an empty stomach, is recommended by Harrison.

**Obstruction of the Ureter** may exceptionally occur from compression in pelvic cellulitis or peritonitis. The pressure of pelvic neoplasms, such as uterine fibromata, and especially carcinomatous disease of the uterus extending into the broad ligaments, may lead to occlusion, with grave and even fatal consequences.

*Symptoms.*—The symptoms produced are pain in the course of the ureter above the point of obstruction, and tenderness on pressure. The kidney on the affected side is generally found to be sensitive on bimanual palpation. The ureteral catheter is arrested at the seat of obstruction, or if, perchance, it can be passed beyond the point of constriction, a quantity of decomposing urine will be evacuated from the distended ureter.

*Treatment.*—When the obstruction is the result of previous pelvic inflammation, ureteral catheterization and gradual dilatation of the ureter with bougies may give relief if the structural changes in the kidneys be not too far advanced. In malignant disease treatment is futile. In case of a myoma impacted in the pelvis, and incapable of dislodgement, myomectomy or hysterectomy is indicated.

**Ureteritis** may occur by extension of the inflammatory process from the bladder, from the kidney, or from the surrounding structures, or may arise from causes which reside in the ureter itself. The disease may be septic, gonorrhœal, or tubercular in character, and may affect one or both ureters. The ureter is thickened and its lumen sometimes irregularly contracted. In severe inflammation the process may extend to the surrounding connective tissue,—periureteritis.

In rare instances the ureters may be injured during the passage of the fœtal head through the pelvis. Vesical injuries during labor are most likely to occur in unskilful forceps or other instrumental deliveries, and especially in primiparæ. If the forceps be applied before the head has engaged and when dilatation of the cervix is incomplete, the bladder and ureters are liable to be carried down in advance of the descending head and to sustain injury from pressure.

In a post-partum case of uretero-pyelitis occurring in the practice of the writer, the cystoscope revealed a fissure of the vesical mucosa at the orifice of the inflamed ureter, the infection of which by a catheter was believed to have been the source of the ureteral inflammation.

*Symptoms and Signs.*—The most constant symptom of ureteritis is frequent micturition. There is sharp, burning pain over the ureter, most commonly on the left side. Pain is increased during menstruation, and is sometimes so intense that the patient is confined to her bed. A curious symptom mentioned by Mann[1] is a distaste for water. The urine is frequently scanty, is of a highly acid reaction in the absence of cystitis, and it contains pus and blood; the presence of pus without excess of mucus is almost diagnostic of ureteritis. On palpation through the vagina, the ureters are found thickened, tender, and sometimes sacculated. The patient complains of severe pain and desire to urinate when the inflamed ureter is pressed under the finger. By cystoscopy or by ureteral catheterization the urine from the affected ureter is shown to be purulent.

According to Skene,[2] the history in cases following obstetric injuries is that of pelvic pain and tenderness in the lower abdomen, which at first may not be severe. Usually the symptoms become more acute after a time, the pain and tenderness increasing rather abruptly. A chill or rigor may occur, with some tympanitic distention of the bowel, and the temperature may rise to 102° or even 105° F., with corresponding acceleration of the pulse. The tenderness is markedly increased on pressure, and bimanual manipulation on the affected side causes distress rather than acute pain. These symptoms increase in severity in from three to five days, and soon thereafter pus and blood may be found in the urine. With the appearance of purulent urine the patient's condition generally improves, pain and tenderness are to some extent relieved, the pulse becomes less rapid, and the temperature falls. Tube-casts may sometimes be found in the urine. The bleeding subsides in a few days, but the pus-discharge continues for a week or more. In other cases the inflammation pursues a different course, and about the time that pus appears in the urine and is discharged from the

---

[1] Transactions of the American Gynæcological Society, 1894.
[2] Ibid., vol. xv.

bladder, acute disease of the kidney supervenes, with diminution of the urinary secretion and varying degrees of uræmic intoxication.

*Treatment.*—The coexisting cystitis should first be treated in the usual manner. Rest in the recumbent posture should be enjoined, the bowels being freely opened with salines, morbid urinary conditions corrected, and the urine rendered antiseptic with salol. Vesical irrigation with hot acidulated water relieves the pain. A restricted diet, largely of milk, and the copious ingestion of mineral waters, like those of Vichy, Ems, and Wildungen, act favorably by flushing the urinary tract. (Skene.) Good results have been obtained by the use of high rectal enemata of water in quantities of one or two quarts. They act by their diuretic effect. (Ford.)

If there is constriction at the ureteral orifices sufficient to cause hydroureter, catheterization, followed by dilatation with bougies, is indicated. Bozeman makes a large opening in the base of the bladder in the region of the ureter and brings it under direct observation; he then passes a catheter, and through it irrigates the ureter and pelvis of the kidney with a bland antiseptic solution. With the use of Kelly's urethral speculum, or by direct catheterization per urethram, the vesico-vaginal incision is unnecessary and the technique of ureteral irrigation greatly simplified. The ureteral injections are repeated at suitable intervals till the urine comes away clear from the ureter.

**Operative and other Injuries.**—The ureter is liable to injury in abdominal operations upon the pelvic viscera and in vaginal hysterectomy. Cushing,[1] while extirpating a soft myoma in the broad ligament, cut one ureter and united the severed ends with two silk sutures and one catgut suture, then packed the wound and drained with gauze. A small fistula remained; it subsequently closed, however, and the patient ultimately made a complete recovery. In a case recently reported, Dr. H. A. Kelly,[2] during an operation for the removal of a large uterine myoma, doubly ligated and cut the right ureter. The tube became enlarged to about four times its normal calibre, forming a well-marked hydro-üreter. He succeeded in re-establishing the ureteral function by Van Hook's method of anastomosis. After ligating the end of the lower segment of the ureter close to its cut extremity, he made a longitudinal slit one centimetre in length in its anterior wall, half a centimetre below the ligature. A fine silk suture was then passed through the posterior wall of the lower portion from without inward, half a centimetre below the lower angle of the slit; this was brought out through the slit and caught in the outer coats of the upper portion of the ureter, two millimetres from its end, and then carried back into the slit, emerging through the wall of the ureter close to the original point of entrance. A second suture was passed at a point directly opposite, catching the upper end in a similar manner. By making traction

---

[1] Boston Medical and Surgical Journal, January, 1894.
[2] Annals of Surgery, January, 1894.

on these sutures while holding the slit open, the upper end of the ureter was readily invaginated into the lower. These sutures were snugly tied, and, in order to avoid the risk of urine backing up through the slit, the edges were sutured to the intussuscepted ureter with about ten fine silk interrupted rectangular sutures, catching only the outer coats.

The general principles of treatment in ureteral injuries, as laid down by Van Hook,[1] are as follows. The extra-pelvic portion of the ureter is most readily and safely accessible for surgical treatment by the retro-peritoneal route ; hence all operations upon the ureters above the crossing of the iliac arteries should be performed retro-peritoneally, except in those cases in which the necessity for the ureteral operation arises during laparotomy.

The intra-pelvic portion may be reached by incision through the abdominal wall, through the bladder, through the vagina, or by Kraske's sacral method, according to the location of the injury.

The chemical composition and reaction of the urine must be studied in all injuries to the ureter, the urine being rendered acid, if possible, and the specific gravity kept low. In all injuries where the urine is septic before the operation, or where the wound is infected during the operation, drainage must be effected.

In aseptic longitudinal wounds of the ureter occurring in the course of cœliotomy, suture may be practised and the peritoneum protected by suture. Transverse wounds of the ureter involving less than one-third of the circumference of the duct should be treated by free drainage (extra-peritoneal), and not by suture. In transverse injuries in the continuity of the ureter involving more than one-third of the circumference of the duct, stricture by subsequent scar-contraction should be anticipated by converting the transverse into a longitudinal wound and introducing longitudinal sutures.

In complete transverse wounds of the ureter at the pelvis of the kidney, sutures may be used if the line of union be made as great as possible. In complete transverse injuries of the ureter in continuity, union must not be attempted by suture. In these cases union without subsequent scar-contraction may be obtained by Van Hook's method of lateral implantation. In complete transverse injuries of the ureter very near the bladder, the duct may be implanted, but with less advantage, into the bladder directly.

At the pelvis of the ureter, continuity after complete transverse injury may be restored by Kuester's method of suture, provided the severed ends can be approximated by slightly loosening the ureter from its attachments. Rydgier's method of ureteroplasty in such injuries may be tried if other methods cannot be utilized. The primary operation should at least fix the ends of the tube as nearly as possible together.

In both trans-peritoneal and retro-peritoneal operations the ureteral ends can be approximated by Van Hook's method, even after the loss of about

---

[1] Transactions of the American Medical Association, 1893.

an inch of its substance. The use of tubes of glass and other materials for the production of channels to do duty in place of destroyed ureteral substance must be rarely satisfactory, and, even if temporarily successful, the duct is almost sure to be choked by scar-contraction.

In injuries of the portion of the ureter within the pelvis, with loss of substance, the ureter should be treated as follows. If possible, the continuity of the ureter should be restored by Van Hook's method. If this be not possible, the ureter, if injured in vaginal operations, should be sutured to the base of the bladder with a covering of mucous membrane so far as possible, with a view to future implantation or formation of vesico-vaginal fistula with kolpokleisis.

In injuries to the pelvic ureter during cœliotomy, where the continuity cannot be restored, and where temporary vaginal implantation cannot be effected, the proximal extremity of the duct should be fastened to the skin at the nearest point to the bladder.

Implantation of one or both ureters into the rectum is absolutely unjustifiable under all circumstances, because (1) the primary risk is too great; (2) there is great liability to stenosis of the duct at the point of implantation; (3) suppurative uretero-nephritis is almost certain to occur either immediately or after the lapse of months or years.

Extirpation of a normal kidney for injury or disease of the ureter is utterly unjustifiable, except where the ureter cannot be restored in one or other of the ways cited.

# CHAPTER XVII.

## DISEASES OF THE RECTUM AND ANUS.

BY EDWARD E. MONTGOMERY, M.D.

*Anatomy.*—The rectum is continuous with the sigmoid flexure. Commencing at the left sacro-iliac synchondrosis, it follows the concavity of the sacrum towards the median line, crosses over the third section of the sacrum to the right side of the pelvis, recrosses the median line and inclines slightly to the left, and again follows the median line down to the anus. Its antero-posterior curvature is like that of an S whose upper concavity is parallel with that of the sacrum and whose lower faces the coccyx. It presents two transverse curvatures, the first looking to the left, the second and smaller to the right. The upper portion of the rectum is completely invested with peritoneum; as it proceeds downward, the mesorectum disappears. Below the cul-de-sac of Douglas there is no peritoneal covering whatever, the rectum being in relation here anteriorly to the wall of the vagina and posteriorly to the coccyx and levator ani, laterally to cellular tissue. The envelopment of peritoneum forming what is known as the mesorectum permits a certain mobility of the superior part of the canal and admits of its possible displacement. As the mesorectum disappears, the union between the rectum and the sacrum becomes more complete, and this portion of the intestine is less distended. In one case under the writer's observation the displacement of the upper part of the rectum produced a condition of obstruction similar to that in an old, weakened garden-hose where a twist or bend occurs, so that the patient would suffer from severe attacks of flatulent distention until the gas would apparently overcome the kinking in the tube. In its lower part the intimate relation of the rectum with the vagina is of great importance in digital examination and diagnosis, since through the anus we may be able to explore indirectly the uterus, vagina, and pelvic cavity, while from a surgical stand-point its close association may be the cause of danger from wounds in operations upon the posterior wall of the vagina and in injuries to the parturient canal.

The rectum consists in its upper part of the peritoneal, muscular, and mucous coats; in its lower part, of the muscular and mucous coats alone. It consists of a double muscular tunic. The first layer is superficial and longitudinal, though the fibres terminate in a reflection at the level of the perineal elevators, increasing the pelvic aponeurosis. Other fibres blend

879

with those of the perineal elevators; the latter finally terminate in the skin at the circumference of the anus. Beneath the longitudinal fibres is a second tunic of circular fibres, which terminate at the level of the anus by a fillet constituting the internal sphincter, essentially distinct from the external sphincter, which is composed of striated fibres. Between the muscular and mucous coats is a cellular layer which is continuous throughout the intestinal tract and renders the mucous layer movable. This movement of the mucous membrane becomes pathological in cases of rectal prolapse. The mucous membrane is destitute of papillæ, and is covered by cylindrical epithelium rich in glands and tubes. At the junction of the inferior and middle thirds is a fold of the mucous membrane, known as Houston's valve, which is recognized by the finger in ano-rectal exploration.

*Anus.*—The anus is the termination of the alimentary canal, and in its description we must take into consideration its orifice and the two sphincters which control it. The orifice is in reality a circular canal with its circumference puckered into folds. Normally, and when not subject to strain, it is closed. A number of folds will be seen radiating from the centre towards the circumference, and are disclosed by gentle traction upon the orifice. The mucous lining is rose-colored, and is found upon close examination to present a number of vertical folds, called the columns of the rectum. Between these are valvular folds which resemble somewhat in appearance the aortic valves. These small pouches may be the starting-point of suppuration due to irritation from the presence of foreign bodies. The external sphincter surrounds the orifice of the anus, and has fixed attachments which correspond to fibrous bands passing from the anal orifice to the tip of the coccyx and anteriorly to the superficial perineal fascia. Its fibres blend with those of the sphincter vaginæ, constituting a figure-of-eight muscle which surrounds the vagina and anus, while the internal sphincter is formed by the lower circular fibres of the muscular coat, which are more developed at this point. The internal sphincter is a little over an inch and a half in breadth, being overlapped by the external. The anus is about three-fourths of an inch in length, presenting a puckered or wrinkled orifice caused by the sphincter. The border-line between the skin and the mucosa is distinguished by a fine white streak indicating the interval between the external and the internal sphincter. The anal branch of the pudic nerve supplies the skin at the verge of the anus: hence pain from anal fissure is due to an exposed filament of this nerve.

*Physiology.*—When at rest the sphincters are constantly on guard and keep the orifice closed. If the patient has a lesion of the dorsal cord, they become relaxed and there is incontinence of fæces. The act of defecation has for its origin a vague sensation of weight, due to the pressure exercised upon the anus by a fæcal mass. This sensation induces a reflex contraction of the muscular tunic of the rectum which tends to force towards the anus the accumulated material. If the sphincters offer resistance, an anti-peristaltic action results, pushing the fæcal matter towards the upper part of the rectum. The tonicity of the sphincter, however, has a limit, which is overcome when the column formed by the fæcal material is high. In such cases a single peristaltic movement of the intestines is sufficient for the act of defecation, by which the latter is accomplished in the ordinary cases. If the material becomes solid, it requires a severe muscular effort for relief.

INJURIES.

Injuries of the rectum are of two kinds, accidental and surgical. The former are generally rare, on account of the protection of the rectum by the sacrum. The causes of injuries vary, as falling from ,a height on a pointed body, sliding off a hay-rick upon the point of a fork or fork-handle, the careless use of a sound or the tip of a syringe. Perforation or rupture of the rectum may occur spontaneously, as in the fœtus; straining at stool may cause partial rupture of the rectal wall. Parturition is a well-known cause. Prolonged use of a metallic or hard-rubber pessary may cause a fissure and finally a wound of the septum; the latter is generally slight or superficial. The symptoms of such an injury are localized pain and discharge of blood and muco-pus.

Peritonitis may sometimes complicate wounds of the rectum. The inflammation is usually circumscribed, and is not serious. When peritonitis occurs, it is apt to be acute in character, and the patient succumbs in a few days. Perirectal phlegmon is a less serious complication, and generally ends in the formation of a fistula. Emphysema has been mentioned, but is rare. The extent and depth of these wounds are exceedingly variable. One may be superficial, while in another there may be considerable destruction of tissue.

The diagnosis is usually determined by the symptoms, as local pain, discharge of blood, and later muco-purulent material, by the anus; and to these signs may be added others, as the passage of fæcal matter through the vagina, or with the urine, or the escape of urine by the rectum. Hemorrhage itself is a symptom of sufficient significance to demand interference. When it is severe, the loss of blood may be sufficient to cause syncope. Such injuries are sometimes complicated by peritonitis. If the inflammation extends gradually, it may be circumscribed and may not be grave, unless the peritoneum has been injured and there is a communication with the bladder or the rectum; peritonitis then becomes of a very acute character, and the patient rapidly succumbs. A much less significant complication is perirectal phlegmon, which generally terminates in the formation of a fistula. The condition described as emphysema is exceedingly rare, and results from perforations of the rectum; it may assume alarming proportions, as in a case reported in the *Lancet*, where it had extended over all the lower portion of the body.

The prognosis will depend entirely upon the situation, extent, and depth of the wound. Recovery in the majority of cases is the rule.

56

Treatment should be directed to relieving pain and possible peritoneal complications. Pain may be allayed by the use of opium; cold applications or an ice-bag may be applied over the affected region with the view of limiting inflammation. If suppuration is established in the perirectal tissue, free incisions should be made, followed by antiseptic irrigation. Hemorrhage at the time of the accident may be severe and even dangerous, requiring that an important vessel should be secured or that the cavity should be firmly packed with gauze.

### FOREIGN BODIES.

Foreign bodies in the rectum may be divided into three classes : 1, those which have been introduced through the anus ; 2, those which have reached the rectum by way of the intestinal canal after they have been swallowed; 3, those which have formed in the rectum.

Where foreign bodies have been introduced through the anus the subjects are usually of depraved habits; pederasty and abnormal sexual impulses afford the motives. The character of the objects introduced is exceedingly variable, such as beer-glasses, mortar pestles, marbles, and pebbles. The length of the body introduced into the rectum has been in some cases phenomenal, and it is difficult to comprehend how an individual could insert a mortar pestle twelve inches long and three inches in thickness without producing a serious lesion. Irregular bodies which have rough, unequal surfaces give rise to erosions and sometimes to lacerations. A misplaced pessary may have produced ulceration and perforation of the recto-vaginal septum, so as to enter the rectum.

The second class of foreign bodies are those which reach the rectum through the intestinal tract. Merlin relates a case in which a fish-bone had perforated the rectal and uterine walls and implanted itself in the fœtus. Other cases of this kind are false teeth, pins, or pieces of money.

The third class of foreign bodies includes those which develop in the intestine or in the rectal pouch. In children these are frequently masses of lumbricoid worms. In some cases, especially in the old or paralytic, an accumulation of excrement may form a hard mass. Such masses are found particularly in aged females, also in the hysterical. The hardened fæcal matter may be covered with a whitish coating and may present the character of a true concretion or calculus. In the middle of such a compact mass may be found smaller portions which have had for their point of origin a biliary calculus or the stone of a cherry or prune. The true cause of the accumulation is the diminished reflex power in the large intestine and the defective contraction of the muscular fibre, with the presence of a retained hard fæcal mass which acts upon the formation of the structure of the rectal surface. Dilatation of the rectum about a fæcal calculus occurs, and finally an ulcerative proctitis constitutes the characteristic lesion.

The symptoms are those which arise from the accumulation of fæces, also the pain produced by proctitis, a sensation of weight on the perineum, sero-sanguinolent diarrhœa which is quite fetid, but, most important of all, constipation.  Lumbar and crural pains are present, with a frequent desire to defecate, which proves fruitless; sometimes dry, almost petrified, scybala are expelled.  Straining and efforts at evacuation are laborious and painful. Prolonged retention of fæcal matter reacts badly upon the general health, causing toxæmia, digestive disturbance, hepatic pain, and nervous irritability.

If the condition arises as the result of a true foreign body in the rectum, the symptoms are more acute and severe.  After about forty-eight hours, or rarely later, the patient is forced to seek surgical intervention, and will complain of pretty severe pain in the belly and a sensation of weight at the level of the anus.  Not infrequently there is inflammation of the bladder and uterus.  If the object has been pushed deeply and roughly into the rectum, the peritoneum may become inflamed.  Prolonged retention of a foreign body in the rectum may cause inflammation or even gangrene of its walls, pelvic cellulitis, hypogastric phlegmon, abortion, and intestinal obstruction.

The diagnosis is sometimes very difficult, and when exact information is wanting, the rectum should be palpated if a patient complains of obstinate constipation, with pain in the region of the rectum, perineum, and base of the bladder.  In some cases two fingers, or the entire hand, if small, may be introduced into the rectum, when a foreign body may be detected as high as the sigmoid flexure.

The prognosis is generally favorable, and will depend somewhat upon the character of the body and how it has been introduced.  If it is fragile or sharp, and has been introduced through the anus, its removal may be attended with difficulty.

The treatment is necessarily varied.  In some cases it requires all the surgeon's ingenuity to accomplish the successful removal of the body.  The celebrated case of Marchetti's should be kept in mind, where a pig's tail, rough with bristles, was pushed into the rectum of a public woman by some students during an orgy.  The more the tail was pulled the more forcibly were the bristles driven into the mucous membrane and the greater was the difficulty of its removal.  It was withdrawn by passing over a string attached to the tail a hollow reed, which pushed the mucous membrane off the surface and permitted the removal of the foreign body.  Where the body is situated high up, it may be necessary to resort to abdominal section and to accomplish its removal by incision of the intestine and subsequent suture.  In some cases a posterior rectotomy may be sufficient.

### ANAL PRURITUS.

Anal pruritus is an intermittent or continuous itching of the anal region. It may be so severe as to produce prolonged insomnia and constitute a most distressing malady.  The itching may be so intense that the patient cannot avoid scratching the parts, even though she may be so situated as to make it extremely annoying. Pruritus may be divided, according to its cause, into parasitic, secondary, and essential pruritus. The most frequent cause is the *oxyuris vermicularis*, a form of intestinal worm about two-fifths of an inch in length, resembling a large white thread. It is readily seen with the naked eye when we examine the anus. The mere exploration is not always sufficient. If it is not observed at the first examination, it is well to make two or three, and even to inspect the fæces. Secondary pruritus is observed as a sequela of hemorrhoids, erythema, eczema, or herpes. In a word, it is the result of any affection which can cause irritation of the anal region. The cause can be readily determined by direct examination. Essential pruritus differs from the others in that there is no trace of any parasite or any pathological lesion. It is, then, due to a simple neuralgia or dermatalgia. It is only in the absence of any appreciable cause that this variety is admitted.

The treatment must necessarily depend upon the cause. In the parasitic form the margin of the anus should be frequently washed with a sublimate solution (1 to 1000), or with equal parts of water and ordinary vinegar, or with carbolic acid one part, glycerin twenty parts, infusion of absinthe one hundred and twenty-five parts. In secondary pruritus the cause of the affection should be treated by the appropriate remedy. In essential pruritus, apply hot lotions several times a day, or use a ten-per-cent. cocaine ointment, or try cauterization of the margin of the anus, morphine suppositories, and, if necessary, dilatation under chloroform anæsthesia.

### FISSURE OF THE ANUS.

By this name is designated a small superficial excoriation seated between the radiating folds, which gives rise to sharp pain and spasmodic contraction of the sphincter. It is produced by habitual constipation. Hard fæcal matter cannot pass over the anal region without causing erosions or tears of the membrane. In some cases, in addition to the fissures and hemorrhoids, eczema and erythema exist, and to these conditions and the reflex contraction of the sphincters has been attributed the constipation; in others, congenital narrowing of the anus has been mentioned as a cause.

Fissures have been divided into two classes, the tolerable and the intolerable, the former being almost devoid of pain, the latter producing acute suffering. The pain attains its most severe paroxysm at the moment of defecation, but gradually subsides at the end of twenty to twenty-five minutes. The patient has an acute lancinating pain at the anus, a pricking, burning sensation with radiating pains in the loins, thighs, and lumbar regions. Patients may be confined to bed, not daring to make a movement. At times they assume the strangest postures in order to compress the anus, sitting on the edge of a chair, etc. In some the distress during defecation is so acute that they avoid going to the closet. As a result, obstinate constipation occurs, with gastralgia, disturbance of the digestive functions, stercoræmia, loss of flesh and appetite, and an alteration of the tissues which may resemble an actual cachexia. The acute stage may be complicated with colic, vesical spasms, and crural and sciatic neuralgia.

It is generally easy to recognize the existence of the fissure by mere inspection. The little muco-cutaneous processes called anal valves, and the pouches behind them, known as the sinuses of Valsalva, are often the sites of fissures. In these cases there will be a small external pile at the bottom of the sinus. It is sometimes called the "sentinel" pile. In some cases we may not be able to discover the fissure. We may then move the finger around the anal orifice and determine its site by the localized pain. If the patient strains, the rectal mucous membrane protrudes and the ulceration is disclosed. When the fissure has existed for some time, anal vegetations may develop in its neighborhood which may conceal it and lead to error. It is difficult to confound a fissure with hemorrhoids or vegetations. The only condition in which there may be the possibility of error is the affection known as neuralgia of the anus. In it, however, the pain appears spontaneously, and does not necessarily occur at the time of defecation.

The treatment may be palliative or curative. The former consists in the use of baths and ointments, particularly iodoform or ichthyol ointment; ichthyol is said to exert a marked curative effect in anal fissure. The radical treatment of fissure, however, is surgical, and consists in dilatation of the sphincter, either by the aid of bougies or by the introduction of the thumbs or two fingers through the sphincter, and their forcible separation, the patient being thoroughly anæsthetized.

### PROCTITIS.

Proctitis is an inflammation of the mucous membrane of the rectum. It is generally concomitant with or consecutive to inflammation of the large intestine, but may appear independently, being sometimes acute and sometimes chronic. Among the causes of proctitis are inflamed hemorrhoids, inflammation of the mucous surface of the anus, blennorrhagia, the abuse of drastics, obstinate constipation, foreign bodies, as fish-bones, biliary concretions, worms, and the practice of pederasty. The condition may be developed by careless methods of examination. Hence, in making a vaginal examination, the rule should always be to wash carefully the finger before inserting it into the rectum, as through any specific discharge from the vagina an infection of the rectum may be very readily accomplished, producing gonorrhœa.

The symptoms are local, being confined to the inferior part of the digestive tube. Little by little the patients experience painful sensations in the region of the sacrum, coccyx, bladder, and uterus. The anus becomes red, hot, very sensitive, and contraction of the sphincter occurs. It is accompanied by constipation, which may persist during several days. Evacuations soon become painful, followed by tenesmus and the expulsion of a glairy mucus or of a mixture of pus and mucus, and sometimes of blood. After this first period comes another, characterized by profuse diarrhœa and mucous or muco-purulent discharge. In neglected or badly treated cases acute proctitis soon becomes chronic, the symptoms being somewhat similar in character to those already described. Diarrhœa alternates with constipation. Examination by the speculum will disclose the presence of multiple points of ulceration, which are rounded and superficial, or extensive vegetations, the latter specially marked in cases of blennorrhagic proctitis. The thick, greenish discharge attending this condition becomes the point of departure for a series of complications. It produces a red appearance, excoriation, and even an eczematous eruption of the perineum ; the mucous membrane itself becomes altered, thickened, sclerosed, and narrowing of the rectum may result. In severe cases we sometimes see phlegmons, abscesses, and fistulæ complicating the intense inflammation of the rectum.

The disease is not usually difficult to recognize. It is characterized by constipation, with sharp pain during defecation, and a rise of temperature, followed by a mucous discharge and tenesmus. In dysentery, the frequency of the stools, hemorrhages, and the expulsion of shreds of mucous membrane are symptoms too characteristic to be confounded with simple proctitis.

The treatment consists in rest, the use of enemata of hot water or astringent injections, such as one-half to one grain of sulphate of zinc to an ounce, nitrate of silver, one-eighth to one-fourth of a grain to the ounce, or some of the vegetable astringents, as tannic acid, fluid extract of hamamelis, or fluid extract of hydrastis. A five-grain iodoform suppository, used twice daily after irrigation of the canal with either hot water or some astringent agent, will be found useful. A combination of extract of belladonna or extract of hyoscyamus with the iodoform is often beneficial, particularly where there is much tenesmus.

### PHLEGMONS OR ABSCESSES OF THE ANUS AND RECTUM.

Phlegmons and abscesses of this region may be divided into three classes : 1, the superficial inflammations of the anal region and of the rectum ; 2, those which have their origin in the ischio-rectal fossa ; 3, those which are developed in the cellular tissue beneath the peritoneum and under the levator ani muscle. The causes of the development or extension of phlegmon are quite various. It may be due to scratching of the anal region, to uncleanliness, or to blennorrhagic discharges from the vaginal cavity. These are not slow in producing excoriations. The passage of hard fæcal matter is also an etiological factor. The cause of the deep ischio-rectal variety is often difficult to determine. Many of these abscesses arise as the result of a local development of tuberculosis. In other cases they may be produced by ulceration, proctitis, cancer, stricture, inflamed hemorrhoids, and, finally, surgical intervention, such as dilatation of the rectum, excision of condylomata, hemorrhoids, or other tumors. Superficial inflammations comprise superficial abscess and phlegmonous abscess, or phlegmon proper. Superficial abscess presents the following appearance. There is generally a tumor the size of a hazel-nut, of a light-red color, which, on examination, is found to be superficial and limited by a circumscribed induration. At the end of a few days the tumor, after the patient has suffered more or less acute pain, becomes soft and fluctuating, the skin reddens and becomes thin, and there is a discharge of very fetid pus. The tension ceases, pain disappears, and all that remains of the abscess is a small induration.

It is only necessary to recall the signs that have been mentioned to enable us to avoid error in diagnosis. The affection is one of slight gravity, and generally disappears quickly. When a small abscess, however, is developed at the expense of tuberculous tissue, it often persists for a long time as a small fistula, from which a serous or sero-purulent liquid is discharged.

The proper treatment before suppuration occurs is the application of cold and the regulation of the bowels. If suppuration is imminent, it may be promoted by the application of starch poultices, and when fluctuation is established the abscess should be incised.

*Phlegmon.*—Phlegmon is situated at the margin of the anus, and is the form which we meet most often. This inflammation occurs in the subcutaneous cellular tissue, but, instead of being circumscribed, it has a tendency to spread over the surface. Later the patient has a sensation of tension in the region of the anus, followed by swelling and painful defecation. Fluctuation will be very clear, with the aid of one finger introduced into the rectum while the other is applied externally. These abscesses are not infrequently followed by fistula.

The abscess should be opened early by a long, deep incision, then irrigated with a strong carbolic solution or with a solution of chloride of zinc. If there is a fistulous opening into the rectum, a director should be introduced into it and all the tissue should be incised, including the sphincter.

*Abscess of the ischio-rectal fossa* is generally obscure at the outset. If a large collection of pus develops in the perineal region, it travels over the anus towards the sacrum and from the anterior part of the perineum towards the coccyx; the integument becomes hard and thickened, and forms a sort of resisting shield. Pus destroys the deep layers of tissue, and spreads along the large ligaments towards the ischial tuberosities. As in all suppurations in close proximity to the intestine, the pus becomes exceedingly fetid. It finds a considerable obstacle in the levator ani muscle and the thick skin, passes towards the rectum, and, after having destroyed the external layers of the gut, may collect under the mucous membrane. The collection may take place in the ischio-rectal fossa, and may communicate with the abscess upon the opposite side. This condition is known as circular or horseshoe abscess, and permits the pus to flow from one sac to the other. In some cases these abscesses may point beneath the skin, and the patient has a high fever, frequent pulse, delirium, sometimes collapse, and the condition terminates fatally after several days. Gangrene of the ischio-rectal fossa may occur, generally due to the infiltration of fæcal matter or urine. The skin rapidly assumes a dark tint, and bluish spots and large blisters cover the surface; from the latter very fetid pus escapes, mixed with bubbles of gas. In certain grave cases the rectal wall is also affected by gangrene, the patient having prostration, delirium, dryness of the tongue, and an extremely profuse and fetid diarrhœa.

The condition is not generally difficult to recognize. Rectal touch discloses perirectal induration, which does not extend much beyond the levator ani.

The condition is very grave. Complications may bring death with but brief delay.

The treatment should be prompt and energetic. A deep incision should be made. This may be accomplished with the thermo-cautery, and should be followed by irrigation with an antiseptic solution, or even by cauterization with chloride of zinc.

*Abscess of the Superior Pelvi-Rectal Spaces.*—We have been discussing inflammation of the cellular tissue beneath the muscular band constituted by the levator ani muscle. We now come to the consideration of phlegmons which are situated in that space, full of cellular tissue, limited above by the pelvic peritoneum and behind by the superior faces of the levator muscle, covered with its aponeurosis. The anatomical relations of the bladder, uterus, and rectum explain the reason of phlegmons in this region, of which some are the result of affections of the genital organs and others may owe their origin to ulceration of the rectum or inflammation of the hemorrhoidal veins. Caries of the anterior face of the sacrum and sacro-iliac arthritis may also be the point of departure for pelvic suppuration.

The symptoms are often obscure. The affection, in its beginning, is insidious. Patients complain of a sensation of weight in the pelvis, sometimes an actual pain which they can hardly localize. They suffer from constipation, difficulty in evacuating the bowels, and a general uneasiness, associated with fever. The progress of the affection varies. Sometimes pus collects in, and separates the fibres of, the levator muscle, and makes its way towards the ischio-rectal fossa. It there forms an abscess, which at a later period opens externally; the resulting fistulous tract may measure from three to five inches. At other times the purulent collection empties into the rectum and thus establishes a symptomatic diarrhœa. Patients who have before complained of obstinate constipation and painful stools have diarrhœa associated with the ejection of a considerable quantity of pus. The evacuation of the pus-cavity, however, is imperfect; the orifice of communication is generally small, and the abscess tends to become chronic. In some cases the pus passes beneath the pelvic aponeurosis and discharges into the vagina or bladder, though it is clear that it originated high up in the perirectal tissues. The only method by which we can approximate its position is by the rectal touch.

The treatment should consist in opening the abscess through the rectum at the site of the enlargement, and the incision should be made as free as possible.

## FISTULA IN ANO.

A fistula is a narrow canal or sinus which connects two neighboring regions that are separated in the normal state. Fistulæ may be divided into—1, complete (Fig. 1, A), or a sinus with an opening upon the mucous membrane and another externally,—in other words, a continuous canal; 2, incomplete (a) blind external (Fig. 1, C), in which there is no communication with the rectum, and (b) blind internal (Fig. 1, B), which open upon the surface of the mucous membrane only. From a pathological stand-point they may be divided into—1, fistulæ which are sequelæ of inflammation of the cellular

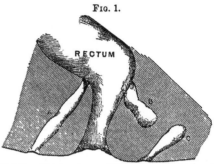

FIG. 1.

Varieties of fistulæ.—A, complete fistula: B, blind internal fistula; C, blind external fistula.

tissue of the pelvi-rectal fossa, as the common anal fistula; 2, fistulæ which have for their source suppuration in the adipose layer of the superior pelvi-rectal space, and are known, consequently, as superior pelvi-rectal fistulæ; 3, fistulæ which have their origin in a bony lesion, and are called osteopathic fistulæ. The latter need not occupy our attention.

The inferior or common anal fistulæ are the most frequent, and form the greater number of those seen in daily practice. In an ordinary fistula the tract is situated immediately beneath the integument of the anus, not involving the fibres of the sphincter muscle. Now, in the description of all fistulæ we must consider the orifices, internal and external, and the intermediate tract. The external or cutaneous orifice is more frequently at one side of the anus, and is generally single. It may be situated near to, or at some distance from, the anus, sometimes in the midst of the radiating folds. In a deep fistula, the external orifice is some distance from the termination of the digestive tube. Generally it is quite narrow, and we see it in the summit of a small projecting pimple of a reddish color or presenting a fungous aspect; at other times the orifice is concealed in the depth of an ulceration. In some cases we find in a prominence a series of straits which sometimes open into the same canal, at other times into a series of tracts communicating with the rectum. The internal or mucous orifice is sometimes situated immediately beneath the point where the skin borders the mucous membrane, but it is not always so: it may open one-fifth of an inch to two inches from the anal orifice. The appearance of the internal orifice also varies. Sometimes it is a simple opening at the level of a projection of moderate dimensions; at other times it is large and irregular.   In some cases we may find that the probe passes upward along-side the rectum, while the opening is lower down.   It can generally be found just above the external sphincter or between the two sphincter mus-cles.   The tract is sometimes straight, sometimes tortuous, having a direc-tion from the cutaneous surface towards the rectum.   When the fistula is incomplete, the canal is arrested midway.   When several orifices are situ-ated about the anus, exploration with the probe will often determine the fact that they communicate with each other.   This crescentic burrowing in the vicinity of the anus has been designated by the name of the "horseshoe" fistula.   In such cases the canal may attain a considerable length.

Superior pelvi-rectal fistulæ have their origin in inflammation and con-secutive abscess of the cellular tissue between the levator ani and the peri-toneum.   The fistulous tracts in this form are often rectilinear, and quite deep,—from three and a half to six inches.   In examining these fistulæ we notice that there is considerable tissue separating the finger introduced into the anus and the probe in the fistulous tract, which fact distinguishes them from ordinary fistulæ.   Probably one of the most frequent causes of fistula is tuberculosis.   Microscopical examination will demonstrate that the condition has arisen from a deposit of tuberculous tissue in the midst of the cellular structure, and its subsequent degeneration or necrosis, which results in the loss of normal tissue and the formation of a purulent collec-tion, which sometimes discharges externally, sometimes into the rectum. Foreign bodies arrested at the level of the folds of the anal region, or rupture of a hemorrhoidal lobe, facilitate infection of the cellular tissue and the subsequent formation of an abscess.   It has often been asked why fistulæ are so slow to heal, and why, in many cases, in spite of skilful treatment, they cicatrize so badly and leave a small tract which has no tendency to close again.   This has been explained by the extreme mo-bility of the rectum ; frequent contractions of the levator ani muscle would render cicatrization impossible or very difficult.   But the tardy healing is due especially to the nature of the affection.   So long as tuberculous granu-lations remain the fistula will not close.

*Symptoms.*—Patients afflicted with fistulæ complain of varying sensa-tions.   Some have pruritus, others a secretion of pus which may not be abundant, but which always has a very penetrating odor.   Eczema or simple erythema may later appear about the external opening ; the latter may be obliterated, and there is then retained pus and an inflammation of the tissues which renders the condition insupportable.   If we examine the anal region, we find one or more small openings, the latter presenting the appearance of the head of a watering-pot.   In cases of blind internal fistula there is a discharge of pus from the anus, associated with a con-gestion of the whole perianal region.

*Diagnosis.*—The patient should be placed in the lateral position, with the upper thigh strongly flexed.   The parts are exposed, the superior buttock is raised, and the anal region inspected. This sometimes suffices to determine the diagnosis of fistula. It is necessary to introduce the finger into the rectum, however, to ascertain the extent and variety of the lesion. A probe is pushed through the small papilla or projection, and is carried gently along the canal, the point being pressed against the finger in the rectum in order to locate the internal opening. This is generally found just within the margin of the external sphincter. The probe will often pass upward alongside the bowel, but if withdrawn and pressed towards the upper margin of the external sphincter it passes through the internal opening and impinges against the finger. In blind internal fistula the touch is very painful; only a small quantity of pus is discharged; the finger meets no induration, ulceration, or fungosities in the lower end of the rectum, which enables us to eliminate the probability of cancer, polypi, or cicatricial stenosis of the gut. An induration surrounding the anus renders the diagnosis of blind internal fistula probable.

*Prognosis.*—Such lesions are always serious; although the affection itself may not be grave, it is an indication of a bad general state, and shows that the subject is predisposed to the development of tubercle-bacilli.

*Treatment.*—The earlier method of treatment of such conditions (which is still preferred by some surgeons) was the application of the elastic ligature. A needle or probe, armed with a thread of caoutchouc, was passed through the internal orifice and out at the anus. The thread was tied, and it gradually cut through the tissues, cicatrization at the same time occurring behind it, so as to fill up the opening. Often after the thread disappeared the fistula persisted. In these cases it was asserted that the affected tissues were not destroyed.

Incision by the thermo-cautery is far more efficacious. The canula sound is introduced into the tract, and the finger into the rectum. Following the direction which the sound travels, the internal orifice is discovered and the canula is brought out. The tissues are then divided by the thermo-cautery, and the bottom of the wound is cauterized and covered with iodoform gauze.

The best method of procedure is to incise the tract with a bistoury, to curette and irrigate it with an antiseptic solution, and then to suture the edges of the wound. This method of procedure is by far the preferable one, particularly in the female, for the reason that the intimate arrangement and association of the sphincter ani and sphincter vaginæ muscles lead to weakening of the sphincter subsequent to incision and granulation, while suturing the wound results in its restoration to a normal condition. To accomplish this operation, however, it is important that any secondary sinuses or fistulæ should be opened up and curetted prior to the closing of the edges of the wound. In some cases where the tissue is depraved the wound fails to unite, and the subsequent condition of the patient is bad. When a number of fistulæ are opened about the anus, it is desirable that they should not be cut through, even if suturing is done, as failure to unite would result in

loss of power of the sphincter. The preferable plan in such cases would be
the incision of the sinus up to the sphincter, careful curettage of the remaining portion of the canal, and packing the cavity with iodoform gauze. This
plan of procedure has resulted, in the hands of the writer, in the cure of
extensive fistulæ without influencing the subsequent action of the sphincter.
It is important at the same time that the general health of the patient
should be improved, and for this purpose cod-liver oil, creosote, phosphate
of lime, iodide of potassium, and various tonics may be employed.

### RECTO-VAGINAL FISTULÆ.

A recto-vaginal fistula is one which connects the rectum and the vagina.
The sinus may be situated in any part of the septum. In women who

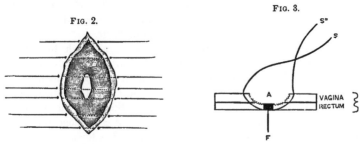

FIG. 2.

FIG. 3.

Denudation of the fistulous edges in the vagina,
with introduction of transverse sutures.

A, freshened edges; S, S, suture; F, fistula.

have borne a number of children there may be one or more openings from
the rectal pouch into the lower part of the vagina. These fistulæ not

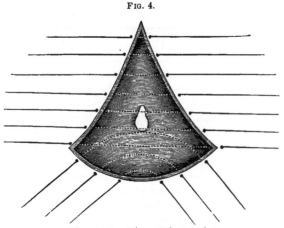

FIG. 4.

Triangular denudation. (After Schauta.)

infrequently result from the lesions of parturition, or they may be due to
the same causes as ordinary fistula in ano. In all cases where the history

FIG. 5.

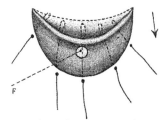

Closure of fistula by transverse crescent-shaped lips.
(After Fritsch.)

FIG. 6.

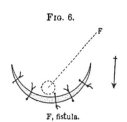

F, fistula.

FIG. 7.

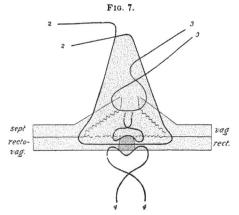

1, 1, Buried suture of the rectal surface of fistula; 2, 2, deep vaginal sutures;
3, 3, superficial vaginal sutures; 4, 4, supporting rectal sutures.

FIG. 8.

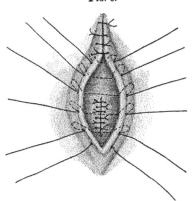

Closure of the vaginal incision by deep sutures, seen from above.

FIG. 9.

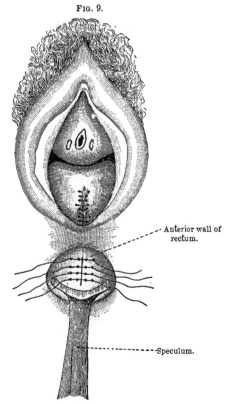

Vaginal incision closed. Introduction of rectal sutures. (After Saenger.)

FIG. 10.

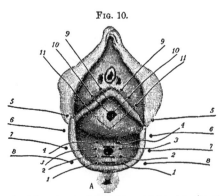

Simple perineal flap. A, anus; 1, 2, 3, 4, Lauenstein's buried sutures for closure of the rectal fistula; 5, 6, 7, 8, perineal sutures; 9, 10, 11, vaginal sutures to close opening in the vaginal flaps.

excludes the possibility of its being a sequela of parturition, the rectum should be carefully examined for stricture.

*Symptoms.*—The discomfort and annoyance of such a lesion must be

**Fig. 11.**

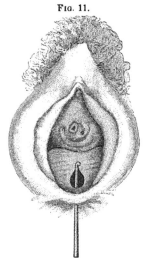

Fistula with only perineal fragment remaining.

**Fig. 12.**

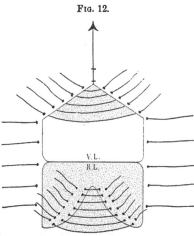

Diagrammatic representation of operation. R.L., rectal flaps, with Lauenstein's sutures; V.L., vaginal flaps.

directly dependent upon its size. The escape of flatus and liquid fæces will continually soil and render offensive the discharges of the vagina.

*Diagnosis.*—The position and size of the fistula will be determined by inspection, by its direction and length, and by the use of the probe. Where the odor of the discharge causes it to be suspected, and inspection does not disclose it, its presence may be revealed by distending the rectum with a colored fluid.

*Treatment.* — The operation for such a lesion must necessarily be dependent upon its size. When it is complicated, or is caused by stricture, no operation for its closure is indicated until the full calibre of the bowel can be restored. When the opening is small, a series of flap operations may be performed (Figs. 2, 3, 4, 5, 6, 7, 8, 9, 10, 11, 12, 13), closing the opening into the rectum by buried sutures and then stitching the flap back in place.

**Fig. 13.**

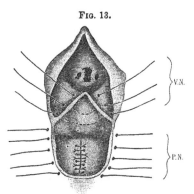

Anterior rectal wall closed by Lauenstein's deep sutures. P.N., perineal sutures; V.N., vaginal sutures.

## HEMORRHOIDS.

The term hemorrhoids signifies the varicose dilatation of the veins of the anus commonly called piles. Hemorrhoids are divided into external and internal, according to their relation to the sphincter. These hemorrhoidal dilatations are ampullary (see Fig. 14), and above the sphincter

FIG. 14.

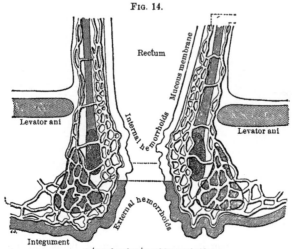

Internal and external hemorrhoids.

the tumor may form at the expense of the capillaries as well as of the veins. Below the level of the external sphincter, however, these ampullæ are often converted into blood-cysts. If the blood is coagulated, the hemorrhoids become hard, forming true blood-clots, which irritate by their presence the neighboring tissue, causing an indurated mass more or less extensive and the formation of small, hard tumors.

*Etiology.*—Hemorrhoids are a frequent affection in men, but still more so in women. They are met with especially in those of a gouty or rheumatic diathesis, and are increased under the influence of rich food, the use of alcohol, and a sedentary life. Among the most prominent exciting causes may be considered habitual constipation, the use of purgatives, and venereal excess. In women they may be developed as a result of serious mitral lesions, from the pressure of ovarian cysts, of uterine tumors, or of tumors in the walls of the pelvis, and from retroversion or retroflexion of the uterus.

*Symptoms.*—A great variety of symptoms may be produced by the presence of hemorrhoids; especially such as a sensation of uneasiness, pressure, twinges, tingling, and intolerable smarting, so that standing or walking becomes distressing. The patient lies in bed, sometimes upon one side, sometimes upon the abdomen, and keeps her muscles in a state of absolute rest. Hemorrhoids are generally complicated with constipation, which aggravates the tendency to headache, vertigo, and buzzing in the ears. The patient becomes pale and loses her appetite. All these phenomena may become exaggerated when she is at the climax of suffering. Little by little the tension of the hemorrhoidal varices becomes less, pain disappears, and the patient enjoys comparative comfort. This tension may be quickly relieved by the rupture of hemorrhoidal varices, or the passage of a hard fæcal mass may cause fissure of the ano-rectal mucous membrane, with more or less abundant discharge. The anus presents a different appearance according to the situation of the lesion. Sometimes the hemorrhoid is scarcely perceptible, appearing as a slightly rounded or prolonged projection, more or less soft, smooth, and bloodless. This is the flabby hemorrhoid. Or, again, it may be tense, resisting, and painful. In some places the mucous membrane and the skin are both involved, the tumor is indurated, and resembles a true condyloma. Besides these external hemorrhoids, there are others, the true character of which can be appreciated only by the use of the speculum, when we see small, soft granular projections which the touch alone may fail to reveal. When the patient strains, these protrude from the anus; and at its level there is a double varicose enlargement, one formed by the external hemorrhoids, the other by the internal. These may be replaced with more or less facility, some without any pain, while others produce severe tenesmus. Internal hemorrhoids, when prolapsed, are grasped by the sphincter and strangulated, becoming the seat of intolerable pain. The patient has the sensation of a red-hot iron at the anus. If we examine a strangulated hemorrhoid, we find it hard and tense, purplish, brown, or even black. This change is due to an interruption of the venous circulation from the spasmodic contraction of the anal sphincter; if this continues sufficiently long, a slough is caused. At the end of some days the slough separates and the symptoms improve. Sloughing of the mass may be complicated with inflammation and suppuration of the surrounding tissue, and even with erysipelas.

The *diagnosis* of hemorrhoids is not difficult. By examination they are distinguished from condylomata, polypi, and other hard and isolated tumors. Prolapse of the rectum is characterized by a symmetrical swelling, and not by unequal projections. In cancer of the rectum there is an ulcerated fungous tumor which secretes an ichorous fluid accompanied by abundant hemorrhages, so that it would rarely be confounded with an ulcerated hemorrhoid. In examining hemorrhoids, it is important, however, always to seek for the true cause of the condition before beginning treatment, and especially to ascertain that it is not due to an affection of the liver, to a tumor of the abdominal cavity, or to a retroflexed uterus.

*Treatment.*—The treatment of hemorrhoids will depend upon the cause. One of the first considerations should be the correction of irregular and injurious habits. The patient should be directed to abstain from wines, liquors, spices, to overcome constipation, and to avoid the employment of

57

drastic purgatives. No operation should be done while the pelvis is occupied by a large fibroid or ovarian tumor, or while the uterus is retrodisplaced. In many cases the treatment of these conditions will be sufficient to relieve the patient of hemorrhoids.

As to the surgical means, there are, in the first place, various drugs which are injected, such as ergot, iron, and carbolic acid. The latter agent is one which has been exceedingly popular among advertising specialists. It affords the advantage that the patients are enabled to continue their duties, and to be about, without a severe and painful surgical procedure. It is, however, proved to have been dangerous in some cases, producing extensive ulceration at the site of the operation, septic infection, and even death, by the formation of emboli. The thermo-cautery has been advocated. The chief methods of operation, however, are: 1. Ligature with incision. 2. Crushing. 3. The clamp cautery. 4. Incision.

Hemorrhoids, according to Allingham, may be divided into two classes. The first group are those which come down at stool, which are almost always in a state of prolapse, and which bleed profusely with each movement of the bowels. The operation to be chosen for such conditions should be one that can be performed as quickly as possible, so that the patient will lose little blood, with the least danger of secondary hemorrhage. The ligature meets these requirements, as it can be applied in five minutes, or even less time, and is practically free from danger of subsequent hemorrhage.

The second class of hemorrhoids are those which are regarded as producing inconvenience chiefly by protruding and preventing the patient from riding or walking. They rarely bleed, and do not impair the health. These may be crushed or cut off, bleeding vessels being ligated. Before ligating a pile, it is drawn down by volsella forceps and is separated with scissors from the muscular and subcutaneous tissues upon which it rests. The incision is made at the junction of the skin and mucous membrane, and is carried up the bowel so that the pile is left attached by its vessels and mucous membrane only. It is then ligated with strong silk at the neck, and the ligated pile is returned within the sphincters. This plan of procedure is applicable to vascular hemorrhoids and to those in patients suffering from kidney, cardiac, or atheromatous disease. It is, without doubt, the safest operation. The objections to this procedure are that it leaves a wound which is slow to heal, and that there is greater pain after the operation and on the first movement of the bowels than after crushing or simple excision. There is more sloughing and greater liability to contraction.

The crushing operation consists in drawing the pile by means of a hook into a powerful screw crusher. This should be applied to the longitudinal aspect of the bowel and be left *in situ*. This method is applicable when the piles are of medium size and are pedunculated. It is contra-indicated when the ligature is most advisable,—that is, when the pile is large and vascular, or when the patient is distant from medical aid and rapidity of operation is necessary. It is not so safe a procedure as the ligature. The advantages claimed for it are that there is freedom from pain after the operation, retention of urine is rare, suppuration is unlikely, there is little or no pain during defecation, and recovery is usually rapid.

In using the clamp and cautery the pile is drawn down into the clamp. This portion is cut off, and the stump and vessels are cauterized until the vessel is thoroughly seared. Statistics, however, show that this is a much more fatal operation than ligation or crushing. The burning gives great pain, hemorrhage is more likely to follow, there is extensive sloughing of the rectal tissues, and more time is required to heal, while there is greater contraction.

Probably the most effective method of procedure is that known as the Whitehead operation, which consists in making an incision clear around the anus, through the junction of the skin and mucous membrane, dissecting up the varicose tissue from about the sphincters, removing the hemorrhoidal mass, bringing the mucous membrane down, and suturing it to the skin. In this way all the hemorrhoidal tissue is removed, and the patient is much less likely to suffer from relapse, pain is not great, there is no inconvenience in the evacuation of the bowels, and in severe cases the writer has found that the patients are far more comfortable after the operation than they had been for months previously. In the external hemorrhoid, where a hard blood-clot is formed, the quickest method of procedure and that which affords most prompt relief is to incise and turn out the clot. This results in a cicatrization which cures the hemorrhoid and prevents the formation of external tags or folds of mucous membrane.

In the treatment of hemorrhoids we must not forget the importance of constitutional measures, the relief of the tendency to the development of rheumatism and gout, and the hygienic measures already indicated.

### POLYPI.

Benign pedunculated tumors are occasionally found in the rectum. They are usually few in number, and in the adult it is rare to find more than one. Though generally of small size, they sometimes become as large as a prune or even a hen's egg. (Figs. 15, 16.) The size of the growth is dependent upon the blood-supply. The tumor is usually of a rounded form, and is dependent by a slender pedicle. Polypi are commonly situated about an inch to an inch and a half above the anus, rarely higher, though occasionally they are found as high as six inches. Their most common seat is the posterior wall of the gut. The pedicle may be round or flattened ; it is large and short in the fibrous varieties, long and slender in the soft ones. With the repeated passage of fæcal matter over the tumor the pedicle stretches and becomes so elongated that it may tear during defecation.

Such a growth may exist for a long time without causing any suspicion of its presence. The patient may be aware of its existence only when a tumor appears at the anus. It may produce a series of phenomena, as severe pain during defecation, tenesmus, twitching, and a sensation of burning of

the anus radiating through the entire pelvis.    Besides such phenomena,
there is a discharge of glairy mucus or blood.    The general health remains
good, unless the hemorrhage is so great that anæmia is induced; in such

FIG. 15.

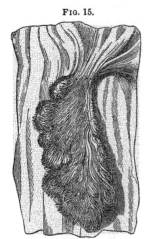

Rectal polypus.  (Esmarch).

FIG. 16.

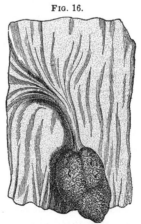

Glandular polypus.  (Esmarch).

cases the patient has vertigo and a tendency to syncope.    Polypi may not
infrequently be associated with fissures, prolapsus, or even fistulæ.    The
progress of the disease is slow in some cases, and may terminate spontaneously by rupture of the pedicle and discharge of the polypus.

The diagnosis is generally easy.    When the tumor protrudes from the
anus, inspection is sufficient to reveal its character.    If it is concealed, the
introduction of the finger may disclose and bring it down.    From hemorrhoids it is distinguished by the fact that the former are small, turgid
projections, disposed like a collar about the anus.    In prolapsus we find,
notwithstanding a considerable projection of the mucous membrane, that its
centre presents an orifice into which the finger can be introduced, and that
no pedicle is present.    Malignant tumors are recognized by the extremely
fetid secretion and the grave alteration of the general health.

The treatment consists in the removal of the tumor.    Some operators
draw it down and twist its pedicle; this should be carefully done, so as to
avoid prolapsus of the rectum.    The elastic ligature may be used, and a
large pedicle should be tied in two sections.    The safest and most expeditious method is to apply a pair of hæmostatic forceps to the base of the
pedicle, to draw it down, and to cut away the tumor, leaving the forceps in
place.

### PROLAPSE OF THE RECTUM.

Prolapse of the rectum is a more or less complete protrusion of the
mucous membrane or of all the tunics of the bowel.    The mucous membrane is so loosely connected with the muscular layer by cellular tissue that

it can slide upon the latter and even protrude from the anus. (Fig. 17.)
A slight straining effort, such as accompanies defecation, may be sufficient

FIG. 17.

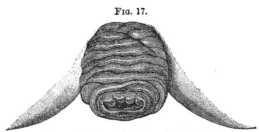

Prolapse of all the coats of the rectum. (Busche.)

to cause such protrusion. This condition can be seen in an exaggerated
state in the horse. Instead of the mucous membrane only, all the layers
sometimes prolapse. (Figs. 18, 19.) A cylindrical tumor from one to three inches in length is then formed. When the tumor is small it has at its inferior extremity a small round orifice, and when large it is often found hollowed out like a horseshoe by the traction of the mesorectum. In the descent the peritoneal cul-de-sac is ordinarily obliterated and a portion of the small intestine may be carried down with it. Notwithstanding the natural predisposition of the tissues to

FIG. 18.

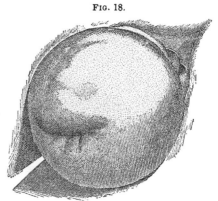

Prolapse of the rectum.

become invaginated, unusual force is necessary to cause extensive prolapse.
The active factors may be diarrhœa or chronic dysentery, the presence of
a polypus or hemorrhoids, repeated pregnancies, tumors of the sacrum, and
the efforts of coughing in cases of chronic bronchitis.

*Symptoms.*—Simple prolapse appears first as a slight eversion of the
mucous membrane when the patient strains, which disappears more or less
when the effort ceases. The swelling does not subside, but increases in size,
forming a small cylinder an inch and a half to two inches long. The
surface is soft, glistening, folded, and of a rosy hue. In the centre is a
contracted orifice by which the intestine is entered. At the level of the
anus the rectal mucous membrane is continuous with the skin. This
degree of prolapse can be easily reduced by slight pressure. Patients
experience discomfort in walking. The cylinder becomes elongated; the
mucous membrane changes to a dark color and is painful to the touch.

Subsequently it is covered with pus, or has a grayish hue, showing superficial ulcerations. The membrane assumes the character of the skin, losing its flexibility and sensibility, while its natural furrows gradually disappear. The tumor may attain the size of an orange. It is difficult to reduce it, on account of the hardening and thickening of the submucous tissue, which prevent it from slipping back. In cases of this degree the sphincters dilate, lose their tonicity, and no longer prevent the escape of fæcal matter. Complete prolapse may result in the formation of a very large mass, which may be more or less globular and of a pink or red color. Its external surface still bears the traces of the transverse folds, which indicate the points

FIG. 19.

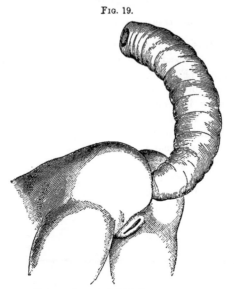

Prolapse of invaginated intestine.   (Esmarch).

at which the membrane was in most intimate relation with the muscular tunic. At the most dependent portion of the tumor an orifice will be found communicating with the intestine. The base of the tumor is surrounded by the anus. The prolapsed intestine tumefies and becomes the seat of an acute inflammation which may continue until it sometimes produces repeated hemorrhages that endanger the life of the patient. Peritonitis may be a complication, and finally symptoms develop which indicate strangulation of the intestine. The progress of prolapse is generally slow but continuous, and if the affection is neglected or is badly treated it becomes excessive, and renders not only walking but even the erect position painful.

*Diagnosis.*—The diagnosis of prolapse is readily determined. In hemorrhoids there are projections more or less independent of one another and separated by small furrows. Polypi are smooth, pedunculated tumors springing from within the internal orifice of the rectum. Epithelioma cannot be confounded with prolapse, as there are neither the induration, the cauliflower masses, nor the ichorous discharge in the latter which are so characteristic of a malignant neoplasm.

*Prognosis.*—The prognosis is dependent upon the extent of the affection ; the condition is curable according as the prolapsus is reducible or irreducible.

*Treatment.*—In the treatment of reducible prolapse we return the bowel to its normal position and endeavor to remove the causes which lead to the condition. As a curative means we may employ the thermo-cautery. With the latter instrument three or four lines of tissue are cauterized. The patient is given bismuth or opium to produce constipation, which is overcome on the eighth or ninth day by a light purgative. In irreducible prolapse a number of methods have been advocated, some of which are purely palliative, while others are supposed to restore the muscular tone of the vessels forming the pelvic floor and serving to support the rectum. Nux vomica, strychnine, and finally hypodermic injections of ergotine have been administered with this purpose. Dupuytren produces a cicatricial narrowing of the anus by removing with curved scissors from two to six radiating folds to the right and left of the anus. Duret removed from the posterior wall of the rectum a triangular piece of the mucous membrane, the base of which included a part of the sphincter. Schwartz excises a large piece of the anterior wall of the anus and rectum. Mikulicz shortens the rectum in the following manner. The intestine is emptied by an injection, and opium is administered to limit peristalsis. The patient is placed in the dorsal position, and the field of operation is rendered aseptic. At a point from two-fifths to four-fifths of an inch from the anus the external cylinder is divided in its anterior half. The next step consists in incising transversely the posterior half of the external cylinder, layer by layer, from three-eighths to six-eighths of an inch from the margin of the anus. Sometimes upon reaching the peritoneum a hernia of the small intestine will be perceived, and will need to be reduced. Should the sphincter prevent reduction, the muscle may be cut and the peritoneal folds united. The bowel is then incised, layer by layer, the vessels met with being tied, and the two edges are reunited by interrupted sutures carried through all the coats, threads being left long enough to serve to steady the rectum during the remainder of the operation. The dissection and suturing of the posterior half are next performed, all the sutures are cut short, and the mass is powdered with iodoform and reduced.

An operative procedure called " rectopexy" was introduced by Verneuil. It consists of three steps, as follows. An incision is made about an inch and a half long upon each side of the anus, extending obliquely from above downward and backward. The portion of the anal circumference included between the anterior extremities of these incisions corresponds to the portion to be contracted; they begin at the point of junction of the skin and the mucous membrane. From their posterior extremities start two other small incisions, which meet at the coccyx. · The included flap is dissected from behind forward, the posterior fourth of the sphincter being removed at the same time, care being taken not to injure the rectal wall. The second step consists in the insertion of four sutures of silkworm-gut, introduced transversely with a curved needle into the posterior wall of the rectum, without injuring the mucous membrane. When the sutures are drawn towards the sacrum, it will be seen that the cavity of the rectum is made decidedly narrower and that the posterior wall is fixed to a certain extent. To make this result permanent, a needle is introduced through the skin near the sacro-coccygeal articulation, about an inch from the median line, and is brought out in the ano-coccygeal wound. The corresponding end of the upper suture is then passed through the needle's eye and is drawn out by withdrawing the needle, which is then introduced at a corresponding point at the opposite side, and the other end is secured. The other sutures are treated in the same way, being tightly drawn and tied one after the other. The third step consists in excision of the cutaneous flap which has been dissected and is adherent by its base. A few sutures are inserted in the vicinity of, and a little higher than, the anus. This operation affects only a limited portion of the rectum either in length or in height.

*Roberts's Operation.*—Roberts recommends the following plan of procedure. The patient is placed in the lithotomy position, and the protruded rectum is reduced. An incision is made in the median line of the perineum, near the coccyx, large enough to admit the point of the finger, and the cellular connections posterior to the rectum are separated. By introducing the knife into the anus a triangular portion of the tissue, consisting of skin,

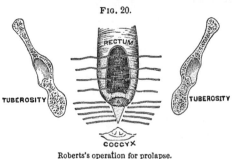

FIG. 20.

Roberts's operation for prolapse.

cellular tissue, and an inch of the sphincter muscle, is incised; the base of the triangle is at the margin of the anus. With scissors a long triangular section is cut out of the posterior wall of the rectum, the apex of which is about three inches up the gut, while its base corresponds with the inch of excised sphincter previously described. (Fig. 20.) Hemorrhage is controlled with catgut ligatures, and the rectal wound is closed with chromicized catgut sutures, which are all tied from the rectal side. The operation renders the lower end of the bowel funnel-shaped, with the small end of the funnel towards the anus.

## STRICTURE OF THE RECTUM.

Stricture of the rectum is a narrowing or stenosis of the canal, which may result from a variety of conditions. One of the most important is cancer, but this form of stricture we shall consider under that heading. The pathology of non-malignant stricture of the rectum is somewhat obscure. While some assert that it is due to syphilis only, there is no question whatever that chronic diarrhœa and dysentery may give rise to inflammation and ulceration of the mucous membrane, which subsequently results in thickening of the submucous tissue and stenosis of the canal. Tuberculous disease is also a not infrequent cause. With tuberculous ulceration there is a tendency after a time to healing of the ulcerated surface, which results in contraction. This may continue until a large extent of the intestine is involved and the stenosis is very marked. The tissue contracts, the bowel above becomes dilated, ulceration takes place around the margin of the stricture, and this subsequently contracts, thus giving increased length to the stricture. In addition to the causes mentioned, stricture may result from the introduction of irritating substances, the presence of foreign bodies, and syphilis. Syphilitic stricture is usually annular in form, is situated at the lower part of the canal, and is quite firm.

*Symptoms.*—The patient complains of distress and great difficulty in evacuating the bowels; she cannot defecate unless the contents are in a fluid condition. She has a sensation of weight and pressure in the pelvis. Fæcal movements, when formed, are thin and ribbon-shaped, and are expelled with marked difficulty; later only fluid can pass the bowel. Strictures are readily recognized by the rectal touch. Situated, as they usually are, at the lowest part of the bowel, they are generally within reach, and there is no difficulty in arriving at an accurate knowledge of the condition.

*Treatment.*—It has long been the rule to treat rectal strictures by divulsion with large bougies. The objection to this, however, is that the use of these instruments only aggravates the stricture by causing an increase of the cicatricial tissue. The bougies must be frequently used, or the patient will suffer a return of the trouble. In an annular stricture the better plan of procedure would seem to be either to incise it posteriorly and then to sew the divided edges together from above downward, which would considerably increase the calibre of the gut, or to cut out a ring involving the diseased tissue and to suture the divided ends of the gut. The entire ring may be excised and the ends of the gut brought in apposition by sutures. The only objection to this procedure is the difficulty with which it is accomplished from within the rectum. If the stricture becomes very tight, and the patient suffers marked inconvenience, we must consider the advisability of forming an artificial anus. It seems to the writer preferable in all such cases to precede the operation by sacral resection, and, after removing the diseased tissue, to make the artificial anus at the end of the resected bone. The advantages that may be claimed for this procedure over inguinal or lumbar colotomy are—1, the patient is enabled to have an evacuation of the bowels without being obliged to assume an unnatural position, and with much less disarrangement of her apparel; 2, she is better able to protect her clothing and person from being soiled with fæcal matter; 3, the situation of the artificial anus near the bone renders it much less likely to undergo cicatricial contraction than when it is situated in the loin. When there is a suspicion of syphilis, the local should be supplemented by anti-syphilitic treatment.

### CANCER OF THE RECTUM.

The usual seat of cancer is at the inferior extremity of the rectum, unless it is secondary to cancer of the uterus, when it is situated higher up. Cancer of the rectum varies greatly in appearance. It may occupy the lateral wall, having an annular form, or it may appear as small disseminated nodules. The recto-vaginal septum is often invaded. When the disease is far advanced it may result in the formation of a recto-vaginal fistula. The exuberant variety has a cauliflower appearance, a soft consistence, and bleeds at the slightest touch. When a great number of these vegetations unite they form actual tumors. The ulcerative form is often met with, especially when the cancer occupies the anal region. The ulcer rests upon an infiltrated base sharply circumscribed. It is not unusual to find at its edges outgrowths similar to those which have been mentioned. As it progresses, rectal cancer results in constriction of the gut, which may be complete. The resulting complications are similar to those referred to in the description of simple stricture; there may be abscesses or fistulæ even more frequently than in the purely cicatricial form.

*Symptoms.*—The onset of cancer is insidious, but it is easily recognized by the general condition of the patient, which is visibly affected. Obscure digestive troubles develop, and repugnance to certain foods, especially meat. The patient complains of constipation, alternating with diarrhœa, and the stools often present the appearance of soot or coffee-grounds. If we do not examine the rectum, we may suspect cancer of the stomach, but later phenomena appear which draw the attention of the patient to the site of the trouble. She has a sensation of weight, burning pain, and tenesmus; defecation becomes painful, and is accompanied with more or less loss of blood and mucus. As the neoplasm extends, the symptoms enumerated in the description of stricture are present. Stercoræmia may exist, to which is added the absorption of septic products, due to breaking down of the growth. Intestinal obstruction seems imminent, and there is a constant burning pain which radiates through the pelvis, so that the patient finds it impossible to sit or lie, and her existence is rendered miserable.

*Diagnosis.*—The diagnosis of rectal cancer presents but few difficulties. The finger recognizes the annular disposition of the growth, the cauliflower vegetations, induration, and other phenomena indicating the character of the disease. On withdrawal, the finger will be found to be covered with blood and epithelial débris, and the examiner will be aware of the extremely fetid odor of the discharge. It is important to note the form, extent, and variety of cancer, and at the same time to make a complete examination of the vulva, vagina, cervix uteri, and cul-de-sac of Douglas. In making a differential diagnosis, it is always well to bear in mind the different tumors which develop at the level of the rectum or in its vicinity. Polypi are smooth and pedunculated, and are implanted upon the unaltered mucous surface. A cicatricial stricture is regular, more circumscribed, and never presents the extensive induration and large vegetations so frequent in epithelioma. In some cases it is difficult to distinguish scirrhous from fibrous strictures, and it is only from the progress of the case that one can decide the diagnosis. Hemorrhoids cannot be readily confounded with epithelioma ; they are small capillary tumors, smooth, rounded, circumscribed, and even when they are the seat of ulceration, the ulcerations are small.

*Prognosis.*—The prognosis is always extremely grave, and the relief, even after the most radical treatment, is generally only temporary.

*Treatment.*—The treatment varies according to the indications. If the disease is rapid, the general state bad, and there are signs of metastasis, it

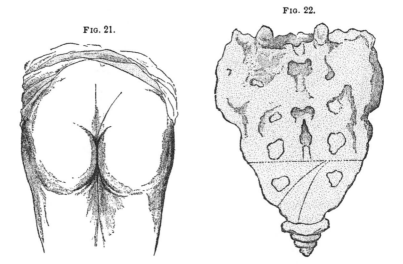

Fig. 21.

Fig. 22.

is better to avoid operation. All that we can do is to relieve the pain with suppositories or injections of morphine, and to overcome constipation with laxatives. The diet should be carefully regulated, being confined to such food as furnishes the largest amount of nourishment with the least amount of solid residue. The palliative procedure, dilatation by bougies, should be rejected. Proctotomy consists in making a posterior median section comprising all the soft parts from the anus to the coccyx. This operation is done for the purpose of facilitating the evacuation of the bowels and saving

the patient from obstruction.  The indications for it, however, are exceptional.  The creation of an artificial anus is the most effective method of
treating the obstruction in some cases.  This should be made in the left iliac
region in those cases in which the disease involves the greater part of the rectum.  When it is limited to the anus or the lower five inches of the rectum,
extirpation should be performed.  This is best done by the sacral method.
The patient is placed upon her left side, and a crescentic incision is made
over the sacrum (Fig. 21), beginning at the right side of the sacro-iliac synchondrosis, the knife being carried across the median line to the left side,
ending to the left of the anus ; the skin and superficial fascia are drawn aside
and the coccyx and sacrum are exposed ; the muscular attachments are dissected from the sacrum and the coccyx is removed.  Then, with bone forceps
or with a chain saw, two lower segments of the sacrum are exsected, the precaution being taken not to extend the resection above the third sacral foramen.  (Fig. 22.)  Bleeding is arrested, and the rectum is then drawn aside

FIG. 23.                                    FIG. 24.

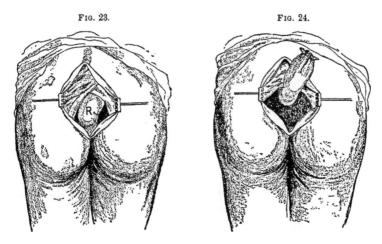

and is dissected completely away.  (Fig. 23.)  If the vagina is already involved, a portion of the vaginal wall may be removed with the rectum.  The
entire gut should be encircled, separated, drawn down, and, if the disease
has extended high up, the gut may be removed within the peritoneal cavity.
(Fig. 24.)  This is performed by opening the peritoneum, detaching its
reflection from the bowel, drawing the latter well down so as to cut beyond
the disease, and stitching the parietal to the visceral peritoneum : we then
proceed to amputate the diseased tissue.  In this way we make sure that
the peritoneal cavity will not be infected by the escape of fæcal matter.
The edges of the divided intestine are then sutured to the skin over the
sacrum, so that a new anus is formed just beneath this bone.  The writer
has performed five sacral resections, with one death.  In the last case in
which it was necessary to perform this operation—in a young woman

FIG. 25.

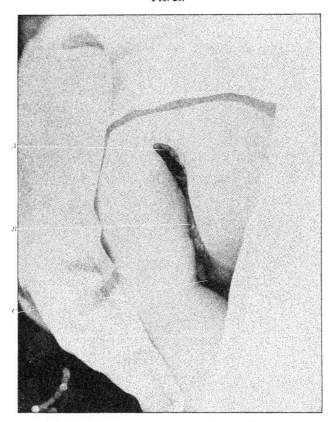

Sacral resection, with removal of a portion of the rectum, the uterus and appendages, and the posterior wall of the vagina and the perineum.—*A*, artificial anus; *B*, anterior wall of vagina; *C*. vulva.

twenty-three years of age—the disease had already involved the vagina and the margin of the perineum, and extended upward along the vagina as high as the cervix uteri. Inguinal colotomy had been done some four months previously. The sacrum was resected; five inches of the bowel, the whole of the posterior wall of the vagina, the perineum, the uterus, ovaries, and tubes, were removed; the intestine was sutured to the anterior wall of the vagina and posteriorly to the skin over the sacrum; the skin of the buttocks was sutured to the edge of the anterior wall of the vagina. After the patient had recovered, the opening in the colon was closed, so that all evacuations now take place through the opening in the bowel at the upper part of the vagina. Fig. 25 shows the extent of the wound.

# CHAPTER XVIII.

## DISEASES OF THE FEMALE BREAST.

BY DUDLEY P. ALLEN, M.D.

THE female breast varies largely in its anatomical, histological, and physiological condition, according to the time of life and the functions which it performs.

Before puberty the breast of the girl differs very little from that of the boy. With the advent of puberty the former enlarges and becomes more prominent. Often from the age of twenty-five to thirty there is a decrease in the size of the female breast, due to a decrease in adipose tissue consequent to a corresponding decrease in the weight of the person, which is not infrequent at that age. During pregnancy and lactation the breast increases largely in size, but after the cessation of lactation it decreases, becoming smaller and more relaxed, as a rule, than before pregnancy. After the menopause the breast atrophies, and is much relaxed. Occasionally the decrease accompanying the cessation of lactation and the menopause may be compensated for by the increase of adipose tissue, so that the contour of the breast is preserved.

In the new-born, according to Orth,[1] there are from ten to fifteen milk-ducts, ending in club-shaped enlargements, and lined with cylindrical epithelium. With puberty multiple buds or diverticuli appear, and the gland takes on an acinous character. These gland-formations push themselves outward into the surrounding fat, being enveloped by hyaline connective tissue.

During pregnancy new acini are developed, each containing a distinct lumen. The membrana propria surrounds the acini and connecting ducts, and is formed of flattened cells. Around this is a connective tissue rich in vessels. In pregnancy the acini increase in number and size and are crowded closely together; they terminate in twelve to fifteen ducts with spindle-shaped enlargements, and end in the nipple, which is surrounded by unstriped muscular fibre. With the end of secretion the glandular elements decrease, though they do not disappear, but the connective tissue increases. After the menopause the glandular portions decrease, the acini disappear, but the ducts remain, being similar to those in the new-born.

---

[1] Lehrb. der Speciel. Path. Anat., 1893.

These ducts may become dilated and pour out a green or brown secretion.

According to Sappey, the breast is very rich in lymph-vessels. They surround the acini and milk-ducts, converging towards the centre of the gland. About the areola there is an abundant convolution of lymph-vessels, and these together enter several large lymph-channels which converge towards the axilla.

Heidenhain suggests that this concentric arrangement of the lymph-vessels may account for the fact that the location of a tumor does not seem to influence the time at which the axillary glands become enlarged. Orth says that the deep lymph-vessels go to the fascia of the pectoralis major and spread themselves out upon it, terminating in the axillary glands, and a small portion of them penetrate the chest-wall near the sternum. Heidenhain says, "So far as I can see, the lymph-vessels of the pectoralis fascia are not connected with those of the muscle itself." Ludwig and Schweigger-Seidel say that the injection of the lymph-channels is easy in the direction away from muscles and tendons, but difficult towards them.

Heidenhain says that, though infection of the muscle is hard to trace, it must come, when it does occur, through the lymph-channels, and he cites one case in which he found an infected lymph-gland close to the sternum, and a second in which he found a gland infected with carcinoma lying upon the pectoralis major.

The breast receives its blood-supply chiefly from the internal mammary and long thoracic arteries. Some branches may come from the intercostal artery.

The nerve-supply is principally from the intercostal nerves, between the fourth and the sixth.

The physiological function of the female breast is the secretion of milk. This may be carried on normally, beginning with the secretion of colostrum sometimes a little before, and at any rate shortly following, parturition. It is followed by the secretion of milk, which continues for a varying length of time. Owing, doubtless, to changes resulting largely from civilization, the amount of milk secreted varies widely in different cases.

### ANOMALIES OF THE BREAST.

Anomalies of the breast may be of different sorts, resulting from retarded development or from increased development. There are also anomalies of function. According to Leichtenstern, increase in the number of nipples, with or without a corresponding increase in the number of breasts, occurs with about equal frequency in both sexes, probably, however, a little oftener among men than among women. In ninety-one per cent. of all cases this increase is upon the anterior wall of the thorax. Cases occurring in the axilla, on the back, over the acromion, and on the thigh, are rare. In ninety-four per cent. of all cases they occur below the normal breast, and usually towards the median line. He observed thirty-four accessory nipples on the left and sixteen on the right side. There was no evidence of heredity. The accessory breast may secrete milk. Orth says that the development of accessory breasts or nipples brings out the question of atavism.

Delbet[1] cites a case in which there were four breasts, from all of which the patient could nurse equally well.

Bland Sutton, as does Orth, suggests that supernumerary breasts and nipples on the anterior part of the thorax correspond to analogous conditions in the lower animals, their location depending on the fact that they receive their blood-supply from the internal mammary and epigastric arteries.

Blanchard and Delbet suggest that all those occurring away from the line of the epigastric and mammary arteries should be regarded as anomalies, produced by the epiblast. Martin[2] says that the irregular location of supernumerary nipples is due to the fact that the milk-line is located in the embryo upon the back, and as it is gradually pushed forward upon the sides and front, irregularities in the arrangement of the nipples may occur, and he thus accounts for their presence on the thigh and over the acromion.

**Microthelia.**—Microthelia is a term applied to conditions in which the nipple is small or sunken. In the case of sunken nipples Kehrer has suggested that an elliptical piece may be removed from the integument above and below the nipple, and that by drawing together the openings thus made in the integument the nipple will be lifted up and made sufficiently prominent.

The nipple may, however, become invaginated, turning inward like the finger of a glove, so that no operation can benefit it.

**Athelia.**—Athelia, or absence of the nipple, according to Williams,[3] is more common than absence of the breast. The breast may be normal in other respects. Microthelia and athelia (Birkett) are common sources of inflammation. In ninety-seven cases of acute mammary abscess Birkett found imperfect development in forty-eight. According to the same author, absence of the nipple is not infrequently ascribable to traumatism occurring in the newly-born.

**Polythelia.**—In polythelia the supernumerary nipples follow a line from the normal nipple downward and inward, or upward and outward. This, according to Wiedersheim, would correspond to the milk-line to be discovered in the embryo of pigs.

Bruce[4] among 207 men found 9.11 per cent. of supernumerary nipples; among 104 women, 4.8 per cent. Ammon[5] among 2189 men found either

---

[1] Duplay et Reclus, vol. vi.

[2] Archiv f. Klin. Chirurg., Band xlv. Heft 4, p 883.

[3] Journal of Anatomy and Physiology, London, 1890 and 1891, p. 304.

[4] Ibid., 1879, p. 425.

[5] Wiedersheim, Bau des Menschen, 1893, p. 17.

distinct nipples or indications of them in 114 cases, or in one out of every nineteen. Bardeleben[1] found among 2430 men 76 cases of multiple nipples on the left side, 44 on the right side, and 31 on both sides,—in all 151 cases, or 6.21 per cent. All supernumerary nipples were below the normal breast. In six or eight cases there were from three to four nipples on one side.

Fig. 1.

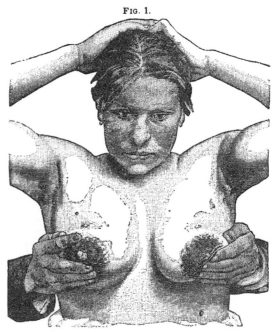

Polÿthelia, showing ten nipples. (F. L. Neugebauer, Warsaw.)

**Micromazia.**—Micromazia, or small breast, is a more frequent defect than absence of the breast. Williams says it may affect one or both breasts, and may or may not be accompanied by malformation of the chest-wall, muscles, or genital organs. According to Orth, it is more common on the right than on the left side.

Delbet (*op. cit.*) says that breasts may remain seemingly normal until puberty, and then fail to develop on one or on both sides. Puech is cited by Delbet as suggesting that small breasts may be associated with an infantile uterus. Cases of this sort are recorded by Virchow, Négreer, and Rokitansky.

**Amazia.**—Delbet says that absence of one breast is extremely rare, and has been observed only in women. It is accompanied at times by

---

[1] Bardeleben, Verhandl. Anat. Gesell., München, 1891, p. 249.

deficiencies of the corresponding arm and pectoral muscles, and in one case there was absence of the corresponding ovary. Williams (*op. cit.*) affirms that amazia is one of the rarest of deformities, and, although commonly accompanied by other defects, may occur in subjects otherwise entirely normal. Orth (*op. cit.*) says that amazia of both sides occurs only in monsters. When single, it is more common on the right than on the left side. Delbet says that amazia on both sides occurs only in monsters, and usually in those having other deformities which render them incapable of existence.

Polymazia.—Polymazia, or multiple breasts, is of more frequent occurrence than some of the other anomalies. They may vary from small

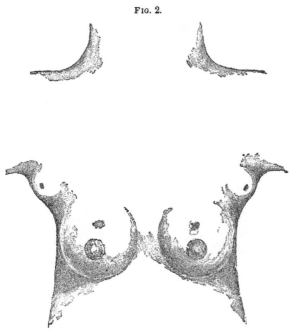

Fig. 2.

Polymazia. Accessory nipples on each breast, and accessory breasts at border of each axilla. (Illustration from Dr. T. Kuroiwa, of Tokyo, Japan.)

nodules to breasts sufficiently developed to suckle infants. Hansemann collected two hundred and sixty-two cases; of these, eighty-one were men, one hundred and four were women, and in seventy-seven cases the sex was not given. Delbet (*op. cit.*) cites Leichtenstern as having found among seventy-two women with multiple breasts only three who bore twins.

Among the interesting cases of polymazia were those of the mother of the Emperor Severus, who was named Julia Mammæ on this account, and Anne Boleyn. A very perfect instance of this condition is cited by Kuroiwa in a medical journal published in Tokyo. The case presented, in addition to the normal breasts, two nipples four centimetres above each breast. On

FIG. 3.

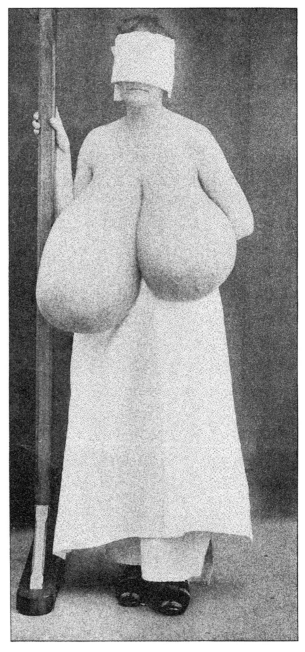

HVpertrophy of the breasts.

the border of each axilla were two small mammary glands with well-formed nipples.

Baraban[1] says that enlargements found on the border of the pectoralis major, as distinguished from those within the axilla, when connected with tumors of the breast, should arouse the suspicion of their being secondary portions of the mammary gland rather than infected lymphatic glands. In connection with lactation the accessory glands may become enlarged, and, as has been said, secrete milk in considerable quantities, although this is by no means universal. An aid to their diagnosis is the fact that in connection with lactation and sometimes with menstruation these accessory nodules become enlarged, as does the normal breast, and at times painful. The importance of recognizing them is that they may be distinguished from what might otherwise be taken to be malignant growths.

Martin holds that portions of breast-tissue in the axilla, without excretory ducts, should be looked upon not as accessory breasts, but as portions of the breast which have become detached in the process of development. He differs from Williams and Bardeleben in holding that these are rarely the seats of malignant growths.

**Hypertrophy.**—Hypertrophy of the breast is a comparatively rare condition. It is usually described as occurring at two periods: first, at the age of puberty; second, in connection with pregnancy. A considerable number of cases are reported as occurring at both these periods. Crawford cites a case of acute hypertrophy in both mammæ in a girl of the age of fifteen. Both were amputated, the second at an interval of sixteen days after the first, the first weighing thirteen pounds and the second weighing eleven and one-half pounds. Delbet (*op. cit.*) has collected twenty-seven cases of hypertrophy of the breast, of which twenty-five appeared before the age of twenty and eleven between the ages of fourteen and fifteen. He considers hypertrophy the result of a simple increase of physiological processes.

Porter[2] reports an interesting case of hypertrophy of both breasts in a woman thirty-seven years of age, whose history is somewhat peculiar, inasmuch as the woman had borne two children, the youngest being ten years old. Three years previous to her entrance to the hospital she had noticed a hard lump in the right breast, which had gradually increased in size and with it the whole breast. Three months later the left breast became similarly affected. At the end of six months the right breast was the size of a baby's head and the left a little smaller. From this time on the growth was gradual until three months before entering the hospital, when the growth became very rapid. Both breasts were removed, with an interval of three weeks between the operations. The weight of the tumors was not given, but they were very large.

---

[1] Revue Médicale de l'Est, 1890, p. 252.
[2] Transactions of the American Surgical Association, 1891.

According to Delbet, in cases occurring at puberty the growth is usually so rapid that in from two to three months the volume becomes considerable. Sometimes it is slower, requiring from one to two years. Of the cases occurring at puberty, Monteils reports one as resulting in recovery.

Orth says that diffused hypertrophy usually begins with the first menstruation, and that the breasts grow rapidly during two to four months. Growth then ceases. He says they are apt to increase again at pregnancy. This is due to the development of the gland structures, since hypertrophied breasts—as, in fact, all maiden breasts—are largely made up of connective tissue. The differential diagnosis between hypertrophy and adenoma may be difficult. Symmetrical enlargement would indicate hypertrophy, while irregular enlargement would indicate adenoma. Histologically, the fact of the acini being lined with cylindrical epithelium would indicate them to be adenoma.

Billroth[1] says that diffuse hypertrophy usually begins with puberty. The breasts grow rapidly for a time, and then growth ceases. They may increase again during pregnancy, but they do not grow to an unlimited degree. As they enlarge, the skin covering them becomes stretched, the nipple flattened, and the patient greatly burdened by the weight.

Delbet says that hypertrophy is the result of augmentation of the gland-tissue, and not of the fat or fibrous tissue. The condition of the gland varies in size according to whether it is observed during pregnancy, lactation, or at some other period. Hypertrophy does not prevent secretion of milk. Billroth (*op. cit.*) cites a case of abortion at the fifth month, the hypertrophied breasts being engorged with milk. Lotzbeck mentions a case of hypertrophy of one breast where there was enormous secretion of milk in the second pregnancy. The case had become hypertrophied at the time of puberty. Delbet says that during gestation and lactation the glandular tissues predominate; at other times, fibrous tissue is most abundant. Various modifications may occur, however, in hypertrophied breasts. Large numbers of fibrous nodules may occur, and cysts may be present. The former may give the aspect of a uterus filled with fibromata, or the latter may break open and suppurate. The prognosis of hypertrophy at the time of puberty is grave, since it weighs down the patient and requires amputation. If this is not performed the patient may become feeble and emaciated and die of intercurrent affections, suppuration, or even gangrene. Billroth (*op. cit.*) says of diffused hypertrophy that the patient is usually worn down by the growth, though she may live a long time. He cites a case of Gräb's where the patient lived eighteen years. Death usually comes from ulceration and intercurrent affections. Treatment by compression and iodide of potassium is of slight value. Amputation is the only cure.

Tarnier and Boudin say that in cases of hypertrophy confinement is

---

[1] Billroth, Deutsch. Chirurg., p. 74.

usually premature or the offspring is small and feeble. Thus it would seem that in the hypertrophy which occurs at puberty the growth is rapid, that recoveries are few,—the tendency of the disease being to wear out the patient,—and that amputation is the only rational treatment. In the hypertrophy of pregnancy the prognosis is much better, since in a considerable proportion of cases the breast again decreases markedly in size. In a case of hypertrophy accompanying pregnancy, affecting one breast, which came under my own observation, within a few months after confinement the breast decreased largely in size, although it did not become reduced entirely to the size of the other breast.

In the hypertrophy of pregnancy the large breast should be supported by a bandage, in the hope that it may later decrease in size. In the hypertrophy of puberty amputation is the only treatment that is of benefit. Hey cites a case of hypertrophy of both breasts, in which, after the amputation of one, the other diminished in size. Usually, however, both breasts must be amputated.

**Agalactia.**—The complete absence of milk after parturition is of rare occurrence. Often, however, the quantity secreted is very little. This seemingly is the result of artificial habits of living accompanying civilization; its occurrence has not been correspondingly observed among primitive races.

A rare case of agalactia is reported by Harlan, of a woman who bore thirteen children without secreting any milk. Her mother bore twenty-five children without secreting any milk.

**Galactorrhœa.**—Galactorrhœa may occur, and cases have been reported where as much as seven litres has been secreted per day. An abundant flow of milk may continue a long time, even for several years. In rare instances milk is found to have been secreted before puberty, and a case is recorded of a little girl in whom the secretion of milk was stimulated by the placing of a baby to her breast. Billroth cites the case of a girl of eight years who thus secreted milk, and also one of a woman fifty-nine years of age who had not borne a child for seventeen years. He says he had never himself seen a case. In connection with this it may be of interest to mention the case of a woman who told me that with each pregnancy she was able to collect in her mouth, by suction, presumably from her parotid glands, a fluid which resembled milk, and that her sister had the same ability. Unfortunately, I had no opportunity of examining the material secreted.

### ECZEMA.[1]

Eczema is of frequent occurrence in the breast. Although it may attack any part, it is most common beneath large and pendulous breasts which hang down and lie upon the chest-wall, and thus, by the retention of secretions and collection of moisture, create irritation of the skin. Its

---

[1] *Vide* chapter on Cutaneous Diseases.

treatment is similar to that of eczema elsewhere, and it is especially important that the surfaces should be kept apart and the irritation thus prevented.

### MOLLUSCUM.

Pendulous tumors may arise from the areola surrounding the nipple, but are of slight importance. There may also be irritation in and suppuration of the glands of Montgomery surrounding the nipple.

### SEBACEOUS CYSTS.

Sebaceous cysts may occur in the breasts. Cahen cites a case of atheroma having its seat over the sternum. Porta says that of three hundred and eighty-four sebaceous tumors three were found in the deep cellular tissue of the gland of the breast. In a case operated on by my assistant, Dr. Nevison, a small sebaceous tumor was found forcing its way down into the tissue of the gland. The tumors are similar to those found elsewhere.

### DERMOID CYSTS.

Dermoid cysts are very rare. Hermann reports a case of dermoid cyst filled with sebaceous material, discovered post mortem, with a distinct cyst-wall which was easily separated from the surrounding tissue. Klebs[1] says that dermoid cysts containing butter-like masses occur rarely in the neighborhood of the breasts. He cites Gussenbauer as saying that several dermoid cysts which he observed in the mammæ were subcutaneous, and, as they enlarged, had pushed their way into the gland rather than developed in the gland itself. The treatment of dermoid cysts in the breast is by enucleation.

### INJURIES OF THE BREAST.

Contusions of the breast follow much the same course as those occurring elsewhere, though in the case of nervous women they may be the seat of much pain subsequently. At times they are followed by ecchymoses which have been supposed to develop into fibroma. Their treatment consists in compressing the breast and sustaining it by a bandage. Contusions may also give rise to mastitis, and when occurring at birth may produce mastitis neonatorum. They rarely give rise to abscess.

Delbet says of wounds of the breast that they are peculiar only during lactation, at which time it may be necessary to stop nursing in order to heal them. Burns attacking the nipple are serious, since they may so damage the milk-ducts as to destroy them. Wounds may produce serious inflammation as a result of the laying open of the complicated structure of the gland-tissue, a tissue which is not favorable to healing.

Spontaneous ecchymoses may occur, and when they do it is usually at the menstrual period. This hemorrhage is generally subcutaneous, but

---

[1] Klebs, Handbuch der Path. Anat , vol. i. p. 99.

rarely is interstitial, and still more rarely may extend into the lumen of the glandular tissue. It may be vicarious in dysmenorrhœa and amenorrhœa. The hemorrhage is, however, usually absorbed. Rokitansky has suggested that these hemorrhages, which may also result from trauma, may be the origin of connective-tissue tumors.

### NEURALGIA AND NEUROMATA.

Billroth (*op. cit.*) says of neuralgia that—first, it may be connected with tumors and be cured by their removal; secondly, it may be a pure neuralgia without tumors, and not benefited by operation; thirdly, it may have its origin in intercostal neuralgia.

Neuralgia may occur with or without tumors, but it usually occurs with tumors that are benign. It may occur in connection with a series of nodules, only one of which is the seat of pain. It may be accompanied by congestion of the breast; but some cases show no appreciable alteration. The pain in these cases may be extreme. When several nodules are present, an excision of a portion of the nodules is of no service, since pain usually follows in others. Compression in connection with soothing applications is of value. Electricity has been suggested as a means of treatment.

Neuromata are said to be almost universally fibromata. Fowler[1] cites seven cases of tumor of the breast occurring in neurotic women, associated with tenderness and irritability of the uterus and ovaries. Massage of the uterus in a portion of the cases, and marriage in others, caused complete disappearance of the tumors. The tumors had the appearance of malignancy, and removal had previously been advised.

Orth says that there may occur in the breasts of hysterical women enlargements varying from a small size to that of an egg, and appearing in all respects like tumors, while they are simply the result of hyperæmia and œdema of nervous origin. A case has recently come under my own observation of a woman, aged forty, with a tumor which reappears from time to time, being painful when present. So far as the patient can observe, it is influenced chiefly by the weather, returning and being painful in stormy weather and disappearing when the weather again becomes clear.

### HYDATIDS OF THE BREAST.

Echinococci are said by Orth (*op. cit.*) to be rare, and cysticerci rarer still. Boecher says that among four thousand seven hundred and seventy cases treated during ten years in the Charité, Berlin, there were thirty-three cases of echinococci. Of these, fourteen were among women. None of them, however, occurred in the breast. Von Bergmann cites one hundred and two cases of echinococci of the surface of the body, fifteen of which occurred in the breast. Birkett, Henry, Le Dentu, and Von Bergmann report cases varying in size from that of a hen's egg to that of a fist. Bill-

---

[1] New York Medical Record, February 15, 1890, p. 179.

roth says there is usually only one mother-cyst, daughter-cysts being rare. They are, as a rule, sterile, and the hooklets are often absent. They appear like other cysts, are painless, and do not have fremitus, which can often be felt in cysts located elsewhere. They are characterized by the fact that the fluid contains no albumen, unless it be the result of inflammation occurring after the death of the parasite. Billroth advises extirpation.

Dubreuil reports a case of a woman, forty-four years of age, who had a tumor in the upper part of the breast during two years, which was at first movable and painless. Becoming painful and increasing in size, it was removed and found to be a suppúrating hydatid cyst. Hydatids, as a rule, are at first small, being of the size of a hickory-nut. They increase slowly to the size of an egg or a small apple, the growth requiring one or perhaps several years. They are usually hard, non-fluctuating, and commonly free from pain. It is difficult to distinguish them from other cysts, and this can be done only by puncture. Dubreuil recommends in place of ablation a wedge-shaped excision of the portion of the breast containing the cyst.

### MASTITIS.

Inflammatory processes in the breast may be superficial, attacking the nipple and the areola with the integument, or may involve the gland itself, or may be situated behind the gland, lifting the gland from the thoracic wall. Mastitis may also occur, involving the entire tissues of the breast.

Inflammation of the skin has already been spoken of under the head of eczema, as well as abscesses of the glands of Montgomery. Erysipelas and phlegmonous abscesses may occur, resulting in antemammary abscesses. Retromammary abscesses are more common from caries of the rib or pleurisy, and may lift the breast so that it floats upon the thoracic wall. In one of my own cases in which the pleural cavity was full of pus, perforation took place between the third and fourth ribs underneath the left breast, lifting it entirely from the wall of the thorax.

Billroth (*op. cit.*) says that mastitis may occur in new-born children, at puberty, and during pregnancy, but that all these conditions are rare. Delbet says of the mastitis of puberty that it is usually slight and disappears of itself. Mastitis in general is most common in primiparæ, blondes, and lymphatic subjects. Delbet remarks that mastitis is much more common among primiparæ than among multiparæ, and is rare after the fourth pregnancy. Koehler found evidences of inflammation in 55.87 per cent. and Deiss in 50.84 per cent. of cases examined among primiparæ. These statistics refer chiefly to cracks and fissures. The cessation of lactation seems to increase the frequency of mastitis; but it is to be remembered that this cessation may be the result rather than the cause of inflammation. Koehler, already cited, considered the first two weeks as the most common time for mastitis, whereas Bryant, Bumm, and Winckel state that it is most common in the third and fourth weeks. Statistics differ as to whether it is the right or the left breast which is the more frequently attacked.

Delbet cites one hundred and fifty cases of mastitis collected by Martin, all but eight or ten of which occurred during lactation ; of fifty by Winckel, all but one occurred during lactation. Koehler, in his Thèse de Bâle, arrived at about the same result. Deiss, in 1889, reports sixteen hundred confinements from the Heidelberg clinic, with 3.6 per cent. of cases of mastitis.

Winckel,[1] in 1869, noted among one hundred and fifty women seventy-two cases in which there were fissures of the nipple; they were about as frequent among multiparæ as among primiparæ.

Pingat gives an account of fifty-three abscesses of the breast,—nineteen during the first month of lactation, fourteen during the second, three during the third, and seventeen during the tenth month. He also cites the statistics of Dr. Barr, from L'Hôpital Saint-Louis, from 1889 to 1891, showing among 1503 nursing women twenty-nine cases of lymphangitis and two of abscess. From Tarnier's ward, during the years 1888 and 1889, among 1235 confinements there were twenty cases of lymphangitis, sixty-three of fissure or engorgements, and four of abscess or galactophoritis. From 1890 to 1891, among 1727 confinements there were fifty-four fissures, fourteen eruptions from bichloride, and three abscesses. In the latter series bichloride was employed in place of boric acid, used in the former series.

The cause and method of infection in mastitis are questions full of interest and involved in much discussion. The opinion used to be strongly held by such eminent authorities as Velpeau, Chassaignac, and others of their time, that infection resulted from engorgement of milk, either from over-secretion, narrowness of the milk-ducts, or insufficient suction.

Orth says that there is no doubt that mastitis results from pathogenic germs, the chief of these being the staphylococcus and streptococcus. Delbet takes the position that mastitis may have its origin through both the milk-ducts and the lymphatics, holding that the milk-ducts are the more common channel, since in the beginning both pus and milk can be pressed from the nipple. He asserts that infection may be lobular without the axillary glands becoming involved. Engorgement alone will not produce mastitis. This is shown by stopping the milk-ducts experimentally with collodion, as has been done by Kehrer, and by ligature of the ducts, as performed in dogs by Delbet. Another evidence that engorgement does not produce abscess is cited by Pingat,[2] in the fact that supernumerary breasts remaining after enucleation of the normal breasts become engorged in subsequent pregnancies, but never give rise to abscess. Pingat further says of the two theories held concerning the entrance of infection, that whereas it may enter through cracks or excoriations along the lymph-channels, in the absence of these (although favored by their presence) the microbes may follow up the milk-ducts to the acini, where they may multiply and finally find their

---

[1] Die Path. und Therap. des Wochenbett, 1869.

[2] Pingat, Thesis on Abscess of the Breast, Paris, 1891.

way into the cellular tissue. This theory is strengthened by the fact that mammary abscesses occur in cases where neither fissure nor ulcer can be discovered.

Speaking of germs, Orth says that they may enter by the milk-ducts (as occurs in infection of the parotid gland), by the lymph-channels, or by the blood-vessels. He says that while it is unquestionably true that infection may enter through fissures in the nipple, it is probable that different germs follow different channels, streptococci entering by the lymph-channels and staphylococci by the milk-ducts. It is no more remarkable that the germs should travel against the milk-stream than it is that they should travel from the bladder to the kidney. He states that staphylococci are found in the milk-ducts of healthy women, and that although retention is not a cause of mastitis, when present it is a condition favoring the multiplication of germs.

Various investigations have been undertaken in order to determine whether bacteria may exist in normal milk. This is rendered probable by the well-known fact that micro-organisms enter the blood in connection with tubercle, typhoid fever, rabies, etc. Escherich made bacteriological and culture examinations of nine normal cases, in all of which he found the milk to be sterile. He examined five cases with fissures or excoriations, accompanied, however, with other slight inflammation of the gland, and healing rapidly under treatment. In four of these he found staphylococci. He believes that the infection commonly takes place through the milk-channels, and says that staphylococci entering the blood through the infection of the genital apparatus may be excreted through the milk as well as through the urine.

Orth says that the staphylococcus albus may gain entrance into the outer milk-ducts and thus be found in the first milk secreted. Pathogenic germs, he says, may unquestionably be secreted with the milk of septic women, but it is still uncertain how deleterious they are to the infant.

Palleski examined twenty-two healthy nursing women and found the staphylococcus albus in ten cases, although every precaution was taken against error. The presence of germs was not dependent upon the length of lactation or the time elapsing after nursing. He says that in the milk of perfectly healthy women perhaps half of the cases contain micro-organisms belonging to the cocci, and he believes them to be the staphylococcus pyogenes albus. He is uncertain whether they gain entrance from the blood or from the external air. He is sure, however, that the staphylococci may be present in milk in considerable quantities without any appearance of mastitis or general disease.

Karlinski[1] states that micro-organisms from the interior of the uterus in the process of involution can be found in the blood; that offspring among animals suckled by infected mothers die in a large percentage of

---

[1] Prager Medicinische Wochenschrift, 1890, p. 279.

cases; and that, as the infection of the mother does not occur until after parturition, the infection of the child must occur through the milk.

It thus becomes evident that in the opinion of a majority of observers micro-organisms may exist normally in the milk, chief among these being the staphylococcus pyogenes albus. It is held that septic germs may gain entrance through the air and probably also through the blood of the general circulation. It seems probable that they are the source of infection in mastitis, and that they may gain entrance in three ways,—viz., through the milk ducts, through the lymphatic channels, and through the blood-vessels.

In mastitis, according to Orth, usually only a part of the breast is affected at a time, although successive portions may become involved. The outer and lower portions are those most commonly affected. The chief disturbance is in the connective tissue surrounding the acini, and when the cells of exudation enter the milk-ducts this is only a secondary manifestation; if the inflammation has its origin in the milk-ducts, with early suppuration, it may be called a purulent galactophoritis. At first small abscesses form, which later enlarge and coalesce; the gland parenchyma may remain longer and give a nodular appearance to the breast. Fistulæ discharging milk may result from the inflammation.

Billroth holds it as probable that the phlegmonous material is carried by the lymph-stream into the breast, and through the medium of the white blood-corpuscles finds its way into the lobulus and acini. He considers this theory more probable than that of stasis or infection of milk-ducts. The origin of infection may come from various sources. Delbet suggests that it may come from the mouth of the infant, from ophthalmia, or from the hands of the mother herself. Pingat suggests the same, and cites an epidemic of lymphangitis occurring in Tarnier's wards which was found to have arisen from a nurse who had a felon. After this had been properly dressed the epidemic ceased.

As to the prognosis in cases of mastitis, Billroth says, *quoad vitiam*, it is not grave: he had observed fifty-six cases, with two deaths. One of these had erysipelas and the other had septic thrombosis of the femoral vein when received into the hospital.

The fistulæ following mastitis are difficult to heal.

One argument in favor of the retention of milk being the source of mastitis has been that in the pus discharged after the incision of abscesses of the breast milk has been present. It seems more probable, however, that the incision itself, while opening the abscess, may at the same time have opened certain of the milk-ducts.

Galactophoritis is an inflammatory condition of the milk-ducts, which is to be distinguished from a general mastitis by the fact that the induration of the breast is less extensive and it is possible to press out from the nipple small quantities of pus. M. Dudin, in his lectures in 1888, recommends as a treatment for galactophoritis to use pressure perhaps twice daily upon the breast, in order to squeeze out carefully as much pus as possible, and, after thorough cleansing, to support the breast by a carefully-applied dressing and bandage. M. Le Groux, of the Hôpital Trousseau, recommends in such cases that a plaster be applied over the entire breast except the nipple, and that the purulent secretion be drawn off with great care by means of the breast-pump.

The methods of treating mastitis which are recommended are both prophylactic and curative.

The method employed by Tarnier is, in the last month of pregnancy, to exert careful traction upon the nipple twice daily, increasing the amount of traction a little each day: one must desist should this cause uterine contractions. Great care must be taken to have the hands clean. Afterwards a pomade of almond oil, cacao butter, and tannin in equal parts is applied to the nipple. Others recommend alcohol or astringent lotions.

Horne says that in all cases of threatened inflammation of the breast, or where it has already taken place, well-regulated pressure by means of an elastic bandage should be applied, and no attempt made to nurse or to withdraw secretion until the subsidence of the inflammation. As to the advantages of the elastic bandage over the ordinary roller, he says its application is more easy, the pressure is more uniform, it is not so likely to slip, it is more comfortable to the patient, it requires less material, and it is not necessary to apply it over the shoulders. During lactation, Tarnier's method is to wash the breast thoroughly with bichloride of mercury and apply a moist dressing saturated in 1 to 20,000 of the same. Before nursing this is washed away with a solution of boracic acid or common salt. If cracks are present, the child is applied to the affected breast less frequently than to the other; if the cracks are painful, a five-per-cent. solution of cocaine is applied before nursing; if they are exceedingly painful or inflamed, nursing is stopped for a time. Assistance may be gained in nursing by means of a shield. The affected breast is bound up and compressed. For fissures Tarnier considers all pomades undesirable.

In the treatment of fissures, Bonnaire recommends the application of nitrate of silver of the strength of 1 to 100 or 150. For fissured nipples, Hirst advises the use of an ointment of equal parts of oleum ricini and bismuthi subnitratis. Before its application the nipple should be thoroughly disinfected. The child may nurse without the removal of this ointment. For engorgement of the breast he applies lead-water and laudanum, giving the breast support by means of equable pressure. When nursing is abandoned, Pingat believes that special care should be taken in protecting the breast against micro-organisms. He suggests for this purpose that the breast be enveloped in cotton.

When mastitis has gone on to the formation of abscesses, the early and complete evacuation of the pus is of the greatest importance. Failure to effect this may result in extensive abscesses which are extremely difficult to heal and which produce serious results. Instead of opening the abscess,

Boeckel has suggested that the entire abscess be excised. He treated six cases of abscess in this way, with healing by first intention under a single dressing. Billroth makes an early opening in cases of ante- and retro-mammary abscess. He says that a difference of opinion exists concerning abscesses of the gland itself, and he recommends an early small incision, with drainage and antiseptic dressing, which can be left in place for three days and then removed. If the pus has decomposed, as it may do on account of the presence of milk, the opening must be more free, and the finger inserted into the abscess so that dividing walls can be broken down and the cavity thoroughly disinfected and drained. Even in such cases healing may go on rapidly. He considers antiseptic dressings, with press-ure, as very valuable, and nursing should be abandoned if it causes much pain or if there is much inflammation. He says that women often object to the opening of abscesses on account of the cost of milk should nursing cease, through fear of pain or of scars, and lest the stoppage of lactation might make possible another pregnancy. There is also a popular belief that a scar made by a knife is more serious than that resulting from a spontaneous opening.

Chronic Mastitis.—As distinguished from acute mastitis, Delbet cites chronic inflammations of the breast as occurring under three forms: the subacute, coming on gradually with more or less pain, and producing a tumor usually more tender on pressure than a malignant growth and with more definite boundaries, accompanied by enlargement and tenderness of the axillary glands; the resolving form, which may exist for a considerable time and then disappear; and the indurated form, which may remain for months or years, varying with each menstruation. As causes he cites, first, lactation, and, second, traumatism. The fact that enlargements come after pregnancy he considers as always significant of inflammatory origin, since malignant growths rarely appear at this time. In a case of my own an enlargement came on during pregnancy which presented many evidences of being inflammatory. The secretion of milk was abundant, and was stopped with difficulty. A little later the growth was so suspicious that it was removed, although signs of inflammation had not passed away, and it was found to be a rapidly growing carcinoma.

Orth says that a diffuse mastitis may occur involving the whole breast, coming on with symptoms of swelling, pain, and tenderness. Later this may result in contraction, which it may be difficult to distinguish from carcinoma. Billroth thinks that most cases of chronic induration and contraction of the breast which have been described as mastitis are really carcinoma. In his own experience he has met but one case of this sort which he thought might be chronic mastitis.

### TUBERCULOSIS.

Orth says that it was formerly supposed that tuberculosis did not occur in the breast. It is now known that it is not uncommon. Billroth, in his classic work, cites only one case, that of a woman who died of general tuberculosis.

MacNamara[1] says that the first case was reported in 1801 by Benjamin Bell, that surgeon stating that abscesses occasionally occurred in breasts which were mistaken for cancer. He also suggests that some cases which have been reported as malignant disease operated upon with cure may have been cases of tuberculosis. He thinks, however, that extirpation is the best treatment for tuberculosis. Orth says that tuberculosis is most common in women, and may begin before puberty or may occur after the menopause; it is most frequent, however, in advanced adult life. Pregnancy and parturition seem to favor its development. It may occur on one or both sides. It may result from tuberculosis of the ribs, and may be primary or secondary to tuberculosis of the axillary glands. Roux[2] cites Virchow as placing the mammary glands among the organs which are exempt from tuberculosis; he says that Cornil and Ranvier do not even mention tuberculous breasts. Velpeau, in his treatise in 1854, says that the breast is rarely the seat of cold abscesses which from their progress and appearance can be considered to be tuberculous. Sir Astley Cooper describes what he calls scrofulous tumor of the breast, saying that it progresses slowly and is confined to one breast. Roux discusses thirty-two cases of tuberculosis among women and two among men, the average age being thirty-one years, the oldest being fifty-two and the youngest sixteen. Of the thirty-four cases, seventeen had borne from one to eight children, in seven there was no record, and eight cases (two of whom were men) had not borne children. He mentions a case of a tuberculous mother who had lost five out of eight children from nursing them. It thus becomes evident that tuberculosis of the breast is a condition which has been fully understood but recently.

Dr. Welch, of Baltimore, in a verbal communication told me that several times he had, on examination, found breasts which were considered malignant, to be tuberculous, and said that he was of opinion that the condition was more common than is ordinarily recognized.

Delbet describes two forms of tuberculosis: the first is that in which there are isolated and distinct points of tuberculosis; the second is the confluent form. Ohnacker considers these two forms to be but different stages of the same process. He says that it is most common between the ages of twenty-five and thirty-five, that it never occurs before puberty nor after fifty, and that it does not depend upon lactation. Among twenty-six patients, twelve had no other tubercular lesion except that of the glands of the corresponding axilla, ten had pulmonary lesions, and four had other tubercular manifestations.

Roux (op. cit.) classifies the disease under three heads: 1, cold abscess; 2, disseminated tubercles; 3, confluent tubercles.

---

[1] Westminster Hosp. Rep., 1889.

[2] De la Tuberculose Mammaire, 1891.

Of the first variety, he says it resembles cold abscess elsewhere. The second begins in an obscure manner, being unaccompanied by pain and being rarely seen at an early stage. In this condition nodules may be felt in the interior of the mammary gland varying in size and number, and these nodules may reach the size of an almond. Enlarged glands in the axilla, and particularly along the border of the pectoralis major muscle, should suggest the presence of this disease.

The third form, he says, is the most common, is painless, and may be unaccompanied by tumor of either breast or axilla. The breast may be pendulous, somewhat enlarged, and the nipple retracted. In the upper and outer portion of the breast one may find an oval elongated tumor, indistinct fluctuation on deep pressure, and there may be little, if any, elevation of temperature. With the progress of the case the axillary glands usually become enlarged and an abscess forms. A considerable abscess may form by the confluence of several tuberculous points, and this may break through the skin and result in sinuses which are difficult to heal. The process begins in the acini with small, slow infiltration, and spreads to the surrounding tissue.

The disease may show itself first either in the breast or in the axilla, and may extend from one to the other. The diagnosis is very difficult, if not impossible, in the beginning, and the disease may be confounded with chronic inflammation. The most characteristic sign is the relatively early enlargement of the axillary glands, with tuberculous infection of the connecting lymphatic vessels. Later, when ulceration occurs, the diagnosis is easy. Tuberculosis has been confounded with suppurating cancer. Professor Welch, of Johns Hopkins University, related to me two such cases.

The effect of tuberculosis on woman's milk has not been fully investigated. Unquestionably, however, the bacilli are secreted with the milk of tuberculous cows and are a source of danger, and Welch suggests that the same may be true with reference to women.

As to the prognosis, it does not in itself threaten life, but leads to a gradual destruction of the breast. There is always danger, however, that it may involve other organs. The progress of the disease is slow in all three varieties, and is liable to be unfavorable without surgical intervention, resulting in long suppuration and general tuberculous infection. The treatment should be the same as in other cases,—conservative if early, radical if late.

The treatment recommended by Delbet is the removal of a wedge-shaped piece in case of local infection, and the removal of the entire breast, together with the axillary glands, if this be necessary to eradicate the disease. He says that injections are of little value, and that incising, curetting, and cauterizing, though they may be attended with considerable benefit, result in long-delayed healing, and are correspondingly objectionable. Dubar,[1] in

---

[1] Tubercules de la Mamelle, Paris, 1881.

speaking of treatment, concludes that in the disseminated form of the disease the treatment should be palliative. In the confluent form there should be total extirpation of the breast, and proper medication should accompany both forms of treatment. Berchtold, working under the supervision of Professors Courvoisier and Socin, concludes that the rational therapy in tuberculosis of the mamma is total extirpation of the entire breast and dissection of the axilla, since a breast which is once tuberculous is always suspicious, and should never be used for lactation. He says that total extirpation of such breast is as clearly indicated as though the case were carcinoma. Lane reports two cases of tuberculosis of the breast, and concludes that it may occur without infection of the axillary glands.

It thus appears that tuberculosis of the breast, though not a common disease, is by no means rare ; that, whereas it may be a local process, there is a tendency to become generalized. Its presence is a contra-indication to nursing, since it is probable that it may induce tuberculosis in the child. When of slight extent, incision, disinfection, and removal are in place ; when the involvement of the breast is large, and is accompanied, as is often the case, with fistulæ and perhaps enlarged axillary glands, the entire breast should be removed and the axillary glands extirpated.

## SYPHILIS.

The breast may be affected by the primary, secondary, or tertiary lesions of syphilis.

Primary lesions occur upon the nipple, where they may present their usual characteristics, and may result in destruction of the nipple itself. Delbet says that chancres may occur at the same time on both breasts, or may be multiple on one breast.

It goes without saying that secondary syphilides may be found upon the breast as well as elsewhere. Mucous patches have been observed upon the nipple as well as under the fold of the breast. Syphilitic papulæ may occur under the breast and may be of large extent. Of gummata nothing definite is known, and Billroth says that he has never seen a case. Gummata of the nipple are rare, but they may occur. Delbet further says that tumors the result of tertiary syphilis may occur in the breast ; that they are round, movable, that the skin is not adherent or tender, and that they grow more rapidly than malignant tumors. The diagnosis is difficult at first, and is suggested only by a syphilitic history. As the tumor grows, it softens, inflames, and finally opens, the axillary glands becoming involved.

Neumann[1] says that syphilitic abscesses of the breast are rare, and that they occur only in the later stages of the disease. Rokitansky does not mention them. Cheever mentions a case in the *Boston Medical and Surgical Journal* which disappeared under iodides. Landreau, in describing the con-

---

[1] Allgem. Wiener Med. Zeitung, December, 1889.

dition, states that there is no special pain ; the breast gradually enlarges, is irregular, dense, and more or less nodular, not being tender upon pressure. After considering fifteen cases, Neumann says that the diagnosis lies between mastitis, neoplasms, and syphilis. Against mastitis is the absence of signs of inflammation. The fact that the tumor diminishes under iodides helps to exclude neoplasms. In favor of the diagnosis of syphilis are the slow development, the painlessness, the reddish color of the skin, the thin, cheesy pus which escapes when the tumor opens, and the fact that the latter is beneficially affected by iodides.

The treatment of syphilitic manifestations in the breast is the same as that of syphilis elsewhere.

The importance of the diagnosis is shown by the fact that syphilis may be contracted through the milk. On the other hand, offspring come under the law of Colles,—namely, that if a mother gives birth to a syphilitic child through the infection of the father, the mother having escaped infection, she is thereby protected against infection in nursing the child, and it is stated by Ehrlich that under these circumstances the nursing of such a child by the mother is without danger to the latter and is of great benefit to the former.

### CHALKY CONCRETIONS.

According to Billroth (op. cit.), these may occur in the breast, but are very rare.

### ANGIOMA.

These may occur in the breast, but are also very rare. I have observed one case presenting superficially the appearance of an angioma; in the tissues beneath it, however, could be felt an enlargement. Upon its removal, the mass beneath was found to be an alveolar carcinoma.

### CYSTS.

Cysts of the breast may be of different sorts, and there is no little difficulty in distinguishing between them ; under certain circumstances it is impossible to do so. A case in point was one in which I operated upon a woman, about thirty-seven years of age, having a cyst containing perhaps six ounces, which, upon being opened, contained a dark fluid resembling a broken-down blood-clot, the cyst having what seemed to be a simple wall, smooth and free from any unusual appearances. The incision healed, except a small sinus which persisted for some time. Gradually the walls of the sinus became indurated. A small piece removed later from this point of induration for examination proved to be carcinoma. The breast was immediately excised and the axilla cleared, and in the axilla were found numerous glands already infected by the carcinoma. This shows the difficulty and importance of diagnosis in case of cysts. Upon this point, Orth (op. cit.) says that it is difficult to distinguish between adeno-cystoma and simple cyst-formation. The former results in the development of cysts in the newly-formed tissue; the latter is caused by the dilatation of the already existing canals by the pushing of tissue into them; thus ducts and even acini become greatly dilated.  Billroth says that cysts come from dilatation of the milk-ducts, and that they may result from a collection of secretion such as sometimes occurs in the newly-born and in old women, or that they may be due to the degeneration of epithelium. They may be single or multiple, and a great many may occur in the same patient.  They are rarely larger than an orange, and may be very tense and, if the patient is fat, difficult of diagnosis.  He also says they may occur in new formations, such as a fibroma, and they are usually at the periphery of a gland, though they may be at its centre.

Among the rare forms of cysts Forbes records a case of papilliferous fibro-cystic adenoma of an aberrant breast-nodule, and remarks that S. W. Gross had a microscopic slide of a similar tumor.

Johnson reports a case of cystic disease of both breasts, the cysts being large and showing polypoid growths.  Both were removed.  In one there was a recurrence two years afterwards of a cyst-growth above the cicatrix. Billroth says that cysts may be accompanied by a discharge of brownish serum from the nipple.  Extirpation is the best treatment; injections he considers unsatisfactory.

Galactocele.—Much was formerly said of galactocele and the importance of the retention of milk in the production of cysts of the breast. It is now considered to be of much less frequency than formerly, and relatively few well-authenticated cases are recorded.  It becomes a question whether the cysts result from the rupture of ducts or from their dilatation. According to Delbet, the ligature of part of the ducts in dogs who still continued nursing caused no cysts.  Most cases are reported as following an injury, and this is an undoubted cause.  They usually grow slowly, with little, if any, pain.  The contents may vary from a milky to a creamy or buttery consistency.  They occasionally come at the close of pregnancy. The tumors are movable; the skin is not adherent.  It may be possible to express milk.  Their course is usually a slow one, and results in different ways.  The cysts may increase with succeeding pregnancies or may be absorbed, or possibly they may suppurate.

According to Orth, galactocele may result from an inflammatory condition, usually coming during the process of involution.  An interesting case of Scarpa's which contained ten quarts of fluid is cited by Billroth. Well-established cases containing large amounts are, however, rare.

Delbet says that galactocele may be confounded with cystic neoplasms, but the latter usually have a solid part in addition to the cystic portion. Should galactocele occur during lactation, nursing should cease; later, extirpation is the best method.  Incision, with or without injection, is undesirable, since it is followed by long suppuration.  Besides galactocele, the contents of cysts have often been described as composed of material resembling cheese or butter.  Billroth doubts if these observations are correct, and in a case of his own which was examined by Ludwig the contents were found to be emulsified fat.

Smita, however, gives the analysis of the contents of a cyst having the appearance of condensed milk, and showing the presence of casein, albumen, and sugar of milk.

It thus becomes evident that cysts of the breast are of various sorts and of various significance; and whereas they may be benign, they may be the beginning of malignant trouble and may occur in malignant tumors. They should always receive careful consideration, and when not multiple and distributed in both breasts they should be removed.

**Cystic Degeneration, or Maladie Cystique of Reclus.**—A disease was described by Reclus[1] in 1883 which was characterized by the appearance of multiple cysts in both breasts. Writing of the same disease in 1893, he says it is characterized by the existence of a number of cavities, large or small, so hard as to seem solid, and it is only by exploration that the presence of liquid can be diagnosticated. These cysts pervade one and often both breasts. The diagnosis lies between the cysts described and those arising from epithelioma. Whereas in his first article he advocated complete extirpation of the breast, in a later one he says that he is inclined to defer operation, unless there be evidences of malignancy, since numerous cases have followed a benign course. Delbet is inclined to consider this disease of inflammatory origin, and thinks it is the same as that which had previously been described and illustrated by Cooper. Koenig holds to the same opinion. Delbet's idea is that the cystic condition is secondary to a chronic inflammatory one.

Schimmelbusch gives Reclus the credit of having described the disease as typical, rather than as a rare condition. The points of diagnosis, as he lays them down, are the multiple small cysts, their almost sure affection of both breasts, and the fact that they are not connected with neighboring tissues, especially the skin. He cites a case in Von Bergmann's clinic in which both breasts were involved. In one of these, in addition to this, there was a small mass the size of a pigeon's egg, the central portion of which was infiltrated with scirrhus. He cites seven cases observed in Von Bergmann's clinic, together with thirty-six collected from other sources; in three of these carcinoma developed itself. As to treatment, he agrees with other authors in holding that partial extirpation is useless, and that if extirpation is performed at all it should be complete. In patients advanced in years extirpation might be advisable; in those younger he would be inclined to keep the case under observation. He says that microscopic examination shows the cysts to result from a proliferation of the epithelium of the gland. The acini increase in number and are finally dilated and united. It differs radically from carcinoma, since the connective tissue is not invaded, but only pushed aside by the development of the cyst.

---

[1] Revue de Chirurgie, 1883, p. 761.

While it is evident that this disease is one which had been observed by other authors, doubtless to Reclus is due the credit of having brought it prominently to notice. Although in the beginning extirpation was recommended as the sole treatment, as it is found that many cases run a benign course the advice of surgeons has become more conservative, being to observe cases for a time, particularly the young, whereas in those who are approaching or have passed the menopause it is questionable whether removal is not the safer plan, even though a certain number of operations be performed needlessly. Partial extirpation has proved of no value, since the disease continues to develop in the portions of the gland left behind.

### THE CLASSIFICATION AND ORIGIN OF TUMORS.

Tumors have been variously classified by different authors. There are also many theories as to their origin. Neither origin nor theories of classification can, however, be looked upon as settled, and there is a constant tendency to add new varieties to those which have already been described. Perhaps no better division can be made than into, first, those having the type of connective tissue; second, those having the type of epithelial tissue; and, third, tumors of a mixed type.

The first class—namely, those having the type of connective tissue—are of two sorts. The first of these are the benign, being analogous to normal tissue, and include the fibromata, lipomata, and chondromata. The other class of connective-tissue formations are atypical, although they have their prototype in the normal connective tissue. To this class belong the sarcomata. Myxomata are variously classed by some under the first and by others under the second division. To the second class of tumors, having their prototype in epithelial tissue, belong the adenomata, which may be regarded as typical, and the carcinomata, which may be regarded as atypical. The mixed tumors are various combinations of those mentioned, as, for instance, fibro-sarcoma and adeno-sarcoma, and cases are reported in which it is believed there is a mixture of sarcoma with carcinoma. In addition to these three classes of tumors are new growths, such as angiomata and neuromata, and there are cysts, formed, first, by retention, second, by degeneration, and third, by parasites, among which is the echinococcus.

The theories as to the origin of tumors vary widely, and the older ones need not be mentioned.

First among the theories which attempted anything like a scientific explanation was that of Johannes Müller. This was that tumors had their origin in the amorphous layer of the embryo called blastem, drawing their nourishment from the blood and lymph. The explanation given by Virchow is that they are the result of local irritation, causing more rapid growth of tissue. Thiersch regards epitheliomata as due to diminished resistance of tissue underlying the epithelium. Cohnheim[1] considered

---

[1] Councilman, Boston Medical and Surgical Journal, 1893, p. 147.

them to be due to the growth of remaining embryological structures through local stimulation.

It cannot, perhaps, be claimed that any of these explanations meets all the requirements of the case. They are, however, the best that have been offered up to the present time. As to the tendency to various tumors, Gross[1] says that the structural perfection of the mamma renders it most obnoxious to fibroma, sarcoma, and adenoma. Atrophy or decay predisposes to myxoma and carcinoma. He further says that the nearer the structures of the mammary tumor approach those of physiological adult tissues, whether they be connective or epithelial, the more innocent the growth, and that the more they depart from the normal standard the more malignant is the new formation.

Dennis[2] says the more embryonic the structure of the tumor the greater the liability to recurrence. Tumors which have structures departing but slightly from the normal correspond in every instance with a group of cases the clinical histories of which are favorable. Tumors which show a great departure from the normal structure correspond to the unfavorable clinical histories.

With regard to the production of epithelial growths, the question has arisen as to the origin of new cells, and opinions have varied as to whether these were the direct production of the epithelial cells already existing or resulted from the small-cell infiltration which surrounds malignant growths. Waldeyer says there is no evidence that the leucocytes found in cancerous tissue are transformed into cancer-cells, and that they are easily distinguished from these. He further says that, according to his observation, cancer-cells, and especially cancer-nests, have their origin in the pre-existing epithelium of the organ, while the stroma has its origin in the connective tissue.

Delbet (op. cit.) says that benign tumors of the breast are of glandular origin, and not pure connective tissue; otherwise, why should they develop more frequently in the breast than elsewhere? He thinks connective tissue and glandular elements develop together; hence he classes them as adeno-fibroma and adeno-myxoma. Williams[3] states that in the whole body 54.5 per cent. of malignant neoplasms spring from the archiblast (epithelium) and only 9.5 per cent. from the parablast (connective tissue). On the other hand, in the breast 77.6 per cent. spring from the archiblast and 4.1 per cent. from the parablast. He holds that inasmuch as the archiblast tissue retains more closely the embryonic type than do other tissues, where stimulated to unnatural physiological development, as in the uterus and mammæ, it is especially prone to take on malignant growths.

He gives the following statistics of 4597 cases of neoplasm. In men

[1] Gross, Tumors of the Mammary Gland, p. 35.
[2] Transactions of the American Surgical Association, 1891, p. 19.
[3] British Medical Journal, September, 1892.

the disease occurred in the mammæ in 0.5 per cent. of cases. Of 9227 cases of neoplasm in women, 26 per cent. were in the breast, 28.7 per cent. in the uterus, and 8.7 per cent. in the ovaries. Thus, the reproductive organs in women are attacked in about 70 per cent. of cases. Throughout the body the proportion of malignant to non-malignant neoplasms is 64 to 36 ; in the breast it is 81.7 to 18.3. He also says the influence of sex in the development of neoplasms is very great, the proportion occurring among males being about one-half that among females, or 33 to 67. In the breast, however, 99 per cent. of all neoplasms occur in females and only 1 per cent. in males. The following table will show the relative proportion of various neoplasms :

|  | Neoplasms in general. | Breast Neoplasms. |
| --- | --- | --- |
| Cancers . . . . . . . . . . . . . . | 54.5 | 77.6 |
| Sarcoma . . . . . . . . . . . . | 9.4 | 4.1 |
| Non-malignant . . . . . . . . . . | 24.7 | 15.7 |
| Cysts . . . . . . . . . . . . . . | 11.4 | 2.6 |
|  | 100.0 | 100 0 |

Various experiments have been made in order to establish whether tumors are contagious or not. All attempts at inoculation made upon human beings thus far have failed, as well as most attempts of the same sort in animals. A few upon animals, however, have succeeded. Among them is one of Wehr's, presented at the German Surgical Congress in 1889. A carcinoma had been produced in a dog by inoculation, and the tumor had grown until it destroyed the dog, presenting unquestionable evidences of carcinoma. As to the contagion between human beings, Guelliot collected twenty-three cases of cancer of the penis among men whose wives had cancer of the uterus. On the other hand, Demarquay collected one hundred and thirty-four cases of cancer of the penis, in only one of which did the wife have cancer of the uterus. In conclusion, Duplay and Gazin are cited as saying that although we have no evidence of the direct contagion of cancer, we are none the less convinced of the infectious nature of cancer through a process of which we are entirely ignorant.

They further say that, from their own results and those obtained by numerous other experimenters, they believe that there does not exist a single fact authorizing us to conclude that cancerous neoplasms are directly transmissible from one species to another.

The possible influence of bacteria in the production of tumors is a subject which has of late attracted wide attention and has been the source of a vast amount of experimentation. The origin of this was the discovery of certain formations, called coccidia, in the liver of the rabbit, where growths are produced resembling epithelial new formations. Their discovery suggested the possibility that carcinoma in general might be the product of bacteria. The present status of opinion concerning this has been admirably summarized by Councilman.[1]  He says that various forms of bacteria may be found in carcinoma as well as in other portions of the body.  They may produce inflammation or necrosis, but there is no evidence that they have any causal relation to the tumor.

In the rabbit's liver is found a species of protozoa or coccidium which produces nodules.  These nodules are of the type of adenoma, and an analogy has been drawn between them and certain parasites found in carcinoma.  That these were parasites and not bacteria was first pointed out by Thoma.  These forms are variously described, and can hardly be considered as established, certainly not as the cause of carcinoma.  Klebs says that experiments up to the present time as to the origin of carcinoma have produced no definite results.  Culture experiments have demonstrated a series of bacterial organisms in carcinoma, but without sufficient constancy to give them pathological significance.

It is, however, by no means demonstrated that there are no carcinoma parasites, since it is possible there may be parasites the nature and cultivation of which are not yet understood.

Coley,[2] in a very interesting article upon the treatment of sarcoma by inoculation with erysipelas, says there is strong evidence of the bacterial origin of malignant growths.  Kruse concludes that one must exercise great caution in accepting coccidia as the cause of malignant disease, since it is easy to mistake changes in the cells themselves, or the presence of normal elements, for what have been termed coccidia or psorosperms.  Councilman (op. cit.) concludes that parasites present in tumors must be considered as accompanying rather than causing them.  He says it seems impossible that carcinoma should arise from parasites, since metastatic growths take on the structure of the original tumor rather than that of the tissues in which they grow.  This would hardly be the case if they were due to parasites.  In this connection it may be remembered that Billroth has pointed out that while in the axilla metastatic growths have the same structure as in the mamma, metastatic growths occurring elsewhere may have a very different structure.

### CONNECTIVE-TISSUE FORMATIONS.

Although chondroma and osteoma have been considered as occurring in the breast, they are extremely rare growths.  Billroth cites one case of Sir Astley Cooper's as the only fairly established observation.  Delbet says of them that they are probably a small amount of cartilaginous material developing in other tissues, or that they may invade the breast from the ribs.  He also says that calcification may occur.  Coen reports a case of "condro-osteo-carcinoma della mammella muliebre." Orth (op. cit.) says that chondroma and osteoma and mixed forms with sarcoma and carcinoma are rare in men, but that the form is not rare in dogs.

---

[1] Councilman, Boston Medical and Surgical Journal, April 20, 1893, p. 393.

[2] American Journal of the Medical Sciences, May, 1893, p. 488.

Cysts having walls with calcareous infiltration may be mistaken for osteoma.

## LIPOMA.

Lipomata when occurring in the vicinity of the breast are usually separate from it. Delbet cites two cases of lipomata interlacing with the tissues of the gland. Billroth thinks that lipomata usually develop outside of the gland and push it to one side. If these are superficial, their diagnosis is easy; if underneath the gland, it may be difficult. Their removal when the growth is isolated is similar to that of lipomata elsewhere. A. P. Dudley reports the removal of a lipoma by an incision below the breast after the method of Thomas, thus avoiding deformity. Orth makes a division which he calls "lipoma capsulare," due to the increase of the fat surrounding the mamma. If the increase of fat follows a chronic mastitis, with contraction, the nipple may be drawn inward and given the appearance of scirrhus.

## ADENOMA.

The classification of tumors belonging to the type of adenoma is attended with considerable difficulty. By some they have been classed as pure adenoma; by others many of them have been considered to be

Fig. 4.

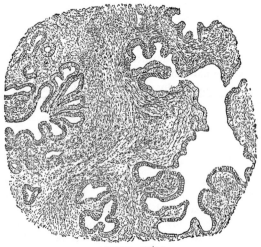

Adenoma. (Orth.)

fibroma. There are probably tumors belonging to both of these classes, but the weight of evidence seems to be that they should be considered as mixed types, and perhaps the best designation for them is adeno-fibroma.

Orth, in speaking of such tumors, says that connective-tissue tumors may develop from the adventitia of the milk-ducts or from the surrounding connective tissue, or there may be combinations of these forms, accompanied also with increase of gland-substance. Pure adenomata are rare; mixed tumors are most common as adeno-fibroma, adeno-myxoma, adeno-sarcoma, etc. Gross (*op. cit.*) says that, when typical, the new acini preserve their natural form, size, and central lumen, containing a relatively small amount of connective tissue. There is a marked tendency for them to become cystic. He further says that adenoma is more rare than any other growth except myxoma, since he found only two among six hundred and forty-nine cases of tumor of the breast. They have their physiological proto-type in the breast preparing for lactation. He elsewhere says they are always solitary. Adenomata are usually ovoid, with nodular outline, and when not cystic are hard. Although limited by a capsule, when of moderate size they are closely united to the breast. Patterson gives excel-lent illustrations of adenoma growing in the breasts of girls aged respec-tively twelve and thirteen years.

Adenoma may be distinguished from cancer by its being more circum-scribed and having a more definite outline; this applies principally to adeno-fibroma.

## FIBROMA.

Fibromata are much more common than pure adenomata. Billroth, in speaking of them, says that he never saw a case before puberty nor after forty. Their most common period is from sixteen to twenty-five, and they are usually small and hard and of slow growth. It is not improbable, however, that certain cases may in later years take on the form of soft sarcoma. Gross says of solid fibromata that the average age for their ap-pearance is twenty-three years, twenty-one per cent. occurring before the sixteenth year and seventy-five per cent. before the thirtieth. Of cystic fibromata, he says that they are never seen before the sixteenth year, the average age being thirty-six years, and that only thirty-five per cent. occur before the thirtieth year. The solid forms grow slowly, whereas the cystic forms may suddenly take on rapid growth.

Schimmelbusch, in speaking of fibro-adenoma, says that in every case which he examined having the appearance of fibroma, glandular elements were found, proving the growth to be fibro-adenoma. These growths never invade surrounding tissue, and never recur. Subsequent tumors, should they recur, must be regarded as new developments. They must be distinguished from sarcomata: sarcomata form cysts in their interior, but do not contain certain gland-elements, while fibro-adenomata have in their interior glandular elements.

According to Gross, adenomata may be confounded with fibromata, but the latter are more movable upon the mamma, more circumscribed, and not so decidedly bossed. Speaking of the openings in tumors of the char-acter of fibromata, Orth says these may be due to a simple dilatation and destruction of the existing ducts. Into these ducts tissues may be pushed having connective-tissue basis covered with epithelium, which gives them,

on cross-section, the appearance of being papillæ.  This gives rise to a
tumor which has been called fibro-adenoma cysticum, arborescent sarcoma,
fibroma intracanaliculare, adenocele, etc.  The openings in these may become so large that they may be seen and followed with the scissors ; the cut
section may resemble a cabbage.  The tissue pushing into the canals may
break into them, and even through the integument.  The cut surface will
vary in appearance according to the preponderance of glandular, connective, or myxomatous tissue.  The cyst contents may be viscid or of a
jelly-like consistence.  The fluid may contain cholesterin or may be tinged
with blood.  Rarely, epithelial pearls are formed from the hardened epithelial masses, coming probably from ducts instead of from the acini.
The mixed adenomata are usually freely movable at first and the skin is
not involved, though later the cysts may break through and cauliflower-like

Fig. 5.

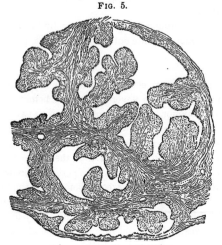

Intracanalicular fibroma.  (Orth.)

masses protrude.  The mixed adenomata must be classed with the benign
tumors, since they cause no metastatic deposits.  They may, however, be
multiple in the same or both breasts, and thus other growths appear after
one has been removed.

An interesting lecture upon adeno-fibroma is given by Duplay.  With
reference to pain, he says that when it is present at the beginning of a
tumor it is characteristic of a benign rather than of a malignant growth.
He classes adeno-fibromata under three heads : 1. Adenoid tumors absolutely distinct from the gland, giving the sensation of a lymphatic gland.
2. Those which have evident connection with the gland.  3. Those which
are surrounded with gland tissue.

It is a question if certain cases may not later develop into sarcomata, and he advises as the sole treatment their removal, saying that the

removal of the entire breast is necessary in those cases in which the surgeon fears transformation of the tumor into a sarcoma. In cases in which the tumor is wholly surrounded by gland tissue it is necessary to remove the entire breast; in cases in which the tumor is nearly or quite independent of the mammary gland a circumscribed operation is indicated. Bennett, in speaking of chronic tumors of the breast, strongly urges the removal of adenomata and fibro-adenomata, since he thinks that there is danger lest they should degenerate into sarcomata, and cites a case of this sort.

In cases of my own of adeno-fibromata of both breasts the growths were removed through curved incisions corresponding to the fold beneath the breast, so that after the operation, when viewed from in front, no scar could be seen. This is a desirable consideration in young ladies, among whom such growths are most common. The operations are usually easy, since the tumors can, as a rule, be enucleated with little destruction of tissue. In another case Dr. I. N. Himes and myself removed the mammary gland from a woman aged fifty-three years. Thirty years before she had been told that the growth was innocent, and was advised to let it alone. She insisted on its removal, on account of the advent of pain and fear lest it might be malignant. The mass proved to be spherical, one and one-half inches in diameter, with a shell of bony hardness having a thickness of from one line to one-eighth of an inch; the interior was composed of friable tissue. Microscopic examination showed this tissue to be made up largely of connective-tissue fibres. Distributed through it were openings filled with lime salts, the arrangement and form of the openings giving to the mass the appearance of an adenoma. My opinion is that the tumor was an old encapsulated adeno-fibroma which had undergone changes from its long enclosure in its bony covering. The wall or shell surrounding the growth, like the shell of an English walnut, showed the following analysis, as made by Professor Perry L. Hobbs: lime, 37.16 per cent.; carbonic acid, 2.98 per cent.; phosphoric acid, 29.86 per cent.; the remainder was organic matter and moisture. The analysis shows the structure to be bone rather than calcareous matter.

A growth called plexiform fibroma is described by Nordmann. It is a condition of increased connective tissue occurring about the milk-ducts, and is most common in women above fifty years of age. He describes fourteen cases, and considers them different from other forms of fibroma heretofore observed. Thirteen cases were gathered from five hundred autopsies performed during two and a half years.

### SARCOMA.

Sarcoma, next to carcinoma, is one of the most important diseases occurring in the breast. Its origin is obscure and has been assigned to many causes, such as traumatism, inflammation, heredity, etc., but none of these is thoroughly established as its cause. It is classed as belonging to the connective-tissue type of tumors, and this has been considered one of its positive characteristics. Exceptions to this have been cited by Billroth. He states that sarcoma, myxoma, and lymphoma may in rare instances have an alveolar formation, so that this formation cannot be looked upon as absolutely characteristic of carcinoma.

This exceptional occurrence in sarcoma is so rare that the rule remains that its chief characteristic is the relation which it bears to connective tissue.

Sarcomata are grouped in various ways. For our purpose the following grouping will answer: Fibro-sarcoma; round-celled and spindle-celled sarcoma, and forms combining the two; soft sarcoma and cysto-sarcoma; giant-celled sarcoma; melanotic sarcoma; osteo-sarcoma.

Before sixteen years of age, Gross says, we find only fibromata and sarcomata, the former being twice as common as the latter. Fibromata are always solid and grow slowly, while sarcomata are cystic in three-fourths of all cases and medullary in the remainder: hence cystic and medullary tumors at this age are sarcomata and nothing else. The youngest age at which they have been observed is nine years, and the oldest seventy-five.

In speaking of fibroma and fibro-sarcoma, Billroth says that there is a layer of hyaline, dense connective tissue, rich in nuclei, surrounding the acini and small excretory duets. It is from this tissue that fibroma and fibro-sarcoma develop. What others have described as adenoma of diffused form he says should come under the head of fibro-sarcoma, the cysts resulting from the dilatation of the excretory ducts.

Gross says that of sixty examples which he had collected of sarcoma, forty-five were spindle-celled and fifteen round-celled. The most common subdivision is the cystic, these forming nearly six-tenths of those operated upon. Next come the myxomatous and telangiectatic. Spindle-celled tumors are more solid than round-celled, but both may be soft and cystic. In a later work he says spindle-celled sarcomata include 68 per cent., round-celled 27 per cent., and giant-celled 5 per cent.; 50 per cent. are cystic and 50 per cent. solid. Of ninety-two cases studied, 64.83 per cent. showed malignant features. Recurrence was most rapid in round-celled sarcoma, being in four months and twenty days; in spindle-celled, recurrence took place in eleven months and twenty-seven days; in giant-celled, in twelve months and ten days; in cystic, in eight months and five days; in simple, in thirteen months and nine days: the average time for recurrence in cystic round-celled sarcoma was three months and four days; in simple round-celled, six months and eight days; in cystic spindle-celled, nine months; in simple spindle-celled, sixteen months. Of twenty post-mortems, twelve showed secondary metastatic deposits. Before the age of thirty-five, small slowly-growing sarcomata do not return, while rapidly-growing and especially cystic ones are liable to do so.

**Round-Celled Sarcoma.**—Round-celled sarcoma is of more rapid growth than adeno-, fibro-, or spindle-celled sarcoma. Poulsen says that among fourteen of his cases the sarcoma was movable under the skin, and the skin was adherent in twelve cases; in two the nipple was retracted, and in two the tumor was adherent to deeper structures.

Gross says that round-celled sarcomata are very malignant and that the prognosis as to their recurrence is grave. Among ten operations, eight had recurrences; of the two remaining, one died in two and one-half years of another affection and the other was alive after ten months.

FIG. 6.

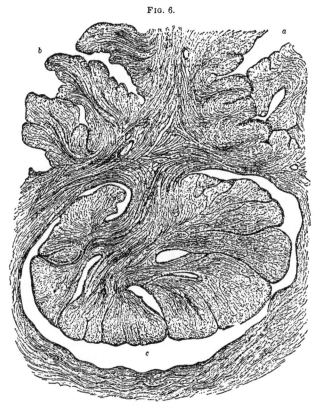

Proliferating cysto-sarcoma.—a, termination of an acinus; b and c, the tissue between the acini taking on increased growth and pushing into and dilating the acini into cysts. (Billroth.)

**Spindle-Celled Sarcoma.**—Billroth says that he never saw a pure and unmixed case of spindle-celled sarcoma and myxo-sarcoma. Steinberger, citing the above from Billroth, says that he observed one case of pure spindle-celled sarcoma. Gross mentions sixteen examples of spindle-celled sarcoma: five patients were living at periods of from a few months to twenty-six months, and one after five years, although the axillary glands were enlarged. The remaining eleven had local or general recurrences.

Thus, of twenty-six cases of round-and spindle-celled sarcoma which Gross cites, six were living free from disease an average of two years, one died without local return of the disease, and nineteen had recurrences.

**Soft Cysto-Sarcoma.**—In speaking of soft sarcomata, Billroth says that they may come at any age, from puberty to the sixties. They appear as small lumps, growing at first slowly and later rapidly. They are difficult to differentiate from cysto-sarcomata. The axillary glands may or may not be involved; recurrences are rapid, and death is usually early, but has been deferred as late as one year. Early writers classed all soft growths, both carcinomata and sarcomata, as encephaloids. Billroth also says that he considers cysto-adenomata as belonging properly with the class of cysto-sarcomata. Speaking of proliferating cysto-sarcomata, he says that they begin in the connective tissue between the terminal acini. This class of growths gradually obliterate the divisions of the acini, thus forming cavities. The epithelial covering may increase and then degenerate, and thus form cysts, and the connective tissue itself may become myxomatous or lymphoid, or, rarely, spindle-celled. Such cases may involve the glands and form metastatic deposits, but this is rare. Thirteen cases of operation for the removal of cysto-sarcomata are reported by Poulsen. In nine of these amputation of the breast alone was made; in two the tumor only was removed; in two there were amputation of the breast and clearing of the axilla; of the last two, the axillary glands were diseased in one and not involved in the other. In neither could the glands be felt before the operation. Of the thirteen patients, nine were living and free from recurrences after two and one-half, six and one-third, seven, nine and one-half, eleven, twelve, and fourteen years, among them being the case mentioned with enlarged glands in the axilla. In two cases recurrent growths were removed; three cases died of metastatic deposits, and one case died of pneumonia ten years after operation. Thus, the prognosis is not unfavorable in cysto-sarcoma, since seventy-five per cent. were living after five years.

**Melano-Sarcoma.**—Melano-sarcomata, though occurring from time to time, are rare. Vieregge reports a case of a melano-sarcoma occurring in a male child. A small nodule the size of a bean, which was present at birth, showed signs of development at two years of age. On removal, it proved to be a melano-sarcoma, and recurred rapidly, being disseminated throughout the body and causing the death of the child.

Cases have also been recorded by Butlin and Billroth, the latter of whom says that he thinks all melanotic growths of the breast are sarcomata and not carcinomata.

**Giant-Celled Sarcoma.**—Orth says that both giant-celled and melanotic sarcomata are extremely rare. Billroth speaks of seeing a case containing giant cells which he thinks was sarcoma, though it was extremely difficult to distinguish it in places from carcinoma.

**Osteo- and Chondro-Sarcoma.**—These are also of very rare occurrence. Gross says that the average age at which they appear is thirty-four, and that the few cases operated upon would indicate them to be the most malignant of sarcomata. Bowlby, in an article on chondro-sarcoma, reports a series of cases recorded by Cooper, Cruveilhier, Müller, and Heur-

FIG. 7.

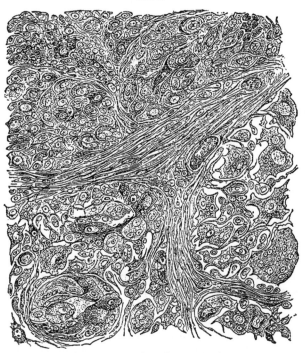

Alveolar sarcoma with giant cells. (Billroth.)

teaux, from the consideration of which he concludes that, while cartilage is very rarely met with in the breast, it may occur as an innocent growth or as a part of a malignant tumor. Professor Welch, of Johns Hopkins University, in an oral communication, says that most of the so-called osseous tumors of the breast are, in his opinion, calcareous infiltrations.

**Growth of Sarcoma.**—The growth of sarcomata seems to vary widely according to the character of the tumors and the age at which they develop. Gross says that their growth may be rapid or slow. Continuous growth indicates freedom from cysts, while sudden increase indicates accumulation of fluid. At a later period they may remain quiescent for years and then grow rapidly, suggesting that a fibrous tumor may take on sarcomatous changes. Sarcomata are usually solitary growths; in only a small proportion are they multiple. They are commonly free from deep attachments, and the skin, as a rule, retains its natural color and texture, the nipple is not retracted, and the lymph-glands are not enlarged.

As sarcomata increase in size cysts may appear and vessels of large size develop, the surface of the breast being rendered irregular by the protrusion of the cysts. The cysts may occasionally burst through the integument, causing a discharge of fluid and at times protrusion of fungous masses. In a case of cysto-sarcoma of my own (of the alveolar round-celled type) the tumor, after removal and the escape of the blood with a large portion of the cyst contents, weighed twenty-one pounds. It was so large as to rest upon the patient's knees before removal, and was equal in size to the largest cases of hypertrophied breasts which have been reported. Unfortunately, I could not secure a photograph. Before its removal, the cysts had burst through the skin and discharged constantly a large amount of fluid, which soaked the patient's clothing, even running down upon the floor. In this case the growth was slow for several years, later becoming rapid, and the development of the vessels from the axilla was very great, some veins being almost as large as the index finger.

As to the tendency of sarcoma to remain local or to become generalized, the statements of different authors vary considerably. Gross says that mammary sarcomata recur locally in 61.53 per cent. of all cases, and that 57.14 per cent. give rise to metastatic deposits. They are less infective locally than carcinoma, recurrence taking place in the proportion of 66 to 88.35 per cent., while they are more prone to produce metastatic infection, this occurring in the proportion of 57.40 to 50 per cent. In a later paper, reporting one hundred and fifty-six cases, he says that the lymphatic glands were enlarged and occasionally tender in nineteen cases. In sixteen of these enlargement was due to irritative hyperplasia, in ten of which there was ulceration of the tumor. The glands were infected in only three cases.

Speaking of the axillary glands, Snow[1] says that he never has seen a sarcoma with these glands infected. Poulsen[2] says that of the more solid sarcomata he had eleven patients, or 58 per cent., living and free from recurrences from four to sixteen and one-half years. In four of them local recurrences were removed. Eight cases of solid tumors, or 42 per cent., died. The axillary glands were involved in three cases; in all three cases swelling of the glands of the axilla could be felt. Two of them died, and in one the outcome was unknown. In none of the cases did the leaving of the axillary glands do harm, or, at any rate, were growths of the axilla removed afterwards. Of thirty-three patients with sarcoma, 63 per cent. were living free from recurrences, and 36.40 per cent. died with recurrences and metastases. Of the three cases of cysto-sarcoma in which he says that axillary glands could be felt, they were removed in but one case, and the patients all remained free from recurrences, so he concludes that the enlargement was a simple hyperplasia. Since, however, a diseased axillary gland was found in one case, and in another an axillary tumor appeared after three

---

[1] Lancet, London, May 6, 1893.
[2] Archiv f. Klin. Chirurg., 1891, p. 637.

years, he concludes that the axilla should be cleared, since the operation is not dangerous. Gould reports having operated on two cases of sarcoma with secondary growths in the axillary glands. Poulsen says, in the same connection, that the axillary glands were involved in only five cases of sarcoma; the remaining cases have either remained well or died of metastatic deposits without involvement of the axillary glands.

The generalization of sarcoma differs from that of carcinoma; for, while the latter extends chiefly through the lymphatic channels, the infection of sarcoma is carried in a greater degree by means of the blood-vessels. It is in this way that the metastatic deposits in distant organs are accounted for. Gross says that the sarcoma may even destroy the blood-vessels, so that the blood is contained in simple cavities in the sarcomatous mass.

Schmidt, reporting the method of operating pursued by Küster, says that in his service sarcomata were removed without clearing the axillary space. In discussing the results following operation upon sarcoma, Gross says that sarcoma occurring in a functionally active breast shows a marked disposition to return after operation, with less disposition to metastasis; while a sarcoma of the declining breast recurs locally less frequently, but is generalized in the greater number of instances. He says that in all varieties, spindle-, round-, and giant-celled, recurrence took place in from 57 to 65 per cent. of cases, the solid recurring in 64.58 per cent. and the cystic in 51.16 per cent. The round-celled had metastatic deposits in 25 per cent., and the spindle-celled in 20.40 per cent. Repeated removals of the recurrent growths seem to prolong life, and the young do not seem to be more subject to recurrence than the old, nor to more rapid growths: thus, in fifteen cases, of from nine to nineteen years, the tumor had been in existence seven and a half years before operation; 28.57 per cent. remained well, 71.43 per cent. recurred, and metastatic deposits were not observed in a single case. After thirty-five years of age, 43.45 per cent. recurred locally and 19.35 per cent. were generalized. Poulsen (*op. cit.*) reports thirty-three cases of sarcoma, or 9.3 per cent. of all mammary tumors. He found that recurrences or metastatic deposits occurred after solid sarcoma in 42 per cent., and after cystic sarcoma in 25 per cent. of the cases. Still, he thinks that the distinction between the two is not very sharp.

Treatment.—It is evident that the only rational treatment for sarcomata is their complete extirpation, on account of their tendency to local recurrence and to form metastatic deposits. Their early diagnosis is of the greatest importance. The operation varies little from that for carcinoma, except with reference to the clearing out of the axilla. While sarcomata have a marked tendency to recur locally, and to invade distant parts by means of metastatic deposits, they do not tend to invade the glands of the axilla, as do carcinomata.

A large number of operations which have proved successful are shown by statistics to have been confined to the removal of the breast, without clearing the axilla.  On the other hand, a considerable number of cases are reported in which the malignant growth has invaded the axilla.  The inability to distinguish certain cases of sarcoma from other malignant growths must necessarily result in their operation by the most radical plan,— viz., that which is recommended in carcinoma.  The only cases in which question will arise as to the method will be those in which the growth is small and seems to be strictly localized, and those in which it is so large and the patient's condition so reduced that it would be unwise to extend the operation more than is absolutely necessary.  In these cases the removal of the breast is all that should be attempted ; in others it is still a question if it is not wiser, for the sake of added certainty, to clear the axilla, as is done in carcinoma.  It is of great importance, however, in the operation to remember the tendency of sarcoma to recur locally, and consequently to make a radical and extensive removal of the tissues surrounding the growth.

### MYXOMA.

Speaking of myxoma, Orth says that pure fibroma and myxoma are very rare.  Gross considers myxoma synonymous with the net-celled sarcoma of Billroth, and places it among the most rare of connective-tissue neoplasms.  He says that pure hyaline myxomata have their prototype in Wharton's jelly of the umbilical cord.  They develop from twenty-nine to fifty-six years of age, the average time being the forty-sixth year, and grow more rapidly than sarcoma, but less rapidly than carcinoma.  One third of the cases recurred, and metastatic deposits were not present.  The growths are soft, and may simulate cysts.  As a rule, myxomata are solitary, and grow continuously and rather rapidly.  They are not bulky, are round or ovoid, are painful, have a limited attachment to the skin, but are movable on deep structures.  They are unattended by enlargement of glands or superficial veins or retraction of nipple.  They should be removed the same as sarcomata.

### CARCINOMA.

The most important neoplasm occurring in the breast is carcinoma.  Of its cause or prevention nothing is known.  The old idea was that carcinoma drew to itself material which existed in the blood, and that the involvement of the axillary glands arose only after the tumor had lost its power thus to purify the blood.  It was upon this idea that the giving of blood-medicines came into vogue, a practice which is still continued.

Various factors have been cited as influencing the development of carcinoma.  Heredity has been considered as of very great importance, and extensive statistics have been collected in order to prove the truth or falsity of this belief.  Winiwarter among one hundred and seventy patients found ten whose parents had had carcinoma.  It must be remembered, however, that probably the records were incomplete, and Billroth, judging from his experience, is of the opinion that the proportion should be much larger.  Gross among 1164 cases found that 8.5 per cent. had a family history of cancer, whereas among the direct ancestors the proportion was 4.72 per cent., and in only one-half of these was the disease in the breast. Dietrich found evidence of heredity in 5.6 per cent. Oldekopf thinks that heredity is entirely overestimated as a cause of cancer, judging from his own cases. Dennis (*loc. cit.*) says that heredity may be assigned as a factor in developing carcinoma in twelve per cent. of all cases.

Fig. 8.

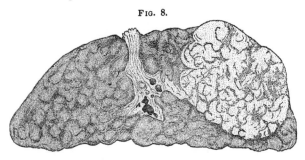

Acinous carcinoma (Markschwamm of Billroth; Encephaloid of Gross). (Billroth.)

Carcinomata of the breast differ considerably in their structure, growth, and malignancy. In the classification of carcinoma we cannot do better

Fig. 9.

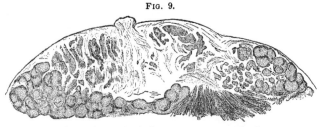

Carcinoma simplex (infiltrating cancer of Gross). (Billroth.)

than follow so eminent an authority as Billroth,—viz.: 1. Acinous carcinoma, partly hard and partly soft (Markschwamm; Gross, encephaloid

Fig. 10.

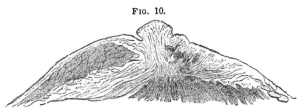

Scirrhus (atrophic scirrhus of Gross). (Billroth.)

or tuberous form of cancer); 2. Carcinoma simplex (Gross, infiltrating cancer); 3. Scirrhus (Gross, atrophic scirrhus); 4. Gallertkrebs (Gross, gelatiniform carcinoma).

Orth says that carcinomata may appear: 1, as isolated nodules; 2, in a diffuse form, involving the entire mamma; 3, they may arise from the nipple and flat epithelium; 4, more rarely they may be formed of cylinder

FIG. 11.

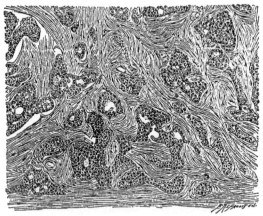

Carcinoma (common form).  (Duplay et Reclus.)

epithelium arising from milk-ducts and bearing close relation to adenoma; 5, they may appear as papillary growths, coming in large solitary cysts, or adeno-cysto-carcinoma.  The beginning of carcinoma is probably usually in

FIG. 12.

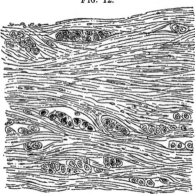

Scirrhus.  (Orth.)

the acini, which are later broken through as the disease extends.  The amount of connective tissue may vary widely from soft carcinoma to scirrhus, the latter being so dense that all epithelial cells disappear and only scar-tissue remains.  In the neighborhood of the carcinomatous tissue is a small-cell infiltration. These cells differ in character from inflammatory cells or leucocytes, since they are simple granulation cells with a single rounded nucleus. The structure of carcinoma is usually alveolar, but may be tubular, or both may be associated in the same tumor. Sometimes the amount of connective tissue is very small and the alveoli are correspondingly large; at other times the reverse is true. Billroth says that carcinoma usually develops when the gland is undergoing atrophy or is already atrophied; this would make it seem improbable that epithelial cells would develop at this time. The epithelium of the milk-ducts is not, however, undergoing a similar degeneration, but at times shows a marked increase and produces an excretion.

Waldeyer says of the structure of carcinoma, that the alveoli are not closed cavities, but communicate with one another, and may be likened to a bathing-sponge. Orth states that the macroscopic appearances of tumors vary; those of acinous structure show on the cut surface projecting portions, and the acinous structure becomes apparent. They are grayish red, and a whitish cancer-milk rich in cells can be scraped from the cut surface. Hard cancer is often infiltrated; it has on section a gray surface, and bundles of connective tissue are plainly visible. On scraping the surface, few, if any, cells are found.

Dennis says that the histological character of the tumor itself influences, more than does any other cause, the recurrence of carcinoma of the breast. The more typical the structure the better the prognosis; the more atypical the structure the more unfavorable the prognosis. Gross says that the size of the tumor depends upon the elements present, it being large when cells predominate and small when the fibrous stroma is in excess.

One of the most important of the divisions of carcinomata is that of scirrhus. Speaking of this, Oldekopf says that it is most common in older subjects, while the alveolar is more common in younger. He states that the average age for the appearance of scirrhus is fifty-one years, and the average length of life with scirrhus is sixty months, while with alveolar carcinoma it is thirty-three and nine-tenths months. Billroth says that in advanced age scirrhus gives the best prognosis.

Ashhurst[1] says, "My own experience is, scirrhus invariably returns sooner or later. Cases in which it has not recurred have been those in which the patients have died of some other affection in the mean time." On the other hand, he says, "I have seen cases in which there has been no recurrence after six or eight years," and that "there are undoubted cases where the period of immunity has lasted as long as ten years."

Butlin[2] concludes that withered scirrhous cancer is not favorable for removal, since the disease almost invariably returns. On the other hand,

---

[1] International Clinics, Philadelphia, July, 1891, p. 114.
[2] Butlin, Operative Surgery of Malignant Disease, 1889.

left to itself, it may pursue a very slow course, and may last for years without producing great local discomfort.

Speaking of gelatiniform carcinoma, or Gallertkrebs, Billroth says that myxomatous tissue may be produced by epithelial cells or may result from degeneration of the connective tissue. Doutrelepont thinks it is a substance poured out by the vessels, usually going to the production of cells, but here producing myxomatous material. Rindfleisch agrees with the last explanation. Orth says of this growth that the central portion is the part usually degenerated, while the periphery may retain its normal characteristics. It is not a simple degeneration from the disturbance of nutrition. Fatty degeneration, however, may occur, and can be distinguished by yellow points and by its structure. This may go on to the breaking down of tissue, or, on the other hand, connective tissue may increase and by contraction retract the nipple. Calcareous degeneration at times occurs. Cholesteatomata are formed from hardened epithelium in the gland-substance, and as such have no connection with cancer.

Hemorrhagic conditions may occur in connection with carcinoma of the breast, presenting the appearance of hæmatoma or of angioma. Willett describes two cases of hemorrhagic carcinoma of the breast, neither of which presented anything unusual before operation, except that the tumors were rather soft. On removal, the cut surface of the tumors was found to be dark red, due to extravasation. This was not generally diffused over the tissues, but was sharply defined by the margin of the malignant growth itself; the microscopic appearances were those of an encephaloid carcinoma. The blood was among the fibrous tissue portions, and not among the cellular elements.

Carcinoma appearing during pregnancy pursues a very rapid course. Cases of this sort are cited by Gross, also by Paget, Henry, and Billroth. In a case of my own the growth appeared two weeks after confinement, presenting in many respects the appearance of inflammation, the whole breast being dense and hard. It was, however, only slightly painful on pressure, and upon removal it was found to be an alveolar carcinoma very rich in cells and with but a small amount of connective tissue. The whole breast was removed and the axilla cleared. Death followed, however, about four months later, the patient complaining of excruciating pain in the region of the liver, which was markedly enlarged, and also of pain in the lumbar portion of the spine. Unfortunately, no post-mortem could be secured; but the evidences of metastatic deposits were unquestionable.

Rapid progress of the disease is indicated by the softening of the tumor, by the rapid infiltration of the whole breast, and also by the infiltration of the infra- and supra-clavicular glands.

Gross says that the average time of the appearance of ulceration in carcinoma is nineteen and nine-tenths months. Immobility on subjacent tissues occurs on an average after twenty-nine and nine-tenths months. Infection of the opposite breast occurred in 2.85 per cent. of cases. The statistics of various observers as to the age at which carcinoma appears with the greatest frequency differ but little. Winiwarter found the age of greatest frequency to be from forty-one to forty-five years, Oldekopf from forty-six to fifty, the youngest being twenty-five years and the oldest seventy years. Oldekopf says that 53.7 per cent. appear during the period of menstrual activity; 31 per cent. appear during the climacteric, or from the ages of forty-nine to fifty-eight; 15.3 per cent. appear after the climacteric, or after the age of fifty-nine. The youngest patient observed by Poulsen was twenty and one-half years old; the oldest was seventy-six; the largest number were from forty to forty-four.

Lücke among one hundred and fifty-seven cases found the age of greatest frequency to be from forty-six to fifty years. Henry among one hundred and eighty-three cases found the greatest frequency to be from forty-six to fifty. Eichels among one hundred and fourteen cases found the greatest number to be between fifty-one and fifty-five. Gross among 1622 collected gives the age of greatest frequency as from forty to fifty; the second period from fifty to sixty. Whereas 18.8 per cent. were during the age of greatest activity, or up to the age of forty, 81.2 per cent. were after that age, or during the period of functional decline. In 1545 women in whom the social condition was given, 85.5 per cent. were or had been married and 14.5 per cent. were single. Of 627 women mentioned, 66.5 per cent. were in excellent health, 20.57 per cent. were in moderate health. Among all these cases collated, Billroth's statistics show his patients to have averaged the youngest. In explanation of this fact, he states that most of his statistics were taken from operations performed upon Poles, Hungarians, and Jewesses, who develop, as a rule, younger than the inhabitants of Northern Europe.

As to the effect of age, Dennis says that the older the patient is, within certain limitations, the more malignant the carcinoma; the nearer the gland is to a healthy functional activity, the less likely it is to assume malignancy.

The great frequency of cancer is shown by the statement of Dennis, that there were 1387 deaths from carcinoma of the breast in this country in the year 1880. Williams says that of eighty-six cases of cancer of the breast, forty-four were in women of dark complexion and forty-two in women of fair complexion. According to the statistics given by Billings, the deaths from cancer in 100,000 whites and blacks were 27.96 of whites and 12.17 of blacks. As to the proportion of carcinoma to other tumors, Billroth states that he had seen in all four hundred and forty tumors of the breast, and of these three hundred and seventy-five were carcinoma. Orth places carcinoma as forming eighty per cent. of all mammary tumors. As to the proportion in the right and left breast, Gross says that of 1664 cases the seat of tumor was 4.54 per cent. more common in the left than in the right breast, and of these it occurred in both breasts in two cases only. Its most common seat was in the upper and outer portion of the breast, or in 46.22 per cent. of cases; its next most common seat was in the neighborhood of the nipple, or 28.17 per cent. Oldekopf places the proportion of cases in the right and left breasts as six to five, being directly the opposite of the observations made by Gross. Dennis says that carcinoma occurs in both breasts in about five per cent. of all cases.

Pick says that recurrence of cancer in the opposite breast cannot be explained on the supposition that the cancer germs remaining have travelled from one breast to the other. He believes that both breasts must have been in a condition of cessation of function favorable to such changes. Terrillon says that he four times removed both breasts for carcinoma, but states that this is a very rare condition, and that the invasion of both breasts by tumor is usually a sign of benignity. The occurrence of carcinoma in both breasts is cited by Segay, Crawford, Nunn, and De Morgan. The location of carcinoma is placed by Dietrich as most common in the upper and outer quadrant, and next to this in the outer quadrant.

Various causes have been assigned for the production of carcinoma. In examining into trauma as a cause, Gross cites 1511 cases in which the trauma was assigned as a cause in 13.36 per cent., but in only about one-fourth of these was it shown that the carcinoma developed from the indurations following the injury. He says that the sole causes predisposing to carcinoma are age, irritation, and inheritance. Jonathan Hutchinson says that advanced age gives proclivity, local irritation excites, and subsequently hereditary transmission may perpetuate. Social condition and childbearing seem to have no influence. Dennis considers marriage as increasing the frequency of carcinoma, and traumatism as having some influence.

The question of lactation has also received extended consideration. Dietrich[1] among sixty-eight cases of carcinoma found that nineteen per cent. had nursed more than six children. On the other hand, twenty-eight per cent. did not nurse at all. Both he and Winiwarter conclude that the failure to nurse children, as well as the nursing of a large number of children, increases the liability to carcinoma.[2]

A comparison made by Dietrich of married and single women shows carcinoma to be relatively more frequent among the former. In speaking of these statistics, Billroth says that statistics do not show that childbearing favors carcinoma, though he does not criticise minute statistics on this subject. All that can be concluded concerning the subject is that the mamma, from the peculiar method of its development and periodical function, is especially liable to the growth of tumors. The statistics as to the influence of married and single life demonstrate little except that single women are not free from carcinoma.

Oldekopf and Dietrich consider mastitis a predisposing cause of cancer. The same they hold to be true of trauma, especially if it results in the extravasation of blood. On this point Gross cites one hundred and twenty

---

[1] Deut. Zeitsch. f. Chirurg., 1892, p. 472.
[2] Archiv f. Klin. Chirurg., 1879, p. 542.

cases of mastitis or abscess, in only forty-nine of which could it be demonstrated that the growth developed from the lump left from inflammation, and in only seven was the inflammation recent.  These facts and the occurrence of carcinoma in sterile females render mastitis a doubtful cause.  Billroth thinks that women who have had mastitis are more likely to have tumors in their breasts than those who have not.

As to the generalization of carcinoma, Billroth says it is probable that both the continuance and the separate points of cancerous infection result from a conveyance of cellular elements, but that this has not been anatomically established.  It is only in the glands of the axilla, as a rule, that the same cancerous structure can be discovered as in the original growth.  He thinks that the corpuscular elements of the small-cell infiltration possess the same power of infection as the epithelial cells, and when carried to other localities produce ulceration and inflammatory processes, without carrying with them epithelial cells.

Among the diagnostic signs of cancer, retraction of the nipple has been considered as classic.  Not only may retraction occur at the nipple, but other portions of the integument may be similarly affected.  Billroth says that when pain is present it should receive consideration, and discharge of a reddish-brown fluid from the nipple may occur not only with carcinoma, but with other tumors as well, and even without any tumor ; so that it cannot be regarded as a positive sign of malignancy.  Of the retraction of the nipple and dimpling of the skin, Gross says that they are important signs ; but these must be distinguished from those cases in which the breast is pushed outward around the nipple, where the latter can be made to project again by pressure.  Retraction of the nipple occurred in 52.17 per cent. of Gross's cases, and, since it occurs in only 5.22 per cent. of non-carcinomatous cases, it is a valuable sign.  Out of two hundred and seven cases, Gross found discharge of a watery or bloody material in only fifteen cases.

A special cachexia has often been described as peculiar to carcinoma.  Oldekopf (*loc. cit.*) does not believe that there is such a cachexia.  Gross, among four hundred and seventeen cases in whom this point is noted, found that 66.55 per cent. were in excellent health, while only 20.57 per cent. were in indifferent or moderate health, and 12.92 per cent. were broken down from the disease.  He says that scarcely one in twenty suffers in health previous to sixteen months after the detection of the disease.  Billroth says that the appearance of the patient is of little significance : in the beginning she looks perfectly well ; the cachexia comes later, with involvement of other organs and septic fever.

The metastatic deposits of carcinoma, as has been stated, occur more commonly through the lymph- than through the blood-channels, differing in this respect from sarcoma.  Gross says that in one out of every seven cases this deposit may occur without infection of the lymph-glands.  He further states that among seven hundred and twenty-eight patients metastatic deposits had formed, or were presumed to have formed, in two hundred and four cases, or 28.02 per cent. As indicated by section, they were present in fifty-one per cent of the cases.

Poulsen (*loc. cit.*) places frequency of metastatic deposits in the following order : 1, pleura ; 2, liver ; 3, lungs.

Speaking of metastatic deposits in the bodies of the vertebræ, Billroth says that they pursue a rapid course, being exceedingly painful, and thus different from caries. He says he knows of no condition causing so much suffering.

Snow states that thickening of the upper end of the humerus and sternum occurs not infrequently in carcinoma mammæ as a result of the disease. He says that the manubrium of the sternum is the most common seat of such involvement, and he thinks the condition would be more frequently observed if examinations were made for it.

Infection.—Infection in cases of carcinoma takes place by direct extension and through the circulation, it being most common through the lymph-channels, towards the axilla and the region below and above the clavicle. Orth says that infection may be carried to the anterior mediastinum. He says that infection of the internal viscera and bone probably takes place through the blood-current. The bones most often affected are the upper end of the humerus, the spinal column, and the upper extremity of the femur.

The growth of carcinoma often infiltrates the integument by direct extension, and may penetrate it, causing open ulceration. These points may become so generalized as to form an indurated mass over the entire front of the thorax, causing what is called cancer *en cuirasse.* It may project internally, involving the pectoralis major and ribs and even the pleura. As has been said, the lymph-vessels play an important part in the spreading of infection. According to Sappey, the lymph-vessels of the breast form two planes : first, a superficial or cutaneous, constituting a net-work which surrounds the breast and nipple ; second, a deep system of prodigious richness surrounding each of the lobes and lobules of the gland ; all the trunks of this net-work direct themselves from the surface and depth of the gland towards the nipple, where they form a plexus remarkable for the large size of the vessels which compose it. From this plexus surrounding the nipple, two, and sometimes three, large trunks direct themselves towards the glands of the axilla.

Heidenhain has written a very interesting paper upon the lymphatics of the breast, and in it cites the above quotation from Sappey, together with the investigations of Sorgius and Langhans. He says that these authors agree in the arrangement of the lymph-vessels, but that Langhans and himself hold that the deeper lymph-channels, instead of being directed towards the nipple, are directed posteriorly, accompanying the veins along the fascia covering the pectoralis major.

He holds that the infection is transmitted by means of the carrying of infected cells along the lymph-channels, and that this is the only means of explaining the distribution of cancerous cells to considerable distances. He further says that in the extremities and in the penis returns of malignant disease are usually in the next-lying glands, and there is no evidence of disease of the lymph-channels lying between them. In the breast this does not seem to be true. This, perhaps, is due to the fact that the channels are not direct, but are bent.

Speaking of infection, Poulsen says that the time when carcinoma becomes adherent to the skin and the pectoralis major varies widely with the character of the growth and the individual case. Oldekopf says that movable carcinoma infects more early the axillary glands, while if fixed to the pectoralis major the glands are infected later. The movable form infects the glands in from twelve to sixteen months; fixed carcinoma in from thirteen to twenty-six months. The conclusions reached by Heidenhain[1] are,—First, the pectoralis fascia is very thin, especially in fat women, and is difficult to separate from the muscle without removing the muscle or portions of it. Second, the mamma of thin women lies directly on the muscle, and in fat women small lobes are similarly situated, so that in amputating above the fascia, portions of the mamma are easily left behind. Third, every breast in which there is a carcinomatous nodule is diseased to a wide extent, perhaps throughout, the epithelium of the acini becoming proliferated with an accompanying pernicious growth of connective tissue, and recurrent foci are perhaps due to the proliferating acini which remain behind in the wound. Fourth, in the retro-mammary fat there are usually accompanying blood-vessels from the glands to the lymph-channels in the fascia; in two-thirds of the cases of carcinoma of the breast there are small microscopic metastases in these lymph-channels; the epithelial growth extends rapidly through these pre-existing channels, even through thick layers of fat, down to the fascia. Fifth, the pectoralis major is, as a rule, undiseased so long as the carcinoma is freely movable upon it; it is diseased first when a metastatic nodule of the fascia grows into the muscle, or when the primary disease, through continuous growth, attaches itself to the muscle. Probably the cancer itself extends into the lymph-channels of the muscle and forces its way from these between the muscle-fibres. Sixth, probably by contractions of the muscle the epithelial cells are pushed with the lymph-stream into the muscle. A cancerous muscle seems in its entire extent to be suspicious.

Volkmann was the first to point out the necessity of removing the fascia covering the pectoralis major, in order to escape recurrence of the disease. Heidenhain says that he is convinced that carcinomata which have reached the lymph-channels—and this is true of the majority of cases—have already reached the surface of the pectoralis major independent of the thickness of the fat. He also pointed out that the muscle itself remained for a long

---

[1] Deut. Gesell. f. Chir., 1889, p. 58.

time unaffected, and it is his belief that the lymph-passages above the pectoralis major run parallel to it, but not into the muscle. He says that from physiological and pathological investigations we may conclude that the muscle remains sound as long as the carcinoma has not grown fast to and into it. He collected sixty-five cases of carcinoma adherent to muscle, the cases being those of Volkmann, Küster, and Helfreich. Among these were only two positive cures, seven relative cures, and fifty-six deaths. He concludes that the attachment of the tumor to the pectoralis major renders the prognosis very bad. Six of the relative cures lasted from one-half to one and three-fourths years. One died after two and one-half years, probably from metastasis. He also thinks that recurrences of carcinoma in the skin from portions remaining behind in it are rare. These secondary infections of the skin he thinks arise from portions of the growth remaining in the deeper tissues.

**Axillary Glands.**—The question of enlargement of the axillary glands, in its relation to carcinoma mammæ, is one which has attracted attention for many years, but its true importance has not been so long recognized. Formerly it was common to advise that operations for carcinoma mammæ should be deferred until all the symptoms belonging to the disease had made themselves clear, such as retraction of the nipple, involvement of the skin, and perhaps enlargement of the axillary glands. If the glands of the axilla were not found to be enlarged, even at a later date, the breast was removed without attention being paid to them; whereas more recently the opinion has rapidly gained credence that in a large majority of cases the axillary glands are involved and demand removal as imperatively as the breast itself. This method was first insisted upon as one universally to be followed by Küster. In 1883, and from time to time thereafter, he made statements as to the large proportion of cases in which the axillary glands were found to be infected after operation, even though they could not be felt before. In 1887 he stated that in operations upon one hundred and sixty-three cases of carcinoma mammæ he found enlarged axillary glands one hundred and fifty-eight times, or in 97 per cent of his cases. Before operation they could be felt in one hundred and seventeen cases, or 71.77 per cent.; in forty-three cases, or 26.25 per cent., they could not be felt before operation, and still they were found at the operation. Rotter, reporting the cases of Von Bergmann's clinic, cites one hundred and fourteen cases operated upon, the axillary glands being found to be involved in all but two cases. Speaking of supra-clavicular glands, Billroth says that while they may be indistinctly observed before operation, after the removal of the breast and axillary glands they may at first enlarge, and later, through fatty degeneration, contract and almost wholly disappear. The infection of the axillary glands follows the beginning of the disease in from fourteen to eighteen months, taking place a little earlier when the primary growth is in the upper and outer quadrant of the breast.

Gross cites one hundred and ninety-two cases of local dissemination noted by Török and Wellalshöps. There was invasion of the glands in 52.6 per cent. and metastasis in 72.9 per cent. Of one hundred and seventy-four cases free from local infection, the glands were affected in 42.5 per cent. and there were metastases in 45.4 per cent. These statistics are from a record of three hundred and sixty-six post-mortem examinations. One-half of the cases had been operated upon. He says that the seat of tumor does not seem to influence the time of the involvement of the axillary glands. Heidenhain quotes Küster as saying that among ninety-five cases of recurrence he saw but one recurrence in the axilla. Gross says recurrences in the axillary glands are more frequent by twenty-seven per cent. in cases in which they were not removed than in those in which they were removed at the same time with the breast. Oldekopf says that in cases requiring extirpation of the axillary glands the patients live less time than those in whom the glands cannot be felt before operation. It must be remembered, however, that the former cases are those of long continuance. Poulsen cites thirteen cases of carcinoma of from one month's to five years' standing, in which the patients died with recurrence in the axilla, no enlarged axillary glands being felt before operation, and hence the axilla not being opened. He also cites twenty-four cases of a similar sort in which the breast was removed and the axilla was not opened. Of these twenty-four cases, twenty were living and free from recurrence for periods varying from five to thirteen and one-half years. Two died of phthisis after four and five and one-half years, showing no signs of recurrence. He records twenty other cases in which recurrence took place in the axillary glands; in all, the return was during the first year. In one-half of these cases the axilla had not been cleared, because the glands could not be felt to be enlarged. His conclusion is that the axilla should always be cleared.

As to the time existing before operation, Gross records one hundred and forty-six cases in which the history of the operation could be followed. The average time of the existence of the disease before operation was thirteen and three-tenths months; the average time of cure was five years and nine months. Dietrich, writing upon this point, says that in the cases which he reports the disease had existed seventeen and two-tenths months before operation. He cites also the cases reported by Schmidt from Küster's clinic, to the effect that while from 1872 to 1880 64 per cent. of cases had existed one year before operation, during the last ten years only 35.5 per cent. had existed over one year.

Kortweg,[1] in comparing the statistics gathered from Winiwarter, Oldekopf, Sprengel, Hildebrand, and Küster,—three hundred and twenty-two cases in all,—in which the length of time before operation and the length of life after the operation were recorded, says the tables show that the longer the time during which a tumor existed before operation the longer the

---

[1] Deut. Zeitsch. f. Chir., 1892, p 480.

patient lived afterward. He concludes from this that the more malignant tumors, through pain and rapid growth, etc., attract attention and come earlier to operation, while the less malignant ones are operated upon later. He believes that some tumors are relatively much more malignant than others, and that in such cases one should be more conservative about operation.

The various opinions which have existed and still exist concerning the curability of carcinoma by operation are very interesting, and may perhaps be explained by the different operative procedures which have been in vogue. The old method was simply to extirpate the malignant nodule from the breast, taking but a small amount of additional tissue and leaving the axilla unopened. If we can trust statistics, the more radical methods now in vogue produce far better results, and it is perhaps due to this difference of method that the different opinions held by able men have come to exist. In this connection it will be of interest to cite the opinions held by eminent surgeons unfavorable to operation.

First among them we shall quote Paget,[1] who says, " In deciding for or against the removal of a cancerous breast in any single case, we may dismiss all hope that the operation will be a final remedy for the disease. I will not say that such a thing is impossible, but it is so highly improbable that the hope of its occurrence in any single case cannot be reasonably entertained." He further says, " I am not aware of a single clear instance of recovery,—that is, with a patient who lived for more than ten years free from the disease or with the disease stationary."

Hodges,[2] a man of wide experience and an acute observer, says, " I have never known but one instance of seemingly prolonged life after removal of cancer of the breast. I cannot expunge the belief that patients with cancer of the breast are, as a rule, better off without than with an operation, or that their cure, if cured they are to be, lies in some as yet undiscovered remedial measure of coming surgery rather than in extending a mutilation which, whether limited or comprehensive, must always remain *immedicabile vulnus.*"

On the other hand, the statistics of many able surgeons must be taken as proof that carcinoma can be cured by operation. Dennis says that the returns three years after removal amount to scarcely two per cent. The celebrated dictum of Volkmann[3] is, that when an entire year has passed after the operation and no symptoms of local recurrence, enlarged glands, or infection of the viscera can be found on the most careful examination, one may begin to hope that a permanent result has been reached. After two years the result is commonly permanent, and after three years it is almost sure to be so.

Billroth, after citing this opinion of Volkmann, says that if after one

---

[1] Paget's Pathology, London, 1876, p. 657.

[2] Boston Medical and Surgical Journal, November, 1888, p. 523.

[3] Volkmann's Beiträge zur Chirurgie, Leipsic, 1875, p. 325.

year a thoroughly experienced surgeon can find absolutely no sign of recurrence of disease, the patient may be looked upon as cured.

Oldekopf (*loc. cit.*) says that recurrences are rare after three years.

As to the length of life of patients with and without operation the following table is given by Dietrich:

|  | No Operation (Months). | Operation (Months). |
|---|---|---|
| Winiwarter . . . . . . . . . . . . . . . . . . . . | 32.9 | 39.3 |
| Henry . . . . . . . . . . . . . . . . . . . . . . | 26 | 39.6 |
| Fink . . . . . . . . . . . . . . . . . . . . . . . | 20.5 | 27.4 |
| Sprengel . . . . . . . . . . . . . . . . . . . . . | 27 (?) | 34.7 |
| Oldekopf . . . . . . . . . . . . . . . . . . . . . | 22.6 | 38.1 |
| Schmidt. . . . . . . . . . . . . . . . . . . . . . | (?) | 32.4 |
| Lücke . . . . . . . . . . . . . . . . . . . . . . | 24 | 31.2 |

It will thus be seen that, so far as we can judge from statistics, operation markedly increased length of life. It must be remembered, however, that the patients who were not operated upon may have been refused operation because of their hopeless condition when observed, and hence the table may not properly represent the length of life under the two conditions.

Gross cites one hundred and seventeen patients dying without operation, with an average length of life of 28.6 months. Of six hundred and sixty-five dying after operation, with recurrence demonstrated or suspected, the average length of life was 38.5 months. Poulsen says that the average length of life for operated cases was 4 years, and for unoperated cases 5.9 years. Omitting cases of slowly growing cancer existing from ten to forty years, the length of life was, for cases operated upon 3.4 years, for cases not operated upon 2.3 years. These represent two hundred cases operated upon and fifty in which no operation was done. Dietrich cites Lücke as saying that cancer can undoubtedly be cured. The prognosis depends upon: 1, early operation; 2, radical removal. Dennis says the earlier the disease can be detected, the better the prognosis as regards recurrence. If a tumor can be radically removed within six months from its incipiency, and the axilla can be thoroughly cleared, the prognosis will yield brilliant results not before realized. Kortweg, notwithstanding his unfavorable opinion concerning the results of operation, advocates the early and complete removal of tumors and glands, as promising more than anything else in good cases and as being the only chance in bad cases.

Dowd[1] cites cases in which carcinoma and sarcoma were developed after many years from what seemed to be benign growths. Similar cases are reported by Oldekopf, Hutchinson, and Pompinel. I have recently had an opportunity of observing such a case in a woman sixty-four years of age. With her second and last lactation, at the age of thirty-one years, she observed a small nodule in the right breast, which remained quiescent

---

[1] New York Medical Record, April, 1892, p. 436.

until within six months, when it began to enlarge with considerable rapidity. A few days ago I found on examination that the lump had attained a diameter of about two inches, with unmistakable evidences of malignancy, and that the axillary glands were extensively enlarged.

Recurrences.—Recurrences may occur either in the axilla or in the internal viscera. Schmidt gives statistics concerning ninety-five patients observed by Küster, all of whom died with recurrence. Fifty-nine had local recurrences in the scar, skin, muscle, or carcinoma en cuirasse.

Of thirty-four recurrences recorded by Rotter, thirty were in the region of the mamma, twelve were complicated later by growths in the supra- and infra-clavicular regions, and in six cases these pushed downward into the axilla. Six recurred in the other breast. Only one had involvement of the axilla alone. Of one hundred and seven cases which he reports as surviving the operation, thirty-four were cured.

Gross collected one thousand and thirty-six cases operated upon, having local reproductions in 66.86 per cent. Recurrence took place in 44.14 per cent. in three months. After one year there were but 15.5 per cent. of recurrences, and after three years there were only 2.32 per cent. Dennis estimates the recurrence of cancer after extirpation as about 75 per cent. of all cases. Poulsen, reporting two hundred and seventy-five patients, says that in one hundred and seventy-four, or in 63 per cent., there was local recurrence. In sixty-eight cases the recurrent growths were extirpated, but in only five of these did there remain immunity from recurrence for three years. In the other cases there was renewed recurrence or the patient died within a short time; 80 per cent. of all recurrences were within the first year. Oldekopf says 46.4 per cent. of recurrences are within three months; after one year only 16 per cent. take place. Küster reports one case of recurrence five years after operation.

In speaking of his cures, Dennis says, " In my list of cases permanently cured all were under fifty excepting one; in all cases in which there was return followed by death the patients were over fifty years." He concludes that there is less malignancy in carcinoma affecting the breast in the early stages of obsolescence of the gland tissue than when the gland has fully completed its degenerative changes. He suggests that the irritation of the cicatrix remaining after the removal of a carcinoma may be a potent factor in causing recurrence, since the recurrent nodules are found near the cicatrix. Consequently, he advises that the cicatrix be carefully protected from irritation.

Rieffel,[1] assistant of Tillaux, speaking of recurrent disease, concludes, " It is caused, first, by imperfect removal of the gland, prolongations of the disease having escaped the operator's notice; second, even if the entire gland has been removed, infection has gone beyond the limits of the gland, either in subcutaneous cellular tissue, the skin, or pectoralis major. Fre-

---

[1] Thèse de Henri Rieffel, Paris, 1890.

quent recurrences of growth in this neighborhood suggest the possibility of their seat being in the pre-muscular tissue." He says that nothing is understood of the late recurrence of the disease.

Terrillon concludes that recurrence seems to be the rule with extirpation of the breast when the axillary glands are involved. Recurrence is most common in early years, and patients do not survive more than six or seven years. He reports from 1880 to 1890 one hundred extirpations of the breast, and concludes that tumors with infected axillary glands have a malignancy almost fatal.

Dennis reports seventy-one cases of tumor of the breast operated upon, with only one death, which occurred in a patient with hæmophilia. Among these were thirty-three pure carcinomata; in two the result was unknown. Of the remaining thirty-one cases, eight, or a little more than 25 per cent., were living after three years. Besides these, there were a number approaching the three-year limit, so that he estimates his cures at about 30 per cent. Gross, uniting his own cases with those of Banks, places the percentage of permanent cures at 20.86. Among Gross's own cases he found the axillary glands involved in 87.5 per cent. Among forty-three operated on by Gross and ten by his colleagues in the same hospital, there was a mortality of 3.7 per cent.

Poulsen says, of two hundred and forty-two operations, twenty-two per cent., or fifty-five cases, lived free from recurrence for three years or more. Of these fifty-five cases, five were without microscopic examination. Of fifty patients living and free from recurrence from three to fifteen and one-half years, there were six that later had recurrence,—namely, in three, three and one-half, four and three-fourths, six, and nine years after operation,—and five cases had died. Of these operations, some were for amputation of the tumor or breast alone and some were connected with clearing of the axilla.

Butlin says, "I am confident that we may regard operations for the removal of mammary cancer as successful in effecting a complete cure in rather more than ten per cent. of all cases treated. I believe that a percentage of twelve to fifteen is nearer true." From a consideration of the more modern statistics, it seems probable that with the awakening of the profession to the necessity of the early recognition and removal of carcinoma mammæ, results heretofore unexpected may be attained, and that instead of ten per cent. of cures after extirpation, even thirty to forty per cent. may be realized.

Paget's Disease.[1]—In 1874, Paget[2] described a condition of the breast characterized at first by eczema and later by carcinoma. To this has been given his name. The disease is described by Wickham[3] as one which always begins in the nipple with small crusts, which form repeatedly upon it. This condition may continue for years. After a time ulceration takes

---

[1] See chapter on Cutaneous Diseases.
[2] St. Barthol. Hosp. Rep., 1874.
[3] Thesis on Paget's Disease, London, 1890, p 232.

place and gradually extends into the tissues beyond the nipple. This has been described as occurring in concentric rings about the nipple and areola. The nipple gradually becomes retracted. The rapidity with which the cancerous condition of the breast appears after the ulceration varies widely. It has been described as occurring within a year or two, and in other cases as not occurring until after years, even up to fifteen or twenty. Barling describes a case of this sort, beginning in an intractable eczema lasting during six months and accompanied by suspicious nodules of the breast. The nipple showed an abraded surface, but no ulcer. Running inward from the nipple was an indurated cord one and one-half inches in length, ending in a nodule the size of a bean. On removal, this enlargement was shown to be a carcinoma.

The effect of coccidia or psorosperms has been extensively studied in connection with this disease. Among those who have called attention to this condition are Darier, Hutchinson, and others. J. Hutchinson, Jr., presented before the London Chirurgical Society specimens of eczema of the breast illustrating various appearances in the surface epithelium, which he believed to confirm Darier's statement that coccidia or psorosperms are to be found in these conditions, sometimes in great numbers. He says that these appearances have not been found in cases of eczema other than the chronic condition known as Paget's disease, neither are they found in all supposed cases of the latter. He observed them in three out of five cases. Duret considers the coccidia to be the cause of the eczema which results in epithelioma. Orth says that the eczema of Paget's disease is supposed to be due to a round parasite. Oldekopf, among his series of cases, cites only one of carcinoma with eczema. Bowlby reports five cases; in two there was eczema of the nipple without tumor, and this went to show that the disease of the nipple might precede disease of the breast. On the other hand, Thin holds the disease to be malignant dermatitis of the epithelium, affecting the mouths of the milk-ducts, and believes the eczema to be secondary rather than primary. Delbet says that the coccidia are not proved to be the cause of Paget's disease. The psorosperm has been studied, especially in rabbits, by Malassez, and these germs are held to be the cause of malignant disease by Darier, Albarran, Wickham, Hutchinson, and O'Neil, especially in Paget's disease. Delbet says that other interpretations of the disease have been given by Cornil, Faber, Domergue, and others. He questions, however, whether there is any such disease, and whether the two conditions—cancer and eczema—may not be coincident. Wickham advises immediate operation as soon as diagnosis is made. Delbet says that one should wait until the cancer is fully developed, since it may never appear.

**Villous-Duct Cancer and Tubular Cancer.**—Under these heads are described forms of growth which by some are considered identical and by others as separate conditions. In speaking of these, Orth says that there are developments of cysts containing villous growths which may be slight or may entirely fill the cyst. The cyst-wall is smooth, and is probably a dilated duct. The villous growths are probably carcinomatous, being due to the development of carcinoma in the wall of a duct, and its subsequent distention. It is possible that the disease described by Reclus, and in some instances followed by carcinoma, may be developed in this manner.

Williams speaks of growths which he describes as "tubular cancers," being conditions which are relatively rare, and says that they are associated with cysts and intra-cystic papillary growths. He questions if they may not be the later development of a villous-duct cancer of many years' standing. He says that from the columnar type of cells and the tubular form assumed by the ingrowths it may be inferred that the growths originate from the mammary ducts. The growths are usually nodular, and the nipple is not retracted nor is the skin involved. He uses the term "tubular" in a different sense from that used by Billroth. Cases have also been described by Shattuck, and one has been described by Butlin. Williams says that the youngest patients are forty and the oldest sixty-five and one-half years; the average age of eighteen cases was fifty-three and one-half years. Williams advises the amputation of the breast exactly as in scirrhous diseases, but the axilla need not be cleared unless absolutely involved, since this variety of cancer is more limited than scirrhus. Williams considers villous-duct cancer identical with Billroth's tubular cysto-adenoma, Gross's true adenoma, and Cornil and Ranvier's *carcinome villeux*. He says that it is composed of a slender framework of fibrous tissue lined by one or more layers of columnar epithelium. It is a perfectly innocent growth, though often multiple, has no tendency to local infection, does not become disseminated into adjacent lymph-glands or into the system at large, and when completely removed never recurs. Villous papillomata develop later than fibro-adenomata and carcinomata, and are most liable to be confounded with scirrhus or sarcoma. When the disease is diffused the whole gland must be removed.

Routier says that if the breast is not attacked throughout by nodules, but only in places here and there a prominent point appears, and if, above all, there is a discharge of blood by the nipple, the diagnosis is *épithéliome dendritique*. There can be no doubt as to the diagnosis, provided that the skin is adherent, the axillary glands are involved, and the nipple is retracted. As to prognosis, if one operates upon a true cyst, the cure is permanent. The prognosis after the removal of an *épithéliome dendritique* is doubtful, the danger being the same as after the removal of cancer, although such growths are to be placed among the least malignant.

Robinson describes, under the head of duct papillomata, what Bowlby calls duct cancer. The name applied by Cornil and Ranvier is *carcinome villeux*. Dubet calls them *épithéliome dendritique*. Labbé and Coÿne call them *épithéliome intra-canaliculaire*. Bowlby[1] cites a case with two recur-

---

[1] Lancet, London, vol. i., 1892, p. 860.

rences, Butlin[1] a case with five, while Robinson reports one. The latter states that duct adenomata and carcinomata are associated with duct cysts. These are growths appearing in dilated milk-ducts, and not filling them as do duct papillomata; they may be sessile or villous forms and extend into the cyst. He says that this pedunculated duct adenoma may be multiple, and the prognosis seems to be favorable. The malignant disease may be implanted on the duct cysts. With its advent there may be pain and retraction of the nipple and the skin becomes involved. The disease progresses more slowly than scirrhus, and the glands are not so frequently involved. He suggests exploratory incision. If the growth is pedunculated, local removal may suffice; if it is nodular, total removal is indicated. He thinks that there is a similarity between duct carcinoma and Paget's disease, and details one case in which the same forms were present in the epithelium that were described by Darier and Wickham as coccidia in Paget's disease. Bowlby[2] reports twenty-one cases of duct cancer, thirteen of which were his own and eight belonged to other surgeons. There were four patients under forty years of age, five between forty and fifty, eight between fifty and sixty, and three between sixty and seventy. In ten of his own cases blood-stained fluid exuded from the nipple, and this was noted also in some of the others. The nipple and areola were not affected, the growths were close to the nipple, and the axillary glands were not involved. In three cases there was return after removal. No case had proved fatal up to the time of writing; one patient had remained well nine years, and others six, five, and four years. The growths are sometimes multiple in the same breast; they are firm and elastic or else knotted to the touch, not hard and nodular like scirrhus. On section, they are found to be encysted, soft and friable, and blood-stained. A portion of the villous growth may even protrude through a dilated nipple. Although the tumors may recur locally, they are not so prone to do so, or to affect the glands, as is scirrhus. They are classed as carcinomata, since they grow from the epithelium of the ducts and infiltrate the tissues around them. They occur, as a rule, in women older than those with sarcoma, and do not grow so rapidly as sarcoma. Their treatment is extirpation.

Diagnosis.—The diagnosis of the various diseases of the breast is often made with great difficulty, but there are signs which are of importance and which may lead to the establishment of the proper conclusion.

Speaking of carcinoma, Gross says that pain occurred in 88 per cent. of all cases. In a series of 1414 cases in which the facts were noted, there were adhesion and discoloration of the skin in 10.44 per cent. of the cases and ulceration in 23.9 per cent. The average time at which infection of the skin takes place is 15.8 months. As to the diagnosis of carcinoma, Billroth says that an error can occur after careful investigation, in mis-

---

[1] St. Barth. Hosp. Rep , vol. xxiv.
[2] Lancet, London, June, 1893, p. 1369.

taking a deep cyst for a carcinoma, and that it is far better in such cases to operate than to fail to remove a carcinoma, since even the cyst may be carcinomatous.  He also says that a solid tumor developing in the breast of a woman over thirty-five years of age, which continues to increase in size, is usually carcinoma.

As to the diagnosis of tumors in general, the same author says that from the age of puberty to thirty or thirty-five years, movable, painless, and rounded tumors growing slowly may be inflammatory due to injury, or fibroids.  If the former, they will disappear or develop abscess; if they continue to grow slowly and then remain hard and nodular, perhaps turgescent and slightly painful at menstruation, they are fibromata.  If they grow slowly and constantly, they are adenomata, adeno-sarcomata, or cysto-sarcomata.  Large cysto-sarcomata are most common from twenty-five to thirty-five, and may reach an enormous size and be followed by recurrences.  Rapidly growing soft tumors (which in the beginning may be confounded with abscess) in young women are usually medullary sarcomata.  Cysts, when deep or small, are difficult to diagnosticate; if superficial, they are easy.  The majority of tumors occurring from twenty to thirty years of age are fibromata; from thirty to forty, cysto-sarcomata; from forty to fifty, carcinomata.  Dr. Welch, in a verbal communication, told me that he had frequently examined growths of the breast supposed to be benign and had found them to be malignant.

Gross says that errors may be made in the diagnosis of cases with a retracted nipple, since an abscess may be present rather than a carcinoma.  In a case of my own there were stony hardness and a retracted nipple, the growth presenting marked resemblance to a scirrhus.  No suggestion of fluctuation was present.  On incision, however, it proved to be a collection of pus, although there had been no symptoms pointing to such a condition.

**Treatment of Cancer.**—It is unnecessary to go into the history of the treatment of cancer.  Innumerable methods have been proposed.  Medication thus far has proved of no service.  There still remain three methods of treatment: first, inoculation by erysipelas; second, removal by the cautery or by caustics; third, extirpation.  The first and second methods demand a few words.

*Treatment by Inoculation with Erysipelas.*—Treatment by inoculation with erysipelas has of late attracted some attention.  An interesting report upon this subject has been made by Coley (*loc. cit.*), who has collected twenty-three cases of malignant disease accidentally inoculated by erysipelas and fifteen cases intentionally inoculated.  Of these, seventeen were carcinomata, seventeen were sarcomata, and four were either one or the other.  Of the cases of carcinoma, three patients were permanently cured, ten were improved, with undoubted lengthening of life, and one died on the fourth day.  Of the seventeen cases of sarcoma, seven patients were permanently cured, the remaining, save one, showed more or less improvement, and one died with erysipelas.  Of two cases of sarcoma treated by the toxine of erysipelas, kindly furnished me by Dr. Coley, one was a melanotic sarcoma, and could not be kept sufficiently long under treatment to allow of any conclusion being reached.   The other case—a large sarcoma of the thigh— is still under treatment, and the growth of the tumor has been markedly retarded.   Coley's conclusions are that the curative effect of erysipelas on malignant tumors is an established fact; that it acts more powerfully on sarcoma than on carcinoma; that the curative action is systemic, and is due to toxic products of the streptococcus.   His belief in the parasitic origin of malignant disease has already been stated.

*Caustics.*—Butlin (*op. cit.*) cites a record of one hundred and sixty-two cases of carcinoma treated by Bougard, in which the glands of the axilla were already involved.   According to Bougard's statement, these operations were performed without a single death, and he claims a larger percentage of cures than that obtained by extirpation.   For the purpose he uses a paste made of

| | |
|---|---|
| Wheat flour . . . . . . . . . . . . . . . . . . . . . . | 60 grammes. |
| Starch . . . . . . . . . . . . . . . . . . . . . . . . . | 60    " |
| Arsenic . . . . . . . . . . . . . . . . . . . . . . . . | 1 gramme. |
| Cinnabar  . . . . . . . . . . . . . . . . . . . . . . . | 5 grammes. |
| Sal ammoniac . . . . . . . . . . . . . . . . . . . . | 5    " |
| Corrosive sublimate . . . . . . . . . . . . . . . . . . | 0.50 gramme. |
| Solution of chloride of zinc (52 per cent.) . . . . . . . . | 245 grammes. |

Butlin, after a study of the work of Bougard, considers it sufficiently successful to require notice, but still holds to the opinion that extirpation is the preferable method.

.To avoid the dangers which formerly attended the extirpation of tumors by the knife, on account of infection, various methods have been devised. Gosselin reports, out of one hundred cases operated upon by the knife, thirty-eight deaths, while in one hundred cases operated upon by caustic arrows (*flèches*) his mortality was only five per cent.   With the knife, he says, erysipelas occurred in forty-six out of one hundred cases.   Labbé and Coÿne[1] cite the experience of Velpeau, who, after operation with the knife, had erysipelas in forty out of one hundred cases, and fourteen out of one hundred died.   His mortality with caustics was nine out of one hundred.   With the advent of aseptic surgery all this has been changed, so that the danger of erysipelas has been entirely overcome.

In this connection, Billroth says that all treatment with salves, by pressure, etc., should be abandoned.   The reasons for the abandonment of caustics are evident, since with the advent of aseptic surgery the risk is less with the knife than with caustics, there is no pain, a definite amount of tissue can be removed, and regions in which caustics would cause serious danger can be invaded by the knife with safety.   We may say that the time for the removal of carcinoma mammæ by the use of caustics

---

[1] Traité des Tumeurs bénignes du Sein.

has passed. The injection of inoperable malignant growths with a 1 to 200 aqueous solution of pyoktanin has been largely tried, having been introduced by Mosetig-Moorhof, of Vienna. Though seemingly retarding the progress of some cases, it has been of little permanent benefit.

*Extirpation.*—We now come to consider the treatment of carcinoma by extirpation. The method formerly employed has already been described, —namely, the simple removal of the tumor,—and to its prevalence is to be ascribed the failure which has attended it. To the more thorough method followed by modern operators is unquestionably due their greater success. It is only fair, however, to say that this success has been made possible less, perhaps, by greater operative skill than by the development of modern surgery. Certain cases present themselves in which positive diagnosis is impossible. Unfortunately, it is still far too common, under such circumstances, to wait until the advent of classic signs, such as retraction of the nipple, ulceration of the skin, and involvement of the axillary glands, before undertaking operation.

In this connection, Schmidt, assistant to Küster, suggests that in case of doubt an exploratory incision should be made. If the growth is malignant, it should be excised ; if it is doubtful, a piece is rapidly placed under the microscope, and if it proves to be malignant it is extirpated. If the growth is thought to be benign, it is enucleated, and is submitted to microscopical examination, and if shown to be malignant is extirpated twenty-four hours later. In the same connection, Poulsen says that every case of tumor of the breast, whether malignant or not, should be extirpated as soon as possible, even if not larger than a hazel-nut, and examined microscopically. If found to be malignant, the radical operation of removing the entire breast and clearing the axilla should be performed. He suggests that the exploratory operation should be made under cocaine. Considerable difference of opinion formerly existed as to whether, in operations upon tumors of the breast, the removal should be partial or entire. Of recent years perhaps the most prominent advocate of partial removal is Butlin (*op. cit.*), who favors it in suitable cases, holding this plan to be as successful as complete operation. He has gathered extensive statistics upon this point. The weight of opinion is, however, strongly in favor of extirpation of the entire breast.

Several extracts from Billroth cannot fail to be of interest in this connection on account of the wide experience and the unquestioned ability of this great surgeon. One cannot read his work upon diseases of the breast without being impressed by the breadth of his knowledge and the candor of his statements. He says that the sooner the diagnosis is positive and is followed by treatment the better. He lays down the principle that every tumor of the breast which continues to grow should be extirpated. He recommends the immediate removal of carcinoma, so long as this is possible without imminent danger to life, since extirpation of the tumor and axillary glands undoubtedly delays the disease. He advises the removal of growths recurring in the scar or in the axilla. While advocating total extirpation, he says he is not able to prove from his own statistics that partial extirpation is followed by earlier recurrence than total, and he believes that solid tumors which are not growing (fibromata) and scirrhus in old women may be let alone; still, there is seldom reason to refuse such patients operation, if desired. As to benign tumors, their removal is desirable, since as years advance they may increase and become malignant. There are many observations to prove that tumors quiescent for years and seemingly benign may later become malignant; besides, a tumor in the breast has a depressing influence on many women.

In the same connection, Waldeyer says, "Partial extirpation of cancerous organs is entirely useless. In cancer of the breast one should remove the entire gland, even though it seems for the most part intact. Here conservative surgery is entirely out of place. It cannot arouse any opposition when I hold that a partial removal of the organs infected with cancer is wholly useless; in fact, it is a dangerous procedure. Thus, one ought never to make a partial amputation of the breast when infected with cancer, but should always remove the entire gland, even though it seems to be not generally diseased."

Heidenhain, after a careful study of carcinoma, says, "I am thoroughly convinced that every cancerous breast is altered through its entire structure. Everywhere and widely distant from the chief seat of the disease one finds the epithelium in the acini increased in size and the lumen of the acini largely absent." Not only the entire breast, but the glands, with the afferent and the efferent vessels, are involved and should be removed.

The removal of the axillary glands is not so modern a method as has been supposed. Billroth states that it was performed by Fabricius ab Aquapendente and Fabry von Hilden, and the method was further developed by J. L. Petit. Whether it should or should not be performed is still a matter of discussion. Butlin, in discussing the subject, cites one hundred and forty-one cases in which the breast alone was amputated, and one hundred and seventy in which it was amputated together with the glands of the axilla. In the three hundred and eleven cases there were fifty-one deaths : thirty-nine were after the operation in which the axilla was opened, and twelve were after simple amputation of the breast. The deaths from the larger operation were about twice as numerous as those from the smaller. He says that it is better to remove the enlarged axillary glands by drawing them out separately or two or three at a time with the fingers, even tearing them out of the fat in which they lie, than to use the knife freely, on account of the proximity of the large vessels and nerves. If distinct cords can be felt running up into the axilla or directly to the glands, they should certainly be removed, and with them the fat and connective tissue in which they lie; but if there are no distinct cords, it is not necessary to search for the line of the lymphatic vessels or to remove a large amount of fat.

Pick[1] does not believe in dissection of the axilla in every case of malignant disease, first, because recurrence takes place in a large majority of cases in the original scar instead of in the axilla, and clearing the axilla adds materially to the mortality of the operation. He estimates this increased mortality at ten per cent. He advises an incision in the axilla and the insertion of the finger to determine the presence or absence of enlarged glands; if these are found, he advises extirpation.

Terrillon[2] says, "I am strongly of the opinion that one should not remove the glands of the axilla unless they are manifestly involved." "It is usually possible to feel them, even in a fleshy woman, upon the border of the pectoralis major on comparison with the other side, and, failing to find these, one may find indurated tissue as characteristic as the glands themselves." On the same subject, Ashhurst (loc. cit.) says, "Unless I find glandular enlargement, I prefer not to open the axilla." Bryant in ordinary cases would open and clear the axilla, but does not do this in feeble or in aged women with ulcerating cancers. He does not open the axilla unless enlarged glands are felt, and he states that in atrophic forms of cancer in people advanced in years he is opposed to operation, since the progress of the disease is usually slow when let alone, whereas when operated upon the process seems to be rendered more active and the disease speedily recurs.

As opposed to the opinions already stated, we record an interesting extract from the work of Volkmann, which is as follows : "One scarcely trusts his eyes when he reads in a recent work on operations that to remove the axillary glands one should lay bare the glands one by one, split the capsule, and shell out the glands without the loss of blood. Whoever operates in this way had better once and forever restrain his hand from carcinoma."

Terrillon[3] says that malignant and mixed tumors should be extirpated and the enlarged axillary glands removed, if they exist. Recurrent growths should be removed when possible. Banks[4] deems the old incomplete operation unscientific and useless ; by the complete operation life is prolonged and recurrences are less common. He does not hesitate to tie or remove portions of the axillary vein, if necessary. Johnston,[5] after examining a large number of amputated breasts, concludes that the entire breast, all overlying skin, and the surface of the pectoralis muscle should be removed. Deaver's[6] method is first to clear the axilla, believing that in this way there is less liability of infection of the tissues of the armpit. He favors the clearing of the axilla in all cases, and says that the dissection, if properly made, does not injure the nerves contained in the

[1] Clinical Journal, London, May 31, 1893.
[2] Bull. de Thérapeutique, Paris, 1891, p. 385.
[3] Loc. cit.
[4] Lancet, London, March, 1887, p. 627.
[5] Ibid., January, 1892, p. 89.
[6] International Clinics, Philadelphia, July, 1891, p. 131.

space and is not followed by impairment of motion such as has been supposed.

Stiles[1] concludes thus : " The principle which should underlie all operations for carcinoma of the mamma should be the complete removal, not only of the tumor and the breast, but also of as much of the surrounding tissues as are likely to contain lymphatic spaces and highways along which the malignant elements of the disease had been disseminated." Dietrich,[2] in a record of ninety-eight cases of carcinoma of the breast, states that in all, except two, not only the entire breast was removed, but the axilla was cleared. In one of the two cases the growth had been observed only two months and the other was characterized by a cyst-formation. One of these patients is still living after eight and the other after five and one-half years. Watson Cheyne,[3] after praising Stiles's method for detecting by nitric acid portions of the disease remaining after operation, concludes that in all cases there should be free removal of the skin, especially over the tumor,—very free, indeed, if the skin is actually the seat of the disease. There should be complete removal of the breast, bearing in mind its great extent, removal of the pectoralis fascia coextensive with the breast and right on to the sternum, along with a thin layer of the muscle behind the tumor and the main part of the breast, and complete clearing out of the axilla, and also of portions of the pectoralis major, if involved.

Extensive citations have thus been given with reference to the importance of removing the axillary glands, because it is only within a few years that this method has received general acceptance. It is beyond question that the great increase in cures reported during the few years past is dependent upon the more extensive and complete removal of the disease than in earlier operations, and this is the reason for the difference in statistics between early and late operators.

The dangers attending the clearing of the axilla, although great in the pre-aseptic period, have almost disappeared, and those dangers which have been feared from injury to vessels and nerves are, in the hands of skilful operators, easily avoided. It has become evident also that injury to these parts is not so serious as was formerly supposed. Billroth says that if the axillary vein is wounded it should receive a double ligature, and that death from entrance of air into the vein has been observed; also that branches of the axillary vein should be ligated two centimetres (three-fourths of an inch) from the vein, to avoid necrosis and hemorrhage. Ligation of the axillary artery does not produce the disturbance in circulation one would suppose. He has often done this, and has seldom observed œdema of the arm as a result. Langenbeck records two cases in which he was obliged to remove five centimetres of the brachial plexus with large vessels. The patients recovered from the operation, but one died one year

---

[1] British Medical Journal September, 1892, p. 673.
[2] Deut. Zeitsch. f. Chir., 1892, p. 479.
[3] Lancet, London, August, 1892, p. 358.

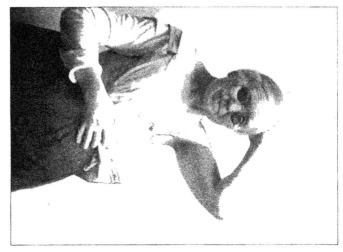

Fig. 13.

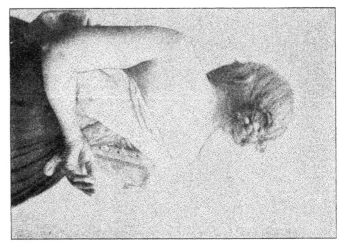

Fig. 14.

Mobility of arm after removal of pectoralis major.

later from recurrence; the other case was living after two years. In a third case he was obliged to divide also the subscapular artery, and in this case gangrene and death resulted. Esmarch, in cases where the removal of the axillary glands is otherwise impossible, advises disarticulation of the humerus, as being a better operation than division of the brachial nerves and vessels.

Von Rotter reports three cases of Von Bergmann's. In one he ligated the axillary vein, in one the axillary artery, and in one both artery and vein, without producing long-standing œdema. In one case he opened the thorax, but closed the opening at once with a moist gauze tampon, and later stitched the muscle over it and secured union by first intention.

Dennis reports a successful case in which it was necessary to remove not only the breast and the contents of the axilla, but also the pectoralis major muscle and ribs. In this same connection, Billroth says that if the pectoralis major is involved the diseased portion should be removed. Resection of the ribs is not advisable. Multiple carcinomata of the skin cannot be successfully removed. If the axillary glands compress the nerves and vessels, operation is not advisable, and amputation of the shoulder-joint is preferable to the division of nerves and vessels.

The question of the removal of the pectoral muscles has also become one of interest. Kiewicz details a case in which, in order to clear the infraclavicular fossa, both the pectoralis major and the pectoralis minor were divided. Poulsen, speaking of removing the entire pectoralis major, says, "The operation seems to me to be so great that one must well consider it." Gould[1] recommends the removal of the entire pectoralis major muscle when infiltrated by disease. Fowler[2] says that the operation is not rendered a much more serious one because of this added feature, and the functional disturbance is scarcely noticeable. Heidenhain thinks that the removal of the pectoralis major, when necessary, should be radical; it does not increase danger or bleeding, and interferes very little with the motion of the arm. In a discussion in London, the removal of the pectoralis, when infected, was recommended by Lane, but was considered inadvisable by Watson Cheyne and Eve.

The degree of mobility remaining after complete removal of the pectoralis major is shown in the accompanying plates of a woman from whom, on account of extensive involvement, it was necessary for me to remove the entire pectoralis major from the sternum to the humerus. She is now able to use the arm freely, and the degree of mobility shows that it is thoroughly satisfactory. After the breast has been removed, it requires but a moment to divide the insertion of the pectoralis from the humerus and to dissect it entire from the front of the thorax, and the hemorrhage is easily controlled.

---

[1] International Clinics, Philadelphia, 1892, vol. i. p. 217.
[2] Brooklyn Medical Journal, 1890, p. 718.

The dangers of operations for carcinoma mammæ, and their character, are illustrated by the following statistics from Billroth's clinic, recorded by Winiwarter:

Among thirty-four deaths from operation, five were due to sepsis, or 14.7 per cent.; one to carbolic-acid poisoning, or 2.9 per cent.; eight to pyæmia, or 24.4 per cent.; three to pyæmia with erysipelas, or 8.6 per cent.; thirteen to erysipelas, or 38.2 per cent.; two to hemorrhage, or 5.8 per cent.; one to pleurisy, or 2.9 per cent.; one to peritonitis, or 2.9 per cent.

These thirty-four deaths occurred in one hundred and forty-three operations at the beginning of the introduction of antiseptic surgery.

Billroth gives the following facts. Up to 1877, before antiseptic methods were introduced, he operated upon three hundred and five cases of carcinoma mammæ, with 15.7 per cent. of deaths. Of these cases, 6.7 per cent. were extirpation of the breast alone; 21.3 per cent. were extirpation of the breast and axillary glands. From 1877 to 1879 he operated upon sixty-eight cases, with 5.8 per cent. of deaths. In cases of extirpation of the breast alone there were no deaths; in those of extirpation of the breast and axilla together there were 10.5 per cent. of deaths. Of these, one was from hemorrhage and three were from sepsis. He says that, deducting deaths from hemorrhage, the percentage of deaths in sixty-eight operations was 4.4, or three cases. He closes by saying that he would not be surprised to learn that an operator might in the future reach one hundred per cent. of successful operations, since much depends upon the experience of surgeons and assistants.

Watson Cheyne,[1] speaking of Lister's operations, says that from 1871 to 1877 he performed thirty-seven excisions of the mamma antiseptically, with two deaths,—one from erysipelas, the other from septicæmia. Between 1877 and 1880, he says, Professor Lister made sixteen excisions of the breast and axillary glands, with two deaths, both operations being very extensive, the patients dying of shock within thirty-six hours.

Butlin (op. cit.), considering the same subject, takes six hundred and five cases. Five hundred and nineteen of these are from Gross, including the cases of Henry, Oldekopf, Winiwarter, and one hundred of his own. Of the six hundred and five, ninety-six, or 15.85 per cent., died from causes referable to the operation. Two or three deaths resulted from bronchitis, not referable to the operation. The majority of deaths were from pyæmia, septicæmia, and erysipelas; some were from gradual exhaustion several days after the operation, and some from pleurisy or pneumonia. He says that there is reason for believing that the latter disease may result directly from exposure during operation. Of thirty deaths reported by Henry out of one hundred and forty-seven operations, 8 per cent. followed amputation of the breast alone, and 22 per cent. followed removal of the breast and axillary glands.

---

[1] Antiseptic Surgery, p. 373.

Dietrich reports from 1870 to 1880, from forty-four operations, nine deaths; from 1880 to 1890, from one hundred and forty operations, only eight deaths. The causes of these deaths were: pneumonia, one; erysipelas, three; metastasis in the brain, one; the remaining deaths were from metastasis in other organs. During the last nine years, he says, there were no deaths from erysipelas.

Rotter reports Von Bergmann's operations as follows. One hundred and fourteen operations, with six deaths. One died from ulcer of the stomach, one from collapse after double amputation, one from embolism of the brain, one from septic pleurisy, and two later from unknown causes.

Schmidt, reporting Küster's cases, says that from 1871 to 1885 there were two hundred and twenty-two cases, with twenty-four deaths (10.81 per cent.); from 1883 to 1885, ninety-six cases, with five deaths (5.2 per cent.). Of these cases, twenty-five were in 1883, with three deaths (12.07 per cent.); twenty-five in 1884, with one death (4.7 per cent.); and forty in 1885, with one death (2.5 per cent.). In 1886 there were no deaths. The large number of deaths in 1883 is ascribed to the much greater extent of operations then undertaken, with the introduction of antiseptic surgery. Terrillon says that the operation is almost without risk. Dennis reports seventy-one cases of extirpation of the breast, with but one death, and that death occurred from hæmophilia.

It thus becomes apparent that, with the increased experience gained in aseptic surgery in operations upon the breast, not only has the percentage of permanent cures increased, but the number of deaths resulting from operation has largely diminished, and it is possible that a time is near at hand when the prophecy made by Billroth may be realized, and some surgeon may extirpate the breast and axillary glands in one hundred cases without a death.

The removal of recurrent growths is widely advocated. Billroth says that in one case he saw a permanent cure follow the third operation. Terrillon reports one in which he performed five successive operations with apparent benefit. The most remarkable is a case of spindle-celled sarcoma, reported by Gross, in which fifty-two tumors were removed by twenty-three distinct operations, and the patient was living eleven years after the last operation.

The method of operating which is most widely in vogue at the present time follows closely that which was first suggested by that great surgeon, Richard Volkmann. Küster[1] describes it as follows:

He makes a long incision below the breast, reaching from near the sternum to the axillary space. He then dissects the breast free from the thorax from below upward, making the incision above the breast last. The borders of the pectoralis major, pectoralis minor, and latissimus dorsi are laid bare. He then locates the axillary vein at the distal extremity of

---

[1] Deut. Gesell. f. Chir., 1883, p. 295.

the axillary space, which is done by cutting carefully down, with the knife laid flat, until the blue color of the vein is distinguished. Next he clears the axillary space from its lower to its upper extremity, and, by keeping the vein constantly in view, avoids injury to the axillary artery and the brachial plexus, since both are underneath the vein. It is important to preserve three nerves,—the subscapularis to the subscapular muscle, the nerve to the teres major, and the nerve supplying the latissimus dorsi. The author thinks that the impaired motion of the arm is due not to the cicatrix, but to changes in these muscles resulting from destruction of the nerve-supply. When these nerves are preserved, the motion of the arm is not hindered. The nerve destroyed is the intercosto-humeral.

One who has not performed the operation by this method can scarcely appreciate its advantages. By laying bare the axilla at its outer extremity and finding the vein, the safest possible guide is obtained to enable one to preserve it and the other important contents of the axilla from injury. Having the vein thus distinctly in view, unless the malignant infiltration of the glands, closely surrounding the vein and its branches, is very great, it is not a difficult matter, even with the sharp edge of a scalpel, rapidly to set free the entire axillary contents without serious injury to any part. If one prefers, or is inexperienced, he would probably do better with curved scissors or with the handle of a scalpel in making the dissection. By this method the axilla may easily be cleared up to the line of the clavicle. The latter part of the dissection is greatly aided by rotating the arm slightly inward and lifting it well upward by the side of the head. It is of advantage, also, to lift the pectoralis major and pectoralis minor muscles upon a blunt retractor, thus gaining space and light. The branches of the axillary vein and axillary artery can thus be easily seen and seized by a pair of hæmostatic forceps before division. It is best either to ligate these at once or to take great care in holding the forceps, lest by pulling upon them the vessels be torn off so close to the main trunks that ligation will be impossible.

In order to enable one to determine whether or not the diseased tissue has been entirely removed, Stiles[1] has recommended the following. The breast, immediately after its removal and the washing away of all blood, is placed in a five-per-cent. solution of nitric acid for about ten minutes, and is then washed in running water from three to four minutes. By this method the connective tissue becomes translucent, homogeneous, and somewhat gelatinous, and is rendered tough and like india-rubber. The parenchyma of the gland remains more or less dull grayish-white and opaque, owing to the coagulation of the highly albuminous epithelial cells; the fat is unaltered. The carcinomatous tissue behaves in the same way as the parenchyma, and is rendered even denser and more opaque. In carcinomata which are quite rich in cells the tissue resembles boiled white

---

[1] Transactions of the Medico-Chirurgical Society, Edinburgh, 1891, 1892, p. 40.

of egg, though of a grayish color. The characteristic arrangement of the parenchyma is generally sufficient to distinguish it from the cancerous tissue.

Stiles suggests that this method may be employed while the axilla is being cleared, and by it any points which have been left behind can be demonstrated on the corresponding surface of malignant tissue upon the removed breast. By marking the position in which the breast was removed, the corresponding point of tissue remaining can be found and extirpated. This method is highly praised by Chiene, of Edinburgh, and other operators.

Ashhurst (loc. cit.) says that it is important that the patient should be kept thoroughly covered during operation, since the exposure of the thorax may cause pleurisy, congestion of the lungs, and even pneumonia. He advises that the wound be kept thoroughly protected. Butlin (op. cit.), in speaking of operation, says that it is very difficult to preserve asepsis in operations on the breast, because of the axilla.

Favoring the clearing of the axilla as the primary part of the operation, upon this account, Duret[1] says partial extirpation of the breast calls for stricter antisepsis and more minute care than total extirpation, because in the former one makes large openings into lymph-spaces and milk-canals, thus giving rise to accidents of retention. These cases especially require careful drainage. He makes occasional partial extirpations in young women with limited disease, but accompanies this with the complete dissection of the axilla. Nancrede[2] says, " I now cut into the axilla first, and, if I cannot remove the glands, I close the wound and let the breast alone."

In removing the breast and clearing the axilla a large amount of tissue is exposed. It is important that this should be protected, both on account of the possibility of infection and because of the danger arising from a long exposure of the thorax, bringing with it the possibility of damage to the respiratory tract. After the breast has been extirpated up to the line of the axilla, and the divided vessels have been thoroughly secured by hæmostatic forceps, it is well to cover the wound with a sterilized towel wrung out in hot distilled water, and then to proceed with the dissection of the axilla. When this is completed the thoracic wound may be again uncovered, all forceps removed, and the few vessels which continue to bleed may be ligated. It will be found, however, that most of them have ceased. As has been previously stated, in dissecting the axilla the immediate branches of the axillary vein and axillary artery should be ligated as soon as possible, else, if the forceps are left hanging from them, they may tear openings into the vessels, causing hemorrhage difficult to control. The remaining vessels on which hæmostatic forceps have been placed may be ligated after those of the axilla have been secured. It is of primary

---

[1] Journal des Sciences Médicales de Lille, 1890, p 558.

[2] Transactions of the American Surgical Association, 1891.

importance to check thoroughly all hemorrhage, for upon this depends the successful healing of the wound.

For the operation from eighteen to twenty-four forceps are of great convenience, especially if the breast is large and very vascular.

Having stopped the hemorrhage, the wound may be united by a continuous suture. The flaps will bear much greater tension than would be supposed by one inexperienced in the operation. In inserting the continuous suture, the lower border of the wound will be found to be longer than the upper one, consequently each stitch must take in more tissue along the lower than along the upper border, and it is easy in this manner to unite the entire wound with little puckering. At times, when the amount of integument is small, it is possible to unite the surface by first stitching together the axillary extremity of the incision for about one-third of its length, then uniting the sternal portion of the incision for a similar distance, and finally uniting the central portions of the lower border of the wound to each other. When united in this manner, the wound has three lines of sutures radiating from a central point. If it is not possible thus to unite the borders of the wound without too great tension, assistance may be gained by retention sutures of silver wire, inserted some distance from the border of the wound and attached to lead plates, thus holding the flaps more firmly together; after this the borders of the wound may be united by ordinary sutures.

In cases where it has been impossible to cover the breast, on account of the large amount of integument removed, I have not hesitated to proceed at once to cover the opening by large grafts of skin taken from the thigh of the patient, after the method of Thiersch. For this purpose a broad-bladed razor is highly desirable. The skin of the thigh should be thoroughly disinfected. By holding the thigh so that the razor shall be in the horizontal position while cutting the grafts, and keeping water dropped carefully upon it, large skin-grafts can be made to lie upon the razor, and flaps be transferred having a breadth of from half an inch to one inch, and any length required, so that for one skilled in the operation but a few moments are necessary to close a large opening. The wound should be completely covered by the skin thus obtained, great care being taken to place the denuded surface of the graft thoroughly in apposition with the denuded surface of the thorax. When the opening is entirely covered, a piece of thin oil-silk protective should be placed over the grafts, extending a quarter of an inch beyond the margin of the wound. If it is not possible thus to cover the open surface at the time of the operation, on account of the feeble condition of the patient, it may be done at a later period, should the opening be sufficiently large to demand it.

In dressing the wound remaining after extirpation of the breast, whether skin-grafts are used or not, an abundant sterilized dressing is required. A good method is first to express from the wound any small amount of blood which may remain after closing it by suture. If this is done, the

FIG 15

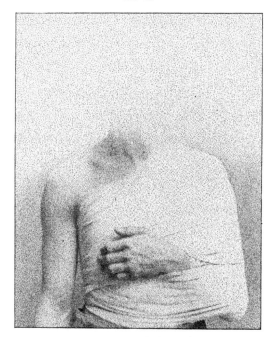

Bandage of the breast after operation.

hemorrhage having first been carefully controlled and the surface of the wound held closely in apposition before and during the application of the dressing, no blood will remain beneath the flaps and no drainage will be necessary. If one has not thoroughly stopped the bleeding, and is not expert in the application of dressings, it would be unwise to omit drainage, since otherwise the retained blood may fail to organize, and suppuration may result. After one has become thoroughly practised in the application of dressings, drainage may be done away with, and in a large proportion of cases the wound will heal through its entire extent by first intention, under the primary dressing. The dressing should cover the surface to a wide distance from the border of the wound, and a firm pad should be placed under the arm, so as to press upward into the axilla. Sufficient gauze and cotton should be put behind the arm, over the elbow, over the front of the chest, and upward above the clavicle, completely to occlude the wound. A bandage may then be placed over the entire thorax and arm, leaving out only the hand of the affected side, and over all a starch bandage, to retain the dressing thoroughly in position, so that any movement on the part of the patient shall be impossible. (Fig. 14.) The first dressing may be left from six to eight or even ten days, provided that there is no evidence of inflammation. Should inflammation arise, it will be necessary to remove the dressing earlier and to inspect the wound. Upon the removal of stitches after from six to ten days, a small strip of iodoform gauze one inch in width and from four to six layers in thickness may be laid over the wound, and long strips of adhesive plaster applied to the thoracic wall to prevent tension upon the newly-formed cicatrix.

# CHAPTER XIX.[1]

## CUTANEOUS DISEASES PECULIAR TO WOMEN.

### BY LOUIS A. DUHRING, M.D., AND MILTON B. HARTZELL, M.D.

SEX exercises an influence upon the production of diseases of the skin through peculiarities of anatomical structure, through physiological functions, and through pathological states of sexual organs. A small number of diseases of the skin occur so much more frequently in women than in men that they may be said to be peculiar to the female sex. Examples of these are Paget's disease of the nipple and impetigo herpetiformis. Other diseases, while common to both sexes, are distinguished in women by special localization and clinical symptoms due to differences in anatomy. Another distinguishing feature of these diseases is to be found in the etiological relationship which they bear to internal organs, being associated with functional and pathological disturbances of the reproductive and nervous systems. Thus, while resembling in their external features cutaneous maladies seen in man, they are noteworthy in that they are dependent upon causes associated with the sex of the subject. Anæmia and chlorosis, so much more frequent in women than in men, whether primary or secondary to disease of other organs, affect the cutaneous system as well as the general nutrition, and give rise to various skin manifestations. The mode of life of woman, while diminishing her liability to certain diseases, particularly those known as professional dermatoses, or diseases of the skin arising from occupation, favors either directly or indirectly the occurrence of others. Owing to the greater impressibility of the nervous system in females, neurotic diseases of the skin occur more frequently than in males, manifesting themselves either as structural alterations or, as is more frequently the case, as disorders of sensation.

DISEASES DUE TO SPECIAL ANATOMICAL STRUCTURE.—The skin covering organs peculiar to females is frequently the seat of disease which in many instances presents features differing from the ordinary type as seen elsewhere. The breasts are not infrequently the seat of eczema,

---

[1] In the preparation of this chapter the writers have endeavored to direct attention to the diseases of the skin which are commoner in women than in men, and to point out the sexual causes which are liable to produce them. No attempt has been made to enter upon the treatment of the diseases incidentally referred to. The aim has been to avoid as much as possible all resemblance to the style of a text-book, or treatise, on diseases of the skin.

978

which begins upon the nipple and extends to the surrounding parts, forming a circular patch having the nipple in the centre. In severe cases the nipple is retracted and covered with crusts. This variety of eczema is apt to be of long duration, and is not readily amenable to treatment. It occurs in most instances in pregnant and nursing women, particularly the latter, but is occasionally seen in the unmarried as well, in the last-named being often confined to the nipple. In this connection it may be proper to recall the fact that the nipples and areolæ are favorite localities for invasion by the itch mite, and a general eczematous eruption, in a woman, in this region more marked than elsewhere should suggest the possibility of the eruption being scabies.

In connection with eczema of the nipple, mention should be made of the malady first described by Sir James Paget, and since called by writers **Paget's disease of the nipple.** This affection usually begins upon the nipple, and spreads thence to the areola and often beyond, in some cases involving the skin over the greater part of the gland. As a rule, it is unilateral, the right side being more frequently affected than the left. It begins with the formation of corneous incrustations upon the nipple, which are firmly adherent to the underlying skin. Upon removing them, the surface beneath is seen to be reddened, superficially excoriated or ulcerated, and fissured. With the progress of the disease the areola becomes involved; its surface, at first red and covered with small scales, becomes excoriated and discharges a yellowish, viscid fluid, which soon gives rise to crusts. When fully developed, the diseased area is bright red and finely granular, oozes abundantly, is more or less circular in shape, with the nipple in the centre, and is sharply circumscribed in outline, the margins in some cases being slightly elevated above the surrounding healthy skin. These features are characteristic of the disease and serve to distinguish it from ordinary eczema of the breast, with which it is apt to be confounded, particularly in its early stages. Soon in the course of the disease parchment-like induration of the superficial tissues takes place, which feels "like a penny felt through a cloth." Retraction of the nipple is a peculiar feature, which, beginning early, sometimes leads to its complete disappearance. Itching and burning in varying degrees of intensity are present from the beginning. The general health remains unaffected until the final stages of the disease. Within a period varying from a few months to many years cancerous degeneration makes its appearance, beginning either superficially upon the ulcerating surface or, what is more commonly the case, in the deeper parts, —in the glandular tissue. When this stage is reached the symptoms are those of ordinary mammary carcinoma, consisting of deep-seated, lancinating pain and extensive ulceration, together with involvement of the lymphatic glands of the axilla.

The treatment in the early stages, while the diagnosis may yet be in doubt, is much the same as in eczema. All irritating applications should be avoided. When, however, the diagnosis of Paget's disease has been established, vigorous measures should be adopted at once. The diseased surface should be thoroughly curetted and afterwards cauterized with pure carbolic acid or diluted caustic potash, or treated with a twenty- to fifty-percent. plaster of pyrogallol. When cancerous degeneration of the deeper structures has taken place, amputation of the breast is demanded.

Eczema frequently attacks the genitalia in women. It may be confined to the labia, but it usually extends to the surrounding parts,—the mons veneris, the inner surface of the thighs, the perineum and anus, and occasionally the vagina. At times there is abundant exudation of serum, the parts being swollen and more or less crusted. In other cases the skin is dry, red, and scaly. The itching is often of the most distressing character, and is apt to occur paroxysmally. A leucorrhœa may act as the direct exciting cause, or it may be a consequence of pregnancy or of tumors of the uterus or the ovaries. Care should be taken to distinguish between eczema vulvæ and pruritus vulvæ, since these two affections are not infrequently confounded. An accurate diagnosis can be made, as a rule, only by a careful ocular inspection of the parts affected. It is of importance to remember that eczema of the genitalia is a frequent complication of glycosuria, or diabetes mellitus. The urine should always be examined for sugar. The treatment of this distressing variety of eczema must be conducted on general principles. If uterine or ovarian disease be present, as is frequently the case, this must be appropriately treated before a permanent cure can be expected. In cases of eczema the result of glycosuria, constitutional as well as local treatment must be employed. Among the local remedies, carbolic acid, applied as a lotion in the strength of ten to fifteen grains to the ounce of water, is extremely useful. Applying a cloth dipped in hot water as hot as can be borne for a few minutes will sometimes relieve the itching for a considerable period. Painting the parts with a solution of nitrate of silver in nitrous ether (five or ten grains to the ounce) is another remedy which may be referred to. Salicylic acid and resorcin are also both valuable remedies.

DISEASES ASSOCIATED WITH PHYSIOLOGICAL FUNCTIONS PECULIAR TO WOMEN.—The performance of the various functions special to the female sex is often accompanied by cutaneous disorders which manifest themselves either as disturbances of function, alteration of sensibility, increased or diminished action of the glands, or structural changes by the formation of the various cutaneous lesions. The two most important functions of the sex, menstruation and gestation, play an important rôle in the causation of affections of the skin. The former is attended by a considerable variety of cutaneous disorders, the most common of which is acne. It is a matter of common observation that this affection is apt to be much worse during the menstrual period. In some cases it occurs mainly at this time, disappearing more or less completely in the interval between the menses. Occasionally it undergoes no decided change during menstruation. In some women herpetic eruptions upon the lips coincide with each menstrual period. Less frequently herpes of the vulva occurs in the same manner. Cutaneous hemorrhage in the form of **purpura** occasionally manifests itself with each menstrual period. E. Morin gives the notes of a case where for ten years purpura appeared two or three days before each menstruation and disappeared at the end of eight or ten days. Certain diseases which have appeared independently of menstruation—*e.g.*, eczema—frequently become worse during the menstrual flow. Besides these structural changes in the skin, functional disturbances are of common occurrence, such as **flushing**, various forms of **erythema**, and **hyperidrosis**, confined to a single region, as the face or the palms. In disorders of the function, as in dysmenorrhœa, amenorrhœa, and irregular menstruation, they are still more frequent. Certain cutaneous maladies are likewise common during the **menopause**, those which are under the influence of the nervous system predominating. Acne rosacea, eczema, and pruritus vulvæ are often seen at this time, the itching in the two latter being usually of the most aggravated character. Abnormal development of hair and deposit of pigment are also observed at the climacteric period.

Various disorders of the skin accompany the function of **gestation**. In addition to the deposit of pigment which occurs in the mammary areola and the linea alba during pregnancy, patches of pigmentation, round, oval, or irregular in shape, varying from a light yellow to a deep brown or even almost black, are frequently observed, situated oftenest upon the face, but in some cases covering considerable areas upon the trunk. This pigmentation continues during the period of gestation and disappears after parturition. An excessive growth of hair has been occasionally observed. Thus, Slocum reports a case in which, during three successive pregnancies, an abnormal growth of hair occurred upon the chin, falling off with the return of menstruation. Eczema of the genitalia and pruritus vulvæ are common during the period of gestation, and are often the source of much annoyance and even great distress, imperatively demanding treatment, and in many cases taxing to the utmost therapeutic resources. Psoriasis is a disease which is sometimes influenced in a striking manner by pregnancy, in some cases being improved, in others distinctly aggravated. The latter occurrence is noted particularly in the case of women who are naturally weak and who are further debilitated by gestation. Pointed condylomata growing luxuriantly upon the vulva have been observed which rapidly disappeared after delivery.

Among the cutaneous disorders of **pregnancy** there is a severe disease which was first described by Hebra, in 1872, with the name **impetigo herpetiformis**. Since that date further knowledge on the subject has been contributed by several writers, notably by Kaposi. The limited number of cases recorded have occurred almost exclusively in women, and, moreover, in the pregnant and puerperal states. All of Hebra's original series of five cases occurred in women, and all but one terminated fatally. While within the past few years it has been shown that the disease may also in rare instances appear in men, it must nevertheless be regarded as being a disease of the skin to which women are particularly prone. It is characterized by numerous superficially seated, pin-head-sized, miliary pustules, which begin as such and remain pustules throughout their course. They are always arranged in clusters and groups, new lesions tending to form on the periphery of older patches, the disease thus creeping onward and gradually invading new territory. The lesions soon become confluent and crusted, considerable crusting often taking place, much as occurs in pustular eczema, but there does not exist the disposition to continual oozing so common in eczema. A series of new pustules form about the original patch, which inclines to heal in the centre. The process thus extends, runs an acute or a subacute course, and may involve large areas, having predilection especially for the genitalia, the abdomen, the trunk generally, and the thighs. In severe cases patches as large as a hand may be found, red and inflamed, discharging a puriform fluid which dries into greenish and brownish foul smelling crusts. The disease is accompanied with chills and marked fever, and is almost invariably fatal.

The symptoms, however, are not always so sharply defined as above described; some cases have been observed (as in one by C. Heitzmann) where the lesions are more vesicular or more bullous in character, as the names herpes impetiginiformis, herpes pyæmicus, herpes vegetans, and herpes puerperalis, given by earlier observers, clearly indicate. One of us (Duhring) has expressed himself in effect that the disease occasionally possesses certain symptoms in common with the more polymorphous disease dermatitis herpetiformis, a view which has been insisted upon by S. Sherwell. The nature of the process must be regarded as being in most cases septic.

The diagnosis in typical cases is not difficult, the pustules and their arrangement and grouping being peculiar. The severe general disturbance, and the course of the disease (in all cases grave and frequently terminating fatally) must also point to impetigo herpetiformis. It is most likely to be confounded with dermatitis herpetiformis, especially the pustular variety; also with pemphigus, and in particular with pemphigus vegetans, the latter being likewise a fatal disease in almost all instances. All these affections have much in common as regards their etiology and pathology, and from such a stand-point might properly be grouped together. The nervous system is profoundly impressed in all of them, but especially so in impetigo herpetiformis and pemphigus. From the unfavorable history of the disease in reported cases, no specific treatment can be recommended. Asepsis locally and general tonic remedies afford the only means known at present of combating the disease.

Another disease met with in women, especially in connection with pregnancy, is dermatitis herpetiformis. It is a multiform, inflammatory, generalized disease of the skin, characterized by puckered, grouped lesions, particularly by erythema of the form common to erythema multiforme;

vesicles, minute, pin-head-sized, or larger; blebs, variously sized and shaped; and pustules similar in form with the vesicles and blebs. The lesions tend to appear in crops, are distinctly herpetic, and do not incline to rupture. The affection is accompanied by intolerable itching, and pursues in most cases a chronic course. It tends to recur. It is intimately associated with the nervous system, as shown by numerous recorded observations. In women it occurs at times in connection with pregnancy, constituting the so-called "herpes gestationis" of some authors. It is most apt to appear during the latter part of pregnancy, and almost invariably continues until after delivery; in some cases it first appears after parturition. In either case the cause may be found in disturbance of the nervous system. The trunk, thighs, and arms are the regions usually invaded; in some cases the eruption becomes universal.

It is liable to be mistaken for vesicular and pustular eczema, and also for pemphigus and impetigo herpetiformis. It differs in its course from the two last-named diseases in not tending to terminate fatally. Occasionally cases show complications. Constitutional symptoms, as malaise, chilliness, and alternate sensations of heat and cold, together with general physical and mental depression, not infrequently exist in the graver cases. As stated, the itching and burning are usually marked, being more severe even than in vesicular eczema of similar development. The disease is of much more frequent occurrence than impetigo herpetiformis, and varies in the degree of its development.

Treatment is unsatisfactory, local remedies in particular having often but little effect in relieving the itching. Frictions with strong sulphur ointment, thus breaking down the lesions, may be employed with the most hope of affording relief. Internally, the nervous system should be treated in chronic cases with appropriate remedies. Arsenic is sometimes of value, but it is not so useful as in pemphigus, and in some cases even proves harmful.

Lactation in some instances calls forth disease of the skin. As has already been mentioned, eczema of the nipple is most frequently seen during this period, for reasons which are obvious. It is often extremely obstinate, resisting the ordinary remedies and demanding treatment of the most vigorous kind: in severe cases nothing short of weaning the child will succeed. Emollient and protective ointments containing zinc, salicylic acid, or carbolic acid may at first be tried, care being taken to remove them thoroughly before nursing; but if these fail to afford relief, stronger and more stimulating applications must be made, such as a strong solution of carbolic acid, resorcin, corrosive sublimate, or nitrate of silver. Another disease sometimes markedly influenced by lactation is psoriasis, the cutaneous manifestation tending in some cases to make its appearance first, in others to become worse, during this period. It may be viewed in most cases as being influenced by debility consequent on the drain upon the general system.

PATHOLOGICAL CONDITIONS OF THE UTERUS AND OVARIES.—These often exert an influence upon the skin similar to that produced by menstruation and pregnancy. Deposits of pigment in various situations—the so-called **chloasma uterinum**—are observed in connection with uterine and ovarian disease, functional and organic. These discolorations are sometimes associated with tumors of the uterus and ovaries. **Acne vulgaris** and **rosacea** are common cutaneous complications in disease of the female sexual apparatus. **Urticaria** is at times dependent upon the same cause. Hebra mentions the case of a woman with a flexion of the uterus in whom the introduction of the uterine sound produced an attack of urticaria, this having occurred fifteen times in succession. **Chromidrosis** and **seborrhœa nigricans**—rare diseases—occur most frequently in unmarried women the subjects of disease of other organs than the skin, the sexual apparatus or nervous system generally presenting evidences of functional or organic disorder. The color of the secretion varies, blue, black, and red being the most common. The face is the region oftenest affected. In cases of supposed colored sweat the utmost care should be exercised to eliminate all possibility of wilful or unintentional deception.

HYSTERIA.—To this peculiar condition of the nervous system, characterized by a variety of symptoms, some of them difficult of definition, must be attributed the manifestation of some of the commoner diseases of the skin as well as certain rare or anomalous affections. In some instances characteristic hysterical symptoms are present, in others indefinable symptoms exist. In some cases the cutaneous disturbance is insignificant, slight, and transient, while, on the other hand, it is occasionally severe or peculiar. Hysteria may produce a profound influence upon the nervous centres, causing varied manifestations to appear on the skin. The cutaneous disease may be connected with the vaso-motors or with nerve-trunks and branches, producing disturbances of nutrition, superficial or deep-seated, more frequently the former. Occasionally they are of reflex origin. Among the commoner affections may be mentioned the superficial congestions which are grouped under the general heading of **erythema**. These may be simply hyperæmic, or congestive, as in flushing, especially of the face and particularly of the cheeks,—the "flush centres,"—or exudative, giving rise to multiform inflammatory erythema. Of the latter there are many forms, the most frequent being a diffuse erythema occupying a small or a large area. **Urticaria** may also be referred to as a not uncommon manifestation. Among the glandular diseases, **chromidrosis** and **seborrhœa**, especially seborrhœa nigricans of the orbital region, may be mentioned. Of the still rarer diseases, those accompanied by hemorrhagic effusions through the glandular ducts (**hæmatidrosis**) into the corium, constituting so-called "bleeding stigmata," as occurred in the well-known case of Louise Lateau, and "neurotic excoriations," as reported by Erasmus Wilson and other observers, are striking and peculiar. Their existence was formerly doubted and even denied by some authors. While in some of the cases the lesions are the result of artifice (with the view to deceive or to excite sympathy) on the part of the woman herself, there is no doubt that the majority of cases are examples of genuine disease.

A series of remarkable cases, similar in their history and clinical manifestations, characterized for the most part by erythematous, vesicular, bullous, and gangrenous localized lesions, pursuing usually a chronic course, and having a resemblance to herpes zoster, have been reported by Kaposi, Kopp, Doutrelepont, Montgomery, and one of us (Duhring). These cases have been described under such titles as "zoster gangrænosus recidivus atypicus hystericus," "pemphigus neurotico-traumaticus," "hysterical spontaneous gangrene," "traumatic neurosal pemphigus," "gangræna cutis acuta multiplex," and "dermatitis vesiculosa neuro-traumatica." The several titles are given here *in extenso* because they express the chief characteristics of the disease. They are peculiar in their mode of origin, which has usually been traumatism, often slight or insignificant, and in itself insufficient to account for the development of the subsequent cutaneous disease. Thus, in some cases the disease has originated from the prick of a pin or needle or from a burn, and a curious feature noted in some cases is that the cutaneous disease did not appear at the site of the traumatism, but near by or even elsewhere. From this observation it would seem that the disease of the skin was reflex in character. In almost all of these cases there is marked hysteria. The possibility of their artificial production is to be excluded.

Cutaneous **hyperæsthesia** frequently occurs in hysterical women, and is in marked cases so extreme that the lightest touch gives shock or pain. This hyperæsthesia is not limited to definite nerve-tracts, and it is distinguished by its trifling character, changing its situation from time to time without perceptible reason. On the other hand, anæsthesia more or less complete may exist. This is usually unilateral, occupying the entire half of the body, or it may be limited to certain areas. In hysterical hemianæsthesia the anæsthetic area is usually sharply limited by the median line of the body, and, like the hyperæsthesia, it often shifts about, passing from one side to the other in the most inexplicable manner. **Analgesia,** or loss of perception of pain, also occurs, tactile sensibility being impaired.

A rare form of disease, characterized by the development of a peculiar, large and bulky, localized and circumscribed, brownish, corrugated, dry, non-offensive crust, arising from an erythematous, non-ulcerated, unbroken skin, accompanied by rapid respiration and other hysterical symptoms, has been described and figured by S. Weir Mitchell. One of us (Duhring) also had the opportunity of observing and studying this case, which might properly be designated as an "hysterical epithelial crust." It was the size of an adult hand, from one-half to three-quarters of an inch in thickness, and resembled the bark of an oak-tree. The lesion had existed for a year or more, and had recurred several times after forcible removal, which operation caused great pain. On one occasion it was removed in large fragments by Dr. Mitchell, under hypnotism. The epithelium beneath the crust was

reddened, thin, dry, without breach of continuity, and the corium was the seat of a chronic, peculiar, cold inflammation. There had never been any discharge or ulceration.

**Factitious diseases** of the skin, also called "artificial" and "feigned" skin-diseases, produced by the patient with various agents, mostly mechanical and chemical, are met with chiefly in hysterical women, more especially in young women. They are produced with the view of exciting sympathy, of deceiving, or of shirking work or some irksome duty, and are induced by scratching or rubbing with the finger-nail or some other instrument, or by friction, or by applying some chemical irritant, discutient or caustic, with the idea of simulating disease. While such productions are rare, they are occasionally met with, and sometimes in women who cannot be regarded as hysterical, but who are rather to be considered as malingerers. The same form of malingering has been noted in the case of healthy men in the army and navy, with the view of shirking duty.

Feigned diseases are usually met with on parts of the body easily accessible to the patient, and in most cases are seen upon the anterior surface and in right-handed persons on the left side. While the appearance of the eruption rarely corresponds to that of any of the ordinary cutaneous diseases, the diagnosis is often perplexing. A conclusion should never be reached hastily.

# INDEX.

THE END.

Lightning Source UK Ltd.
Milton Keynes UK
UKHW012030110119
335429UK00010B/772/P

9 780243 325603